PERIOPERATIVE NURSING PRACTICE

PERIOPERATIVE NURSING PRACTICE

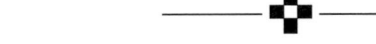

Mark L. Phippen, R.N., M.N., CNOR
Manager, OR/PACU
The Methodist Hospital
Houston, Texas

Maryann Papanier Wells, R.N., M.S., CNOR
Perioperative Nurse Manager, Perioperative Nursing
Hospital of the University of Pennsylvania
Philadelphia, Pennsylvania

W.B. SAUNDERS COMPANY
A Division of Harcourt Brace & Company
Philadelphia   London   Toronto   Montreal   Sydney   Tokyo

W.B. SAUNDERS COMPANY
A Division of
Harcourt Brace & Company

The Curtis Center
Independence Square West
Philadelphia, Pennsylvania 19106

Library of Congress Cataloging-in-Publication Data

Perioperative nursing practice / [edited by] Mark L. Phippen,
Maryann Papanier Wells.

    p.   cm.

ISBN 0–7216–7233–7

1. Operating room nursing.   I. Phippen, Mark L.
   II. Wells, Maryann M. Papanier.   [DNLM: 1. Operating
   Room Nursing.   Preoperative Care. WY 162 P4445]

RD32.3.P47 1993

610.73′677—dc20

DNLM/DLC   92-24341

Perioperative Nursing Practice   ISBN 0–7216–7233–7

Last digit is the print number: 9   8   7   6   5   4   3   2   1

Dedication

*To Cristina, my very understanding wife and friend,
and my daughters, Maria, Sara, and Catalina.
Thank you for your love and support
during this long and exciting adventure.*

Mark L. Phippen

*To life's rarest commodities—family, friends, and
colleagues. Thank you for your endurance.*

Maryann Papanier Wells

Contributors

Cynthia A. Abbott, R.N., Ph.D., CNOR
Lieutenant Colonel, Army Nurse Corps
Patient Assessment and Diagnosis: A Functional Health Patterns Approach; Planning Patient Care: A Functional Health Patterns Approach; Evaluating Patient Care: A Functional Health Patterns Approach

Jean M. Allen, R.N., B.S.N., CNOR
Nurse Manager, Central Processing, Ben Taub General Hospital, Houston, Texas
Providing Instruments, Equipment, and Supplies

Juan A. Bonilla, M.D.
Assistant Clinical Professor, Department of Otolaryngology, University of Texas Health Science Center; Chief, Otolaryngology (Pediatrics), Santa Rosa Children's Hospital, San Antonio, Texas
Otolaryngologic Surgery

Jeannie Botsford, R.N., M.A., CNOR
Administrative Director, Surgical Services, Scripps Memorial Hospital, La Jolla, California
Financial Management for the Perioperative Nursing Manager

Mary Bradley, R.N., M.S.N., CNOR
Clinical Coordinator, Perioperative Nursing, Hospital of the University of Pennsylvania, Philadelphia, Pennsylvania
Patient and Family Teaching; Perioperative Nursing Job Descriptions and Performance Appraisals

Linda Brazen, R.N., M.S.N., CNOR
Center for Perioperative Education, Association of Operating Room Nurses, Inc., Denver, Colorado
Perioperative Nursing Staff Development

Marc Cendron, M.D.
Assistant Professor, Tufts University School of Medicine; Pediatric Urologist, New England Medical Center, Boston, Massachusetts
Urological Surgery

Barbara Diomede, R.N., M.S.N., CNOR
Clinical Nurse Specialist, DePaul Health Center, St. Louis, Missouri
Pediatric Surgery

Beverly W. Ejsing, R.N., M.S., CNOR
Staff Nurse, Perioperative Nursing, Hospital of the University of Pennsylvania, Philadelphia, Pennsylvania
Vascular Surgery

Dietra A. Evans, R.N., M.S., CNOR
Clinical Nurse Specialist, Perioperative Nursing, Hospital of the University of Pennsylvania, Philadelphia, Pennsylvania
Gynecological Surgery

Rebecca P. Fairly, C.R.N.A., B.S.N.
Nurse Anesthetist, Mississippi Methodist Rehabilitation Center, Jackson, Mississippi
Assisting the Anesthetist

Susan K. Fisher, R.N., M.S.N., CNOR
Staff Nurse, Perioperative Nursing, Hospital of the University of Pennsylvania, Philadelphia, Pennsylvania
Cardiac Surgery

Vicki J. Fox, R.N., M.S.N., CNOR
Clinical Nurse Specialist, Specialty Nursing Services, PC, Tyler, Texas
Providing Hemostasis; Facilitating Postoperative Care

Patricia S. Fritz, R.N., B.S., CNOR
Nursing Supervisor, Jefferson Surgical Center, Thomas Jefferson University Hospital, Philadelphia, Pennsylvania
Plastic Surgery

Susan A. Garruto, R.N., M.S., CNOR
Staff Nurse, Perioperative Nursing, Hospital of the University of Pennsylvania, Philadelphia, Pennsylvania
Transplantation Surgery

Nancy Girard, R.N., Ph.D., C.S.
Assistant Professor, University of Texas Health Science Center, School of Nursing; Nursing Consultant, Audie Murphy Veteran's Hospital, and Nursing Clinical Associate; Medical Center Hospital, San Antonio, Texas
Geriatric Surgery

Rosemary Grandusky, R.N., B.S.N., CNOR
Operating Room Manager, Highland Hospital, Rochester, New York
Performing Sponge, Sharps, and Instrument Counts

Alexia Green, R.N., Ph.D.
Chairperson, Department of Nursing, Lamar University, Beaumont, Texas
Legislative Trends in Nursing: Implications for the Perioperative Nurse

Michael Griswold, R.N., M.S.N., CNOR
Major, Army Nurse Corps
Transferring the Patient

Carolyn Grous, R.N., M.S.N., CNOR
Perioperative Nurse Manager, Perioperative Nursing, Hospital of the University of Pennsylvania, Philadelphia, Pennsylvania
Urological Surgery

Candice Hawley, R.N., CNOR
Manager, Pediatric Medical-Surgical Unit, St. Louis Children's Hospital, St. Louis, Missouri
Pediatric Surgery

Sharon Hendricks, R.N., B.S.N., CNOR
Clinical Educator, Perioperative Services, Santa Rosa Children's Hospital, San Antonio, Texas
Handling Cultures and Specimens

Barbara Jeane Kalman, R.N., B.S.N., CNOR, R.N.F.A.
Assistant Nurse Manager, Perioperative Nursing, Hospital of the University of Pennsylvania, Philadelphia, Pennsylvania
Orthopedic Surgery

Elaine Thomson Keith, R.N., B.S.N., CNOR
Manager, Neurosensory Perioperative Nursing, The Methodist Hospital, Houston, Texas
Quality Assessment and Improvement

Joseph A. Kinnaman, R.N., B.S.
Director, Surgical Services, Missouri Baptist Medical Center, St. Louis, Missouri
Handling Tissues with Instruments

Frances A. Koch, R.N., M.S.N., CNOR
Associate Administrator, Operating Room Services, Henry Ford Hospital, Detroit, Michigan
Developing Perioperative Nursing Department Policies and Procedures

Angela M. Martinelli, R.N., M.S.N., CNOR
Doctoral Student, The Catholic University of America, Washington, D.C.
A Conceptual Model for Perioperative Nursing Practice; Administering Drugs and Solutions; Physiologically Monitoring the Patient

Noreen E. McHugh, R.N., M.S., CNOR
Clinical Director, Perioperative Nursing, Hospital of the University of Pennsylvania, Philadelphia, Pennsylvania
Perioperative Nursing Job Descriptions and Performance Appraisals

Patricia A. Mews, R.N., M.A., CNOR
Nurse Consultant, Baxter Convertors/Custom Sterile, Baxter Healthcare Corporation, McGaw Park, Illinois
Creating and Maintaining a Sterile Field

Robin Moushey, R.N., M.S.N.
Clinical Instructor, St. Louis University School of Nursing for Nursing of Children; Clinical Specialist, Pediatric Surgery, St. Louis Children's Hospital, St. Louis, Missouri
Pediatric Surgery

Lori Ominsky, R.N., B.S.N., CNOR, R.N.F.A.
Staff Nurse, Perioperative Nursing, Hospital of the University of Pennsylvania, Philadelphia, Pennsylvania
Preparing the Patient for Surgery

Steven L. Perry, M.S.N.
Major, Army Nurse Corps
Positioning the Patient

Mark L. Phippen, R.N., M.N., CNOR
Manager, OR/PACU, The Methodist Hospital, Houston, Texas
A Conceptual Model for Perioperative Nursing Practice; Patient and Family Teaching; Providing Instruments, Equipment, and Supplies; Preparing the Patient for Surgery; Perioperative Nursing Job Descriptions and Performance Appraisals; Quality Assessment and Improvement

Susan Puterbaugh, R.N., M.B.A., CNOR
Instructor, University of Phoenix; Executive Director, National Certification Board: Perioperative Nursing, Inc., Denver, Colorado
Neurosurgery

Leana Revell, R.N., M.S.N., CNOR
Associate Professor, Department of Nursing
Education, San Antonio, Texas
Monitoring and Controlling the Environment

Jane C. Rothrock, R.N., D.N.Sc., CNOR
Professor and Program Coordinator, Perioperative
Nursing, Delaware County Community College,
Media, Pennsylvania
*Professional Involvement: An Issue of Survival for
Perioperative Nursing*

Dan Sandel
Chairman of the Board and Chief Executive Officer,
Devon Industries, Inc., Chatsworth, California
The Entrepreneurial Nurse

Ruth P. Shumaker, R.N., B.S.N., CNOR
Clinical Director, Surgical Services, Mississippi
Methodist Rehabilitation Center, Jackson, Mississippi
Assisting the Anesthetist

Gwendolyn Singleton, R.N., B.S.N.
Staff Nurse, Neurosensory Operating Rooms, The
Methodist Hospital, Houston, Texas
Otolaryngologic Surgery

Joyce M. Stengel, R.N., B.S.N., CNOR
Nurse Manager, General, Plastics, and Oral Surgery,
Perioperative Nursing, Hospital of the University of
Pennsylvania, Philadelphia, Pennsylvania
General Surgery

Rosalie Stewart, R.N., CNOR
Staff Nurse, Perioperative Nursing, Hospital of the
University of Pennsylvania, Philadelphia, Pennsylvania
Handling Tissues with Instruments

**Inez E. Tenzer, R.N., M.S., B.S.N., CNOR,
C.N.A.A.**
Assistant Regional Nurse Consultant, Kaiser
Foundation Hospitals, Southern California, Los
Angeles, California
Staffing and Scheduling

Suzanne Ward, R.N., M.S., M.N., CNOR
Consultant, Perioperative Nursing, Los Angeles,
California
*Encroachment of Practice: Implications for the
Perioperative Nurse*

Donna S. Watson, R.N., M.S.N., CNOR
Doctoral Student, University of Colorado Health
Sciences Center, Denver, Colorado
Vascular Surgery

Maryann Papanier Wells, R.N., M.S., CNOR
Perioperative Nurse Manager, Perioperative Nursing,
Hospital of the University of Pennsylvania,
Philadelphia, Pennsylvania
*A Conceptual Model for Perioperative Nursing
Practice*

Linda Dickey White, R.N., M.S., CNOR
Barnes Hospital, St. Louis, Missouri
Dealing with Regulatory Bodies

Carla Willis, R.N., M.S., CNOR
Director of Surgery Services and Director of the
Center for Educational Services, Memorial Hospital
Southeast, Houston, Texas
*Legislative Trends in Nursing: Implications for the
Perioperative Nurses*

Preface

In the United States there are over 80,000 perioperative nurses. Yet the number of textbooks available to perioperative nurses is very small. *Perioperative Nursing Practice* was developed to start the chain reaction for a literary explosion in the perioperative arena.

Perioperative Nursing Practice is intended for an audience of perioperative nursing clinicians, administrators, researchers, and educators. It is also a valuable resource for general nursing students.

The book is organized into five sections with a total of 42 chapters. Section I, Basic Competencies, includes a new conceptual model for perioperative nursing practice in Chapter 1 and describes the basic competencies (the knowledge, skills, and abilities) the perioperative nurse should demonstrate in order to provide safe, effective, and efficient nursing care during the patient's surgical experience in Chapters 2 through 14. The Association of Operating Room Nursing, Inc. (AORN) *Competency Statements in Perioperative Nursing* were used as a framework for this section (AORN, 1992, II:2-4–2-12).

Two competencies—positioning the patient and handling cultures and specimens—were added to the list identified by AORN. We believe these additional competencies are critical and thus should become part of the nursing competencies recognized by the perioperative nursing community.

The systems-in-contingency model for perioperative nursing presented in Chapter 1 is a nursing model in evolution. It reflects what we believe to be *perioperative nursing reality.* We invite the reader to explore the model, debate the concepts reflected in the model, and use it as a framework for practice.

Chapters 2 and 3 present the nursing process components of assessment, diagnosis, and planning from the functional health patterns approach. In Chapter 2, the author describes 54 diagnoses from the North American Nursing Diagnosis Association (NANDA) approved list of approved diagnoses and discusses the perioperative nursing implications for these diagnoses.

Chapters 4 through 13 provide a step-by-step discussion of how to

- transfer a patient during the perioperative period
- provide patient and family education
- create and maintain a sterile field
- perform sponge, sharps, and instrument counts
- provide instruments, equipment, and supplies
- administer drugs and solutions
- physiologically monitor the patient
- monitor and control the environment
- position the patient
- handle cultures and specimens

The competencies described in Chapters 4 through 13 are presented in a nursing process format. When the chapters were being written, the authors were asked to answer the following questions: *What are the implications to the patient if the perioperative nursing team does not perform activities described in the chapter?* and *What types of patients are likely to experience problems if the activities described in the chapter are not performed by the perioperative nursing team?* From their answers, the authors identified one or more nursing diagnoses for each chapter. All but one of the nursing diagnoses identified by the authors of Chapters 4 through 13 were identified as potential (high-risk) diagnoses. Most of these diagnoses cannot be found on the approved NANDA list. The diagnoses, however, incorporate terminology from the approved NANDA list to identify potential patient problems frequently seen in the perioperative patient population. These diagnoses will assist the practitioner in identifying patients at risk for experiencing alterations in functional health patterns during the perioperative period. We also believe the nursing diagnoses identified by the contributing authors provide a focus for clinical perioperative nursing research.

The format for Chapters 4 through 13 includes a definition of the competency presented in the chapter, identification of the measurable criteria for the competency, and a discussion of specific considerations having an impact on the competency. The nursing diagnoses for each chapter follow the introductory material. Diagnoses include a definition, identification of risk factors or defining characteristics, and expected outcomes. The nursing diagnoses are categorized under a functional health pattern according to the format described by Gordon (1987, pp. 431–434). Perioperative nursing interventions needed to achieve the expected outcomes for which the perioperative nurse is accountable follow the discussion of nursing diagnoses.

Chapter 14 completes the discussion of basic competencies by describing the evaluation of patient care from a functional health patterns approach.

Section II identifies and describes competencies for the registered nurse first assistant (RNFA). The competencies include

- preparing the patient for surgery
- handling tissues with instruments
- providing hemostasis
- facilitating postoperative care

Like Chapters 4 through 13, the chapters for this section use the nursing process format when describing competencies for the RNFA. The authors for this section have identified actual and potential (high-risk) nursing diagnoses frequently seen in their practices as RNFAs. The content in this section is also intended for perioperative nurses who have limited their practice to the scrub nurse and circulating nurse roles. Surgeon practice patterns are evolving because of changes in the parameters for reimbursement. Consequently, more perioperative nurses will be called on to provide first assistant services in the future. This section will provide the perioperative nurse with some of the knowledge necessary for acquiring the skills and abilities to function as a first assistant.

Sections III and IV integrate the perioperative nursing knowledge, skills, and abilities described in Sections I and II with clinical applications (anesthesia and surgical procedures, described in Chapters 19 through 29) and special surgical populations (pediatric and geriatric patients).

Section III, Clinical Applications, includes Chapters 19 through 29.

Chapter 19, *Assisting the Anesthetist,* describes the activities performed by the perioperative nurse when assisting the anesthetist in administering anesthesia. The authors discuss monitoring of patients receiving local anesthesia, positioning, emergency surgery, and blood component therapy. In the section on anesthesia complications, the author describes how the perioperative nurse can assist the anesthetist during episodes of patient hypotension and hypertension, patient coughing and laryngospasm, difficult intubations, cardiac arrest, and malignant hyperthermia.

Chapters 20 through 29 discuss common surgical procedures performed in general surgery, vascular surgery, cardiac surgery, transplantation surgery, plastic surgery, neurosurgery, urological surgery, orthopedic surgery, gynecological surgery, and otolaryngologic surgery. Each chapter has an introductory format that presents surgical anatomy and the instruments, supplies, and equipment used in the surgical service. For each operation described, the reader will find

- a definition of the operation
- indications for the operation
- perioperative nursing implications (type of anesthesia, position commonly used, aspects of creating and maintaining the sterile field, equipment and supplies used, drugs and solutions used, aspects of physiological monitoring, typical physicians orders, and common laboratory and diagnostic studies ordered by the physician)
- a description of the procedure (incision and exposure, details of the procedure, and closure)
- aspects of postoperative care
- potential surgical complications

Chapters 30 and 31 compose Section IV. These chapters focus on the perioperative care of pediatric and geriatric patients. The authors present an in-depth discussion about these special patients.

Chapters 32 through 42 compose Section V. This section presents an eclectic overview of education, management, and other issues pertinent to perioperative nurses. Topics discussed include

- perioperative nursing staff development
- perioperative nursing policies and procedures
- financial management
- staffing and scheduling
- perioperative nursing job descriptions and performance appraisals
- quality assessment and improvement
- strategies for dealing with regulatory bodies
- legislative trends
- encroachment issues
- strategies for promoting professional involvement
- entrepreneurship

Notes

Association of Operating Room Nurses. (1992). *Standards and recommended practices for perioperative nursing.* Denver.
Gordon, M. (1987). *Nursing diagnosis: Process and application* (2nd ed.). New York: McGraw-Hill.

Acknowledgments

Like many other textbooks, *Perioperative Nursing Practice* was not the work of a single person. It was the work of many dedicated professionals within the perioperative nursing and publishing communities. We thank you for your collective efforts, knowledge, and commitment of time.

A genuine thanks to Christopher Shawne Webster for his unending enthusiasm in manuscript preparation and revision of many of the contributing authors' very long chapters.

We extend special thanks to Baxter Healthcare Corporation, McGaw Park, Illinois, and Ethicon Incorporated, Somerville, New Jersey, for their assistance in procuring illustrations for the book.

A very sincere thanks to our W.B. Saunders nursing editor and friend, Daniel T. Ruth. His unending guidance and attention to detail made this book happen. Also, many thanks to Danni Morinich and Amy Norwitz. Without their assistance and organization the book could have never gotten off the ground.

Perioperative Nursing Practice has been a long time coming. We have worked many long and hard hours. But it has been a labor of love for our profession. We are privileged for this wonderful opportunity to share our knowledge with our nursing colleagues and to promote the advancement of the nursing profession.

MARK L. PHIPPEN
Houston, Texas

MARYANN PAPANIER WELLS
Philadelphia, Pennsylvania

Contents

BASIC COMPETENCIES

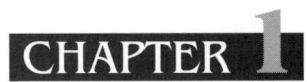

CHAPTER 1

A Conceptual Model for Perioperative Nursing Practice

Mark L. Phippen, Maryann Papanier Wells, and Angela M. Martinelli

Nursing is establishing itself as a scientific discipline. Its thrust toward scientifically sound social usefulness includes the development of conceptual models. The nursing model provides the basis for selecting knowledge to be transmitted in nursing education, the framework for nursing practice, and the impetus and direction for nursing research.

RIEHL AND ROY, 1980, p. 1.

As the perioperative nurse's responsibilities become more complex and challenging, the need for a conceptual model for perioperative nursing practice becomes apparent. The systems-in-contingency model for perioperative nursing meets that need. The model presents a "mental image of the realm of [perioperative] nursing—how it is put together and how it works" (Riehl and Roy, 1980, pp. 6–7).

Like other models, the systems-in-contingency model for perioperative nursing practice is made up of a set of interrelated core concepts. These core concepts, which are person, environment, health, and nursing, abstractly describe patient-environment interaction, nursing goal, and nursing intervention (Fawcett, 1980, p. 11; Gordon, 1987b, p. 69). The core concepts provide the focus for nursing process. They give direction to the perioperative nurse in

- collecting patient health data
- analyzing health data and determining diagnoses
- identifying expected outcomes
- planning care that prescribes interventions to achieve expected outcomes
- implementing interventions

- evaluating the patient's progress toward achievement of outcomes (AORN, 1992, *II*:4–1—4–4)

The following discussion examines the elements of the systems-in-contingency model—assumptions, values, goal of action, patiency, actor's role, source of difficulty, intervention focus and mode, and intended and unintended consequences. Refer to Table 1–1 for a description of these terms.

ASSUMPTIONS

Assumptions, which are statements accepted as true without proof, are fundamental to all nursing models (Riehl and Roy, 1980, p. 180). The assumptions supporting the systems-in-contingency model are based on the model's concepts of the person as a contingency system interacting with the environment and the process of establishing and sustaining system equilibrium during the perioperative period.

Assumption 1 The person is a holistic system composed of physical, psychological, sociocultural, and spiritual components

The theory of holism describes the universe in terms of interacting wholes that are more than the mere sum

4

TABLE 1–1. ESSENTIAL UNITS OF CONCEPTUAL MODEL FOR NURSING

Unit	Description
Assumptions	Statements accepted as true without proof; fundamental to all models of nursing.
Values	Intrinsically desirable qualities that describe the utility of the model's goal.
Goal of action	The ideal purpose of the profession. The goal of action is expressed as a desired state, condition, or situation.
Patiency	A descriptive term for the patient.
Actor's role	How the nurse interacts with the patient.
Source of difficulty	The originating point of deviations from the desired state or condition.
Intervention focus	The types of problems found when deviations from the desired state occur; the disturbances in the patiency that are prevented or treated by the nurse.
Intervention mode	The major means of preventing or treating deviations from the desired state or condition.
Intended consequences	The outcomes of desired action.
Unintended consequences	Outcomes that are not intended but that might follow and that may or may not be desirable.

Adapted from Riehl, J. P., Roy, C. (1980). *Conceptual models for nursing practice* (2nd ed.). New York: Appleton-Century-Crofts.

of elementary particles. The person, when viewed from a holistic perspective, is seen as an interacting system that is more than the total of the components of the system. Like other nursing models, the systems-in-contingency model for perioperative nursing views the person as having a physical (biological) nature, a psychological nature, and a sociocultural nature. The model goes a step further, however, to describe the spiritual nature of the person (Fig. 1–1).

Specifically, the physical component describes the anatomical parts of the person and how they function physiologically, whereas the psychological component,

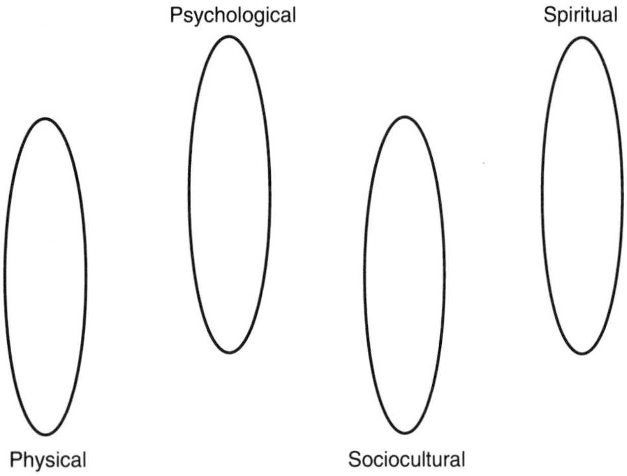

FIGURE 1–1. Components of the person.

the psychic organization of the person that produces behavior, describes the "perceiving, learning, and acting part" of the person (Roy, 1976, p. 3). The sociocultural component describes the behaviors common to all members of human society and those required for successful functioning in a particular segment of human society. Social behaviors refer to the interactions of a person with a group of people such as the family, a community, or a work group, and cultural behaviors refer to the customary beliefs, values, symbols, knowledge, attitudes, and habits of a specific social group. The spiritual component describes the incorporeal presence, the animating principle, or the actuating cause of a person's life. A person's view of the spiritual component is influenced by religious and philosophical beliefs.

Assumption 2 The physical, psychological, sociocultural, and spiritual components of the system exist in a state of contingency

The physical, psychological, sociocultural, and spiritual components of a person are interrelated, are dependent, and are conditioned by one another (Fig. 1–2). Furthermore, each component receives sustenance from the others, which leads to a state of interdependence.

Assumption 3 The spiritual component of the person is the unifying force of the system

The spiritual component is the element that holds the system together (Fig. 1–3). In this model, the spiritual component continues to exist after biological death. For example, for some it may exist in the form of a soul; for others it exists through reincarnation. For still others, one's spirit may continue to exist in one's family, church, work, community, or school.

Assumption 4 The person exists in a state of contingency with other systems in the environment

For each person, there are intrinsic and extrinsic environments. The intrinsic originates within the person, whereas the extrinsic originates outside the person. Because a person constantly interacts with the environment, the person does not exist in a vacuum but in a state of contingency with other systems in the environment (Fig. 1–4). Examples of systems that interact with the person are a spouse, the family, the community, the hospital, and the surgical team (perioperative nurse, surgeon, anesthetist, and perioperative nursing assistant). The person is also a component of other systems and therefore exists in a state of interdependence with the other components that compose the larger system.

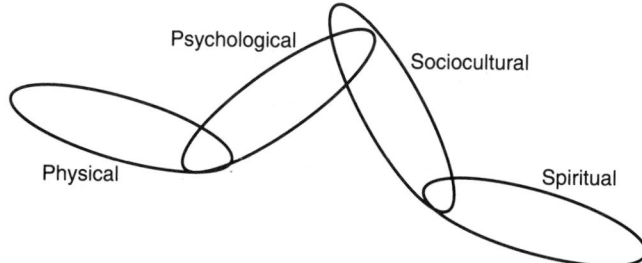

FIGURE 1–2. Components of the person exist in contingency.

The relationships between the person and the systems of his or her environment are dynamic.

Assumption 5 Health is dependent on the person's ability to cope with intrinsic and extrinsic environmental stressors

A stressor is a variable that has the potential for causing disequilibrium within the person and between the person and his or her environment. Intrinsic stressors originate within the person; extrinsic stressors originate outside the person (Fig. 1–5). Examples of intrinsic stressors are incontinence, sensorimotor loss, and cognitive impairment. Prolonged pressure, friction, shearing force, and immobility owing to traction are examples of extrinsic stressors.

Health is a relative concept. A person is well if his or her physical, psychological, sociocultural, and spiritual

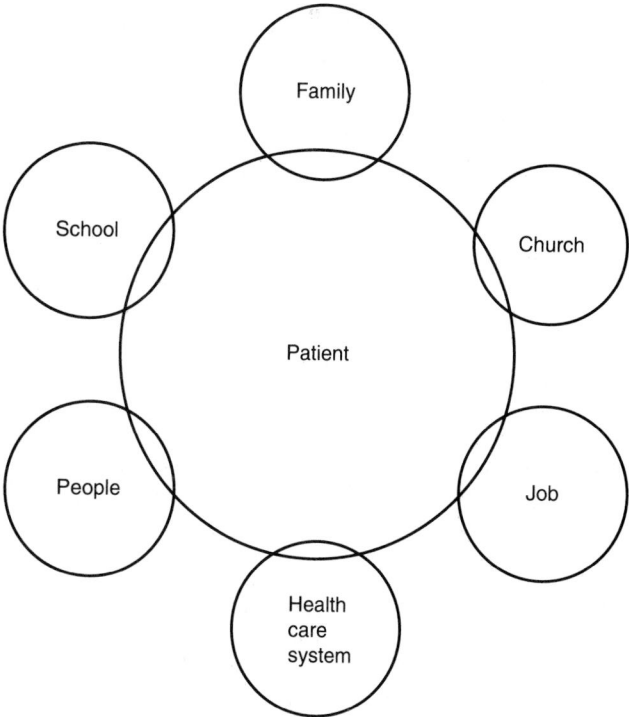

FIGURE 1–4. People exist in contingency with other systems.

components are united and if each of the components is successfully coping with intrinsic and extrinsic stressors, and if the person is in a state of equilibrium with the environment. She or he becomes ill, however, when one or more of the physical, psychological, sociocultural, or spiritual components fail to cope adequately with intrinsic or extrinsic stressors, leading to a state of disequilibrium with the environment.

Illness is not limited to the physical and psychological components of the person. As an example, a person

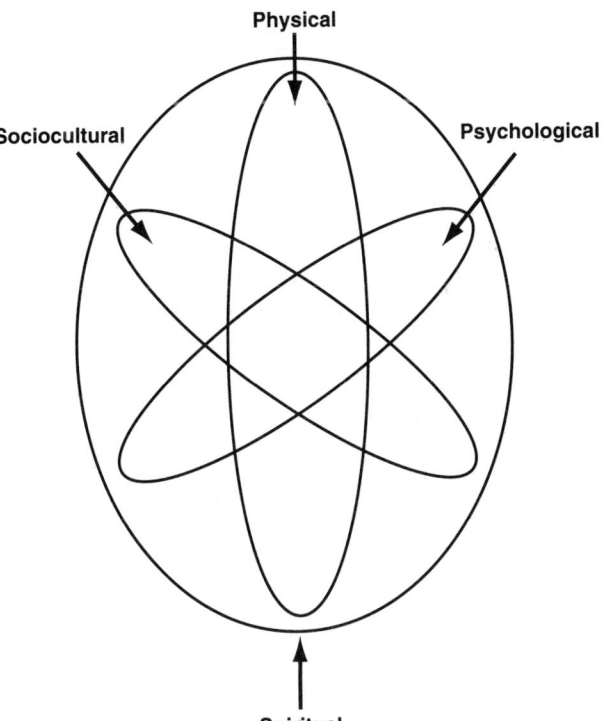

FIGURE 1–3. Holistic system unified by the spiritual component.

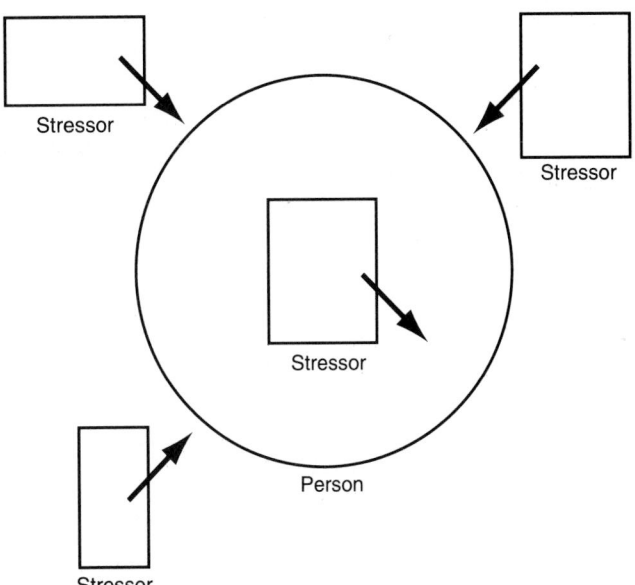

FIGURE 1–5. Intrinsic and extrinsic stressors.

who is physically and psychologically fit but experiencing a severe disturbance in role performance because of the loss of a job is not in a state of integrated wellness; she or he is socioculturally ill.

Assumption 6 The person is in a constant state of movement along a life continuum

The person is always moving along the life continuum toward biological death (Fig. 1–6). Movement along the continuum is dynamic and is characterized by fluctuations between wellness and illness. Wellness or illness can occur at conception, at birth, during life, or at death. For some, illness can occur in the afterlife. Spiritual illness may occur when a person biologically dies with bad memories, thoughts, or feelings toward family members, the community, or other significant people or systems who were part of the person's life experiences. Exit from the continuum can occur at any time. Furthermore, depending on the person's state of physical, psychological, sociocultural, and spiritual health, the person may exit in a state of wellness or illness. As an example, a healthy young woman killed in an automobile accident by a drunk driver exits the continuum in a state of wellness. A person dying of cancer, however, exits the continuum in a state of illness.

Assumption 7 The surgeon and the anesthetist are therapeutic stressors

Failure to cope adequately with intrinsic or extrinsic stressors can lead to conditions (stressors) that necessitate surgical intervention. In this case, the patient may seek a surgeon, who operates to eliminate, attenuate, or modify the stressor. In doing so, however, the surgeon becomes a stressor for the patient (Fig. 1–7). As an example, cigarette smoking (an extrinsic stressor), if not eliminated, can lead to the formation of a tumor in the respiratory tract. The tumor is an intrinsic stressor, which if not eliminated (removed) can lead to death. When the surgeon operates to remove the tumor, she or he becomes a stressor because she or he orders and

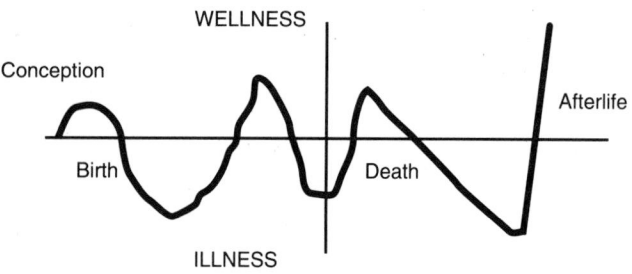

FIGURE 1–6. Illness and wellness can occur at any time on the continuum.

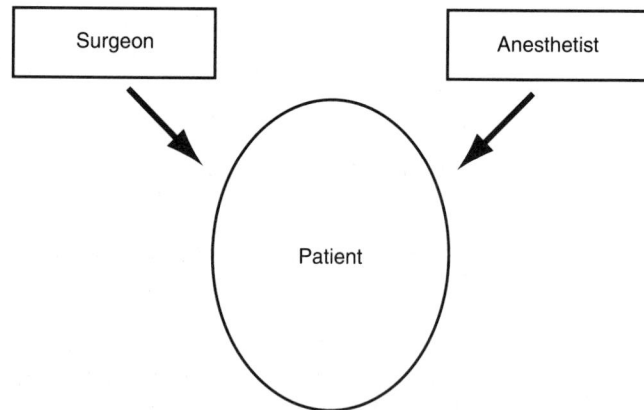

FIGURE 1–7. Therapeutic stressors.

performs tests and procedures that cause the patient pain and anxiety.

Surgical intervention causes system disequilibrium (pain and alteration in body processes). The anesthetist initiates anesthesia to maintain system equilibrium. In doing so, however, like the surgeon, the anesthetist becomes a stressor for the patient (see Fig. 1–7). As an example, when the anesthetist performs a regional nerve block to anesthetize an extremity, he or she becomes a stress inducer because the nerve block causes the patient pain, discomfort, and anxiety.

VALUES

Values are intrinsically desirable qualities that describe the utility of the model's goal. Like assumptions, values are accepted as true without proof (Riehl and Roy, 1980, p. 183). Four basic values support the systems-in-contingency model's goal:

1. Perioperative nursing is a socially significant specialty component of professional nursing practice that provides essential services needed by patients and families experiencing surgical intervention.
2. Establishing and sustaining system equilibrium during surgical intervention is essential for the patient's welfare.
3. Establishing and sustaining equilibrium during surgical intervention is assumed to facilitate the rehabilitation process after surgery.
4. Perioperative nursing is unique because it focuses on the patient as a holistic system interacting with other systems in the surgical environment.

GOAL OF ACTION

The *goal of action* describes the purpose of nursing activity (Riehl and Roy, 1980, p. 183). The goal of perioperative nursing activity is to establish and sustain

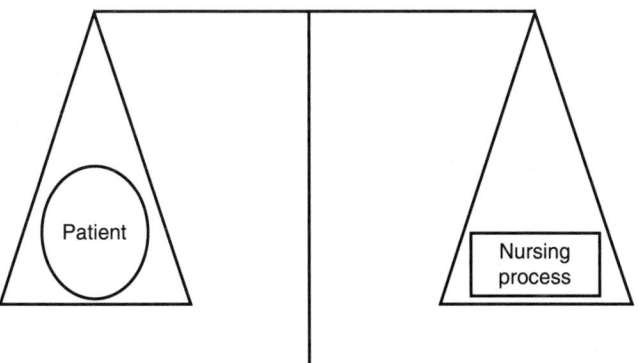

FIGURE 1–8. The nursing process establishes and sustains patient equilibrium during the perioperative period.

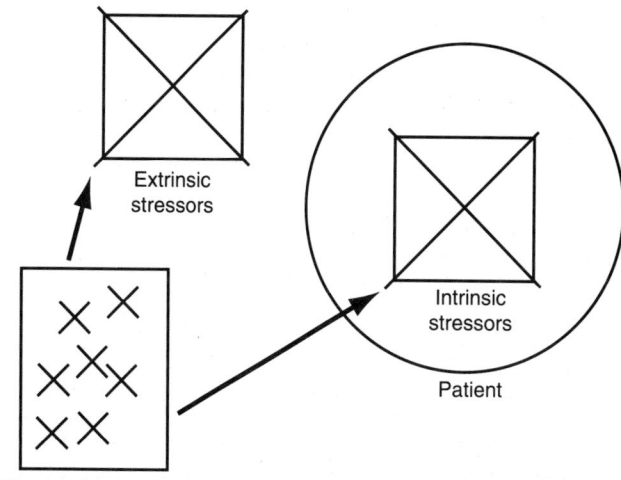

FIGURE 1–9. The nurse helps the patient cope with stressors.

system equilibrium during the perioperative period (Fig. 1–8). All perioperative nursing activities (assessment, diagnosis, outcome identification, planning, implementation, and evaluation) focus on establishing and sustaining the patient's equilibrium with the preoperative, intraoperative, and postoperative surgical environment.

PATIENCY

The term *patiency* describes who receives the nursing activity (Riehl and Roy, 1980, p. 184). The systems-in-contingency model for perioperative nursing describes the recipient of perioperative nursing activity (the patient) as a holistic system composed of interrelated and interdependent physical, psychological, sociocultural, and spiritual components; the goal is to enhance, preserve, or achieve unity and equilibrium among the system components.

ACTOR'S ROLE

The role of the perioperative nurse is to establish and sustain system equilibrium during the perioperative period by assisting the patient in coping with the intrinsic and extrinsic stressors of the surgical environment (Fig. 1–9) and by facilitating the work of the surgeon and the anesthetist during surgery (Fig. 1–10). Specifically, the perioperative nurse assists the patient with coping by identifying the extrinsic and intrinsic stressors of the patient's surgical environment, formulating actual and potential nursing diagnoses, identifying expected outcomes, planning appropriate interventions, implementing the interventions, and evaluating the care given.

To illustrate, consider electrosurgery. Preoperatively, the perioperative nurse identifies electrosurgery as a potential extrinsic stressor because improper application of the dispersive electrode may cause system disequilibrium (impaired skin integrity at the application site of the dispersive electrode). Next, the patient is assessed for intrinsic stressors such as excessive hair, scar tissue,

bony prominences, and metal implants that indicate his or her potential for experiencing injury related to electrical hazard, and then the nurse plans appropriate interventions. Intraoperatively, equilibrium is established by applying the dispersive electrode to a site free from hair, scar tissue, bony prominences, and metal implants. Equilibrium is sustained by the perioperative nurse's periodically checking the dispersive electrode to ensure that it remains attached to the patient and by preventing tension on the electrode cord. Postoperatively, the patient is assessed for signs of impaired skin integrity at the site of electrode application. If signs of impaired skin integrity are found, the perioperative nurse starts the process of reestablishing system equilibrium by referring the patient to the surgeon for treatment.

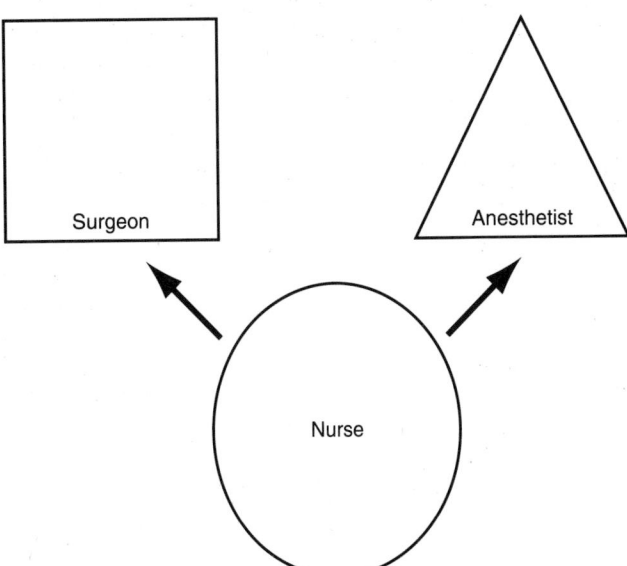

FIGURE 1–10. The nurse facilitates the work of the surgeon and the anesthetist during the perioperative period.

Another component of the perioperative nurse's role is to facilitate the work of the surgeon and the anesthetist during surgery, which is essential for the patient's welfare. This role is derived from the assumption that the person exists in a state of contingency with other systems in the environment. During surgery, the patient, as a holistic system, temporarily becomes a component of the system identified as the surgical team: surgeon, anesthetist, circulating nurse, and scrub nurse. An operation that proceeds smoothly is performed by a surgical team in a state of equilibrium with one another and the patient. The key to this equilibrium is the perioperative nursing team. The scrub nurse facilitates the work of the surgeon at the sterile field. The circulating nurse facilitates the work of the surgeon and the anesthetist from outside the sterile field.

SOURCE OF DIFFICULTY

The *source of difficulty* is "the originating point of deviations from the desired state or condition" (Riehl and Roy, 1980, p. 184). The systems-in-contingency model for perioperative nursing defines the source of difficulty as the patient's failure to cope with the intrinsic and extrinsic stressors during the perioperative period, which can lead to system disequilibrium (Figs. 1–11 and 1–12). As an example, when an area of the body is exposed to prolonged pressure, such as when a person sits in one position for too long, the person adjusts by changing his or her position, which relieves the pressure. The patient under general or spinal anesthesia cannot change position; she or he loses the ability to cope and becomes vulnerable to system disequilibrium.

INTERVENTION FOCUS

The *intervention focus* describes the types of problems found when deviations from the desired state occur (Riehl and Roy, 1980, pp. 184–185). It delineates the potential and actual types of disequilibrium (described by nursing diagnoses) in patiency that are prevented or treated by the perioperative nurse.

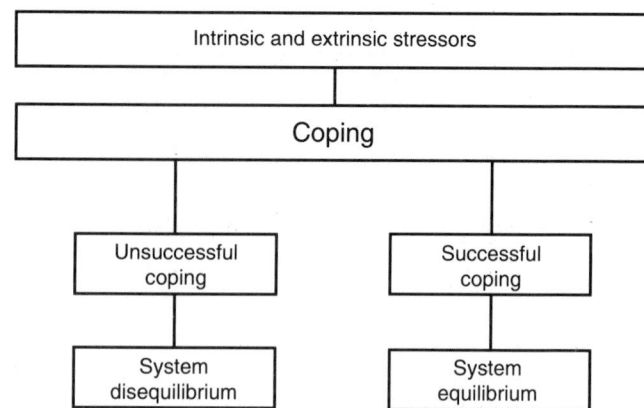
FIGURE 1–12. Coping with stressors.

The systems-in-contingency model for perioperative nursing implies the following:

● The person is a holistic system composed of physical, psychological, sociocultural, and spiritual components.
● The physical, psychological, sociocultural, and spiritual components of the system exist in a state of contingency.
● In a contingency system, no one component of the system can be understood without knowledge of the other components; the system must be viewed as a whole.
● The person exists in a state of contingency with other systems in the environment.

The *functional health patterns* framework (Table 1–2), because it also focuses on the integration of the physical, psychological, sociocultural, and spiritual components of the system, implies that "no one pattern can be understood without knowledge of the other patterns," emphasizes system-environment interactions, and is used as an approach for identifying the potential and actual types of disequilibrium in patiency frequently observed in perioperative nursing practice (Gordon, 1987a, p. 10).

According to Gordon (1987b, p. 92), functional patterns contribute to a person's health, quality of life, and achievement of potential. Patterns, defined as sequences

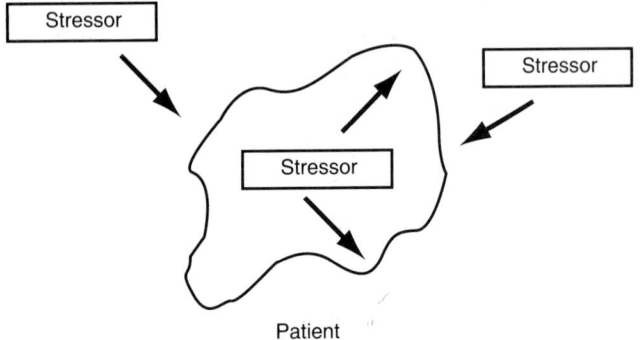
FIGURE 1–11. Failure to cope with stressors leads to illness.

TABLE 1–2. FUNCTIONAL HEALTH PATTERNS
Health perception–health management pattern
Nutritional-metabolic pattern
Elimination pattern
Activity-exercise pattern
Sleep-rest pattern
Cognitive-perceptual pattern
Self-perception–self-concept pattern
Role-relationship pattern
Sexuality-reproduction pattern
Coping–stress tolerance pattern
Value-belief pattern

Modified from Gordon, M. (1987). *Nursing process: Process and application* (2nd ed.). (p. 93). New York: McGraw-Hill.

of behavior across time, are therefore the focus of nursing assessment. Functional health patterns are used to measure the equilibrium of the system. If the perioperative nurse identifies functional patterns (patient strengths) during the assessment, it is an indication that the patient is in a state of equilibrium. If, however, the perioperative nurse identifies potential or actual dysfunctional patterns (nursing diagnoses) during the assessment, it is an indication that the patient is susceptible to, or in an actual state of, disequilibrium.

Gordon (1987b, pp. 431–434) arranged all diagnostic categories approved by the North American Nursing Diagnosis Association according to health patterns. She also included diagnoses not currently accepted by NANDA. These are indicated by an asterisk (*). Listed below are a description of the health patterns and the diagnostic categories identified by the authors as pertinent to perioperative nursing practice and thus the suggested focus of intervention by the perioperative nurse.

The *health perception–health management pattern* describes the patient's "perceived pattern of health and well-being and how health is managed" (Gordon, 1987a, p. 10). This pattern provides insight into the patient's ability and desire to adhere to surgical and nursing prescriptions and participate in the rehabilitation process. The intervention focuses are

Health maintenance alteration
Noncompliance
High risk for infection
High risk for injury

The *nutritional-metabolic pattern* describes the patient's pattern "of food and fluid consumption relative to metabolic need and pattern indicators of local nutrient supply" (Gordon, 1987a, p. 11). This pattern provides information about the patient's tissue repair process, heat-regulating mechanism, and fluid volume. The intervention focuses include

High risk for fluid volume deficit
High risk for impairment of skin integrity
High risk for alteration in body temperature
Hyperthermia
Hypothermia

The *elimination pattern* describes the patient's "patterns of excretory function (bowel, bladder and skin)" (Gordon, 1987a, p. 11). The intervention focus is

Altered urinary elimination pattern

The *activity-exercise pattern* describes the patient's "pattern of exercise, activity, leisure, and recreation" (Gordon, 1987a, p. 11). This pattern provides information about the patient's ability to tolerate and recover from the stressors of surgery. The intervention focuses include

High risk for activity intolerance
Self-care deficit
Impaired physical mobility
Ineffective airway clearance
Ineffective breathing pattern

Alteration in tissue perfusion
*Altered growth and development: self-care skills

The *sleep-rest pattern* describes the patient's "patterns of sleep, rest, and relaxation" (Gordon, 1987a, p. 12). This pattern provides information about the patient's ability to engage in restful sleep during the rehabilitation process. The intervention focus is

Sleep-pattern disturbance

The *cognitive-perceptual pattern* describes the patient's pattern of auditory, visual, kinesthetic, gustatory, tactile, and olfactory senses, as well as cognitive abilities such as language, memory, and decision making (Gordon, 1987a, p. 12). This pattern provides information about the patient's ability to understand instructions and teaching objectives related to the surgical experience. The intervention focuses include

Alteration in comfort: pain
*Uncompensated sensory deficit
Sensory/perceptual alteration: input excess
Sensory/perceptual alteration: input deficit
Knowledge deficit
*Uncompensated short-term memory deficit
*High risk for cognitive impairment
*Decisional conflict

The *self-perception–self-concept pattern* describes the patient's attitudes about body image, identity, sense of worth, emotional pattern, and cognitive and psychomotor abilities (Gordon, 1987a, p. 12). This pattern provides information about the patient's ability to deal with psychological stressors such as fear, anxiety, the inability to control a situation, and the disruption of body image and personal identity. The intervention focuses are

Fear
*Anticipatory anxiety (mild, moderate, severe)
Anxiety
Hopelessness
Powerlessness
Self-esteem disturbance
Body image disturbance

The *role-relationship pattern* describes the patient's "role engagements and relationships." This pattern provides information on how surgery will affect the patient's "perception of the major roles and responsibilities" in his or her current life situation (Gordon, 1987a, p. 12). The intervention focuses are

Anticipatory or dysfunctional grieving
Altered role performance
Social isolation
Impaired social interaction
Alteration in family processes
High risk for alteration in parenting
Impaired verbal communication

The *sexuality-reproduction pattern* describes the patient's "satisfaction or dissatisfaction with sexuality" as well as the reproductive pattern. This pattern provides information on how surgery will affect the patient's "perceived satisfaction or disturbances in" sexuality and reproductive stage (Gordon, 1987a, p. 13). The intervention focuses are

Sexual dysfunction
Altered sexuality patterns

The *coping–stress tolerance pattern* describes the patient's "general coping pattern and effectiveness of the pattern in terms of stress tolerance." This pattern provides information on how surgery will affect the patient's ability to "resist challenge to self-integrity, modes of handling stress, family or other support systems, and perceived ability to control and manage situation" (Gordon, 1987a, p. 13). The intervention focuses include

Ineffective individual coping
Ineffective family coping: compromised or disabling
*Avoidance coping
Impaired adjustment
Post-trauma response

The *value-belief pattern* describes the patient's "patterns of values, goals, or beliefs . . . that guide choices or decisions." This pattern provides information on how surgery will affect the patient's perceptions of what "is important in life and any perceived conflicts in values, beliefs, or expectations" caused by surgery (Gordon, 1987a, p. 13). The intervention focus is

Spiritual distress

INTERVENTION MODE

The *intervention mode* is the primary method of preventing the potential problems or treating the actual problems identified in the intervention focus (Riehl and Roy, 1980, p. 186). The mode of intervention is the elimination, attenuation, or modification of the intrinsic and extrinsic stressors confronting the patient.

Elimination refers to the process of removing the stressor from the patient's environment. Removal of the stressor negates the potential or actual effect of the stressor on the patient. As an example, foreign bodies are potential stressors. If items such as sponges, sharps, and instruments are retained, the patient experiences system disequilibrium after surgery. Sponge, sharps, and instrument counts ensure that these potential stressors are eliminated from the immediate surgical environment (wound) before closure.

Attenuation refers to the process of weakening the stressor. By weakening the stressor, the perioperative nurse decreases the potential or actual effect of the stressor on the patient. As an example, the surgical patient has the potential for wound infection because of the presence of microorganisms in the immediate surgical environment, but complete elimination of microorganisms from the patient's surgical environment is impossible. The effect of microorganisms on the patient, however, can be minimized by decreasing their numbers.

The perioperative nurse accomplishes the desired effect by preparing the patient's operative site with an antimicrobial solution and ensuring that the surgical team members adhere to aseptic practices.

Modification refers to the process of altering how the stressor affects the patient during the perioperative period. The stressor remains the same; the effect, however, is altered. As an example, an elderly emaciated patient scheduled for a 6-hour surgical procedure is confronted with the intrinsic stressors of inadequate adipose tissue, protruding bony prominences, and poor skin turgor. This patient is also confronted with the extrinsic stressors of a lengthy surgical procedure, extended immobility while under anesthesia, and the surface of the operating room bed. The perioperative nurse cannot eliminate these stressors. She or he can, however, modify the effect of the stressors by padding the operating room bed and the bony prominences.

Because perioperative nurses have traditionally focused on the prevention of potential health problems, such as potential infection and injury, the primary aim of the intervention mode in the systems-in-contingency model for perioperative nursing practice is the prevention of potential alterations in system equilibrium during the perioperative period. This does not mean, however, that perioperative nurses ignore actual health problems. On the contrary, treatment of actual health problems falls within the practice domain of perioperative nursing. Examples of perioperative nurses' treating actual health problems are interventions implemented for anxiety, anticipatory grieving, and body image disturbance; correction of knowledge deficit; and preoperative teaching of postoperative breathing and splinting techniques and dressing change technique (particularly for the ambulatory surgery patient).

CONSEQUENCES

The intended consequence of the systems-in-contingency model is system equilibrium during the perioperative period.

There are no unintended consequences.

SUMMARY

The patient is a holistic system interacting with other systems in the surgical environment. The perioperative nurse is a strategic component of that environment. The systems-in-contingency model for perioperative nursing practice provides direction for the practice of nursing in the complex reality of the inpatient or outpatient surgical suite. This approach to the perioperative nursing paradigm provides a stimulus and direction for the development of perioperative nursing curriculum, clinical practice, and research.

Bibliography

Association of Operating Room Nurses. (1992). *Standards of perioperative clinical practice*. Denver.

Fawcett, J. (1980, November-December). A framework for analysis and evaluation of conceptual models of nursing. *Nurse Educator,* pp. 10–14.

Gordon, M. (1987a.) *Manual of nursing diagnosis: 1986–1987.* 2nd ed. New York: McGraw-Hill.

Gordon, M. (1987b.) *Nursing process: Process and application.* New York: McGraw-Hill.

Riehl, J.P., Roy, C. (1980). *Conceptual models for nursing practice* (2nd ed.). New York: Appleton-Century-Crofts.

Roy, C. (1976). *Introduction to nursing: An adaptation model.* New Jersey: Prentice Hall, Inc., p. 3.

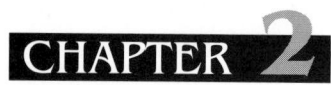

Patient Assessment and Diagnosis: A Functional Health Patterns Approach

Cynthia A. Abbott

Assessment is one of the four phases in the nursing process performed by the perioperative nurse during the patient's surgical experience. As the initial step in the nursing process, an accurate assessment is the most critical component because it is the foundation for the planning, implementation, and evaluation phases of perioperative nursing care. The functional health patterns approach is an exciting method of patient assessment. The use of functional health patterns enables perioperative nurses to perform comprehensive patient assessments in a holistic manner.

DEFINITION OF ASSESSMENT

Assessment is a systematic and deliberate process of collecting and interpreting data concerning a patient's health status. For the perioperative nurse, assessment entails preoperative, intraoperative, and postoperative

---

The views expressed in this chapter are those of the author and do not reflect the official position or policy of the Department of the Army, the Department of Defense, or the U.S. Government.

patient evaluation. Data may be used to develop, revise, or discard a nursing diagnosis, which directs nursing plans, interventions, and evaluations. Data not used to formulate nursing diagnoses are documented in the patient's record as a health status evaluation (Gordon, 1987).

MEASURABLE CRITERIA

The perioperative nurse demonstrates competency to perform a patient assessment and nursing diagnosis by

- evaluating the patient's health patterns
- interpreting assessment data
- clustering data
- making nursing diagnoses using the eleven functional health patterns
- supporting nursing diagnoses with scientific knowledge
- documenting and communicating the assessment data and nursing diagnosis

PHYSIOLOGICAL DATA

The perioperative nurse uses the following diagnostic tests and procedures during data collection:

Blood Studies. Common laboratory tests ordered for the surgical patient are found in Table 2–1.

Vital Signs. Respirations, pulses, blood pressure, and body temperature are measured with the patient in the sitting or the supine position. The perioperative nurse uses observation, palpation, and auscultation skills to assess the patient's vital signs. Normal values for vital signs for adults include the following:

Respiration rate of 12 to 18 breaths/minute
Pulse rate of 50 to 100 beats/minute in a regular and strong pattern (Fig. 2–1)
Blood pressure of 120/80
Body temperature
   Oral: 98.6°F (37°C)

Axillary: 97.6°F (36.5–36.6°C)
Rectal: 99.6°F (37.4–37.5°C) (Luckmann and Sorenson, 1987)

Table 2–2 describes the effect of abnormal vital signs on the patient's perioperative experience.

Serological Studies. Serological blood determinations reflect heart and thyroid alterations as well as the presence of syphilis and infectious mononucleosis (Kneedler and Dodge, 1987).

Toxicological Studies. Blood or urine values reflect poison or drug levels, including the presence of barbiturates and anticonvulsants (Kneedler and Dodge, 1987) (Table 2–3).

Microbiological Studies. Cultures are taken of sputum, urine, blood, spinal fluid, stool, and throat, eye, ear, nasopharyngeal, vaginal, and urethral areas to identify pathogens and specific microorganisms (Kneedler and Dodge, 1987).

TABLE 2–1. COMMON PREOPERATIVE BLOOD TESTS

Test	Normal Range	Abnormal Findings Increase	Abnormal Findings Decrease
Potassium	3.5–5 mEq/L	Dehydration Renal failure	Excessive use of diuretics Nausea, vomiting, hypotension, malnutrition, cardiac arrhythmias
Sodium	136–145 mEq/L	Cardiac or renal failure Hypertension Excess amounts of intravenous fluids containing normal saline Edema	Nasogastric drainage Vomiting, diarrhea Excessive use of laxatives and/or diuretics
Chloride	96–106 mEq/L	Alkalosis Dehydration Renal failure	Excessive nasogastric drainage Vomiting Excessive use of diuretics
Carbon dioxide	22–34 mEq/L	Chronic obstructive pulmonary disease Respiratory acidosis Intestinal obstruction Vomiting or nasogastric suctioning	Hyperventilation Diabetic acidosis Diarrhea
Glucose (fasting)	60–100 mg/dl	Hyperglycemia Excess amounts of intravenous fluids containing glucose Pancreatic and/or hepatic disease	Hypoglycemia
White blood cell count	4500–11,000 cells/mm³	Infection	Immune deficit
Hemoglobin	12–15 g/dl (women) 14–16.5 g/dl (men)	Fluid overload	Dehydration Excessive blood loss Anemia
Hematocrit	37–45% (women) 42–50% (men)		
Creatinine	0.6–1 mg/dl (women) 0.8–1.7 mg/dl (men)	Renal damage with destruction of large number of nephrons	Atrophy of muscle tissue
Blood urea nitrogen	5–15 mg/dl	Dehydration Renal failure Excessive protein in diet	Overhydration Liver failure Malnutrition
Prothrombin time	12–14 s (2–2.5 times normal is a therapeutic range)	Coagulation defect Increased chance of hemorrhage Too high a dose of anticoagulant (aspirin, heparin, warfarin)	Increased chance of embolus (thrombophlebitis, pulmonary emboli)
Partial thromboplastin time	28–44 s (results are compared with aging laboratory control)		

Adapted from Ignatavicius, D., Bayne, M. V. (1991). *Medical-surgical nursing: A nursing process approach* (pp. 435–437). Philadelphia: W. B. Saunders.

TABLE 2–2. ASSESSING ALTERATIONS IN VITAL SIGNS

Vital Sign	Normal Finding	Abnormal Finding	Possible Indication	Possible Postoperative Complication
Temperature	Oral: 98.6°F (37°C) Axillary: 97.6°F (36.5–36.6°C) Rectal: 99.6°F (37.4–37.5°C)	Fever (temperature > 101°F [38.3°C] in an adult)	Infection Dehydration (when accompanied by decreased skin turgor)	Systemic infection Wound infection, dehiscence, or evisceration Fluid imbalance Shock
Pulse	50 to 100 beats/min in a regular and strong pattern	Tachycardia (>100 beats/min)	Pain Fever Dehydration Anemia Hypoxia Shock	Poor tissue perfusion Vascular collapse Cardiac arrhythmias Renal failure Anesthetic complications
		Bradycardia (<60 beats/min)	Drug effects (e.g., of digitalis) Spinal injury Head injury	Spinal shock Increased intracranial pressure (see also complications for tachycardia)
Respiration	12 to 18 breaths/min	Tachypnea (>24 breaths/min)	Atelectasis Pneumonia Pain or anxiety Pleurisy Infection Renal failure	Tissue hypoxia Anesthetic complications Pneumonia Atelectasis
		Bradypnea (<10 breaths/min)	Brain lesion Respiratory center depression	See complications for tachypnea
Blood pressure	120/80	Hypotension (<90 mm Hg systolic)	Shock Myocardial infarction Hemorrhage Spinal injury	Poor tissue perfusion Renal failure Vasodilation Shock
		Hypertension (>140 mm Hg systolic and/or 90 mm Hg diastolic)	Anxiety or pain Renal disease Coronary artery disease	Stroke Hemorrhage Myocardial infarction

Adapted from Ignatavicius, D., Bayne, M. V. (1991). *Medical-surgical nursing: A nursing process approach* (p. 432). Philadelphia: W. B. Saunders.

TABLE 2–3. ASSESSING DRUG LEVELS

Drug	Effective Concentrations*	Nursing Actions
Alcohol ethanol	Legal toxicity varies, may begin at 0.05–0.15 g/100 ml	
Acetaminophen	Therapeutic: 10–20 μg/ml Toxic: >300 μg/ml	

Barbiturate	Therapeutic: adult and child: phenobarbital:
	  1.5–4 mg/100 ml
	  Others: 0.05–0.3 mg/100 ml
	Toxic: adult and child:
	  Short acting: 3 mg/100 ml
	  Moderate acting: 6 mg/100 ml
	  Long acting: 9 mg/100 ml	

Cadmium
  Serum
  Urine
	Normal:
	  Negative
	  <15 μg/24 h	

Carbamazepine	Therapeutic: 3–9 μg/ml	
Carbon monoxide	0–2% saturation. Symptoms appear with levels over 20%	
Chlordiazepoxide	Therapeutic: 1–3 μg/ml	

Chlorpromazine	Therapeutic:
	  Adult: 30–50 ng/ml
	  Children: 40–80 ng/ml	

Clonazepam	Therapeutic: 5–70 ng/ml	
Desipramine	Therapeutic: 40–60 ng/ml Toxic: >1 μg/ml	
Diazepam	Therapeutic: 300–400 ng/ml	
Diphenhydramine	Therapeutic: >25 ng/ml Toxic: >100 μg/ml	
Doxepin	Therapeutic: 30–150 ng/ml	
Ethosuximide	Therapeutic: 40–100 μg/ml	
Haloperidol	Therapuetic: 1 ng/ml Toxic: >15 ng/ml	
Imipramine	Therapeutic: 100–300 ng/ml Toxic: >1 μg/ml	
Indomethacin	Therapeutic: 0.3–3 μg/ml Toxic: >5 μg/ml	

Lead
  Serum
  Urine
	Normal: negative
	Toxic: >0.08 mg/100 ml
	    >0.08 mg/24 h
		Collection container must contain preservative or be kept on ice

Lithium	Therapeutic: 0.6–1.2 mEq/L Toxic: >2 mEq/L	
Meperidine	Therapeutic: 0.4–0.7 μg/ml	
Methanol	May be fatal when as low as 10 mg/100 ml	
Methsuximide	Therapeutic: 10–100 μg/ml	
Naproxen	Therapeutic: >50 μg/ml	
Nitrazepam	Toxic: >200 ng/ml	
Nortriptyline	Therapeutic: 50–140 ng/ml	
Phensuximide	Therapeutic: 40–80 μg/ml	
Phenylbutazone	Therapeutic: 50–150 μg/ml	
Phenytoin	Therapeutic: 10–20 μg/100 ml	
Primidone	Therapeutic: 4–12 μg/ml	
Protriptyline	Therapeutic: 100–200 ng/100 ml	
Pyridostigmine	Therapeutic: 50–100 ng/ml	
Salicylate	Therapeutic: 150–300 μg/ml	Draw specimen 2 h after dose
Trimethadione	Therapeutic: 20–40 μg/ml	
Valproic acid	Therapeutic: 50–100 μg/ml	

*Please note, these values are guidelines. Check with the laboratory performing the test.
From Brenner, Z. R. (1987). *Diagnostic tests and procedures applying to nursing.* East Norwalk, CT: Appleton & Lange.

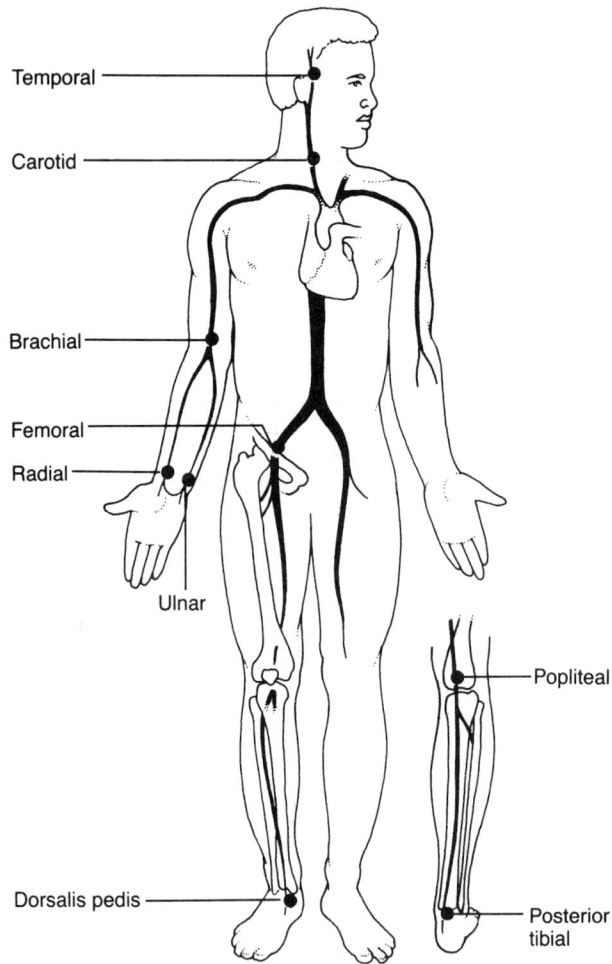

FIGURE 2–1. Assessing arterial pulses. (From Ignatavicius, D., Bayne, M. V. [1991]. *Medical-surgical nursing: A nursing process approach* [p. 2102]. Philadelphia: W. B. Saunders.)

Gastrointestinal System Studies. Radiological examination of the gastrointestinal tract includes an upper gastrointestinal series, a barium swallow, small bowel series, and double-contrast study. An upper gastrointestinal series assesses the presence of celiac disease, regional enteritis, or malabsorption syndrome. In addition, an upper gastrointestinal series assesses esophageal varices, gastric spasm, ulcerations, and other abnormalities. A lower gastrointestinal series using a radiopaque contrast medium, fluoroscopy, and serial timed radiographs assesses the contour of the colon, the cecum, and the appendix. This procedure is useful to examine polyps, small nonobstructing carcinomas, or inflammatory bowel disease (Brenner, 1987).

Cardiovascular Examinations. Cardiovascular system studies that the perioperative nurse commonly encounters include ECG, chest radiography, ultrasonography, magnetic resonance imaging (MRI), and scintigraphy. The three-lead ECG effectively screens most patients preoperatively. Patients with known cardiac disease often undergo a 12-lead ECG to thoroughly evaluate electrical impulses in the heart. The 12-lead ECG also detects the presence of right ventricular infarction and the effects of chemical imbalances or drug therapy on cardiac function. As discussed above, the chest x-ray film provides information about the size and condition of vessels and cardiac muscle. Ultrasonography permits noninvasive assessment of the heart's structure, valves, vessels, and blood flow by analyzing sound wave patterns. MRI is another noninvasive method of assessing the function and tissue composition of the heart. This procedure is often used for patients with suspected vascular disease. MRI is contraindicated for patients with aneurysm clips or pacemakers because of their interference with the magnetic field. Scintigraphic studies are noninvasive and involve the uptake of a radiopaque solution to assess the cardiovascular system. Common scintigraphic tests include (1) thallium scanning, which identifies areas of myocardial fibrosis and ischemia; (2) technetium scanning, which identifies damaged tissues and is often used in patients with an altered ECG; and (3) iodine-125–labeled fibrinogen uptake test,

Chest Radiography. Chest x-ray films screen patients preoperatively for diseases such as carcinoma, tuberculosis, and heart disease. Chest x-ray films provide information on the heart's position, the extent of calcium deposits (calcification), and the size of the chambers and great vessels (Brenner, 1987). In addition, chest x-ray films reflect alterations in the chest wall, the pleural spaces, the tracheobronchial tract, and the diaphragm (Kneedler and Dodge, 1987). Chest x-ray films are used to determine the location of central venous pressure catheters, arterial catheters, pacemaker wires, and so on (Brenner, 1987).

Electrocardiography. Electrocardiograms (ECGs) reflect the heart's electrical activity. Alterations in the normal ECG pattern may indicate previous cardiac ischemia or infarction. A normal ECG does not eliminate the possibility of cardiac pathological changes because the heart's muscle strength is not measured in this study (Kneedler and Dodge, 1987). Figure 2–2 shows a normal ECG pattern. Figures 2–3 through 2–9 show examples of ECG alterations that the nurse might observe during the perioperative period.

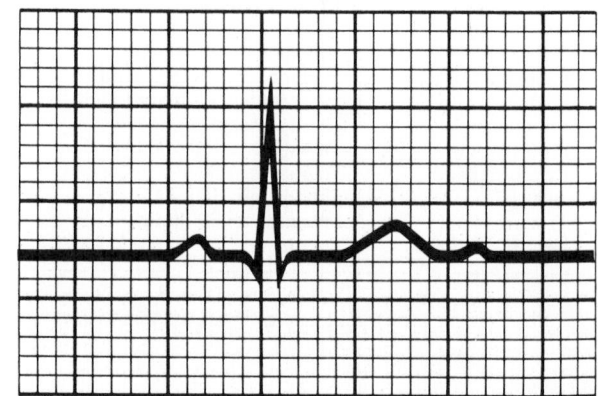

FIGURE 2–2. Normal ECG pattern. (From Ignatavicius, D., Bayne, M. V. [1991]. *Medical-surgical nursing: A nursing process approach* [p. 2102]. Philadelphia: W. B. Saunders.)

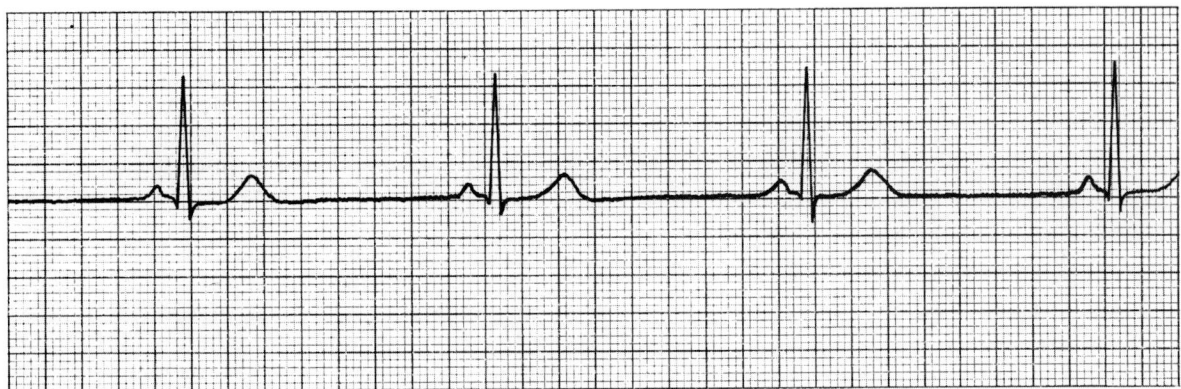

FIGURE 2–3. Sinus bradycardia. This condition occurs in well-conditioned athletes or is caused by parasympathetic stimulation resulting from excessive vagal stimulation (carotid massage, Valsalva maneuvers, suctioning, and spinal cord injury); pharmacological agents such as digitalis, beta-adrenergic blocking agents, opiates, and tranquilizers; and hypothyroidism, hyperkalemia, or inferior myocardial infarctions. (From Ignatavicius, D., Bayne, M. V. [1991]. *Medical-surgical nursing: A nursing process approach* [p. 2120]. Philadelphia: W. B. Saunders.)

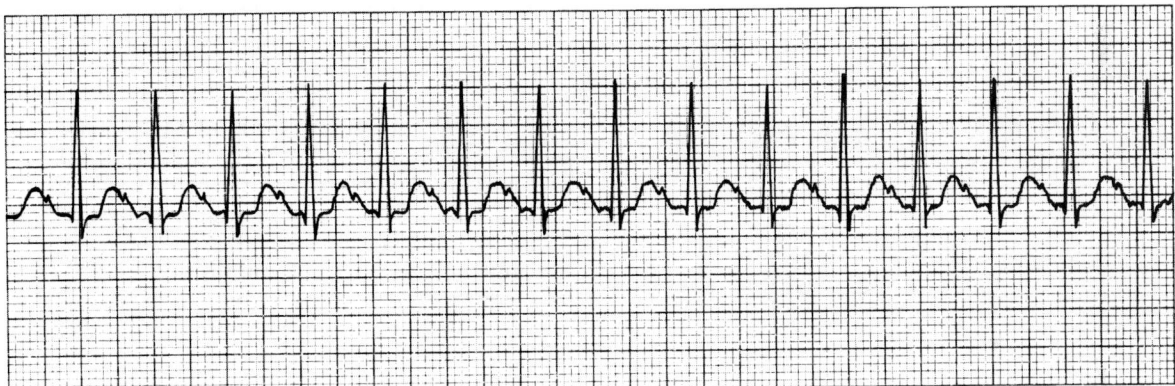

FIGURE 2–4. Sinus tachycardia. Causes include central nervous system–mediated sympathetic stimulation caused by anxiety, pain, fright, or stress; and increased heart beat in compensation for decreased stroke volume related to fever, alcohol ingestion, hypovolemia, heart failure, hyperthyroidism, and anemia. (From Ignatavicius, D., Bayne, M. V. [1991]. *Medical-surgical nursing: A nursing process approach* [p. 2119]. Philadelphia: W. B. Saunders.)

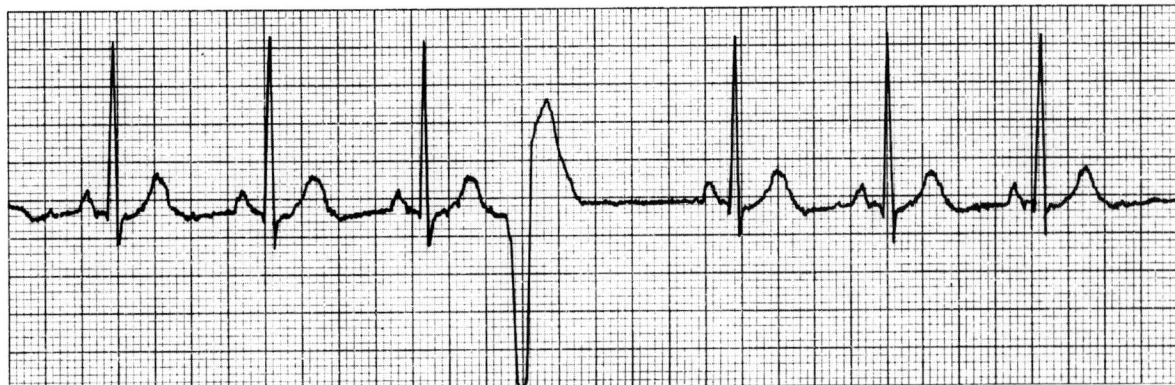

FIGURE 2–5. Premature ventricular contraction. It can be caused by cardiac ischemia, digitalis toxicity, increased catecholamine release, edema at the tissue level, hypoxia, electrolyte imbalance, overuse of stimulants such as caffeine or nicotine, lack of sleep, anxiety, or stretching of the myocardia fibers secondary to fluid overload, heart failure, or valvular disorders. (From Ignatavicius, D., Bayne, M. V. [1991]. *Medical-surgical nursing: A nursing process approach* [p. 2121]. Philadelphia: W. B. Saunders.)

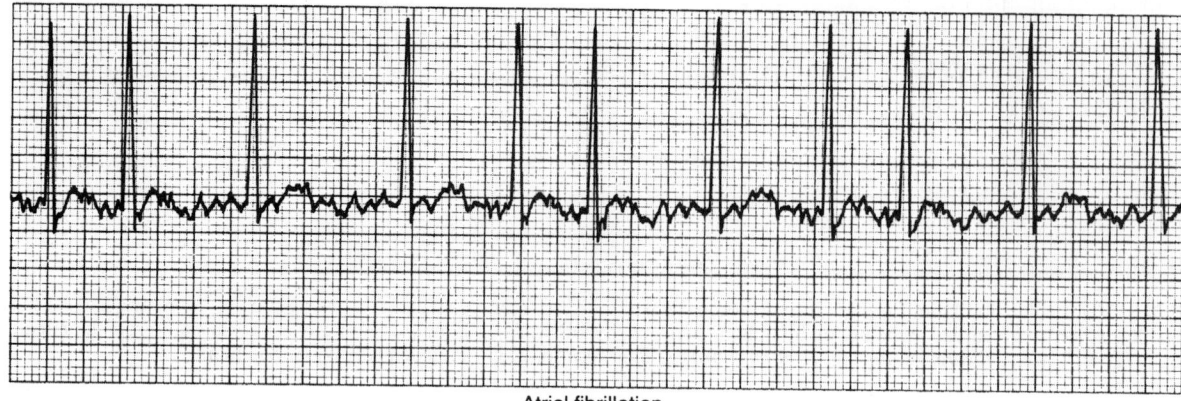

Atrial fibrillation

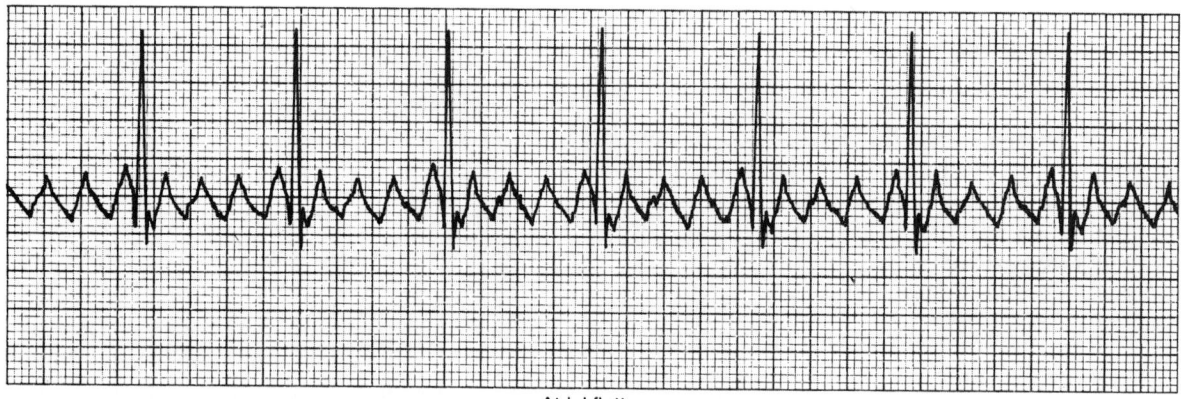

Atrial flutter

FIGURE 2–6. Atrial fibrillation and atrial flutter. Causes include vagal stimulation with carotid massage, Valsalva maneuvers, or prolonged suctioning resulting in pauses in sinus node discharge; and hyperkalemia or digitalis toxicity. (From Ignatavicius, D., Bayne, M. V. [1991]. *Medical-surgical nursing: A nursing process approach* [p. 2124]. Philadelphia: W. B. Saunders.)

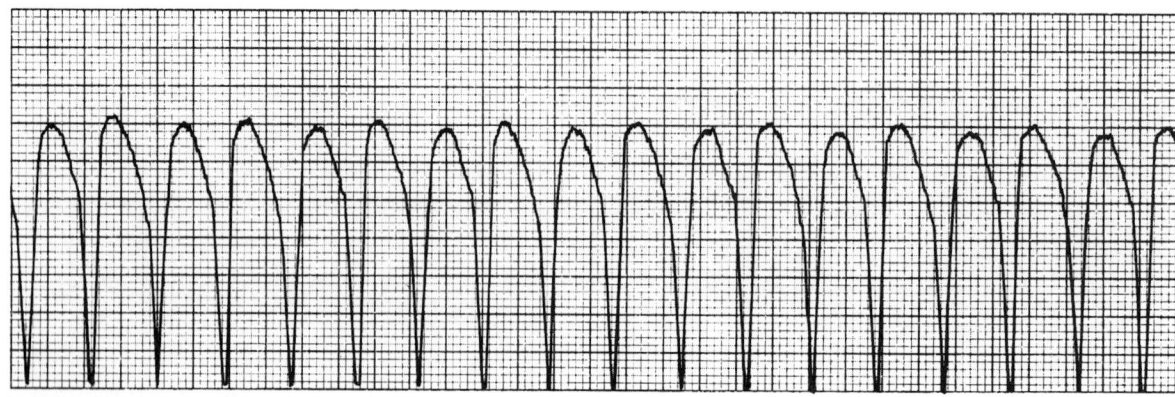

FIGURE 2–7. Ventricular tachycardia. This condition results from myocardial ischemia or infarction, digitalis toxicity, mitral valve prolapse, cardiomyopathy, myocarditis, hypokalemia, prolonged QT interval, or excessive circulating catecholamines. (From Ignatavicius, D., Bayne, M. V. [1991]. *Medical-surgical nursing: A nursing process approach* [p. 2129]. Philadelphia: W. B. Saunders.)

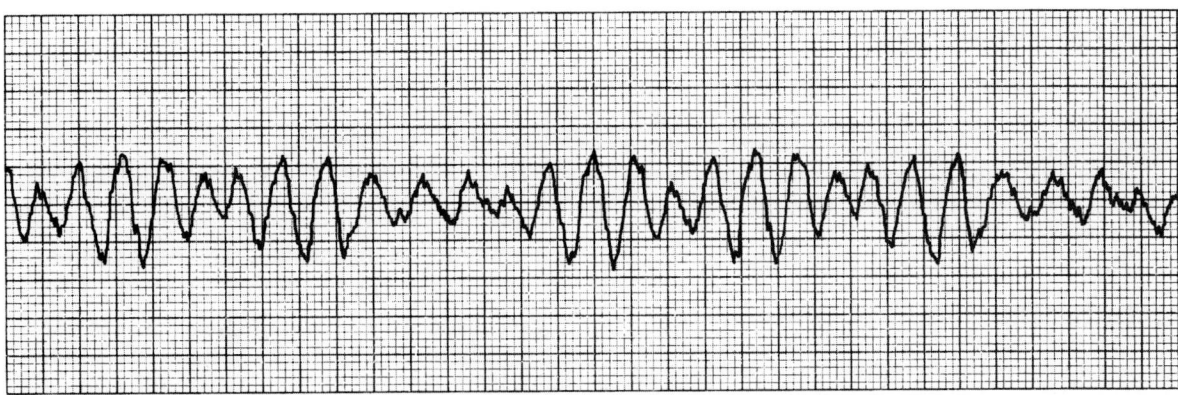

FIGURE 2–8. Ventricular fibrillation. Causes include coronary artery disease (can be initiated by single premature ventricular contraction or ventricular fibrillation), myocardial ischemia or infarction, hypoxia, hypothermia, acidosis, or electrolyte imbalance. (From Ignatavicius, D., Bayne, M. V. [1991]. *Medical-surgical nursing: A nursing process approach* [p. 2130]. Philadelphia: W. B. Saunders.)

which is used for patients with suspected deep venous thrombosis (Brenner, 1987).

Neurological System Studies. Examinations commonly performed for the patient with neurological alterations include ultrasonography, measurement of electrical activity (i.e., electroencephalography), MRI, scintigraphy (brain scan), computed tomography (CT), and contrast studies. Echoencephalography is a type of ultrasonography that assesses movement of the lateral ventricles seen in cerebral lesions. This procedure evaluates the presence of subdural hematomas, intracerebral hemorrhage, and neoplasia. It is effective in infants because the infant brain has a higher water content and more subarachnoid fluid than the brain of adults. Electroencephalography provides graphic readings of electrical activity within the brain. This procedure detects the presence of epilepsy, organic brain syndrome, and brain death by assessing the frequency, amplitude, and type of brain waves present. MRI is a noninvasive procedure for patients with suspected intracranial disease, hemorrhage, mass, or lesion. This procedure identifies disease, lesions, and trauma involving the spinal cord and the pituitary gland. Brain scans identify the presence of subdural hematomas, cerebral thrombosis, and intracranial tumors when CT is not available. CT identifies the presence of soft tissue tumors and injury in severely traumatized children. CT differentiates among intracranial hemorrhage, ischemia, and infarction by identifying variations in tissue density. This procedure is used to determine developmental defects of the central nervous system in infants. Myelograms identify abnormalities and obstructions of central spinal fluid flow in the vertebral subarachnoid space. This invasive procedure is performed with a contrast medium, fluoroscopy, and serial timed radiographs for patients with suspected intervertebral disk disorders, neoplasms, or abscesses (Brenner, 1987).

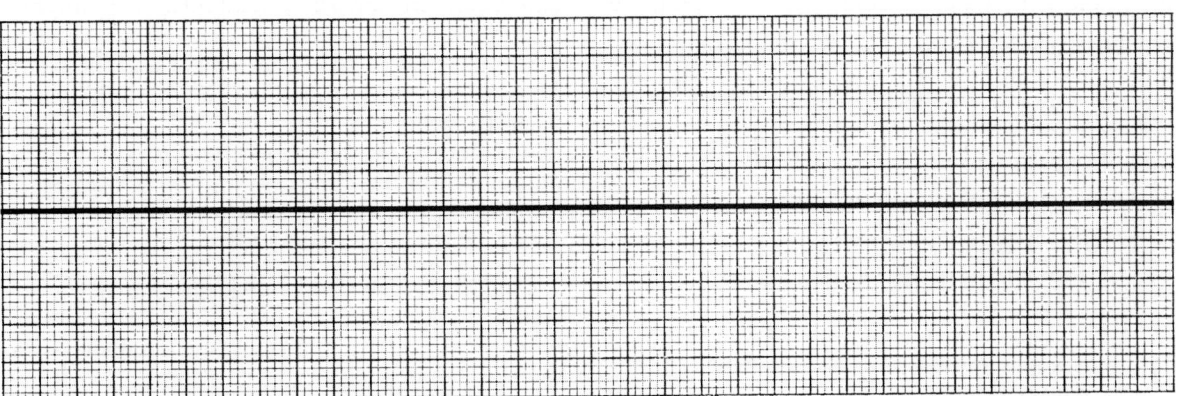

FIGURE 2–9. Asystole. Causes include extensive myocardial ischemia from prolonged periods of inadequate coronary perfusion and severe metabolic disorders, such as hyperkalemia and acidosis. (From Ignatavicius, D., Bayne, M. V. [1991]. *Medical-surgical nursing: A nursing process approach* [p. 2130]. Philadelphia: W. B. Saunders.)

GROWTH AND DEVELOPMENT PROCESS

Growth and development are dynamic processes built into the health patterns assessment framework (Gordon, 1987). *Growth* refers to physical changes and an increase in size that occur during the first 20 years of life. *Development* is the behavior that reflects a patient's mastery of skills (Kozier and Erb, 1983).

Perioperative Nursing Implications

The perioperative nurse uses growth and development concepts to establish a baseline assessment and to identify problems or needs that the patient may encounter during the surgical experience (Gordon, 1987). The preoperative assessment later serves as a point of reference for intraoperative and postoperative behavioral evaluation. The perioperative nurse looks for the behavioral patterns associated with each of five concepts within a specific age group. Alterations in physiological, cognitive, psychosocial, moral, or spiritual concepts cue the perioperative nurse to potential or actual patient problems within the 11 functional health patterns (see Table 2–4).

Key Concepts

The five concepts of growth and development that the perioperative nurse assesses are (1) *physiological*, (2) *cognitive*, (3) *psychosocial*, (4) *moral*, and (5) *spiritual* elements. The physiological component refers to the patient's anatomical size and structure. The psychosocial component describes the quality and type of social interactions the patient has with others. This component also includes the motor skills attained to interact with the environment. Erikson's eight stages of development and Havighurst's developmental tasks describe the psychosocial behaviors of patients. The moral component covers the values, attitudes, and beliefs the patient associates with right and wrong. Erikson's virtues depict moral development. The cognitive component refers to the intellectual and reasoning abilities of the patient. Piaget's phases of cognitive development describe significant behaviors to assess. The spiritual component represents the relationship the patient has with the universe and his or her philosophy about life. Fowler's stages of spiritual development describe an approach to spiritual assessment (Kozier and Erb, 1983).

Application of Key Concepts to Stages of Development (Kozier and Erb, 1983)

Generalities about growth and development are presented here. The perioperative nurse must evaluate the significance of the patient's variation in development when determining whether there are alterations in health patterns.

Infant (Birth to 1 Year)

Physiological. Growth is rapid in the infant. Movements are initially reflexive and gradually become more purposeful. Meeting oral needs is more important at this age. The trunk of the body grows rapidly. The urinary system is completely developed at the end of the first year. Eye muscles function, and the infant differentiates simple shapes. The final number of brain cells is present by age 1 year (Kozier and Erb, 1983).

Psychosocial. The infant develops a sense of trust versus mistrust with others and learns to trust or mistrust himself or herself. Sufficient parenting and caregiving are important to meet the infant's needs. Motor skills include learning to walk, to take solid foods, and to talk (Kozier and Erb, 1983).

Cognitive. Initial perceptions center on physical states (wetness, dryness, hunger, and so on). Next, the environment is recognized; then the infant actively attempts to change the environment (Kozier and Erb, 1983).

Moral. The infant develops hope or confidence in achieving desires or wishes from the environment (Kozier and Erb, 1983).

Spiritual. The infant is unable to draw philosophical conclusions about herself or himself or the environment until 4 years of age (Kozier and Erb, 1983).

Toddler (1 to 3 Years)

Physiological. The growth rate decreases in this age group. The chubby toddler's fat deposits decrease as muscle tissue development increases (Kozier and Erb, 1983; Wolf et al., 1983). Farsightedness increases in toddlers until age 8 years, when the eye becomes adult size (Kozier and Erb, 1983). The abdomen protrudes until abdominal muscles develop. Most deciduous teeth are present by age 2 years (Wolf et al., 1983).

Psychosocial. Erikson describes this age as seeking autonomy versus doubt and shame (Kozier and Erb, 1983). To move into this phase, the child must have confidence in himself or herself and in others in the environment. This developmental phase is characterized by exploration of the environment and the frequent use of "no." A common conflict for the toddler is learning what to keep and when to let go of objects in the environment. The prominent motor skill involves learning to control the elimination of body wastes. The child enjoys playing alone or alongside others without interaction (Wolf et al., 1983).

Cognitive. The child perceives that he or she is the center of the universe. Everything in the environment relates to "me." Language development is rapid and the child associates words with things (Kozier and Erb, 1983).

Moral. The toddler seeks to control the environment. She or he learns to balance personal desires and self-restraint during this phase of autonomy development (Kozier and Erb, 1983).

Spiritual. The infant is unable to draw philosophical conclusions about herself or himself or the environment until 4 years of age (Kozier and Erb, 1983).

Preschooler (3 to 6 Years)

Physiological. The preschool child experiences rapid growth. Muscle size increases slowly. Permanent teeth begin to replace deciduous teeth (Kozier and Erb, 1983). Increased development of the eye allows the child to begin reading late in this phase (Wolf et al., 1983).

Psychosocial. Erikson describes this age according to the development of initiative and the resolution of guilt (Kozier and Erb, 1983). The child is aware of gender differences and sexual modesty. This is the phase critical to sexual identity development. Playing with other preschoolers is meaningful, as increased language skills facilitate interaction with others. Intrusive behavior typifies this age as the child asserts himself or herself in the environment of others and enters the world of fantasy and dreams (Wolf et al., 1983).

Cognitive. The self-centered "me" thinking of the toddler diminishes. The child thinks of one idea at a time, and language reflects personal thoughts of the child (Kozier and Erb, 1983).

Moral. The child begins to distinguish between right and wrong. This development of a conscience is the foundation for values and morals later in adult life (Wolf et al., 1983). Erikson sees the preschooler as developing a purpose for action and courage in pursuing valued goals (Kozier and Erb, 1983).

Spiritual. The preschooler organizes various images and beliefs given by trusted others. The child interprets the images and beliefs according to her or his life experiences and personal imagination. This stage is known as the intuitive-projective phase of spiritual development (Kozier and Erb, 1983).

School-Age Child (6 to 12 Years)

Physiological. The child is strong and lean by the time he or she enters school. Growth generally slows and physical stability is developed by age 12 years (Wolf et al., 1983). Growth spurts in girls occur at about 10 years of age, and strength at puberty is greater than in boys. The immune system is functionally mature in this age group (Kozier and Erb, 1983).

Psychosocial. Erikson describes this phase as a time of industry and developing a sense of competence and perseverance about manipulating and creating objects in the environment. The developmental task of the school-age child is to develop a sense of industry rather than mediocrity. A sense of mediocrity develops when a child is unable to effectively create and manipulate

items in the environment. To achieve a feeling of industry, the child must learn physical skills necessary for games, get along with children of similar age, and learn the appropriate masculine or feminine social role (Kozier and Erb, 1983). In addition, the child attains a feeling of personal independence and learns that adults are not perfect (Wolf et al., 1983).

Cognitive. The child develops fundamental skills for reading, writing, and calculating. These skills assist the child to solve concrete problems, understand the concept of right and left, be aware of differing viewpoints, and understand relationships such as size, volume, and weight (Kozier and Erb, 1983). An interest in categorizing items is present. The child likes to collect things, which promotes the development of concrete thought processes (Wolf et al., 1983).

Moral. A feeling of competence arises in the school-age child. The feeling of competence or incompetence affects the child's attitudes towards social institutions such as educational, religious, political, and economic groups. The child develops a conscience, a sense of morality, and a scale of values based on a feeling of competence (Kozier and Erb, 1983).

Spiritual. This is the mythical-literal age of spiritual development. Religious symbols take on specific meanings. Children use their private world of fantasy and wonder to interpret dramatic stories and myths depicting spiritual meanings (Kozier and Erb, 1983).

Adolescent (12 to 20 Years)

Physiological. Rapid development typifies adolescence (Wolf et al., 1983). Rapid growth in boys begins about 13 years of age, and muscle strength is greater than in girls. The heart reaches mature size by age 16 years. The reproductive organs mature at puberty and hair distribution changes. There is an increase in basal metabolic rate, adrenal gland growth, and sebaceous gland activity (Kozier and Erb, 1983).

Psychosocial. Erikson describes adolescence as the period of attaining self-identity versus identity role confusion (Kozier and Erb, 1983). Peer relationships often are more significant than family relationships during adolescence. Peers foster self-identity in the adolescent by defining the "in thing to do" until a more secure self-identity is found. Adolescents seek independence and an identity outside of the parental sphere. Peers are the support system adolescents use when testing parental reaction to new behaviors. Testing parental reactions and identifying with a peer group assists the adolescents in resolving self-identity issues. In addition, adolescents seek to achieve new and more mature relations with peers of both sexes, accept their physical appearance, achieve socially responsible behavior, prepare for a career, and prepare for family and marriage or other life style choices (Wolf et al., 1983).

Cognitive. The ability to deal with abstract concepts and the ability to perform deductive, reflective, and hypothetical reasoning begin at 12 to 15 years of age. This final stage in Piaget's cognitive development theory describes the mind as having the capacity for continuous learning and the ability to organize concepts for the future (Wolf et al., 1983).

Moral. Adolescents develop the ability to sustain personal loyalties despite contradictions between their value systems and those of others (Kozier and Erb, 1983). These value systems serve as a guide for adolescent behavior as well as social, political, and philosophical ideologies. Highly altruistic movements supported by personal ideologies motivate the adolescent toward responsible involvement in the community to improve society (Wolf et al., 1983).

Spiritual. The adolescent views the environment and the world in terms of the expectations and judgments offered by others (Kozier and Erb, 1983).

Young Adult (20 to 40 Years)

Physiological. Although adulthood is perceived as a physiological plateau, this period includes many changes between 20 and 65 years of age. Between 20 and 30 years of age, the young adult achieves maximum physiological maturity. Physiological decline begins shortly after physiological maturity (Wolf et al., 1983).

Psychosocial. Erikson describes this phase according to achievement of intimacy with another versus isolation. Intimacy is commonly experienced with mutual trust and cooperation in a marital relationship. As intimacy develops, the couple become involved with community activities to promote a good environment for their children. Developmental tasks such as selecting a mate, learning to live with a spouse, starting a family, rearing children, managing a home, starting a career, assuming civic responsibilities, and finding a congenial social group describe accomplishments of this age group (Wolf et al., 1983).

Cognitive. Reasoning and intellectual abilities are well developed but often peak later in life (Wolf et al., 1983).

Moral. The virtue of love and mutual devotion develop during the phase of intimacy versus isolation (Kozier and Erb, 1983).

Spiritual. During this phase the adult constructs his or her own belief system according to his or her individual needs and perceptions. The adult has obtained a high degree of self-consciousness (Kozier and Erb, 1983).

Adult (40 to 65 Years)

Physiological. Physiological functioning gradually declines and changes in physical appearance occur during this phase. An increase in weight and redistribution of body fat make the adult structure appear narrow at the ends and heavy in the middle. Receding hairlines and thinning and graying of hair are typical of this age

group. The skin loses elasticity and wrinkles appear. The cumulative effects of these changes lead to disappointments for those adults who derive feelings of worth from physical beauty. In general, this age group experiences fewer acute illnesses, fewer accidents, and more chronic illness (Brunner and Suddarth, 1988).

Psychosocial. Erikson describes this age group as dealing with the choices of generativity versus stagnation (Kozier and Erb, 1983). Generativity relates to the nurturing and guiding of the next generation. These adults often increase their involvement in social and civic responsibilities to create a better environment and world for the next generation. Stagnation occurs when the individual becomes bored, dissatisfied, and uncaring about the future (Wolf et al., 1983). The adult strives to achieve an adequate standard of living, develop new leisure time activities, and assist teenagers to become responsible and satisfied adults (Kozier and Erb, 1983).

Cognitive. Intellectual skills and creative thought processes are often at their peak (Wolf et al., 1983).

Moral. The adult of 40 to 65 years experiences care and concern for those who promote creativity for others (Kozier and Erb, 1983).

Spiritual. After the age of 30 years, the adult becomes aware of the many truths associated with a variety of viewpoints and spiritual philosophies (Kozier and Erb, 1983).

Older Adult (65 Years and Older)

Physiological. Increased fragility in homeostatic processes typifies older adults. The external signs of aging are apparent, but the internal changes have the greatest impact on body functioning. Temperature regulation and pain sensitivity become less efficient. A decrease in the central nervous system's functioning results in slower reactions and labored movements. The older adult's sense of balance becomes disturbed and the ability to perform fine motor movements lessens. The skeleton changes as the head sits forward, the back arches, and the hips and knees flex. Skeletal bones become porous and brittle owing to mineral losses. Tissues in joints stiffen, which results in less flexible movement. Mobility decreases unless exercise continues. Plaque deposits line the blood vessels, which decreases the size of the vessels and increases the pressure resistance on the heart. Decreased flexibility of tissues in the heart, the vessels, and the respiratory system results in decreased metabolic efficiency, less mobility, and decreased exertion. A decrease in the production of digestive juices, the absorption of food nutrients, and peristalsis leads to changes in nutrient intake, constipation, and indigestion. Approximately 75% of men older than 65 years experience hypertrophy of the prostate gland. In addition, stress incontinence commonly occurs in this age group owing to relaxed muscles of the urinary opening. Tooth decay and loss lead to the necessity for dentures, which may become ill fitting over time (Wolf et al., 1983).

Psychosocial. Erikson describes this phase as integrity versus despair. The mature adult faces the task of accepting his or her worth, uniqueness, and death. Indicators of negative adaptation to this stage include feelings of loss and contempt for others (Kozier and Erb, 1983). Issues that the mature adult faces include adjustments to decreased physical strength and health, retirement and reduced income, loss of a spouse, inadequate socialization with one's age group, and living arrangements that primarily need to be quiet, warm, maintenance free, and relatively inexpensive in a location accessible to churches, medical facilities, transportation, and family members (Wolf et al., 1983).

Cognitive. Cognitive functioning does not decrease unless disuse occurs. Reasoning and rational thinking do not decline unless disease intervenes. Thinking is slower, but the mature adult has the ability to learn when given sufficient time, empathy, and patience by family and health care team members (Wolf et al., 1983).

Moral. The mature adult develops intense wisdom in dealing with life issues. This phase includes the acceptance of death and a peaceful perspective on life (Kozier and Erb, 1983).

Spiritual. The principle of universalizing may never be experienced by the adult. Universalizing may be seen in the mature adult's acceptance of death. Believing that principles of love and fairness justify the adult's reason for living is an example of universalizing (Kozier and Erb, 1983).

POTENTIAL ALTERATIONS IN FUNCTIONAL HEALTH PATTERNS

A *functional health pattern* is a sequence of health behaviors that occur over time (Gordon, 1987). Gordon (1987) identified functional health patterns as the strengths in a patient's life style.

Dysfunctional health patterns are health care problems resolved by nursing activities and are known as nursing diagnoses (Gordon, 1987). The perioperative nurse seeks a description from the patient of past and present changes in health patterns to identify potential or actual problems that could occur during the surgical experience. The perioperative nurse must correctly identify the health problem before forming a nursing diagnosis.

The 11 functional health patterns described in Table 2–4 provide a framework for the perioperative nurse to identify potential or actual patient problems. This framework includes assessment of cultural, developmental, and disease phenomena. In addition, the health patterns framework ensures a holistic assessment, regardless of a patient's age, level of care, or medical disease (Gordon, 1987).

A medical diagnosis is concerned with only the patient's disease state. Other problems not associated with pathophysiology may exist for the patient. These prob-

TABLE 2–4. **TYPOLOGY OF ELEVEN FUNCTIONAL HEALTH PATTERNS***	
Health perception– health management pattern	Describes client's perceived pattern of health and well-being and how health is managed
Nutritional-metabolic pattern	Describes pattern of food and fluid consumption relative to metabolic need and pattern indicators of local nutrient supply
Elimination pattern	Describes patterns of excretory function (bowel, bladder, and skin)
Activity-exercise pattern	Describes pattern of exercise, activity, leisure, and recreation
Cognitive-perceptual pattern	Describes sensory-perceptual and cognitive pattern
Sleep-rest pattern	Describes pattern of sleep, rest, and relaxation
Self-perception– self-concept pattern	Describes self-concept pattern and perceptions of self (e.g., body comfort, body image, feeling state)
Role-relationship pattern	Describes pattern of role-engagements and relationships
Sexuality-reproductive pattern	Describes client's patterns of satisfaction and dissatisfaction with sexuality pattern; describes reproductive patterns
Coping–stress tolerance pattern	Describes general coping pattern and effectiveness of the pattern in terms of stress tolerance
Value-belief pattern	Describes patterns of values, beliefs (including spiritual), or goals that guide choices or decisions

*The pattern areas were identified by the author about 1974 for purposes of teaching assessment and diagnosis at Boston College School of Nursing. Colleagues have suggested some minor changes in labels and content. Faye E. McCain's (1965) and Dorothy Smith's (1968; Becknell and Smith, 1975) assessment concepts were particularly influential, as were the comments of clinical specialists and students who reviewed and tried out the categories in practice.
Modified from Gordon, M. (1987). *Nursing diagnosis: Process and application* (2nd ed.). New York: McGraw-Hill.

lems need to be identified by the perioperative nurse. Assessment using functional health patterns ensures that problems unrelated to the medical problems are identified, thereby allowing a holistic approach to perioperative nursing care.

Prioritizing Health Patterns Assessment

Professional nurses often report that there is insufficient time to perform complete patient assessments. The perioperative nurse prioritizes questions in patient's functional health patterns assessment according to two criteria. First, the perioperative nurse must determine the *critical nature* of the patient's condition (Gordon, 1987). Patients in a critical physiological or psychological condition may be able to focus their attention only on questions related to the immediate surgical experience or concern. An example of decreased patient attention is a new adolescent mother undergoing an emergency cesarean section. The new mother is likely to have a high level of psychological and physical anxiety before surgery. The perioperative nurse makes a briefer assessment of the patient's 11 functional health patterns before surgery for this patient than for the mother who is scheduled for a planned cesarean section on a subsequent day. The perioperative nurse uses primarily examination and observation skills to collect data when the patient does not have the energy, capacity, or attention span to provide a health history.

The second criterion used to prioritize functional health patterns assessment questions is time. The perioperative nurse prioritizes assessment time according to the *degree of risk* the patient may experience if a nursing diagnosis is missed. Insufficient data collection by the perioperative nurse resulting in an omitted diagnosis or a misdiagnosis may cause patient discomfort, distress, or injury (Gordon, 1987). To direct the patient assessment in a time-efficient manner, the perioperative nurse uses open-ended questions that start with the interrogatives "who," "what," "when," "where," or "how." The perioperative nurse is responsible for providing a standardized assessment of the patient's condition to adequately communicate the patient's problems to other health care team members.

Patient Problems

Actual or Potential Health Problems

Gordon (1987) described two types of health problems or dysfunctional patterns. The perioperative nurse must be able to differentiate between an actual and a potential health problem because they necessitate different approaches to nursing intervention. An actual health problem is an existing problem. The perioperative nurse directs nursing care to remove or decrease environmental and patient-related risks that contribute to or maintain the health problem. A potential health problem is a problem that may develop into an actual problem as a result of a change or a dysfunction in a health pattern. The perioperative nurse provides preventive nursing care to reduce the risk factors that make the patient susceptible to a dysfunctional health pattern or health problem (Gordon, 1987). The perioperative nurse uses this knowledge about actual or potential health problems to direct nursing interventions in the clinical setting.

Definition of Nursing Diagnosis

A nursing diagnosis is an actual or potential health problem that is resolved through nursing intervention. A nursing diagnosis is not a medical diagnosis. A nursing diagnosis comprises three elements: (1) the problem statement, (2) the cause of or reason for the health problem (related factor), and (3) a cluster of signs and symptoms (defining characteristics). For potential health problems, the perioperative nurse describes a set of risk factors for a dysfunctional pattern. Risk factors are elements within the patient environment that increase the patient's susceptibility to acquire a health problem. The words "high risk for" are used when defining potential health problems (e.g., *high risk for infection*) (Gordon, 1987).

The patient's description of the dysfunctional health pattern and problem cues the perioperative nurse to the

problem statement, which refers to an alteration in one or more of the 11 functional health patterns. Next, the perioperative nurse explores with the patient possible causes of the change or existing health problem. The causes or reasons for the problem are known as etiological factors, or *related factors*. In addition, the perioperative nurse clusters both objective and subjective data from the patient interview, the chart, and discussions with significant others, family members, and additional health care team members to substantiate the existence of the health problem. These information clusters are known as signs and symptoms, or *defining characteristics*. Defining characteristics validate the perioperative nurse's selection of the problem statement.

The following discussion defines health problems in the context of health patterns and presents problem statements in terms of nursing diagnoses. Next, this section lists some possible related factors and defining characteristics associated with each nursing diagnosis. Risk factors are listed for potential nursing diagnoses (high-risk diagnoses). The preoperative, intraoperative, and postoperative implications regarding each nursing diagnosis follow the defining characteristics or risk factors. After the nursing diagnoses within the health pattern are discussed, the section entitled Preoperative Assessment Focus may be used by the perioperative nurse to guide the patient assessment. The formula to develop a nursing diagnosis using the 11 functional health patterns will be given later in this chapter.

Health Perception–Health Management Pattern

Definition

The health perception–health management pattern evaluates the patient's perceptions about health management (Gordon, 1987). It is necessary to obtain insight into the patient's ability and desire to participate in the perioperative care plan. The perioperative nurse uses information about this health pattern to identify the potential for injury, infection, and noncompliance.

Perioperative Nursing Objective

Identify the actual or potential alterations in health perception and health management patterns, the potential for or actual noncompliance with nursing and medical interventions, and unrealistic perceptions about health and illness (Gordon, 1987). Alterations in the health perception–health management pattern are evaluated according to the patient's ability to identify health needs, to comply with the prescribed nursing and medical regimen, and to prevent injury.

Nursing Diagnoses

(1) Altered health maintenance, (2) noncompliance, (3) high risk for infection, and (4) high risk for injury

Altered Health Maintenance

Definition

Inability to identify, to learn, or to maintain health (Kim et al., 1987)

Related Factors (Kim et al., 1987)

- Dysfunctional health beliefs
- Difficulty with communication skills (e.g., does not speak the primary language of the health care team)
- Poor judgment; inability to make a deliberate or thoughtful decision (e.g., Alzheimer patients and adolescent mothers)
- Cognitive impairment of health or life style
- Loss of gross or fine motor skills
- Dysfunctional coping or grieving
- Insufficient financial resources to seek care (e.g., no telephone, transportation, or health insurance)
- Inadequate personal support system (e.g., no one to care for the children while the patient seeks health care)

Defining Characteristics (Lederer et al., 1986)

Subjective

- Verbalizes limited use of health care agencies (e.g., avoids hospitals, clinics, physicians, and nurses)
- Expresses a desire to improve health behaviors (e.g., exercise, stop smoking, lose weight, and lower blood pressure)
- Verbalizes limited use of preventive health practices (e.g., avoids periodic dental and physical examinations)
- Reports a history of untreated symptoms of the disease (e.g., fainting spells, shortness of breath, headaches, and blurred vision)
- Reports infrequent exercise

Objective

- Hypertension
- Obesity
- Smoking
- Disheveled appearance
- Elevated glucose level
- Blurred vision
- Inactive life style

Perioperative Nursing Implications

Preoperative. Beliefs about health care and personnel are based on previous experiences and information from others. When the perioperative nurse encounters a patient with altered health maintenance, it is important for the nurse to identify the patient's beliefs and myths about the health care system. The perioperative nurse uses this information to work with the patient and to facilitate patient and family participation during the surgical experience. The perioperative nurse coordinates information about health care agencies for significant others to facilitate the patient's entering the health care system. For example, while assessing a Hispanic woman who is scheduled for a hysterectomy, the perioperative nurse learns that the patient is the mother of four children younger than 7 years of age, is geographically separated from her family, and has not sought out vaccinations for her children because of poor English skills, lack of a telephone, and lack of readily available transportation. The perioperative nurse tells the patient about the availability of vaccinations from a public health nurse. The perioperative nurse ascertains the time and location of the public health van's next stop in the patient's home neighborhood, so she can provide immunizations and health maintenance for her children.

Intraoperative. The patient with misconceptions and myths about the health care system is likely to translate these beliefs into fears, which increase the patient's anxiety intraoperatively. The perioperative nurse uses touch and soothing words to reassure the patient before intubation and after extubation. In addition, the patient's fears are assuaged by providing continuity of nursing care for the patient. For example, the perioperative nurse making the preoperative assessment should provide intraoperative care to promote a sense of trust between the nurse and the patient.

Postoperative. The perioperative nurse evaluates the patient's beliefs about maintaining a level of wellness for himself or herself and family members. The perioperative nurse calls and coordinates with a significant other who can assist the patient in making a follow-up appointment or receiving assessment by telephone after discharge from the hospital.

Noncompliance

Nonadherence to a recommended treatment plan following informed decision and expressed intention to achieve the goals specified in the plan (Gordon, 1987)

Related Factors (Kim et al., 1987; Lederer et al., 1986)

- Discordant health, cultural, or spiritual value system of a patient (e.g., Scientology or Native American culture): cultural or spiritual values conflict with the treatment plan
- Dysfunctional relationship with health care providers
- Negative outcome of the treatment plan
- Negative perception of the treatment plan

Defining Characteristics (Kim et al., 1987; Lederer et al., 1986)

Subjective

- Patient or a family member reports nonadherence to the treatment plan (e.g., smokes, drinks, or eats after midnight when on nothing by mouth [NPO] status)

- Patient expresses that a suggested treatment opposes cultural or spiritual beliefs (e.g., receiving blood)
- Complains of negative side effects of prescribed medications or treatment plan (e.g., NPO status prevents patient from enjoying morning coffee or cigarette the day of surgery)
- Verbalizes an insufficient desire to follow the treatment plan
- Verbalizes a dissatisfaction with health care providers or the facility

Objective

- Failure to keep health care appointments
- Development of complications
- Failure to complete short or simple instructions associated with the treatment plan

Perioperative Nursing Implications

Preoperative. Patients unwilling to follow past or present treatment plans are at risk for noncompliance. Elements of the care plan with potentially undesirable effects (e.g., NPO status, which prevents the intake of a traditional morning beverage) may be violated by the surgical patient. The perioperative nurse describes the possible consequences of noncompliance to encourage patient compliance with the treatment plan. For example, the perioperative nurse reviews the meaning of NPO status if the patient is unable to describe its intent. Next, the nurse tells the patient the reason for maintaining NPO status (i.e., the stomach must be empty to prevent gastric contents from going into the patient's lungs during intubation). The perioperative nurse emphasizes that aspiration can be potentially dangerous for the patient. Finally, the nurse solicits the patient's willingness to inform the unit nurse or an operating room (OR) team member of an inability to adhere to this regimen. The perioperative nurse may solicit help from a significant other who can support the patient in following the prescribed plan. This is effective for patients who report an unwillingness to follow the plan and have a history of noncompliance. The significant other's objective is to provide support for the patient and to tell the unit nurse or the perioperative nurse of noncompliant behavior.

Intraoperative. The perioperative nurse asks the patient if the specific element of the prescribed plan was adhered to. The nurse evaluates the consistency between verbal and nonverbal behavior (e.g., eye contact) when the patient answers.

Postoperative. The perioperative nurse reinforces the importance of follow-up evaluations to maintain the patient's health. The nurse identifies with the patient potential obstacles to making follow-up appointments and coordinates the resources of a significant other to assist the patient in meeting follow-up appointments.

High Risk for Infection

Definition

The state in which a patient has the potential for being invaded by pathogenic organisms (Gordon, 1987)

Risk Factors (Kim et al., 1987)

- Surgical intervention that alters tissue and skin integrity
- Inadequate secondary defenses (e.g., decreased hemoglobin concentration, leukopenia, suppressed inflammatory response, and immunosuppression)
- Inadequate acquired immunity (e.g., acquired immunodeficiency syndrome [AIDS])
- Chronic disease leading to suppressed immunity (e.g., lupus erythematosus)
- Invasive drains and monitors (e.g., intravenous pressure catheters, hyperalimentation catheters, nasogastric tubes, Foley catheters, and chest tubes)
- Malnutrition that interferes with tissue repair
- Chemotherapeutic agents
- Blood abnormalities such as sickle cell anemia, thrombocytopenia, and thalassemia
- Inadequate tissue perfusion
- Broken skin integrity (e.g., traumatic wound, abrasion)

Perioperative Nursing Implications

Preoperative. Preoperative nursing actions taken to reduce the potential for infection include proper preparation of instruments and supplies, adherence to principles of aseptic technique when creating a sterile field, and adequate patient preparation. The *Standards and Recommended Practices for Perioperative Nursing* (Association of Operating Room Nurses [AORN], 1992) provides specific guidelines for instrument and supply sterilization. Creation of a sterile field according to the principles of aseptic technique decreases the chance of contaminating the sterile field and infecting the patient. Patient preparation reduces the amount of pathogenic organisms. NPO status reduces the amount of gastric contents capable of being aspirated by the patient during intubation or extubation. Preoperative scrub preparations by the patient with a bacteriostatic soap on the unit or at home reduce the amount of transient flora on the patient's skin before the patient enters the OR.

Intraoperative. The perioperative nurse reduces the potential for infection by using sterile technique and following recommended practices. Intraoperative nursing actions that reduce the patient's potential for infection include maintaining a sterile field, monitoring and controlling the environment, and performing sponge, sharps, and instrument counts (AORN, 1992). In addition, equipment and supplies are provided in a timely manner to decrease operative time, thus reducing the amount of time a patient has an open surgical wound. The presence of pathogenic microorganisms is verified by processing intraoperative aerobic and anaerobic cultures for laboratory analysis.

Postoperative. The perioperative nurse evaluates the patient's temperature and incision for signs of infection. An elevated temperature indicates an increase in body metabolism, which may be a sign of the body's mobilizing its defenses to fight pathogenic microorganisms. An elevated white blood cell count verifies the body's attempt to fight infection. The perioperative nurse checks the incision site for purulence, redness, and swelling. These signs indicate wound infection. Before the patient's discharge from the hospital, the perioperative nurse instructs the patient or a significant other on wound care, dressing changes, and signs indicating infection.

High Risk for Injury

Definition

Presence of risk factors for the patient to experience bodily harm during the perioperative period related to positioning, extraneous objects, or chemical, physical, and electrical hazards (AORN, 1992, *II*:7–2)

Risk Factors (AORN, 1992, *III*:5–2, 7–1—7–5)

- Impaired hand-eye coordination
- Weakness or unsteadiness when ambulating
- Poor vision with inability to read newsprint
- Impaired fine motor or gross motor skills
- Cognitive or emotional impairment
- Inability to sense coldness, sharpness, or warmth
- Failure to implement adequate safety precautions in the home
- Exposure to dangerous equipment, chemicals, or gases
- Exposure to malfunctioning equipment
- Neuromuscular impairment
- Musculoskeletal impairment
- Inappropriate placement of dispersive electrodes
- Body surface that increases risk (hairy surface, excessive scar tissue)
- Internal metal prosthetic devices or pacemaker
- Allergies or sensitivities to drugs and chemicals
- Obesity or emaciation

Perioperative Nursing Implications

Preoperative. During the perioperative period the patient is exposed to a variety of variables that place him or her at risk. The perioperative nurse determines the patient's risk during the preoperative assessment. Of particular importance is the patient's risk for injury related to positioning, extraneous objects, or chemical, physical, and electrical hazards. The perioperative nurse anticipates the position that will be used, the type of preparation employed, and special or routine equipment

that will be used during surgery, such as the laser or electrosurgical unit. See Chapters 6 through 17 for further discussion concerning the patient's risk for injury during the perioperative period.

Intraoperative. The perioperative nurse employs and directs many safety interventions to prevent accidental injury to the patient during the intraoperative phase. The nurse ensures that the transfer gurney is locked in place and that personnel are located at the side of the bed and the gurney to prevent a fall by the patient. Safety straps are applied to secure the patient to the OR bed to prevent a fall if the patient moves in an unexpected manner. A grounding pad is applied to the patient to ensure that electrical current passing from the electrosurgical unit is properly grounded. Hypothermia or hyperthermia blankets are covered with a linen sheet to prevent burns to sensitive skin. Electrical cords are checked for fraying or damage to ensure that excessive current is not delivered to the patient. During laser use, sponges are moistened to prevent accidental fires and an ensuing explosion (AORN, 1992, *III*:7–4, 10–3).

Postoperative. After surgery, the perioperative nurse evaluates the patient for possible injury that might have occurred during the intraoperative period related to positioning, extraneous objects, or chemical, physical, and electrical hazards. See Chapters 4 and 6 through 17 for criteria that can be used when evaluating the patient for possible injury. Prior to discharge, the patient is also assessed for the risk for injury in the home. The perioperative nurse determines if the patient will be able to implement self-care treatment regimens, particularly self-medication. Patients discharged with casts or other immobilization devices or with impaired ambulation are at risk for injury, particularly if the home environment is not suitable for or conducive to convalescence or rehabilitation.

Preoperative Assessment Focus
(Gordon, 1987)

Subjective: From Patient

- Describe health, in a general sense.
- Describe how health or illness interferes with life style.
- Describe strategies to keep healthy. Do these strategies work?
- Is cigarette, alcohol, or drug use a part of the patient's life style?
- What does the patient believe is the cause of the illness?
- What did the patient do when he or she became aware of symptoms? What resulted?
- Describe allergies and reactions.
- Describe the employment history.
- Describe the neighborhood and the living environment.

- What form of transportation is used?
- What is important to the patient before, during, and after surgery?

Objective: From Perioperative Nurse or Chart

- Describe the general health status of the patient.

Nutritional-Metabolic Pattern

Definition

Assessment of the nutritional-metabolic pattern evaluates the pattern of food and fluid intake needed for metabolic functions (Gordon, 1987). It provides the perioperative nurse with information about the patient's tissue repair process, heat-regulating mechanism, and fluid volume. The perioperative nurse uses this information to identify potential problems in nutritional intake, impaired tissue repair, inefficient temperature control, and hypovolemia and hypervolemia.

Perioperative Nursing Objective

Identify actual or potential alterations in patterns concerning food and fluid intake, tissue healing, child growth, and actions taken to solve health pattern problems (Gordon, 1987). The perioperative nurse determines the success of resolving the actual or potential problems by considering the patient's knowledge of the five basic food groups, the patient's knowledge of healing of the surgical incision, and the patient's plan to maintain or improve his or her nutritional-metabolic pattern.

Nursing Diagnoses

(1) Altered nutrition: less than body requirements, (2) altered nutrition: more than body requirements, (3) impaired tissue integrity, (4) impaired skin integrity, (5) fluid volume deficit, (6) fluid volume excess, (7) high risk for altered body temperature, (8) hyperthermia, and (9) hypothermia

Altered Nutrition: Less Than Body Requirements

Definition

Inadequate absorption or ingestion of nutrients necessary to meet metabolic needs owing to a decreased desire or an inability to tolerate food or fluids (Lederer et al., 1986)

Related Factors (Kim et al., 1987; Lederer et al., 1986)

- Varices, ulcerations, or tumors inside the alimentary canal

- High metabolic states such as hyperthyroidism and hyperactivity
- Knowledge deficit of balanced nutritional needs
- Inadequate nutrition
- Loss of appetite due to stress or nausea
- Alcoholism
- Drug abuse
- Vomiting
- Ill-fitting dentures
- Dental caries

Defining Characteristics (Lederer et al., 1986)

Subjective

- Complains of nausea, indigestion, cramping, or vomiting
- Verbalizes that certain odors activate or increase nausea
- Requests an antiemetic
- Verbalizes a loss of appetite
- Expresses a disinterest in food
- Verbalizes an inability to eat
- Significant other expresses concern about the patient's food intake
- Complains that ill-fitting dentures cause pain while chewing food

Objective

- Vomitus
- Limited intake of food or fluids
- Failure to eat
- Weight loss
- Weight 20% less than norms for his or her height
- Abnormal levels of electrolytes, transferrin, or albumin

Perioperative Nursing Implications

Preoperative. Identifying the problem of inadequate nutritional intake is the initial focus of the perioperative nurse. After identifying the cause of the altered pattern, the perioperative nurse initiates patient teaching for those with inadequate knowledge. For the patient who is unaware of the cause of nausea or vomiting, the perioperative nurse explores the types of food, odors, or activities that may cause disinterest in food. The perioperative nurse discusses nausea or vomiting tendencies with anesthesia personnel to ensure that an appropriate antiemetic is considered for the preoperative medication. An emesis basin should accompany the patient with nausea or vomiting tendencies during patient transfers.

Intraoperative. Additional warm coverings may be necessary for the patient who weighs 20% or less than ideal body weight. Adipose tissue serves as an insulator. Patients with less than required nutritional intake are likely to have insufficient adipose tissue to conserve their body heat. In addition, the perioperative nurse should be prepared to assist anesthesia personnel with a vomiting patient by ensuring that the suction apparatus is activated and by moving the OR bed to the Trendelenburg position when emesis occurs. An emesis basin to contain the vomitus and a dry towel to clean the patient should be readily accessible.

Postoperative. The perioperative nurse evaluates the efficacy of preoperative teaching by assessing the amount and quality of foods that the patient consumes after the surgery. This evaluation can be performed by telephone for patients in the home. The perioperative nurse reinforces the importance of adequate nutrient intake to promote tissue healing and quality of life.

Altered Nutrition: More Than Body Requirements

Definition

Excessive intake of nutrients relative to metabolic needs whereby the patient weighs 10 to 20% more than the ideal body weight (Lederer et al., 1986)

Related Factors (Lederer et al., 1986)

- Use of eating as coping mechanism (oral gratification) for depression, stress, or loss
- Low metabolic rate
- Endocrine disorders (e.g., hypothyroidism)
- Inactivity, sedentary life style
- Intake of frequent (more than three times a day) meals and high-calorie snacks

Defining Characteristics (Lederer et al., 1986)

Subjective

- Reports emotional satisfaction with food intake
- Verbalizes depression and feelings of stress
- Expresses unhealthy eating habits

Objective

- Large portions of food at meals
- Frequent snacks of high-calorie foods or drinks
- Exercise less than 20 minutes, three times a week
- Excess body weight

Perioperative Nursing Implications

Preoperative. The perioperative nurse assesses the patient's knowledge of the five basic food groups to determine if a knowledge deficit is the nutrition problem. The nurse obtains a nutritional history to determine if the problem is frequent intake of high-calorie foods. Next, the perioperative nurse assesses the patient's metabolic needs to determine if a reduction in intake and an increase in exercise would resolve the patient's altered nutrition problem. The perioperative nurse then evaluates the patient's desire and ability to reduce caloric intake and to alter the present pattern of ingesting excessive nutrients relative to his or her metabolic requirements. The nurse reviews with the patient the potential negative effects of excessive weight on maintaining health (e.g., hypertension, edema, and increased stress on cardiovascular and musculoskeletal systems). The perioperative nurse plans nutritional teaching with the patient and the family if the patient desires to initiate a change in weight status. The abdominal girth of a patient exceeding 250 pounds should be measured to determine if the OR bed will hold the patient safely. Patients exceeding 300 pounds do not need to be measured because they are often too wide for the bed. The patient should move himself or herself onto the gurney during patient transfers, or equipment should be available to safely move the patient.

Intraoperative. The perioperative plans for the patient with excessive weight include having extra preparation solutions or preparation sets available for a large body mass such as the abdomen. Assistance may be needed in moving the anesthetized patient's legs to a froglike position for catheterization. Two OR beds placed side by side should be available before the patient enters the OR for the patient whose abdominal girth exceeds the width of the bed.

Postoperative. Patient transfer equipment such as a patient roller should be used to move the immobilized patient from the OR bed to the litter. The patient or family members are reminded postoperatively to call the perioperative nurse if any questions regarding nutritional intake arise.

Impaired Tissue Integrity

Definition

Damage to mucous membranes or corneal, subcutaneous, and internal tissues (Kim et al., 1987)

Related Factors (Kim et al., 1987)

- Altered tissue perfusion (e.g., atherosclerosis, cardiac arrest), prolonged tourniquet use
- Inadequate nutrition (e.g., in alcoholics, drug addicts, indigent persons, and the elderly)
- Inadequate fluid volume (e.g., caused by dehydration or hemorrhage)
- Prolonged inactivity (e.g., impaired physical mobility)
- Chemical irritant (e.g., povidone-iodine [Betadine] irrigation and antibiotic irrigation)
- Therapeutic radiation
- Physical irritant (e.g., endotracheal and nasogastric tubes)
- Mechanical irritant (e.g., instruments for cutting, stretching, and retracting tissues, pneumatic tourniquet)
- Chemotherapy medication
- Increased evaporation of moisture from tissues during surgery
- Crushing or penetrating injury
- Infection

Defining Characteristics (Kim et al., 1987)

Subjective

- Complains of pain
- Verbalizes dryness and irritation in corneal and mucous membranes
- Verbalizes problems with wound healing

Objective

- Gunshot, stabbing, or other puncture wound
- Crushing injury as seen in patients thrown against a steering wheel in an automobile accident or pedestrians hit by a car
- Swollen, red, taut skin with purulent drainage
- Infection

Perioperative Nursing Implications

Preoperative. Each patient undergoing surgery is at risk for impaired internal tissue integrity. The perioperative nurse identifies the specific cause of possible tissue impairment to prioritize preoperative and intraoperative nursing actions. If internal tissue impairment is related to a crushing or penetrating injury with internal or external hemorrhage, the perioperative nurse prepares for fluid administration. The nurse prepares copious amounts of irrigation solutions for patients with infected internal tissues. If impaired tissue integrity is related to a fluid or nutritional deficit, the perioperative nurse assesses the patient's knowledge of the basic food groups and the patient's state of wellness.

Intraoperative. Many intraoperative nursing actions are performed to prevent or correct impaired tissue integrity. Sutures appropriate to the size and strength of tissue are available to repair impaired tissue. Sponges are used to improve visualization of the wound by removing pooled blood from the wound. In addition, sponges protect internal tissues from hard metal retractor surfaces. Copious amounts of irrigation solution are delivered to the sterile field to dilute and remove pathogenic organisms and foreign objects from internal tissues.

Postoperative. The perioperative nurse evaluates the damage of internal tissue according to the patient's ability to resume activities at preinjury levels.

Impaired Skin Integrity

Definition

Damage to the skin surface that alters the skin's protective barrier (Lederer et al., 1986)

Related Factors (Lederer et al., 1986)

- Inadequate grounding of an electrosurgical unit
- Inadequate circulation of oxygenated blood to the site because of pressure (e.g., tourniquet use and bed rest without adequate turning)
- Nutritional deficit that prevents repair of broken skin

- Nutritional excess of immobilized patient leads to pressure ulcer
- Impaired physical mobility resulting in pressure ulcers
- Radiation treatments
- Inadequate self-care whereby urine and feces break down skin tissue
- Infection of broken tissue site
- Diabetes
- Surgical incision
- Puncture wound such as a knife stabbing, a gunshot, or open fracture
- Prolonged use of corticosteroids

Defining Characteristics (Lederer et al., 1986)

Subjective

- Complains of pain, discomfort, or tenderness
- Requests medication or intervention for pain

Objective

- Surgical incision
- Visualization of internal tissues such as adipose tissue, muscle, and bones
- Draining wound
- Chest tubes, Hemovac drains, and so on
- Open skin lesion
- Necrotic skin tissue
- Rash
- Poor skin turgor
- Reddened area from pressure site or electrosurgical ground site

Perioperative Nursing Implications

Preoperative. The perioperative nurse identifies all alterations in skin integrity before surgical intervention to establish a baseline for comparison postoperatively. The approximate size, color, and location of the skin breakdown is noted to determine if impaired skin integrity remained at preoperative levels or increased during surgery. In addition, data collection should indicate whether the skin impairment is dry or draining. The color, amount, and viscosity of any drainage should be described.

Intraoperative. Most patients undergoing surgery are at risk for actual impairment of skin integrity related to the surgical incision. In addition, various patient positions exert shearing pressure on the patient's skin. This pressure interferes with circulation of adequate oxygenated blood to the pressure point, and pressure ulcers develop if inadequate padding is available to protect the pressure point. Another cause of skin breakdown is the pooling of preparation solutions under the skin during the surgical procedure. The perioperative nurse places absorbent sterile towels under the patient during the surgical preparation to collect any solutions that may otherwise pool under the patient. The towel collecting the preparation solutions is carefully removed before draping is performed, and the underlying surface in contact with the patient's skin is checked for dryness. The electrosurgical unit subjects the patient to electrical burns and impaired skin integrity if the unit is improperly grounded. The nurse prevents burns by selecting a fleshy area, such as the thigh, that is void of hair, scar tissue, and tissue breakdown for the grounding pad of the electrosurgical unit. The perioperative nurse shaves the site if necessary to remove thick hair because hair is an insulator for electrical current. The perioperative nurse ensures that the cotton webril placed between the patient's arm and the tourniquet is smooth and without wrinkles to avoid compressing tissue unevenly. In addition, the patient is subject to thermal burns from plaster splints or casts when plaster is moistened in hot water rather than tepid water.

Postoperative. The perioperative nurse evaluates the size, color, and drainage of preoperative skin impairments. In addition, the skin around ECG leads is assessed for discoloration. The ECG leads are possible exit sites of improperly grounded electrosurgical units. The site of tourniquet application is assessed for possible skin impairment. The color and amount of drainage on the dressing is evaluated. The incision is evaluated for purulence, redness, and swelling, which indicate possible infection and interference with the establishment of skin integrity. The perioperative nurse provides postoperative instruction regarding dressing changes and incision care in the home for the ambulatory surgery patient.

Fluid Volume Deficit

Definition

Vascular, cellular, or intracellular dehydration related to inadequate fluid intake or excessive loss of body fluids (Lederer et al., 1986)

Related Factors (Lederer et al., 1986)

- Diaphoresis, diarrhea, and vomiting
- Preoperative, intraoperative, or postoperative hemorrhage
- Fluid loss through indwelling drainage tubes
- Problem with the hypothalamus
- Prolonged NPO status

Defining Characteristics (Lederer et al., 1986)

Subjective

- Expresses fatigue or thirst
- Verbalizes confusion and disorientation

Objective

- Hemoglobin and hematocrit concentrated
- Hemorrhage
- Increased urinary output, then urinary output less than 30 ml/hour and increased specific gravity of urine
- Fluid output greater than intake

- Poor skin turgor
- Hot, dry skin
- Hypotension
- Increased pulse rate
- Altered levels of electrolytes (sodium, potassium, and blood urea nitrogen)

Perioperative Nursing Implications

Preoperative. The perioperative nurse prepares the patient with a fluid volume deficit for fluid volume replacement. A large-bore IV catheter is inserted while the patient is in the holding area to enable rapid fluid replacement. The nurse evaluates the patient's hematocrit, hemoglobin, and electrolyte results to anticipate whether whole blood, packed blood cells, or volume expanders should be prepared by the laboratory for intraoperative administration. The nurse also determines the type of surgery planned and how invasive and lengthy the procedure will be. Long invasive procedures such as those involving vital organs, long bones, and large vascular beds often necessitate the administration of blood components. The adult patient experiencing preoperative hemorrhage greater than 1500 ml of blood needs to have blood components prepared preoperatively for intraoperative infusion.

Intraoperative. The perioperative nurse prepares for fluid administration and measures fluid loss. The nurse provides two large-bore IV catheters if blood components are to be administered. The IV catheter inserted preoperatively is for infusion of anesthetic agents. The second catheter is for the administration of blood components. A pressure cuff and a blood warmer are also needed for blood administration. In addition, the perioperative nurse assists anesthesia personnel in correcting the fluid volume deficit by monitoring the fluid loss to prevent fluid volume excess. The stomach contents from the nasogastric tube suction container, blood loss in the suction apparatus, and urine output in the collection bag are measured. The perioperative nurse measures blood and fluid loss to assist anesthesia personnel, who are often unable to see the suction apparatus adequately from behind the anesthesia screen. Sponges are weighed intraoperatively by the circulating nurse to provide additional information about the patient's total fluid loss. The scrub nurse tabulates the amount of irrigation fluid used. The circulating nurse subtracts the amount of irrigation fluid from the total amount of fluid in the suction apparatus to determine the actual amount of blood loss from the sterile field. The fluid loss, urine output, and nasogastric contents totals are subtracted from the amount of IV fluids infused to determine the actual amount of fluids needed to correct the fluid volume deficit.

Postoperative. The perioperative nurse compares blood values, skin turgor, and vital signs with preoperative and intraoperative values to determine if the fluid volume deficit was corrected. Vital signs taken while the patient is lying down, sitting up, and standing indicate whether the hypotension from a fluid volume deficit is resolved. The perioperative nurse teaches the patient and significant others concerning interventions to correct future instances of fluid volume deficit if the volume deficit was caused by diaphoresis, vomiting, or diarrhea.

Fluid Volume Excess

Definition

Increased fluid retention (Lederer et al., 1986)

Related Factors (Lederer et al., 1986)

- Corticosteroid therapy
- Excessive fluid intake
- Excessive sodium intake
- Renal disease
- Intake greater than output
- Problem with the hypothalamus

Defining Characteristics (Lederer et al., 1986)

Subjective

- Complains of extremities swelling
- Reports puffiness of the fingers, toes, and face
- Expresses difficulty with movement and ambulation

Objective

- Edema
- Weight gain
- Shortness of breath
- Vital signs values indicative of hypertension
- Decreased urine output
- Abdominal distention (ascites)
- Neck vein distention
- Pulmonary congestion on x-ray film
- Abnormal breath sounds such as rales
- Mental confusion
- Altered electrolyte values

Perioperative Nursing Implications

Preoperative. The perioperative nurse determines the potential source of the patient's weight gain, such as high sodium intake, corticosteroid therapy, and renal disease. The nurse works with the patient to develop a low-sodium dietary plan if appropriate. The perioperative nurse notes the patient's weight preoperatively for postoperative evaluation of fluid retention. Sufficient personnel or equipment should be available for moving the patient who experiences shortness of breath after minimal exertion or who is unable to move himself or herself and is heavy.

Intraoperative. The pressure points of patients with edema are checked for sufficient padding to avoid inadequate tissue perfusion during the surgical procedure. Calculation of fluid administration and fluid loss is performed intraoperatively to ensure that the risk of fluid volume excess does not increase. A urinary catheter may be inserted intraoperatively.

Postoperative. The patient's preoperative and postoperative weights are compared to determine if the fluid volume excess was maintained or increased during surgery. Vital signs are also compared to determine the status of the patient's hypertension. The nurse reviews the low-sodium diet plan and the patient's understanding of foods high in sodium with a significant other if fluid volume excess is related to excessive sodium intake.

High Risk for Altered Body Temperature

Definition

The state in which the patient is at risk for failing to maintain body temperature within a normal range (Kim et al., 1987; Gordon, 1987)

Risk Factors (Kim et al., 1987)

- Surgical patients
- Extremes of age
- Extremes of weight
- Family history of malignant hyperthermia
- Patients with endocrine disorders
- Problem with the hypothalamus

Perioperative Nursing Implications

Preoperative. All surgical patients have the potential for altered body temperature. The cool environment of the OR subjects patients to hypothermia. Anesthesic agents may interfere with the body's temperature-regulating mechanism and metabolic rate. Patients may have significant anxiety about impending surgery, which may raise their temperature preoperatively. The perioperative nurse provides an overview of the surgical process and provides factual information that lessens the patient's anxiety to prevent possible spikes in temperature extremes. Preoperative sedation may lower the metabolic rate and temperature before the patient's arrival in the OR. The perioperative nurse assesses the patient for trends in high and low temperature extremes to determine the potential for altered body temperature intraoperatively.

Intraoperative. The perioperative nurse provides warm covers for the patient's body, extremities, and head during the surgical procedure to prevent hypothermia. A rectal temperature probe may be prescribed to determine accurate temperature readings during surgery. This is often used for pediatric patients because their temperatures may change quickly and dramatically during surgery. A hypothermia or hyperthermia blanket is covered with protective linen and placed on the OR bed before the patient enters the OR. The hypothermia or hyperthermia blanket is not used for intraoperative temperature control for patients requiring anteroposterior intraoperative x-ray films (e.g., cholangiograms) because the blanket interferes with the diagnostic films. Additional intraoperative heating and cooling techniques are discussed below under the hyperthermia and hypothermia patterns.

Postoperative. The perioperative nurse compares the temperature ranges during surgery with those after surgery to determine if temperature alterations were prevented intraoperatively. The perioperative nurse evaluates the patient postoperatively for temperature spikes, which may indicate infection.

Hyperthermia

Definition

Body temperature above normal range (Kim et al., 1987)

Related Factors (Kim et al., 1987)

- Exposure to hot environments
- Dehydration
- Inability to perspire or cool
- Vigorous activity
- Medications causing vasoconstriction or increased metabolic rate
- Inadequate shelter from environmental heat
- Illness or trauma involving temperature-regulating organs such as the hypothalamus

Defining Characteristics (Kim et al., 1987)

Subjective

- Complains of fever or feeling hot
- Expresses an inability to cool self

Objective

- Body temperature elevated above normal range
- Hot dry skin
- Flushed color
- Increased respiratory rate
- Tachycardia

Perioperative Nursing Implications

Preoperative. The perioperative nurse assesses the cause of hyperthermia before forming a plan or providing interventions. Hyperthermia caused by environmental heat, exposure, and exercise is resolved with shelter from the heat, fluid administration, and the application of a hypothermia blanket preoperatively. Malignant hyperthermia is a deadly form of hyperthermia if not effectively managed intraoperatively. The population at risk for malignant hyperthermia includes patients with bulky large muscles and with muscular defects as seen in inguinal hernias and ptosis. Malignant hyperthermia is most often seen in children and men. A muscle biopsy is taken for those with suspected malignant hyperthermia who do not need immediate anesthetic intervention. The patient with suspected malignant hyperthermia is given dantrolene sodium preoperatively to avoid complications under anesthesia.

Intraoperative. The patient with undetected malignant hyperthermia is often identified intraoperatively. Succinylcholine is often the anesthetic agent that triggers the contracture response of the masseter muscle. Masseter muscle contraction makes extension of the jaw and visualization of the vocal cords difficult for anesthesia intubation. During a malignant hyperthermia crisis, the perioperative nurse assists anesthesia personnel by preparing dantrolene sodium and exchanging the sodium lime canister and anesthesia circuits. Administration of dantrolene sodium is the definitive treatment to resolve a malignant hyperthermia crisis. Dantrolene sodium causes muscle relaxation, a decrease in metabolism, and fever. This medication moves the high concentration of calcium ions causing muscle contractions back into the sarcoplasmic reticulum of the muscle cell. Placement of a hypothermia blanket, ice packs to the groin area, and wet cold towels assists in body cooling. The perfusion team is called when temperatures continue to rise above 104°F. If the malignant hyperthermia crisis arises after an incision has been made, the scrub nurse prepares suture for a rapid closure.

Postoperative. The perioperative nurse evaluates the patient's temperature postoperatively to determine the progress of the rehabilitation phase. Hyperthermia within the first 48 hours after surgery may indicate potential infection. The perioperative nurse contacts the surgeon or refers the patient for further evaluation by the physician if hyperthermia is a recurrent cycle.

The hypermetabolic state of malignant hyperthermia caused by extensive muscular contractions sensitizes the patient to touch. The patient is likely to feel excruciating pain during movement. The perioperative nurse arranges for a smooth transfer of the patient from the OR bed to a stretcher by ensuring that sufficient personnel and equipment are available.

Hypothermia

Definition

Body temperature below normal range (Kim et al., 1987)

Related Factors (Kim et al., 1987)

- Inadequate protection from a cold environment
- Submersion
- Inactivity in a cold environment
- Administration of medications causing vasodilation and lowered metabolic rate such as preoperative medication or spinal anesthesia
- Illness or trauma involving temperature regulators such as the hypothalamus
- Impaired skin integrity as seen in extensive body burns
- Trauma surgery involving extensive skin preparation and body exposure; an absence of sterile drapes to retain body heat
- Decreased metabolic rate caused by general anesthesia coupled with the cool temperature of the OR

Defining Characteristics (Kim et al., 1987)

Subjective

- Expresses an inability to feel warm
- Verbalizes sensations of feeling cold or freezing

Objective

- Body temperature below normal range
- Shivering, goose flesh, cyanotic nail beds and lips, chattering of teeth, cool pale skin
- Decreased respiratory rate
- Bradycardia

Perioperative Nursing Implications

Preoperative. The perioperative nurse assesses the patient's skin temperature and color preoperatively to determine if inadequate perfusion of peripheral tissues predisposes the patient to hypothermia. The patient's body temperature is recorded to establish a baseline for intraoperative and postoperative evaluation. During preoperative teaching, the perioperative nurse discusses the cool environment of the OR and the use of warm coverings for the body, head, and feet. If the patient is receiving local anesthesia, the nurse alerts the patient to the use of warm and cool preparation solutions to avoid surprising the patient intraoperatively. Blankets are offered during patient pickup, and heated coverings are offered while the patient waits in the holding area. Hypothermia blankets with a linen cover are placed on the OR bed and under the patient to provide continuous warmth for the patient intraoperatively. A hypothermia blanket is contraindicated if intraoperative anteroposterior x-ray films are to be taken. The OR thermostat is raised preoperatively to increase the ambient temperature and decrease heat loss for infants and young children.

Intraoperative. Each patient undergoing surgery has the potential for intraoperative hypothermia. The cool OR temperature, the patient's inactivity and lack of clothing, extensive and invasive surgical procedures, and decreased metabolic rate related to anesthetic medications lower the patient's body temperature. The perioperative nurse performs several nursing actions to preserve or increase the patient's body temperature intraoperatively. Warm coverings are placed next to the patient's skin to provide immediate warmth. An outer blanket should be placed on top of the warm covering to insulate the heat provided to the patient. Warm towels are placed on the feet and head to provide warmth and prevent additional heat loss and energy expenditure. Warm saline irrigation is used to decrease the amount of heat evaporating from warm body core tissues to the cool external OR environment. A temperature probe is inserted rectally or applied externally to monitor body temperature accurately. Heat lamps located a safe distance from the patient provide additional external heat and warmth.

Postoperative. To promote warming, the perioperative nurse provides warm coverings for the patient's torso, feet, and head before transfer from the OR. The perioperative nurse compares the patient's preoperative temperature and color of the skin with postoperative levels to determine the effectiveness of intraoperative nursing actions.

Preoperative Assessment Focus
(Gordon, 1987)

Subjective: From Patient

- Describe typical daily intake of food, vitamins, and snacks.
- Describe daily fluid intake (amount and type).
- Describe weight loss or gain.
- Describe height loss or gain.
- Describe appetite.
- Describe healing process (good or poor healing).
- Describe the skin condition. Is there dryness, swollen areas, or lesions?
- Are there dental problems?
- Is there a history of sudden fevers or problems with anesthesia in the patient or family members?

Objective: From Perioperative Nurse or Chart

- Describe the skin condition (bony prominences, moistness, lesions, and nail bed flush).
- Describe the condition of oral mucous membranes (moistness, color, and lesions).
- Describe the teeth (missing or broken, general appearance, or dentures).
- Describe the hair (thick, thin, balding, or presence of a hairpiece).
- What is the patient's actual weight and height?
- What is the patient's temperature?
- Is feeding intravenous or parenteral?

Elimination Pattern

Definition

Assessment of the elimination pattern evaluates excretory functioning involving the bowel, the bladder, and skin (Gordon, 1987). The perioperative nurse uses information about the patient's elimination pattern to plan for alterations in bowel, bladder, and skin excretions related to surgical intervention.

Perioperative Nursing Objective

Identify actual or potential problems of controlling and regulating the elimination of wastes (Gordon, 1987). The perioperative nurse designs a plan to resolve problems related to excretory functions and evaluates the plan according to the improvement or maintenance of elimination patterns.

Nursing Diagnoses

(1) Constipation, (2) diarrhea, (3) altered patterns of urinary elimination, (4) incontinence, and (5) urinary retention

Constipation

Definition

Alteration in normal bowel habits characterized by decreased frequency or passage of hard, dry stools (Lederer et al., 1986)

Related Factors (Lederer et al., 1986)

- Inadequate fluid intake
- Inadequate dietary intake of bulk and fibrous foods
- Inadequate physical activity or immobility
- Use of medications such as iron sulfate and vitamin supplements
- Chronic use of stool softeners, laxatives, and enemas
- Gastrointestinal obstruction
- Painful defecation
- Inadequate privacy
- Weak abdominal muscles related to surgical incision

Defining Characteristics (Lederer et al., 1986)

Subjective

- Reports decreased appetite
- Complains of painful defecation
- Reports feeling of fullness or pain in the rectum or abdomen
- Reports straining during stool elimination
- Reports a less frequent pattern of stool elimination
- Reports a decreased quantity of stool
- Complains of headache
- Reports frequent use of laxatives

Objective

- Hard formed stool
- Palpable mass
- Decreased or absent bowel sounds

Perioperative Nursing Implications (Lederer et al., 1986)

Preoperative. The perioperative nurse asks the patient to describe her or his usual bowel pattern to establish the patient's routine and bowel activity level. In addition, the nurse asks the patient to describe typical daily food and fluid intake to assess the dietary pattern. The perioperative nurse assesses the patient's abdominal quadrants for the presence or absence of bowel sounds and palpates the abdomen for abdominal distention. If the patient reports infrequent bowel movements and suspected impaction, the nurse assesses the rectum for stool impaction after checking the color, integrity, and tautness of perianal skin. The perioperative nurse arranges for the patient to receive increased fiber in the diet, copious amount of preferred fluids, stool softeners, and laxatives and to optimize physical activity to stimulate bowel activity. A bowel preparation may be ordered preoperatively to promote the evacuation of bowel contents for bowel surgery. Immobilized patients, especially the elderly, are often at risk for constipation.

Intraoperative. Bowel surgery such as a colon reanastomosis often necessitates a preoperative bowel evacuation to empty the bowel of feces. Feces contaminate the sterile field and may leak out of the bowel into the patient's abdominal cavity, causing postoperative peritonitis. Bowel impaction or constipation interferes with intraoperative bowel repair if it is not corrected before the intraoperative period.

Postoperative. The perioperative nurse arranges a bowel elimination plan for the patient experiencing constipation postoperatively. Mild constipation is a common problem in patients undergoing general anesthesia because anesthetic agents often reduce normal peristalsis. A diet high in fiber, intake of fluids, and exercise are often prescribed for the patient experiencing constipation. The perioperative nurse instructs the patient on the function and use of bowel elimination aids to promote an optimal bowel pattern at home. In addition, the nurse teaches the patient to observe the frequency of bowel elimination at home, as well as to note the color and consistency of the stool.

Diarrhea

Definition

Alteration in normal bowel habits characterized by frequent passage of loose, fluid, unformed stools (Lederer et al., 1986)

Related Factors (Lederer et al., 1986)

- Stress and anxiety
- Dietary intake
- Inflammation, irritation, or malabsorption of the bowel

Defining Characteristics (Lederer et al., 1986)

Subjective

- Complains of abdominal pain or cramping
- Complains of inadequate control of stool elimination

Objective

- Increased frequency of bowel sounds
- Loose, liquid stools
- Weight loss
- Fluid and electrolyte imbalances

Perioperative Nursing Implications

Preoperative. Ask the patient to describe the frequency, color, and consistency of the stool. Ask the patient to describe the normal bowel elimination pattern. Assess the perianal skin for redness and indications of a breakdown in skin integrity. Check fluid electrolyte levels for imbalances indicative of dehydration. Assess the patient's weight and the frequency of urine output to determine the extent of dehydration. The perioperative nurse assists the patient in identifying stressors that may contribute to diarrhea. The perioperative nursing care plan should direct transportation personnel to apply several disposable absorbable pads or linen under the patient's buttocks in case loose stool is involuntarily eliminated on the gurney en route to the OR. Patients experiencing preoperative diarrhea are often concerned about experiencing diarrhea intraoperatively. Reassure the patient that provisions are made to contain diarrhea intraoperatively and that the patient will be cleaned of stool before transfer to the recovery room.

Intraoperative. The perioperative nurse applies several disposable pads that can absorb loose stool if the patient involuntarily eliminates stools intraoperatively. Anesthetic agents causing smooth muscle relaxation may relax sphincter control and allow stool elimination.

Postoperative. The perioperative nurse assists the patient in identifying potential causes of diarrhea. The nurse explores areas such as dietary patterns, fluid intake, and stressors. The nurse provides guidelines for change, including nutritional information and relaxation techniques, to the patient and the family.

Altered Patterns of Urinary Elimination

Definition

Disruption in the urine elimination pattern (Lederer et al., 1986)

Related Factors (Lederer et al., 1986)

- Sensory motor impairment
- Neuromuscular impairment
- Bladder irritation due to infection
- Preoperative anxiety
- Smooth muscle relaxation affecting the bladder related to anesthetic agents

Defining Characteristics (Lederer et al., 1986)

Subjective

- Complains of bladder spasms
- Complains of pain or burning during urination
- Reports urinary frequency
- Complains of hesitancy with urinary stream
- Reports urinary frequency at night

Objective

- Incontinence
- Urinary retention

- Hematuria
- Presence of a urinary catheter

Perioperative Nursing Implications
(Lederer et al., 1986)

Preoperative. The perioperative nurse requests a description of the patient's urinary elimination pattern to establish a preoperative baseline. The nurse solicits a description of urine color and urinary frequency during the day and night. The nurse documents the incidence of reported burning or pain with urination. After the patient has urinated, the perioperative nurse palpates the bladder just above the patient's symphysis pubis to determine if urinary retention is a problem.

Intraoperative. The perioperative nurse assesses the catheterized patient's potential for altered patterns of urinary elimination by draining the urinary collection bag. The collection bag is drained of preoperative urine to determine if the patient is producing a minimum of 50 ml of urine per hour. Output less than 50 ml/hour may indicate a fluid volume deficit, inadequate tissue perfusion, or alterations in cardiac output.

Doses of anesthetic muscle relaxants alter the muscle control of the bladder sphincter and interfere with the patient's ability to urinate postoperatively. Insertion of a urinary catheter intraoperatively may be expected for the patient undergoing extensive or invasive procedures. The perioperative nurse prepares a sterile urine sample immediately after catheterization to establish a baseline for urine microbiological studies later.

Postoperative. The perioperative nurse documents and reports to recovery personnel the amount of urine eliminated in the collection bag intraoperatively if this is not done by anesthesia personnel. The perioperative nurse designs a program with the patient and the family to improve the patient's elimination patterns in the home. The nurse reviews intake and output calculations and has the patient perform a return demonstration of the procedure. The nurse assists the patient in identifying potential obstacles to improving urinary elimination. The nurse recommends that the patient seek privacy during urination, establish a daily voiding routine at regular intervals, and drink a significant amount of fluids unless contraindicated. The patient is told of techniques that facilitate urination such as running water in the sink, running warm water over the hands, and providing a warm towel or cover over the pelvis. The family should be encouraged to support the patient's dignity and to provide nonjudgmental assistance while caring for the patient at home.

Incontinence

Definition

Unpredictable or involuntary passage of urine (Lederer et al., 1986)

Related Factors (Lederer et al., 1986)

- Immobility or mobility deficit
- Decreased awareness of need to pass urine

- Aging process
- Loss of sphincter control
- Weak or stretched pelvic muscles from pregnancy
- High intraabdominal pressure (obesity, gravid uterus)
- Fistula
- Trauma or disease causing injury to the spinal cord nerves

Defining Characteristics (Lederer et al., 1986)

Subjective

- Complains of inability to control urinary elimination
- Complains of dribbling urine with increased abdominal pressure
- Reports lack of awareness of a full bladder

Objective

- Urge to void that results in a loss of urine before reaching an appropriate receptacle
- Urinary frequency
- Elimination of urine occurring at unpredictable times
- Reddened perineal skin
- Stoma

Perioperative Nursing Implications

Preoperative. The perioperative nurse discusses the patient's usual regimen of urinary elimination to establish a baseline before surgical intervention. If the patient reports incontinence preoperatively, the perioperative nurse assesses the patient's skin around the site of elimination (e.g., perineal skin or stoma). The patient with a stoma and collection bag is encouraged to wear the collection bag to the OR where it is removed just before the surgical preparation during abdominal surgery.

The incontinent patient may be concerned about involuntary urination during patient transfer and in the holding area. The perioperative nursing care plan directs transportation personnel to apply disposable absorbent pads on the gurney under the patient's buttocks. In addition, a urinal or bedpan accompanies the patient gurney during patient transfers.

Intraoperative. The amount of urine in the collection bag surrounding the stoma is documented. The collection bag needs to be discarded for an abdominal surgical preparation. The skin surrounding the stoma is evaluated for alterations in skin integrity as the collection bag is removed. Depending on the type of procedure, the surgical preparation is initiated around the exterior of the stoma and moves outward in concentric circles. The face of the stoma is the last area prepared for most procedures involving stomas (e.g., bowel anastomosis).

Postoperative. (Lederer et al., 1986) The perioperative nurse develops a plan with the patient and the family to establish bladder control. First, the perioperative nurse assesses the patient's willingness to learn.

Next, the nurse designs a plan to achieve a state of dryness by scheduling voiding every 2 hours and teaching techniques that facilitate voiding such as drinking water or running water in the sink before urination. In addition, the nurse teaches the patient urinary internal or external catheterization techniques. The teaching plan includes information concerning maintenance of skin integrity. Teaching points include assessment signs of poor skin integrity (e.g., redness and abrasions), use of protective clothing and protective bed pads, and information about continence aids.

Urinary Retention

Definition

The state in which the patient experiences incomplete emptying of the bladder (Gordon, 1987)

Related Factors (Lederer et al., 1986)

- Blockage in the urinary tract
- Early morning wake-up for the administration of preoperative medication and an inability to void without morning fluid intake (NPO status)
- Bladder spasm or muscle constriction related to preoperative anxiety
- Postoperative pain

Defining Characteristics (Lederer et al., 1986)

Subjective

- Reports bladder fullness
- Complains of pain or burning during urination

Objective

- Bladder distention
- Frequent voiding of small amounts of urine or absence of urine output
- Dribbling
- Residual urine

Perioperative Nursing Implications

Preoperative. The perioperative nurse asks the patient to describe the usual pattern of urination to identify problems with urinary retention. If urinary retention is noted preoperatively, the perioperative nursing care plan indicates that an in-and-out red Robinson catheter or Foley catheter be available for the intraoperative phase of patient care.

Intraoperative. The symphysis pubis is palpated to determine if the bladder is full. A Foley catheter is inserted or an in-and-out red Robinson catheter may be used for patients undergoing intestinal, genitourinary, obstetrical, and gynecological surgery. It is important for the bladder to be empty and decreased in size during these procedures to avoid nicking the bladder when the surgeon is working in the pelvic region. The perioperative nurse documents in the intraoperative notes if the patient voided during surgery.

Postoperative. Postoperative patients are catheterized to remove residual urine if the patient is unable to void within the first 12 to 24 hours after surgery. The perioperative nurse informs recovery nurses if the patient voided during surgery. The perioperative nurse initiates the teaching plan for urinary retention, which includes the following teaching points: recognizing the signs and symptoms of urinary tract infection, introducing techniques to precipitate voiding (e.g., running water, maintaining privacy, and placing a warm cover across the pelvis), developing health practices to prevent urinary tract infection (e.g., 2000 to 2500 ml of fluid intake unless contraindicated and intake of ascorbic acid or cranberry juice to maintain acidic urine), and increasing the activity level to four or five assisted walks per day.

Preoperative Assessment Focus
(Gordon, 1987)

Subjective: From Patient

- Describe the bowel elimination pattern (frequency, character, discomfort, problem to control, or use of laxatives or enemas). If a problem exists, what is the perceived cause?
- Describe urinary elimination pattern (frequency, problem to control, or discomfort).
- Is excessive perspiration or odor problematic?
- Is excretion from a body cavity, tubes, ostomy bag, suction, and so on?

Objective: From Perioperative Nurse or Chart

- Review laboratory or pathology reports of specimens.
- Examine drainage or feces for color and consistency.

Activity-Exercise Pattern

Definition

Assessment of the activity-exercise pattern evaluates exercise, activity, and recreation (Gordon, 1987). It is necessary to obtain information about the patient's ability to tolerate and recover from the stressors of surgery. The perioperative nurse uses information about this pattern to identify potential alterations in mobility, self-care activities, airway clearance, breathing patterns, gas exchange, cardiac output, tissue perfusion, and growth and development.

Perioperative Nursing Objective

Identify actual or potential alterations in this pattern related to energy expenditure for exercise, mobility, leisure (diversionary activity), and daily activities (home management) by obtaining a description of the problem, the patient's perception of the problem, actions taken to solve the problem, and the perceived efficacy of those actions (Gordon, 1987). Alterations in the activity-exercise patterns are evaluated according to the patient's preoperative respiratory status, ability to move without pain, ability to perform self-care activities, and growth and development indicators.

Nursing Diagnoses

(1) Activity intolerance, (2) impaired physical mobility, (3) self-care deficit, (4) impaired home maintenance management, (5) ineffective airway clearance, (6) ineffective breathing pattern, (7) impaired gas exchange, (8) decreased cardiac output, (9) altered tissue perfusion, and (10) altered growth and development

Activity Intolerance

Definition

Inadequate physiological or psychological energy to sustain or increase activity (Kim et al., 1987)
The perioperative nurse identifies the probable causes and symptoms indicative of activity intolerance to maintain or move the patient toward a state of wellness.

Related Factors (Kim et al., 1987)

- Pain related to injury or disease process
- Administration of preoperative medication or other sedation
- Imbalance between oxygen supply and demand (impaired gas exchange)
- Arrhythmias
- Generalized weakness or fatigue
- Sedentary life style
- Bed rest or immobility
- Psychological discomfort or personal anxiety
- Aphasia

Defining Characteristics (Kim et al., 1987)

Subjective

- Verbalizes feeling fatigued or weak
- Expresses discomfort on exertion (shortness of breath when climbing stairs)
- Expresses feeling faint
- Verbalizes a decreased activity level

Objective

- Inability to begin activity
- Exaggerated and slow fine or gross motor movements
- Abnormal increase in heart rate, pulse rate, or blood pressure with activity
- Rapid, shallow respirations on exertion
- Arrhythmias or ischemia noted on ECG
- Diaphoresis after minimal exertion
- Skin pallor

Perioperative Nursing Implications

Preoperative. The perioperative nurse ensures that assistance is provided in moving the patient during bed and stretcher transfers. This assistance saves the patient's energy reserves to cope with other perioperative stressors. Physical assistance increases the patient's comfort level when he or she is weak or fatigued.

Intraoperative. The perioperative nurse ensures that sufficient personnel and equipment are available to transfer the patient to and from the OR bed.

Postoperative. The perioperative nurse encourages the patient to increase activity tolerance with assistance or supervision as appropriate to the rehabilitation regimen.

Impaired Physical Mobility

Definition

Limited ability for independent physical movement
The perioperative nurse identifies the level of mobility impairment to determine the type of assistance needed to move the patient during patient transfers and if mobility impairment resulted during the intraoperative phase of the surgical experience. The patient's mobility is assessed according to one of the following levels:

Level I: Requires use of assistive equipment or device (e.g., an elderly patient needing a cane for support during ambulation)

Level II: Requires assistance, supervision, or teaching from others (e.g., a patient with a broken ankle needing crutches for ambulation)

Level III: Requires assistance from others and the use of assistive equipment or device (e.g., paraplegics using a wheelchair during automobile transfer)

Level IV: Is dependent on others and does not participate in movement (e.g., quadriplegics) (Gordon, 1987)

Related Factors (Kim et al., 1987)

- General or spinal anesthesia
- Preoperative medication or other sedation
- Activity intolerance; reduced strength and endurance
- Chronic or acute pain associated with an injury or a disease process
- Perceptual, cognitive, or sensory impairment (e.g., Alzheimer disease and impaired vision)
- Neuromuscular impairment (e.g., insufficient padding for lateral, lithotomy, or prone positions for surgery or long procedures in the spine position, resulting in neuropathy; spinal cord injury)
- Musculoskeletal impairment (e.g., patients restricted to bed rest without adequate exercise, resulting in a breakdown of muscle tissue; broken or frozen bones and joints)
- Bulky and heavy plaster casts on the extremities
- External traction devices
- Depression or severe anxiety
- Mechanical assistive devices (e.g., respirator, oxygen tank, suction for drainage tubes)

Defining Characteristics (Kim et al., 1987)

Subjective

- Expresses weakness or instability with movement
- Verbalizes a fear of falling during ambulation
- Expresses pain during movement

Objective

- Impaired gross motor coordination
- Inability to move independently in the physical environment (movement into and out of bed, transfers from bed to stretcher to bed, ambulation)
- Hesitancy or reluctance to move
- Limited range of motion
- Limited movement related to prescribed bed rest for conditions such as edema
- Exaggerated slow and incomplete motions

Perioperative Nursing Implications

Preoperative. The perioperative nurse ensures that safety and comfort measures are used during patient transportation. The perioperative nursing care plan should direct transportation personnel to move the affected extremity (e.g., with heavy leg or shoulder plaster casts) or to assist in patient movement on the affected side (e.g., frozen shoulders or hips). Extremity movement occurs in unison with movement of the patient's torso and follows body alignment principles. The patient with external traction devices is often moved to the OR in the ward bed with traction devices, such as weights, attached. The patient with external traction may be anesthetized in the unit bed equipped with traction devices and moved after intubation to the OR bed.

Preoperative teaching should inform the patient of the potential for activity intolerance related to the effects of preoperative medication. Instruct the patient about safety precautions including the patient's remaining in bed, side rails' being raised, and the nurse call button's being accessible if the patient has a request or question after receiving the preoperative medication.

Intraoperative. Positioning the patient in lithotomy, lateral, prone, and upright sitting positions leads to strained muscles, nerve damage, and tissue hypoxia if inadequate safety measures are not provided by the perioperative nurse. Knowledge of human anatomy and correct body alignment enables the perioperative nurse to provide sufficient padding and positioning equipment for the patient to prevent the occurrence of or an increase in impaired physical mobility.

Postoperative. Postoperative patient assessment evaluates whether the potential for impaired physical mobility was prevented or if the existing level of physical mobility was maintained or increased postoperatively. The change in impairment is determined by comparing the preoperative level of mobility with the postoperative level.

Self-care Deficit

Definition

Impaired ability to perform or complete bathing and personal hygiene activities, grooming activities, feeding activities, or toileting activities for oneself (Kim et al., 1987)

These behaviors are known as activities of daily living (ADL). The perioperative nurse identifies the functional level for each area of limitation according to the amount of assistance required to complete ADL. The perioperative nurse can then determine the assistance required to prepare the patient for surgery. In the outpatient setting, the perioperative nurse uses this information to promote or coordinate the recovery needs of the rehabilitating patient in the residential setting. The perioperative nurse or a significant other provides assistance to complete ADL according to the following three levels of dependence:

Level I: Provides equipment to perform ADL
Level II: Provides equipment and completes ADL
Level III: Performs ADL without patient involvement

Related Factors (Kim et al., 1987)

- Neuromuscular impairment (e.g., patient with one-sided paralysis may be unable to complete ADL on opposite side of body)
- Musculoskeletal impairment (e.g., muscle degeneration may limit movement, which interferes with the completion of ADL)
- Developmental lag (e.g., a mentally handicapped child may require more assistance from an adult than do children of the same age without a handicap)
- Pain or discomfort may interfere with completion of ADL (e.g., arthritic joints may prevent adults from performing grooming and ill-fitting dentures may interfere with mastication and feeding)
- Perceptual, sensory, or cognitive impairment (e.g., interference with awareness of the need to complete ADL)
- Activity intolerance; decreased strength and endurance (e.g., patients debilitated by disease or inadequate nutrition and patients restricted to long-term bed rest)
- Impaired mobility (e.g., prescribed bed rest and inadequate ambulation assistive devices)
- Inaccessible or inadequate assistive devices available to move the patient with musculoskeletal or neuromuscular impairment to a mirror, toilet, bath, and so on.
- Loss of an extremity

Defining Characteristics (Kim et al., 1987)

Subjective

- Expresses feeling of fatigue
- Complains of immobility
- Verbalizes lack of muscle strength
- Complains of pain
- Expresses feelings of depression

Objective

- Inability to perform or complete purposeful movements (e.g., comb hair and wash self)
- Restricted activity such as bed rest
- Paralysis
- Confusion
- Sensory deficit (e.g., olfactory, visual, kinesthetic, tactile, and perceptual)
- Inability to wash body or body parts
- Inability to obtain or get to water source
- Inability to regulate temperature or flow of water
- Body odor, dental caries, foul breath
- Absence of personal hygiene items in the patient's room or the home
- Inability to put on or remove necessary clothing
- Inability to fasten clothing
- Inability to maintain a satisfactory appearance
- Inability to bring food from a receptacle to the mouth
- Inability to arrive at the toilet
- Inability to sit on or rise from the toilet
- Inability to manipulate clothing for toileting
- Inability to perform proper toilet hygiene
- Inability to flush toilet or empty commode

Perioperative Nursing Implications

Preoperative. Disease states such as paralysis, arthritis, and loss of an extremity may interfere with the patient's ability to complete preoperative preparations such as washing of the surgical site the night before surgery or replacing personal sleep wear for a hospital gown. The perioperative nurse coordinates with the unit nurse to ensure that the patient has assistance in completing preoperative wound site preparation.

Intraoperative. The patient with an identified self-care deficit may need assistance intraoperatively to prepare the surgical incision site. The perioperative nurse may be the first health care team member to remove dirt from under the fingernails of a patient preparing for hand surgery, old skin collected in the umbilicus for the patient undergoing a laparoscopy, or foul body odor caused by the patient's inability to maintain body hygiene because of increasing joint pain experienced each time body hygiene is attempted.

Postoperative. The perioperative nurse identifying a self-care deficit is often concerned with the patient's rehabilitation in the home. The patient with one-sided paralysis may have difficulty changing a dressing on the affected and unaffected side. After eliciting the cooperation of the patient, the perioperative nurse contacts a family member or a close friend to instruct him or her in wound care and dressing changes. The perioperative nurse also acts as a resource to determine what equipment or self-care aids would benefit the patient's rehabilitation in the home.

Impaired Home Maintenance Management

Definition

Inability to independently maintain a safe and growth-promoting environment owing to physical, financial, emotional, or psychological obstacles (Kim et al., 1987)

The perioperative nurse identifies the obstacles that interfere with maintaining safety in the home for the rehabilitating patient. This is especially important for the outpatient whose only contact with nursing expertise is the perioperative nurse.

Related Factors (Kim et al., 1987)

- Injury to a family member other than the patient (e.g., a new mother undergoing a cesarean section has a spouse with debilitative arthritis who cannot assist with the care of the infant)
- Disease or injury of the patient (e.g., the patient's condition interrupts family functioning such as meal preparation and budget planning)
- Inadequate family organization or planning (e.g., inability to assimilate the role and responsibilities of an injured family member, such as meeting financial, nutritional, and emotional needs)
- Insufficient finances
- Unfamiliarity with neighborhood resources to obtain assistance
- Impaired cognitive or emotional functioning that interferes with effective decision making about home maintenance
- Knowledge deficit about home maintenance
- Lack of role modeling
- Inadequate support systems

Defining Characteristics (Kim et al., 1987)

Subjective

- Expresses difficulty in maintaining the home
- Requests assistance with home maintenance
- Family describes outstanding debts or financial crises
- Reports household temperatures that are inappropriate for the season
- Family expresses an inability to care for the patient at home
- Verbalizes difficulty maintaining a hygienic or clean home environment (e.g., water, sewage, rodent, insect, refrigeration, and food preparation problems)
- Family requests assistance to care for the patient at home
- Overburdened family members (anxious, exhausted)

Objective

- Preventable falls, burns, and accidents related to disorderly surroundings or absence of needed equipment and aids
- Unwashed or insufficient clothing
- Repeated infections
- Frequent reports of missing school or work related to minor illnesses

Perioperative Nursing Implications

Preoperative. The perioperative nurse provides guidance and serves as a resource to assist the patient and the family in managing alterations in home maintenance. A disruption in home maintenance often occurs owing to an injury, an illness, or hospitalization of the patient. If family members are unable to assume the multiple roles involved in home maintenance, impaired home maintenance management interferes with the patient's recovery. The perioperative nurse identifies actual or potential problems in home maintenance to increase the patient's ability to recover in the home environment.

Intraoperative. The patient experiencing impaired home maintenance management is likely to have anxiety about insufficient finances or inadequate support systems to care for children. The perioperative nurse uses therapeutic communication techniques such as active listening and empathy to help allay the patient's feelings of anxiety concerning the surgery.

Postoperative. The perioperative nurse employs the problem-solving process to help the patient identify support systems available at home. The new mother recovering from a cesarean section who cares for a dependent family member in addition to the new baby with no help has the potential for impaired home maintenance management related to inadequate physical resources resulting from her surgery.

Ineffective Airway Clearance

Definition

Inability to clear secretions or obstructions from the respiratory tract to maintain airway patency (Kim et al., 1987)

The perioperative nurse identifies the patients at risk, the probable causes, and the symptoms indicative of ineffective airway clearance to prevent the patient from experiencing potential respiratory problems.

Related Factors (Kim et al., 1987)

- Decreased energy and fatigue
- Tracheobronchial infection
- Tracheobronchial obstruction and secretions
- Irritants (anesthetic agents and endotracheal tube)
- Perceptual or cognitive impairment (e.g., in patients with stroke and cerebrovascular accident)
- Trauma (e.g., injury resulting in bleeding and the presence of a foreign object)
- Supine position with the patient's head not elevated during transport

Defining Characteristics (Kim et al., 1987)

- Abnormal breath sounds (e.g., rales or crackles, and rhonchi or wheezes)

- Increases in respiratory rate with shallow breath sounds
- Spontaneous coughing with or without sputum
- Inability to expectorate
- Cyanosis of mucous membranes
- Audible, labored, or difficult breathing
- Absent or decreased breath sounds in posterior chest
- Distressed facial expression and flared nostrils
- Restlessness
- Shortness of breath
- Abnormal blood gas values

Perioperative Nursing Implications

Preoperative. Airway clearance is the first pattern to assess for in the trauma or critically injured patient. The perioperative nurse follows trauma management: assessing airway, breathing, and circulation. The perioperative nurse ensures that the patient's airway is clear so that breathing patterns and gas exchange can provide adequate oxygenation for tissues.

Intraoperative. The perioperative nurse promotes effective airway clearance patterns by assisting the anesthetist with the induction process. The perioperative nurse ensures that the suction apparatus is activated and functional to remove secretions blocking the airway. The perioperative nurse holds the endotracheal tube to the side of the patient's face within the peripheral vision of the anesthetist. In addition, cricoid pressure is applied when requested to facilitate passage of the endotracheal tube. The perioperative nurse prepares for extubation by ensuring that the suction is operational. The nurse stands to the right side of the patient to assist the anesthetist in the event of laryngospasm or vomiting after extubation. The nurse helps prevent aspiration of vomitus by preparing to move the OR bed to the Trendelenburg position.

Postoperative. The perioperative nurse promotes effective airway clearance postoperatively by assisting the anesthetist during transport of the patient to the recovery area. The nurse is alert for indications of patient vomiting during this time and responds immediately by helping the anesthetist place the patient on his or her side and clearing the mouth. Postanesthesia nurses are alerted to initiate immediate suctioning if the patient vomits during transport to the recovery area. In addition, if the patient had extensive secretions during the procedure, the postanesthesia nurse is alerted for the possible need of suctioning.

Ineffective Breathing Pattern

Definition

Inhalation and exhalation pattern that provides inadequate movement of air through the alveoli (Kim et al., 1987)

The perioperative nurse identifies the probable causes and the symptoms associated with ineffective breathing patterns to promote effective respiratory patterns and optimal gas exchange.

Related Factors (Kim et al., 1987)

- Neuromuscular impairment such as neuropathy of the phrenic nerve innervating the diaphragm and one-sided paralysis as seen in the stroke patient
- Pain from injury or postoperative incisional pain
- Musculoskeletal impairment as seen in a broken rib cage
- Anxiety causing shallow breaths and a rapid respiration rate
- Tracheobronchial obstruction such as secretions or blood that cannot be expectorated
- Increased resistance of lung expansion related to the dependent position of the chest wall with the patient in the lateral, prone, Kraske, and sitting positions

Defining Characteristics (Kim et al., 1987)
Subjective

- Complains of fatigue or generalized weakness
- Reports an inability to breathe effectively
- Expresses a need for supplemental oxygen
- Verbalizes an inability to get sufficient sleep

Objective

- Audible labored or difficult breathing
- Distressed expression and flaring nostrils
- Shortness of breath
- Abnormal increase in respiratory rate (e.g., greater than 40 beats/minute for adults) that leads to hyperventilation if not stopped
- Fremitus (vibrations and tremors felt through the chest wall when palpating the chest) often found over the right apex of the lung
- Abnormal arterial blood gas results
- Cyanosis of the mouth and lips
- Cough
- Shallow depth of respiration
- Pursed-lip breathing and prolonged expiratory phase
- Straining of the neck muscles during inspiration
- Increased anteroposterior diameter of the chest wall
- Visible straining of accessory muscles
- Unequal expansion of the chest during inspiration

Perioperative Nursing Implications

Preoperative. The perioperative nurse specifies in the perioperative nursing care plan that the head of the bed should be elevated 45 degrees during patient transfers for the patient experiencing problems with breathing patterns. Instruct the patient taking shallow and rapid breaths to take slow deep breaths to prevent hyperventilation. Assess and document rib cage expansion and breath sounds bilaterally to compare the preoperative status with intraoperative and postoperative breathing patterns.

Intraoperative. The perioperative nurse compares the patient's rib expansion and breath sounds intraoperatively with the preoperative status to ensure that adequate breathing patterns occur under local anesthesia. Apply principles of correct body alignment and provide adequate positioning aids for the prone, Kraske, and lateral positions. These positions cause increased resistance of lung expansion owing to the dependent position of the chest wall.

Postoperative. The perioperative nurse compares the preoperative status of rib cage expansion and the depth of breath sounds with the postoperative results to determine if the preoperative status was maintained or improved.

Impaired Gas Exchange

Definition

Imbalance between oxygen uptake and carbon dioxide elimination from the alveoli to the vascular system (Kim et al., 1987)

The perioperative nurse identifies the symptoms of impaired gas exchange and reviews the probable causes to prioritize the nursing activities that promote gas exchange for the patient.

Related Factors (Kim, et al., 1987)

- Altered oxygen supply related to changes in altitude, removal of mechanical assistive devices, decreased cardiac output, and so on
- Alveolocapillary membrane changes related to respiratory disease
- Alveolocapillary membrane impairment (pulmonary inflammation, decreased tissue elasticity, nicotine deposits, infection)
- Altered blood flow (e.g., hypovolemia, hemorrhage, or decreased cardiac output)
- Altered oxygen-carrying capacity of the blood related to blood anemia or hypovolemia

Defining Characteristics (Kim et al., 1987)

Subjective

- Reports fatigue
- Verbalizes shortness of breath
- Expresses need for supplemental oxygen

Objective:

- Disorientation to time, place, and person
- Restlessness
- Irritability
- Inability to expectorate secretions
- Continuous drowsiness or sleepiness
- Abnormally high levels of carbon dioxide in the blood
- Abnormally low levels of oxygen in the blood

Perioperative Nursing Implications

Preoperative. The perioperative nurse establishes a baseline assessment preoperatively to compare gas exchange during the intraoperative and postoperative phases. The nurse evaluates the patient's smoking. Smoking decreases tissue elasticity by serving as an irritant to the pulmonary tissues. Filaments of nicotine deposits on lung tissues decrease the alveolar tissue's capacity to exchange gases. The perioperative nurse checks the hematocrit, hemoglobin, and blood gas results preoperatively to determine the blood's capacity to carry oxygen and remove carbon dioxide. The physician's orders are reviewed to determine if blood components are ready for administration in case of intraoperative hemorrhage.

Intraoperative. The perioperative nurse provides supplemental oxygen per nasal cannula to decrease the patient's potential for impaired gas exchange when monitoring patients under local anesthesia. The perioperative nurse assists the anesthetist in monitoring impaired gas exchange by drawing or processing blood samples to be taken to the laboratory for immediate analyses. The nurse provides small bags of ice for the transport of arterial blood gas samples to the laboratory to facilitate an accurate analyses of the sample. The nurse anticipates the administration of blood on the basis of an estimation of intraoperative fluid loss and blood analyses. The perioperative nurse may be responsible for preparing the blood administration setup and assisting with blood administration by verifying the identification of blood component units with the anesthetist.

Postoperative. The perioperative nurse compares the preoperative and intraoperative blood values with postoperative blood results to evaluate the level of gas exchange postoperatively. The perioperative nurse may be responsible for collecting and logging in the empty blood component containers for blood bank analyses to ensure that blood compatibility was provided intraoperatively. After surgery involving inhalation anesthesia, the perioperative nurse coordinates the instruction and evaluation of the patient's wound splinting, coughing, and deep breathing exercises. As appropriate, the perioperative nurse offers counsel concerning the dangers of smoking.

Decreased Cardiac Output

Definition

Blood pumped by the heart insufficient to meet the needs of the body's tissues (Kim et al., 1987)

The perioperative nurse identifies the patient at risk for decreased cardiac output according to the defining characteristics. The nurse also reviews the related factors to prioritize nursing activities and to move the patient toward a more normal cardiac output pattern.

Related Factors (Kim et al., 1987)

- Air embolism in arterial blood during a craniotomy
- Changes in the cardiac muscle strength (e.g., drug side effects such as those in chemotherapy drug recipients)
- Electrical alterations in rate, rhythm, and conduction leading to arrhythmias

- Structural weaknesses in cardiac tissue
- Overexertion during physical exercise
- Overwhelming psychological stressors perceived as threats

Defining Characteristics (Kim et al., 1987)

Subjective

- Complains of chest pain
- Reports dizziness
- Complains of fatigue
- Reports weakness
- Verbalizes difficulty in breathing

Objective

- Arrhythmias or ECG changes
- Jugular vein distention
- Decreased peripheral pulses indicating decreased circulation to the extremities
- Cyanosis or skin pallor
- Cool, clammy skin
- Abnormal blood study results
- Low blood pressure, indicating hypotension
- Audible labored or difficult breathing with flaring of the nostrils
- Moist rales (crackling sounds) indicating the presence of secretions, which interfere with gas exchange
- Decrease or absence of urine eliminated (e.g., less than 30 ml/hour)
- Fatigue and lethargy
- Decreased level of consciousness

Perioperative Nursing Implications

Preoperative. The perioperative nurse ensures that sufficient personnel and equipment are available during patient transfers to avoid undue physical exertion by the patient with decreased cardiac output. Preoperative teaching includes an overview of the surgical experience for the patient and the family to allay psychological stressors concerning fear of the unknown. The perioperative nurse assesses the patient's vital signs, breathing pattern, mucous membrane color, and peripheral pulses to determine the effectiveness of cardiac output in delivering blood and oxygen. Blood results are reviewed to check for fluid and electrolyte imbalances and cardiac tissue damage. The ECG is checked for previous arrhythmic patterns.

The patient should be told if there will be a change in rooms and who will care for his or her belongings. The patient's family should know where to wait, the length of the surgery, and who will notify them when the patient is ready for transfer to the recovery area.

Intraoperative. The perioperative nurse assists in monitoring the patient's cardiac output by observing the ECG pattern for cardiac arrhythmias, monitoring peripheral pulses, and checking the skin color during surgery. The circulating nurse compares intraoperative vital signs with preoperative values to determine if the patient experiences decreased cardiac output. The perioperative nurse can anticipate that patients with a history of decreased cardiac output may need a Foley catheter inserted before the surgical incision. Urine production is measured to determine the heart's ability to pump sufficient blood to vital organs such as the kidney.

Postoperative. The perioperative nurse assesses the patient's vital signs, urine output, breathing patterns, mucous membrane color, and ECG readings to determine if the patient's cardiac output status was maintained or improved during surgery.

Altered Tissue Perfusion

Definition

Decrease in nutrition and oxygenation at the cellular level due to a deficit in capillary blood supply (Kim et al., 1987)

The perioperative nurse identifies the defining characteristics of the tissue perfusion pattern and reviews the related factors. The nurse uses this information to plan care and prioritize the nursing activities that will resolve the problem of inadequate tissue perfusion most effectively.

Related Factors (Kim et al., 1987)

- Interruption of arterial or venous blood flow related to the severance of vessels and caused by preoperative injury or intraoperative surgical intervention
- Gas exchange problems related to pulmonary disease
- Hypovolemia related to hemorrhage
- Blood shunting to the body core related to the shock phenomenon
- Atherosclerosis

Defining Characteristics (Kim et al., 1987)

Subjective

- Verbalizes a loss of sensation
- Reports numbness
- Complains of pain in the lower extremities when walking
- Verbalizes a tingling sensation
- Complains of severe pain in the calf muscles when walking that subsides with rest (intermittent claudication)

Objective

- Absent or faint peripheral pulses
- Cool skin
- Cyanosis
- Edema
- Necrotic tissue
- Skin lesions
- Pale skin color: the elevated extremity is pale on elevation, and the color does not return when the extremity is lowered

- Lack of lanugo in the infant
- Gangrene
- Slow-growing, thick, brittle nails
- Bruits
- Slow healing of lesions

Perioperative Nursing Implications

Preoperative. The perioperative nurse establishes a tissue perfusion baseline to assess the adequacy of tissue perfusion during the intraoperative and postoperative phases of the surgical experience. The nurse assesses the skin for lesions, pressure ulcers, edema, cyanosis, and skin pallor. These conditions indicate inadequate peripheral tissue perfusion with oxygenated blood. The perioperative nurse performs a simple perfusion test by checking the nail bed flush in the patient's toes or fingers. The nurse presses the nail bed for 5 seconds. The time needed for the pink color to replace the blanched color indicates the degree of tissue perfusion in the extremities. Adequate tissue perfusion is related to sufficient cardiac output and fluid volume.

Intraoperative. The perioperative nurse determines the adequacy of peripheral tissue perfusion by comparing the nail bed flush with the preoperative flush refill. Tissue perfusion of the vital organs is assessed by measuring the amount of urine produced in the catheterized patient. Urine production should be greater than 30 ml/hour to ensure that sufficient oxygenated blood is circulated through the body core to perform vital functions. The perioperative nurse may assist anesthesia personnel in monitoring tissue perfusion by measuring the hourly urine output from the urine collection bag.

Postoperative. The perioperative nurse evaluates tissue perfusion by comparing the skin condition, nail bed flush, and urine output with preoperative and intraoperative levels. Incisional and wound healing indicate adequate tissue perfusion. The skin around the incision should be the same color as the surrounding skin to indicate that adequate oxygenated blood is available at the site for tissue repair.

Altered Growth and Development

Definition

Deviations from the cognitive and psychomotor norms of an age group (Kim et al., 1987)

The perioperative nurse identifies the characteristics of altered growth and development to plan patient needs such as family teaching, referrals for community assistance, and stress management for overburdened parents.

Related Factors (Kim et al., 1987)

- Inadequate caretaking; indifference, inconsistent responsiveness, and multiple caregivers
- Separation from significant others
- Environmental and stimulation deficiencies
- Effects of physical or genetic disability
- Prescribed dependence on caregiver

Defining Characteristics (Kim et al., 1987)

Subjective

- Family reports inactivity and social isolation by the patient
- Family reports feelings of guilt about an inability to care for the patient as desired
- Family reports stress in caring for the patient
- Family reports a high dependency level by the patient
- Family reports that the patient's behavior is inappropriate for the situation

Objective

- Delay or difficulty in performing motor, social, or expressive skills typical of the age group
- Altered physical growth
- Inability to perform self-care or self-control activities typical of the age group
- Flat affect
- Listlessness, avoidance of interaction with others

Perioperative Nursing Implications

Preoperative. The elderly, children, and mentally handicapped persons are at risk for altered growth and development. The perioperative nurse plans for continuity of nursing care for the patient experiencing social isolation by having the same perioperative nurse care for the patient during the preoperative and intraoperative phases. The same perioperative nurse should evaluate the patient postoperatively to decrease the amount of social stimulation experienced by the socially isolated patient. The child or mentally handicapped patient may have a high level of dependency.

Arrangements should be made to allow the caretaker to accompany the patient into the OR suite if the caretaker or the patient desires. If this is impossible, the amount of time the dependent patient is in the holding area should be minimal and a familiar perioperative nurse should be present to decrease the degree of unfamiliarity. The elderly, young, or handicapped patient should be allowed to bring a familiar pillow, picture, or personal item to the OR if the patient must be separated from the significant other.

An overview of intraoperative activities to be performed is discussed and demonstrated for the patient and the caretaker as appropriate. Intraoperative activities include the application of the ECG leads, the use of an inhalation mask, and the process of closing the eyes, breathing deeply, and thinking pleasant thoughts. The caretaker or the patient is asked what words are used to wake the patient in the morning in the home environment.

Intraoperative. The perioperative nurse alerts the surgical team to the patient's developmental or growth alteration. The perioperative nurse completes the majority of intraoperative tasks before the patient enters the OR to increase the time the nurse is available to provide empathetic support. In addition, the perioperative nurse monitors the noise and traffic level of the room to decrease environmental stimulation.

Postoperative. The perioperative nurse compares the patient's level of altered growth and development with preoperative levels because developmental lags may be related to a temporary anxiety associated with surgery, separation, and environmental stimulation. If the nurse determines that the developmental alteration is not temporary, the significant other is contacted to determine if the patient's pattern has been recognized as being a problem for the patient. This intervention is most appropriate for social and expressive skill deficits as seen in children or isolated elderly patients. If the problem has not been identified by the patient or the significant other, the perioperative nurse refers the patient to resources available in the community to resolve the problem.

Preoperative Assessment Focus
(Gordon, 1987)

Subjective: From Patient

- Is there sufficient energy to perform desired or required activities?
- Describe the type and regularity of exercise pattern.
- Describe the time for leisure activities. Describe play activities [for child].
- On scale of 1 (low—dependent on someone else) to 3 (high—complete self-care), what is the ability concerning

  1. Cooking and feeding oneself meals?
  2. Bathing?
  3. Toileting?
  4. Achieving mobility to get in and out of bed?
  5. Dressing?
  6. Grooming and performing personal care?
  7. Achieving general mobility?
  8. Managing home maintenance?
  9. Home housekeeping?
  10. Shopping?

Objective: From Perioperative Nurse or Chart

- Describe gait and posture. Is a prosthesis or assistive device used for an absent body part? Specify on a scale of 1 (requires support device) to 4 (does not participate in movement or is quadriplegic) the level of assistance needed for movement.
- What is the range of motion and muscle firmness (hand grip)? Can the patient pick up a pencil?
- Describe the pulse (rate, rhythm, and strength).
- Describe respirations (rate, rhythm, and depth of breath sounds).
- What is the blood pressure reading?
- Describe the patient's overall appearance (grooming, hygiene, and energy level).

Cognitive-Perceptual Pattern

Definition

Assessment of the cognitive-perceptual pattern evaluates auditory, visual, kinesthetic, gustatory, tactile, and olfactory senses as well as the patient's cognitive abilities such as language, memory, and decision making (Gordon, 1987). It provides the perioperative nurse with information about the patient's ability to follow instructions and comprehend the teaching objectives related to the surgical experience. The perioperative nurse uses information about this pattern to identify learning needs and comprehension problems of the patient and teaching modalities. The nurse focuses the assessment of this pattern by reviewing potential or actual problems with patient comfort, deficient thought processes, self-neglect, knowledge deficits, and sensory and perceptual alterations.

Perioperative Nursing Objective

Identify actual or potential alterations in language, cognitive, and perceptual skills (Gordon, 1987). Alterations in cognitive-perceptual patterns are evaluated according to the patient's level of comfort; the ability to see, hear, smell, touch, and taste; the ability to perform self-care; and the level of information acquired and thought processes demonstrated during the preoperative, intraoperative, and postoperative phases of the surgical experience.

Nursing Diagnoses

(1) Alterations in comfort: pain; (2) sensory/perceptual alteration: visual, auditory, kinesthetic, gustatory, tactile, and olfactory; (3) unilateral neglect; (4) knowledge deficit; and (5) altered thought processes

Alterations in Comfort: Pain

Definition

Verbal or nonverbal indicators of severe discomfort (Gordon, 1987)

The perioperative nurse identifies the characteristics indicative of alterations in comfort and reviews the related factors to prevent increased patient discomfort.

Related Factors (Lederer et al., 1986)

- Bone, skin, and organ injury
- Incisional pain
- Stretched muscles and tissues from intraoperative retraction and manipulation
- Coughing and vomiting from inhalation anesthesia
- Prolonged surgery in the lithotomy, lateral, prone, and sitting positions

- Decreased tolerance level for pain related to additional physical, social, or psychological stressors associated with injury
- Decreased effectiveness of pain medication with chronic illness or long-term hospitalization for tissue repair
- Decreased activity level with increased focus on the comfort level
- Change in life style and increased adjustments in personal, familial, and community roles

Defining Characteristics (Lederer et al., 1986)

Subjective

- Complains of pain, discomfort, or nausea
- Requests medication for pain relief

Objective

- Grasps the injured area with a grimace
- Splints the pain site when coughing or taking deep breaths
- Pale skin and diaphoresis
- Limited slow movement
- Crying, restlessness
- Grimace
- Lack of eye contact, fixed gaze, or scattered eye movement
- Increased blood pressure and respiratory rate
- Increased pulse rate above patient's normal level

Perioperative Nursing Implications

Preoperative. The perioperative nurse explores with the patient effective coping mechanisms used to manage pain such as medications, back rubs, relaxation, biofeedback, and warm moist or dry heat applied to the painful site. The nurse asks the patient to rate the pain level on a scale of 0 to 10 (0 is no pain and 10 is unbearable pain) to compare with pain levels experienced postoperatively. The perioperative nurse discusses postoperative pain management during preoperative teaching. The nurse informs the patient that pain medication will be available (if appropriate) to assist the patient with pain management postoperatively. The patient is encouraged to use the pain medication as often as needed to achieve an optimal activity level postoperatively.

Intraoperative. The perioperative nurse arranges for sufficient personnel to assist with gurney to OR bed transfers when a patient is unable to move herself or himself owing to a broken extremity or severe back pain. A lift sheet or patient roller may be used to facilitate a smooth patient transfer. In addition, the perioperative nurse ensures that one individual supports and moves the broken extremity as the patient is moved. Warm covers are offered to decrease the cool temperature effects of the OR environment and to increase the patient's comfort level.

Postoperative. The perioperative nurse asks the patient to rate the level of postoperative pain on the 0 to 10 scale used preoperatively to compare the patient's perception of preoperative and postoperative pain levels. The nurse evaluates the frequency and amount of pain medication used with the activity level of the patient by reviewing the patient's chart. Next, the nurse evaluates the patient's perception of effective pain management to determine if alternative methods of pain relief (e.g., warm heat and massage) would benefit the patient. Before the patient is discharged from the hospital, the perioperative nurse designs a pain management regimen with the patient and the family to promote maximal comfort and an increased activity level at home.

Sensory/Perceptual Alteration: Visual, Auditory, Kinesthetic, Gustatory, Tactile, and Olfactory

Definition

Decreased sensory input related to the process of aging, excessive stimuli, a physiological imbalance, or disorientation (Lederer et al., 1986)

The perioperative nurse identifies the characteristics that indicate alterations in the patient's senses or perceptions and reviews the possible factors causing the sensory/perceptual alteration to assist the patient in managing environmental stimuli associated with the surgical experience (e.g., bright overhead lights and speaking clearly).

Related Factors (Kim et al., 1987; Lederer et al., 1986)

- Isolation or protection from a stimulating sensory environment (e.g., isolation, intensive care, bed rest, traction, an illness confining the patient to home, and the use of an infant incubator)
- Partial or total loss of hearing
- Partial or total loss of vision
- Disease or injury involving sensory organs
- Physiological changes related to aging
- Altered consciousness
- Sensory overload
- Chemical alteration: endogenous (electrolyte imbalance, hypoxia, elevated blood urea nitrogen, and ammonia levels) or exogenous (central nervous system stimulants and depressants or mind-altering drugs)

Defining Characteristics (Kim et al., 1987; Lederer et al., 1986)

Subjective

- Expresses anxiety or fear
- Demonstrates ineffective problem solving
- Verbalizes limited understanding of the environment
- Complains of severe pain

- Reports substance abuse
- Expresses fear, anxiety, or depression

Objective

- Deficits in visual, auditory, kinesthetic, gustatory, tactile, or olfactory senses
- Erratic sleep pattern
- Limited concentration
- Apathy, labile affect
- Inappropriate responses to questions
- Abnormal levels of electrolytes, blood urea nitrogen, and creatinine
- Regular intake of prescription or over-the-counter medications
- Disorientation to person, place, or time
- Limited understanding of the environment
- Withdrawal from the environment
- Noncompliance with instructions
- Uncoordinated fine motor movements (e.g., difficulty with handwriting)

Perioperative Nursing Implications

Preoperative. The perioperative nurse assesses the patient's orientation to time, place, and person. Next, the perioperative nurse assesses the patient's neurological status by observing pupil dilation and constriction, the ability to move an injured extremity, and the ability to sense cold, sharp, and dull sensations on the injured body part. The nurse assesses the patient's level of concentration and adjusts the information given to the patient according to his or her attention span. In addition, the perioperative nurse increases or decreases the voice tone, visual aids, room lighting, and other environmental stimuli to facilitate patient communication and learning. The perioperative nurse reminds the patient to leave hearing aids, glasses, and other health aids on the patient's unit or at home to avoid losing these valuables intraoperatively.

Intraoperative. The perioperative nurse checks the OR for potential environmental stressors. Bright overhead OR lights are often stressful for patients looking up from the OR bed. The scrub nurse arranges major instruments on the sterile field before the patient enters the OR to avoid clanging of instruments and stressful noise. In addition, sterilizing of instruments should be completed before the patient enters the OR to prevent noise of autoclave buzzers and alarms from disturbing the patient. The nurse speaks in a clear, low-pitched tone to patients with a hearing deficit.

Postoperative. The perioperative nurse compares the patient's preoperative levels of orientation to time, place, and person and neurological status with postoperative levels. The perioperative nurse assists the patient in identifying factors that contribute to altered sensory perceptions after surgical intervention. The perioperative nurse designs a plan for rehabilitation with the patient and the family to facilitate the adaptation or recovery process.

Unilateral Neglect

Definition

Perceptual unawareness or inattentiveness to one side of the body (Kim et al., 1987)

The perioperative nurse identifies the side of neglect to plan for safety measures related to transferring, positioning, and communicating with the patient.

Related Factors (Kim et al., 1987)

- Disturbed perceptual abilities (hemianopia) related to cerebrovascular accident
- One-sided blindness
- Neurological illness or trauma
- Alterations in mental health

Defining Characteristics (Kim et al., 1987)

Subjective

- Verbalizes unawareness of people, inanimate objects, or senses on the affected side
- Reports lack of awareness of or interest in the affected side

Objective

- Consistent inattention to stimuli on the affected side (e.g., does not turn the head in response to touch on the affected side)
- Inadequate self-care (e.g., does not brush teeth or comb hair on the affected side)
- Does not look toward the affected side
- Leaves food on plate on the affected side

Preoperative Nursing Implications

Preoperative. The perioperative nurse communicates and establishes eye contact on the patient's unaffected side during assessment. In the perioperative nursing care plan, the perioperative nurse directs safe transfers between the bed and the gurney for patients experiencing unilateral neglect. The perioperative nurse directs transportation personnel to assist with patient movement on the affected side and ensures that sufficient personnel are available to assist on the unaffected side during bed to gurney transfers. The care plan may specify that a patient movement device such as a roller be used, depending on the extent of unilateral neglect. In addition, the care plan should specify that the patient's extremities on the affected side be safeguarded during transfer, as the patient may be unable to express pain. For example, a hand on the affected side that extends beyond the edge of a gurney is subject to injury during passage through narrow areas such as an elevator door. Avoid confusing the patient by providing a scenario of events to expect in the preoperative, intraoperative, and postoperative phases.

Intraoperative. The perioperative nurse communicates and provides therapeutic touch on the unaffected side of the patient. The nurse ensures that sufficient padding and safety straps for safe positioning are provided during local anesthesia because the patient is unable to voice discomfort about the affected side. Inform the patient of affected limb placement when moving or positioning the patient.

Postoperative. The perioperative nurse continues to communicate with the patient on the unaffected side and ensures that sufficient personnel are available to assist in OR bed to gurney transfers. The perioperative nurse evaluates the pressure points on the affected side to determine if skin integrity was maintained intraoperatively. The perioperative nurse assesses the patient's support system to determine if adequate assistance is available for a smooth rehabilitation in the home. If insufficient assistance is available, the perioperative nurse arranges a patient care conference with the family and community resource personnel to coordinate patient rehabilitation.

Knowledge Deficit

Definition

Inability of the patient or the family to learn and comprehend information about the surgical experience or health care to improve the patient's level of wellness (Lederer et al., 1986)

The perioperative nurse identifies learning needs to focus teaching interventions on areas with the greatest impact on the patient's adaptation to the surgical experience.

Related Factors (Lederer et al., 1986)

- First surgical experience
- Differences in inpatient and outpatient surgical experiences
- Differences in preoperative, intraoperative, and postoperative surgical experiences among surgical specialties
- Lack of consistent and accurate information from the health care team and the community
- Inability to understand information concerning the surgical experience related to the mode of presentation (e.g., the nurse speaks faster than the learner comprehends)
- Lack of desire to learn about the surgical experience (e.g., denial of the illness or injury)

Defining Characteristics (Lederer et al., 1986)

Subjective

- Expresses a limited understanding of the injury or disease process
- Expresses a limited knowledge of the surgical experience
- Expresses a desire to learn about the surgical experience
- Expresses a lack of understanding about the surgical

experience related to psychosociological barriers in accepting the health situation and the impending surgical experience
- Refuses or is reluctant to learn about the surgical experience

Objective

- Cognitive deficit
- Sensory deficit that interferes with learning
- Inability to relay knowledge about the surgical experience when asked

Perioperative Nursing Implications

Preoperative. The perioperative nurse assesses the patient's level of understanding and willingness to learn before implementing preoperative teaching. The perioperative nurse provides teaching about the upcoming surgical experience in portions and at levels appropriate to the patient's understanding. Teaching should include topics such as the importance of NPO status; the removal of personal clothing, dentures, and hearing and visual aids; and voiding before receiving preoperative medication. In addition, a description of the surgical process starting with patient pickup and ending with postoperative routines decreases the potential for surprises, fear, and anxiety. Include a description of the OR such as bright overhead lights, cool temperature, and a narrow OR bed. The nurse then explains that warm coverings will be offered and safety straps applied to ensure patient safety. In addition, the patient should be informed of tubes (e.g., catheters and drains), bulky dressings, and casts that will be in place when the patient leaves the OR. The family should be included in preoperative teaching and given guidelines concerning the approximate time when the patient will enter the recovery area, where the family is to wait, and the surgeon's routine for speaking with family members (e.g., between cases or at the end of the day). Provide auditory or visual aids for the patient and the family to reinforce teaching points. Request verbal or written feedback of the information given.

Intraoperative. The perioperative nurse tells the patient which nursing action is being performed before touching the patient (e.g., preparation, placement of safety straps, and application of a grounding pad). A simple reminder of the purpose of safety or comfort measures may be necessary for the patient whose memory may be clouded by the preoperative medication.

Postoperative. The perioperative nurse evaluates the effectiveness of preoperative teaching by asking the patient if he or she experienced any surprises or if anything occurred that he or she would have liked to have been informed about preoperatively. The perioperative nurse also assesses the patient's and the family's level of understanding and ability to care for the patient at home. The nurse has the patient and the family perform return demonstrations of dressing changes and wound care to facilitate tissue healing in the home environment.

Altered Thought Processes

Definition

Inability to understand reality, solve problems, or perceive reality (Lederer et al., 1986)

The perioperative nurse identifies altered thought processes to assess whether a family member should assist in allaying the patient's fears or if psychotherapeutic intervention from another health care team member is recommended.

Related Factors (Lederer et al., 1986)

- Psychological changes related to aging
- Psychological changes related to tissue changes (e.g., Alzheimer disease and drug overdose)
- Traumatic psychological events
- Dysfunctional family patterns

Defining Characteristics (Lederer et al., 1986)

Subjective

- Expresses fearful thoughts
- Describes hallucinations
- Family complains of patient's irritability
- Verbalizes memory loss

Objective

- Preoccupation with self
- Restlessness
- Easy distractibility
- Inappropriate affect or responses
- Verbalization of incomplete thoughts
- Inaccurate interpretation of environmental stimuli
- Disorientation
- Inability to solve problems
- Regressive behavior (e.g., pouting, shouting, crying, throwing tantrums, and throwing objects)
- Inability to follow simple directions (e.g., maintain NPO status and stay in bed after the administration of preoperative medication)

Perioperative Nursing Implications
(Lederer et al., 1986)

Preoperative. The perioperative nurse assesses and documents the patient's orientation to time, person, and place. The perioperative nurse uses visual aids to orient the patient to the surgical process. The nurse uses the family to assist in patient orientation. The nurse ensures that the safety strap is secured and the side rail is raised if the patient is on a gurney.

Intraoperative. The nurse explains the reason for performing nursing actions before touching the patient to avoid surprise. The nurse does not acknowledge or support a patient's hallucinations; rather, the nurse orients the patient to time, person, place, and purpose.

Postoperative. The perioperative nurse assesses the patient's support system to determine if adequate assistance is available to facilitate the patient's rehabilitation.

The nurse continues to orient the patient to time, person, and place as necessary. The perioperative nurse provides supports to the family during periods of patient disorientation. The nurse explains the role of the disease process, hospitalization, and the effects of anesthesia in altering the patient's thought processes. The perioperative nurse offers positive feedback and reinforcement of appropriate patient behavior. The nurse instructs the family or the significant others to reorient the patient during periods of confusion or hallucinations.

Preoperative Assessment Focus
(Gordon, 1987)

Subjective: From Patient

- Is there difficulty in hearing? Does the patient use a hearing aid?
- Describe vision. Does the patient wear glasses?
- Has there been a recent change in memory?
- Is the patient an auditory or visual learner? Are there learning difficulties?
- Is there pain or discomfort? If yes, what is the level of pain experienced on a scale of 0 (no pain) to 10 (unbearable pain)? How does the patient manage it?

Objective: From Perioperative Nurse or Chart

- Is the patient oriented to time, place, and person?
- Does the patient hear whispers?
- Does the patient read newsprint?
- Does the patient grasp ideas and questions (abstract, concrete)?
- What is the patient's speech ability?
- What is the vocabulary level and attention span?

Sleep-Rest Pattern

Definition

Assessment of the sleep-rest pattern evaluates sleep, rest, and relaxation. The perioperative nurse uses information about this pattern to identify potential alterations during the surgical experience that result from disturbed sleep or rest.

Perioperative Nursing Objective

Identify actual or potential alterations in sleep or rest as perceived by the patient. This pattern is evaluated according to the patient's perceived satisfaction with sleep or rest.

Nursing Diagnosis

Sleep Pattern Disturbance

Definition

Disruption of the sleep pattern that causes discomfort or interferes with the desired life style or required activities (Gordon, 1987)

Related Factors (Lederer et al., 1986)

- Psychological stress
- Illness
- Environmental changes such as sleeping in the hospital
- Stressful life style leading to sleep deprivation
- Medications causing drowsiness or sleep during the day and disrupting nocturnal sleep

Defining Characteristics (Lederer et al., 1986)

Subjective

- Complains of difficulty falling asleep
- Complains of waking earlier or later than desired
- Verbalizes interrupted sleep
- Complains of not feeling well-rested
- Reports increased irritability

Objective

- Daytime napping
- Yawning
- Restlessness
- Disorientation
- Lethargy
- Ptosis of eyelid
- Expressionless face
- Dark circles under eyes

Perioperative Nursing Implications

Preoperative. The perioperative nurses assesses the patient's usual pattern of sleep and the use of sleeping aids. Each surgical patient has the potential for experiencing a sleep disturbance related to preoperative anxiety. Anxiety about the surgical procedure may cause interrupted sleep several nights before surgery. The perioperative nurse may request a sleeping aid for the patient experiencing extreme preoperative anxiety. The preoperative patient may be tired, irritable, and impatient, which may affect the patient's ability to comprehend preoperative teaching plans. In addition, the presence of a hospital roommate or family members or inadequate privacy may interfere with the patient's ability to achieve sufficient sleep. The perioperative nurse adjusts the teaching plan and communication according to the patient's attention span and interest level.

Intraoperative. Local or general anesthesic agents interrupt the patient's sleep pattern by promoting or initiating sleep during the day.

Postoperative. The patient often recovers from anesthesia with additional daytime rest, which interferes with the patient's ability to sleep at night. In addition, the hospital environment and the therapeutic regimen may disturb the patient's ability to sleep. Ordering vital signs four times per 24 hours often interferes with the patient's ability to achieve deep sleep.

Preoperative Assessment Focus

Subjective: From Patient

- Is the patient rested and ready for daily activities after sleep?
- Are there problems with sleep onset? Need for aids? Nightmares? Early awakening?
- Describe rest or relaxation periods.
- Describe the pattern of promoting sleep when restless.
- Describe the pattern of awakening activities.

Objective: From Perioperative Nurse or Chart

- What sleep medications were taken during hospitalization?

Self-perception–Self-concept Pattern

Definition

Assessment of the self-perception–self-concept pattern evaluates the patient's attitudes about self-image, identity, sense of worth, emotional responses, and cognitive and psychomotor abilities (Gordon, 1987). The perioperative nurses uses information about this pattern to identify patient problems in dealing with psychological stressors such as fear, anxiety, the inability to control a situation, and the disruption of body image and personal identity.

Perioperative Nursing Objective

Identify actual or potential alterations of psychosocial stressors concerning body image, social self, self-competence, and moods; whether the patient is experiencing a psychosocial change, loss, or threat concerning these psychosocial stressors; and possible solutions to resolve problems of the self-concept and self-perception pattern (Gordon, 1987). The perioperative nurse evaluates this pattern according to the patient's preoperative responses concerning feelings of safety and security and perceptions about the surgical experience and rehabilitation.

Nursing Diagnoses

(1) Fear, (2) anxiety, (3) hopelessness, (4) powerlessness, and (5) self-esteem disturbance

Fear

Definition

Feeling of dread by the patient related to an identifiable source such as surgery. The patient perceives the source as a threat or danger to himself or herself (Gordon, 1987)

Related Factors (Lederer et al., 1986)

- Lack of control over the surgical experience
- Lack of control over the hospital environment and routine
- Use of general anesthesia
- Invasive surgical procedures
- Unidentified feelings of powerlessness
- Real or imagined threat to personal safety, privacy, roles, and image related to hospitalization and surgery

Defining Characteristics (Lederer et al., 1986)

Subjective

- Expresses fear
- Expresses feelings of panic
- Verbalizes feelings of helplessness
- Expresses a decrease in self-assurance
- Identifies a source of threat
- Complains of dry mouth
- Expresses a need to withdraw from the situation

Objective

- Restlessness
- Short attention span, easy distractibility
- Sweaty palms
- Dilated pupils
- Concentration on identified threat (e.g., anesthesia, surgical incision, and length of hospitalization)

Perioperative Nursing Implications (Lederer et al., 1986)

Preoperative. Each patient undergoing surgery faces a potential threat to her or his well-being. The perioperative nurse observes the patient's behavior to assess the patient's level of fear. Next, the nurse conveys an accepting attitude to promote communication. The nurse assists the patient in differentiating between a real and an imagined threat by discussing potential causes of the fear in a therapeutic manner. The perioperative nurse reduces the patient's level of fear by providing empathetic verbal and nonverbal communication and relaying factual information to soothe fears. The nurse arranges a patient care conference with the surgeon, the family, the perioperative nurse, and the patient if continuity of information is a problem among health care team members or if the patient is considering cancelling surgery because of a high level of fear. Fears frequently experienced by surgical patients include being unable to awaken from anesthesia, saying something embarrassing under general anesthesia, and undergoing body mutilation.

Intraoperative. Continuity of care is important for the patient experiencing preoperative fear. The trusting relationship between the nurse and the patient established during the preoperative phase is maintained by having the same perioperative nurse provide care for the patient intraoperatively. Otherwise, documenting information in the care plan concerning effective methods of reassuring the patient should be available for the nurse providing care during the intraoperative period. A soothing voice, therapeutic touch, and an empathetic attitude help promote a nurturing atmosphere in the OR's high-technology environment. In addition, providing information concerning what to expect before performing a nursing action decreases the patient's fear of the unknown.

Postoperative. The perioperative nurse evaluates the patient's level of fear and the effectiveness of therapeutic actions by comparing the preoperative and intraoperative signs and symptoms of fear with postoperative levels. In addition, the nurse assesses the presence of new fears that may have developed after the patient dealt with preoperative and intraoperative concerns.

Anxiety

Definition

Feelings of uneasiness that threaten self-worth and self-esteem (Lederer et al., 1986)

Related Factors (Lederer et al., 1986)

- Removal from a familiar environment and routine
- Lack of involvement in decision making concerning the health care regimen
- Uncertainty about surgical benefits and outcome
- Change in roles and relationships resulting from the surgical experience
- Uncertainty about a successful or enjoyable future

Defining Characteristics (Lederer et al., 1986)

Subjective

- Verbalizes tension
- Expresses insecurity
- Verbalizes concern about personal safety or future plans
- Expresses vague apprehension
- Expresses powerlessness
- Verbalizes ambivalence regarding impending surgery
- Expresses concern about unmet expectations and future health outcomes (e.g., ability to work and parent)
- Anticipates a change in the life situation resulting from the illness or the surgical experience
- Verbalizes feelings of regret
- Focuses on the outcome of previous surgical experiences

Objective

- Restlessness
- Lack of eye contact
- Continuous activity (e.g., drumming fingers, biting nails, pacing, and frequently adjusting position when sitting in a chair)

- Increased pulse rate
- Hand tremors
- Perspiration
- Facial flushing
- Crying
- Wringing of hands
- Urinary frequency
- Insomnia
- Inability to learn

Perioperative Nursing Implications

Preoperative. The perioperative nurse identifies anxiety in a patient by looking for the objective signs and listening for the subjective cues of anxiety. The nurse assesses the patient's unmet expectations of the surgical experience by encouraging open expression and communication of thoughts and feelings. The perioperative nurse helps the patient identify anxiety-reducing techniques successfully used in the past to cope with uncomfortable situations. The nurse helps the patient focus on the upcoming preoperative period to prevent the patient from feeling overwhelmed with the numerous possible outcomes. The perioperative nurse encourages the patient to express feelings and provides an empathetic, private environment for the patient to cry and express anger. The patient is provided preferred music, television, or a familiar personal object in the holding area to soothe anxiety. The perioperative nurse arranges a patient care conference for the patient with anesthesia personnel, the surgeon, and the support system such as a family member or a chaplain to promote continuity of information and to facilitate problem solving for the patient experiencing high levels of anxiety.

Intraoperative. The perioperative nurse provides empathetic verbal and nonverbal communication to lessen a patient's anxiety intraoperatively. Therapeutic touch such as gently holding the patient's hand or lightly patting an arm relay concern and care for the patient. The perioperative nurse assesses the patient's acceptance of touch to determine if this technique is reassuring for the patient. If the patient becomes tense or pulls away from touch, the nurse should discontinue this nursing action for the anxious patient.

Postoperative. The perioperative nurse compares the patient's preoperative and intraoperative levels of anxiety with the postoperative level to determine the effectiveness of nursing actions. The perioperative nurse assesses the patient for new areas of concern causing anxiety, employs anxiety-reducing techniques used successfully in the preoperative and intraoperative phases, and arranges for a follow-up evaluation of nursing actions with the patient at home or by telephone.

Hopelessness

Definition

Perception of insufficient alternatives available to the individual, resulting in the inability to mobilize energy for himself or herself (Kim et al., 1987)

Related Factors (Kim et al., 1987)

- Prolonged activity restriction resulting in isolation (e.g., bed rest and prolonged intensive care)
- Deteriorating physical condition (e.g., uncontrolled or insulin-dependent diabetes and AIDS)
- Long-term stress with limited financial and support resources (e.g., long-term care of a parent or child with a debilitating illness such as Alzheimer disease or cystic fibrosis)
- Inadequate support systems
- Lost belief in a higher being (e.g., God)

Defining Characteristics (Kim et al., 1987)

Subjective

- Expresses "I can't," sighing
- Expresses difficulty in making decisions regarding health care, family matters, and personal goals
- Expresses "what's the use" regarding the health care plan

Objective

- Withdrawal
- Absence of eye contact
- Unfocused staring
- Closure of the eyes to leave the environment
- Turning from a speaker
- Shrugging when asked a question
- Decreased appetite, increased sleep

Perioperative Nursing Implications (Kim et al., 1987)

Preoperative. The perioperative nurse provides empathetic support and promotes independence for the patient experiencing hopelessness. The hopeless patient may be difficult to care for because the patient often appears unresponsive to nursing actions taken to nurture the patient. The perioperative nurse's focus is to establish a relationship of trust with the patient and to provide factual information regarding the upcoming surgical experience. The nurse encourages the expression of feelings by the patient through active listening, open-ended questions, writing, or drawings. The perioperative nurse is alert for clues of suicidal intent and arranges crisis counseling for patients at risk. The nurse works with the patient and significant others to identify with whom the patient feels comfortable sharing feelings and works with this support system to communicate with the patient if he or she remains unresponsive. The perioperative nurse assists the hopeless patient without a support system by identifying the consequences of decisions made and not made. The patient experiencing hopelessness is often soothed with a preferred type of music preoperatively during patient pickup and in the holding area.

Intraoperative. Continuity of perioperative nursing care is important for the hopeless patient. The hopeless patient often experiences low self-esteem and does not easily establish trust with others. The perioperative nurse conducting the preoperative assessment should provide intraoperative nursing care to promote communication and trust with the patient. The hopeless patient often rejects, withdraws from, and appears uncaring of nurturing gestures made by the perioperative nurse because of inadequate feelings of self-worth. The nurse relays empathy and understanding when communicating with the hopeless patient.

Postoperative. The perioperative nurse contacts the patient's support system to assist the hopeless patient postoperatively. The perioperative nurse works with the patient and the significant other to design a plan that increases the patient's influence over her or his environment. The plan includes realistic goals that enable the patient gradually to assume responsibility for her or his well-being.

Powerlessness

Definition

Feelings of inadequate control and influence over the immediate environment (Lederer et al., 1986)

Related Factors (Kim et al., 1987; Lederer et al., 1986)

- Removal from familiar environment and routine during hospitalization
- Absence of involvement in perioperative decision making
- Preoperative trauma and multisystem injuries, whereby nurses are so busy with tasks that the patient's need for information is unmet
- Lack of information and preoperative education
- Personal belief system that does not allow patient to be responsible, to control, or to affect his or her own destiny

Defining Characteristics (Kim et al., 1987; Lederer et al., 1986)

Subjective

- Complains of decreased independence
- Expresses anger
- Verbalizes an inability to accept the situation
- Expresses a lack of control over the environment
- Verbalizes a lack of control over the illness and the recovery process
- Expresses a lack of control over self-care

Objective

- Wringing of hands
- Withdrawal
- Disinterest in perioperative education and contribution to the outcome of the surgical experience

Perioperative Nursing Implications (Kim et al., 1987)

Preoperative. Every surgical patient preparing for surgery is at risk for feelings of powerlessness. The OR is a highly controlled environment and there is little opportunity for the patient to exercise control or to make decisions preoperatively; therefore, it is important for the perioperative nurse to provide the patient an opportunity to express feelings about his or her illness, impending surgery, or other stressors. Encourage the patient to express his or her viewpoint or questions before providing directions or information. During preoperative teaching, break information into small segments and offer the patient an opportunity to ask frequent questions. This teaching technique decreases the patient experiencing powerlessness from feeling overwhelmed.

The nurse helps the patient to identify situations during the surgical experience that the patient is able or unable to control. Identifying the difference between patient-controllable and uncontrollable situations increases the patient's opportunity to make decisions about the surgical experience. For example, maintaining an NPO status before surgery is a patient-controlled situation. The time of morning when the patient is to be picked up for surgery is not a controllable event unless the patient violates the NPO status and the procedure is cancelled. Preoperative teaching should include a description of the events or stages that the patient will experience during the preoperative, intraoperative, and postoperative phases. For example, a description of the patient pickup process should include an explanation for removing all personal clothing and wearing a hospital gown. This familiarization decreases the patient's feeling of powerlessness over the surgical experience. The perioperative nurse assesses the patient's familiarity with medical terminology and avoids using unfamiliar language. Unfamiliar language further alienates the patient from a participative approach in perioperative nursing care delivery.

Intraoperative. The perioperative nurse decreases feelings of powerlessness in the patient by telling the patient what to expect before performing a nursing action (e.g., moving the patient from a gurney to the OR bed, placing safety straps, applying a grounding pad, and performing surgical preparation). The perioperative nurse is careful to provide for the privacy needs of patients experiencing powerlessness. Protecting the patient's privacy needs such as placing a folded bath towel across exposed breasts is an indication of the concern demonstrated for the patient's privacy.

Postoperative. The postoperative phase is an ideal period to facilitate the patient's active participation in self-care. The perioperative nurse increases the patient's confidence and involvement in the recovery process by providing factual information about dressing changes, wound care, exercise, and so on to the patient and a significant other before the patient's discharge from the hospital. Patients experiencing high levels of powerlessness may need a written structured plan provided in small increments to avoid being overwhelmed.

Self-esteem Disturbance

Definition

Experience of one of the following:

1. Body image disturbance, which is viewing oneself differently as a result of actual or perceived changes in body structure or function
2. Personal identity disturbance, which is a disturbed perception of "who am I?"
3. Disruption in role performance, which is the inability to fulfill activities expected of a particular role in a community
4. Disturbance in self-confidence, which is the lack of confidence to accomplish one's goals (Lederer et al., 1986)

Related Factors (Lederer et al., 1986)

- Perceived mutilation of body part or function
- Cultural importance associated with appearance and performance of specific roles with success, usefulness, and one's worth
- History of unsuccessful surgical or medical attempts to correct an illness or injury
- Lack of confidence in the health care team
- Inadequate support system related to internal anger projected outward to significant others
- Absence of significant others

Defining Characteristics (Lederer et al, 1986)

Subjective

- Expresses "why me?"
- Verbalizes concern about a significant other's response to body alteration (e.g., mastectomy, scarring from burns, hysterectomy, penile implant, loss of a limb, and stoma)
- Expresses anger, depression, despair, or grief
- Family expresses concern about substance abuse
- Defers self-care activities to others (e.g., wound care, dressing changes, taking prescribed medication, and ADL)
- Verbalizes difficulty in accepting positive reinforcement and encouragement

Objective

- Labile affect
- Withdrawal from health care team members or significant others
- Unkempt appearance
- Apathy
- Substance abuse
- Avoidance of discussion of the recovery process, the surgical experience, or future role adjustments
- Reluctance to touch or look at the surgical incision, an amputated limb, or the face or affected body part involved in injury or surgical intervention

Perioperative Nursing Implications

Preoperative. Each surgical patient undergoing surgery is at risk for self-esteem disturbance. Disturbances in family roles related to separation from the family in the perioperative period and a disturbance in body image related to removal of a body function or part may cause problems in the patient's perception of self. The perioperative nurse assists the patient in coping with self-esteem disturbances by identifying the problem, exploring reasons for the disturbance, and encouraging the patient to verbalize his or her feelings about the problem. The nurse clarifies inaccuracies about the patient's concerns, surgical outcomes, and life style changes. For example, a common misconception for women having a hysterectomy is that sexual intercourse is no longer possible. The perioperative nurse clarifies that intercourse may continue as desired but the ability to conceive children no longer exists. The perioperative nurse conveys concern to the patient with eye contact, therapeutic touch, and active listening while designing a perioperative nursing care plan.

Intraoperative. The perioperative nurse provides care in a nonjudgmental manner while maintaining the patient's privacy and dignity. Privacy is maintained by communicating the patient's concern in the nursing care plan. The perioperative nurse controls traffic of curious onlookers in the OR while the procedure is in progress. Additionally, the perioperative nurse keeps the patient's body covered during the surgical preparation to preserve personal dignity.

Postoperative. The perioperative nurse discusses with the family potential changes of self-esteem and role performance that the patient may experience as a result of surgical intervention. Next, the nurse develops a plan of care with the patient that encourages family participation in the rehabilitation process. The nurse assists the patient and the family to identify new coping mechanisms needed to deal with changes in body image, personal identity, role disruption, and self-esteem disturbance.

Preoperative Assessment Focus
(Gordon, 1987)

Subjective: From Patient

- Describe how the patient feels about the self most of the time.
- Describe problems concerning changes in the body or things the patient does.
- Describe changes in perceptions since the onset of illness or the realization of impending surgery.
- Is the patient frequently annoyed, angry, fearful, or depressed?
- After surgery, when does the patient believe that life will return to normal?
- What does the patient do to gain control of stressful situations?

Objective: From Perioperative Nurse or Chart

- Does the patient maintain eye contact? Is the patient easily distracted?
- Does the patient's voice tremble? Is there a regular rhythm to the speech pattern? Is speech monotone and labored or inflectional and expressive?
- Does the patient sit erect or are the shoulders and head bent?
- Are the patient's body movements labored or quick and jerky?
- On a scale of 1 to 5, with 1 being calm and 5 being exceptionally nervous, does the patient appear nervous?
- On a scale of 1 to 5, with 1 being active and 5 being exceptionally passive, does the patient appear passive?

Role-Relationship Pattern

Definition

Assessment of the role-relationship pattern evaluates the roles and responsibilities that reveal satisfaction or disturbances in family, work, or social relationships (Gordon, 1987). The perioperative nurse uses information about this pattern to identify alterations in the patient's roles and relationships in the family and the community.

Perioperative Nursing Objective

Identify actual or potential alterations in this pattern related to the expenditure of emotional energy to perform family and social roles, to achieve satisfactions or experience dissatisfactions in relationship patterns, and to resolve problems (Gordon, 1987). Alterations in role-relationship patterns are evaluated according to the patient's preoperative grieving responses, alterations in communication, the potential for family violence, and adjustments to role performance and parenting responsibilities in the family.

Nursing Diagnoses

(1) Anticipatory grieving, (2) social isolation, (3) impaired social interaction, (4) altered family processes, (5) altered parenting, and (6) impaired verbal communication

Anticipatory Grieving

Definition

Grieving response that occurs before the actual loss (Lederer et al., 1986)

Related Factors (Lederer et al, 1986)

- Biopsy scheduled for a suspicious growth (e.g., breast biopsy and testicular biopsy)

- Impending removal of body part or function (e.g., amputation, hysterectomy, and mastectomy)
- Poor prognosis of family member (cancer of the pancreas)
- Medical diagnosis of chronic or terminal illness (e.g., paralysis and cancer)
- Surgery outcome resulting in significant change in the life style or goals (e.g., loss of a job, loss of a family role, loss of self-worth, and loss of security)

Defining Characteristics (Lederer et al., 1986)

Subjective

- Expresses anger
- Verbalizes depression
- Expresses an inability to accept the situation
- Expresses grief
- Expresses sorrow or extreme sadness
- Verbalizes a need to bargain with a higher being
- Verbalizes an acceptance of loss

Objective

- Withdrawal
- Change in eating behavior
- Loss of an extremity or body part
- Loss of body function (e.g., from hysterectomy)
- Crying
- Poor prognosis
- Medical diagnosis of chronic or terminal illness

Perioperative Nursing Implications

Preoperative. The perioperative nurse identifies that the patient is experiencing anticipatory grieving. Many patients verbalize feelings of anger, depression, or sadness but are unable to identify the cause of those feelings. The perioperative nurse explores the possibility of anticipatory loss with the patient. The perioperative nurse contacts a significant other to provide a support system for the patient. The nurse also assesses the significant other's perception of the anticipated loss to ensure that the significant other can provide adequate and healthy support for the patient.

Intraoperative. Continuity of care is important for the patient. The perioperative nurse making the initial assessment and identification of the patient's anticipatory loss should be with the patient intraoperatively if possible. This promotes trust and communication between the patient and the perioperative nurse.

Postoperative. The perioperative nurse evaluates the patient's level of grief, sadness, or depression by asking the patient how he or she feels about the loss. This feeling is compared with preoperative feelings. Eye contact, level of activity, and tone of speech are compared. The perioperative nurse making the initial assessment provides the most accurate evaluation of the patient's grief response.

Social Isolation

Definition

Inability to establish or maintain relationships with others despite a desire for socialization (Lederer et al., 1986)

Related Factors (Lederer et al., 1986)

- Elderly patients living alone
- Chemical dependence
- Inadequate or undeveloped social skills appropriate for the chronological age
- Debilitating medical condition that limits the patient to his or her home
- Physical handicap that prompts a negative reaction and rejection from the community
- Dysfunctional family relationships resulting in rejection
- Inadequate role modeling of socialization by the adult of the same sex during youth

Defining Characteristics (Lederer et al., 1986)

Subjective

- Verbalizes an inability to establish or maintain relationships with others in the community
- Verbalizes loneliness
- Verbalizes a fear of others
- Verbalizes anger toward others
- Expresses a negative self-image

Objective

- Inability to interact with health care team members during assessments and data collection
- Indecisiveness
- Unwillingness to make a decision
- Restlessness
- Sleep disturbance
- Withdrawal

Perioperative Nursing Implications

Preoperative. The focus for the perioperative nurse is to identify the presence of social isolation. The perioperative nurse may choose to interview a significant other for the preoperative assessment if the patient is unable or unwilling to communicate. Using a significant other lessens the patient's stress of interacting with numerous and different health care team members preoperatively. The perioperative nurse provides the patient or the significant other with information about the upcoming surgical experience such as patient transfers, a description of the holding area, and the nursing activities to anticipate in the OR. The perioperative nurse caring for the patient intraoperatively should interview the patient preoperatively, when possible, to promote a sense of trust between the patient and the nurse.

Intraoperative. The perioperative nurse should have a majority of nursing activities completed before the patient enters the OR (e.g., counting sponges, sharps, and instruments). This preparation increases the time that the perioperative nurse is available to provide support for the patient. The perioperative nurse ensures that bright overhead lights not yet needed are turned off, warm coverings are available for the patient's body and feet, and environmental noise is reduced to a minimum when the patient enters the room. The nurse also provides appropriate measures of touch and soothing communication to lessen anxiety. In addition, the perioperative nurse tells the patient what will occur before performing the activity. For example, the patient is reminded of the need for and application of safety straps, the placement of a grounding pad, and the use of preparation solution before the nursing activity is performed.

Postoperative. Continuity of perioperative nursing care is important to decrease the number of new personnel and interpersonal stressors experienced by the patient. The perioperative nurse verifies the patient's desire to change his or her state of social isolation. If decreased social isolation is desired, the perioperative nurse works with the patient and the significant other to design a plan to change the extent of social isolation through family and community resources.

Impaired Social Interaction

Definition

Participation in an abnormal amount of social interaction or an ineffective quality of social interaction (Kim et al., 1987).

Related Factors (Kim et al., 1987)

- Loss of self-worth
- Low self-esteem
- Social isolation
- Cognitive and developmental deficit concerning verbal and nonverbal communication skills
- Limited physical mobility
- Absence of significant others
- Lack of understanding about appropriate cultural responses

Defining Characteristics (Kim et al., 1987)

Subjective

- Verbalizes discomfort with social interactions
- Expresses a lack of belonging, caring, or interest in social situations
- Family expresses changes in the style of interaction (e.g., withdrawal, abruptness in group communication, and frequent interruption of conversation)

Objective

- Unsuccessful social interactions (e.g., poor verbal

and nonverbal communication and frequent exclusion from conversation by group)
- Sweating, frequent rubbing of the hands and shifting of position, no eye contact, restlessness, and standing at the edge of a group during social interaction
- Inappropriate responses and behaviors in social interactions

Perioperative Nursing Implications

Preoperative. Impaired social interaction is important to identify preoperatively. Postoperative responses during rehabilitation can be evaluated more appropriately when the baseline for responses and behaviors is established preoperatively. The preoperative nurse requests the cooperation of a significant other to collect data and understand the patient's responses. The patient with a cognitive and developmental delay such as a mentally handicapped patient may have impaired verbal and nonverbal communication skills, which contribute to impaired social interaction. The perioperative nurse may choose to communicate with the patient through simple pictures and music to illustrate a teaching point or convey a question or idea for patients with impaired social interaction. In addition, the perioperative nurse asks the significant other to bring to the hospital a familiar and soothing object from the home environment, such as a toy, a blanket, and a tape of music.

Intraoperative. The perioperative nurse ensures that the patient is transported to the OR with the familiar object from home. If the significant other provides support for the patient, he or she should accompany the patient to the holding area and OR to stand at the patient's side as desired.

Postoperative. The perioperative nurse communicates to recovery room personnel the importance of the familiar object from home to ensure that the object is not lost. If the patient or the significant other is unaware that help is available for the patient with impaired social skills, the perioperative nurse serves as resource for assistance and activities available in the community.

Altered Family Processes

Definition

Inability of the family unit to maintain a normal degree of physical, emotional, or psychological support for each other because of actual or perceived changes in the family brought about by the patient's surgical intervention (Lederer et al., 1986)

Related Factors (Lederer et al., 1986)

- Permanent or temporary disability related to the surgical intervention that results in changes in family roles
- Increased economic burden related to hospitalization

- Permanent or temporary role changes related to the rehabilitation process
- Inadequate coping mechanisms related to changes in role expectations during the surgical experience and rehabilitation
- Perceived threat to family integrity related to a poor prognosis, hospitalization, and the surgical experience
- Changes in family roles related to life stressors such as divorce, retirement, first child, and death of a family member

Defining Characteristics (Lederer et al., 1986)

Subjective

- Expresses concern regarding disruption of the family unit during hospitalization
- Expresses concern regarding a change in family role expectations during postoperative rehabilitation
- Complains of altered eating habits
- Expresses disruption in the sleep pattern unrelated to health care regimen (e.g., not caused by vital signs monitoring)
- Expresses concern that the postoperative prognosis and rehabilitation process differ from the preoperative explanation
- Expresses anger, anxiety, hostility, or depression
- Verbalizes an inability to accept the situation
- Family members express concerns about somatic complaints
- Verbalizes an inability to cope with changes in family integrity

Objective

- Verbal hostility between the family and the hospital staff
- Verbal hostility between the family and the patient
- Verbal hostility between family members
- Absence of family interaction
- Manipulative behavior (e.g., "I won't drink anything after midnight if you won't tell my wife I had this cigarette.")
- Physical or emotional neglect of the patient by the family

Perioperative Nursing Implications

Preoperative. The perioperative nurse determines if the family unit is experiencing alterations in family functions by assessing communication patterns. The nurse explores negative references made by the patient about another family member or a family situation. The perioperative nurse supports communication that clarifies the specifics about who, what, where, and when in a family interaction. Often, a life stressor such as retirement, a divorce, or the death of a significant other precipitates alterations in family function. The perioperative nurse assesses the family unit for flexibility in assuming roles of the disabled family member.

Intraoperative. The perioperative nurse notifies the appropriate support system to assist the family while the patient undergoes surgery. A chaplain, family member, or significant other should assist the family with group cohesion and provide individual support of family members during the surgical experience.

Postoperative. The perioperative nurse assists the patient in identifying potential or actual alterations in family functions postoperatively. The nurse may call a significant other to assist in home maintenance or parenting during the patient's postoperative rehabilitation. The perioperative nurse assists the family to reframe the stressful situation in more favorable terms (e.g., surgery prolonged the patient's life and a fund is established to assist with medical costs). In addition, the nurse assists the family in exploring options for problem solving and serves as a sounding board regarding the consequences for the proposed solution.

Altered Parenting

Definition

Inability of nurturing figures to create an environment that promotes optimum growth and development of a child or another human being (Kim et al., 1987)

Related Factors (Kim et al., 1987)

- Inadequate role modeling
- Physical or psychological abuse received from nurturing figure
- Inadequate support from significant others
- Separation from support systems due to relocation
- Inadequate social or emotional maturational needs of parenting figures (e.g., adolescent parents)
- Interruption in parent bonding process (e.g., hospitalized child or parent and critically ill parent or child)
- Perception of a child as a threat to the achievement of future needs
- Mental illness of a child
- Absence of responses from a child to the parent's nurturing behaviors
- Presence of stress (e.g., financial or legal problems, living in an unfamiliar culture, personal or family crises, and divorce)
- Inadequate knowledge of the nurturing role
- Lack of role identification (e.g., adolescent mothers or fathers may identify more with peer relationships than with the parental role)
- Multiple children without adequate financial and support resources
- Unrealistic expectations of the self, the child, and significant others

Defining Characteristics (Kim et al., 1987)

Subjective

- Expresses inappropriate negativeness of a child's characteristics (e.g., the child is perceived as "stupid" by the parent when not answering questions during a nursing assessment)
- Continuous verbalization of disappointment in the child's gender or physical characteristics
- Expresses resentment of the child for interruptions in life goals (e.g., career objectives not met)
- Verbalizes inadequacy in parenting role (e.g., unable to meet the child's needs and the needs of the self)
- Verbalizes disgust at the child's inability to achieve toilet training schedule
- Verbalizes that cannot control child

Objective

- Lack of parental attachment behaviors (e.g., absence of caressing the child, lack of appropriate use of touch, lack of expressed or demonstrated pride in the child, exclusion of the child from interactions, and no visual contact with the child)
- Neglect of the child's psychosocial or physical needs (e.g., inadequate or excessive nutritional intake, lack of parental contact with child, and lack of interaction with others)
- Inability to make health appointments for self or a child
- Inappropriate or inconsistent discipline practices
- Frequent accidents involving the child (e.g., scalding, broken limbs, excessive bruises in unusual areas)
- Frequent illnesses of the child (e.g., pneumonia and bronchitis)
- Delay in growth and development of the child
- History of child abuse or abandonment by primary caregiver
- Seeks continuous approval from others concerning parenting role
- Evidence of physical or psychological trauma

Perioperative Nursing Implications

Preoperative. The perioperative nurse assists the parent in identifying areas of inadequate knowledge and unrealistic role expectations. The nurse assesses the parent's readiness and ability to learn. The perioperative nurse assists the parent in identifying parenting expectations of himself or herself, the spouse, and the child. The nurse provides the parent an opportunity to express his or her feelings about unmet expectations. In addition, the nurse encourages the parent to think of reasons for unmet expectations. In addition, the perioperative nurse may assist the parent in arranging for child care during the surgical experience.

Intraoperative. During surgery the perioperative nurse keeps the parents informed of the child's status, as appropriate. If the parents need additional support, the perioperative nurse arranges to have a chaplain, social worker, or other specialist familiar with family dynamics visit the parents.

Postoperative. The perioperative nurse provides information about parenting skills at a level appropriate to the patient's level of interest and understanding. The perioperative nurse assists the patient in creating a positive learning situation to test new parenting information. The nurse assists the patient in developing new strategies to meet parenting expectations successfully. The nurse may also arrange individual or group counseling for the patient to further examine her or his parenting role.

Impaired Verbal Communication

Definition

Inability to express thoughts, feelings, and needs so that they are understood by others and to understand others (Lederer et al., 1986)

Related Factors (Lederer et al., 1986)

- Primary language different from that of the health care team members
- Inability to speak
- Impaired hearing
- Acute disorientation
- Motor or sensory aphasia
- Infants with undeveloped speech or cognitive skills
- Disease process such as a cardiovascular attack and Down syndrome
- Interventions such as a tracheotomy and endotracheal tube placement

Defining Characteristics (Lederer et al., 1986)

Subjective

- Complains that others do not understand him or her
- Expresses an inability to answer questions
- Expresses inability to follow directions

Objective

- Sign language as the primary mode of communication
- Incomplete thoughts expressed
- Communication in a foreign language
- Garbled, not understandable speech
- Exaggerated length of words so that several breaths are needed to complete one sentence
- Absence of audible speech

Perioperative Nursing Implications

Preoperative. The perioperative nurse encourages the patient with impaired verbal communication to express his or her thoughts and feelings. Encouragement is offered through active listening, maintaining eye contact, and allowing sufficient time for the patient to complete his or her thoughts. The nurse assists the patient in identifying impaired verbal communication by pointing out the discrepancies in verbal and nonverbal communication. In addition, the nurse alerts the patient to discrepancies between the words and the tone of voice used to communicate.

Intraoperative. The perioperative nurse maintains eye contact with the patient and employs appropriate use of touch. These nonverbal forms of communication convey a meaning of presence and caring to the patient.

Postoperative. The perioperative nurse encourages interaction with others who will increase the patient's self-esteem. The nurse teaches the patient about communication techniques that promote a healthy expression of feelings. For example, the patient should be encouraged to request feedback when communicating, to use active listening skills, and to provide positive and negative feedback about communication with others.

Preoperative Assessment Focus
(Gordon, 1987)

- Does the patient live alone? What is the nuclear family composition? Are there extended family members living with the patient?
- What, if any, family problems is the patient having difficulty handling?
- What things do family members depend on the patient for? What plans have been made to manage these responsibilities?
- Is there difficulty handling problems with children [if appropriate]?
- Is income sufficient to meet needs?
- Does the patient feel a part of the community where he or she is living?

Sexuality-Reproductive Pattern

Definition

Assessment of the sexuality-reproductive pattern evaluates the satisfaction or dissatisfaction with sexuality and sexual identity to include the female patient's reproductive state (e.g., premenopause or postmenopause) (Gordon, 1987). The perioperative nurse uses data to identify potential alterations in the patient's sexuality and reproductive pattern.

Perioperative Nursing Objective

Identify concerns, changes, and emotional needs of the patient regarding his or her sexuality. The perioperative nurse evaluates this pattern according to the patient's ability to identify personal conflicts and to obtain information about sexuality.

Nursing Diagnoses

(1) Sexual dysfunction, (2) altered sexuality patterns, and (3) rape-trauma syndrome

Sexual Dysfunction

Definition

Inadequacy, dissatisfaction, or incompatibility related to sexuality (Lederer et al., 1986)

Related Factors (Lederer et al., 1986)

- Familial history of Down syndrome, mental retardation, cystic fibrosis, and so on
- Career priorities above family and parenting interests
- Inadequate division of roles and responsibilities between working spouses
- Altered bladder control
- Body image disturbance such as stoma appearance or absence of a breast
- Depression
- Impotence
- Loss of touch sensation
- Medications for hypertension
- Loss of sexual drive
- Painful coitus

Defining Characteristics (Lederer et al., 1986)

Subjective

- Verbalizes a change in sexual relationships
- Expresses a decrease in sexual desire
- Verbalizes difficulty in sexual performance (e.g., erection and climax)
- Expresses discontent with sexual role
- Expresses a fear of pregnancy
- Expresses a fear of infectious disease (e.g., venereal disease and AIDS)
- Expresses limitations imposed by disease, medications, surgery, and fatigue
- Verbalizes misinformation regarding sexuality
- Expresses sexual exploitation or abuse
- Verbalizes overwhelming family or career roles and responsibilities, resulting in fatigue

Objective

- Inadequate division of roles and responsibilities between working spouses
- Altered bladder control
- Body image disturbance such as stoma appearance or absence of a breast
- Depression
- Impotence
- Loss of touch sensation
- Effects of medications

Perioperative Nursing Implications (Lederer et al., 1986)

Preoperative. The perioperative nurse discusses the potential for disinterest in sexual activity based on cues provided by the patient. Examples of patient cues are listed above under defining characteristics. The periop-

erative nurse must be aware of his or her own feelings about sexuality before discussing this pattern with a patient. If the perioperative nurse feels uncomfortable discussing this pattern, the nurse arranges for another nurse to conduct patient teaching rather than cutting the patient off from needed information. In addition, the nurse allows sufficient time and privacy to answer the patient's questions concerning sexual dysfunction because this issue may be difficult for patients to discuss. Often, a preoperative discussion of this pattern is short unless an immediate threat of sexual dysfunction exists. The preoperative discussion may lead to further discussion postoperatively as the trust relationship between the nurse and the patient increases.

Intraoperative. The perioperative nurse maintains control of communication in the OR including discussion, jokes, or comments with a sexual connotation. After the induction of general anesthesia, the patient's hearing is the last sense to leave. Also, anesthetized patients have been known to overhear conversations between team members during a surgical procedure.

Postoperative. Factual information about sexuality and communication between the patient and a sexual partner are teaching points to be included in a postoperative discharge plan for patients with the potential for sexual dysfunction due to surgical intervention. Patients may be unwilling to discuss sexual dysfunction with the perioperative nurse, but reading written information at home may provide the type of privacy needed to explore sexuality issues.

Altered Sexuality Patterns

Definition

The patient or significant other expresses concern about his or her sexuality (Kim et al., 1987)

Related Factors (Kim et al., 1987)

- Inadequate knowledge about sexuality patterns related to a change in body function or an alteration of a body part
- Fear of pregnancy or acquiring a sexually transmitted disease
- Lack of privacy
- Dysfunctional relationship with a significant other
- Lack of a significant other
- Absence of or dysfunctional role models

Defining Characteristics (Lederer et al., 1986)

- Expresses difficulties, limitations, or changes in sexual activities
- Expresses a decrease in sexual drive
- Verbalizes dissatisfaction with the sexual role
- Reports a fear of pregnancy or sexually transmitted disease
- Expresses incorrect information about sexuality
- Reports a history of sexual abuse

Perioperative Nursing Implications
(Lederer et al., 1986)

Preoperative. The perioperative nurse assesses the patient's comfort level in discussing sexual activity. The perioperative nurse notes if there is a difference in comfort level when the patient is alone or with the sexual partner.

Intraoperative. The perioperative nurse maintains control of communication, including jokes with a sexual connotation. The perioperative nurse protects the patient's dignity and privacy by providing protective coverings for the patient during gurney transfers and surgical preparation.

Postoperative. The perioperative nurse arranges a planning conference with the patient and the surgeon to discuss resuming sexual activity. The perioperative nurse designs a program with the patient to increase progressively the activity level and activity tolerance. In addition, the discharge teaching program includes information about the side effects of antihypertensives, tranquilizers, and ganglion blocking agents, which may affect the patient's libido and sexual performance. The patient should be informed of times to avoid intercourse such as when fatigued, when stressed, after a heavy meal, and during environmental heat and cold extremes. The perioperative nurse should advise the patient of signs and symptoms that indicate heart strain.

Rape-Trauma Syndrome

Definition

Effects of involuntary, violent intercourse occurring against the victim's will

The trauma syndrome that follows an attack or attempted attack includes an immediate disorganization of the victim's life style and a long-term reorganization of the life style (Lederer et al., 1986).

Related Factors (Lederer et al., 1986)

- Assault to victim's soul, self-esteem, body image, and personal identity

Two weeks to three months after rape crisis (the intermediate phase):

- Inadequate emotional intervention after crisis
- Inadequate support system
- Inability to connect rape crisis with current physical and emotional status

Defining Characteristics (Lederer et al., 1986)

Subjective

- Expresses feelings of anger
- Expresses feelings of blame
- Verbalizes a fear of violent death
- Verbalizes feelings of humiliation and shame
- Verbalizes thoughts of revenge

- Complains of sleep pattern disturbances (e.g., repetitive nightmares)

Objective

- Gastrointestinal irritability (e.g., nausea, cramps, and diarrhea)
- Muscle tension
- Genitourinary discomfort

Perioperative Nursing Implications (Kim et al., 1987)

Preoperative. The perioperative nurse provides the rape victim the opportunity to express her feelings. The nurse also allows the patient the privacy associated with silence. The perioperative nurse provides nonverbal support for the patient through therapeutic touch and eye contact. The nurse asks the patient if she would like to be alone or talk to a chaplain. The nurse provides a quiet and private holding area for the patient awaiting family or significant others. The nurse asks the patient if she would like to be alone or talk to a chaplain, social worker, or therapist. The perioperative nurse verifies with the patient the need for family counseling if the patient is in the intermediate phase of the rape-trauma syndrome (see above).

Intraoperative. The perioperative nurse ensures that the patient's privacy is protected by assisting with the transfer of covers during patient movement from the OR bed to a gurney. Warm coverings are offered to the patient, and the nurse tells the patient about the nursing activity to be performed before initiating the activity (e.g., the placement of safety straps, surgical preparation, and the application of a grounding pad). The patient is spoken to in a gentle, soothing, and clear voice. Therapeutic touch is offered and continued only if a positive response is returned by the patient. For example, the perioperative nurse would not continue to use therapeutic touch if the patient removed her hand from the perioperative nurse's hand.

Postoperative. The perioperative nurse encourages and facilitates family counseling for the patient. The nurse provides support opportunities by calling the patient after discharge from the hospital to determine the adequacy of support systems and the patient's mental and physical health. The nurse discusses with the patient strategies to avoid future assaults. In addition, the perioperative nurse provides instruction on progressive relaxation techniques. Later, during follow-up telephone consultations, the perioperative nurse designs a plan to pace social activities and arranges for sexual counseling with a significant other as desired.

Preoperative Assessment Focus
(Gordon, 1987)

Subjective: From Patient

- Are sexual relationships satisfying? Are there changes? Problems? [Ask if appropriate to the age and situation. For example, this is an inappropriate assessment for a child.]

- Does the patient use contraceptives? Are there problems with contraceptive use [if appropriate]?
- Do sexual relationships involve multiple partners? Are condoms used?
- Female patients: When did menstruation start? When was the last menstrual period? Are there menstrual problems? Is the woman para? Gravida?

Objective: From Perioperative Nurse or Chart

- Have adolescents developed secondary sexual characteristics?

Coping–Stress Tolerance Pattern

Definition

Assessment of the coping–stress tolerance pattern evaluates the capacity to resist threats to self-integrity and the family and other support systems, including mechanisms of handling stress, and the perceived ability to control and manage situations (Gordon, 1987). The perioperative nurse uses information about this pattern to identify potential alterations in effective coping mechanisms and adaptive responses to stressors.

Perioperative Nursing Objective

Identify actual or potential alterations in patterns requiring energy for adjusting to the environment and maintaining support systems (Gordon, 1987).

Nursing Diagnoses

(1) Ineffective individual coping, (2) impaired adjustment, (3) post-trauma response, (4) family coping: potential for growth, and (5) ineffective family coping

Ineffective Individual Coping
Definition
Inability to maintain a normal level of functioning in physical, emotional, or psychological areas because of actual or perceived changes in the environment (Lederer et al., 1986)

Related Factors (Lederer et al., 1986)
- Alterations in body image
- Anger
- Denial
- Depression
- Grief

Defining Characteristics (Lederer et al., 1986)
Subjective
- Expresses feelings of anger
- Expresses feelings of depression

- Verbalizes difficulty in coping
- Reports alterations in appetite
- Verbalizes disruptions in sleep patterns

Objectives
- Restlessness
- Manipulative behavior
- Lack of desire to plan or participate in care
- Withdrawal from or hostility toward family members or hospital staff
- Absence of eye contact

Perioperative Nursing Implications

Preoperative. The perioperative nurse seeks to identify with the patient the possible cause of ineffective coping. Next, the nurse discusses with the patient, the family, or a significant other when symptoms of ineffective coping first appeared. The perioperative nurse assesses the patient's potential for self-destructive behaviors. Without judging, the nurse encourages the patient to express his or her feelings to promote a trusting relationship with the patient and the family. The perioperative nurse asks the patient, the family, or a significant other about the most effective method of communicating and supporting the patient. If no information is available, the perioperative nurse uses a technique such as role playing to determine the patient's ability to problem solve and to assist the patient in making a decision. The nurse uses open-ended questions as follows: What options do you have after this decision is made? What consequences do you face after choosing this option? By starting questions with the interrogative "what" and using an open-ended approach, the perioperative nurse assists the patient experiencing ineffective coping with decision making throughout the perioperative period.

Intraoperative. The perioperative nurse uses a technique identified with patient during the preoperative phase to communicate with the patient (e.g., speaking softly, holding a hand in silence, and active listening). The patient who withdraws from the environment should not be forced to interact if she or he is unwilling to participate in nursing care. Instead, allow the patient to maintain distance from others. Recognizing the patient's need for separateness from the health care team is most therapeutic after attempts to involve him or her are made. However, do not ignore the patient. Gently inform the patient of nursing activities that involve him or her to avoid surprising the patient (e.g., performing the surgical shave preparation and applying safety straps and a grounding pad).

Postoperative. The perioperative nurse discusses the preoperative behavior with the patient. The nurse identifies the defining characteristics and seeks validation of these from the patient. If the patient acknowledges the problem of preoperative ineffective coping, the perioperative nurse explores with the patient the desire for counseling during the rehabilitation phase. If the patient denies these preoperative behaviors, the perioperative nurse discusses the patient's response with the family or a significant other. The nurse refers the significant other to a counselor or chaplain to seek assistance.

Impaired Adjustment

Definition

Inability to modify behavior needed to support a change in mental or physical health status (Kim et al., 1987)

Related Factors (Kim et al., 1987)

- Disability caused by disease (e.g., lung cancer) or injury (e.g., traumatic amputation)
- Insufficient support from significant others
- Impaired problem solving caused by an unexpected life style change
- Injured self-esteem (e.g., resulting from layoff or relief from a job)
- Incomplete grieving

Defining Characteristics (Kim et al., 1987)

Subjective

- Denies change in health status (e.g., "I'll continue to smoke. Nothing is wrong with my lungs.")
- Verbalizes an inability to resolve issues or meet goals
- Expresses feelings of anger and disbelief about the health status change
- Expresses an inability to set goals or make plans for the future

Objective

- Continues to perform unhealthy behavior (e.g., smokes two packs of cigarettes a day)
- Depends on others for ADL and decision making with no desire to increase independence

Perioperative Nursing Implications (Kim et al., 1987)

Perioperative. The perioperative nurse assesses the extent of the patient's adjustment by encouraging the expression of feelings. The nurse avoids critical attitudes and judgment about the patient's feelings to promote a trusting relationship with the patient. The perioperative nurse provides the patient the opportunity to express fears of death and disease. The nurse clarifies misinformation with facts about the patient's surgical procedure, prognosis, and rehabilitation. The perioperative nurse helps the patient identify past support systems used successfully to cope with a threatening situation. The nurse coordinates this support (e.g., spouse, chaplain, and friend) with the patient if possible.

Intraoperative. The perioperative nurse encourages a sense of control for the patient by allowing the patient to make decisions related to nursing care. For example, the patient may choose which hand the intraoperative IV cannula is placed, whether warm sheets are desired

on the feet, or what color of cap to wear on the head. In addition, the perioperative nurse recognizes the patient's right to emotions such as helplessness, withdrawal, and sadness. The nurse supports the patient with gentle touch and soft voice tone when speaking with the patient. The perioperative nurse does not personalize the patient's rejection of these comfort measures.

Postoperative. The perioperative nurse evaluates the patient's thoughts about the manner in which the surgical intervention will change the patient's life style. The nurse assists the patient in identifying roles and activities that will remain unchanged. This reminds the patient of the consistencies and strengths in the patient's life. In addition, the perioperative nurse assists the patient in developing a plan to adjust stressors during rehabilitation. The plan may include relaxation exercises, methods necessary to perform ADL independently (e.g., use of public transportation if without a car), and support systems to use in the community during a crisis.

Post-trauma Response

Definition

Pain associated with a traumatic event (Kim et al., 1987)

Related Factors (Kim et al., 1987)

- Accident
- Explosion
- Assault
- Rape
- Inhumane treatment
- War
- Earthquake or other disaster

Defining Characteristic (Kim et al., 1987)

Subjective

- Flashbacks of the event
- Verbalizes excessively about the traumatic event
- Reports repeated nightmares related to the event
- Expresses guilt associated with survival of the event
- Expresses an inability to remember the event
- Reports difficulty with interpersonal relationships

Objective

- Self-destructive behavior, such as drug abuse
- Explosive behavior
- Inability to control impulses

Perioperative Nursing Implications (Kim et al., 1987)

Preoperative. The perioperative nurse assists the patient in establishing a support system preoperatively. The nurse arranges contact with a significant other by telephone or a personal visit. The nurse arranges for the patient and the significant other to have a private area for interaction. After the need is validated with the patient, the perioperative nurse calls a chaplain or counselor to assist the patient in coping with extraordinary feelings of guilt. In addition, music preferred by the patient is offered to assist with relaxation. Answer patient's questions about the traumatic event but avoid graphic descriptions and pictures.

Intraoperative. The perioperative nurse provides therapeutic touch guidance to the patient intraoperatively. The nurse reminds the patient that significant others will see the patient postoperatively. A continuity of care providers is important throughout the perioperative period to promote a sense of trust with the patient. The perioperative nurse performs a thorough assessment of skin and tissue integrity because the patient experiencing a traumatic event may refuse a preoperative assessment or may not accurately report feelings of pain and injury.

Postoperative. The perioperative nurse requests that family members bring in familiar clothing, pictures, and other items for inhospital patients. In addition, the family is asked to prepare a list of telephone numbers of friends and family for easy access by the patient. The family is reminded of the importance of frequent short visits to the patient by family and friends. In addition, the patient should be praised for small strides in managing ADLs.

Family Coping: Potential for Growth

Definition

Family member's readiness to learn new tasks that facilitate growth and development of the patient and the self (Kim et al., 1987)

Related Factors (Kim et al., 1987)

- Sufficient basic needs are met to promote growth and self-actualization

Defining Characteristics (Kim et al., 1987)

Subjective

- Family member expresses the positive impact of patient's health crisis on his or her own goals, values, and relationships
- Family member reports the performance of activities that promote wellness
- Family member expresses interest in a self-help group with those experiencing a similar situation (e.g., Teen-Anon)

Objective

- Initiates health-promoting activities such as performing regular aerobic exercises, stopping smoking, and stopping drinking alcoholic beverages

Perioperative Nursing Implications (Kim et al., 1987)

Preoperative and Postoperative. The perioperative nurse assists the family in identifying changes in family dynamics related to the crisis of death, loss, or surgical intervention. The nurse identifies the family's readiness to receive support from sources outside the family. If the family does not want support from external sources, the perioperative nurse is wasting time; the nurse's attempt to intervene may increase the family's resistance to support. The nurse provides information to the family to facilitate the formulation of new goals and new techniques for achieving growth. The perioperative nurse evaluates the effectiveness of the assistance provided and further assesses the family member's potential for growth.

Ineffective Family Coping

Definition

Inability of a primary family member or friend to provide sufficient or effective support needed by the patient to adapt to the health challenge (Kim et al., 1987)

Related Factors (Kim et al., 1987)

- Temporary preoccupation with emotional conflicts which interferes with the ability to offer support to others (e.g., loss of a child interferes with a spouse's ability to support another)
- Temporary family disorganization associated with role changes
- Insufficient support of the primary family member by the patient

Defining Characteristics (Kim et al., 1987)

Subjective

- Expresses concern about a family member's response to his or her health problem
- Family member expresses concern about his or her reaction to the patient's health problem (e.g., protracted fear, anticipatory grief, and guilt)
- Expresses feelings of emotional abandonment

Objective

- Neglectful care of the patient
- Rejection of the patient (e.g., not visiting the patient)
- Physical abandonment by family
- Assuming illness signs and symptoms of the patient
- Neglecting relationships and needs of other family members

Perioperative Nursing Implications (Kim et al., 1987)

Preoperative. The perioperative nurse assists the family in crisis with support and communication. The nurse calls additional family members or significant others who may want to join the family and offer support. A chaplain is called if family members desire spiritual support to regain family unity.

Intraoperative. The perioperative nurse provides objective information on the patient's surgical progress to the family or supporting chaplain as much as possible.

Postoperative. The perioperative nurse encourages the family members and significant others to express their feelings such as loss, guilt, anger, and relief. The nurse decreases anxiety of family members by supporting the legitimacy to own positive and negative feelings about the patient's crisis. In addition, the perioperative nurse advises the family of the need to recognize changes in roles and relationships resulting from the patient's illness or injury. The nurse assists the family in prioritizing the roles necessary to maintain family integrity. Lastly, the perioperative nurse encourages family members to seek counseling regarding changes in family functioning.

Preoperative Assessment Focus
(Gordon, 1987)

- Are there significant changes in patient's life in the past year or two? Crises?
- Who is most able to take on the patient's responsibilities? Is that person available now?
- Is the patient tense or relaxed most of the time? What does the patient do to relieve tension? Does the patient use medication or alcohol?
- Is the primary family member tense or relaxed most of the time? What does the primary family member do to relieve tension? Does the primary family member use medication or alcohol?
- When (or if) problems occur, how are the problems resolved?
- Are these activities usually successful?

Value-Belief Pattern

Definition

Assessment of the value-belief pattern evaluates the values, goals, or beliefs (including spiritual) that guide choices and decisions concerning health and life (Gordon, 1987). The perioperative nurse uses information about this pattern to identify potential alterations in the patient's philosophical values and religious beliefs.

Perioperative Nursing Objective

Identify actual or potential alterations in patterns requiring psychological energy to cope with stressors challenging the patient's values, beliefs, goals, and health-related outcomes during the surgical experience (Gordon, 1987).

Nursing Diagnosis

Spiritual Distress (Distress of the Human Spirit)

Definition

Disruption of a value system that serves as a source of security and strength (Lederer et al., 1986)

Related Factors (Lederer et al., 1986)

- Threat to spiritual well-being related to poor prognosis or invasive surgical intervention
- Threat of death
- Test of spiritual beliefs
- Disruption in spiritual practices

Defining Characteristics (Kim et al., 1987)
Subjective

- Expresses concern with the meaning of life-and-death issues (e.g., "I don't know if there's anything to live for.")
- Verbalizes concern about values and beliefs system (e.g., "What good is money if I'm not healthy enough to enjoy it?")
- Expresses anger toward a higher being (e.g., God)
- Verbalizes an inner conflict about beliefs
- Expresses doubts about relationship with a higher being (e.g., God)
- Verbalizes confusion about the meaning of his or her existence (e.g., "I don't know why I survived when the others did not.")
- Expresses concern about the moral and ethical implications of surgical intervention (e.g., prolonging life with a decrease in the quality of life)
- Displaces anger toward a religious representative
- Regards illness as punishment
- Expresses self-blame (e.g., "The reason I have lymphoma is because I've cared only for myself and not others all these years.")
- Expresses a lack of responsibility for problems (e.g., "It's not my fault I smoke three packs a day—that boss of mine drives me to smoke. . . .")

Objective

- Inability to choose to or failure to participate in usual religious practices
- Request for spiritual assistance
- Nightmare or sleep disturbances with a spiritual overtone
- Changes in mood behavior (e.g., anger, crying, withdrawal, preoccupation, anxiety, hostility, and apathy)

Perioperative Nursing Implications

Preoperative. The perioperative nurse identifies the patient's usual pattern of spiritual practices. The patient's response attunes the nurse to potential or actual disruptions in spiritual beliefs. The perioperative nurse explores the type of spiritual strength most beneficial to the patient (e.g., visit with a chaplain and spiritual reading). The nurse arranges for intervention by the chaplain or the patient's spiritual/religious leader in a private setting if desired.

Postoperative. The perioperative nurse reassesses the patient's spiritual status with the patient after surgery to determine if spiritual intervention would promote physical and psychological wellness.

Preoperative Assessment Focus
(Gordon, 1987)

- Is the patient generally satisfied with the life style?
- Does the patient have future plans?
- Is religion an important element in the patient's life?
- Does religion help when difficulties arise [if appropriate]?
- Does the patient expect any interference with religious practices during the surgical experience [if appropriate]?

HEALTH PATTERN ASSESSMENT SUMMARY

The health patterns approach assists the perioperative nurse in identifying the health problem and related factors (e.g., probable causes) and in defining characteristics (e.g., signs and symptoms) or risk factors that support the existence of a patient problem. Data collected according to the functional health patterns framework systematically result in nursing diagnoses. Each nursing diagnosis represents a category of related health problems and a cluster of signs and symptoms (Gordon, 1987) or risk factors. The purpose of making nursing diagnoses is to organize the planning, implementation, and evaluation phases of perioperative nursing care delivery (Gordon, 1987). Nursing diagnoses may be formulated for the preoperative, intraoperative, and postoperative phases of the patient's surgical experience.

INTERPRETING ASSESSMENT DATA

Collecting a wide range of data is useless unless the data are interpreted. The perioperative nurse compares all assessment data with developmental, cultural, and physiological norms. Variances from these norms are cues for the perioperative nurse that a health problem exists. The perioperative nurse uses cognitive inference and decision-making skills to explain his or her findings.

Clustering Data

The perioperative nurse uses reasoning and judgment skills to organize interpreted data into groups, or clusters. The memory stores of education and clinical experience enable the perioperative nurse to cluster cues from the assessment into meaningful categories. These meaningful categories of clustered signs and symptoms allow the perioperative nurse to formulate nursing diagnoses. The clustering of signs and symptoms facilitates communication of the patient's perioperative health problem in a concise format (Gordon, 1987). Use of a data collection tool based on the functional health patterns (see Table 2–4) assists the perioperative nurse in categorizing data. After two or three probable diag-

noses are formulated with related factors, the defining characteristics are reviewed for each possible nursing diagnosis until the correct diagnosis is identified.

Making Nursing Diagnoses Using the Eleven Functional Health Patterns

The formula for making a nursing diagnosis is as follows:

Problem statement + "related to" + related factor = nursing diagnosis

FORMULATING A NURSING DIAGNOSIS

EXAMPLE:

Problem statement: Altered peripheral tissue perfusion

Related factor: Impaired circulation

Defining characteristics: Absence of peripheral pulses, cool skin, cyanosis of the nail bed, edema, patient complaints of a tingling sensation in the extremities, and patient complaints of pain, numbness, and loss of tactile sensations

Nursing Diagnosis: Altered peripheral tissue perfusion related to impaired circulation

A case study is presented to demonstrate the process of formulating nursing diagnoses for the surgical patient.

Case Study

A 75-year-old woman admitted at 2:30 AM is scheduled for a repair of a fractured right hip. The medical history reports emphysema. Laboratory values and vital signs fall within normal ranges, and arterial blood gas values will be determined intraoperatively. The chest x-ray film reveals generalized cloudiness of lung tissue indicative of emphysema.

Health Perception–Health Management Pattern: The patient reports that she is "good about following doctor's orders. Just tell me what to do to get well again. I try to take good care of myself now. Sometimes, I'm a little dopey-headed in the morning. Sometimes I can't find my walker right away—that's how I fell—couldn't find my walker this morning."

Discussion: The patient expresses a desire to participate in her plan of care. The patient has a *high risk for infection* related to several factors. The surgical incision breaks the patient's first line of defense against pathogens. The broken head of the femur and entrance into the bone during surgery exposes a part of the patient's immunological system to the environment, resulting in possible infection. In addition, the length of the surgical procedure and the extent of surgical retraction expose tissues to environmental pathogens. Further investigation entails identification of defining characteristics of "dopey-headed." If the patient became confused or disoriented from a pain medication administered postoperatively and she wanted to leave the unit bed, the patient has a *high risk for injury* related to an unsteady gait. Although additional defining characteristics are needed to validate this potential nursing diagnosis, the perioperative nurse would document the information pertaining to the unsteady gait (i.e., the patient uses walker for ambulation and may be confused) to communicate with the unit nurses postoperatively.

Nutritional-Metabolic Pattern: The patient's height is 5 feet 6 inches and her weight is 235 pounds. Bruises approximately 5 to 7 cm in size appear approximately 1 inch above the elbow and 3 inches below the elbow on the dorsal aspect of the right arm. The skin of the right hip appears reddened and taut. No other skin lesions, rashes, or cuts are apparent.

Discussion: The perioperative nurse documents the presence of the skin condition preoperatively to determine if tissue integrity is maintained intraoperatively. The patient has a *high risk for impaired skin integrity* in the coccyx area and ankles, depending on the type of fracture table used. Preparation solutions run down into the coccyx area from the leg if insufficient absorbable pads or nonabsorbable protective sheets are used during the surgical skin preparation. The potential for altered tissue perfusion related to shearing forces of patient positioning may occur if inadequate padding around ankles is used because the patient is overweight. Supplies or equipment used to secure the ankle to a fracture table may inhibit adequate tissue perfusion.

The patient is overweight for her height. The perioperative nurse would explore the related factors for *altered nutrition: more than body requirements* postoperatively. The nurse looks for cues related to low self-esteem, problems in role-relationships, knowledge deficit, grieving, anxiety, and so on.

Elimination Pattern: "I have a BM [bowel movement] every day at 9:30 [AM]. It's my morning constitution." The patient takes an over-the-counter stool softener every other day. There is no regular use of laxatives.

Discussion: The patient has the potential for *constipation* related to decreased mobility during the 3 to 5 day expected stay in the surgical intensive care unit postoperatively. The perioperative nurse would encourage fluid intake and validate this potential nursing diagnosis postoperatively.

Activity-Exercise Pattern: "I take complete care of myself, except when I get sick, then my daughter comes over to help me. I get around pretty good with my walker. I have my groceries delivered. My daughter takes me shopping. I really slowed down when I got emphysema 5 years or so ago. Smoked over a pack a day for 55 years—doctor told me to

stop. I can hardly take a set of stairs now without wheezing and gagging on the stuff [secretions] in my windpipe."

Discussion: The patient states that she is able to fulfill her self-care needs. However, the patient is "sick" and, considering the impending surgery, there is an impending *self-care deficit* related to the musculoskeletal impairment of the fractured hip and pain and discomfort resulting from surgery. The fractured hip decreases the patient's physical mobility. Thus, the patient has *impaired physical mobility* related to a fractured hip. In addition, the patient experiences *ineffective airway clearance* related to tracheobronchial secretions. An ineffective airway clearance is validated by the patient's description of secretions while climbing stairs. Additional data are needed to validate the presence of impaired gas exchange and ineffective breathing patterns. A description of the patient's breathing sounds and patterns as well as the nail bed flush would be objective data needed to validate additional nursing diagnoses. Vital signs fall within normal ranges in this patient.

Cognitive-Perceptual Pattern: The patient reports that she is able to read the newspaper without glasses and has "pretty good hearing—I can hear better than my daughter." The patient reports difficulty tolerating bright lights. "Ever since I had that car accident, bright lights are unbearable! My grandkids make me crazy if they don't turn off those glaring lights when we watch TV. I can tolerate the noise, not the lights."

Discussion: The perioperative nurse confirms the patient's visual and hearing abilities. The patient has a *high risk for sensory/perceptual alteration* related to visual sensory overload of the bright lights in the OR. This nursing diagnosis is validated by the patient's reported reaction to bright lights in the home environment.

Sleep-Rest Pattern: The patient reports no problem with the onset of sleep or interrupted sleep, "except for the last couple of nights—I thought someone was trying to break into my house."

Discussion: The patient was admitted at 2:30 AM. It is unlikely that the patient had sufficient sleep before surgery. A change of sleep habits related to time of admission is noted. In addition, a *sleep pattern disturbance* is related to fear of potential physical injury in the home. The perioperative nurse would return to the health perception–health management pattern to document a *high risk for injury*. During the postoperative visit, the perioperative nurse would identify with the patient and significant others the potential for physical injury in the patient's home.

Self-perception–Self-concept Pattern: "I'm counting on the Lord and my daughter to take care of me—plus you folks [health care team], of course. My body is getting so old, I'm unable to do much except to ask for help."

Discussion: Several cues are given here. The reference of calling the daughter made in the health perception–health maintenance pattern assessment verifies the patient's hint of dependence on the daughter. The reference to having others such as the health care team, the religious being, and daughter "help" the patient compensate for an "old" body infers an inability to change her condition. The inability to change the patient's condition implies a sense of *powerlessness.* The perioperative nurse must decide if the potential for powerlessness related to the physical injury is a dysfunctional health problem, considering the patient's situation. As the perioperative nurse collects additional data and cues, she or he determines whether the powerlessness interferes with the patient's ability to move toward wellness. A degree of powerlessness may be the coping mechanism needed to deal with hospitalization and provide compliance with the health care regime. In addition, the perioperative nurse validates with additional data whether the powerlessness contradicts the patient's desire to participate in her care as noted in the health perception–health management pattern assessment. The perioperative nurse continues to collect and clarify defining characteristics to validate the powerlessness diagnosis.

Role-Relationship Pattern: The daughter is with the patient. The daughter states that she will be with patient throughout the hospitalization. The mother does not ask the daughter to leave.

Discussion: The daughter appears to be a primary support system for the patient. The patient depends on the daughter during sickness and with some self-care activities as reported in the health perception–health management pattern, the activity-exercise pattern, and self-perception–self-concept pattern assessments. The patient and the daughter are following their family support processes in the hospital, similar to the pattern described when the patient is "sick" at home. Thus, given the data, *altered family processes* is not a problem. A withdrawal of or change in the daughter's existing support would indicate a potential problem for the patient in the role-relationship pattern.

Sexuality-Reproductive Pattern: The patient's spouse died 9 years ago. Significant others include the daughter and a family of three grandchildren. The patient enjoys being by herself when she is not with her family.

Discussion: No changes or problems in the sexuality-reproductive pattern are reported by patient. The perioperative nurse evaluates this health pattern primarily by the subjective data reported by the patient.

Coping–Stress Tolerance Pattern: The patient states that she talks about stressful issues with her daughter. She reads novels and knits to work through problems. She has approximately two glasses of wine with her evening meal. These activities prove to be successful stress management activities. The daughter states that she will bring in a novel and knitting for her mother during the hospitalization.

Discussion: No change in coping strategies is suggested. Wine may not be available with the patient's meals, but pain medication will be offered postoperatively. Pain medication may interfere with the patient's ability to read. More data are needed postoperatively to determine if a potential health problem exists.

Value-Belief Pattern: The patient's record states that the patient is Protestant. No chaplain is desired. Religion is a "private matter" in patient's life.

Discussion: In the self-perception–self-concept pattern assessment, the patient stated that she expected "the Lord" to take care of her during the surgical experience. This reference denotes belief in a higher being. The perioperative nurse listens for cues postoperatively that reflect whether the patient's expectations of a higher being or of her quality of life were met or unmet. These data would validate whether the patient experiences a dysfunctional health problem in the value-belief pattern.

Supporting Diagnoses with Scientific Knowledge

The classification of nursing diagnoses is an evolving process. Nursing diagnoses must not only be developed by expert opinion, but also supported by scientific knowledge through nursing research. Each perioperative nurse has the opportunity to contribute to nursing's body of knowledge by critiquing existing nursing diagnoses and determining if the defining characteristics and related factors for actual nursing diagnoses and risk factors for potential nursing diagnoses consistently occur for the identified diagnosis in the perioperative nursing setting. New nursing diagnoses must be developed to capture the myriad patient responses evident in ORs today. In addition, nursing research is needed to support or improve the identification of nursing diagnoses, related factors, and defining characteristics. This research will assist the perioperative nurse in preoperative, intraoperative, and postoperative decision making and nursing care delivery.

DOCUMENTATION AND COMMUNICATION PROCEDURES

Perioperative nurses have a professional and legal responsibility to document patient findings and communicate professional decisions. The Association of Operating Room Nurses and the Joint Commission on Accreditation of Health Care Organizations support this professional responsibility (Kneedler, 1987). Professional competency standards for perioperative nursing identify documentation as an expectation of professional practice (AORN, 1992). In addition, the nursing diagnoses are communicated in writing to promote continuity of information and care for the perioperative patient. The perioperative nurse follows the standards for documentation identified by individual facilities.

Documentation that follows standards identified by the facility can be excellent legal protection for patients and perioperative nurses. Written description of patient findings during assessment should clearly note the patient's condition: good documentation describes specifics, not generalities (Kneedler and Dodge, 1987). The specifics are the objective and subjective findings (signs and symptoms) known as defining characteristics for actual nursing diagnoses and risk factors for potential nursing diagnoses. Generalities (e.g., good, bad, big, little) should be avoided; broad descriptors have different meanings for many people. Therefore, perioperative nursing documentation should reflect objective behavior and physiological signs as well as direct subjective patient statements. This information enables accurate communication among health care team members.

Bibliography

Association of Operating Room Nurses (1992). *Standards and recommended practices for perioperative nursing.* Denver.

Brenner, Z. R. (1987). *Diagnostic tests and procedures applying to nursing.* East Norwalk, CT: Appleton & Lange.

Brunner, L. S., Suddarth, D. S. (1988). *Textbook of medical-surgical nursing* (pp. 132–139). Philadelphia: J. B. Lippincott.

Gordon, M. (1987). *Nursing diagnosis: Process and application* (2nd ed.). New York: McGraw-Hill.

Kim, M. J., McFarland, G. K., McLane, A. M. (1987). *Guide to nursing diagnoses* (2nd ed.). St. Louis: C. V. Mosby.

Kneedler, J. A., Dodge, G. H. (1987). *Perioperative patient care* (2nd ed.). Boston: Blackwell Scientific.

Kozier, B., Erb, G. (1983). *Fundamentals of nursing: Concepts of growth and development* (2nd ed.) (pp. 233–294). Menlo Park, CA: Addison-Wesley.

Lederer, J. R., Marculescu, G. L., Gallagher, J., Mills, P. (1986). *Care planning pocket guide: A nursing diagnosis approach.* Menlo Park, CA: Addison-Wesley.

Luckmann, J., Sorenson, K. C. (1987). *Medical-surgical nursing: A psychophysiologic approach.* Philadelphia: W. B. Saunders.

Wolf, L., Weitzel, M. H., Zornow, R.A., Zsohar, H. (1983). *Fundamentals of nursing* (7th ed.) (pp. 57–89). Philadelphia: J. B. Lippincott.

CHAPTER 3

Planning Patient Care: A Functional Health Patterns Approach

Cynthia A. Abbott

Planning perioperative nursing care enables the perioperative nurse to individualize care in a systematic and comprehensive manner. Patient-centered care prioritizes nursing actions during the surgical experience to meet the goals for the patient and the patient's needs for nursing care. If used, the nursing care plan promotes continuity of information and solicits the patient's cooperation in achieving a higher state of wellness.

DEFINITION

Planning is the development of a course of action that moves the patient toward wellness by resolving health problems (nursing diagnoses). The planning phase begins when the perioperative nurse reviews the nursing diagnoses to formulate, prioritize, and implement patient goals and expected outcomes. The planning phase ends with the development of a nursing care plan (Yura and Walsh, 1983).

MEASURABLE CRITERIA

The perioperative nurse demonstrates competency to plan perioperative nursing care by

The views expressed in this chapter are those of the author and do not reflect the official position or policy of the Department of the Army, the Department of Defense, or the U.S. Government.

- developing patient goals
- developing outcome statements
- developing criteria to measure the achievement of outcome statements
- identifying nursing activities to meet expected patient outcomes
- setting priorities for nursing care
- sequencing nursing activities
- communicating and coordinating patient care needs
- making patient care assignments
- preparing for patient care emergencies
- planning for the patient's discharge
- documenting and communicating the nursing care plan (AORN, 1992, *I*:2–6—2–7)

THE PLANNING PROCESS

Developing Patient Goals

Recommended standards for perioperative nursing practice direct the perioperative nurse to develop goals for the plan of nursing care (Association of Operating Room Nurses [AORN], 1992). The perioperative nurse develops goals using health problems identified in the nursing diagnosis (Gordon, 1987). The perioperative nurse collaborates with the patient, significant others, and other health care personnel during goal development (AORN, 1992). The perioperative nurse provides the patient with an opportunity to voice his or her agreement or disagreement about the goals to solicit the patient's support and cooperation in developing the perioperative nursing care plan.

To obtain the patient's participation in goal achievement, the perioperative nurse involves the patient during goal formation. Patient goals consist of four components. The first component of the goal is the patient. The patient is the *subject* because perioperative nursing care and rehabilitation center on the patient. The next component to include in goal formulation is the *verb phrase*. Examples of verb phrases useful in goal formulation include "explains," "demonstrates," "is free from," and "maintains." The final elements of the goal statement address *when* and *where* the goal is measured (Kneedler and Dodge, 1987). The postoperative day should be specified to determine whether goal attainment was achieved when expected. Goals guide nursing actions to improve or maintain the patient's state of wellness described by the health problem-nursing diagnosis (AORN, 1992).

FORMULATING GOAL STATEMENT

Step One: Identify the functional health pattern containing the nursing diagnosis (Table 3–1).

Step Two: Identify the nursing diagnosis describing the health problem (see Table 3–1).

Step Three: State the patient goal according to the desired level of wellness, such as absence of alterations in the health pattern, freedom from alterations in the health pattern, and maintenance of the functional health pattern.

Step Four: State the time or perioperative phase when the goal is to be measured (e.g., intraoperatively, 24 hours postoperatively, 48 hours postoperatively, and when the patient is discharged from the hospital)

Example: A 57-year-old man is scheduled for an inguinal hernia repair. He is blind in one eye from congenital optic nerve damage. Blood studies indicated a decreased hemoglobin concentration.

Nursing Diagnosis 1: High risk for infection related to interruption of skin integrity by the surgical incision

Step One: Health perception–health management is the functional health pattern.

Step Two: High risk for infection is the health problem.

Step Three: The patient's health perception–health management pattern is free from alterations.

Step Four: This is noted postoperatively.

Nursing Diagnosis 2: Sensory/perceptual alteration (visual) related to optic nerve damage

Step One: Cognitive-perceptual pattern is the functional health pattern.

Step Two: Sensory/perceptual alteration (visual) is the health problem.

Step Three: The patient's cognitive-perceptual pattern is maintained.

Step Four: This occurs during the intraoperative phase.

Goals are broad statements that describe the desired state of patient wellness. More specific descriptions of the desired wellness are required to plan nursing actions. More specific descriptions of the patient's wellness are known as patient outcomes (Gordon, 1987).

Developing Outcome Statements

Outcomes are observable patient behaviors used to measure goal achievement. A behavioral objective is another term used to describe patient outcomes. The perioperative nurse uses patient outcomes to guide decisions about planning care. Additionally, well-written outcomes serve as a framework for measuring the effectiveness of nursing care delivery postoperatively. Expected patient outcomes indicate when the health problem is resolved and the patient is ready for discharge from the hospital (Gordon, 1987).

The perioperative nurse reviews the nursing diagnosis and converts the wording of the health problem into a statement of the desired patient outcome. The nurse develops an expected patient outcome by identifying the opposite of the health problem in the nursing diagnosis. Converting the health problem stated in the nursing diagnosis into a description of the desired state of wellness is an efficient and precise method of developing patient outcome statements (Gordon, 1987).

FORMULATING OUTCOME STATEMENTS

Step One: Identify the health problem and review the nursing diagnosis.

Step Two: Convert the health problem into an outcome statement by using wording such as "absence of alterations in," "freedom from alterations in," and "maintenance of."

Example: A 57-year-old man is scheduled for an inguinal hernia repair. He is blind in one eye from congenital optic nerve damage. Blood studies indicate a decreased hemoglobin concentration.

Nursing Diagnosis 1: High risk for infection related to interruption of skin integrity by the surgical incision

Step One: High risk for infection is the health problem.

Step Two: The patient is free from infection postoperatively.

Nursing Diagnosis 2: Sensory/perceptual alteration (visual) related to optic nerve damage

TABLE 3–1. NURSING DIAGNOSIS IN A FUNCTIONAL HEALTH PATTERN FRAMEWORK

Health Perception–Health Management Pattern

Altered health maintenance
Noncompliance
High risk for infection
High risk for injury

Nutritional–Metabolic Pattern

Altered nutrition: less than body requirements
Altered nutrition: more than body requirements
Impaired tissue integrity
Impaired skin integrity
Fluid volume deficit
Fluid volume excess
High risk for altered body temperature
Hyperthermia
Hypothermia

Elimination Pattern

Constipation
Diarrhea
Altered patterns of urinary elimination
Incontinence
Urinary retention

Activity-Exercise Pattern

Activity intolerance
Impaired physical mobility
Self-care deficit
Impaired home maintenance management
Ineffective airway clearance
Ineffective breathing pattern
Impaired gas exchange
Decreased cardiac output
Altered tissue perfusion
Altered growth and development

Cognitive-Perceptual Pattern

Alterations in comfort: pain
Sensory/perceptual alteration: visual, auditory,
    kinesthetic, gustatory, tactile, and olfactory
Unilateral neglect
Knowledge deficit
Altered thought processes

Sleep-Rest Pattern

Sleep pattern disturbance

Self-perception–Self-concept Pattern

Fear
Anxiety
Hopelessness
Powerlessness
Self-esteem disturbance

Role-Relationship Pattern

Anticipatory grieving
Social isolation
Impaired social interaction
Altered family processes
Altered parenting
Impaired verbal communication

Sexuality-Reproductive Pattern

Sexual dysfunction
Altered sexuality patterns
Rape-trauma syndrome

Coping–Stress Tolerance Pattern

Ineffective individual coping
Impaired adjustment
Post-trauma response
Family coping: potential for growth
Ineffective family coping

Value-Belief Pattern

Spiritual distress

Step One: Sensory/perceptual alteration (visual) is the health problem.

Step Two: The patient's tactile, olfactory, kinesthetic, auditory, and gustatory senses and perceptions are maintained postoperatively.

Discussion: Because the congenital optic nerve damage causing visual alterations cannot be resolved with nursing activities, the outcome statement focuses on maintaining the remaining senses and perceptions. The perioperative nurse evaluates the viable senses and perceptions that are measurable postoperatively.

The perioperative nurse evaluates whether the patient's behavior, statements, and demonstrations are consistent with the outcome statement written during the planning phase. The perioperative nurse compares the expected outcome with the patient's signs and symptoms, verbalizations about level of wellness, and demonstrations of self-care skills needed for rehabilitation. This comparison indicates whether the patient goal and projected outcomes were achieved. The health pattern format guides the perioperative nurse in formulating criteria to measure the attainment of patient outcomes.

Developing Criteria to Measure the Achievement of Outcome Statements

Defining characteristics (signs and symptoms) or risk factors of the nursing diagnosis are useful in recognizing solutions to patient problems and identifying criteria to measure the achievement of outcome statement (Gordon, 1987). The perioperative nurse reviews the defining characteristics or risk factors of the nursing diagnosis in the assessment phase (see Chapter 2). The opposite condition of each defining characteristic is known as a *criterion* of the expected outcome. A criterion is used to measure the achievement of outcome statements (Kneedler and Dodge, 1987). The perioperative nurse uses criteria derived from defining characteristics or risk factors to measure the achievement of outcome statements.

EXAMPLE OF PLANNING PROCESS

Nursing Diagnosis: High risk for infection related to interruption of skin integrity by the surgical incision

Goal: The patient's health perception–health management pattern is free from alterations postoperatively.

Expected Outcome: The patient is free from infection within 48 hours postoperatively.

Outcome Criteria:

1. The incisional site is free from redness, swelling, or drainage.
2. The wound edges are approximated with no evidence of dehiscence.
3. Oral temperature is less than 100°F.
4. Vital signs remain within normal limits.
5. Laboratory values remain normal.

Identifying Nursing Activities to Meet Expected Outcomes

The perioperative nurse uses patient goals to identify nursing actions needed to achieve expected outcomes (AORN, 1992). Statements of nursing activities are written for each criterion. Nursing activities assist the patient in moving from his or her present state of health problems to achieve a level of wellness described in the expected outcomes (Gordon, 1987).

The statement of the nursing activity often begins with verb to describe the action to be performed by the perioperative nurse (Kneedler and Dodge, 1987). For example, "*maintain* sterility during opening of supplies," "*monitor* sterile field," and "*implement* operating room sanitation protocols" are nursing actions taken to prevent the potential for infection intraoperatively.

Kneedler and Dodge (1987) stated that the written nursing activity, which is also known as a nursing order, includes several elements of information. The nursing activity designates *what* nursing activity is to occur to achieve the patient goal. For example, "Identify the patient by *checking* the identification band during patient transfer and in the preoperative holding area." The nursing activity statement indicates *how* the patient is to be identified (by checking the patient's identification bracelet). *When* and *where* the patient's identity is to be verified are included (during patient transfer and in the perioperative holding area). *Who* is the final element to be included in the nursing order. The nursing order specifies whether a registered nurse, a licensed practical nurse, a surgical technician, or a nursing assistant is to perform the nursing activity (Kneedler and Dodge, 1987). This element is excluded from the above example. Specifying who is to perform the nursing activity directs accountability and responsibility for the care provided. Whether it is specified in the nursing order or initialed after completion of the nursing activity, documentation should indicate who performed the nursing action.

Gordon (1987) recommended that perioperative nurses focus on the factors related to the health problem. The perioperative nurse reduces the risk of a potential problem and the significance of an actual problem by planning nursing activities that resolve the cause or remove the potential cause of the health problem (Gordon, 1987). After the cause of the problem is attenuated by nursing actions, the patient moves to a higher level of health. Examples of preoperative, intraoperative, and postoperative nursing actions performed for each health problem are found in Chapter 2.

Prioritizing Nursing Care

The functional health patterns approach assists the perioperative nurse in organizing and prioritizing nursing diagnosis and patient outcome statements. A patient may have a myriad of nursing diagnoses. Solving all health problems at one time is impractical, unreasonable, and not necessary.

The perioperative nurse prioritizes nursing diagnoses according to immediate, intermediate, and long-term categories. Immediate priorities include nursing diagnoses that could injure the patient if left untreated (Gordon, 1987). Examples of immediate priorities in the activity-exercise pattern include ineffective airway clearance, decreased cardiac output, and ineffective breathing pattern (see Table 3–1). These health problems are more critical to the patient's immediate well-being than alterations in growth and development; however, altered growth and development increases in priority after life-threatening problems subside.

Alterations in growth and development may be seen as intermediate or long-term priorities, depending on the cause of the health problem. For example, altered growth and development related to inconsistent parenting skills by caregivers is an example of an intermediate priority. The caretaker can increase the quality of parenting (e.g., by setting limits consistently). Expecting limits in behavior improves the child's social behaviors and acceptance by others. The perioperative nurse's expected outcome of increased peer acceptance for the child occurs by performing the following nursing actions: (1) arranging counseling for the child and the caretakers, (2) providing a reference list of recommended readings and addresses and telephone numbers of community resources, and (3) scheduling a follow-up evaluation by telephone or by another health care team member. The growth and development health problem may also be a long-term problem. The growth and development issues of physically or mentally handicapped children may have a long-term priority.

The perioperative nurse uses consultation with colleagues, nursing experience, educational preparation, and reasoning and analytical skills to determine whether the related factors indicate that the health problem is an immediate, intermediate, or long-term priority. In addition, the perioperative nurse validates the decision concerning health problem priorities with the patient. When differences in priority setting arise, the perioperative nurse works with the patient to identify the patient's priorities, to negotiate a mutual agreement of priorities, and to obtain cooperation in resolving health problems.

Sequencing Nursing Activities

Nursing activities are the psychomotor and cognitive behaviors that the perioperative nurse performs to meet criteria, expected outcomes, and patient goals. The perioperative nurse performs nursing activities according to the priorities established for the nursing diagnoses (Gordon, 1987). Nursing activities associated with immediate-priority nursing diagnoses are performed before nursing activities associated with nursing diagnoses of intermediate and long-term priorities. The perioperative nurse reviews the nursing diagnosis that must be addressed immediately and sequences the nursing activities according to goals and expected outcomes.

For example, the perioperative nurse uses primarily two actions in assembling supplies after reviewing goal priorities and expected outcomes. First, the perioperative nurse checks and collects supplies and equipment in the most time- and motion-efficient manner. Supplies are checked for sterility and equipment for proper functioning before the patient enters the operating room (OR) to prevent delays in surgery and increased anesthesia exposure. Equipment and supplies are collected before the patient enters the OR to avoid problems associated with incorrect equipment. Second, information sources such as the perioperative nursing care plan, the surgeon's preference card, and the OR request slip are reviewed to identify all nursing activities needed. The perioperative nurse ensures that items required for the surgical procedure function properly and are readily available.

The most immediate goals common to surgical patients, such as absence of infection, maintenance of skin integrity, and maintenance of effective airway, are performed for all surgical patients. The perioperative nurse often performs nursing activities associated with these patient goals first. Examples of routine nursing activities are to perform and monitor OR sanitation procedures to ensure a clean environment, to ensure that anesthesia's suction is connected and ready for operation, to check the package integrity and expiration date of sterile supplies, to create and maintain a sterile field, to provide adequate padding and accessories for pressure points during patient positioning, and to substitute an appropriate surgical preparation solution for the iodine-allergic patient. Next, the perioperative nurse checks and collects supplies and equipment and performs nursing actions associated with goals and expected outcomes individualized for the patient. All nursing activities are performed with a minimum of effort, expense, and waste, in concern for the patient's and the institution's financial resources (Kneedler and Dodge, 1987).

Communicating and Coordinating Patient Care Needs

The care plan for the perioperative patient ensures that the goals and expected outcomes for the patient's surgical experience are met. The purpose of the perioperative nursing care plan is to communicate with other health care team members and coordinate responses to the patient's needs in a consistent manner. Communication of the perioperative nursing care plan during surgery is achieved by giving it to the patient care coordinator or the perioperative nurse providing care for the patient or by placing the care plan in the OR where the surgery is scheduled (Kneedler and Dodge, 1987). In addition to the perioperative nursing care plan, other methods may be used to coordinate patient care needs.

Patient care conferences before the surgical procedure involve intraoperative team members. The perioperative nurse may use time at change of shift, between cases, or when opening a sterile setup to relay special patient care needs to others. In addition, a review of the literature pertinent to the patient's health problem adds an educational dimension to the patient care conference and lends itself to an inservice session later.

Two methods of reporting patient care needs facilitate coordination of nursing actions. The written format of communication is seen in perioperative nursing care plans and preoperative, intraoperative, and postoperative nursing notes. The nursing actions completed during the patient's surgical experience should support the goals, expected outcomes, and criteria of the care plan.

The verbal mode of communication can be accomplished as change-of-shift reports. Verbal reports include information about the equipment and supplies, the type of surgery, and the expected patient needs. Reports are usually performed when one shift of nurses begins perioperative care and the another shift ends. Tape recorders facilitate continuous communication and coordination of perioperative care when one nurse relieves another in the OR. Communication and coordination of patient care needs is a continuous process needed to complete or update the perioperative nursing care plan throughout the patient's surgical experience (Kneedler and Dodge, 1987).

Making Patient Care Assignments

The perioperative nursing care plan is an excellent tool for making patient care assignments. The care plan provides an overview of the patient's health. The care plan indicates the patient's acuity level and the amount of nursing care needed by the patient, which are vital for making decisions about who provides perioperative nursing care to each patient (Kneedler and Dodge, 1987).

The perioperative nurse is the health care team member legally accountable and responsible for the provision of perioperative nursing care (Kneedler and Dodge, 1987). The perioperative nurse is able to identify which nursing activities are appropriate for delegation to paraprofessionals such as licensed practical nurses, nursing assistants, and transportation aides by reviewing the care plan.

The care plan includes all nursing actions required for goal and expected outcome attainment in one location. This information provides valuable insight for the perioperative nurse when paraprofessionals are used to supplement nurses owing to limited nursing resources. By initialing the completion of nursing actions performed by others, the perioperative nurse is able to measure and account for nursing actions delivered when multiple team members assist with perioperative nursing care.

Preparing for Patient Care Emergencies

The perioperative nurse follows the same process of identifying the patient's needs and coordinating supplies and equipment for the patient with a life-threatening emergency as for the patient requiring scheduled surgery, with a few exceptions. First, the entire care planning process is much briefer for the former. Time is critical for the patient requiring emergency surgery. Experienced perioperative nurses agree that documentation of nursing activities for an upcoming patient care emergency is one of the most important and difficult challenges of nursing practice. The perioperative nurse is unable to account for judgments and decisions made for patient care during emergency surgeries without documenting the planning process. Standardized care plans for patient care emergencies with common nursing diagnoses, goals, expected outcomes, and nursing actions are effective tools for facilitating perioperative nursing accountability.

A standardized care plan is acceptable if it can be altered or expanded according to the patient's needs. A standardized care plan must be individualized to identify and resolve unique health problems in addition to common life-threatening health problems that arise in emergency situations. Examples of life-threatening health problems to address in a standardized emergency care plan include ineffective airway clearance, ineffective breathing pattern, decreased cardiac output, and altered tissue perfusion. In addition, impaired skin integrity may be identified as a common health problem for patient care emergencies. Health problem trends should be ascertained among the population the facility serves to determine which health problems should be included in a standardized nursing care plan for patient emergencies.

Supplies and equipment necessary to perform emergency nursing care are often located in a central area and checked regularly for outdated items. Some facilities collect supplies needed for patient care emergencies in a case cart or supply cart with wheels. Facilities that commonly manage emergencies designate and supply an

OR with items needed for trauma management. Regardless of the location, supplies and equipment that are collected before a nursing care emergency arises and a standardized care plan with common health problems assist the perioperative nurse in managing emergencies. The standardized care plan guides the new perioperative nurse in preparing for patient emergencies and in prioritizing health problems and nursing actions. The standardized care plan assists the experienced perioperative nurse in documenting and accounting for perioperative nursing care during chaotic patient care emergencies.

Discharge Planning

The decisions and nursing activities involved in measuring and communicating patient care needs are known as *discharge planning*. Discharge planning starts when nursing diagnoses are entered on the nursing care plan and patient outcomes are projected. Documentation by the perioperative nurse of the patient's movement from a lower state to a higher state of wellness is necessary for health care team members in the community. The care plans provide the information needed to understand the patient's surgical experience and to develop realistic goals and patient outcomes for rehabilitation. Ensuring continuity of nursing care between acute care facilities, such as surgical settings, and the community, such as the patient's home, is difficult. If patient needs and resolution of health problems are not communicated clearly from the acute care setting to the rehabilitation setting, fragmented care results (Gordon, 1987).

The perioperative nursing care plan, reflecting the identification and resolution of patient health problems, is an effective method of communicating the patient's needs to health care providers in the community. Health care consumers have noted the importance of communicating patient needs and resolved health problems in the form of discharge planning. Federal and state law and hospital policies have frequently required that discharge planning be documented for patients (Gordon, 1987).

Before the patient is discharged from the hospital, the perioperative nurse assesses the status of immediate, intermediate, and long-term health care problems. The perioperative nurse reviews with the patient or significant other the patient's capabilities as well as the personal, family, and community resources available to facilitate rehabilitation after discharge of the patient from the hospital. Differences between the perioperative nurse's assessment and the patient's perception of capabilities and resources should be identified. The perioperative nurse arranges for support in the community until the patient's confidence level of providing for or seeking assistance with rehabilitation needs increases (Gordon, 1987).

The nursing care plan provides information concerning the patient's progress and changes in health status through different levels of acuity. Documenting the patient's progress and changes in health status is needed to make decisions about referrals and follow-up during rehabilitation. Discharge-planning decisions are critical to the quality and safety of the patient's life (Gordon, 1987). The nursing care plan provides data needed to continue behaviors associated with health promotion and wellness in the rehabilitation phase of the surgical experience.

DOCUMENTATION AND COMMUNICATION PROCEDURES

Perioperative nurses often follow the assessment and planning aspects of nursing process and nursing care plan formulation. The difficulty in planning perioperative nursing care lies in having insufficient time to document the care provided. Perioperative nurses also realize that they are responsible and legally accountable for directing patient care (Kneedler and Dodge, 1987). Frustration results when documentation and communication procedures appear to interfere with the delivery of care. Standardized care plans that can be individualized are a great asset to perioperative nurses with limited time.

Documentation is the recording of patient data and responses to nursing actions provided by the perioperative nurse in the patient's record. The purpose of documentation is to communicate to other health care team members the type of nursing actions delivered to the patient by the perioperative nurse. Documentation of the care plan is a quality assurance tool used to measure retrospectively the effectiveness of perioperative nursing care. In addition, documented care describes the level of nursing care provided for the patient and answers legal questions concerning the patient's responses. Accurate documentation of nursing actions reflects accountability by the perioperative nurse. Finally, documentation of perioperative nursing care can be used in teaching and research settings. Documentation of nursing care for the surgical patient is a contribution to perioperative nursing's body of knowledge (Kneedler and Dodge, 1987).

The perioperative nursing care plan provides consistency and continuity of nursing care delivery. The care plan ensures that priorities of physiological and psychosocial patient needs are met by resolving the health care problems experienced by the patient. Goals, expected outcomes, and criteria measure the extent of health care problem resolution. The functional health patterns framework provides a systematic approach to practical nursing care plan design.

Bibliography

Association of Operating Room Nurses. (1992). *Standards and recommended practices for perioperative nursing.* Denver.
Gordon, M. (1987). *Nursing diagnosis: Process and application* (2nd ed.). New York: McGraw-Hill.
Kneedler, J. A., Dodge, G. H. (1987). *Perioperative patient care* (2nd ed.). Boston: Blackwell Scientific.
Yura, H., Walsh, M. (1983). *The nursing process: Assessing, planning, implementing, evaluation* (4th ed.). East Norwalk, CT: Appleton-Century-Crofts.

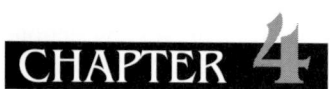

CHAPTER 4

Transferring the Patient

Michael Griswold

DEFINITION

Transferring the patient during the perioperative period is the act of moving the patient to and from the surgical suite.

MEASURABLE CRITERIA

The perioperative nurse demonstrates competency to transfer the patient by

- correctly identifying the patient
- performing or directing the transfer of the patient from the nursing unit to the surgical suite holding area
- admitting the patient to the surgical suite
- performing or directing the transfer of the patient from the surgical suite holding area to the operating room (OR)
- assisting with the transfer of the patient from the OR to the postanesthesia care unit (PACU)
- performing or directing the transfer of the patient

from the OR to the nursing unit after local anesthesia
- performing or directing the transfer of the patient with special needs
- performing or directing necessary documentation and verbal communication

ROLE OF THE PERIOPERATIVE NURSE

Transferring the surgical patient is the responsibility of the perioperative nurse. Others, such as the surgical technologist or the orderly, participate, especially during transfer between the nursing unit and the surgical suite. It is, however, the perioperative nurse who has ultimate responsibility for the welfare of the patient during the preoperative transfer process. This responsibility continues into the postoperative transfer process, when the patient is returning to the nursing unit from the surgical suite after a procedure under local anesthesia or when the patient is transferred to the PACU.

The perioperative nurse assesses the patient to identify needs and problems related to the transfer process. Planning for patient transfers includes the identification of needed transfer equipment and the assignment of trained personnel to perform transfer activities. After the implementation of transfer activities, the perioper-

The views expressed in this chapter are those of the author and do not reflect the official position or policy of the Department of the Army, the Department of Defense, or the U.S. Government.

ative nurse evaluates the patient's response to transfer activities.

CONSIDERATIONS

Transferring the patient to and from the surgical suite is often viewed as a simple but tedious task that anyone can perform. Taking the transfer process lightly can lead to a disastrous outcome for the patient. Because each patient is unique and has different needs, the perioperative nurse must ensure the following:

- Only qualified personnel, such as the perioperative nurse, the surgical technologist, and the orderly, who are trained to implement appropriate safety measures perform transfer activities.
- All transfer equipment is functioning according to manufacturer's specifications.
- Transfer personnel have knowledge of proper body mechanics.
- Transfer activities are performed safely without injury to personnel doing the transfer.

OUTCOME STANDARD

Preoperative and postoperative transfer activities do not compromise or cause injury to the patient.

Criteria

The patient is free from evidence of

- tissue injury
- altered body temperature
- ineffective breathing pattern
- altered tissue perfusion
- discomfort or pain
- fear

POTENTIAL ALTERATIONS IN FUNCTIONAL HEALTH PATTERNS

Health Perception–Health Management Pattern

Diagnosis

High risk for injury related to transfer to and from the surgical suite

Definition

Presence of risk factors that may cause the patient to experience bodily injury while being transported to and from the surgical suite and during transfer activities

Risk Factors

- Neuromuscular impairment
- Musculoskeletal impairment
- Vascular impairment
- Cognitive impairment
- Sensory/perceptual impairment (vision, hearing)
- Speech impairment
- Safety violations by the transporter
- Equipment malfunction
- Extraneous objects (hanging intravenous [IV] bags, patient drainage devices)

Expected Outcome

The patient shows no subjective or objective evidence of injury. There is an absence of

- patient or family verbal or nonverbal complaint of injury
- broken or bruised skin or other signs of injury

Nutritional-Metabolic Pattern

Diagnosis

High risk for altered body temperature related to transfer to and from the surgical suite

Definition

Presence of risk factors that may cause the patient to experience a decrease in body temperature (hypothermia) during preoperative and postoperative transfer activities

Risk Factors (Gordon, 1987)

- Extremes in age (neonate, elderly)
- Extremes in weight
- Fluid deficit (dehydration)
- Altered metabolic rate
- Impaired temperature regulation secondary to illness or injury
- Vasoconstriction or vasodilation secondary to medication
- Cold environmental temperature
- Inadequate covering

Expected Outcome

The patient shows no subjective or objective evidence of a decrease in body temperature during preoperative and postoperative transfer. There is an absence of

- verbal or nonverbal statements of discomfort due to cold
- signs of temperature decrease (shivering or chattering teeth)

Activity-Exercise Pattern

Diagnosis

High risk for ineffective breathing pattern related to transfer to and from the surgical suite

Definition

Presence of risk factors that may cause the patient to experience respirations that are insufficient to maintain adequate oxygen supply for cellular requirements during preoperative and postoperative transfer activities (Gordon, 1987)

Risk Factors (Gordon, 1987)

- Obesity
- Neuromuscular impairment
- Musculoskeletal impairment
- Perceptual or cognitive impairment
- Anxiety
- Preoperative sedation
- Pain
- Improper position of the patient during transfer
- Pregnancy

Expected Outcome

The patient shows no subjective or objective evidence of breathing difficulty. There is an absence of

- verbal or nonverbal statement of breathing difficulty
- orthopnea, dyspnea, shortness of breath, use of accessory muscles, altered chest excursion, tachypnea, cough, and nasal flaring (Gordon, 1987)

Diagnosis

High risk for altered tissue perfusion related to transfer of the pregnant patient to and from the surgical suite

Definition

Presence of risk factors that may cause the pregnant patient to experience a decrease in blood supply to vital organs during preoperative and postoperative transfer activities

Risk Factors

- Interruption of venous flow (e.g., gravid uterus compressing the inferior vena cava)
- Supine position of the patient

Expected Outcome

The pregnant patient shows no subjective or objective evidence of altered tissue perfusion. There is an absence of

- verbal or nonverbal statements of discomfort, especially in the lower extremities
- edema in the lower extremities

Cognitive-Perceptual Pattern

Diagnosis

High risk for discomfort or pain related to transfer to and from the surgical suite

Definition

Presence of risk factors that may cause the patient to experience discomfort or pain during the preoperative or postoperative transfer activities

Risk Factors

- Existing injury
- Chronic physical disease such as osteoarthritis
- Neuromuscular impairment
- Musculoskeletal impairment
- Cognitive or perceptual impairment
- Anxiety
- Surgical wound
- Presence of traction devices
- Equipment malfunction (imbalanced gurney wheels, which cause an uneven ride)
- Careless maneuvering of the gurney or the patient's bed by the transporter

Expected Outcome

The patient shows no subjective or objective evidence of discomfort or pain during the transfer process. There is an absence of

- verbal statements indicating discomfort or pain
- nonverbal expressions such as facial masks of pain, guarded movement, crying, or moaning indicating discomfort or pain

Self-perception–Self-concept Pattern

Diagnosis

High risk for fear related to transfer to the surgical suite

Definition

Presence of risk factors that may cause the patient to experience a feeling of dread related to the impending surgical procedure; the patient who experiences fear related to surgery perceives surgery as a threat or a danger (Gordon, 1987)

Risk Factors (Gordon, 1987)

- Knowledge excess or deficit
- Perceived inability to control an event
- Anticipation of a negative surgical outcome or prognosis
- Stressful or frightening preoperative preparation routines
- Surgical suite environment
- Stressful interpersonal communications with health care workers
- Stressful interpersonal communications with family members and significant others

Expected Outcome

The patient shows little or moderate subjective or objective evidence of fear. There is an absence of

- verbal statements describing feelings of dread, nervousness, or concerns about the impending surgical procedure
- increased questioning or information seeking, restlessness, voice tremors, pitch changes, increased verbalization, hand tremors, increased muscle tension, narrowing focus on the impending surgical procedure, diaphoresis, and increased heart and respiratory rate (Gordon, 1987)

PERIOPERATIVE NURSING INTERVENTIONS

Transferring the Patient to the Surgical Suite Holding Area

This section describes the nursing activities used to transfer the patient to the surgical suite. The supplies and equipment needed are a gurney (wheeled stretcher) with functional side rails and safety strap, an IV pole, an emesis basin, a cover sheet, a head cover for the patient, and a patient pickup slip (Fig. 4–1).

Preparing for the Transfer

After receiving the patient transfer assignment, the transporter reviews the perioperative nursing care plan to check nursing orders concerning transportation equipment requirements and planned patient care activities during the transfer. The transporter obtains the transfer slip (pickup slip), which identifies the patient by name, hospital number, and location. A cover gown is donned by the transporter, and head gear and shoe covers are removed. The time when the transporter leaves the surgical suite is noted according to institutional policy and procedure. After obtaining the needed transporta-

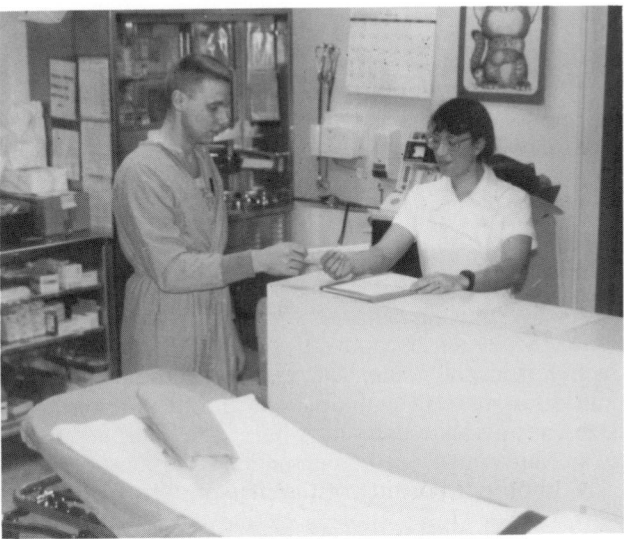

FIGURE 4–2. Personnel assigned to pick up patients announce their arrival with the charge nurse of the nursing care unit and identify the patient to be transferred to the OR.

tion equipment and checking for proper functioning, the transporter proceeds to the designated nursing unit.

Arriving on the Nursing Unit

After arriving on the nursing unit, the transporter reports to the charge nurse (Fig. 4–2), asks if the patient is ready to go to surgery, and requests assistance from unit personnel.

Reviewing the Patient's Chart

Before entering the patient's room, the transporter reviews the patient's chart. The consent is checked to ensure that it is signed and witnessed according to hospital policy and procedure. The preoperative check list is reviewed to ensure that jewelry has been removed, the patient has voided and has had nothing by mouth, and all prostheses have been removed (dentures, hearing aid). The chart is also checked for x-ray films, electrocardiogram, and laboratory reports. Other routine preoperative reports specific to the institution are also checked.

Arriving at the Patient's Room

Unit nursing personnel should accompany the transporter to the patient's room to identify the location of the patient on the unit, perform the preliminary identification of the patient, and assist with the transfer process. After arriving in the patient's room, the transporter should allow the unit nurse to tell the patient that the transporter is to take him or her to the surgical suite.

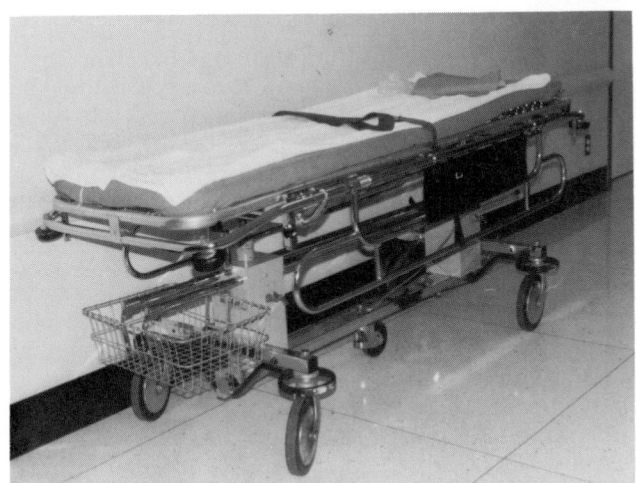

FIGURE 4–1. Gurney used for transporting patients to the OR. Included on the stretcher are a safety strap, side rails, IV pole, blanket, emesis basin, cover sheet, head cover, and patient pickup slip.

Identifying the Patient

The patient should be identified before transport to the surgical suite. This is done to ensure that the correct patient is transported to the surgical suite at the appropriate time with all necessary paperwork completed and in the chart.

Alert and Oriented Patient

As the unit nursing personnel and the transporter enter the patient's room, they should greet the patient by her or his full name. The transporter should introduce himself or herself to the patient and ask the patient to state her or his name and what surgical procedure she or he is having done. Open-ended questions should be asked. Questions such as "Are you Mr. Smith?" or "Are you having a cholecystectomy?" may elicit a yes response without the patient's thinking about what is being asked. Patients are frequently anxious when being prepared for surgery and this can impair their thought processes. The open-ended question requires the patient to think about the answer and allows the transporter to determine if the patient is alert and oriented.

As the patient states her or his name, the transporter reads the name on the transfer slip obtained from the surgical suite (Fig. 4–3). A second identity check is made by comparing the name and hospital number on the transfer slip with the name and number on the patient's identification bracelet. A third check is made between the transfer slip and the patient's chart. The consent is checked again to ensure that the procedure identified on the consent form is the same as that identified by the patient. Discrepancies should be corrected before the patient is transferred from her or his bed to the gurney. The transporter should call the

surgical suite for guidance when a discrepancy is discovered.

Child

The same steps performed for identifying an alert and oriented adult patient must be followed when identifying a child. The difference is to whom the questions are directed, which is based on the development of the child. The transporter should establish initial contact simultaneously with the child and the parents or legal guardian. The parents or legal guardian signed the consent authorizing the surgical procedure; therefore, the transporter should ask the parents or legal guardian the child's name and the procedure being done. If the child's development permits, the transporter should also ask the child questions. The child can effectively be made a participant in the preparation for a surgical procedure by the method of interaction chosen by the transporter.

If the parents or legal guardian is unavailable, the transporter relies on the unit nursing staff to identify the patient. This does not negate the need to check the transfer slip against the patient's hospital bracelet and chart.

Comatose and Disoriented Patient

With modifications, the same steps followed for identifying an alert adult should be followed for the comatose and disoriented patient. If present, family members or a significant other should be asked to identify the patient. In the absence of family members or a significant other, the transporter relies on the unit nursing staff or other personnel, such as a surgeon or a police officer if the patient is in the emergency room, to identify the patient. Again, it is important to compare the transfer slip with the patient's hospital bracelet and chart.

Transferring the Patient to the Gurney

After explaining to the patient what is going to happen, the transporter covers the patient with a sheet or blanket. Next, the gurney is positioned adjacent to the bed and the wheels of the bed and the gurney are locked. The transporter stands next to the gurney and the unit nursing personnel stand opposite, next to the bed (Fig. 4–4). After the bed is raised to the level of the gurney, the patient is told to move from the bed to the gurney, buttocks first, shoulders second, and feet last. During the transfer, the unit nursing personnel stabilize the bed by leaning against it. At the same time, the transporter leans against the gurney. After the patient is on the gurney, the transporter raises the side rails and fastens the safety belt across the patient's thighs. The possibility of side rails' becoming dislodged and falling is an ever present danger; therefore, the patient is instructed to keep fingers, hands, arms, and legs, to include the knees, away from the side rails.

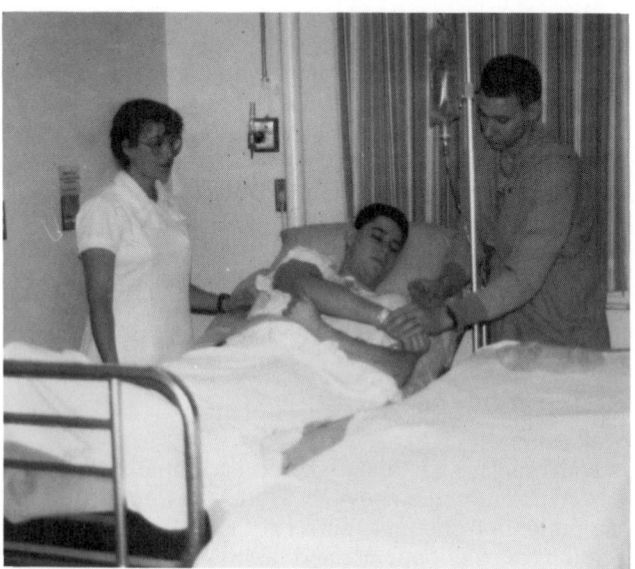

FIGURE 4–3. Identification of the patient to be transferred to the OR is done using a pickup slip initiated by the floor coordinator of the OR.

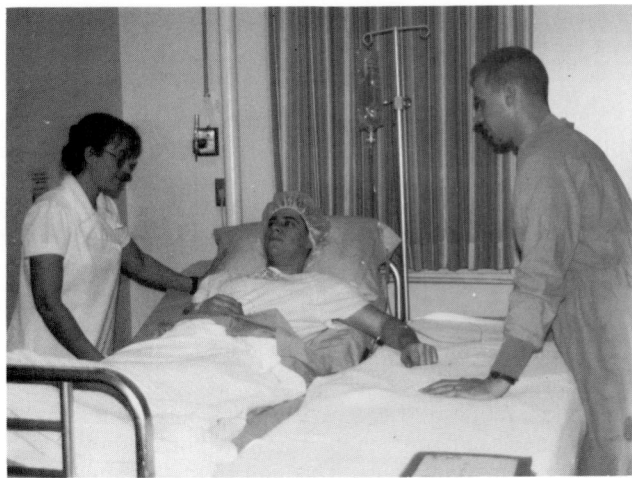

FIGURE 4–4. The patient is provided with a head cover and prepared to be transferred to the gurney.

Transporting the Patient to the Surgical Suite

If family members or significant others are present, they should accompany the patient to the surgical suite (Fig. 4–5). This may help minimize the patient's anxiety about the impending surgery.

The gurney should be pushed with the patient's feet first through corridors. This allows the patient to see where he or she is going. Some patients may experience motion sickness if they are moved backward. When turning corners, the transporter should ensure that obstacles or people are not unexpectedly encountered. If an elevator is used, the transporter should pull the gurney in head first. After arriving at the designated floor, the gurney should be pulled out of the elevator by the transporter. This maneuver allows the transporter to hold the elevator doors back and prevent inadvertent closure on the gurney.

On arrival in the surgical suite, visitors, if not permitted in the holding area, should be allowed to interact with the patient before he or she enters the suite. The transporter should tell, or if possible show, the significant others where to wait while the patient is having surgery. They are also told that the surgeon will be informed that they are in the waiting room so that he or she may speak to them after surgery.

Before entering the surgical suite, the transporter removes his or her cover gown and dons shoe covers and headgear. If the surgical suite doors are not automatic, the transporter should open one of the doors, lean against it, and pull the gurney foot first through the doorway. If the doors are automatic, the doors should be allowed to open completely before the gurney is moved through the doorway.

When in the holding area, the transporter locks the wheels of the gurney and tells the holding area nurse and patient care coordinator of the surgical suite that the patient has arrived. Before leaving the patient, the transporter should document on the patient's chart the

method of transfer, who transported the patient, safety measures used, and the time when the patient arrived in the surgical suite. In some ORs, the time when the patient arrived in the surgical suite is noted on the master surgical schedule.

Admitting the Patient to the Surgical Suite Holding Area

This section describes the nursing activities used to admit the patient to the surgical suite. The supplies required are perioperative documents, laboratory requests slips, and the patient's hospital card. Admitting equipment includes the following: blood pressure cuff and sphygmomanometer; temperature probes and recording devices; oxygen and associated delivery devices; suction devices; emesis basins, urinals, and bedpans; warm blankets; preparation equipment such as depilatory, shaving cream, and razors; and IV needles, tubing, and bags. Some holding areas also have electrocardiographic monitors and pulse oximeters. For pediatric patients, one or two rocking chairs, storybooks, and safe toys are appropriate. Adult and adolescent patients appreciate headphones and cassette players.

Reviewing the Patient's Chart

After the patient has arrived in the surgical suite holding area, responsibility for care is assumed by the holding area nurse. After greeting the patient and putting him or her at ease, the nurse reviews the chart for completeness and the patient data card for accuracy. A review of the preoperative check list determines if the patient has voided, removed jewelry and prostheses, and received prescribed preoperative medications. The

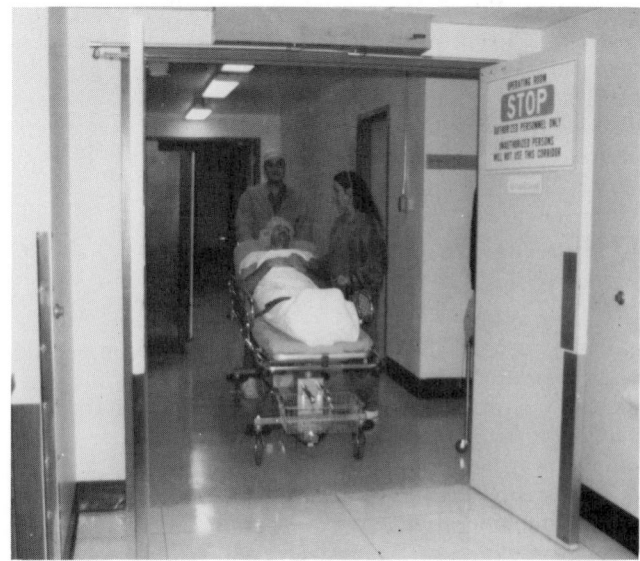

FIGURE 4–5. During the patient's transfer to the OR, family members or significant others are encouraged to accompany the patient.

nurse checks the chart for prescribed test reports and the history and physical examination findings. The patient is questioned about and the chart is checked for information regarding allergies. Nothing by mouth status is validated by asking the patient the last time he or she had something to eat or drink. Items on the check list not initialed as completed before the transfer to the surgical suite must be investigated immediately and corrective action taken.

Careful review of the consent form is essential. It should be completed according to hospital policy. Every effort should be made to ensure that legal and informed consent has been obtained. If hospital protocols have not been followed, barring emergency situations, surgery should be postponed until consent can be obtained. Patients under the influence of preoperative medication should be lucid before giving consent; the patient should be counseled again by the surgeon and requested to sign a new consent form when the patient is no longer under the influence of the preoperative medication.

The holding area nurse should review the preoperative orders to determine if blood or blood products have been ordered for the patient. If blood has been ordered, the nurse should check with the patient care coordinator to ensure that the blood is present in the surgical suite blood refrigerator. If the blood is not present, the nurse should call the laboratory to ensure that the order has been received and to check blood availability.

Performing a Holding Area Assessment

If the perioperative nurse has the opportunity to do a preoperative assessment before the patient arrives in the surgical suite, the holding area nurse reviews the assessment data. Additional assessment data are added to the record as necessary.

If a preoperative assessment has not been done, the holding area nurse does an assessment. Refer to Chapters 2 and 15 for information on performing a preoperative assessment. After completing the preoperative assessment, the holding area nurse gives the assessment data to the perioperative nurse assigned to give intraoperative care.

Preparing the Intraoperative Paperwork

Paperwork for intraoperative documentation should be prepared before the patient is transferred to the OR. Depending on the surgical procedure and hospital policy and procedure, the following should be stamped with the data card and placed in the chart: anesthetic record, operative report, intraoperative nursing record (if separate from operative report), charge slips, labels, and slips from pathology, laboratory, and radiology departments.

Transferring the Patient from the Holding Area to the Operating Room

This section describes the nursing activities used to transfer the patient from the surgical suite holding area to the OR. The supplies and equipment needed are the OR bed, a draw (lift) sheet, arm boards, safety straps for the legs and arms, IV poles, warm sheets, and a head rest (Fig. 4–6).

Preparing for the Transfer

The circulating nurse, after ensuring that all surgical team members are ready to receive the patient, proceeds to the holding area and checks with the nurse about the status of the patient. The holding area nurse reports pertinent findings from the patient assessment. Next, the circulator greets the patient and tells her or him that she or he is to be transported to the OR. After verifying the patient's identity, allergies, and nothing by mouth status and the planned procedure, the circulating nurse checks the chart for the consent form and the presence of laboratory and radiology department reports.

Transporting the Patient to the Operating Room

The wheels of the gurney are unlocked and the patient is transported to the OR feet first (Fig. 4–7). On entering the OR, the circulating nurse announces to the surgical team that the patient is entering the room to ensure that noise is kept to a minimum. The circulator should introduce the patient to the staff in the room. After lowering the side rail next to the OR bed, the circulating nurse positions the gurney adjacent to the bed and locks the wheels of the gurney. The wheels of the OR bed should have already been locked; however, they should be checked before the patient is moved. The other side rail is then lowered.

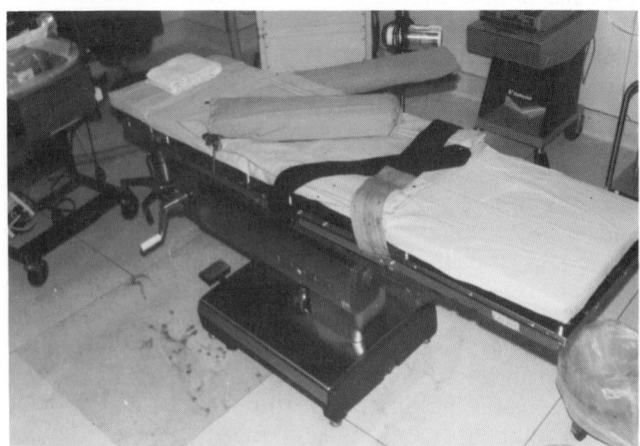

FIGURE 4–6. OR bed used during the surgical procedure. Included on the table are two arm boards, a draw sheet, and a safety strap.

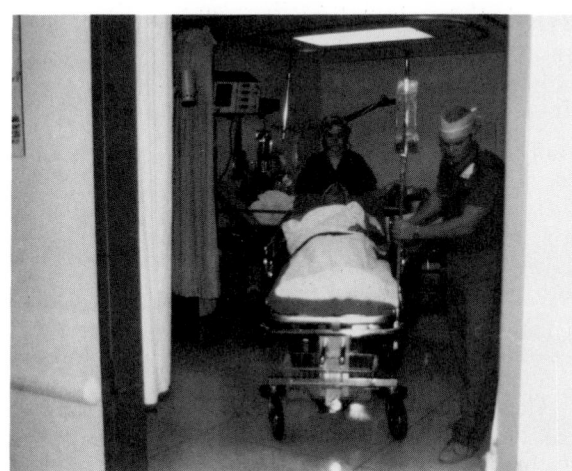

FIGURE 4–7. When the room is prepared for the patient, he or she is transferred to the surgical suite.

Mobile Patient

The circulating nurse stands next to the gurney and asks the anesthetist or the orderly to stand on the opposite side of the OR bed to protect the patient from falling off the bed during transfer (Fig. 4–8). If a blanket was placed around the patient during transfer to the surgical suite, it is removed, leaving only the cover sheet over the patient. IV bags are secured to the IV pole located at the head of the bed. If the patient has drainage devices, these are detached from the gurney and placed on the patient or held by the nurse. The patient is asked to move to the OR bed, moving buttocks first, shoulders second, and feet last. The patient's modesty is maintained by keeping the cover sheet in place during the transfer.

Immobile Patient

Depending on the patient's size, at least four people are needed to move the immobile patient. The lifters (the circulating nurse and assistants) place themselves on each side of the OR bed and one at the foot of the bed (Fig. 4–9). The anesthetist remains at the head of the bed. The patient's arms are then placed across the chest. The side lifters position themselves as close to the OR bed and gurney as possible. Their legs should be apart, one ahead of the other. The side lifters roll the draw sheet up against the patient's side and grasp the sheet up against the patient.

The anesthetist directs the transfer and controls the patient's head. Movement is not initiated until the patient's airway is stabilized. The anesthetist counts aloud to ensure that all lifters begin the transfer in a synchronized motion.

The foot lifter crosses the patient's legs at the ankles and grasps the ankles with both hands. The lifter stands erect at the foot of the gurney and prepares to lift the legs. On the count of the anesthetist, the lifter moves one step in the direction the patient is being moved.

The patient's ankles are lifted and gently lowered onto the OR bed.

The side lifter next to the gurney places her or his dominant leg approximately 6 to 8 inches behind the nondominant leg. Both legs should be slightly bent. Because the dominant leg is usually stronger, the lifter's own body weight should be shifted to the dominant leg. This makes it easier for the lifter to bear the patient's weight during the transfer. The lifter maintains her or his upper torso in a straight upright position. When the transfer begins, the lifter lifts the patient by straightening the legs, lifting the draw sheet under the patient, and slightly walking forward or shifting the weight from her or his back leg (the dominant leg) to the front leg. During the maneuver, the lifter bends slightly at the waist as the patient moves away from her or him, simultaneously keeping the upper torso straight. The patient is gently lowered onto the OR bed.

The side lifter next to the OR bed places her or his dominant leg approximately 6 to 8 inches in front of the nondominant leg. Both legs should be slightly bent. As the transfer begins, the side lifter lifts the patient by straightening her or his legs, lifting the draw sheet, and taking one step backward or shifting the weight from her or his front leg (the dominant leg) to the back leg. Simultaneously while shifting the weight, she or he straightens at the waist and keeps the upper torso in an upright position. The patient is gently lowered onto the OR bed.

Securing the Patient on the Operating Room Bed

After the patient is on the OR bed, the circulating nurse centers the patient's hips and checks the body alignment of the patient's shoulders, abdomen, and feet along the length of the bed. A safety strap is placed across the patient's thighs, approximately 2 inches above

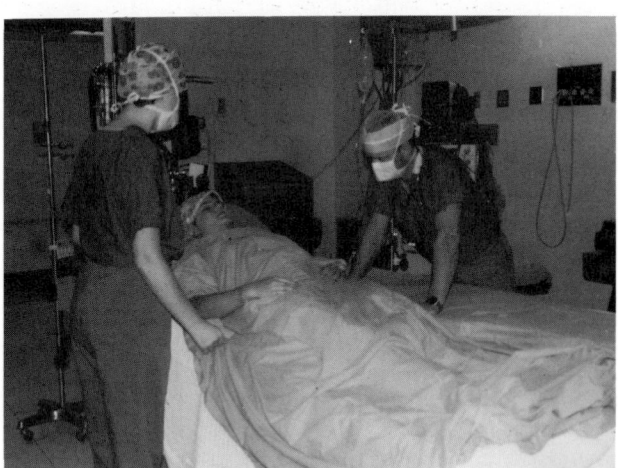

FIGURE 4–8. In the operative suite, the gurney is moved next to the OR bed, the wheels are locked, and preparations to transfer the patient are completed.

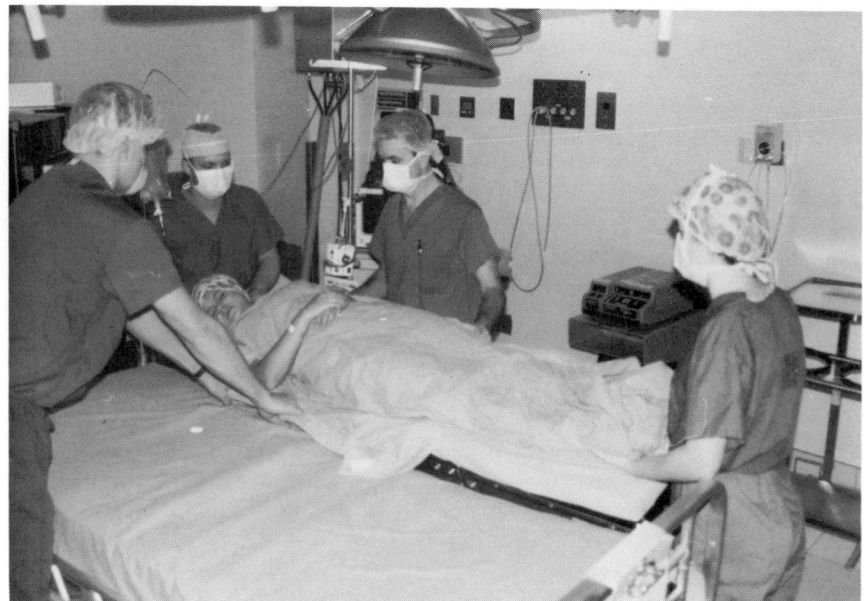

FIGURE 4–9. Preparations are made to transfer the patient from the OR bed to the gurney using a four person lift. Note the number of personnel required to move the patient and their locations.

the knees and secured (Fig. 4–10). The circulating nurse checks to ensure that the strap is not too tight nor too loose by placing one hand between the thighs and the strap. The strap should not be so tight as to prevent the hand's being placed between the thighs and the strap. Securing the strap is crucial, especially as the patient enters the excitement phase of anesthesia and emerges from anesthesia at the end of the case. Typically, pa-

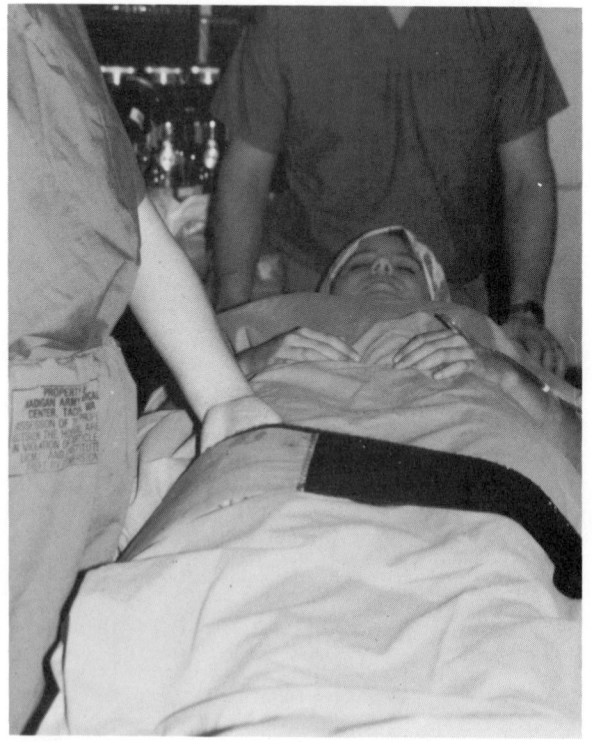

FIGURE 4–10. A safety strap is placed approximately 2 inches above the patient's knees and is fastened loosely enough to allow one hand between the thigh and the strap.

tients who are employed in physically demanding occupations or aggressive hobbies (police officers, football players, soldiers, marines) respond more combatively during the excitement phase than do other patients. Improperly securing the safety strap on these individuals could result in patient injury. The patient's hands and arms are placed on the arm boards and secured with arm straps.

Transferring the Patient from the Operating Room to the Postanesthesia Care Unit

This section describes the nursing activities used to transfer the patient from the OR to the PACU. This is potentially the most dangerous time for the patient during the transfer process. The patient may not be fully recovered from the effects of the anesthetic agents and thus is dependent on the surgical team members for basic physiological functions such as airway management. The supplies and equipment needed are a recovery bed with an IV pole and functional side rails, an oxygen tank with delivery valve and tubing and at least 500 to 1000 pounds/square inch in the tank, an oral airway, a warm sheet and blanket, and a patient body roller.

Preparing to Transfer the Patient from the Operating Room Bed

Four people are needed as described for transferring the immobile patient to the OR bed. The patient's arms are placed across the chest. The side lifter on the side opposite the recovery bed holds the patient's arms across the chest. The arm boards are removed from the bed and the circulating nurse moves away from the bed, thus enabling the recovery bed to be placed adjacent to the OR bed. The wheels of the recovery bed are locked. If the patient is unresponsive or unable to control his or her arms, the lifter on the opposite side of the OR bed from the recovery bed ensures that the patient's arms remain across the chest. Ensuring that the IV solutions are not lowered below the level of the patient's heart, the circulating nursing moves the IV bags to the IV pole on the recovery bed. Next, drainage tubes are moved to the recovery bed. Care is exercised to ensure that IV bags are not elevated above the tube exit sites. The safety strap is removed by the circulating nurse.

Transferring the Patient to the Recovery Bed

Mobile Patient

If the patient is alert, the anesthetist directs the patient to move to the bed, buttocks first, shoulders second, and feet last. The circulating nurse leans against the recovery bed and assists the patient as he or she moves and ensures that modesty is maintained. After the patient moves to the recovery bed, he or she is centered and properly aligned, and the side rails are raised. If indicated, the anesthetist opens the valve on the oxygen tank and secures the mask or nasal cannula.

Immobile Patient

OR Bed Tilt Technique

For this transfer technique, personnel stand next to the OR bed and recovery bed as described for transferring the immobile patient to the OR bed. The OR bed is raised above the level of the recovery bed. The side lifter standing next to the OR bed reaches across the patient and grasps the draw sheet. The sheet is wrapped over the patient and the lifter holds the patient in position while the OR bed is tilted.

The recovery bed is slightly moved away from the OR bed to allow the anesthetist to operate the lever and thus tilt the bed. The bed is tilted toward the recovery bed. After the OR bed is tilted as much as possible, the recovery bed is moved back against the OR bed. The circulating nurse stands next to the recovery bed.

The side lifter holding the patient releases the end of the draw sheet that was used to hold the patient in place. The circulating nurse reaches across the recovery bed to grasp the free end of the draw sheet and places one foot in front of the other. During this maneuver, the circulating nurse bends slightly at the waist and keeps the upper torso straight (Fig. 4–11). On the anesthetist's count, the circulating nurse pulls the draw sheet and the patient toward the recovery bed. While doing this, the circulating nurse shifts her or his body weight from the front foot to the back foot and simultaneously raises the upper torso, which is kept straight.

The side lifter on the opposite side places one foot in front of the other and shifts his or her weight to the back foot. He or she pulls the draw sheet taut under the patient and positions his or her hands against the patient, one at the shoulders and the other at the hips. On the anesthetist's count, the lifter shifts his or her weight to the front foot, bends slightly at the waist while keeping the upper torso straight, and moves the patient down the incline created by the tilted OR bed to the recovery bed. During this maneuver, the anesthetist moves the patient's head and the lifter at the foot of the bed moves the patient's legs and feet (see Fig. 4–9).

Roller Technique

Transfer personnel stand next to the recovery bed and OR bed as described for transferring the immobile patient to the OR bed. The safety strap is removed by the circulating nurse. The side lifter next to the OR bed reaches across the patient and grasps the draw sheet. With permission from the anesthetist, the sheet is pulled up and the patient rolls toward the lifter (Fig. 4–12). After the patient is placed on his or her side, the

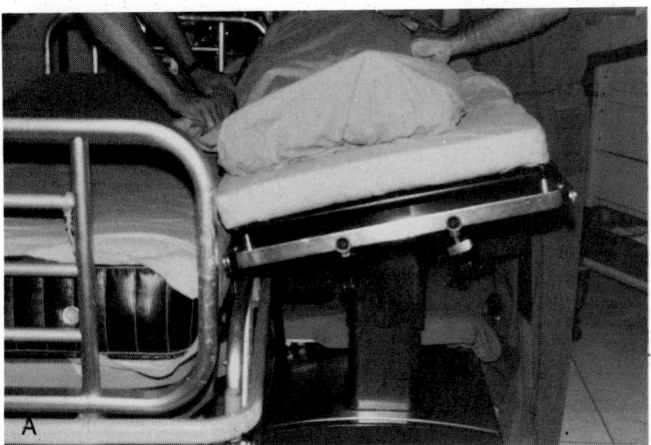
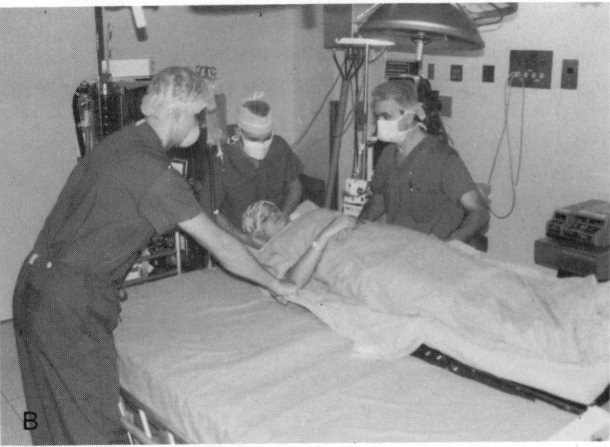

FIGURE 4–11. *A,* The bed tilt transfer affords a slope, or gradient, between the OR bed and the gurney where the patient is being transferred. *B,* This gradient facilitates the patient transfer with minimal impact on the lifters and the patient (see Fig. 4–9).

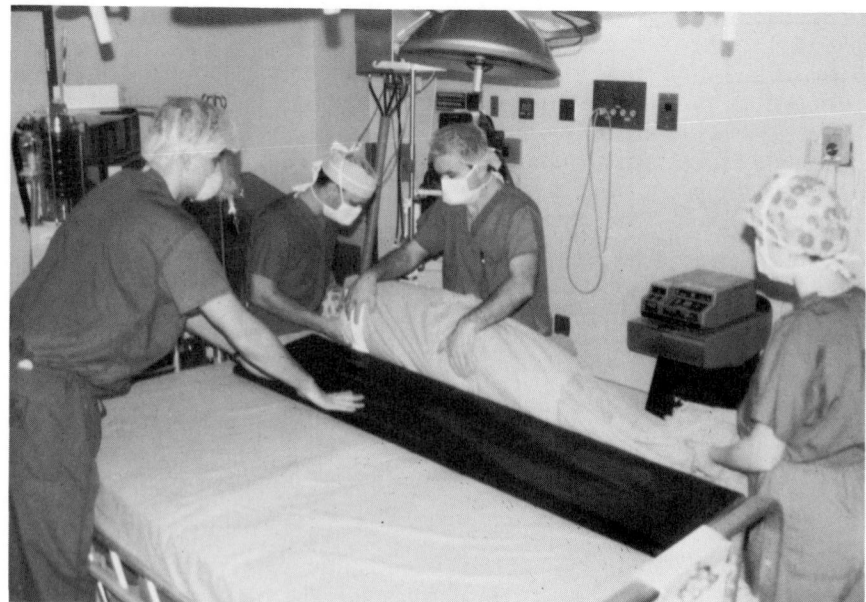

FIGURE 4–12. Patient transfer using the full body roller technique facilitates the transfer of the patient from the OR bed to the gurney without lifting the patient. Instead, the patient is rolled onto one side and a roller is placed underneath the patient.

circulating nurse, who is standing next to the recovery bed, places the body roller under the draw sheet as far as possible. The roller should not extend above the head or foot of the recovery bed. It should be placed between the patient's shoulders and thighs. The patient is then lowered onto the roller.

The circulating nurse stands with one leg slightly ahead of the other and reaches across the recovery bed and grasps the draw sheet. Care should be exercised to ensure that the circulator's upper torso remains straight and does not bend along the spine during the transfer process. On the anesthetist's count, the circulator steps backward and slightly raises her or his upper torso while pulling the draw sheet toward her or him. The lifter on the other side of the OR bed also moves the patient on

the anesthetist's count. This lifter takes one step forward while bending slightly at the waist. Like the circulating nurse, the lifter keeps his or her torso straight. The lifter then moves the patient at the shoulder and hip over the roller to the recovery bed. The anesthetist moves the patient's head while the lifter at the foot of the OR bed moves the patient's feet (Fig. 4–13).

After the transfer is complete, the lifter next to the OR bed positions himself or herself next to the recovery bed, opposite the circulating nurse. On the anesthetist's count, the roller is removed by the lifter as the circulating nurse rolls the patient toward her or him with the draw sheet. After the roller is removed, the draw sheet is pushed under the patient as far as possible. The circulating nurse then rolls the patient back on her or

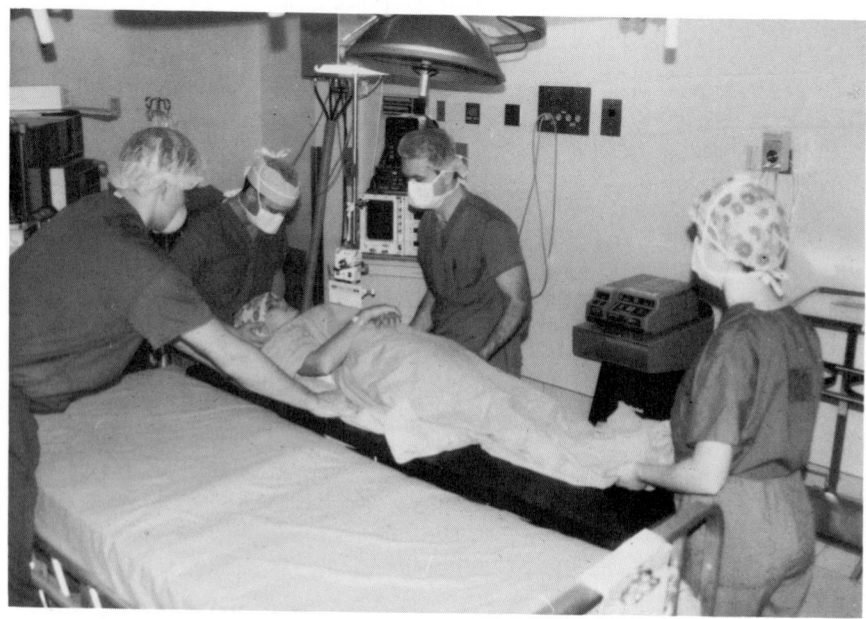

FIGURE 4–13. A roller is used to transfer the patient from the OR bed to the gurney.

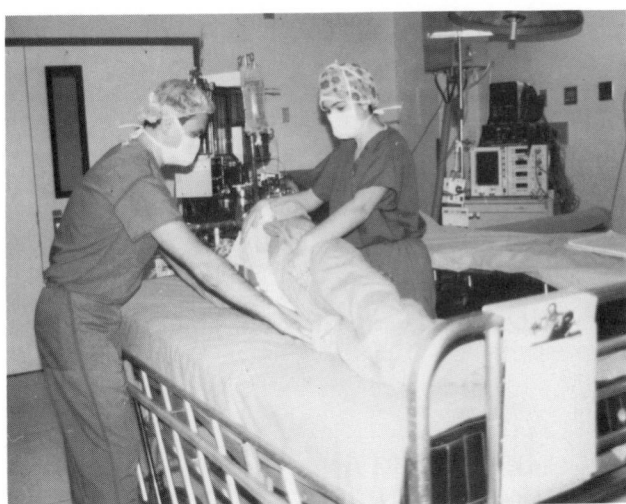

FIGURE 4–14. A soiled draw sheet is removed from under the patient by rolling the patient toward the circulator and sliding the sheet under the patient. The patient is rolled onto the other side and the draw sheet is removed and deposited in a soiled linen hamper.

his back and the draw sheet is removed (Fig. 4–14). At this time, residue of preparation solution, blood, and other secretions is removed with a warm wet towel or sponge. The patient is then dried and covered with a warm blanket. Side rails are raised and the patient is transferred to the PACU.

Transferring the Patient to the Postanesthesia Care Unit

After collecting the chart, nursing notes, and x-ray films, the circulating nurse accompanies the patient to the PACU. The patient is transported feet first. During the transfer, the circulating nurse pulls the recovery bed and helps the anesthetist to maneuver the bed. In the PACU, the circulating nurse gives a report to the postanesthesia nurse. At a minimum, the report should include the patient's condition, the intraoperative nursing care provided, and the location of dressing and drainage devices.

Transferring the Patient from the Surgical Suite to the Nursing Unit After Local Anesthesia

This section describes the nursing activities used to transfer the patient from the surgical unit to the nursing unit after receiving local anesthesia. The supplies and equipment needed are a gurney with functional side rails and safety straps, an IV pole, an emesis basin, and a warm covering for the patient.

Preparing for the Transfer

After transferring and securing the patient to the gurney, the circulator collects the chart, nursing notes, and x-ray films and unlocks the gurney wheels. If transport to the nursing unit is delayed, the patient is transported to an appropriate holding area to await transfer back to the nursing unit.

Giving a Patient Status Report to the Nursing Unit Nurse

The circulating nurse contacts the unit nurse by telephone. Information given to the unit nurse includes the patient's condition, an overview of vital signs during the procedure, the medications given during surgery and the dosage, drainage devices, and physician's orders that must be implemented immediately after the patient returns to the nursing unit.

Transferring the Patient to the Nursing Unit

Before departure, the circulating nurse must assess the patient to determine if a registered nurse should accompany the patient to the unit. The patient is transferred as described for transporting the patient to the surgical suite holding area. After arrival on the nursing unit, the transporter ensures that nursing personnel know that the patient has returned to the unit.

Transferring the Patient with Special Needs

This section describes the nursing activities used to transfer patients with special needs to the surgical suite. Supplies and equipment needed are a gurney with functional side rails and safety strap, an IV pole, a cover sheet and a head cover for the patient, a warm infant transport vehicle for neonates, a crib for young children, oxygen tanks with delivery devices, and portable monitor and defibrillator unit.

Intensive Care Patient

A perioperative nurse or intensive care nurse should accompany all patients from the intensive care unit. If the patient requires respiratory assistance, an anesthetist or a respiratory therapist should also accompany the critically ill patient to the surgical suite.

Before transporting the patient from the intensive care unit, the perioperative nurse contacts the intensive care unit nurse to determine transfer needs. After collecting the appropriate equipment and ensuring its proper functioning, the perioperative nurse proceeds to the intensive care unit with an orderly and an anesthetist or a respiratory therapist, if warranted. Before departing from the intensive care unit, the perioperative nurse coordinates with the surgical suite patient care coordinator to ensure that patient will immediately be taken into the designated OR on arrival. The transfer should not begin until the OR is ready.

Patient with Major Orthopedic Injuries

Before transporting the patient with an orthopedic injury, the perioperative nurse makes an assessment to determine the extent of injury, the traction or immobilization devices in use, and the appropriate vehicle for transfer. Generally, patients with extensive injuries and multiple skeletal support devices are transported to the surgical suite in their orthopedic bed. This minimizes disruption in the skeletal traction being used.

Orthopedic beds with traction devices are not designed for transporting patients to the surgical suite and therefore are not easy to handle. Additional personnel are needed to move the bed through hospital corridors and onto elevators. When transferring the patient with traction devices, the transporter must ensure that the transfer is accomplished without compromise of the patient's traction-induced skeletal alignment.

Neonate

Like the intensive care patient, the neonate is taken directly to the OR. This necessitates prior coordination with the surgical suite patient care coordinator. The perioperative nurse does a preoperative assessment to determine the extent of care required. A warmed infant transport vehicle provides a protective environment for the neonate during the transfer. Depending on the condition of the patient, the perioperative nurse, the pediatrician, or the anesthetist accompanies the patient to the surgical suite. Equipment needed for the neonate may include an oxygen tank with the appropriate delivery equipment, a portable monitor and defibrillator, and IV infusion device. The perioperative nurse should ensure that the neonate's parents know that they may accompany the patient to the surgical suite if they desire. The neonate is not transferred until the OR is warmed and prepared for surgery.

Toddlers

Toddlers and other children who are difficult to restrain should be transported in a crib with a bubble top and side rails up. Parent should accompany the child to the surgical suite and, if possible, may carry the child while the transporter pushes the crib. On arrival in the surgical suite holding area, parents may stay with the patient until the circulating nurse is ready to take him or her into the OR. In some hospitals, parents may enter the OR and stay with the child during the induction of anesthesia.

DOCUMENTATION AND COMMUNICATION PROCEDURES

Documentation begins with the preoperative assessment. The perioperative nurse records assessment data in the chart, identifies nursing diagnoses that pertain to transferring the patient, and develops a nursing care plan. Transporters are informed by the perioperative nurse about the patient's needs during the transfer. The transporter documents transfer activities according to hospital policy and procedure. At a minimum, documentation by the transporter must include the method of transfer, the time of arrival in and departure from the surgical suite, and the identification of who transported the patient.

Bibliography

Carpenito, L. J. (1985). *Handbook of nursing diagnosis*. Philadelphia: J. B. Lippincott.

Gordon, M. (1991). *Manual of nursing diagnosis: 1986–1987*. New York: McGraw-Hill.

McKeller, N. B., Shaw, H. (1986, December). Back breaking work: Lifting patient in the operating theatre. *NATN News*, pp. 14–16.

Scholey, M. (1983). Back stress: The effects of training nurses to lift patients in a clinical situation. *International Journal of Nursing Study, 20*(1), 1–13.

Saunders, H. D. (1985). *Evaluation, treatment, and prevention of musculoskeletal disorders* (2nd ed.). Edina, MN: Educational Opportunities.

Snook, S., Campanelli, R., Hart, J. W. (1978). A study of three preventive approaches to low back injury. *Journal of Occupational Medicine, 20*, 478–481.

Snook, S., Cirello, V. (1974). Maximum weights and work loads acceptable to female workers. *Occupational Medicine, 16*, 527–538.

Wright, B. (1982, July). Lifting and moving patients: An investigation and commentary. *The New Zealand Nursing Journal*, pp. 8–11.

CHAPTER 5

Patient and Family Teaching

Mary Bradley and Mark L. Phippen

DEFINITION

Patient and family *teaching* refers to those activities performed by the perioperative nurse to provide information to the patient and the family regarding the perioperative environment, the potential physical and psychological effects of surgery, coping mechanisms that can be used in response to surgical intervention, and how to participate in the rehabilitation process after surgery.

MEASURABLE CRITERIA

The perioperative nurse demonstrates competency to provide patient and family teaching by

- identifying the patient's and the family's learning needs
- assessing the patient's and the family's readiness to learn
- providing instruction on the basis of identified needs
- determining the effectiveness of teaching
- communicating and documenting teaching (AORN, 1992).

ROLE OF THE PERIOPERATIVE NURSE

The perioperative nurse implements teaching according to the measurable criteria. Patient and family teaching should not be delegated or assigned to assistive personnel. Accountability and responsibility for patient and family teaching rest with the perioperative nurse.

CONSIDERATIONS

Importance

The perioperative nurse's responsibility to participate in patient and family teaching cannot be overlooked. In September 1981, the American Hospital Association's House of Delegates approved the Policy and Statement on the Hospitals' Responsibility for Patient Education Services:

The hospital has a responsibility to provide patient education services as an integral part of high-quality, cost-effective care. Patient education services should enable patients, and their families and friends, when appropriate, to make informed decisions about their

91

health; to manage their illnesses; and to implement follow-up care at home. Effective and efficient patient education services require planning and coordination, and responsibility for such planning and coordination should be assigned. The hospital should also provide the necessary staff and financial resources.

DEVINE, 1985

Reduction of the Stress of Surgery

Without question, surgery creates both physical and psychological stress for patients and their families. Preoperatively, it is a source of fear and anxiety. According to Carnevali (1966), patients fear

- pain and discomfort
- the unknown
- destruction of body image
- separation from the normal environment
- recurrence of prior negative experience
- death
- loss of control
- impact of surgery on finances

A review of the literature reveals that giving information to patients preoperatively reduces patient anxiety and promotes the postoperative course of recovery (Healy, 1968; Flaherty and Fitzpatrick, 1978; Lindeman and Van Acrnam, 1971). It is also shown that family members can better support postsurgical patients if "the family's" fears are alleviated (Moss, 1986). One way to reduce fear and anxiety among patients and their families is to provide them with knowledge and information.

Benefits

It is generally accepted that the benefits derived from patient and family education make this practice an essential component of patient care.

Research and experience demonstrates that the patient and the family benefit from educational programs. Consequently, perioperative nurses should view this process as a routine role function. Educational programs benefit the patient and the family by potentially

- diminishing fear and anxiety
- decreasing the incidence of postoperative complications
- increasing compliance with health care regimens
- increasing the ability to select coping strategies
- shortening the recovery time
- reducing pain
- improving the preparation for surgery
- assisting in the preparation for changes resulting from surgery
- increasing family support
- assisting with the return to normal daily activities

Points to Consider When Teaching the Patient and Family

When preparing to teach the patient and family, the perioperative nurse should consider the following points:

- Environmental conditions should facilitate learning. Choose a time when learning can occur. An undisturbed environment is conducive to learning.
- Because language is a fundamental teaching tool, use simple terms when talking to the patient and the family. Avoid medical terminology.
- Do not assume that a low educational level equates with a low intelligence level.
- Break down instruction into manageable steps.
- Put content in a sequence of activities to facilitate learning. For example, instruct the patient to deep breathe, then to cough.
- Explain the reasons for and the benefits of expected behaviors. For example, postoperative movement of the legs and toes, unless contraindicated, aids circulation and prevents venous stasis.
- Individualize teaching to the specific situation. For example, if the patient is scheduled for an inguinal hernia repair under spinal anesthesia and has a low risk for ineffective breathing patterns or ineffective airway clearance, do not teach how to deep breathe and cough. The patient will not use these skills.
- Avoid overburdening the patient with multiple facts.
- When appropriate, provide written instructions. Go over written material with the patient. Validate the patient's comprehension by asking questions. Factors such as pain, anxiety, and medication can interfere with comprehension (Atkinson and Kohn, 1986)

OUTCOME STANDARD

The patient and/or family members demonstrate knowledge concerning surgical intervention.

Criteria

The patient and/or family members demonstrate knowledge of

- the perioperative environment and pertinent aspects of the surgical procedure
- the potential physical and psychological effects of surgery
- coping mechanisms that can be used in response to surgical intervention
- how to participate in the rehabilitation process after surgery

POTENTIAL ALTERATIONS IN FUNCTIONAL HEALTH PATTERNS

Cognitive-Perceptual Pattern

Diagnosis

Knowledge deficit related to surgical intervention

Definition

The patient and/or family members cannot state or explain information regarding the perioperative environment and pertinent aspects of the surgical procedure and the potential physical and psychological effects of surgery, cannot demonstrate the coping mechanisms that can be used in response to surgical intervention, and cannot demonstrate the cognitive, motor, and affective skills necessary to participate in the rehabilitation process after surgery (Gordon, 1987).

Defining Characteristics (Gordon, 1987)

The patient and/or family members

- demonstrate less than adequate recall of information about past surgical or invasive procedure experiences, or demonstrate misunderstanding, misinterpretation, or misconceptions
- inaccurately follow through with previous instruction
- inadequately perform a self-care skill
- demonstrate inappropriate or exaggerated behaviors such as hysteria, hostility, or apathy

Related Factors (Gordon, 1987)

- Low readiness for reception of information (anxiety)
- Lack of interest or motivation to learn
- Cognitive limitations
- Uncompensated short-term memory loss
- Inability to use materials or information resources owing to factors such as cultural or language differences
- Unfamiliarity with information resources

Expected Outcome

The patient and/or family members demonstrate

- knowledge concerning the perioperative environment and pertinent aspects of the surgical procedure
- knowledge concerning the potential physical and psychological effects of surgery
- coping mechanisms that can be used in response to surgical intervention
- the cognitive, motor, and affective skills necessary to participate in the rehabilitation process after surgery

PERIOPERATIVE NURSING INTERVENTIONS

Identifying the Learning Needs

Patient and family learning needs may be identified through open-ended questioning or direct observation of verbal and nonverbal cues. Patients and families should be asked what they know about the impending surgical intervention. Assumptions should not be made, however, that a lack of questions by the patient or family members signal their understanding of the impending surgical procedure. Minimally, knowledge concerning surgical routines, nothing by mouth status requirements, deep breathing, expansion breathing, splinting of the wound site, coughing, postoperative leg exercises, and discharge instructions should be identified.

Assessing the Readiness to Learn

The perioperative nurse assesses readiness to learn by determining the patient's and the family's

- knowledge, attitudes, and self-care skills concerning surgical intervention
- past experiences related to the health problem
- obstacles to health learning
- level of anxiety (low levels of anxiety enhance learning, whereas moderate and high levels inhibit learning)
- educational background (an individual's use of vocabulary and ability to communicate can provide clues to the educational background)
- orientation and memory
- physical condition (levels of discomfort, energy, alertness, and so on)
- developmental level (intellectual and emotional)
- mental, physical, or educational handicaps (language barrier, sensory deficits)
- motivation and attitude (consider the patient's perception of disease or condition and its seriousness) (Toth, 1983)

Motivation is one of the critical factors in determining if an individual is ready to learn. According to Toth (1983), motivation is affected by the patient's and the family's

- acceptance of a health risk or problem
- awareness of the need to change a health attitude or behavior
- estimation of the level of control that can be exercised in a particular situation

If the individual has not yet accepted his or her condition, it would be useless to attempt learning or behavior change. Rather, Toth (1983) suggests that the perioperative nurse emphasize a trusting, warm, and open relationship and help the patient work through his or her denial. Consideration must also be given to the religious and cultural influences that may have an effect on patient or family learning.

Providing Instruction Based on Identified Needs

After the patient's ability and readiness to learn has been assessed, an individualized teaching approach can be planned on the basis of the identified needs. The perioperative nurse should consider the following points when planning patient and family teaching:

- Provide an overview of expected procedures and events, such as a description of the environment, the sequence of events, and procedures that the patient will experience.
- Describe behaviors that the patient is expected to demonstrate, such as a preoperative shower and nothing by mouth status.
- Describe probable alterations in comfort level such as wound pain, soreness from retractors, and sore throat after general anesthesia with endotracheal intubation.
- Provide strategies for reducing pain and discomfort such as requesting pain medication and ice chips.
- Describe probable tactile, auditory, and visual sensations that the patient will experience while in the operating room.
- Explain potentially frightening equipment that the patient will see or hear while in the operating room.
- Describe postoperative behaviors that the patient is expected to demonstrate such as passive exercises, ambulation, deep breathing and coughing, dressing care, and resumption of diet.
- Teach the patient to perform skills such as deep breathing (Fig. 5–1), expansion breathing (Fig. 5–2), wound splinting and coughing (Fig. 5–3), passive leg exercises (Fig. 5–4), and ambulation.

Research has shown that a maximal effect can be obtained when the skills-teaching session includes a return demonstration from the patient before surgery and a follow-up demonstration after surgery (Devine, 1985). Information and skills training may also have a positive effect on the patient by providing him or her with a sense of predictability and control. Such training identifies for the patient the normal occurrences of surgical intervention. The patient is less likely to identify a normal occurrence as a sign that something is wrong or cause for alarm (Devine, 1985).

Providing the Opportunity to Ask Questions

Comprehension of instructional material is enhanced if the patient and family members are provided an opportunity to ask questions. Questions facilitate patient, family, and perioperative nurse interaction; may alleviate anxiety; and reinforce coping mechanisms. Questions enable the nurse to provide reassurance and, if needed, additional informention.

Teaching During the Postoperative Period

Although most patient and family teaching is done preoperatively, there are some logical extensions of patient and family teaching into the postoperative period (Devine, 1985). Postoperative teaching content depends on the type of surgery done, the recovery progress, the patient's level of discomfort, the prognosis, and the availability of support systems. The perioperative nurse should reinforce preoperative teaching by checking the patient's ability to cough and deep breathe, do passive exercises, and ambulate. Praise and encouragement at this time reinforce the patient's motivation to participate in the rehabilitation process.

During the postoperative period, the patient and family members should be taught how to manage the patient's convalescence after discharge from the hospital. This teaching is particularly important for the outpatient. Written instructions serve as an excellent teaching tool. After the teaching is done, the patient and/or a family member signs the written instructions and is given the original instruction sheet for use at home. The copy is retained in the patient's record as a verification that teaching was done. Figures 5–5 through 5–38 provide examples of English and Spanish outpatient surgery and endoscopy teaching tools.

Determining the Effectiveness of Teaching

The perioperative nurse uses the outcome standard criteria to determine the effectiveness of teaching.

Teaching has been effective if the patient and/or family members can demonstrate knowledge of the perioperative environment and pertinent aspects of the operative procedure. The patient and/or family members should be able to

- state the time when surgery is scheduled
- state the unit to which the patient will return after surgery
- list monitoring and therapeutic devices or materials most likely to be used during the postoperative period
- state the location of family waiting areas
- ask questions about the impending surgery
- perform expected behaviors such as taking a preoperative shower and maintaining nothing by mouth status (Kneedler, 1987)

Teaching has been effective if the patient and family members can demonstrate knowledge of the potential physical and psychological effects of surgery. The patient and/or family members should be able to

- describe in their own words the anticipated physical and psychological effects of surgical intervention
- express their feelings regarding surgical intervention and its expected outcomes (Kneedler, 1987)

Text continued on page 133

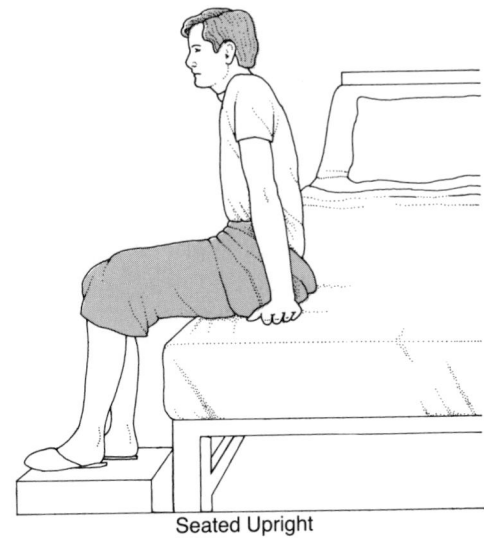

Seated Upright

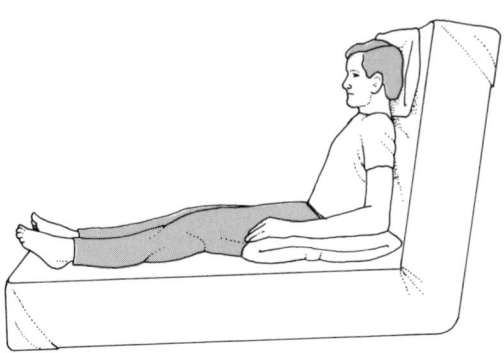

Fowler's Position

1. Instruct the client to sit upright on the edge of the bed or in a chair. (After surgery, deep breathing is done with the client in Fowler's position or in semi-Fowler's position.)
2. Instruct the client to take a gentle breath through the mouth.
3. Instruct the client to breathe out gently and completely.
4. Instruct the client to take a deep breath through the nose and mouth. The client holds this breath to the count of 5.
5. Instruct the client to exhale through the nose and mouth.

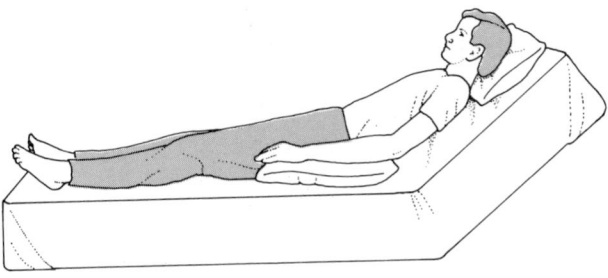

Semi-Fowler's Position

FIGURE 5–1. Teaching deep breathing. (From Ignatavicius, D., Bayne, M. V. [1991]. *Medical-surgical nursing: A nursing process approach* [pp. 443–444]. Philadelphia: W. B. Saunders.)

1. Place the client in a comfortable upright position, with the client's knees slightly bent. (Bending the knees decreases tension on the abdominal muscles and decreases respiratory resistance and discomfort.)
2. Have the client place his or her hands on each side of the lower rib cage, just above the waist.
3. Instruct the client to take a deep breath through the nose, using the shoulder muscles to expand the lower rib cage outward during inhalation.

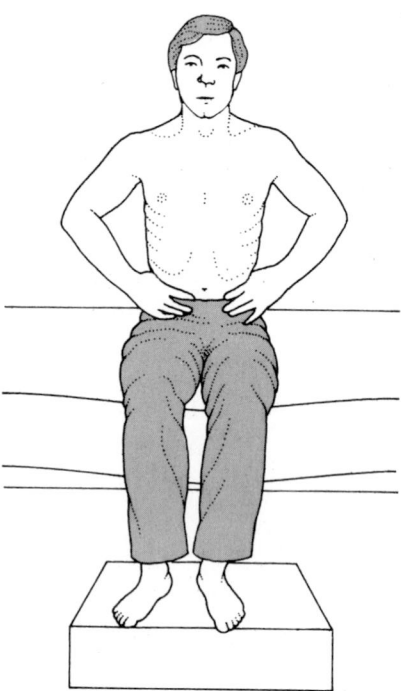

4. Instruct the client to exhale and to concentrate on the inward movement of first the chest and then the lower ribs while gently squeezing the rib cage and forcing air out of the base of the lungs.

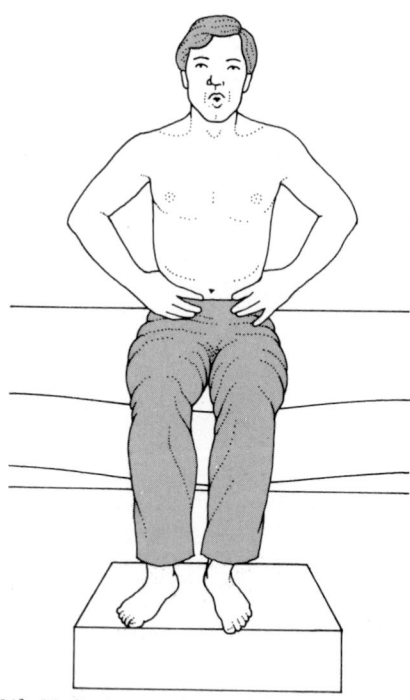

FIGURE 5–2. Teaching expansion breathing. (From Ignatavicius, D., Bayne, M. V. [1991]. *Medical-surgical nursing: A nursing process approach* [p. 444]. Philadelphia: W. B. Saunders.)

1. Place a pillow, towel, or folded blanket over the surgical area and have the client hold it firmly in place.

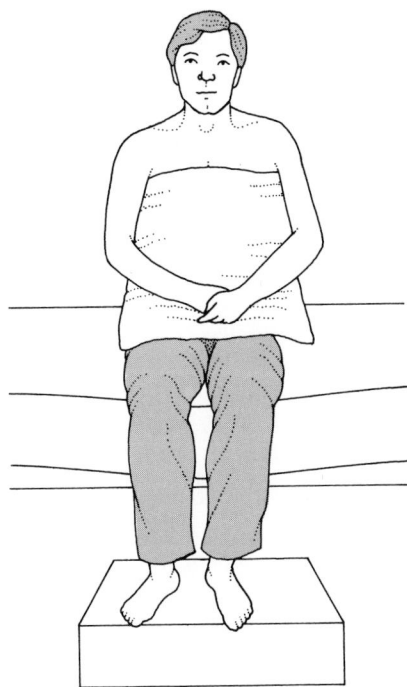

2. Have the client stimulate the cough reflex by taking three slow, deep breaths.
3. Instruct the client to inhale through the nose and exhale through the mouth.
4. On the third deep breath, instruct the client to cough to clear secretions from the lungs.

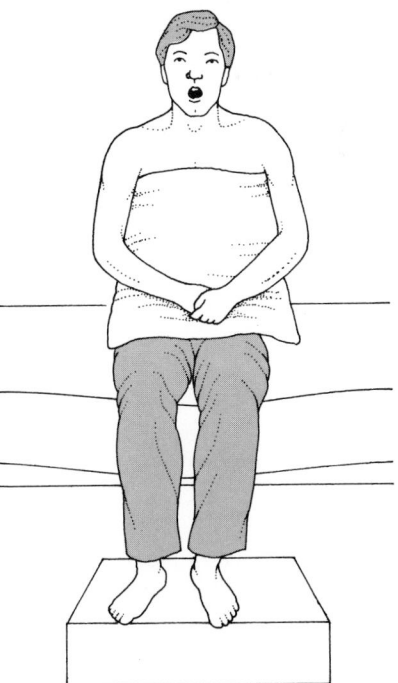

FIGURE 5–3. Teaching splinting of the surgical site and coughing. (From Ignatavicius, D., Bayne, M. V. [1991]. *Medical-surgical nursing: A nursing process approach* [pp. 444–445]. Philadelphia: W. B. Saunders.)

1. Have the client lie in semi-Fowler's position when performing leg exercises to improve peripheral circulation, prevent thrombus formation, and strengthen muscles.
2. Instruct the client to bend the knee, raise the foot, and hold this position for a few seconds. The client then extends the leg and lowers it to the bed. The client should repeat this sequence five times with each leg.

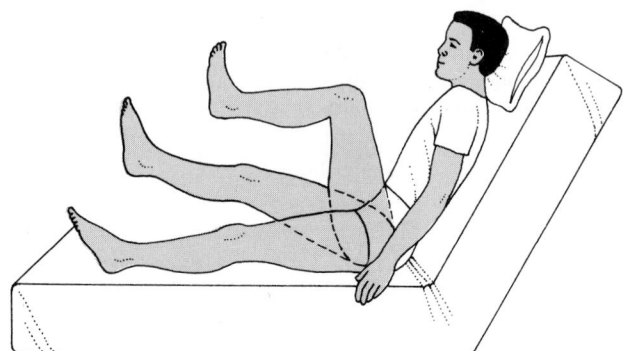

3. Instruct the client to extend the foot toward the bottom of the bed, then flex it toward the face. The client should repeat this exercise several times.

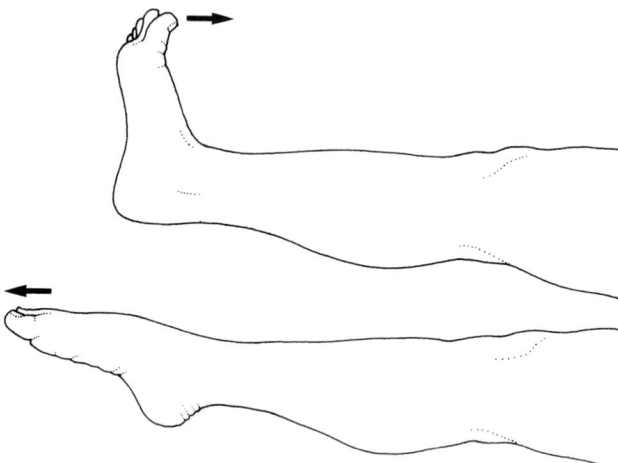

4. Instruct the client to make circles with the ankles, first to the left, then to the right. The client should repeat this exercise several times.

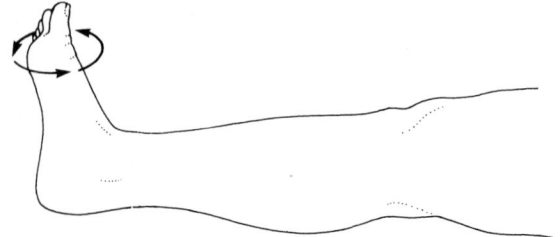

FIGURE 5–4. Teaching postoperative leg exercises. (From Ignatavicius, D., Bayne, M. V. [1991]. *Medical-surgical nursing: A nursing process approach* [p. 447]. Philadelphia: W. B. Saunders.)

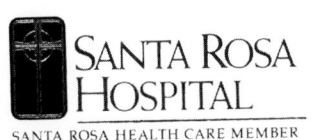
SANTA ROSA HOSPITAL
SANTA ROSA HEALTH CARE MEMBER

Adult Outpatient Surgery

DISCHARGE INSTRUCTIONS FOR PATIENTS WHO RECEIVED GENERAL ANESTHESIA OR IV SEDATION

☐ For your surgery you had
  ☐ general anesthesia,
  ☐ local anesthesia with IV sedation.

☐ If you had general anesthesia, you may have a sore throat for the first 24 hours following surgery due to an airway placed inside your windpipe during your operation. Immediately telephone your doctor if you have difficulty with breathing, swallowing, or swelling of your throat.

☐ You may experience dizziness, drowsiness or light-headedness after general anesthesia or IV sedation.

  ☐ You must have a responsible person drive you home.
  ☐ You should have a responsible person stay with you for 24 hours.
  ☐ Bed rest and limited activity is necessary for 24 to 48 hours following general anesthesia or IV sedation.
  ☐ You should not drive a motor vehicle, ride a bicycle, or engage in other activities that require coordination and the ability to respond quickly.
  ☐ You should not operate machinery and power tools or handle dangerous items such as hot grease, boiling water, smoking, etc.
  ☐ You should not consume alcoholic beverages.
  ☐ You should not sign legally binding documents.
  ☐ You should not engage in sports, perform heavy work, or lift heavy objects.

☐ When you go home, you may have a light-diet.

  ☐ Begin with liquids and light foods such as crackers, JELL-O®, soup, and 7-UP®.
  ☐ Progress to your normal diet if you are not nauseated.
  ☐ You may eat as much as you can tolerate.
  ☐ Avoid spicy, greasy, and fried foods for 24 hours.
  ☐ Tomorrow, you may begin your regular diet, unless otherwise instructed by your doctor.

OTHER INSTRUCTIONS:
_____
_____
_____
_____
_____
_____

I HAVE READ AND RECEIVED THE ABOVE INSTRUCTIONS.

_____
Patient

_____
Significant Other

_____
Nurse
_____
Date

FIGURE 5–5. Discharge instructions for patients who received general anesthesia or IV sedation. (Courtesy of Santa Rosa Hospital, San Antonio, TX. Copyright 1990, Santa Rosa Health Care Corporation, 519 West Houston Street, San Antonio, TX 78207. All rights reserved.)

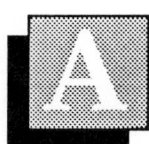

Adult Outpatient Surgery
Cirugía Externa Para Adultos

INSTRUCCIONES POSTOPERATORIAS PARA LOS PACIENTES QUE RECIBEN ANESTESIA GENERAL O SEDANTE INTRAVENOSO

Llamaré al Dr. _____ al
_____ (consultorio) o al
_____ (central telefónica) de inmediato
si se presenta cualquier de los síntomas siguientes:

- salida de sangre extraordinaria o excesiva
- dolor fuerte
- dificultad al respirar
- enrojecimiento o hinchazón
- calentura arriba de 100 grados F.

❏ Si no puedo conseguir al médico por teléfono, iré a la sala de emergencia del hospital más cercano.

❏ Entiendo que mi dieta después de la anestesia general o del sedante intravenoso debe ser ligera (gelatina/sopa/7UP) y que debo evitar la comida grasosa, picosa y frita por 24 horas a partir de la intervención quirúrgica.

❏ Comprendo que no he de tomar bebidas alcohólicas por 24 horas después de la anestesia general o del sedante intravenoso.

❏ Entiendo que despues de la anestesia general o del sedante intravenoso, que puedo sentir mareo, sueño o aturdimiento y que alguna persona responsable tiene que llevarme a casa y acompañarme por 24 horas a partir de la intervención quirúrgica.

❏ Comprendo que después de la anestesia general o del sedante intravenoso que NO he de conducir ningún vehículo; manejar maquinaria ni herramientas mecanicas; hacer decisiones importantes; firmar documentos legales por 24 horas a partir de la operación.

❏ Entiendo que me es preciso guardar cama y limitar mis actividades por 24 horas después de la anestesia general o del sedante intravenoso.

❏ Comprendo que una enfermera del departamento de Cirugía Externa me llamará unos días después de la intervención quirúrgica (ésta es una llamada ordinaria para saber cómo estoy).

❏ Llame al Dr. _____ para fijar una cita en _____ días/semanas.

OTRAS INSTRUCCIONES:

_____

_____

_____

DIETA:

_____

MEDICAMENTOS:

Nombre/Dosis	Cantidad	Frecuencia	Ruta

He leído y he recibido una copia de las instrucciones de arriba y entiendo muy bien cómo cuidarme en casa.

_____
Firma del paciente

_____
Testigo

_____
Fecha

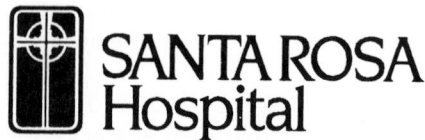

SANTA ROSA Hospital

519 West Houston Street
San Antonio, Texas 78207

FIGURE 5–6. Instrucciones postoperatorias para los pacientes que reciben anestesia general o sedante intravenoso. (Courtesy of Santa Rosa Hospital, San Antonio, TX. Copyright 1990, Santa Rosa Health Care Corporation, 519 West Houston Street, San Antonio, TX 78207. All rights reserved.)

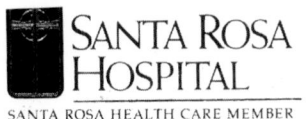

SANTA ROSA
HOSPITAL
SANTA ROSA HEALTH CARE MEMBER

Adult Outpatient Surgery

DISCHARGE INSTRUCTIONS FOR BREAST BIOPSY PATIENTS

☐ **The following instructions tell you how to care for your surgery wound.**

  ☐ Keep your bra on for **24 hours,** unless otherwise instructed by doctor.
  ☐ Change your wound bandage according to the following instructions:

  _____
  _____
  _____
  _____

  ☐ Keep your wound bandage dry and clean.
  ☐ Do not get your wound stitches wet.

☐ **Telephone your doctor if you have**

  ☐ redness, soreness, or swelling around your wound stitches,
  ☐ a fever over 100°F,
  ☐ drainage from your surgery wound,
  ☐ bleeding or oozing from your surgery wound,
  ☐ pain that is not relieved by the medication prescribed by your doctor.

☐ **You may return to your normal activity or employment on _____, unless otherwise instructed by your doctor.**

☐ **If you have an emergency and you cannot reach your doctor by telephone, go to an emergency room nearest your home.**

☐ **Follow the labeled instructions on the prescription medications ordered by your doctor.**

OTHER INSTRUCTIONS:

_____
_____
_____
_____

☐ A nurse from the Outpatient Surgery Unit will telephone you a few days after surgery. The nurse will ask you questions about how you are feeling.

☐ Call Dr. _____ in _____
  ☐ day(s) ☐ week(s) ☐ month for an appointment.
  Your doctor's telephone numbers are:

  Office_____
  Exchange_____

I HAVE READ AND RECEIVED THE ABOVE INSTRUCTIONS.

_____
Patient

_____
Significant Other

_____
Nurse

_____
Date

FIGURE 5–7. Discharge instructions for breast biopsy patients. (Courtesy of Santa Rosa Hospital, San Antonio, TX. Copyright 1990, Santa Rosa Health Care Corporation, 519 West Houston Street, San Antonio, TX 78207. All rights reserved.)

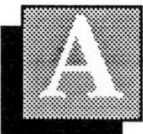

Adult Outpatient Surgery
Cirugía Externa Para Adultos

BIOPSIA DEL SENO

Siga las instrucciones marcadas:

1. No se quite el brassiere por 24 horas, a menos que su médico indique al contrario.
2. Cambie el vendaje según las instrucciones.
3. No cambie el vendaje hasta que Ud. vea a su médico.
4. Mantenga el vendaje seco y limpio.
5. No permita que se mojen las puntadas.
6. Comunique a su médico los sintomas siguientes:

   ● enrojecimiento de la zona alrededor de las puntadas
   ● hinchazón
   ● calentura arriba de 100 grados F.
   ● salida de pus de la incisión
   ● derrame de sangre o supuración de la incisión
   ● dolor que no se alivia con medicamento

7. Siga las indicaciones de la etiqueta de la medicina recetada por su médico.

OTRAS INSTRUCCIONES: _____

_____

Llame al Dr. _____ para una cita en _____ días/semanas/meses; o par comuncar
signos o síntomas anormales al consultorio _____ o a la central telefónica
_____.

He leído y he recibido una copia de las instrucciones de arriba:

_____   _____
Firma del paciente   Fecha

_____
Testigo

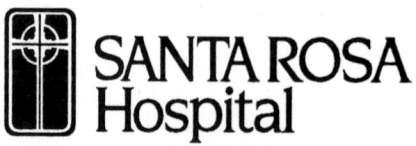

SANTA ROSA
Hospital
519 West Houston Street
San Antonio, Texas 78207

FIGURE 5–8. Instrucciones postoperatorias para biopsia del seno. (Courtesy of Santa Rosa Hospital, San Antonio, TX. Copyright 1990, Santa Rosa Health Care Corporation, 519 West Houston Street, San Antonio, TX 78207. All rights reserved.)

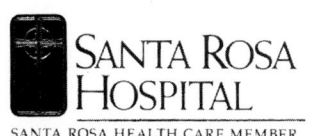

Adult Outpatient Surgery

DISCHARGE INSTRUCTIONS FOR CATARACT PATIENTS

☐ Telephone your doctor if you

- ☐ have pain, redness, or swelling in or around your eye,
- ☐ have discharge coming from your eye,
- ☐ the vision in your operated eye suddenly becomes more blurred.

☐ Things you may do after surgery.

- ☐ After the first office visit to your doctor, you may be up and about and go outside.
- ☐ You may look down as much as you like.
- ☐ You may read, sew, watch TV, brush your teeth and gently comb your hair. Wash your hair in 2 to 3 days. You may cook after 24 hours.

☐ Things you must not do after surgery. Your doctor will tell you when you can resume these activities.

- ☐ Do not bend over or lift heavy objects (over _____ pounds).
- ☐ Do not exercise, push, or pull in anyway.
- ☐ Do not drive your car until your doctor says it is o.k.

☐ Follow the eye care instructions listed below.

- ☐ Do not lie or sleep on the same side as your operation.
- ☐ Do not rub your eye or put pressure on the operated side.
- ☐ Wear your glasses during the day.
- ☐ Wear your plastic eyeshield while napping or sleeping for 2 weeks or until your doctor tells you to stop.

☐ Follow the medication instructions listed below.

- ☐ You may resume taking any medications prescribed by your family doctor.
- ☐ You may take 2 Tylenol® tablets every 4 hours as needed for discomfort.
- ☐ You may take a laxative of your choice to avoid constipation which could lead to straining.
- ☐ Do not use eye drops until your doctor instructs you on use.

☐ Follow your doctor's instructions on using eye drops. Begin _____

☐ CAUTION. You are "seeing" with one eye only. Be careful around stairs, the stove, fans, or other dangerous appliances. Extra lights or help may be needed at night. Be careful getting in or out of bathtub or bed.

☐ If you have an emergency and you cannot reach your doctor by telephone, go to an emergency room nearest your home.

☐ Follow the labeled instructions on the prescription medications ordered by your doctor.

OTHER INSTRUCTIONS:

_____

_____

_____

_____

☐ A nurse from the Outpatient Surgery Unit will telephone you a few days after surgery. The nurse will ask you questions about how you are feeling.

☐ Call Dr. _____ in _____
   ☐ day(s) ☐ week(s) ☐ month for an appointment.
   Your doctor's telephone numbers are:

   Office_____
   Exchange_____

I HAVE READ AND RECEIVED THE ABOVE INSTRUCTIONS.

_____
Patient

_____
Significant Other

_____
Nurse

_____
Date

FIGURE 5–9. Discharge instructions for cataract patients. (Courtesy of Santa Rosa Hospital, San Antonio, TX. Copyright 1990, Santa Rosa Health Care Corporation, 519 West Houston Street, San Antonio, TX 78207. All rights reserved.)

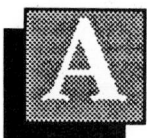dult Outpatient Surgery

Cirugía Externa Para Adultos

OPERACION PARA CATARATAS

1. Ud tiene una cita para ver a su médico mañana a las/entre _____.
2. Si tiene complicaciones, llame a su médico de inmediato al consultorio _____, central telefónica _____.
3. Comunique a su médico cualquiera de los sínto mas siquientes: **mucho dolor, más enroje cimiento, crecimiento de la inflamación, aumento de derrame, la visión del ojo operado de repente se pone más empañada.**

ACTIVIDADES

<u>Ud. Puede:</u>

❑ Estar levantado y salir para afuera sólo después de la primera visita al consultorio

❑ Mirar para abajo cuanto quiera

❑ Leer, coser, ver televisión, cocinar

❑ Lavarse los dientes y peinarse suavemente

<u>No Puede:</u>

❑ Agacharse

❑ Levantar cosas pesadas (más de _____ libras)

❑ Hacer ejercicio, jalar ni empujar de ninguna forma

❑ Conducir su carro hasta que su médico lo autorice

❑ Otro: _____

<u>Cuidado Del Ojo:</u>

❑ No se acueste ni duerma en el lado operado

❑ No se frote el ojo

❑ No ponga presión al lado operado

❑ Al echarse gotas, no toque el párpado ni el ojo con el frasquito

❑ Para protegerse el ojo: puede usar sus anteojos de día; debe usar el protector de plástico al dormir la siesta o al acostarse

❑ Otro: _____

<u>Medicamento:</u>

❑ Puede volver a tomar todo medicamento recetado por su médico personal

❑ Puede tomar Tylenol: dos tabletas cada 4 horas como sea necesario para la molestia

❑ Puede tomar un laxante de su selección para evitar el estreñimiento, que podría llevarlo a hacer un esfuerzo bastante enérgico

❑ No use gotas hasta que el médico le instruya en su uso

❑ Siga las instrucciones del médico con respecto a usar las gotas: Comience _____

OTRAS INSTRUCCIONES:

_____
_____

PRECAUCION: Ud está viendo con un ojo solamente. Tenga especial cuidado al subir y bajar la escalera, al cocinar en la estufa, al meterse a o al salirse de la tina, y con los abanicos y otros aparatos peligrosos. Le será útil poner luces extras y tener quien le ayude de noche.

He leído y he recibido una copia de las instrucciones de arriba.

_____
Firma del paciente

_____
Fecha

_____
Testigo/enfermera

_____
Fecha

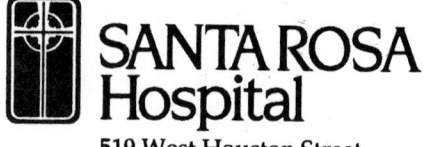

519 West Houston Street
San Antonio, Texas 78207

FIGURE 5–10. Instrucciones postoperatorias para operacion para cataratas. (Courtesy of Santa Rosa Hospital, San Antonio, TX. Copyright 1990, Santa Rosa Health Care Corporation, 519 West Houston Street, San Antonio, TX 78207. All rights reserved.)

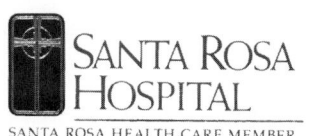

SANTA ROSA
HOSPITAL
SANTA ROSA HEALTH CARE MEMBER

Adult Outpatient Surgery

DISCHARGE INSTRUCTIONS FOR RHINOPLASTY AND SEPTOPLASTY PATIENTS

☐ Immediately telephone your doctor if any of the following occur:

  ☐ bleeding;
  ☐ fever or chills;
  ☐ loose dressing or displacement of nasal packing (cloth stripe inside of nostrils;)
  ☐ severe pain not relieved by pain medication;
  ☐ excessive swelling (some swelling or bruising is to be expected);
  ☐ difficulty in breathing or swallowing.

☐ Do not remove the surgery wound bandage or packing.

☐ Your doctor will give you instructions on when to change and reinforce your drip pad (small gauze under bottom of nostrils).

☐ Keep your head elevated.

☐ Do not get your dressing wet.

☐ If you have an emergency and you cannot reach your doctor by telephone, go to an emergency room nearest your home.

☐ Follow the labeled instructions on the prescription medications ordered by your doctor.

OTHER INSTRUCTIONS:

_____
_____
_____
_____

☐ A nurse from the Outpatient Surgery Unit will telephone you a few days after surgery. The nurse will ask you questions about how you are feeling.

☐ Call Dr. _____ in _____
  ☐ day(s) ☐ week(s) ☐ month for an appointment.
  Your doctor's telephone numbers are:

  Office_____
  Exchange_____

I HAVE READ AND RECEIVED THE ABOVE INSTRUCTIONS.

_____
Patient

_____
Significant Other

_____
Nurse

_____
Date

FIGURE 5–11. Discharge instructions for rhinoplasty and septoplasty patients. (Courtesy of Santa Rosa Hospital, San Antonio, TX. Copyright 1990, Santa Rosa Health Care Corporation, 519 West Houston Street, San Antonio, TX 78207. All rights reserved.)

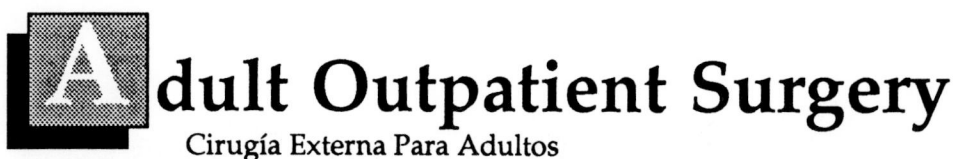

Adult Outpatient Surgery

Cirugía Externa Para Adultos

INSTRUCCIONES POSQUIRURGICAS PARA LOS PACIENTES RINOPLASTIA, SEPTOPLASTIA

LLAME AL MEDICO SI TIENE ESTOS SINTOMAS:

❑ 1. Salida excesiva de sangre
❑ 2. Calentura o escalofrío
❑ 3. Vendaje suelto o aflojamiento del empaque de las narices
❑ 4. Dolor fuerte que no se alivia con medicamento
❑ 5. Hinchazón excesiva (es de esperarse una cierta hinchazón o contusión)
❑ 6. Dificultad al respirar o tragar.

NO SE QUITE NADA del vendaje.

La gasa pequeña bajo las narices ha de cambiarse/reforzarse según indique el médico.

ACTIVIDAD: Mantenga la cabeza elevada.

Baño: No se lave el pelo ni se moje el vendaje.

OTRAS INSTRUCCIONES: _____

_____

Llame al Dr. _____ para fijar una cita en _____ dias/semanas/ meses o para comunicar todo signo o síntoma raro al:

_____ consultorio _____ central telefónica.

He leído, he entendido y he recibido una copia de las instrucciones de arriba.

_____
Firma del paciente

_____
Fecha

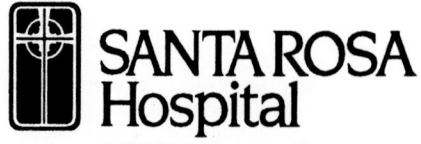

SANTA ROSA Hospital

519 West Houston Street
San Antonio, Texas 78207

FIGURE 5–12. Instrucciones posquirurgicas para los pacientes rinoplastia septoplastia. (Courtesy of Santa Rosa Hospital, San Antonio, TX. Copyright 1990, Santa Rosa Health Care Corporation, 519 West Houston Street, San Antonio, TX 78207. All rights reserved.)

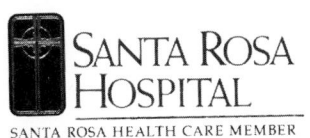

Adult Outpatient Surgery

DISCHARGE INSTRUCTIONS FOR TONSILLECTOMY PATIENTS

☐ When you go home, you may have a light-diet. Disregard diet instructions listed on instruction sheet *Discharge Instructions for Patients Who Received General Anesthesia and IV Sedation.* Follow the instructions listed below.

    ☐ Fluids are very important. Drink mild, non-acidic juices such as apple or apricot juice, and soft drinks. Popsicles may be eaten.

    ☐ Eat soft foods such as JELL-O®, ice cream, custards, pudding, and mashed foods. Keep to this type of diet for the first week after your operation or until the your doctor tells you otherwise.

    ☐ Do not eat hot, spicy, rough, and scratchy foods such as fresh fruits, toast, crackers and potato chips should be avoided since they may scratch your healing throat and cause bleeding.

    ☐ Do not use straws or other hard objects that can stick back in the throat.

☐ Telephone your doctor if any of the following occur:

    ☐ spitting or vomiting of bright red blood or blood clots (blood tinged and pink saliva is normal);

    ☐ severe pain unrelieved by prescribed medication;

    ☐ difficulty with breathing;

    ☐ severe swelling;

    ☐ fever over 100°F.

☐ You will have a moderate amount of throat and ear discomfort following surgery, especially while eating. If the doctor has ordered medication, it will help you swallow more comfortably if you take the medication ½ hour before eating.

☐ If you have an emergency and you cannot reach your doctor by telephone, go to an emergency room nearest your home.

☐ Follow the labeled instructions on the prescription medications ordered by your doctor.

OTHER INSTRUCTIONS:

_____

_____

_____

_____

☐ A nurse from the Outpatient Surgery Unit will telephone you a few days after surgery. The nurse will ask you questions about how you are feeling.

☐ Call Dr. _____ in _____
  ☐ day(s) ☐ week(s) ☐ month for an appointment. Your doctor's telephone numbers are:

Office_____
Exchange_____

I HAVE READ AND RECEIVED THE ABOVE INSTRUCTIONS.

_____
Patient

_____
Significant Other

_____
Nurse

_____
Date

FIGURE 5–13. Discharge instructions for tonsillectomy patients. (Courtesy of Santa Rosa Hospital, San Antonio, TX. Copyright 1990, Santa Rosa Health Care Corporation, 519 West Houston Street, San Antonio, TX 78207. All rights reserved.)

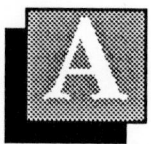

Adult Outpatient Surgery

Cirugía Externa Para Adultos

INSTRUCCIONES POSTOPERATORIAS PARA LA AMIGDALECTOMIA

Llamaré al Dr. _____
en el número _____ (consultorio)
o al _____ (central telefónica)
si se presenta cualquiera de los síntomas siguientes:

● Expectoración o vómito de sangre de color rojo
subido o de coágulos de sangre (la saliva té
ñida de sangre y la de color de rosa son normales).
● Dolor intenso que no se alivia con medicamento
● Dificultad al respirar
● Mucha hinchazón
● Calentura arriba de 100 grados F.

Si no puedo conseguir al médico por teléfono, iré a la
sala de emergencia más cercana.

Entiendo que los fluidos son muy importantes. Los
jugos suaves y no acídicos (jugo de manzana, de chab-
acano), los refrescos y las paletas se recomiendan. Los
alimentos suaves tales como la gelatina, helado, flan,
pudin y purés sirven para mantener la buena nutrición.
Esta clase de dieta deberá observarse la primera semana
después de la operación o hasta que el médico indique
de otra manera. La comida caliente, picosa y rugosa y la
que rasca deben evitarse, puesto que pueden irritar la
garganta y provocar la salida de sangre. También deben
evitarse los popotes u otros objetos duros que pueden
pegarse a la garganta. Esta clase de dieta deberá
observarse la primera semana después de la operación o
hasta que el médico indique de otra manera.

Comprendo que no he de tomar bebidas alcohólicas
hasta que el médico me dé permiso.

Comprendo que me es preciso guardar cama durante
las primeras 24-48 horas, y que puedo levantarme
únicamente para ir al cuarto de baño. Tengo que limitar
mis actividades en casa hasta la primera visita posto-
peratoria.

Comprendo que es de esperarse una cierta molestia en
la garganta y dolor en los oídos. Si el médico ha recetado medicamento, le ayudará a tragar más comoda-
mente si lo toma media hora antes de comer.
Un medicamento que comúnmente se utiliza después de

la intervención quirúrgica es un jarabe que se llama
ACETAMINOFENA. Se puede comprar en su farmacia
bajo los nombres TYLENOL, DATRIL, TEMPRA o
LIQUIPRIN. La acetaminofena funciona como la
aspirina, pero se utiliza en su lugar porque la aspirina
tiene el efecto de provocar la salida de sangre. Al tomar
este medicamento, tómelo solamente según le han
instruido.

OTRAS INSTRUCCIONES:

_____

_____

Llame al Dr. _____
para una cita en _____ días/semanas.

*He leído y he recibido una copia de estas instrucciones
y entiendo muy bien cómo cuidarme en casa.*

_____
Paciente

_____
Testigo

_____
Fecha

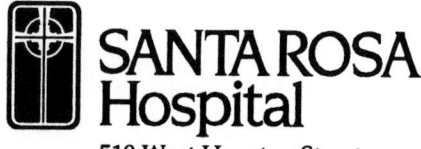

SANTA ROSA Hospital
**519 West Houston Street
San Antonio, Texas 78207**

FIGURE 5–14. Instrucciones postoperatorias para la amigalectomia. (Courtesy of Santa Rosa Hospital, San Antonio, TX. Copyright 1990, Santa Rosa Health Care Corporation, 519 West Houston Street, San Antonio, TX 78207. All rights reserved.)

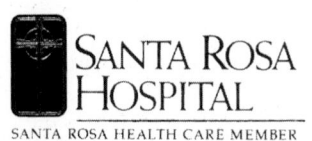
SANTA ROSA
HOSPITAL
SANTA ROSA HEALTH CARE MEMBER

Adult Outpatient Surgery

DISCHARGE INSTRUCTIONS FOR MINOR SURGERY PATIENTS

☐ Check your bandage(s) for signs of excessive bleeding (slow oozing that saturates bandage completely or heavy flow of bright red blood).

   ☐ If bleeding occurs, apply pressure to area.
   ☐ Elevate the area if possible.
   ☐ Contact your doctor at once.

☐ Telephone your doctor if any of the following occur:

   ☐ redness, soreness, or swelling around your wound stitches;
   ☐ fever over 100°F;
   ☐ drainage from your surgery wound;
   ☐ bleeding or oozing from your surgery wound;
   ☐ your pain is not relieved by the medication prescribed by your doctor.

☐ The following instructions tell you how to care for your surgery wound. Follow the instructions for the boxes checked:

   ☐ change your wound bandage according to the following instructions

   _____
   _____
   _____
   _____
   _____

   ☐ keep your wound bandage dry and clean;
   ☐ do not get your wound stitches wet.
   ☐ Keep operative site elevated for the next _____ hours.

☐ If you have an emergency and you cannot reach your doctor by telephone, go to an emergency room nearest your home.

☐ Follow the labeled instructions on the prescription medications ordered by your doctor.

OTHER INSTRUCTIONS:

_____
_____
_____
_____
_____

☐ A nurse from the Outpatient Surgery Unit will telephone you a few days after surgery. The nurse will ask you questions about how you are feeling.

☐ Call Dr. _____ in _____
   ☐ day(s) ☐ week(s) ☐ month for an appointment.
   Your doctor's telephone numbers are:

   Office_____
   Exchange_____

I HAVE READ AND RECEIVED THE ABOVE INSTRUCTIONS.

_____
Patient

_____
Significant Other

_____
Nurse

_____
Date

FIGURE 5–15. Discharge instructions for minor surgery patients. (Courtesy of Santa Rosa Hospital, San Antonio, TX. Copyright 1990, Santa Rosa Health Care Corporation, 519 West Houston Street, San Antonio, TX 78207. All rights reserved.)

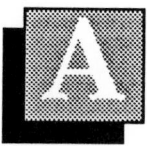dult Outpatient Surgery

Cirugía Externa Para Adultos

INSTRUCCIONES POSTOPERATORIAS PARA EL CUIDADO EN CASA - CIRUGIA MENOR

Se ruega que Ud. siga las instrucciones cuidadosamente.

❑ Haga una cita para ver a su médico en _____.
Llame al consultorio para hacerla.

❑ Observe la(s) region(es) operada(s) por signos de una salida excesiva de sangre: (un exudado que empapa el vandaje por completo o un flujo abundante de sangre de color rojo subido) Si ocurre esto, aplique presión a la región; elévela si sea posible y: llame a su médico en seguida!

❑ Observe la región operada por signos de infección; dolor aumentado, enrojecimiento, inflamación, olor desagradable o derrame. Si se presenta cualquiera de éstos: llame a su médico en seguida!

❑ Entere a su médico de todo dolor que no se alivia con medicamento.

❑ Debe cuidarse la herida así:

❑ Cambie el vendaje según se le ha instruido

❑ No cambie los vendajes hasta que su médico lo vea a Ud.

❑ Mantenga los vendajes secos y limpios.

❑ Aplique hielo a la región operada según se le instruye.

❑ Evite la tensión en la línea de sutura; ni estire ni apriete la herida.

❑ Mantenga elevada la región operada por las próximas _____ horas.

❑ Otras instrucciones:

_____

_____

POSTOPERACION: Una enfermera le llamará unos días después de la intervención quirúrgica (ésta es una llamada ordinaria para saber cómo está).

DIETA:

❑ Comience con líquidos y alimentos ligeros (gelatina, sopa, &7UP, etc.) Progrese a su dieta normal si no siente náuseas. Evite las comidas grasosas, picosas y fritas por 24 horas.

❑ Otras instrucciones:

_____

MEDICAMENTO PARA EL DOLOR:

❑ No conduzca ningún vehículo, ni maneje maquinaria ni herramientas mecánicas mientras está tomando el medicamento. El mareo y el sueño no son raros.

OTRAS INSTRUCCIONES:

_____

_____

_____

Si siente dificultad en respirar, si tiene una salida de sangre que Ud. cree que sea excesiva, si siente náuseas o vómito persistentes, cualquier dolor que sea raro, inflamación o fiebre, se ruega que llame a su médico de inmediato. Si no puede conseguir a su médico, y cree que sus síntomas exigen la atención medica, vaya a la sala de emergencia del hospital más cercano.

He leído y he repasado las instrucciones de arriba y entiendo bien cómo cuidarme en casa.

_____
Testigo

_____
Paciente o tutor

_____
Fecha

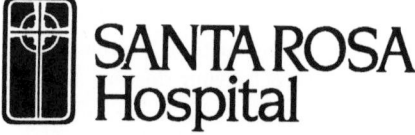

519 West Houston Street
San Antonio, Texas 78207

FIGURE 5–16. Instrucciones postoperatorias para el cuidado en casa cirugia menor. (Courtesy of Santa Rosa Hospital, San Antonio, TX. Copyright 1990, Santa Rosa Health Care Corporation, 519 West Houston Street, San Antonio, TX 78207. All rights reserved.)

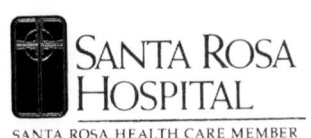
SANTA ROSA
HOSPITAL

SANTA ROSA HEALTH CARE MEMBER

Adult Outpatient Surgery

DISCHARGE INSTRUCTIONS FOR ORTHOPEDIC SURGERY PATIENTS

☐ The following instructions tell you how to care for your surgery wound. Follow the instructions for the boxes checked:

    ☐ elevate affected extremity;
    ☐ apply ice to affected area;
    ☐ wear sling continuously;
    ☐ use crutches as directed.

    _____
    _____
    _____

    ☐ change your wound bandage according to the following instructions

    _____
    _____
    _____
    _____
    _____

    ☐ keep your wound bandage dry and clean;
    ☐ do not get your wound stitches wet.

☐ Telephone your doctor if any of the following occur:

    ☐ *your leg or arm becomes cold, turns a bluish color, feels tingly or numb, or if you have excessive swelling or pain;*
    ☐ redness, soreness, or swelling around your wound stitches;
    ☐ fever over 100°F;
    ☐ drainage from your surgery wound;
    ☐ bleeding or oozing from your surgery wound;
    ☐ your pain is not relieved by the medication prescribed by your doctor.

☐ If you have an emergency and you cannot reach your doctor by telephone, go to an emergency room nearest your home.

☐ Follow the labeled instructions on the prescription medications ordered by your doctor.

OTHER INSTRUCTIONS:

_____
_____
_____
_____

☐ A nurse from the Outpatient Surgery Unit will telephone you a few days after surgery. The nurse will ask you questions about how you are feeling.

☐ Call Dr. _____ in _____
    ☐ day(s) ☐ week(s) ☐ month for an appointment.
    Your doctor's telephone numbers are:

    Office_____
    Exchange_____

I HAVE READ AND RECEIVED THE ABOVE INSTRUCTIONS.

_____
Patient

_____
Significant Other

_____
Nurse

_____
Date

FIGURE 5–17. Discharge instructions for orthopedic surgery patients. (Courtesy of Santa Rosa Hospital, San Antonio, TX. Copyright 1990, Santa Rosa Health Care Corporation, 519 West Houston Street, San Antonio, TX 78207. All rights reserved.)

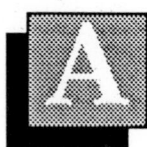

Adult Outpatient Surgery
Cirugía Externa Para Adultos

CIRUGIA ORTOPEDICA

Marque únicamente las frases que le aplican a Ud.:

Haga una cita para ver a su médico en _____.
Llame a su consultorio.

DIETA: Empiece con líquidos y un alimento ligero, tal como la gelatina/sopa/7UP, etc. Progrese a su dieta normal si no tiene náusea.

❑ Recetas mandadas a casa con el paciente. Use según las indicaciones. Al tomar medicamento para el dolor, no maneje maquinaria ni herramientas mecánicas, ni conduzca ningún vehículo, ni tome bebidas alcohólicas, porque éstas pueden causarle mareo y sueño.

ACTIVIDADES:

❑ Es preciso que Ud. guarde cama y que limite sus actividades por 24 a 36 horas después de su operación.
❑ Puede reanudar sus actividades normales.

CUIDADO DE SU HERIDA: Debe cuidar su herida de la manera siguiente:

❑ Cambie el vendaje según las instrucciones
❑ No cambie el vendaje hasta que vea a su médico.
❑ Mantenga el vendaje seco y limpio.

INSTRUCCIONES ESPECIALES: Llame a su médico si la extremidad está fría al tocarla, si se pone azul, si hay entumeciemiento u hormigueo.

❑ Eleve la extremidad afectada.
❑ Aplique hielo a la zona afectada.
❑ Aplique calor a la región afectada.
❑ Use muletas según le instruye el médico.

OTRAS INSTRUCCIONES:
_____
_____
_____

En caso de que tenga dificultad en respirar, derrame de sangre que Ud. considera excesive, náusea o vómito persistente, dolor raro o intenso, hinchazón o fiebre arriba de 100 grados F., se ruega que llame a su médico inmediatamente. Si no puede conseguir a su médico y todavía cree que sus síntomas exigen la atención médica, vaya a la sala de emergencia más cercana.

He leído y he recibido una copia de las instrucciones de arriba, y entiendo muy bien cómo cuidarme en casa.

_____
Testigo

_____
Paciente

_____
Fecha

SANTA ROSA Hospital
519 West Houston Street
San Antonio, Texas 78207

FIGURE 5–18. Cirugia ortopedica. (Courtesy of Santa Rosa Hospital, San Antonio, TX. Copyright 1990, Santa Rosa Health Care Corporation, 519 West Houston Street, San Antonio, TX 78207. All rights reserved.)

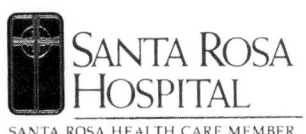

SANTA ROSA HEALTH CARE MEMBER

Adult Outpatient Surgery

DISCHARGE INSTRUCTIONS FOR CYSTOSCOPY PATIENTS

☐ In addition to following the diet instructions listed in the *Discharge Instructions for Patients Who Received General Anesthesia or IV Sedation,* drink plenty of fluids, especially cranberry, water, or tea.

☐ Immediately telephone your doctor if any of the following occur:

   ○ heavy bleeding;
   ○ urine that is bright red (pinkish urine is normal);
   ○ large amounts of blood clots;
   ○ unable to urinate in 6 hours after surgery;
   ○ severe pain during urination (a certain amount of burning and stinging during urination the first few times after your procedure is normal);
   ○ fever over 100°F.

☐ If you have an emergency and you cannot reach your doctor by telephone, go to an emergency room nearest your home.

☐ Follow the labeled instructions on the prescription medications ordered by your doctor.

OTHER INSTRUCTIONS:

_____
_____
_____
_____

☐ A nurse from the Outpatient Surgery Unit will telephone you a few days after surgery. The nurse will ask you questions about how you are feeling.

☐ Call Dr. _____ in _____
   ☐ day(s) ☐ week(s) ☐ month for an appointment.
   Your doctor's telephone numbers are:

   Office_____
   Exchange_____

I HAVE READ AND RECEIVED THE ABOVE INSTRUCTIONS.

_____
Patient

_____
Significant Other

_____
Nurse

_____
Date

FIGURE 5–19. Discharge instructions for cystoscopy patients. (Courtesy of Santa Rosa Hospital, San Antonio, TX. Copyright 1990, Santa Rosa Health Care Corporation, 519 West Houston Street, San Antonio, TX 78207. All rights reserved.)

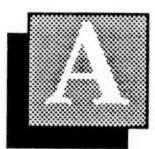 **dult Outpatient Surgery**

Cirugía Externa Para Adultos

INSTRUCCIONES POSTOPERATORIAS PARA LA CISTOSCOPIA

Llamaré inmediatemente al Dr. _____ en su consultorio _____
o a la central **telefónica.** _____ si se presenta cualquiera de los síntomas siguientes:

1. Derrame de sangre extraordinario o abundante
2. Orina de color rojo subido (la orina de color de rosa es normal)
3. Gran cantidad de coágulos
4. Incapacidad de orinar dentro de seis (6) horas después del examen
5. Dolor intenso (es normal una sensación de quemazón o picazón al orinar las primeras pocas veces)
6. Dificultad al respirar
7. Calentura arriba de 100 grados F

Si no puedo conseguir al médico por teléfono, iré a la sala de emergencia del Hospital Santa Rosa o a la sala de emergencia más cercana.

Necesito tomar una taza de fluido cada hora-jugo de arándano agrio (cranberry), agua, té, jugo de manzana, etc.

Comprendo que una enfermera me llamará a unos días después del examen (ésta es una llamada ordinaria para saber cómo anda Ud.)

OTRAS INSTRUCCIONES: _____

_____

_____

_____

Llame al Dr. _____ para una cita en _____ días/semanas.

_____   _____
Firma del paciente   Testigo

_____   _____
Otro   Fecha

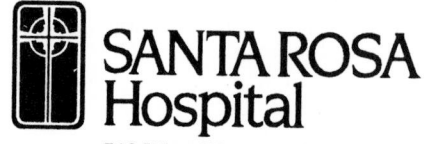

519 West Houston Street
San Antonio, Texas 78207

FIGURE 5–20. Instrucciones postoperatorias para el paciente cistoscopia. (Courtesy of Santa Rosa Hospital, San Antonio, TX. Copyright 1990, Santa Rosa Health Care Corporation, 519 West Houston Street, San Antonio, TX 78207. All rights reserved.)

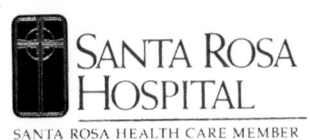

SANTA ROSA
HOSPITAL
SANTA ROSA HEALTH CARE MEMBER

Adult Outpatient Surgery

DISCHARGE INSTRUCTIONS FOR DILATATION AND CURETTAGE PATIENTS

☐ Use sanitary pads only.

☐ Do not use tampons for _____ weeks.

☐ Do not have intercourse for _____ weeks.

☐ Do not take a tub bath for 1 week or go swimming. Showers are acceptable.

☐ Do not douche.

☐ Immediately telephone your doctor if any of the following occur:

    ☐ vaginal bleeding heavier than 1 pad per hour;
    ☐ spot bleeding lasting longer than 2 weeks.
    ☐ foul smelling vaginal discharge;
    ☐ severe abdominal pain (unlike menstrual cramps);
    ☐ fever over 100°F.

☐ If you have an emergency and you cannot reach your doctor by telephone, go to an emergency room nearest your home.

☐ Follow the labeled instructions on the prescription medications ordered by your doctor.

OTHER INSTRUCTIONS:

_____
_____
_____
_____

☐ A nurse from the Outpatient Surgery Unit will telephone you a few days after surgery. The nurse will ask you questions about how you are feeling.

☐ Call Dr. _____ in _____
    ☐ day(s) ☐ week(s) ☐ month for an appointment.
    Your doctor's telephone numbers are:

    Office_____
    Exchange_____

I HAVE READ AND RECEIVED THE ABOVE INSTRUCTIONS.

_____
Patient

_____
Significant Other

_____
Nurse

_____
Date

FIGURE 5–21. Discharge instructions for dilatation and curettage patients. (Courtesy of Santa Rosa Hospital, San Antonio, TX. Copyright 1990, Santa Rosa Health Care Corporation, 519 West Houston Street, San Antonio, TX 78207. All rights reserved.)

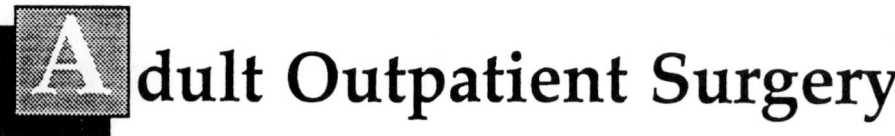

Adult Outpatient Surgery

INSTRUCCIONES POSQUIRURGICAS PARA EL PACIENTE: DILATACION Y RASPADO

❏ 1. Use solamente toallas sanitarias. NO use tampones por _____ semanas.

❏ 2. No tenga relaciones sexuales por _____ semanas.

❏ 3. No se bañe en tina por una (1) semana, y no nade. Se puede regar.

❏ 4. No se duche la vagina.

❏ 5. Comunique a su médico de inmediato cualquiera de los síntomas siguientes:

  ● Derrame de sangre de la vagina que empapa más de una toalla sanitaria por hora.
  ● Salida de sangre que dura más de dos (2) semanas.
  ● Derrame de sangre que despide un olor desagradable.
  ● Dolor fuerte abdominal distinto de los calambres menstruales.
  ● Calentura arriba de 100 grados F.

❏ 6. No vuelva a su régimen de ejercicio ni cargue cosas pesadas sin permiso de su médico.

❏ 7. Cuando vaya a casa hoy, debe guardar cama y levantarse únicamente con ayuda para ir al baño. Mañana puede estar levantada pero todavía debe descansar todo lo posible.

❏ 8. En caso de emergencia, si no puede conseguir a su médico por teléfono, vaya a la sala de emergencia del Hospital Santa Rosa, o a la del hospital más cercano.

Llame al Dr. _____ para fijar una cita en _____
días/semanas/meses, o para enterarle de todo signo o síntoma irregular en el número _____
(consultorio) o en el _____ (central telefónica.)

_____
Firma del médico

_____
Fecha

_____
Firma del paciente

_____
Fecha

_____
Testigo/enfermera

_____
Fecha

May 1989

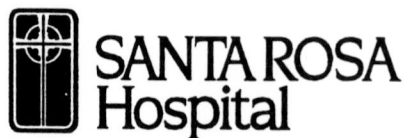

SANTA ROSA
Hospital
519 West Houston Street
San Antonio, Texas 78207

FIGURE 5–22. Instrucciones posquirurgicas para el paciente dilatacion y raspado. (Courtesy of Santa Rosa Hospital, San Antonio, TX. Copyright 1990, Santa Rosa Health Care Corporation, 519 West Houston Street, San Antonio, TX 78207. All rights reserved.)

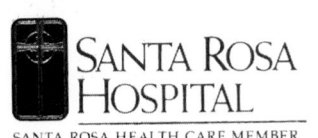

SANTA ROSA HOSPITAL

SANTA ROSA HEALTH CARE MEMBER

Adult Outpatient Surgery

DISCHARGE INSTRUCTIONS FOR CAST PATIENTS

☐ Your cast will take 24 to 48 hours to completely dry. Protect your cast during the drying time. The cast is weak until completely dried.

☐ Prevent swelling of your leg or arm by elevating the leg or arm with the cast to/or above level of your heart for 24 hours and exercising your fingers or toes.

☐ Immediately telephone your doctor if any of the following occur:

  ☐ your toes or fingers swell;
  ☐ you cannot wiggle your toes or fingers;
  ☐ your toes or fingers feel cold or look pale (look at your fingers or toes on your opposite leg or arm to compare);
  ☐ you have pain, numbness, or tingling in your casted leg, arm, fingers, and toes;
  ☐ you smell a bad odor from the cast;
  ☐ you have drainage of fluid or blood from the cast;
  ☐ your cast feels too tight, rubs, or presses against your skin;
  ☐ your cast feels loose, cracks, or breaks;
  ☐ your pain is not relieved by the medication prescribed by your doctor.

☐ Cast care instructions.

  ☐ Do not stick anything under cast to scratch your leg or arm. This may injure your skin and lead to infection.
  ☐ Do not put powder inside your cast.
  ☐ Do not use your cast as a baseball bat. Physical abuse of your cast can prolong healing time.
  ☐ Do not pull out padding from inside your cast.
  ☐ Do not get your cast wet. The plaster will melt if it gets wet. You will have to have your cast changed, thus healing will be slowed.

☐ If you have an emergency and you cannot reach your doctor by telephone, go to an emergency room nearest your home.

☐ Follow the labeled instructions on the prescription medications ordered by your doctor.

OTHER INSTRUCTIONS:

_____
_____
_____
_____

☐ A nurse from the Outpatient Surgery Unit will telephone you a few days after surgery. The nurse will ask you questions about how you are feeling.

☐ Call Dr. _____ in _____
  ☐ day(s) ☐ week(s) ☐ month for an appointment. Your doctor's telephone numbers are:

  Office_____
  Exchange_____

I HAVE READ AND RECEIVED THE ABOVE INSTRUCTIONS.

_____
Patient

_____
Significant Other

_____
Nurse

_____
Date

FIGURE 5–23. Discharge instructions for cast patients. (Courtesy of Santa Rosa Hospital, San Antonio, TX. Copyright 1990, Santa Rosa Health Care Corporation, 519 West Houston Street, San Antonio, TX 78207. All rights reserved.)

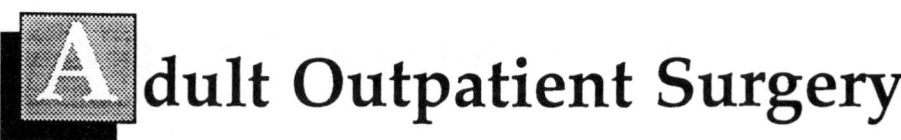

Adult Outpatient Surgery

INSTRUCCIONES PARA EL CUIDADO DEL PACIENTE ENYESADO

Permita que se seque el yeso de 24 a 48 horas. El yeso no alcanza su fuerza máxima hasta que esté completamente seco, y debe protegerse.

Mantenga la pierna o brazo operado elevado al nivel del corazón por 24 horas para prevenir la hinchazón. También, haga ejercicios con los dedos de la mano o pie afectado para reducir la hinchazón.

OBSERVE Y COMUNIQUE A SU MEDICO DE INMEDIATO CUALQUIERA DE LOS SINTOMAS SIGUIENTES:

● Hinchazón de los dedos de la mano o del pie afectado. Incapacidad de mover los dedos afectados.
● Frialdad o palidez de los dedos de la mano o del pie afectado (observe los dedos normales para comparar).
● Dolor, entumecimiento u hormigueo.
● Un olor desagradable o derrame del yeso.
● Un yeso demasiado apretado, o uno que roza la piel. Yeso flojo, partido o quebrado.
● Derrame excisivo de sangre.
● Dolor intenso que no se alivia con medicamento.

LO QUE NO DEBE HACER:

● No meta nada por debajo del yeso para rascarse. Esto puede hacerle daño a la piel.
● No eche polvo para adentro de yeso.
● No use el yeso como un bate de béisbol. El abuso del yeso puede retrasar la curación.
● No saque el relleno del yeso.
● No deje que se moje el yeso. Cuando está mojado, el yeso se derrite y tendrá que cambiarse, así retrasando la curación.

HAGA LO SIGUIENTE: Siga las indicaciones de las recetas que le dio su médico.

OTRAS INSTRUCCIONES:

_____

_____

_____

Llame al consultorio del Dr. _____
para fijar una cita en _____
días/semanas/meses, o para comunicar sus síntomas al
_____ o a la central telefónica
_____.

He leído y he recibido una copia de las instrucciones de arriba.

_____
Firma del paciente

_____
Fecha

_____
Testigo/Enfermera

_____
Fecha

May 1989

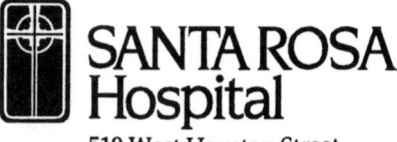

SANTA ROSA
Hospital
519 West Houston Street
San Antonio, Texas 78207

FIGURE 5–24. Instrucciones para el cuidado del paciente enyesado. (Courtesy of Santa Rosa Hospital, San Antonio, TX. Copyright 1990, Santa Rosa Health Care Corporation, 519 West Houston Street, San Antonio, TX 78207. All rights reserved.)

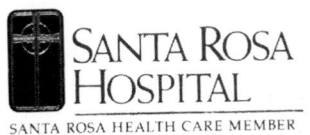

Adult Outpatient Surgery

DISCHARGE INSTRUCTIONS FOR LAPAROSCOPY PATIENTS

☐ Your shoulders and chest may ache the first few days after surgery because carbon dioxide was placed inside your abdomen during surgery. This harmless gas will disappear in a few days. A frequent change in position will help relieve the ache.

☐ After surgery, you should

   ☐ shower at home _____,
   ☐ avoid sexual intercourse for _____ weeks,
   ☐ not douche for _____ weeks,
   ☐ not use tampons for _____ weeks.

☐ Generally, there is no change in menstrual pattern. If you were taking birth control pills, finish your present package before stopping them.

☐ You may have slight vaginal bleeding following the surgery due to the mechanics of the operation. If needed, use a sanitary pad at home.

☐ Telephone your doctor if you

   ☐ have heavy vaginal bleeding (soaking of 1 pad in an hour) or spot bleeding that lasts longer than 2 weeks;
   ☐ have severe abdominal pain;
   ☐ have redness, soreness, or swelling around your wound stitches;
   ☐ have a fever over 100°F;
   ☐ have drainage of fluid or pus from your surgery wound;
   ☐ smell a bad odor from your wound;
   ☐ have bleeding or oozing from your surgery wound;
   ☐ have pain that is not relieved by the medication prescribed by your doctor.

☐ The following instructions tell you how to care for your surgery wound.

_____
_____
_____
_____
_____
_____

☐ If you have an emergency and you cannot reach your doctor by telephone, go to an emergency room nearest your home.

☐ Follow the labeled instructions on the prescription medications ordered by your doctor.

OTHER INSTRUCTIONS:

_____
_____
_____
_____

☐ A nurse from the Outpatient Surgery Unit will telephone you a few days after surgery. The nurse will ask you questions about how you are feeling.

☐ Call Dr. _____ in _____
   ☐ day(s) ☐ week(s) ☐ month for an appointment.
   Your doctor's telephone numbers are:

   Office_____
   Exchange_____

I HAVE READ AND RECEIVED THE ABOVE INSTRUCTIONS.

_____
Patient

_____
Significant Other

_____
Nurse

_____
Date

FIGURE 5–25. Discharge instructions for laparoscopy patients. (Courtesy of Santa Rosa Hospital, San Antonio, TX. Copyright 1990, Santa Rosa Health Care Corporation, 519 West Houston Street, San Antonio, TX 78207. All rights reserved.)

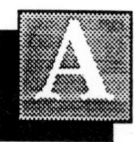# **A**dult Outpatient Surgery

INSTRUCCIONES PARA EL CUIDADO DESPUES DE LA LAPAROSCOPIA

❏ 1. Cuando vaya Ud. a casa hoy, debe guardar cama excepto para ir al baño con ayuda. Mañana puede estar levantado pero todavía debe descansar todo lo posible. Puede reanudar sus actividades normales con inclusión del ejercicio en _____ semanas.

❏ 2. Puede sentir dolor de garganta las primeras 24 horas (debido al tubo que le pasaron por la garganta durante el examen.)

❏ 3. Entere a su médico inmediatamente de cualquier dificultad en respirar o tragar, o de una hinchazón de la garganta.

❏ 4. Pueden haber dolores en los hombros y en el pecho a causa del dióxido de carbono que se le metió al abdomen; este gas no hace daño y desaparacerá en unos días. Los dolores pueden aliviarse cambiándose de posición con frecuencia.

❏ 5. Puede ducharse en casa _____.

❏ 6. Es preferible evitar las relaciones sexuales por _____ semanas.

❏ 7. Por lo general, no hay cambio en el ciclo menstrual. Si estaba tomando píldoras anticonceptivas, acabe con las que quedan antes de dejar de tomarlas.

❏ 8. Algunas veces hay una escasa salida de sangre de la vagina después de la intervención quirúrgica; si es necesario, continúe usando una toalla sanitaria en casa.

❏ 9. No se duche la vagina. No use tompones por _____ semanas.

❏ 10. Comunique calquier salida excesiva de sangre de la vagina (que empapa más de una toalla sanitaria por hora) o salida de sangre que dura más de dos semanas.

❏ 11. Informe al medico de todo dolor fuerte abdominal

❏ 12. Las puntadas ordinariamente se cubren con vendaje o curita. Siga estas instrucciones para el cuidado de las puntadas:

_____

_____ .

❏ 13. Entere al médico de todo signo de infección: pus, inflamación notable o enrojecimiento; calentura arriba de 100 grados F.; olor o derrame desagrables.

❏ 14. Si se presenta una emergencia y no puede conseguir al médico por teléfono, vaya a la sala de emergencia del Hospital Santa Rosa o a la más cercana.

Llame al Dr. _____
para fijar una cita en _____
días/semanas/meses, o para comunicar signos o
síntomas: _____
(consultorio) o _____ (central
telefónica).

_____
Firma del médico   Fecha

He leído y he recibido una copia de las instrucciones de arriba.

_____
Firma del paciente   Fecha

_____
Testigo/enfermera   Fecha

May 1989

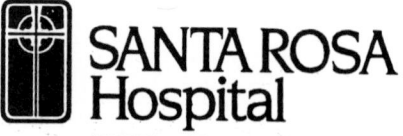
SANTA ROSA Hospital
519 West Houston Street
San Antonio, Texas 78207

FIGURE 5–26. Instrucciones para el cuidado después de la laparoscopia. (Courtesy of Santa Rosa Hospital, San Antonio, TX. Copyright 1990, Santa Rosa Health Care Corporation, 519 West Houston Street, San Antonio, TX 78207. All rights reserved.)

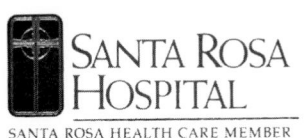

SANTA ROSA
HOSPITAL
SANTA ROSA HEALTH CARE MEMBER

Adult Outpatient Surgery

DISCHARGE INSTRUCTIONS FOR UPPER ENDOSCOPY PATIENTS

☐ During the procedure, in order to prevent gagging, your throat was sprayed with a "numbing" medication. DO NOT eat or drink for 1 or 2 hours and until you can feel yourself swallowing. Accidental choking may occur if you attempt to eat or drink before this medication wears off.

☐ Common side-effects of your examination include the following:

    ☐ sore throat;
    ☐ mild belching;
    ☐ mild abdominal soreness and bloating;
    ☐ mild tenderness at your IV site;
    ☐ spitting of small amounts of blood tinged saliva.

☐ Immediately telephone your doctor if any of the following occur:

    ☐ severe abdominal bloating, cramps, or pain;
    ☐ constant chest discomfort;
    ☐ fever or chills;
    ☐ body rash, hives, itching;
    ☐ nausea or vomiting;
    ☐ vomiting of bright red blood clots, or coffee ground material;
    ☐ pain with swelling, heat, and redness at your IV site or up your arm.

☐ If you have an emergency and you cannot reach your doctor by telephone, go to an emergency room nearest your home.

☐ Follow the labeled instructions on the prescription medications ordered by your doctor.

OTHER INSTRUCTIONS:

_____
_____
_____
_____

☐ A nurse from the Outpatient Surgery Unit will telephone you a few days after surgery. The nurse will ask you questions about how you are feeling.

☐ Call Dr. _____ in _____
    ☐ day(s) ☐ week(s) ☐ month for an appointment.
Your doctor's telephone numbers are:

    Office_____
    Exchange_____

I HAVE READ AND RECEIVED THE ABOVE INSTRUCTIONS.

_____
Patient

_____
Significant Other

_____
Nurse

_____
Date

FIGURE 5–27. Discharge instructions for upper endoscopy patients. (Courtesy of Santa Rosa Hospital, San Antonio, TX. Copyright 1990, Santa Rosa Health Care Corporation, 519 West Houston Street, San Antonio, TX 78207. All rights reserved.)

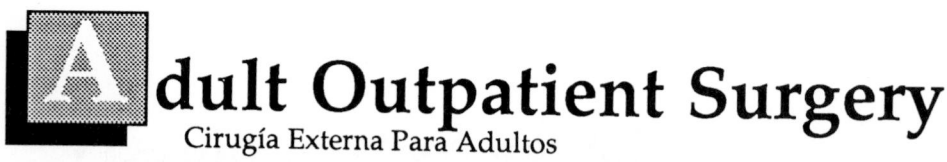

dult Outpatient Surgery

Cirugía Externa Para Adultos

INSTRUCCIONES PARA EL CUIDADO DEL PACIENTE DESPUES DE LA GASTROSCOPIA/ENDOSCOPIA/ DILATACION DEL ESOFAGO

Puede volver a sus actividades normales o al trabajo en _____ a menos que el médico indique de otra manera.

A causa del medicamento entumecedor que se le aplicó a la garganta para prevenir la náusea, no coma ni beba nada hasta que se le regrese la sensibilidad a la garganta. Puede sofocarse accidentalmente si trata de comer o beber antes que los efectos del medicamento hayan desaparecido.

Puede volver a su dieta normal en_____ _____ a menos que su médico le instruya de otra forma, p.ej.:

_____

_____

_____

Después del examen son muy comunes el dolor de garganta, el eructo, un leve dolor abdominal y un poco de hinchazón, un dolor en el sitio de la intravenosa, la expectoración de un poco de sangre y la saliva teñida de sangre.

Si se presenta cualquiera de los síntomas siguientes, llame al Dr. _____ inmediatamente o vaya a la sala de emergencia del Hospital Santa Rosa:

● intensa distensión abdominal o dolor o los dos
● molestia persistente en el pecho
● dificultad al respirar
● fiebre/escalofrío
● erupción general de la piel/urticaria/ comezón
● náusea/vómito
● vómito de sangre de color rojo subido, coágulos de sangre o de materia parecida al sedimento del café
● dolor acompañado de inflamación, calor y enrojecimiento en el sitio de la intravenosa

Llame al Dr. _____
par fijar una cita en _____.

OTRAS INSTRUCCIONES:

_____

_____

_____

He leído y he entendido las instrucciones de arriba para cuidarme en casa:

_____

Paciente
Tutor/otro (especifique):

_____

Fecha

_____

Enfermera

_____

Fecha

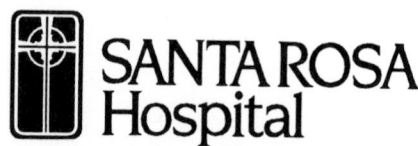

SANTA ROSA
Hospital
519 West Houston Street
San Antonio, Texas 78207

FIGURE 5–28. Instrucciones para el cuidado del paciente después de gastroscopia, endoscopia, o dilatacion del esofago. (Courtesy of Santa Rosa Hospital, San Antonio, TX. Copyright 1990, Santa Rosa Health Care Corporation, 519 West Houston Street, San Antonio, TX 78207. All rights reserved.)

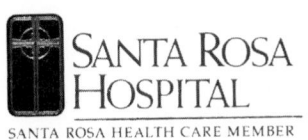

SANTA ROSA HOSPITAL
SANTA ROSA HEALTH CARE MEMBER

Adult Outpatient Surgery

DISCHARGE INSTRUCTIONS FOR COLONOSCOPY PATIENTS

☐ Common side-effects of your examination include the following:

   ☐ sore rectum;
   ☐ passing of flatus or gas from your rectum;
   ☐ mild abdominal bloating;
   ☐ passing of a small amount of blood, tinged mucous or stool;
   ☐ mild tenderness at your IV site.

☐ Immediately telephone your doctor if any of the following occur:

   ☐ severe abdominal cramping, pain, or bloating;
   ☐ fever or chills;
   ☐ nausea or vomiting;
   ☐ body rash, hives, or itching;
   ☐ passage of bright red blood, blood clots, or large amounts of dark or black stools;
   ☐ sudden constant diarrhea;
   ☐ pain with swelling, heat, and redness at your IV site or up your arm.

☐ If you have an emergency and you cannot reach your doctor by telephone, go to an emergency room nearest your home.

☐ Follow the labeled instructions on the prescription medications ordered by your doctor.

OTHER INSTRUCTIONS:

_____
_____
_____
_____
_____

☐ A nurse from the Outpatient Surgery Unit will telephone you a few days after surgery. The nurse will ask you questions about how you are feeling.

☐ Call Dr. _____ in _____
  ☐ day(s) ☐ week(s) ☐ month for an appointment.
Your doctor's telephone numbers are:

Office_____
Exchange_____

I HAVE READ AND RECEIVED THE ABOVE INSTRUCTIONS.

_____
Patient

_____
Significant Other

_____
Nurse

_____
Date

FIGURE 5–29. Discharge instructions for colonoscopy patients. (Courtesy of Santa Rosa Hospital, San Antonio, TX. Copyright 1990, Santa Rosa Health Care Corporation, 519 West Houston Street, San Antonio, TX 78207. All rights reserved.)

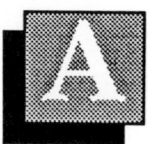

Adult Outpatient Surgery
Cirugía Externa Para Adultos

INSTRUCCIONES PARA EL CUIDADO DESPUES DE UNA COLONSCOPIA/POLIPECTOMIA/SIGMOIDOSCOPIA FLEXIBLE

Puede volver a sus actividades normales o al trabajo en _____ a menos que su médico le instruya de otra manera.

Puede volver a su dieta normal a menos que su médico le instruya de otra forma, p.e.j. _____

_____

_____

Después de este examen, Ud. puede sentir dolor en el recto, pasar flato o gas del recto, tener un poco de hinchazón abdominal, pasar un poco de sangre, mocos o excremento teñidos, y sentir un leve dolor en el sitio de la intravenosa.

Si se presenta cualquiera de los síntomas siguientes, llame al Dr. _____
de inmediato, o vaya a la sala de emergencia del Hospital Santa Rosa:

- ● calambres abdominales, dolor o distensión fuertes
- ● fiebre/escalofrío
- ● náusea/vómito
- ● erupción general de la piel/urticaria/comezón
- ● derrame de sangre de color rojo subido, coágulos de sangre o mucho excremento oscuro o negro
- ● diarrea repentina/persistente
- ● dolor/calor/enrojecimiento/inflamación en el sitio de la intravenosa o por la parte superior del brazo

Llame al consultorio del Dr. _____ para una cita complementaria en _____
_____.

Otros datos: _____
_____
_____.

He leído y entiendo las instrucciones de arriba pertinentes al cuidado en casa.

_____   _____
Paciente   Fecha
Tutor/otro (especifique):

_____   _____
Enfermera   Fecha

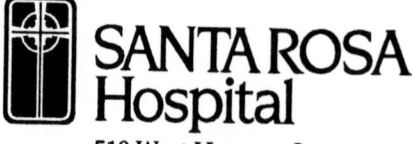

SANTA ROSA Hospital
519 West Houston Street
San Antonio, Texas 78207

FIGURE 5–30. Instrucciones para el cuidao después de una colonscopia, polipectomia, sigmoidoscopia flexible. (Courtesy of Santa Rosa Hospital, San Antonio, TX. Copyright 1990, Santa Rosa Health Care Corporation, 519 West Houston Street, San Antonio, TX 78207. All rights reserved.)

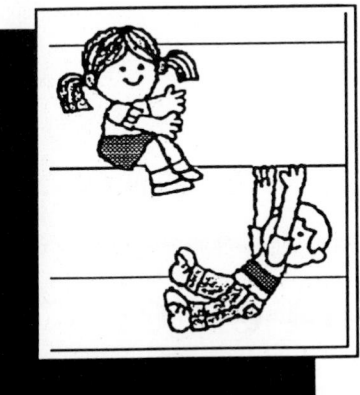

Children's
Out-Patient Surgery ©

HOME INSTRUCTIONS: DENTAL REHABILITATION

Your child has had dental surgery today under general anesthesia at Children's Hospital. We hope the following information and suggestions will be helpful to you as you care for your child at home.

Care of your child's mouth:

- Rinse mouth with tepid water after food and drink. May have difficulty with very cold or hot foods.
- May gently brush teeth tomorrow morning.
- Do not put straws or any foreign objects in the mouth as this may dislodge the clot that begins the healing process.
- Avoid spicy and hard/crunchy foods for 2-3 days.

Observe your child:

- Pink-tinged saliva is normal for about 2 days after the surgery. Notify your doctor for any bright red bleeding.
- Some swelling of the face or lips is normal for about 2 days after surgery. Notify your doctor for any swelling that does not subside.
- Your child may complain of a headache or soreness of the mouth or throat.
- Your child may be sleepy and fussy or complain of an upset stomach from the anesthesia today.

Pain, soreness of the mouth, irritability or a temperature over 102° rectally or 101° orally can be relieved with Tylenol. If pain or temperature is not relieved with Tylenol, or if it lasts longer than 48 hours, notify your doctor. DO NOT USE ASPIRIN PRODUCTS.

See Dr. _____ on _____ at _____ AM/PM.

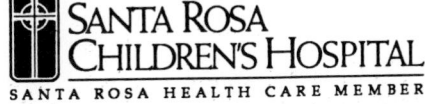

SANTA ROSA
CHILDREN'S HOSPITAL
SANTA ROSA HEALTH CARE MEMBER

519 West Houston Street San Antonio, Texas 78207
(512) 228-2011

© 1990, Santa Rosa Health Care Corporation, San Antonio, TX. All rights reserved.

078600 (8/92)

FIGURE 5–31. Home instructions for dental rehabilitation for pediatric patients. (Courtesy of Santa Rosa Children's Hospital, San Antonio, TX. Copyright 1990, Santa Rosa Health Care Corporation, 519 West Houston Street, San Antonio, TX 78207. All rights reserved.)

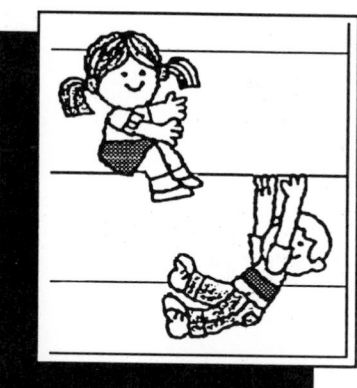

Cirugía Externa en el Hospital de Niños©

INSTRUCCIONES PARA EL CUIDADO EN CASA: RESTABLECIMIENTO DENTAL

Hoy se le hizo una cirugía dental a su niño bajo anestesia local en el Hospital de Niños. Esperamos que los datos y consejos siguientes le sirvan de ayuda con el cuidado de su niño en casa.

Cuidado de la boca de su niño:
● Enjuague la boca con agua tibia después de que coma o beba el niño. Puede tener dificultad con la comida muy caliente o muy fría.
● Puede lavarse suavemente los dientes mañana por la mañana.
● No le metan popotes ni otros objectos a la boca, porque pueden soltar el coágulo que inicia la curación.
● Evite la comida picosa/quebradiza por 2-3 días.

Observe a su niño:
● La saliva teñida de sangre es normal por más o menos 2 días a partir de la intervención quirúrgica. Avise a su médico en caso de cualquier salida de sangre de color rojo subido.
● Es normal cierta hinchazón de la cara o de los labios por aproximadamente 2 días a partir de la cirugía. Avise a su médico en el caso de toda hinchazón que no se resuelva.
● Su niño puede quejarse de un dolor de cabeza o de la boca o de la garganta.
● Su niño puede tener sueño y estar irritado o puede quejarse de tener el estómago trastornado después de la anestesia de hoy.

Pueden aliviarse con Tylenol los dolores de la boca, irritabilidad o la fiebre de 102° rectal o de 101° oral. En caso de que no se alivien el dolor y la fiebre con Tylenol, o si ésta dura más de 48 horas, avise a su médico. NO DEJE QUE SU NIÑO TOME ASPIRINA NI OTROS MEDICAMENTOS QUE TIENEN ASPIRINA.

Vea al Dr. _____ el _____ a la(s) _____ AM/PM.

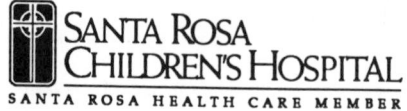

SANTA ROSA HEALTH CARE MEMBER

519 West Houston Street San Antonio, Texas 78207
(512) 228-2011

FIGURE 5–32. Instrucciones para el cuidado en casa restablecimiento dental para los niños. (Courtesy of Santa Rosa Children's Hospital, San Antonio, TX. Copyright 1990, Santa Rosa Health Care Corporation, 519 West Houston Street, San Antonio, TX 78207. All rights reserved.)

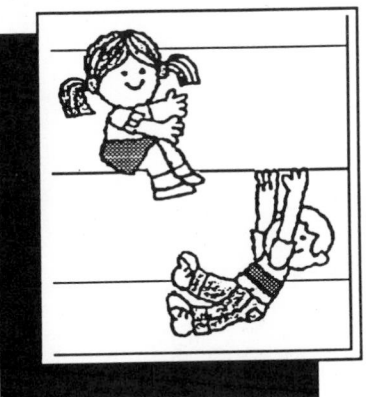

Children's Out-Patient Surgery ©

HOME INSTRUCTIONS: MYRINGOTOMY WITH TUBES

Your child had surgery today at Children's Hospital. The purpose of the tubes are:

- To prevent accumulation of fluid in the middle ear.
- To prevent recurring ear infections.
- To prevent hearing loss.
- To enable air to pass back and forth behind the eardrum and relieve pressure.

Care of your child:
- DO NOT let water get into the child's ears.
- When bathing, shampooing hair, or washing face, use ear plugs or cotton balls covered with vasoline to protect the inner ear.
- NO SWIMMING, until tubes are removed after 6-12 months.
- DO NOT allow your child to place fingers or objects in ears.
- Your child may continue normal activity such as school the next day following surgery.
- Cortisporin Optic Solution may also be prescribed for ears (3-4 drops as specified by your doctor.)

Observe your child:
- A slight amount of blood tinged or purulent drainage may occur the first two days after surgery. Notify your doctor if this drainage occurs longer than two days after surgery.

Pain, irratability or temperature over 102° rectally or 101° orally can be relieved with Tylenol. If pain or temperature is not relieved with Tylenol, or if it lasts longer than 48 hours, notify your doctor.
DO NOT USE ASPIRIN PRODUCTS.

See Dr. _____ on _____ at _____ AM/PM.

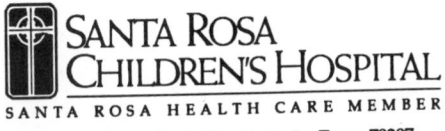

SANTA ROSA CHILDREN'S HOSPITAL
SANTA ROSA HEALTH CARE MEMBER
519 West Houston Street San Antonio, Texas 78207
(512) 228-2011

078650 (8/92)

FIGURE 5–33. Home instructions for myringotomy with tubes for pediatric patients. (Courtesy of Santa Rosa Children's Hospital, San Antonio, TX. Copyright 1990, Santa Rosa Health Care Corporation, 519 West Houston Street, San Antonio, TX 78207. All rights reserved.)

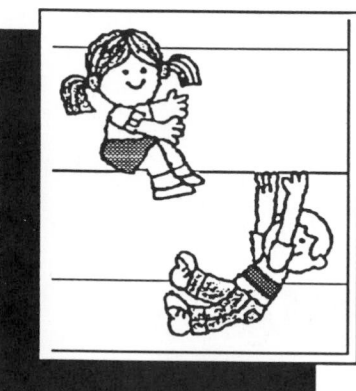

Cirugia Externa en el Hospital de Niños©

INSTRUCCIONES PARA EL CUIDADO EN CASA: MIRINGOTOMIA CON TUBOS

Hoy se le operó a su niño en el Hospital de Niños. El fin de los tubos es:
- prevenir la acumulación de fluido el oído medio.
- prevenir las infecciones crónicas del oído.
- prevenir la pérdida del sentido del oído.
- permitir que el aire tenga paso por detrás del tímpano para aliviar la presión.

Cuidado de su niño:
- NO DEJE meterse el agua a los oídos de su niño.
- Al bañarse o al lavarse el pelo con champú, o al lavarse la cara, utilice tapones o bolitas de algodón cubiertas de vaselina para proteger el oído interno.
- NO PUEDE NADAR hasta que se le quiten los tubos a los 6-12 meses después de la intervención quirúrgica.
- NO DEJE que su niño se meta los dedos o otros objectos a los oídos.
- Su niño puede continuar con sus activitades normales tales como la escuela a partir del día siguiente de la cirugía.
- Es posible que se recete la solución ótica Cortisporin para los oídos (3-4 gotas según especifica su médico).

Observe a su niño:
- Puede haber un desagüe teñido de sangre o un desagüe purulento durante los primeros dos días a partir de la intervención quirúrgica. Avise a su médico en caso de que continúe por mas de dos días después de la operación.

Pueden aliviarse el dolor, irritabilidad o fiebre arriba de 102° rectal o 101° oral con Tylenol. Si no se alivia el dolor ni la fiebre con Tylenol, o si ésta dura más de 48 horas, avise a su médico. NO DEJE QUE SU NIÑO TOME ASPIRINA NI OTROS MEDICAMENTOS QUE TIENEN ASPIRINA.

Vea al Dr. _____ el _____ a la(s) _____ AM/PM.

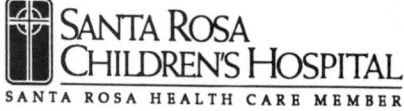

SANTA ROSA HEALTH CARE MEMBER

519 West Houston Street San Antonio, Texas 78207
(512) 228-2011

FIGURE 5–34. Instrucciones para el cuidado en casa miringotomia con tubos para los niños. (Courtesy of Santa Rosa Children's Hospital, San Antonio, TX. Copyright 1990, Santa Rosa Health Care Corporation, 519 West Houston Street, San Antonio, TX 78207. All rights reserved.)

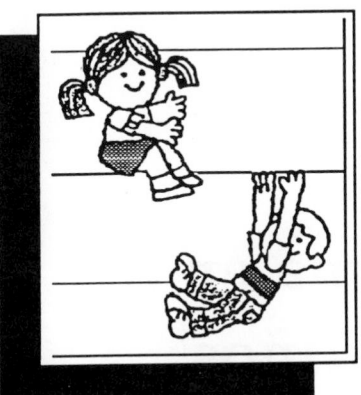

Children's
Out-Patient Surgery©

HOME INSTRUCTIONS: CIRCUMCISION

Your child had surgery today at Children's Hospital. We hope the following information and suggestions will be helpful for you as you care for your child at home.

C are of your child:
- Keep the surgical area clean. The penis will be swollen and reddened. Put diapers on baby loosely. Older children should wear loose fitting clothes such as pajamas or jogging pants. When holding your child carry him sideways with legs spread apart.
- Remove the original dressing after the first voiding (may be soaked off) on the day of operation.
- Wash the incision after each diaper change or after each voiding and apply the antibiotic ointment to the incision and the entire "head" of the penis, for at least 7-10 days.
- The "crusting" that occurs around the sutures is usual and expected. This will go away with continued cleaning after several days. Do not try to remove it all at one time.
- There are no sutures to be removed - the special sutures will begin to "dissolve" sometime after 7-10 days.

O bserve the wound as it heals:
- Call your doctor if it appears red, warm, puffy, or has any odor or drainage (white, green or yellow liquid).
- Call your doctor for any active bleeding from the penis. Firmly press sterile gauze around the penis for 10 minutes, then release pressure. If bleeding persists, call the doctor and keep applying pressure. Blood may ooze from the penis when clotted blood is disturbed by clothing or bed linen.

P ain, irritabilty or a temperature over 102˚ rectally or 101˚ orally can be relieved with Typenol. If pain or temperature is not relieved with Tylenol, or if it lasts longer than 48 hours, notify your doctor. DO NOT USE ASPIRIN PRODUCTS

S ports activities:
- He may engage in normal, level, on-the-ground activity for his age.
- Do not engage in sports activities for at least 4 weeks after the operation; he may swim after 1 week (no diving).
- He should NOT ride a bike, tricycle, or skateboard for at least 4 weeks after the operation.

Your next appointment with Dr. _____ is: _____ at _____ AM/PM.

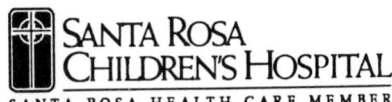

SANTA ROSA HEALTH CARE MEMBER

519 West Houston Street San Antonio, Texas 78207
(512) 228-2011

078750 (8/92)

FIGURE 5–35. Home instructions for circumcision for pediatric patients. (Courtesy of Santa Rosa Children's Hospital, San Antonio, TX. Copyright 1990, Santa Rosa Health Care Corporation, 519 West Houston Street, San Antonio, TX 78207. All rights reserved.)

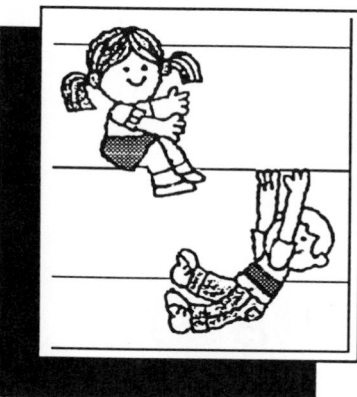

Cirugia Externa en el Hospital de Niños©

INSTRUCCIONES PARA EL CUIDADO EN CASA: CIRCUNCISION

Hoy se le operó a su niño en el Hospital de Niños. Esperamos que los datos y consejos siguientes le sirvan de ayuda con el cuidado de su niño en casa.

Cuidado de su niño:

● Mantenga limpia la región operada. El pene va a estar hinchado y colorado. Póngale los pañales al bebé de manera que le queden flojos. Los niños mayores deben usar ropa floja como piyamas o pantalones de ejercicio. Al cargar a su niño llévelo de lado con las piernas abiertas.

● Quite la venda original después de la primera orinada (puedee mojarse para que se quite más fácilmente el día de la operación).

● Lave la incisión después de cada cambio de pañal o después de cada orinada y aplique el ungüento antibiótico a la incisión y a la cabeza del pene, al menos por 7-10 días.

● La costra que aparece alrededor de las suturas es de esperarse y es normal. Desaparecerá dentro de varios días con la limpiada continua. No trate de quitarla toda de una vez.

● No hay ningunas suturas que quitarse-las suturas comenzarán a disolverse después de un período de 7-10 días.

Observe la herida conforme que se vaya sanando:

● Llame al médico si está colorada, caliente al tocarse, hinchada, o si hay olor o desangüe (líquido blanco, verde o amarillo).

● Llame al médico en caso de que haya una salida constante de sangre del pene.Apriete una grasa esterilizada alrededor del miembro por 10 minutos, luego alfoje la presión. Si persiste la salida de sangre, llame al médico y continúe aplicando presión. La sangre puede exudar del pene cuando la ropa o las sábanas agitan los coágulos.

Pueden aliviarse con Tylenol el dolor, irritabilidad o fiebre arriba de 102° rectal o 101° oral. Si el dolor o fiebre no se alivia con Tylenol, o si ésta dura más de 48 horas, avise al medico. NO DEJE QUE SU NIÑO TOME ASPIRINA NI OTROS MEDICAMENTOS QUE TIENEN ASPIRINA.

Actividades deportivas:

● Puede participar en actividades apropiadas para su edad.

● No puede participar en actividades deportivas por un mínimo de 4 semanas después de un semana (sin hacer clavados).

● NO debe andar en bicicleta, tricicleta o patines por un mínimo de 4 semanas después de la operacíon.

Vea al Dr. _____ el _____ a la(s) _____ AM/PM

SANTA ROSA CHILDREN'S HOSPITAL
SANTA ROSA HEALTH CARE MEMBER
519 West Houston Street San Antonio, Texas 78207
(512) 228-2011

FIGURE 5–36. Instrucciones para el cuidado en casa circuncision para los niños. (Courtesy of Santa Rosa Children's Hospital, San Antonio, TX. Copyright 1990, Santa Rosa Health Care Corporation, 519 West Houston Street, San Antonio, TX 78207. All rights reserved.)

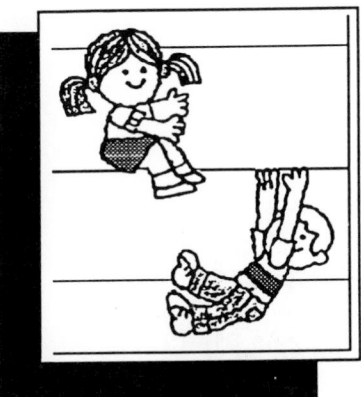

Children's Out-Patient Surgery ©

HOME INSTRUCTIONS: CYSTOSCOPY

Dr. _____ has examined the inside of your child's bladder today by cystoscopy while your child was under general anesthesia at Children's Hospital.

Care of your child:

- Your child may be more comfortable urinating into a tub of clean warm water.

- Perineal care for girls: Clean around the urethra after each urination. Wipe in the direction of front to back and discard paper. Use a clean toilet paper each time you wipe.

Observe your child for:

- Slight bleeding on urination due to the stretching of the urethreal wall by the cystoscopy. Call your doctor if there is an increase of blood in the urine, or if there is still blood in the urine after 2 days.

- A burning sensation with urination due to the cystoscopy, which may persist for 1-2 days.

- Sleepiness and fussiness or complaints of an upset stomach from the anesthesia today.

Pain, irritability or a temperature over 102° rectally or 101° orally can be relieved with Tylenol. If pain or temperature is not relieved with Tylenol, or if it lasts longer than 48 hours, notify the doctor. DO NOT USE ASPIRIN PRODUCTS.

See Dr. _____ on _____ at _____ AM/PM.

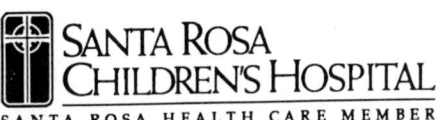

SANTA ROSA CHILDREN'S HOSPITAL
SANTA ROSA HEALTH CARE MEMBER

519 West Houston Street San Antonio, Texas 78207
(512) 228-2011

078550 (8/92)
FIGURE 5–37. Home instructions for cystoscopy for pediatric patients. (Courtesy of Santa Rosa Children's Hospital, San Antonio, TX. Copyright 1990, Santa Rosa Health Care Corporation, 519 West Houston Street, San Antonio, TX 78207. All rights reserved.)

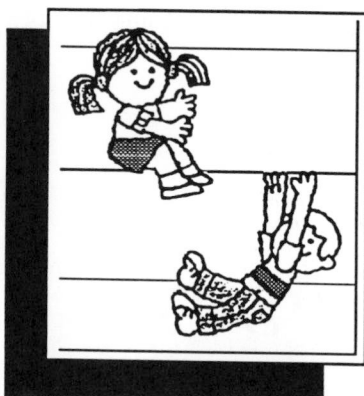

Cirugia Externa en el Hospital de Niños©

INSTRUCCIONES PARA EL CUIDADO EN CASA DESPUES DE LA CISTOSCOPIA

El Dr. _____ ha examinado el interior de la vejiga de su niño hoy mediante la cistoscopia mientras su niño estaba bajo anestesia general en el Hospital de Niños.

Cuidado de su niño:

● Su niño puede estar más a gusto orinando en una tina de agua clara tibia.
● Cuidado perineal de las niñas: Limpie alrededor de la uretra después de cada vez que orina la niña. Frote de adelante para atrás y deseche el papel. Utilice siempre un trozo limpio de papel sanitario al frotar.

Esté atento para estos signos:

● Una salida de sangre al orinar debido a la dilatación de la pared uretral mediante la cistoscopia. Llame a su médico si hay aumento de sangre en la orina, o si todavía hay sangre en la orina después de dos días.
● Una sensación de quemazón al orinar debido a la cistoscopia, que puede durar de 1-2 días.
● Sueño y irritabilidad o quejitas de tener el estómago trastornado después de la anestesia de hoy.

Pueden aliviarse el dolor, irritabilidad o fiebre arriba de 102° rectal o 101° oral con Tylenol. En caso de que el dolor o la fiebre no se alivien con Tylenol, o si ésata dura más de 48 horas, avise al médico. NO DEJE QUE SU NIÑO TOME ASPIRINA NO OTROS MEDICAMENTOS QUE TIENEN ASPIRINA.

Vea al Dr. _____ el _____ a la(s) _____ AM/PM.

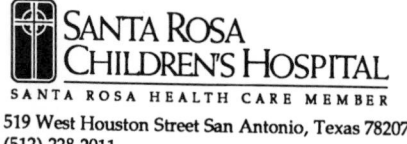

SANTA ROSA CHILDREN'S HOSPITAL
SANTA ROSA HEALTH CARE MEMBER
519 West Houston Street San Antonio, Texas 78207
(512) 228-2011

FIGURE 5–38. Instrucciones para el cuidado en casa después de la cistoscopia para los niños. (Courtesy of Santa Rosa Children's Hospital, San Antonio, TX. Copyright 1990, Santa Rosa Health Care Corporation, 519 West Houston Street, San Antonio, TX 78207. All rights reserved.)

Teaching has been effective if the patient and family members can demonstrate knowledge of coping mechanisms that can be used in response to surgical intervention. The patient and/or family members should be able to

- verbalize expectations about pain relief
- state the measures that can be taken to alleviate pain
- identify family and community support systems (Kneedler, 1987)

Teaching has been effective if the patient and family members can demonstrate knowledge about how to participate in the rehabilitation process after surgery. The patient and/or family members should be able to

- cite the reasons for each of the preoperative instructions provided and exercises explained or practiced
- demonstrate turning, coughing, deep breathing, incision splinting, passive leg exercising, and ambulating
- describe anticipated steps in postoperative activity resumption (Kneedler, 1987)

DOCUMENTATION AND COMMUNICATION PROCEDURES

Patient and family teaching is communicated to appropriate health care team members and documented in the patient's record. Special attention should be paid to informing nursing unit personnel about teaching activities for surgical patients. Subsequent teaching by nursing unit personnel should reinforce teaching activities by the perioperative nurse.

Bibliography

Association of Operating Room Nurses (1992). Basic competency statements. In *Standards and recommended practices for perioperative nursing.* (I:2–8 and II:7–1) Denver.

Atkinson, L. J., Kohn, M. L. (1986). *Berry and Kohn's introduction to operating room technique* (6th ed.) (pp. 72–73). New York: McGraw-Hill.

Carnevali, D. (1966). Preoperative anxiety. *American Journal of Nursing, 1,* 1536–1538.

Devine, E. (1985). Recommended elements of surgical patient education based on current research. In *Surgical patient education does make a difference* (Vol. 4, pp. 21–25). Chicago: American Hospital Association.

Flaherty, J., Fitzpatrick, J. (Nov/Dec 1978). Relaxation technique to increase comfort level of postoperative patients. *Nursing Research* (27), 352–355.

Gordon, M. (1987). *Manual of nursing diagnosis.* New York: McGraw-Hill.

Healy, K. (1968). Does preoperative instruction make a difference? *American Journal of Nursing 68*(1), 62–67.

Kneedler, J. A., Dodge, G. H. (1987). *Perioperative patient care* (2nd ed.) (p. 132). Boston: Blackwell Scientific.

Lindeman, C., Van Acrnam, B. (1971). Nursing intervention with the presurgical patient: The affects of structured and unstructured preoperative teaching. *Nursing Research, 20*(1), 35–42.

Moss, R. (1986). Overcoming fear: A review of research on patient and family instruction. *AORN Journal, 43*(5), 1107–1114.

Toth, S. (1983). *Patient teaching: A nursing process approach instructors guide.* Westport, CT: J. B. Lippincott.

CHAPTER 6

Creating and Maintaining a Sterile Field

Patricia A. Mews

DEFINITION

Creating and maintaining a sterile environment during the surgical procedure minimizes the patient's risk of acquiring a postoperative wound infection. A patient's first line of defense against infection is the skin. Surgery or trauma compromises that line of defense by creating an entry for microorganisms. The most important measure in preventing postoperative wound infection is the application of flawless aseptic technique principles. It is crucial that the entire surgical team be responsible for maintaining asepsis during surgical intervention. The perioperative nursing team reduces or eliminates microorganisms from the patient's immediate surgical environment by establishing and maintaining a sterile field. During surgery, the perioperative nursing team performs actions aimed at preventing the introduction of microorganisms that are present in the environment surrounding the patient. Diligent application of the principles of asepsis and the nursing actions listed as measurable criteria for this competency reduce the patient's risk of acquiring a postoperative wound infection.

134

MEASURABLE CRITERIA

The perioperative nurse demonstrates competency to create and maintain a sterile field by

- donning surgical attire
- performing the surgical hand scrub
- donning sterile gown and gloves
- preparing a sterile field
- performing preoperative skin preparation
- draping the patient and equipment

ROLE OF THE PERIOPERATIVE NURSE

Creating and maintaining the sterile field is the responsibility of the perioperative nurse. All members of the surgical team must be knowledgeable of and adhere to aseptic technique principles. Depending on the circumstances of a particular institution, others, such as the surgeon, may participate in this activity during the preparation or draping procedures. However, the perioperative nurse monitors the implementation of aseptic technique principles by all surgical team members and ensures that breaks in technique are corrected.

CONSIDERATIONS

The *Standards and Recommended Practices for Perioperative Nursing* (Association of Operating Room Nurses [AORN], 1992) provides guidelines for creating and maintaining a sterile field. Knowledge of these recommended practices facilitates performance of this competency. Specific recommended practices that address issues germane to creating and maintaining a sterile field are those related to

- basic aseptic technique
- traffic patterns in the surgical suite
- evaluation of aseptic barrier materials for surgical gowns and drapes
- sterilization and disinfection
- selection and use of packaging materials
- preoperative skin preparation of patients
- surgical attire
- surgical hand scrub

The perioperative nurse approaches the creation and maintenance of a sterile field from a holistic point of view. In addition to ensuring accessibility of the operative site and preventing the transfer of microorganisms from the surgical team and the surrounding environment to the sterile field, the perioperative nurse ensures that the process of creating and maintaining the sterile field does not adversely affect the patient's respiratory patterns, skin integrity, body temperature, and self-esteem.

OUTCOME STANDARD

Creating and maintaining a sterile field does not compromise or cause injury to the patient.

Criteria

The patient is free from evidence of

- postoperative wound infection
- impaired skin integrity
- hyperthermia
- hypothermia
- ineffective breathing patterns
- disturbed self-esteem

POTENTIAL ALTERATIONS IN FUNCTIONAL HEALTH PATTERNS

Health Perception–Health Management Pattern

Diagnosis

High risk for wound infection

Definition

Presence of risk factors for the patient to acquire a postoperative wound infection

Risk Factors (Gordon, 1987, p. 50)

- Impaired skin integrity
- Impaired tissue integrity
- Altered tissue perfusion
- Decreased hemoglobin concentration, leukopenia, and suppressed inflammatory response
- Immunosuppression
- Inadequate acquired immunity
- Existing infection
- Increased environmental exposure due to the length of surgery
- Break in aseptic technique
- Improper wearing of surgical attire resulting in shedding of or spraying of microorganisms from the surgical team into the sterile field

Expected Outcome

The patient is free from wound infection 72 hours postoperatively.

Criteria

Depending on the patient's physical status and the designated wound classification at the time of surgery, the patient shows no evidence of

- cellulitis
- abscess
- lymphangitis
- gas gangrene
- Meleney ulcer
- dehiscence (Rothrock, 1987, pp. 191–192)

Nutritional-Metabolic Pattern

Diagnosis

High risk for impaired skin integrity

Definition

Presence of risk factors for skin disruption or breakdown, particularly around the operative site

Risk Factors (Gordon, 1987, p. 84)

- Impaired tissue perfusion at the operative site
- Allergy or sensitivity to the prepping solution
- Allergy or sensitivity to an adhesive agent in the draping materials
- Obesity
- Gross underweight
- Poor skin turgor
- Pooling of prepping solutions
- Improper application of towel clips

Expected Outcome

The patient's skin integrity is not impaired by the creation and maintenance of the sterile field.

Criteria

The patient is free from evidence of

- puncture of the skin surface by towel clips
- disruption of the skin surface by adhesive drapes
- breakdown of the skin surface related to pooled prepping solution

Diagnosis

High risk for hyperthermia during the surgical procedure

Definition

Presence of risk factors for the patient to experience an elevated body temperature during the intraoperative period

Risk Factors (Gordon, 1987, p. 96)

- Existing hyperthermia (fever)
- Patient illness or trauma
- Dehydration
- Low tolerance for heat-retaining devices (blankets)
- Decreased ability to perspire
- Ineffective air-conditioning system in the operating room
- Overapplication of sterile plastic drapes

Expected Outcome

The patient's body temperature is maintained within normal limits during the intraoperative period.

Criteria

The patient is free from evidence of

- an intraoperative increase in body temperature, above the normal range

- flushed skin during the intraoperative period
- increased intraoperative respiratory rate, particularly in nonventilated patients
- intraoperative tachycardia
- intraoperative seizure or convulsions (Gordon, 1987, p. 96)

Diagnosis

High risk for hypothermia during the surgical procedure

Definition

Presence of risk factors for the patient to experience a decreased body temperature during the intraoperative period

Risk Factors (Gordon, 1987, p. 98)

- Existing hypothermia
- Impaired skin integrity
- Low body weight (malnutrition)
- Age—very young or very old
- Inability to shiver
- Decreased metabolic rate
- Low temperature in the operating room (OR)
- Limited application of covers
- Cold solutions such as intravenous fluids, skin preparation solutions, and wound irrigation solutions
- Medication causing vasodilation

Expected Outcome

The patient's body temperature is maintained within normal limits during the intraoperative period.

Criteria

The patient is free from evidence of

- low temperature
- shivering
- cold skin
- mental confusion
- decreased pulse and respirations (Gordon, 1987, p. 98)

Activity-Exercise Pattern

Diagnosis

High risk for ineffective breathing patterns

Definition

Presence of risk factors that affect the patient's respiratory efforts to maintain sufficient oxygenation of the lungs, particularly in the nonventilated patient

Risk Factors (Gordon, 1987, p. 154)

- Type of anesthesia (local, regional, spinal, or general)
- Neuromuscular impairment
- Musculoskeletal impairment
- Anxiety related to surgery
- Intraoperative pain secondary to the incision or positioning
- Perceptual or cognitive impairment
- Claustrophobia
- Drapes covering a nonventilated patient's face
- Nonfunctioning oxygen delivery devices (masks, nasal prongs)

Expected Outcome

The patient's breathing patterns are maintained during the intraoperative period.

Criteria

The patient is free from evidence of

- shortness of breath or dyspnea
- use of accessory muscle to breathe
- altered chest excursions
- tachypnea
- nasal flaring
- pursed-lip breathing or a prolonged expiration phase
- patient statements indicating respiratory difficulty (Gordon, 1987, p. 154)

Self-perception—Self-concept Pattern

Diagnosis

High risk for self-esteem disturbance

Definition

Presence of risk factors for the patient to experience negative feelings or conception of self related to body exposure, particularly during the preparation and draping procedure (Gordon, 1987, p. 218)

Risk Factors

- Cultural or religious beliefs (i.e., prohibitions against nudity in presence of opposite sex)
- Location of operative site such as genitalia or breasts for female patients
- Type of anesthesia (local, regional, or spinal)
- Derogatory comments or joking by the staff concerning the patient's appearance, weight, or physical condition
- Mixed gender of the staff
- Unnecessary traffic flow in the OR

Expected Outcome

The patient is free from negative feelings or conception of self during the preparation and draping for the surgical procedure.

Criteria

The patient shows no evidence of

- verbal expressions of anxiety or shame during the operative preparation or draping procedure
- restlessness, increased perspiration, facial tension, clenched hands, or shakiness in the extremities (Gordon, 1987, p. 202)

PERIOPERATIVE NURSING INTERVENTIONS

Donning Surgical Attire (AORN, 1992, III:3–1—3–5)

The surgical team is an environmental risk factor in the patient's potential for acquiring a postoperative wound infection. Microorganisms are constantly being shed from exposed skin, hair, and mucous membranes, therefore head covers, masks, scrub attire, and gowns are used as barriers to decrease shedding into the air and prevent wound contamination. Wearing proper surgical attire attenuates the risk of microorganism shedding and spraying by placing a physical barrier between the patient and the surgical team, thus reducing the amount of microorganisms introduced into the sterile field. Donning proper surgical attire is a requirement for all personnel entering the semirestricted and restricted areas of the OR. The surgical suite is divided into three designated areas. The *unrestricted area* includes a control point where both OR personnel and other members of the health care facility communicate. Street clothes are permitted in this area. The *semirestricted area* includes the peripheral support areas (i.e., hallways, storage areas, processing areas, OR offices). Scrub attire and caps are required in semirestricted areas. The *restricted area* includes the area where surgical procedures are performed and where unwrapped supplies are sterilized (i.e., clean core, substerile areas). Scrub attire, caps, and masks are required in this area. (AORN, 1992, III:3–1 and 22–1—22–3).

The perioperative nurse is responsible for ensuring that personnel in these areas comply with the policies governing surgical attire. In this role, the perioperative nurse intervenes on behalf of the patient to meet the expected outcomes identified for the potentially dysfunctional health patterns associated with this competency.

Considerations

Good hygiene, including daily bathing and frequent hair washing, by surgical team members is an essential variable in controlling the amount of microorganisms introduced into the patient's immediate surgical environment. Team members with an infectious disease, such as an upper respiratory tract illness, skin lesions, boils, and infected lesions, should not participate in direct patient care activities and should be prohibited in the restricted area of the surgical suite.

Supplies and Equipment

Dressing properly for the OR requires a scrub top and pants that are easy to don and remove, a long-sleeved warm-up jacket for unscrubbed personnel to minimize shedding from bare arms, a disposable bouffant hat or hood, shoe covers, protective eyewear, and a disposable mask (Figs. 6–1 and 6–2). Surgical attire should be made of fabrics that meet or exceed the requirements of the National Fire Protection Agency regulations and be laundered after each use in the hospital's laundry facilities (AORN, 1992, *III*:3–1). Disposable surgical hats and hoods should be comfortable, lint free, and made of a soft fabric. Protective eyewear should be worn during all surgical procedures owing to the uncontrollability of body fluid splashes.

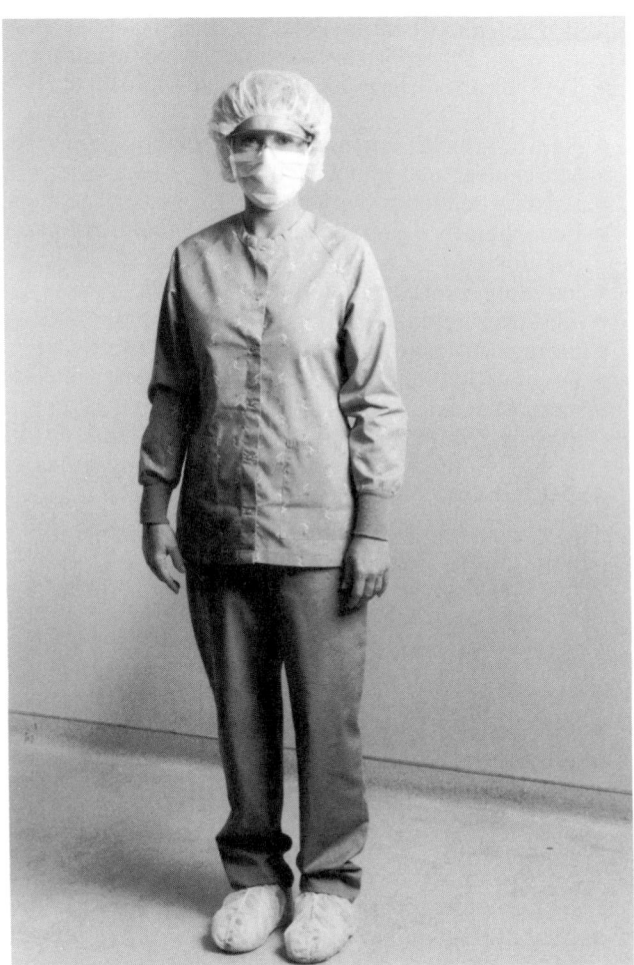

FIGURE 6–2. Female OR attire.

The perioperative nurse should select a mask on the basis of the documented quality of microorganism filtration and comfort. An acceptable mask has at least a 95% efficiency rating. Mask designs include the pleated mask with pliable nosepiece, the cone-shaped mask with elastic band, the antifog mask that is worn with glasses, the laser mask that helps protect against laser plume contaminants, and the fluid shield mask with a splash guard visor to protect the wearer against body fluid splashes and aerosolization.

Procedure

1. Obtain a clean scrub top, pants, and a disposable hat or hood. Select a top and pants for proper fit and comfort (see Figs. 6–1 and 6–2). Tight-fitting OR attire rubs against the body surfaces and may increase the dispersal of body scurf.
2. Remove jewelry, cracked or chipped nail polish, and street clothes. Jewelry, nail polish, and street clothes may harbor microorganisms, thus increasing the patients' risk for acquiring a postoperative wound infection. Cover hair with the bouffant hat or hood before donning the scrub top to prevent the possible dispersal of microorganisms and scalp hair onto the

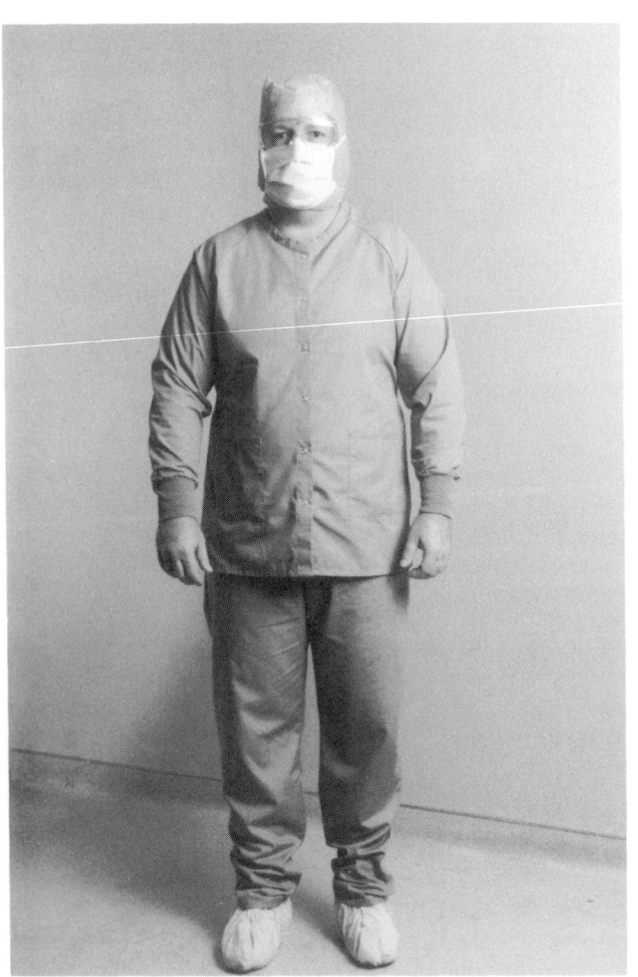

FIGURE 6–1. Male OR attire.

scrub attire. Adjust the hat or hood to cover all scalp hair. Individuals with beards or long sideburns should obtain a beard cover to contain all facial hair (Fig. 6–3).

3. After donning the pants, tuck the top and pants' ties into the pants to prevent the possible dispersal of body scurf from beneath the shirt. Pants should not come in contact with the floor during dressing. Change scrub attire when it is soiled or wet.

4. Change to comfortable, supportive, protective footwear to protect the feet against falling items such as sharps and heavy instruments and to allow one to move quickly and safely in an emergency. Place disposable shoe covers over the shoes to protect footwear from gross contamination. If shoe covers become moist or contaminated with body fluids or tissue during surgery, the wearer should remove them before leaving the OR and thus avoid tracking blood and debris throughout the surgical suite.

5. On entering the restricted area of the surgical suite and other designated areas such as the substerile area, the sterile center core, and the scrub sink area when team members are scrubbing, apply a surgical mask. Form the pliable nosepiece of the mask over the bridge of the nose; tie the mask at the back of the head and behind the neck, allowing the mask to fit securely and preventing venting at the sides. The transmission of nasopharyngeal and respiratory bacteria from the surgical team to the patient can be minimized by the proper wearing of a surgical mask. Masks should be changed between procedures and be removed by handling them by the strings only. Avoid touching the filter portion of the mask and discard in an appropriate receptacle. Masks are either on or off; they are not to be worn around the neck, nor on top of the head, nor in a pocket.

6. Before scrubbing, apply protective eyewear or a mask with a protective splash guard visor to protect against uncontrolled body fluid splashes (OSHA Occupational exposure to bloodborne pathogens, 1991). During laser procedures, laser masks and protective eyewear specified for the type of laser in operation should be worn. Eyewear should be cleansed with an antimicrobial agent between surgical procedures.

7. Surgical scrub attire should not be worn outside the surgical suite. If laboratory coats or cover gowns are worn, they should have long sleeves, be completely closed, and fall below the knees.

8. Written policy and procedure should be established and followed by all members entering the surgical suite.

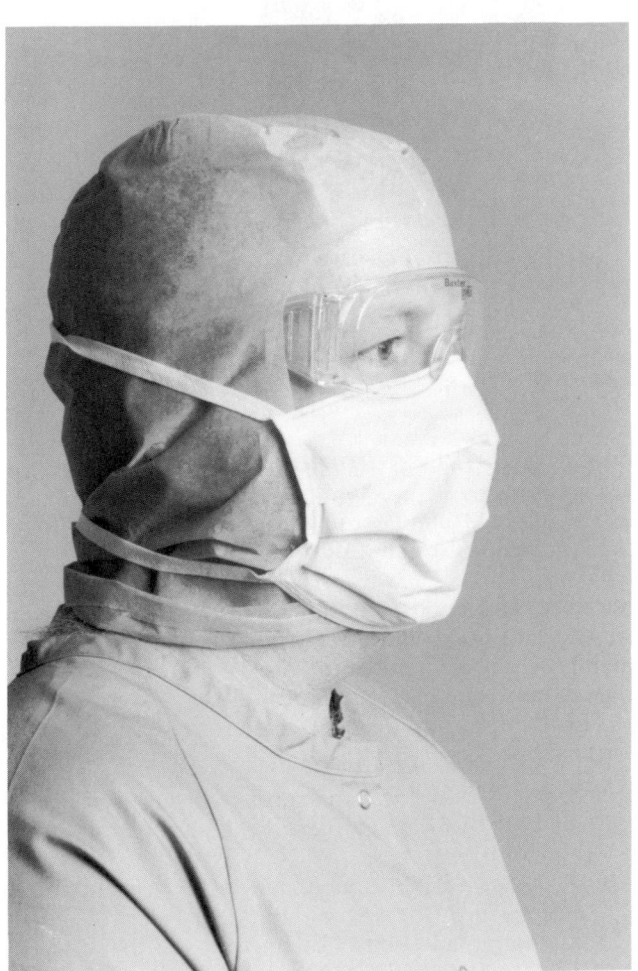

FIGURE 6–3. Hood and beard cover.

Performing the Surgical Hand Scrub
(AORN, 1992, *III*:8–1—8–5)

Before the sterile gown and gloves are donned, the surgical hand scrub is performed. The objectives are to remove gross contaminants, dirt, skin oil, and microbes from the skin; to eliminate transient bacteria while reducing the resident colony count; and to leave an antimicrobial residue on the skin to inhibit the regrowth of microorganisms. This is accomplished during the hand scrub by applying mechanical and chemical action with an antimicrobial agent, thereby inhibiting microbial growth during surgical intervention.

Considerations

There are two types of microorganisms present on the skin: transient and resident. Transient microorganisms are loosely attached to the skin surface and are easily removed by hand washing with soap and water (Garner, 1985, p. 7). Resident microorganisms survive and multiply in superficial skin layers and hair follicles and can be repeatedly cultured and cause wound infections when allowed to enter deep tissues during the surgical procedure. Scrubbing with an antimicrobial agent inhibits or kills them.

There are two methods of surgical hand scrubs: the anatomical timed scrub and the counted brush stroke (Fig. 6–4). When performed correctly both ensure sufficient exposure of all skin surfaces to friction and an antimicrobial agent. The anatomical timed scrub speci-

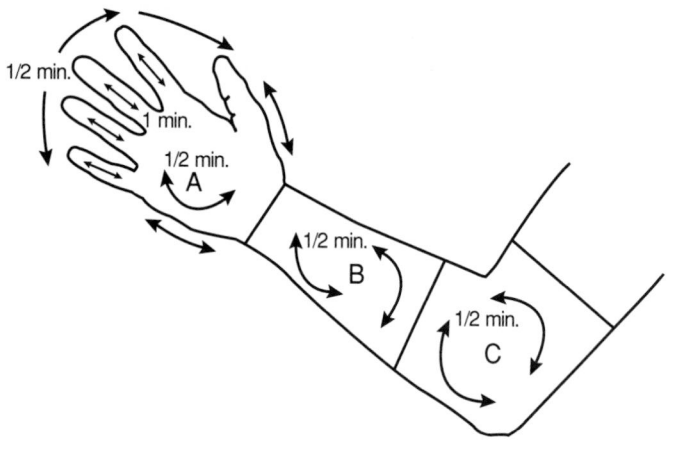

ANATOMICAL TIMED SCRUB METHOD

AREA	TIME
1. Nails (A)	30 seconds w/brush
2. Fingers, each side and web space (A)	1 minute w/sponge
3. Palmar surface (A)	15 seconds w/brush
4. Dorsal surface (A)	15 seconds w/sponge
5. Forearm, divided in half to 2" above elbow (B and C)	1 minute w/sponge (30 seconds each half)
6. Repeat process for other hand	

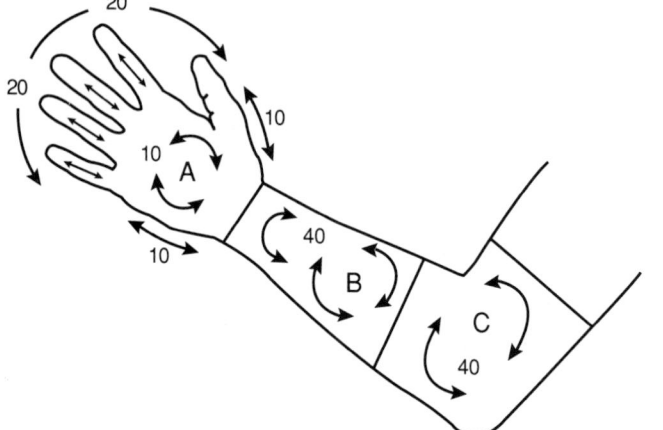

COUNTED BRUSH STROKE METHOD

AREA	TIME
1. Nails (A)	20 strokes w/brush
2. Fingers, each side and web space (A)	10 strokes w/brush
3. Palmar surface (A)	10 strokes w/brush
4. Dorsal surface (A)	10 strokes w/sponge
5. Forearm, divided in half to 2" above elbow (B and C)	40 strokes each half (10 strokes each side w/sponge)
6. Repeat process for other hand	

FIGURE 6–4. Surgical hand scrub techniques.

fies a prescribed amount of time for each anatomical area. The counted brush stroke denotes a set number of brush strokes to each surface of the fingers, hands, and forearms. Numerous studies indicate that there is no significant difference between a 5-minute and a 10-minute scrub (Dineen, 1969, p. 1182). The same scrub procedure should be repeated for all subsequent surgical hand scrubs during the day because the moist, warm environment of the gloved hand can cause bacteria to multiply rapidly.

The surgical team should be in appropriate surgical attire, including a high-filtration mask, to provide a barrier against bacterial contamination and to minimize postoperative wound infections. Protective eyewear or face shields should be applied to protect against uncontrolled splashes or aerosolization of body fluids (OSHA Occupational exposure to bloodborne pathogens, 1991).

Jewelry, chipped nail polish, and artificial or sculptured nails allow a reservoir for microorganisms and are therefore prohibited. The hands and forearms should be free from cuts and abrasions because of the potential danger of wound contamination. Written policy and procedure should be established and posted for those participating in the surgical hand scrub.

Supplies and Equipment

The surgical hand scrub should be performed in an area adjacent to the OR at a scrub sink with foot controls, where the water is set at a comfortable temperature and moderate flow to prevent spraying of surgical attire. High-filtration masks, scrub brushes, metal or plastic nail files, and antimicrobial agents should be within easy reach of the sink.

The antimicrobial agent selected for the surgical hand scrub should be

broad-spectrum and capable of reducing and inhibiting both transient and resident microorganisms (Table 6–1)

fast acting, easily applied, and able to maintain its effectiveness for several hours

nonirritating and nonsensitizing

TABLE 6–1. CHARACTERISTICS OF SIX TOPICAL ANTIMICROBIAL AGENTS

Agent	Mode of Action	Rapidity of Action	Residual Activity	Usual Concentration (%)	Affected by Organic Matter	Safety/ Toxicity	Activity Against				
							Gram-Positive Bacteria	Gram-Negative Bacteria	Mycobacterium Tuberculosis	Fungi	Viruses
Alcohols	Denaturation of protein	Most rapid	None	70–92	No data	Drying, volatile	Excellent	Excellent	Good	Good	Good
Chlorhexidine gluconate	Cell wall disruption	Intermediate	Excellent	4.2 in detergent base; 0.5 in alcohol	Minimal	Ototoxicity, keratitis	Excellent	Good	Poor	Fair	Good
Hexachlorophene	Cell wall disruption	Slow to intermediate	Excellent	3 by prescription only	Minimal	Neurotoxicity	Excellent	Poor	Poor	Poor	Poor
Iodine and iodophors	Oxidation/ substitution by free iodine	Intermediate	Minimal	10, 7.5, 2, 0.5	Yes	Absorption from skin with possible toxicity, skin irritation	Excellent	Good	Good	Good	Good
Chloroxylenol	Cell wall disruption	Intermediate	Good	0.5–3.75	Minimal	More data needed	Good	Fair	Fair	Fair	Fair
Triclosan	Cell wall disruption	Intermediate	Excellent	0.3–1	Minimal	More data needed	Good	Good except for *Pseudomonas*	Fair	Poor	Unknown

Adapted from Larson, E. (1988). APIC Guidelines for infection control practice, guideline for use of topical antimicrobial agents. *American Journal of Infection Control, 16,* 253–266.

not rendered ineffective by soaps, detergents, organic matter or alcohol and approved by the U.S. Food and Drug Administration (Garner, 1985, p. 5).

Procedure

1. Inspect the OR attire by adjusting the hat or hood to cover and contain all hair. The mask should completely cover both the nose and mouth and fit securely to prevent venting at the sides. All loose scrub attire and strings should be tucked in the scrub pants. Replace or adjust shoe covers to completely protect shoes.
2. Examine the hands and forearms for good skin integrity; remove all jewelry. Nails should be free from polish and short, and cuticles should be in good condition.
3. Open the sterile scrub brush package and position it for easy access.
4. Turn on the water, adjusting the temperature and spray so that scrub attire does not become wet.
5. Wash and rinse the hands for the initial wash with water and a small amount of antimicrobial agent to remove transient flora and gross contaminants (Fig. 6–5).
6. Remove the plastic nail stick and the scrub brush from the package and add an antimicrobial agent from a dispenser or squeeze an impregnated sponge to generate lather (Fig. 6–6). Clean nails and cuticles under running water with the plastic nail stick.
7. Clean the nails and cuticles under running water while holding the scrub brush in the opposite hand; repeat for the other hand (Fig. 6–7).
8. Select either the anatomical timed scrub or the counted brush stroke method (see Fig. 6–4). Each takes about 5 minutes to complete.
9. Beginning at the fingertips, scrub vigorously with

vertical strokes using the scrub brush. Proceed to the palm and the back of the hand. Scrub all four sides of each digit, including the web space (Fig. 6–8).

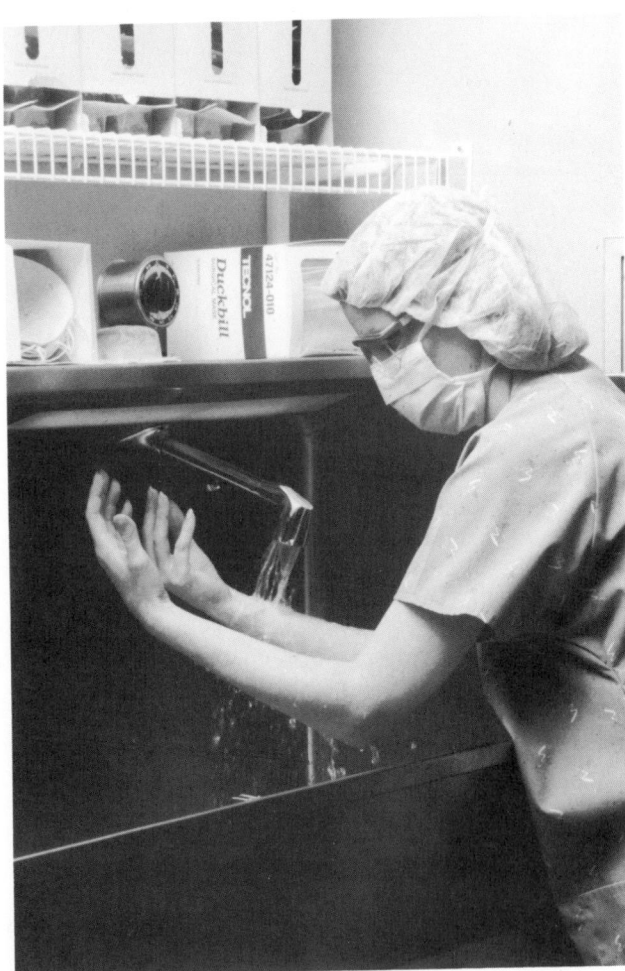

FIGURE 6–5. Initial wash at the scrub sink.

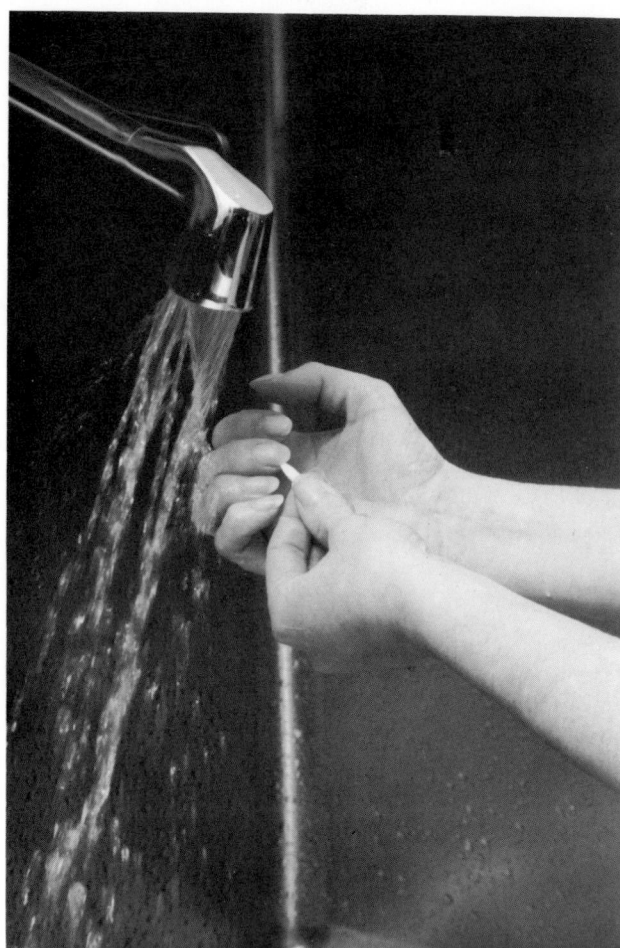

FIGURE 6–6. Clean under each nail using the plastic nail stick.

FIGURE 6–7. Scrub the nails and cuticles with a scrub brush.

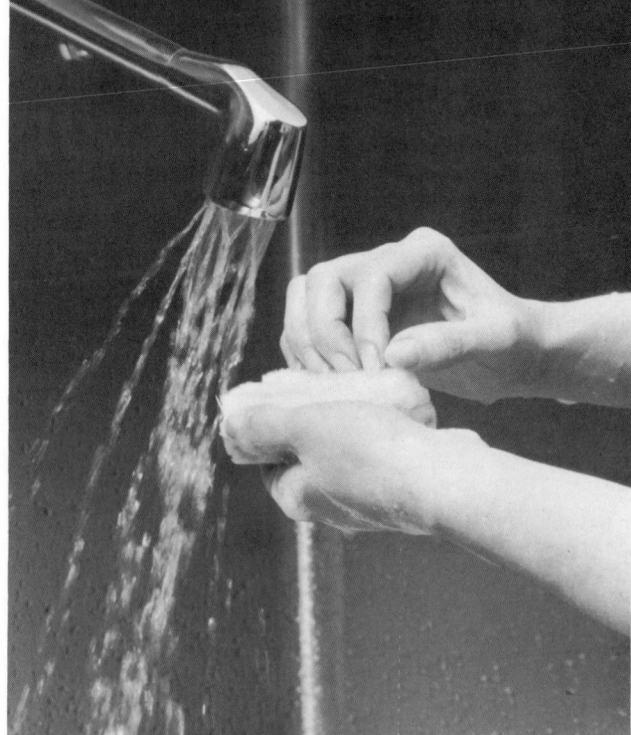

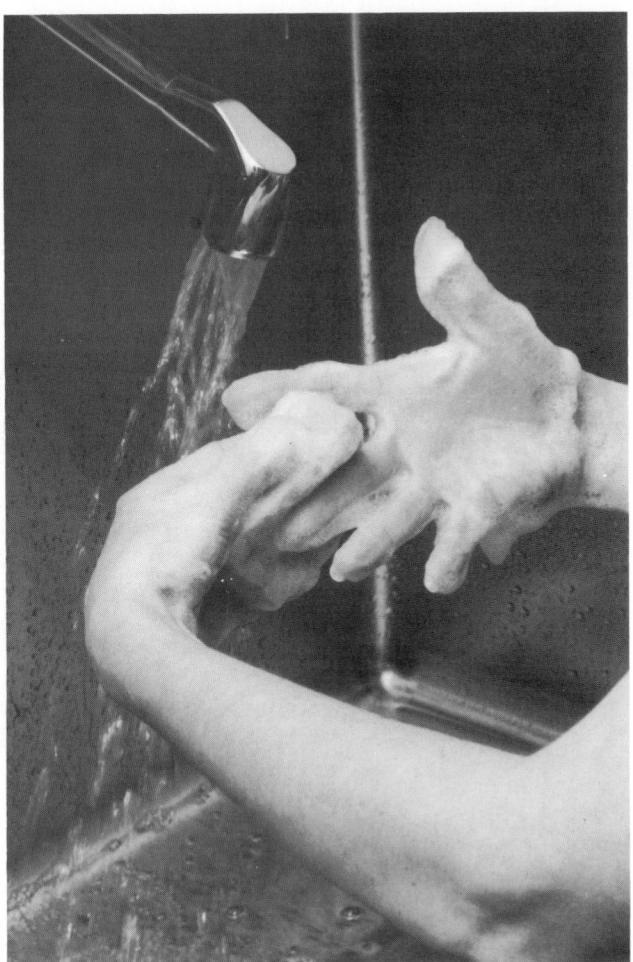

FIGURE 6–8. Scrub all four sides of each digit, including the web space.

10. Proceed to the wrist; with a circular motion continue up the forearm to 2 inches above the elbow (Fig. 6–9).
11. Scrub each anatomical area to ensure that all surfaces are sufficiently exposed to friction and an antimicrobial agent; repeat for other hand, and discard the scrub brush in an appropriate receptacle.
12. Rinse the hands and arms thoroughly under running water, keeping the hands elevated to allow the water to drain off the flexed elbows (Fig. 6–10).
13. Take special care not to touch the faucet, clothing, or other objects and not to splash water onto the OR scrub attire. If the hands or forearms are touched, repeat the scrubbing procedure to correct the contamination.
14. Proceed to the OR, with the hands held upward to allow water to drip off the elbows (Fig. 6–11).

Donning Sterile Gown and Gloves
(AORN, 1992, III:2–1)

Gowning and gloving are essential parts of aseptic practice. The surgical team members don gowns and gloves to protect the patient and themselves from cross-contamination. Gowns and gloves provide a barrier and prevent the transfer of microorganisms from the skin and clothing to the surgical incision. Considerable skill and attention to detail are required in the process of donning a sterile gown and gloves to ensure flawless aseptic technique. The sterile gown is donned after the surgical hand scrub and drying of the hands and arms with a sterile towel and is immediately followed by donning of sterile gloves.

Considerations

Unassisted gowning and gloving should be performed in a separate sterile area because of the possibility of water's dripping off the arms and onto the sterile field, thereby contaminating it.

Surgical gowns are made of disposable nonwoven or reusable materials. An effective barrier must be maintained even when the gown becomes wet to prevent the passage of microorganisms from nonsterile to sterile areas (Garner and Favero, 1985, p. 6). Gown materials should meet recommended standards (AORN, 1992, p. III:6–1) and be a wraparound-style, "sterile back" gown.

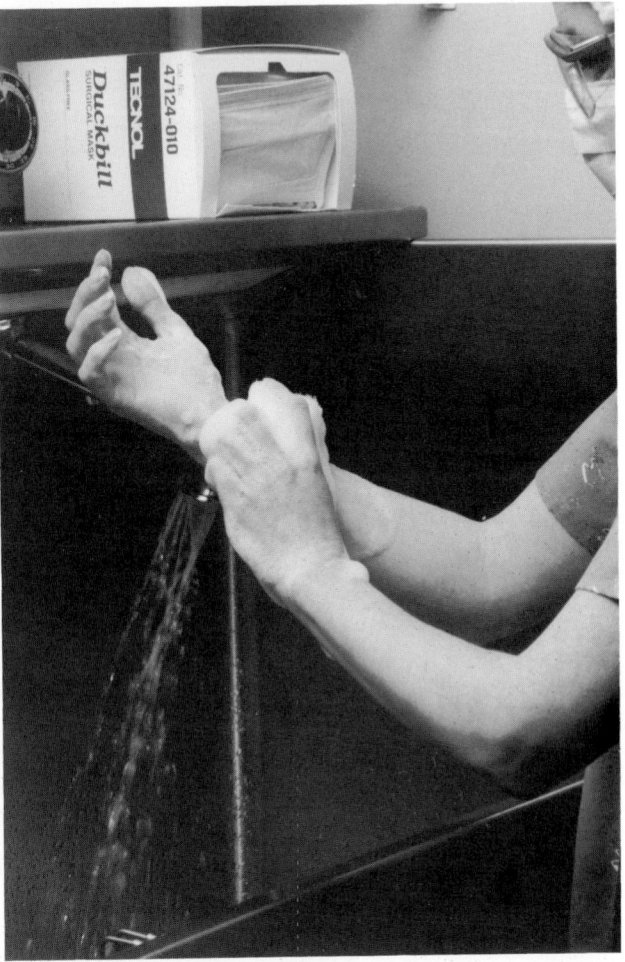

FIGURE 6–9. With a circular motion, scrub the wrist and forearm.

Supplies and Equipment

Sterile surgical gowns, wraparound style with sterile backs; sterile absorbent towels; sterile disposable surgeon's gloves; and separate sterile area for the procedure are needed.

Procedure

Unassisted Gowning

1. After the team member has completed the surgical hand scrub, the folded towel is grasped near the corner with one hand and pulled straight up (Fig. 6–12). Pay careful attention not to drip water onto the sterile field.
2. Step back from the sterile field, extend the arms, and lean slightly forward at the waist to prevent the towel from touching surgical attire.
3. Unfold the towel, begin drying the hand using half the towel, and proceed to the wrist and forearm using a rotating motion, being careful not to retrace any surface.
4. Grasp the untouched end of the towel with the dry hand and repeat the process on the other hand and

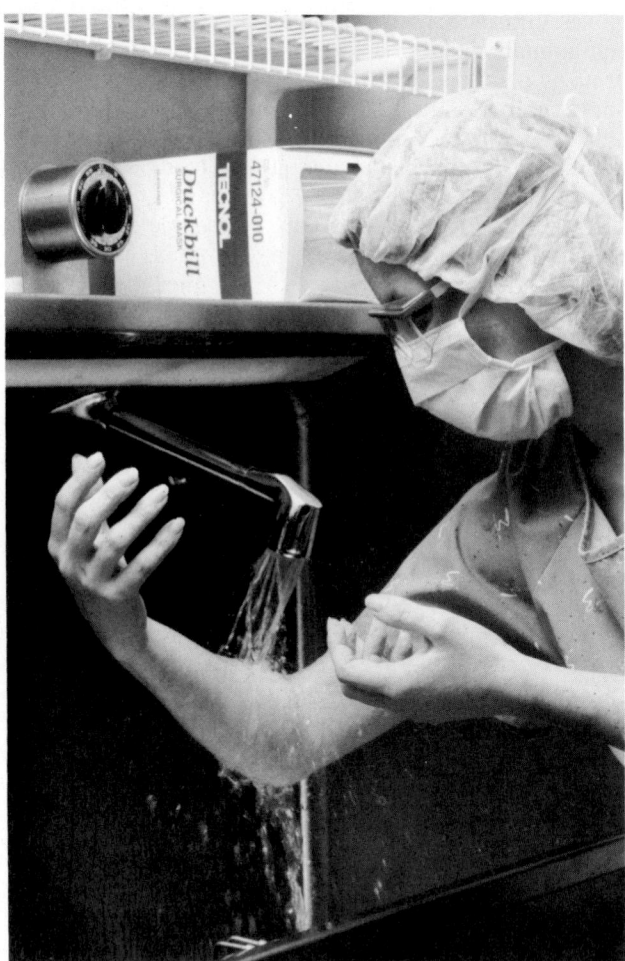

FIGURE 6–10. Rinse the hands and arms.

Gowns are made of materials that are either fluid proof or fluid resistant. Fluid-proof materials provide completely impervious barriers, therefore preventing the gown from becoming soaked with blood or other potentially infectious fluids. Fluid-resistant materials provide an effective barrier and should be worn if there is a possibility of splashing or spraying of blood or other potentially infectious fluids (OSHA Occupational exposure to bloodborne pathogens, 1991). The type of gown material chosen depends on the proposed surgery and the degree of blood and fluid splashing inherent in the procedure.

Surgical gloves should be disposable. Surgical gloves may be donned by either the closed glove technique or the open glove technique. The advantage of the closed glove technique is that it prevents bare skin exposure during gowning and donning of sterile gloves, thereby lessening the chance of contamination. The closed glove technique is preferred, except when donning sterile gloves for procedures not requiring sterile gowns. The open glove technique is used when only sterile gloves are donned for a sterile procedure (e.g., the insertion of a bladder catheter and the insertion of invasive venous or arterial catheters). Written policy and procedure should be established and followed by all members of the surgical team.

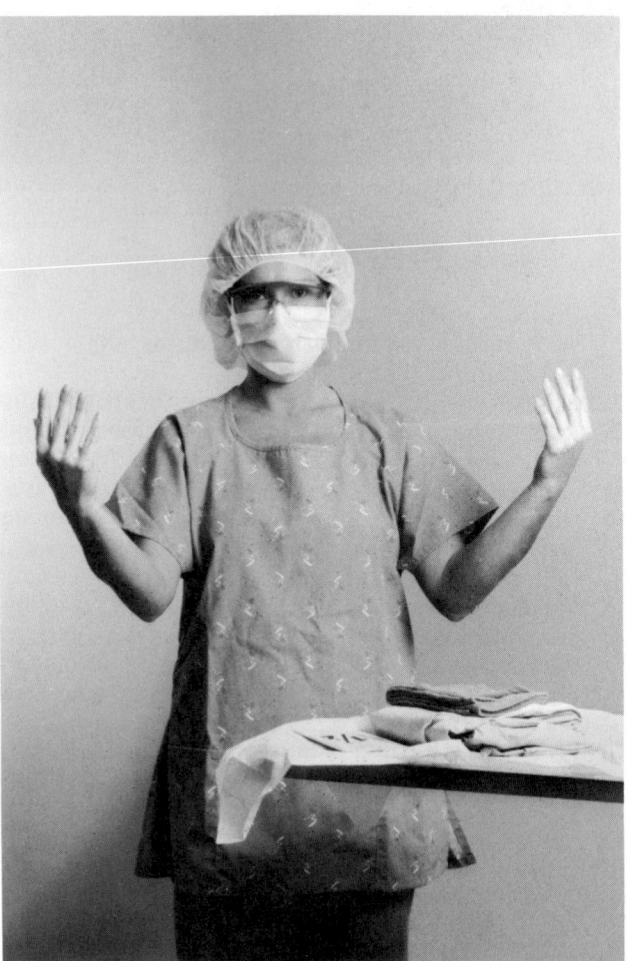

FIGURE 6–11. Hands held up to allow water to drip off the elbows.

a. Grasp the belt tie and hand it to other sterile team member.
b. For a disposable gown, hand the prepackaged card securing the belt tie to the circulating nurse (Fig. 6–18).
c. Secure the belt tie with an instrument and hand it off to the circulating nurse.

11. The circulating nurse holds the prepackaged card or sterile instrument while the sterile team member pivots to the left, thereby completing the back closure of the gown. The sterile team member pulls the belt tie free and ties it while the circulating nurse retains the cardboard or instrument.

12. The arms should be flexed at the elbows and held in front with both hands in sight at all times (Fig. 6–19). Sterile hands should never be dropped below table or waist level.

13. Gowns are considered sterile in the front from shoulder to table level; sleeves are sterile from 2 inches above the elbow to the wrist, excluding the stockinet cuff. The back of a wraparound, sterile back gown is not considered sterile because it cannot be observed by the scrubbed person (AORN, 1992, III:2–1).

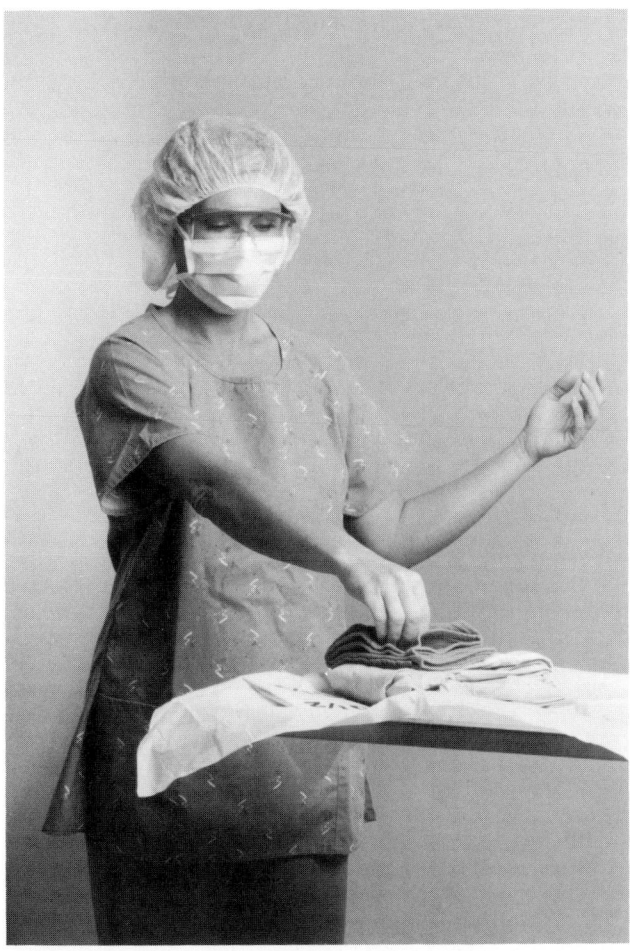

FIGURE 6–12. A scrubbed surgical team member with wet hands grasps a towel.

forearm. Discard the towel in an appropriate receptacle.

5. If the sterile towel touches the scrub attire, discard the contaminated towel and begin with another sterile towel.

6. Grasp the folded gown at the neckline and step back from the sterile field, allowing the gown to unfold completely, with the inside toward the wearer (Fig. 6–13).

7. Holding the arms at shoulder level, slide both arms simultaneously into the armholes (Fig. 6–14).

8. The circulating nurse assists by reaching inside and pulling the gown up over the shoulders for proper sleeve adjustment. The cuffs are left extended over the hands for the closed glove technique, (Fig. 6–15) and the cuffs are pulled up to expose the hands for the assisted gloving technique.

9. The circulating nurse ties the inside tie at the waist and secures the gown at the neckline (Figs. 6–16 and 6–17). The final tie on a wraparound gown is completed after the sterile gloves have been donned.

10. Complete closure on a sterile back gown in one of three ways:

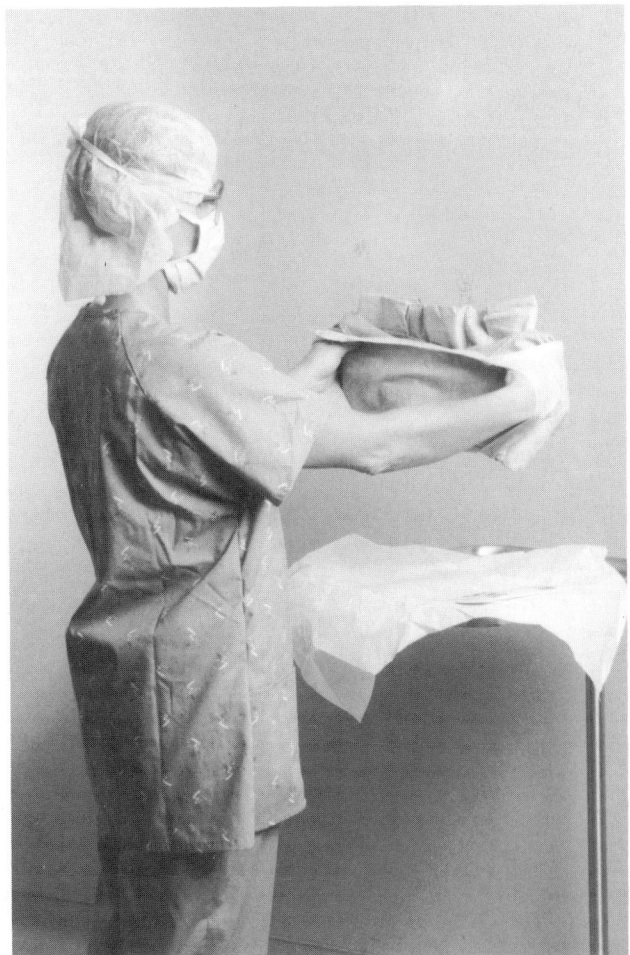

FIGURE 6–13. The folded gown is grasped at its neckline.

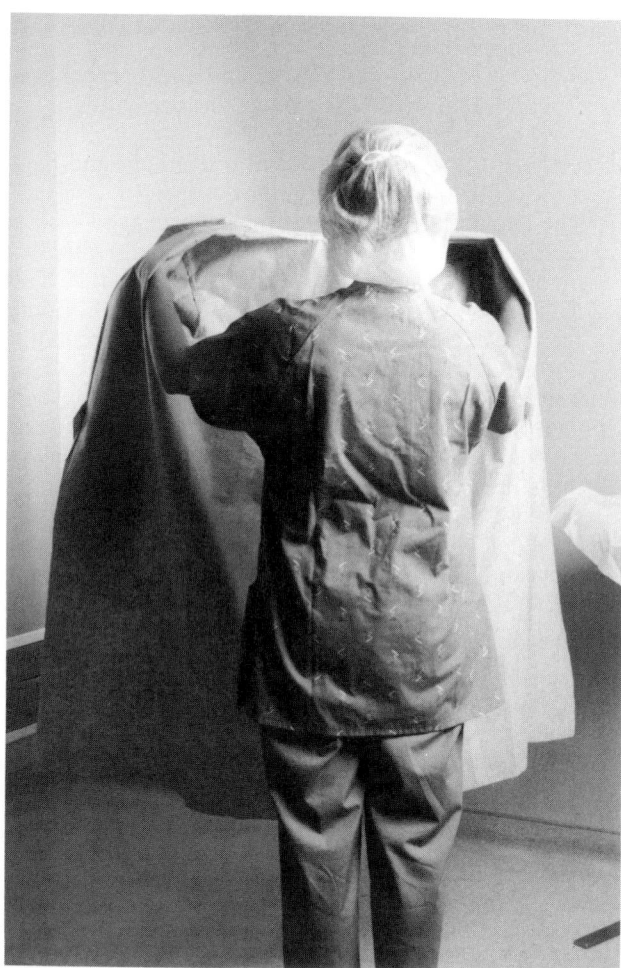

FIGURE 6–14. Both arms are slid into the gown.

FIGURE 6–15. The gown cuffs remain extended over the hands for the closed gloving technique.

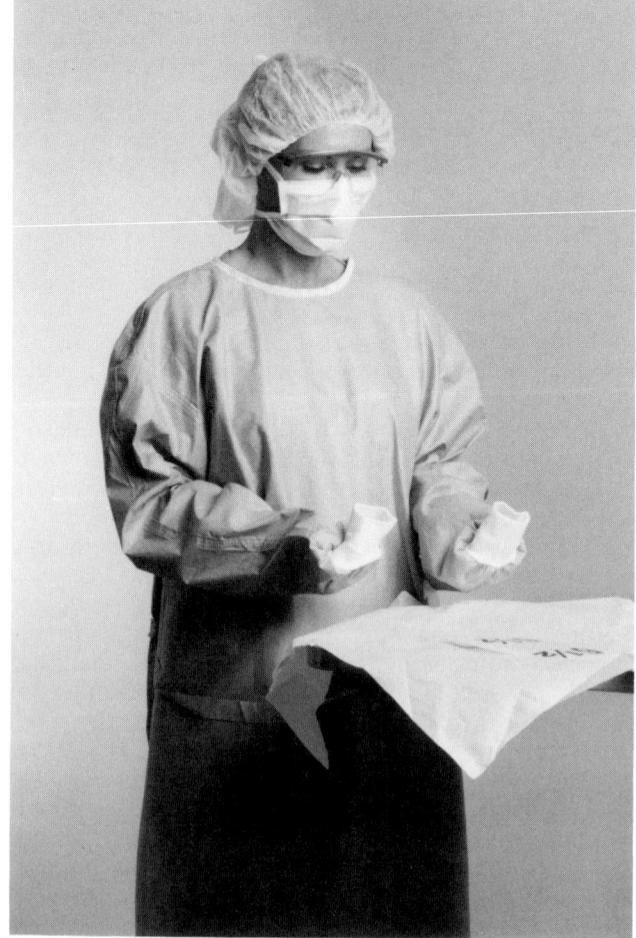

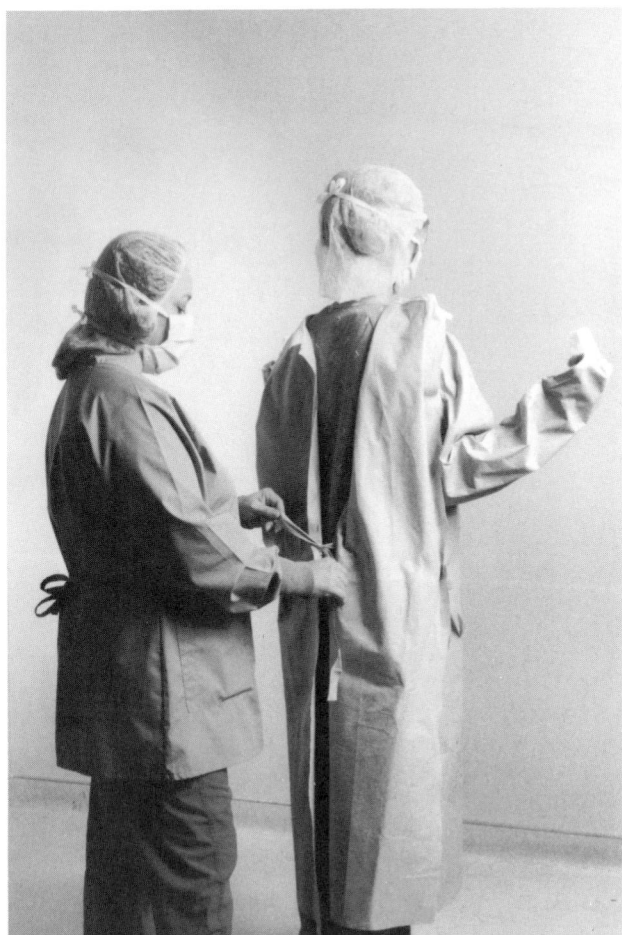

FIGURE 6–16. The circulating nurse fastens the inside tie of the gown.

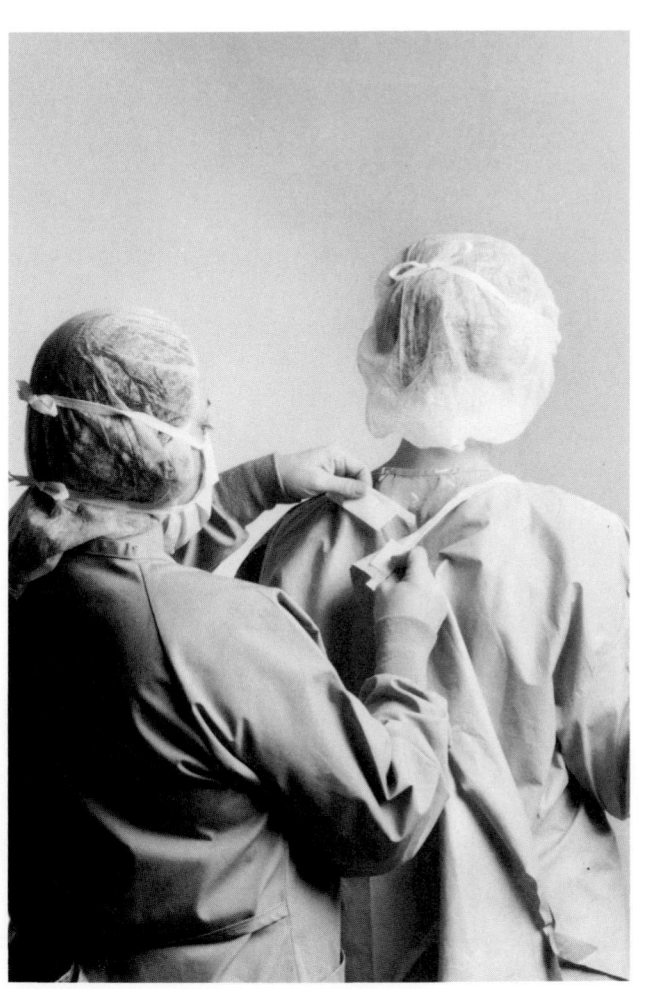

FIGURE 6–17. The circulating nurse fastens the gown at the neckline.

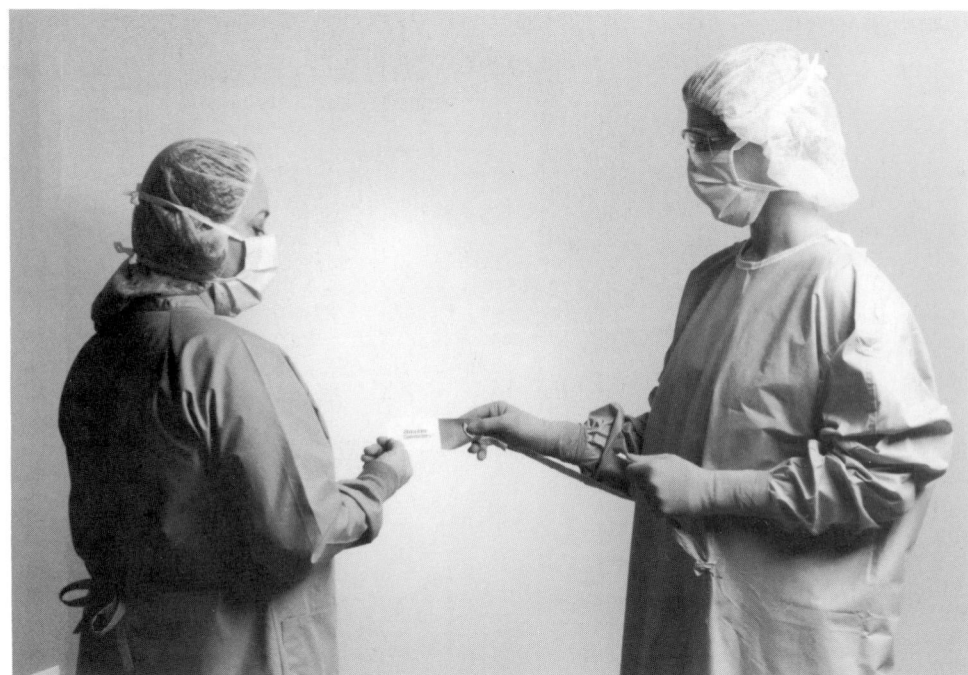

FIGURE 6–18. A prepackaged card securing the belt tie is handed to the circulating nurse.

FIGURE 6–19. Hold arm and hand above waist level to maintain sterility.

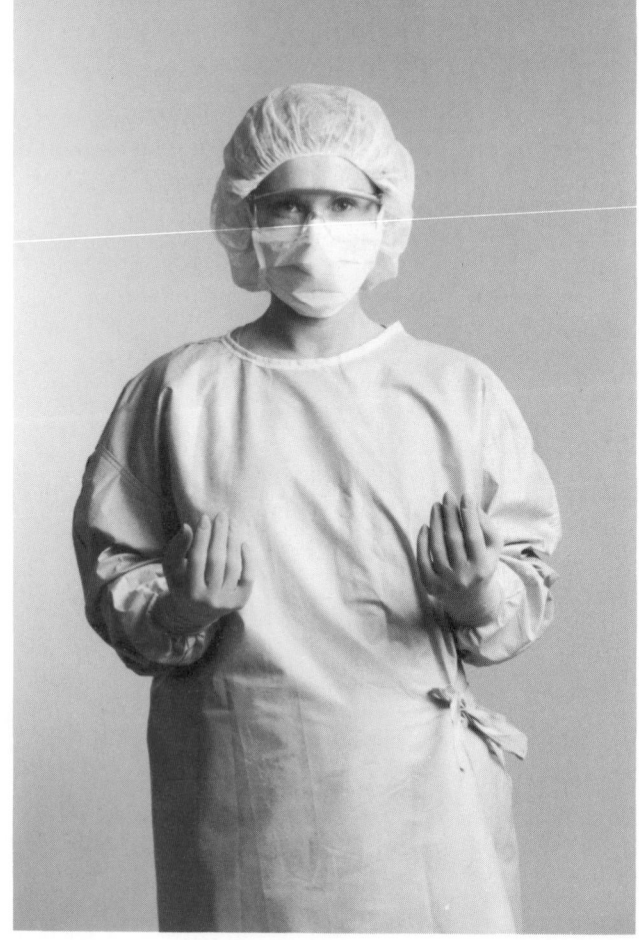

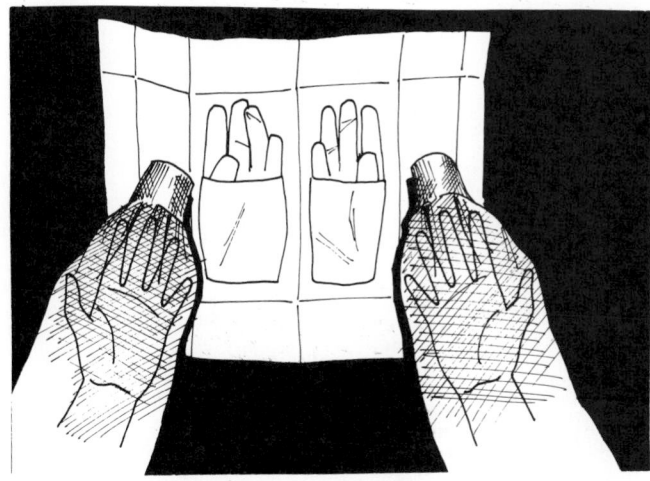

FIGURE 6–20. Open the glove wrapper on a sterile table.

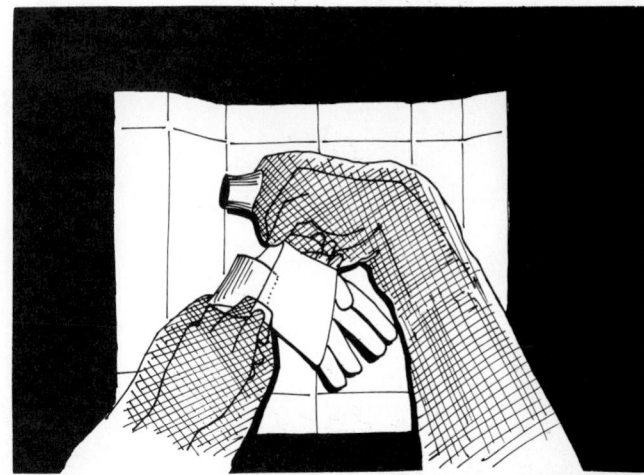

FIGURE 6–22. Grasp the left glove cuff.

Unassisted Gloving

Closed Glove Technique

1. While donning a sterile gown, slide the fingers into the sleeves until the cuff is reached. Open the inner glove wrapper on a sterile field. The gloves should be palm side up, with the glove labeled L on the left and R on the right (Fig. 6–20).
2. Don the left glove first, turn the left hand palm side up, and flip the left glove onto the left palm. Place the folded glove cuff even with the gown cuff seam; the thumb of the glove is on the thumb side of hand and the fingers on the lunar side of the wrist, with the glove finger tips pointing toward the elbow (Fig. 6–21).
3. Grasp the lower edge of the glove cuff with the left thumb and index finger. Secure the upper edge of the glove cuff with the right thumb and index finger and stretch the entire glove cuff over the stockinet opening, being careful not to touch the edge of the stockinet cuff (Fig. 6–22).

4. Work the fingers into the glove, then grasp the left glove and gown at the seam with the right hand and pull up over the wrist (Fig. 6–23).
5. Turn the right hand palm side up, flip the right glove on the right palm. Place the folded glove cuff even with the gown cuff seam; the thumb of the glove is on the thumb side of the hand and the fingers on the ulnar side of the wrist, with the glove finger tips pointing toward the elbow (Fig. 6–24).
6. Grasp the lower edge of the glove cuff with the right thumb and index finger. Secure the upper edge of the glove cuff with the left thumb and index finger and stretch the entire glove cuff over the stockinet opening, being careful not to touch the edge of the stockinet cuff (Fig. 6–25).
7. Work the fingers into the glove, then grasp the right glove and gown at the seam with the left hand and pull up over the wrist (Fig. 6–26).
8. Adjust both gloves for comfort and fit (Fig. 6–27).
9. Remove powder from gloves; its residue has been associated with the development of granulomas and peritonitis.

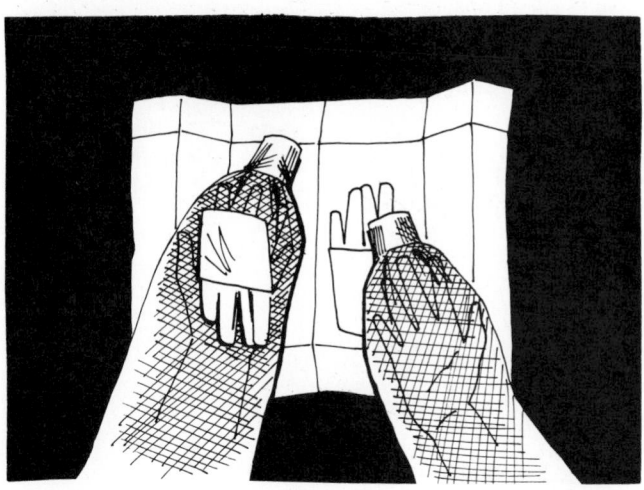

FIGURE 6–21. Place the left glove on the left palm.

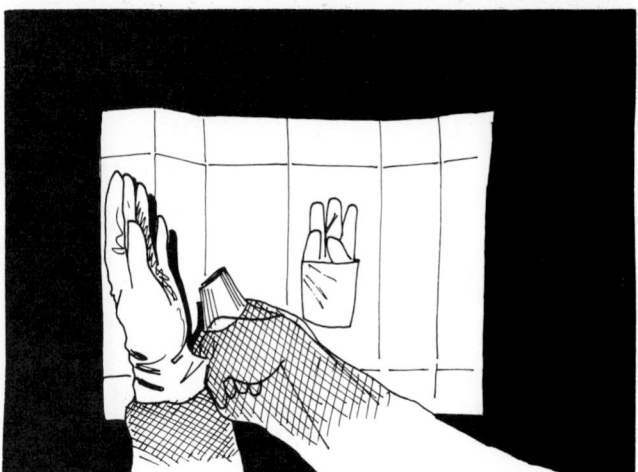

FIGURE 6–23. Pull the left glove up over the wrist.

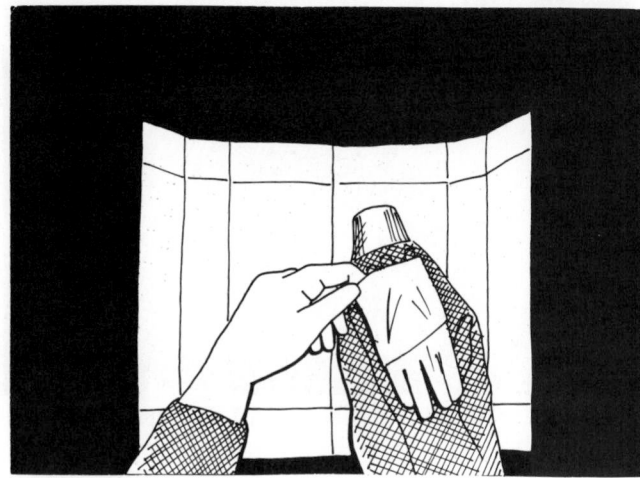

FIGURE 6–24. Place the right glove on the right palm.

FIGURE 6–25. Stretch the entire right glove cuff over the stockinet opening.

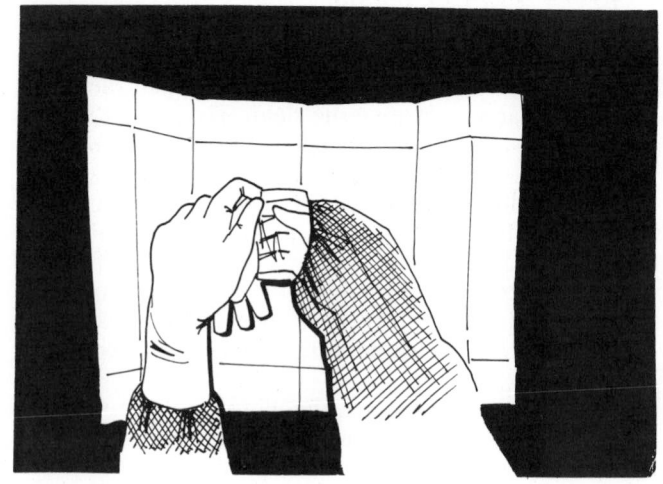

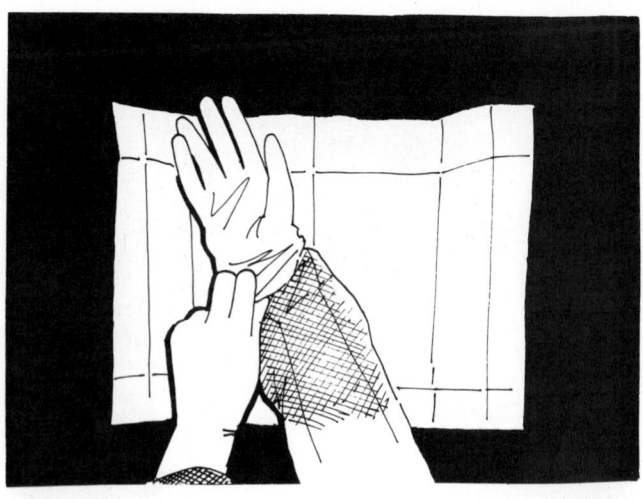

FIGURE 6–26. Pull the right glove up over the wrist.

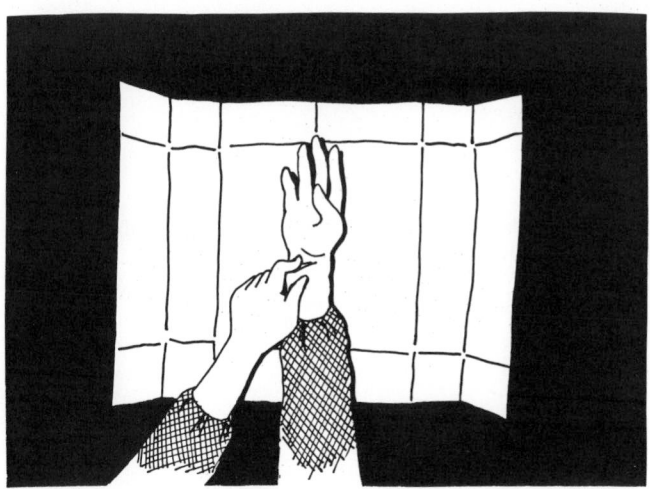

FIGURE 6–27. Adjust the gloves.

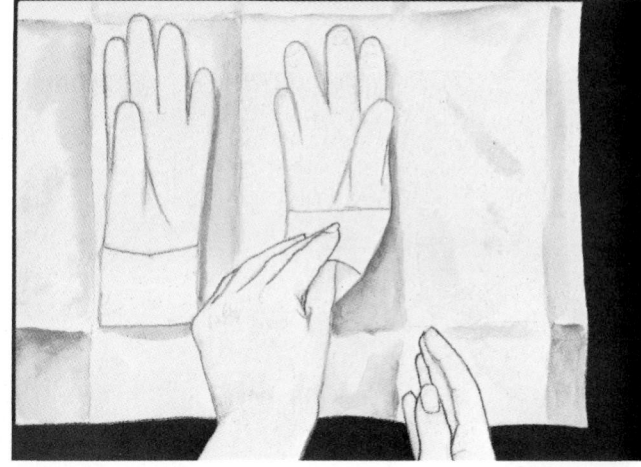

FIGURE 6–29. Grasp the right glove cuff. (Drawing provided by Baxter Pharmaseal.)

Open Glove Technique

1. Extend the hands through the sterile gown cuff. Exposed skin, although scrubbed, is not sterile and should never come in contact with the exterior of the sterile gloves.
2. Open the inner glove wrapper carefully to expose the gloves, making sure that the wrapper does not flip back and contaminate the gloves (Fig. 6–28).
3. Grasp the right glove cuff on the fold with the left thumb and index finger, touching only the *interior* of the glove (Fig. 6–29).
4. Insert the right hand into the glove and gently pull it on, leaving the cuff turned down (Fig. 6–30).
5. Slide the fingers of the gloved right hand under the fold of the left cuff, touching only the *exterior* of the glove and insert the left hand (Fig. 6–31).
6. Gently pull it on and stretch the cuff over the stockinet cuff, avoiding inward rolling of the glove cuff (Fig. 6–32).
7. Slide the fingers of the left gloved hand under the fold of the right cuff and stretch the glove cuff over

the stockinet cuff, avoiding inward rolling of the glove cuff.

Because the open glove technique provides a greater chance that the scrub person's hands come in contact with the sterile glove, thereby becoming contaminated, the closed glove method is recommended.

Assisted Gowning

1. Place an open sterile towel over the outstretched hand of the newly scrubbed team member (Fig. 6–33).
2. Pick up the gown at the neck, step back from the sterile field, and allow the gown to unfold completely.
3. Form a protective cuff by placing the hands at shoulder level exterior side of the gown and drape the gown over the gloves.
4. Identify the armholes and place the gown on the outstretched hands of the scrubbed team member (Fig. 6–34).

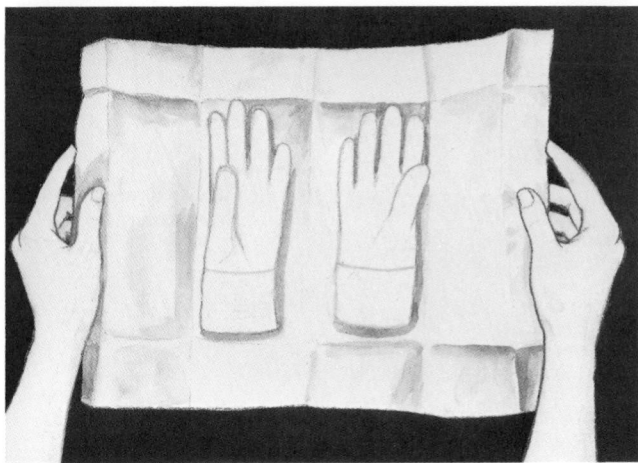

FIGURE 6–28. Open the glove wrapper. (Drawing provided by Baxter Pharmaseal.)

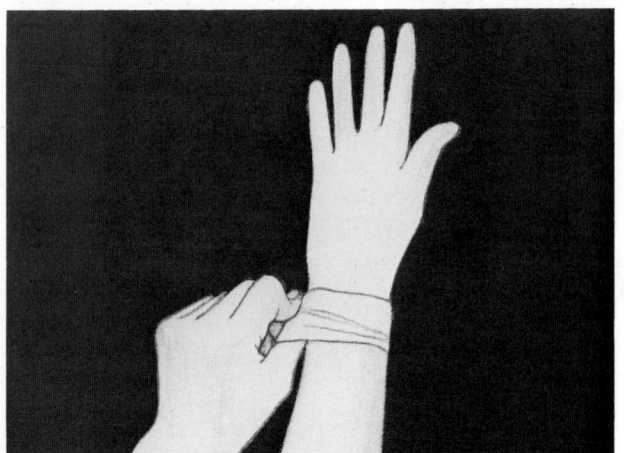

FIGURE 6–30. Pull on the right glove. (Drawing provided by Baxter Pharmaseal.)

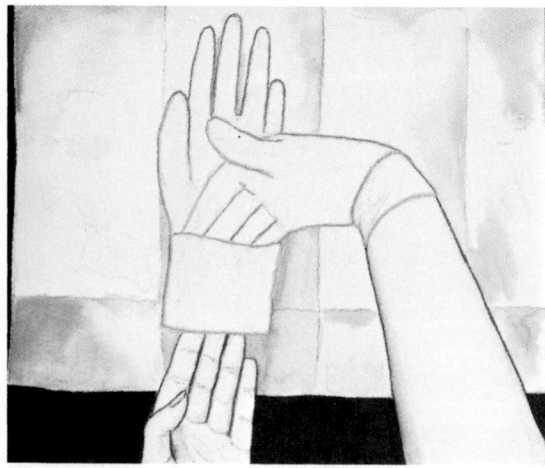

FIGURE 6–31. Slide the right fingers under the left glove cuff. (Drawing provided by Baxter Pharmaseal.)

FIGURE 6–32. Pull on the left glove. (Drawing provided by Baxter Pharmaseal.)

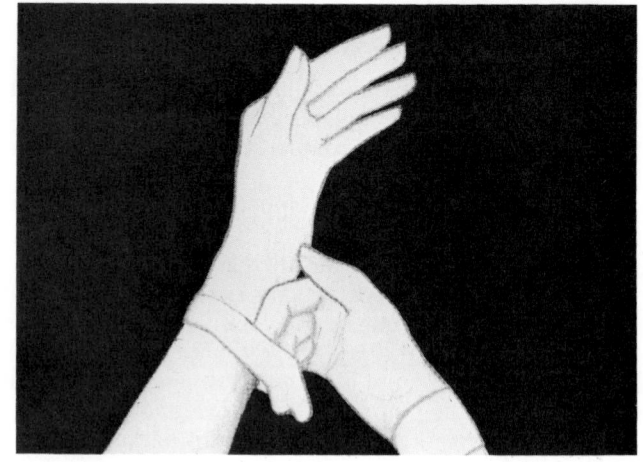

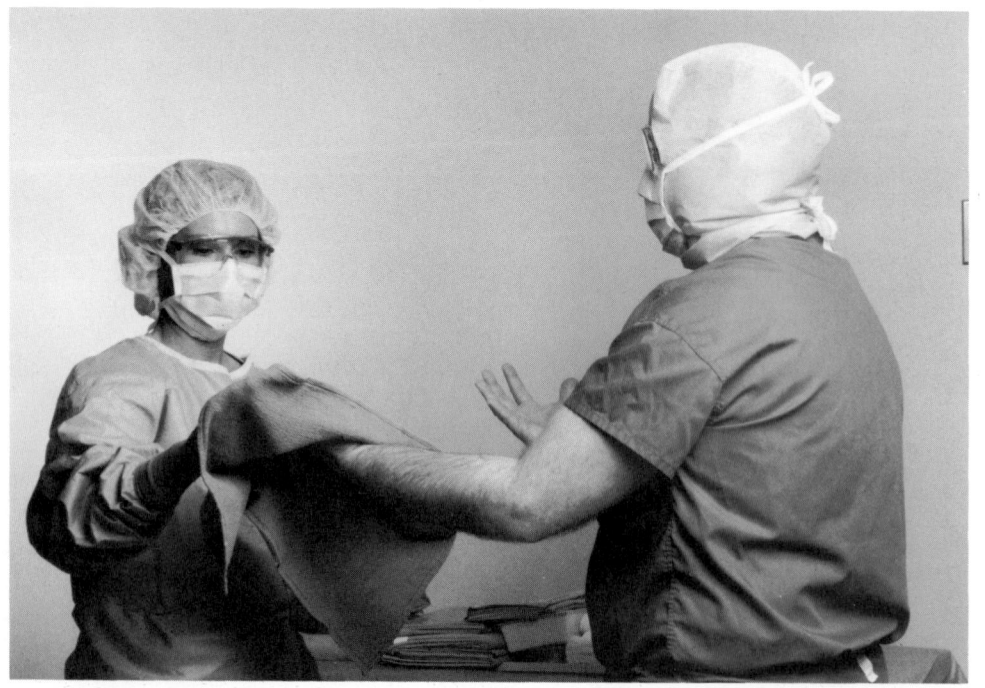

FIGURE 6–33. A towel is placed over the outstretched wet hands of the scrubbed surgical team member by the scrub nurse.

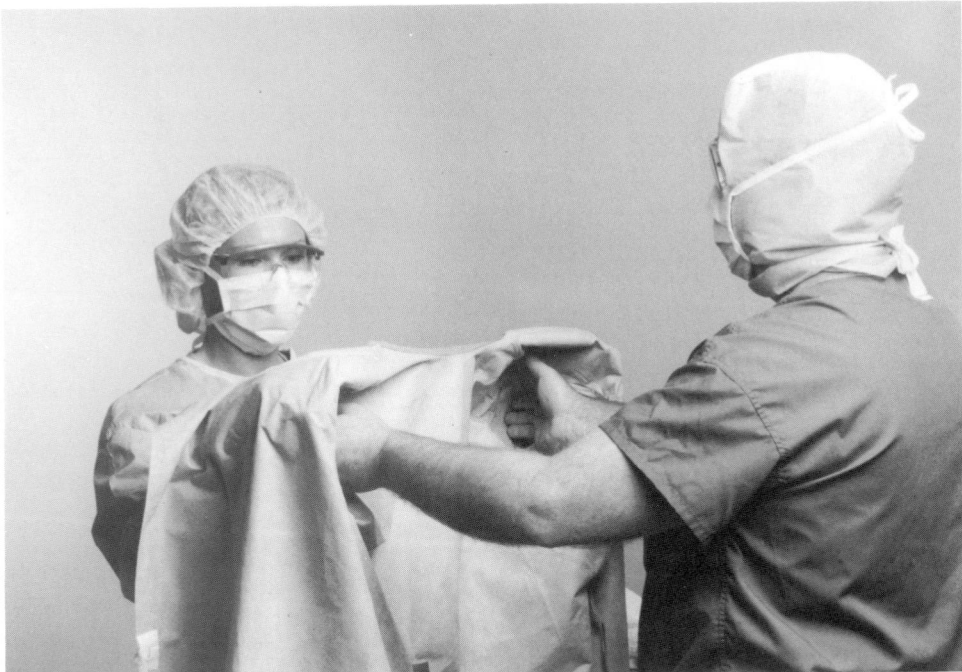

FIGURE 6–34. The gown is placed over the outstretched hands.

5. Release the gown. The circulating nurse assists by reaching inside and pulling the gown up over the shoulder and securing it at the neck and at the waist with the inside tie.

Assisted Gloving

1. Grasp the right glove under the inverted cuff (the right hand is usually gloved first in assisted gloving).
2. Stretch the cuff while protecting the sterile thumbs and fingers by placing them under the cuff on the exterior side of the glove.
3. Hold the stretched glove open, palm side toward the team member being gloved. Assist the team member's hand into the glove by gently pulling the glove upward as the team member pushes his or her hand into the glove (Fig. 6–35).
4. Cover the gown stockinet cuff completely with the sterile glove.
5. Repeat the process for the other hand.

Regowning and Regloving

1. When a glove becomes contaminated, there are three options for regloving:
   a. Ask for assistance from a sterile team member in regloving.
   b. Remove both gown and gloves and regown and reglove.
   c. Apply a sterile glove over the contaminated glove.
2. To remove a contaminated glove, extend the glove out of the sterile field. The circulating nurse wearing protective gloves pulls off the contaminated glove, leaving the stockinet cuff in place (Fig. 6–36).
3. The closed glove technique cannot be used for regloving because the stockinet cuff is contaminated.

4. Ask a sterile team member to assist in gloving; if this is impossible, apply a sterile glove over the contaminated glove.
5. When a gown becomes contaminated, the circulating nurse unties the gown, then faces the scrubbed team member and grasps the gown at the shoulders while inverting the gown as it is being taken off.
6. The circulating nurse removes the gloves by touching the interior of the glove without touching the scrubbed hands, turning the gloves inside out as they are removed. The circulating nurse dons protective gloves before removing the gloves of the scrubbed person.
7. The scrubbed team member is ready to regown and reglove.
8. Contaminated gown and gloves are not to be worn outside the OR.

Preparing a Sterile Field (AORN, 1992, *III*:2–1—2–6)

Creating and maintaining a sterile field, free from microorganisms, are essential to ensure maximal safety for the surgical patient. Proper application of aseptic technique principles is crucial to the success of any surgical intervention. The overall goal of asepsis is to minimize contamination of the surgical wound. Constant inspection and regulation of the patient, the environment, and the equipment is necessary to control and monitor the sources of infection so that the outcome standards for surgical intervention are not altered.

Aseptic technique is practiced to prevent contamination of the open wound, isolate the operative site from the surrounding nonsterile physical environment, and create and maintain a sterile field in which surgery can

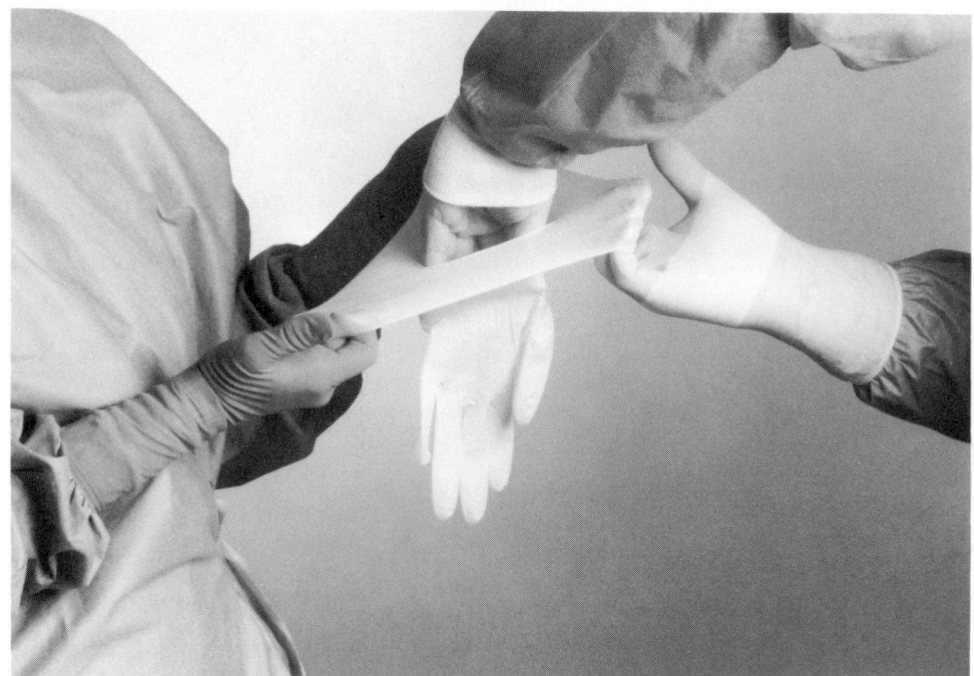

FIGURE 6–35. The glove is held open and upward pressure is exerted.

FIGURE 6–36. Removal of a contaminated glove.

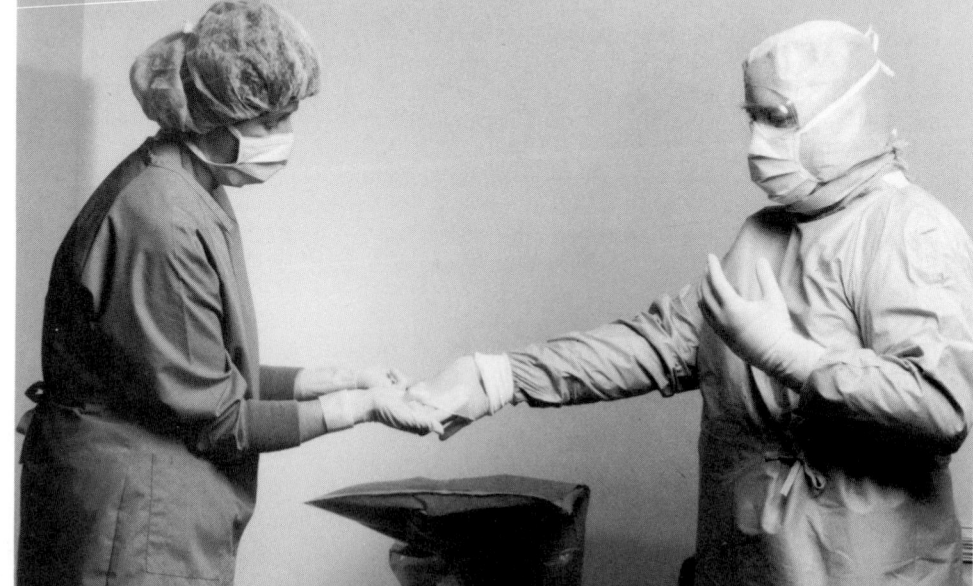

be performed safely (Gruendemann and Meeker, 1983, p. 46). The patient makes up the center of the sterile field, with emphasis on the areas of the body around the site of the incision. The balance of the sterile field includes the Mayo stand, the back table, the ring stand, and any other furniture or equipment covered with sterile drapes and any surgical team member wearing sterile surgical attire.

Because freshly incised tissue can easily become infected, it is imperative that all contact with patient's body tissue during a surgical procedure be sterile. Postoperative infection is serious and a single break in technique can lead to potentially fatal complications for the patient.

In a less extreme case, infection is a health hazard of great expense and significant effect on the final outcome of operative treatment. The patient's quality of life can be altered dramatically, in terms of discomfort, emotional distress, and delayed healing, as well as economic hardship. A longer patient hospital stay can prove costly to patient and hospital alike.

The perioperative nurse plays a key role in the ongoing maintenance of aseptic technique during surgical intervention. As an overseer of the patient's care, the perioperative nurse must be able to meet the requirements of both the patient and the members of the surgical team.

Care must be taken by the perioperative nurse to ensure that the patient is not adversely affected, either physically or emotionally, by the process of creating and maintaining the sterile field. Specifically, a patient should remain free from postoperative wound infection, impaired skin integrity, hyperthermia or hypothermia, ineffective respiratory patterns, and a disturbed self-esteem.

The perioperative nurse must also remain alert to the needs of the members of the surgical team. They should be able to anticipate the instruments, surgical supplies, and equipment needed according to the patient and the procedure, as well as knowing where and how to obtain those items. Additionally, the preferences of a particular surgical team should be noted and acted on when that team is performing a surgical intervention.

The perioperative nurse may function as the circulating or scrub nurse during the intraoperative phase. The scrub nurse maintains the integrity, safety, and efficiency of the sterile field throughout the operation, wearing a sterile gown and gloves and assisting the surgeon and assistants by providing the sterile instruments and supplies required for the surgical procedure.

The circulating nurse is responsible for the coordination and documentation of all activities in the OR during surgical intervention, manages the patient's nursing care in the OR, and controls the physical and emotional atmosphere of the room. Because the circulating nurse is able to view the sterile field from a distance, she or he is better able to observe the entire field and must be on the alert to catch any breaks in aseptic technique that others may not have seen.

The circulating nurse must have an automatic response to any break in aseptic technique during surgery.

No compromise can be made concerning sterility, and as advocates for the patient, the circulating nurse and every other member of the surgical team are responsible to maintain both an individual and a collective surgical conscience.

Surgical conscience involves a concept of self-inspection coupled with moral obligation. Involving both scientific and intellectual honesty, it is self-regulation in practice according to a deep personal commitment to the highest values (Atkinson and Kohn, 1986, p. 98).

Practicing aseptic technique in preparing and maintaining a sterile field should be automatic for all members of the surgical team. Team members should be attentive to the activities of everyone else in the OR and should observe the events that may compromise the sterile field and initiate corrective action (AORN, 1992, III:2–1). The goal of the collective surgical conscience is not to excuse error, but to admit readily and rectify any break in technique to serve the patient better.

Considerations

Maintaining a sterile field necessitates comprehensive attention to detail before and during the surgical procedure. In preparation for an operation, necessary equipment and supplies to be used must be checked to verify their sterility. The operating team is gowned and gloved before handling sterile supplies or having contact with the wound. The sterile field must be created, including skin preparation and draping of the patient to prevent contamination, and then maintained throughout the surgical procedure. Finally, the OR must be kept clean using three main methods: concurrent cleaning, end-of-case cleaning, and terminal cleaning.

Because many postoperative wound infections can be traced to the OR, strict aseptic techniques should be followed at all times. *Sterile* is defined as being maximally free of all microorganisms. Perfect asepsis, the absence of disease-causing microorganisms, is an ideal toward which members of the surgical team should strive.

Sources of infection can be either endogenous or exogenous. Endogenous infection comes from the patient, from the large number of microorganisms found in and on the body. After the skin is incised, certain factors or conditions, including age, nutritional status, impaired defense mechanisms, preexisting disease, and length and type of surgery, can influence a patient's risk of infection.

To control endogenous infection, a number of steps may be taken. Patients are often asked to bathe with an antimicrobial soap before surgery. Before the patient enters the surgical suite, the patient's hair is covered with a cap and any hair at the incision site is removed, either by shaving or using a depilatory cream.

Before draping is performed, the operative area is scrubbed with antimicrobial solution. Gastrointestinal preparations with laxatives and enemas are given before any intestinal surgery. Prophylactic antibiotics may be administered both before and during the operation to a high-risk patient or for specific procedures.

Exogenous infection is acquired from organisms outside the patient's body. People are a major source of contamination. Restricting personnel to the minimum necessary for the surgical procedure and limiting talking minimize the spread of microorganisms. It is imperative that OR personnel be responsible for maintaining good personal hygiene. In addition, to protect the patient from bacteria, all personnel must don proper surgical attire to minimize the chance of spreading microorganisms, including a surgical hat or hood, scrub attire, shoe covers, and masks.

Although the OR is considered a clean environment, it may contain microorganisms in the air and on any permanent structures in the room, such as floors, walls, cabinets, and overhead lights. All are potential sources of infection. Chapter 11 describes the procedures for creating and maintaining a clean environment.

Supplies and Equipment

Supplies, drapes, gowns, gloves, instruments, equipment, OR furniture, fluid containers, and any items used within the sterile field must be sterile.

Procedure

Knowledge of the basic principles that make up aseptic technique is essential to maintain the sterile field during a surgical procedure (Table 6–2). As mentioned above, the surgical conscience of each person on the surgical team compels him or her to follow these principles and to correct any break in sterile technique immediately.

Principles of Aseptic Techniques

Only sterile items are used within the sterile field.

Wrapping and sterilizing items to be used during a surgical procedure is done before surgery. Sterile agents used to kill microorganisms include steam, ethylene oxide gas, liquid chemicals, dry heat, and radiation. Sterile items are kept in appropriate closed storage areas. Packaged materials must allow sterilizing agents to penetrate the contents during sterilization while providing a barrier to microorganisms during transfer and storage.

The shelf life of sterile packages is event, not time, related and is dependent in part on the type of packaging used (AORN, 1992, *III*:12–2). It is the responsibility of the circulating nurse and the scrub nurse to ensure that all sterile packages are inspected before use. The type of packaging, as well as the handling and storage methods used, must be sufficient to maintain sterility. Each package must be inspected for holes, tears, punctures, or moisture to make sure its contents have not been compromised. Container system filters should remain intact, and valves or gaskets should remain sealed after sterilization. Manufacturers' guidelines should be fol-

---

TABLE 6–2. **PRINCIPLES OF ASEPTIC TECHNIQUE**
1. Only sterile items are used within the sterile field.
2. A sterile barrier must be considered contaminated after it has been penetrated.
3. The edges of a sterile package or container are considered contaminated after it is opened.
4. Gowns are considered sterile only in front from shoulder level to table level and the sleeves to 2 inches above the elbow.
5. Only the horizontal surface of a table is considered sterile.
6. Sterile persons and items touch only sterile areas. Nonsterile persons or items touch only nonsterile areas.
7. Movement within or around the sterile field must not contaminate that field.
8. All items and areas of doubtful sterility must be considered contaminated.

Association of Operating Room Nurses, (1992). *Standards and recommended practices for perioperative nursing. III:2–1—2–5*, Denver.

---

lowed. Expiration dates should be checked, as well as any sterilizing chemical process indicators. Packaging materials and methods of storage and handling should meet prescribed standards (AORN, 1992, *III*:12–1).

Flash sterilization of unwrapped instruments and porous items should be done only when time does not permit sterilization by the preferred wrapping method. Speed reduces the margin of safety, in terms of both operator error and the reliability of the sterilizer. Implantable items should not be flash sterilized. They should be monitored with a biological indicator test result that is normal for 48 hours. AORN recommended practices for sterilization and disinfection (1992, *III*:20–1) should be used in selecting types of sterilization.

A sterile barrier must be considered contaminated after it has been penetrated.

Integrity of sterile packages or items, including wrapped items, packages, gowns, gloves, and drapes, can be destroyed by perforation, puncture, or strike through (the soaking of moisture from a sterile or to nonsterile area or vice versa).

If a hole occurs, or a package becomes wet or is dropped, it should be discarded immediately. Packages freshly removed from the sterilizer must be allowed to cool thoroughly to prevent steam condensation and contamination. Any dry stain should be considered contaminated and appropriate action taken.

To prevent strike through in gowns in the critical performance zones (front panel and sleeves) and the critical areas of draping where soaking of blood and body fluids is a risk, a fluid-proof fabric with impervious barriers must be used. In the case of strike through, the contaminated area should be covered with impervious sterile drapes or towels.

The edges of a sterile package or container are considered contaminated after it is opened.

Careful judgment must be used to maintain safety margins between sterile and nonsterile boundaries to prevent accidental contamination of the sterile field.

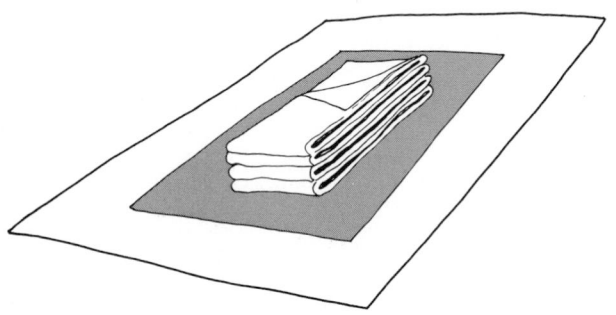

FIGURE 6–37. The shaded area indicates the sterile area.

The area inside linen or nonwoven wrappers that is considered sterile is the area immediately surrounding the sterile item (Fig. 6–37). A sterile package should be opened from the far side first and the near side last (Fig. 6–38). Any loose flaps should be secured so they do not spring back and contaminate the sterile contents.

The wrapper of small peel-back packages must be pulled back and the sterile contents within either flipped onto the sterile field (Fig. 6–39) or exposed away from the nonsterile person and retrieved by the sterile scrub person who pulls the contents straight up and out of the wrapper (Fig. 6–40). If the contents touch the edge of the package or the package tears during opening, it must be considered contaminated and discarded.

Larger packs may be opened on a separate table by opening first the back, then the front flaps, and then the side flaps. Care must be taken to walk around the pack,

rather than reach over the sterile field. When a sterile wrapper also serves as a table cover, only the interior and surface level are considered sterile. After the cap has been removed from a container of sterile fluids, its entire contents must be poured or discarded (Fig. 6–41). The solution receptacle should be placed close to the edge of the table or held by the scrub person. The circulating nurse should be careful not to splash any liquid or let it run down the sides of the container.

Gowns are considered sterile only in front from shoulder level to table level and the sleeves to 2 inches above the elbow.

Gowns are considered completely sterile until put on. The neckline, the shoulders, and the area under the arms may become contaminated by perspiration and are therefore considered nonsterile. The back of the gown is also considered nonsterile because it cannot be observed by the scrubbed person.

Donning of the gown is done on another sterile surface other than the sterile field to avoid dripping water onto the sterile field. Stockinet cuffs are considered contaminated after being touched by the hands and must be covered by gloves. Gloved hands must be held at or above waist level and kept in sight at all times. Scrubbed persons must be careful to keep gloved hands away from the face and from under the axillary areas, as well as to keep their elbows close to their sides.

Any item that is dropped below the waist is considered

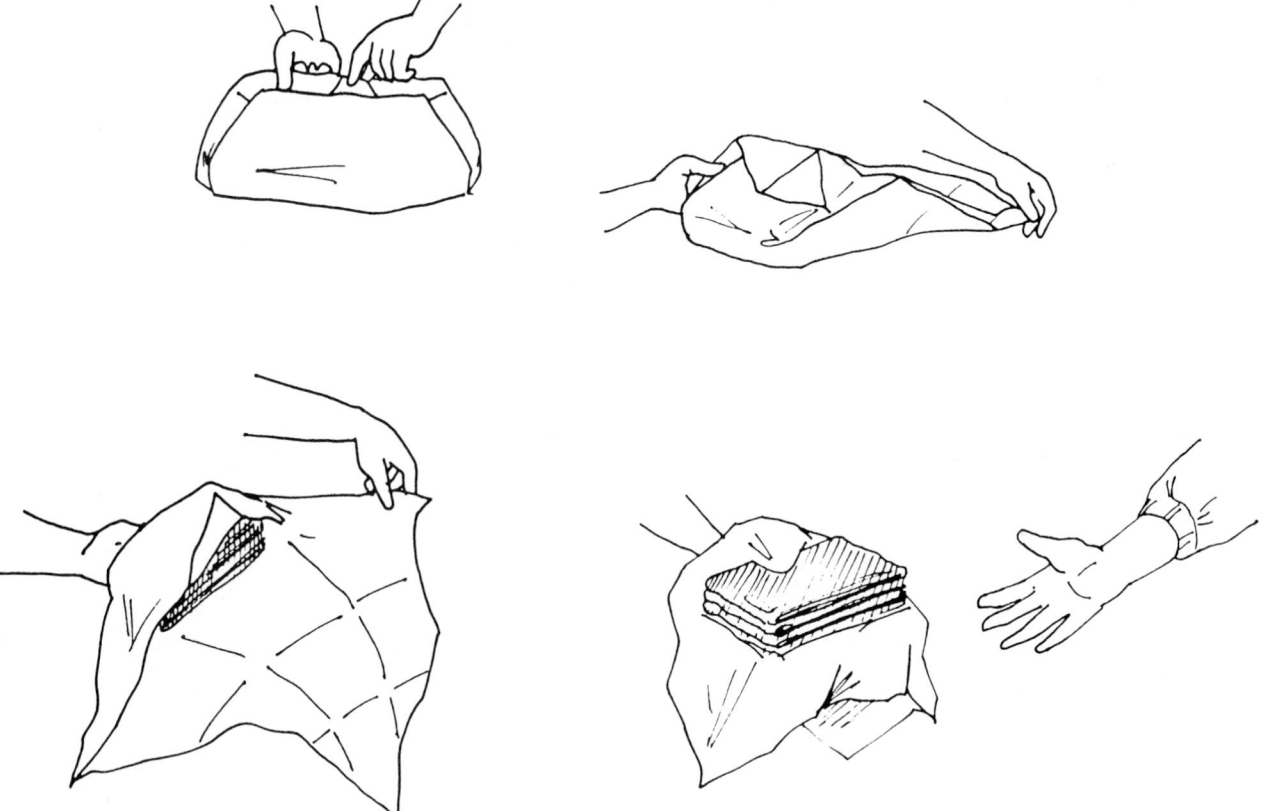

FIGURE 6–38. Open a sterile package from the far side first; secure any loose flaps so they do not contaminate the sterile contents.

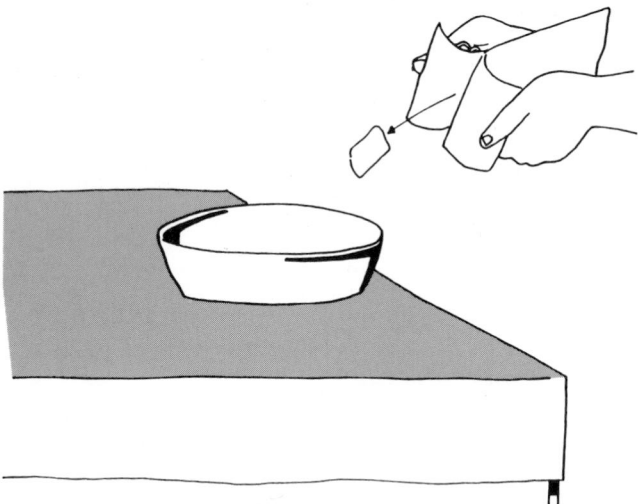

FIGURE 6–39. Contents of a peel-back package deposited onto the sterile field.

contaminated and is discarded. Changing table heights is to be avoided, as is sitting, unless the entire surgical procedure is to be performed sitting.

Only the horizontal surface of a table is considered sterile.

The edges and sides of table drapes are considered nonsterile because they are out of sight and cannot be monitored (Fig. 6–42). When a sterile drape is unfolded, the part that drops below the table surface is not brought back up to table level.

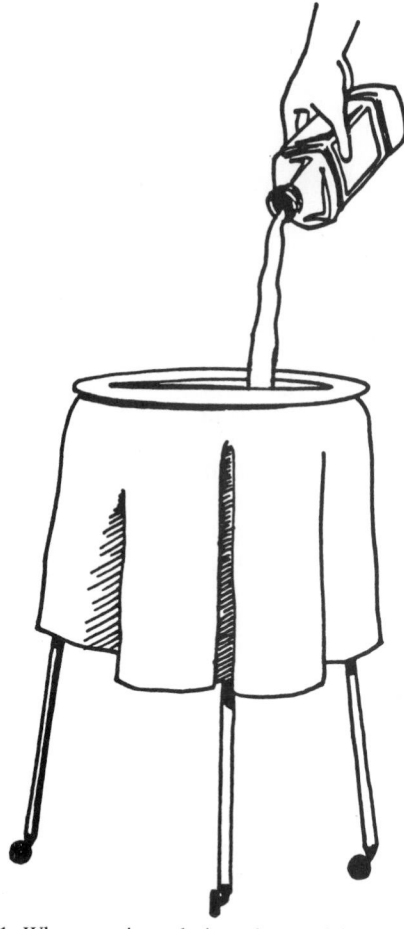

FIGURE 6–41. When pouring solutions, be careful not to splash any liquid or let it run down the sides of the container.

Scrubbed persons should not allow their hands to fall below the sterile field and any item that falls over the edge of the table is considered contaminated. Items that remain on the drapes during the surgical procedure are secured to prevent them from sliding below the level of the sterile field, such as cords and tubings.

Sterile persons and items touch only sterile areas. Nonsterile persons or items touch only nonsterile areas.

Surgical team members must be aware of sterile and nonsterile items and areas in the OR and maintain a safety margin, either by space or by the use of an instrument for extension.

The patient is the center of the sterile field. All sterile equipment is grouped around the patient and within view of scrubbed personnel, who must stay as close as possible to and face the sterile field. Sterile team members maintain contact with the sterile field by wearing sterile gown and gloves.

Nonsterile persons must maintain enough distance from the sterile field to prevent accidental contamination but should always face the sterile field. Nonsterile team members should not lean or reach over the sterile field and should never walk between two sterile fields.

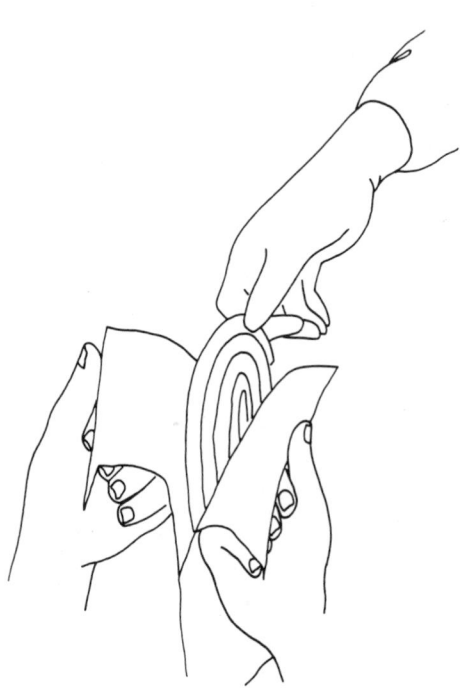

FIGURE 6–40. Contents of a peel-back package grasped by the scrub person.

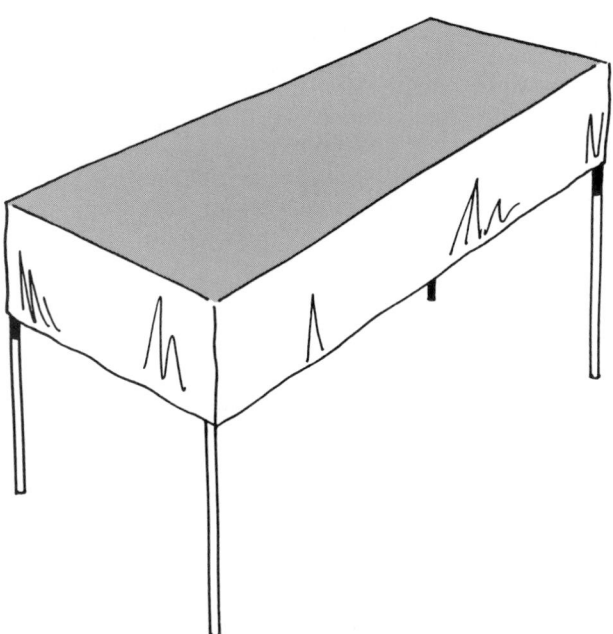

FIGURE 6–42. Only the top of a table is sterile.

When contact between a scrubbed person with a nonsterile person or item is necessary, such as during draping procedures, the sterile scrubbed person's gloves are protected by cuffing a portion of the sterile drape over the gloves, forming a barrier between the glove and the nonsterile person or item contacted.

When passing an item to the scrub nurse, the non-sterile circulating nurse pulls the wrapper of items back over the hand so that only sterile surfaces are presented, making it possible for the sterile scrub person to touch only the sterile item. The circulating nurse never directly

contacts the sterile field, but it is her or his responsibility to open sterile wrappers and packages for sterile team members.

Movement within or around the sterile field must not contaminate that field.

Movements and air currents must be kept to a minimum to avoid contamination of the sterile field. Establishing traffic patterns within and around the sterile field helps to prevent any spread of microorganisms.

The motions of the scrubbed surgical team are from sterile to sterile areas and from nonsterile to nonsterile areas. For example, when two gowned persons must pass each other, it is done face to face, sterile to sterile areas, and back to back, nonsterile to nonsterile areas (Fig. 6–43).

A sterile person should turn his or her back to a nonsterile person or item when passing. A sterile person may ask a nonsterile person to step aside to avoid risk of contamination.

All items and areas of doubtful sterility must be considered contaminated.

If the sterility of any item is in doubt, it should be discarded. Even though a sterile package may not appear to be damaged, for the safety of the patient it must be assumed to be contaminated.

Sterile fields should be prepared as close to the time of use as possible. The longer any sterile item is exposed to the environment, the greater is its chance for contamination. A sterile field left unattended should be considered contaminated, because there is no way to ensure sterility (Kneedler, 1987, p. 439).

Sterile fields should not be covered, because removing

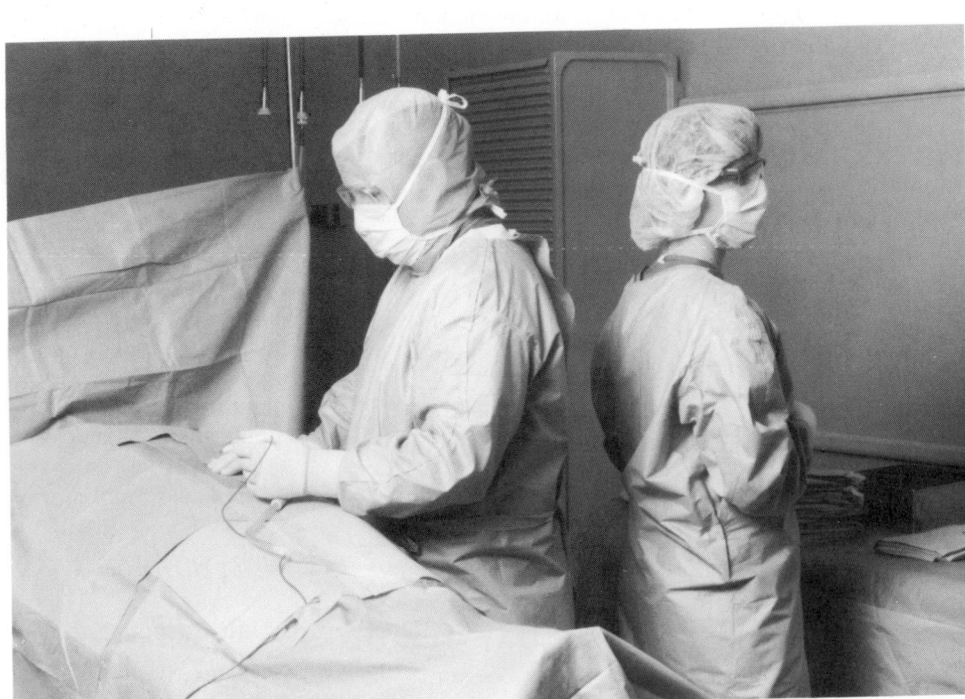

FIGURE 6–43. Gowned persons pass back to back.

the cover later allows a part of the cover that was below table level to be drawn up above the table. Additionally, covered sterile fields are often left unobserved and it is important to monitor constantly all sterile areas and items for any possible contamination.

Performing Preoperative Skin Preparation (AORN, 1992, *III*:18–1—18–5)

Preparing the patient's skin is an important step that can help reduce the risk of postoperative wound infection. When performed correctly, the preparation removes gross contaminants, dirt, skin oil, and microbes from the skin and eliminates transient bacteria while reducing the resident colony count in the shortest period of time with the least amount of tissue irritation. An antimicrobial residue should be left on the skin to inhibit rebound growth of microorganisms during the surgical procedure. Skin preparation may include a patient shower or bath, the removal of hair, the removal of foreign substances (adhesives, tar, grease), and the cleansing of the incision site and surrounding area with an antimicrobial agent.

Considerations

Maintaining the surgical patient's skin integrity should be a major focus during the preoperative skin preparation. The skin acts as a mechanical barrier to infection and is composed of three layers: the epidermis, the dermis, and the subcutaneous tissues (Fig. 6–44). The most superficial layer, the epidermis, is thin, devoid of blood vessels and divided into two layers: an outer horny layer of dead keratinized cells and an inner cellular layer in which both melanin and keratin are formed. The transient flora resides on the epidermis and is easily removed with soap and water. The epidermis depends on the underlying dermis for its nutrition. The dermis is well supplied with blood. It contains connective tissue, the sebaceous glands, and some of the hair follicles. The resident flora survives and multiplies in the dermis and can be repeatedly cultured and causes wound infection when allowed to enter deep tissues

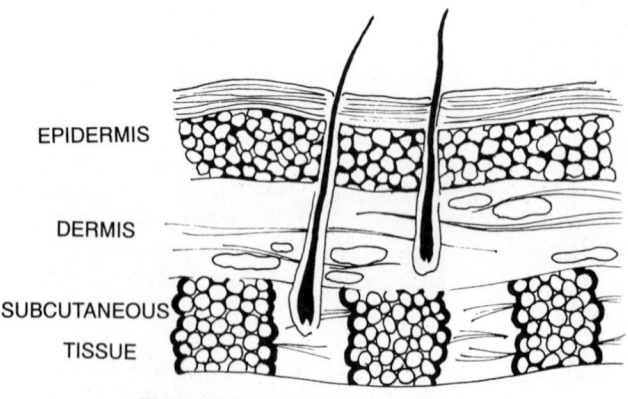

FIGURE 6–44. Layers of the skin.

during the surgical procedure. The dermis merges below with the subcutaneous tissues, which contain fat, the sweat glands, and the remainder of the hair follicles. The skin has many functions: it protects the deeper tissues from drying and injury, regulates body temperature, maintains fluid balance, and houses the sensory nervous system (Price and Wilson, 1986, pp. 1005–1008).

To maintain skin integrity when preparing the patient's operative site, a number of factors must be considered. These include the patient's overall physical condition, allergies, and skin sensitivities; whether the patient showered or bathed with an antimicrobial agent prior to hospital admission; the degree of bioburden within the operative site; the anatomy involved during the surgical procedure; the patient's skin condition in and around the operative site; whether the patient will be awake or anesthetized during the skin preparation; the types of supplies and antimicrobial agents available; and whether extra personnel will be required to help stabilize fractures, support an extremity, or assist with multiple trauma or an extensive preparation.

Hair should not be removed unless it interferes with the incision. If shaving is deemed necessary, it should be performed directly before the surgical procedure. The time between the preoperative shave and the surgery has a direct effect on wound infection rate; the longer the delay between the shave and the surgery, the greater is the risk of postoperative infection (Cruse and Foord, 1973, p. 208).

However, shaving should not be done in the OR because the airborne hair and skin debris could contaminate the sterile field. Clipping hair with electric clippers or scissors and using depilatories lowers the risk of postoperative wound infection (Willford, 1984, p. 301). Most pediatric and female facial procedures do not require shaving because of the relative lack of body hair. Hair removal around the eye area must be approached with caution. Shaving of the eyebrows is avoided if possible because they often do not grow back completely.

Supplies and Equipment

A shave preparation kit, nonsterile gloves, a disposable or terminally sterilized reusable razor, skin solvents, and an antimicrobial detergent are used for a wet shave. A depilatory cream and terminally sterilized electrical clippers and/or scissors can also be used. A small separate movable table; a sterile preparation tray, including bowls, or a plastic tray with compartments; sponges; sponge sticks; cotton-tipped applicators; sterile gloves; sterile absorbent towels; a sterile nail cleaner; a sterile brush; and antimicrobial agents are needed.

Procedure

Hair Removal

1. Check the patient care area for adequate lighting and patient privacy. Explain the procedure to the patient.

Inquire about allergies, scars, or moles that may interfere with hair removal.

2. To perform a wet shave, prepare towels, detergent, a sharp disposable or terminally sterilized razor, and a container with warm water. Expose the incisional area, and assess the patient's skin condition. Don nonsterile gloves and place an impervious towel beneath the area to be shaved. Lather the skin in the incisional area and let it set for a few minutes. Hold the skin taut and shave by moving the razor in the direction of hair growth, avoiding cutting or making nicks in the skin. Shave only the hair in the incisional area that interferes with the surgical procedure. After shaving, clean, rinse, and dry the skin and make the patient comfortable.

3. When removing hair with a depilatory cream, a skin sensitivity test should be performed before application. Apply the cream according to manufacturer's instructions. After the specified time, remove the cream and the hair. Clean, rinse, and dry the skin.

4. To remove hair with electrical clippers or scissors, clip hair in the prescribed area to prevent contamination of the incisional area with hair. Long hair surrounding the incisional area may need to be trimmed so that it does not interfere with the surgical procedure.

5. Document the patient's skin condition before and immediately after the hair removal, noting any redness, razor nicks, or skin abrasions.

Patient Skin Scrub

The surgical skin preparation is a sterile procedure and should incorporate aseptic technique.

1. Prepare sterile supplies for skin preparation on a separate, small movable table.

2. Select broad-spectrum antimicrobial agents capable of reducing and inhibiting both transient and resident microorganisms. They should be fast acting; easily applied and able to maintain effectiveness for several hours; nonirritating and nonsensitizing; not rendered ineffective by soaps, detergents, organic matter, or alcohol; and approved by the U.S. Food and Drug Administration. When using an antimicrobial agent, always read the manufacturer's instructions because some can be neurotoxic and some may be toxic or harmful at various body sites. Eye injury associated with chlorhexidine gluconate has been reported, and chlorhexidine gluconate can cause ototoxicity if instilled directly into the middle ear (Larson, 1988, p. 258).

3. If the patient is awake, explain the procedure and provide privacy and comfort. Make every effort to allay fears, and answer questions in a reassuring manner.

4. If the patient has been anesthetized, check with the anesthetist before starting the preparation.

5. After the patient has been positioned, move the small table with the sterile skin prepping supplies close to the patient. Expose the area to be prepared, assessing the skin condition and the effectiveness of hair removal.

6. Don sterile gloves and arrange supplies for the procedure. Place absorbent towels on each side of patient to absorb excess solution and to prevent pooling under the patient, electrodes, and the electrosurgical dispersive pad. To prevent pooling under tourniquets, seal off with an impervious U-drape or towel. Pooling of solutions may result in skin burn or irritation owing to chemical action. Also place impervious pads under the extremities to prevent solutions from saturating the patient's linen.

7. Begin cleansing at the incision site in a circular motion, moving out toward the periphery. When the edges of the preparation site have been reached, discard the used sponge, and with a new sterile sponge, repeat the process. Never bring a soiled sponge back toward the incisional site. Prepare at least 6 to 8 inches beyond the incisional site in all directions unless otherwise stated for a specific procedure (see below). The cleansing of the operative site should last long enough to thoroughly cleanse the skin. Cotton-tipped applicators should be used to clean thoroughly the umbilicus and hard-to-reach areas.

8. Cleansing should proceed from clean to dirty, scrubbing an area of high bioburden last and discarding the sponge. Areas of high bioburden are the umbilicus, the axillary area, the vagina, the anus, open skin lesions, soiled traumatic wounds, and stomas.

9. If the incisional site includes a stoma as an integral part of the procedure, cover the stoma with a sterile gauze, and cleanse the area surrounding the stoma, and cleanse the stoma last. If the stoma is in the operative area, yet not included in the incision, isolate the stoma with a clear plastic adherent drape and then begin the preparation.

10. Most open traumatic wounds, burns, or denuded areas necessitate copious amounts of sterile solutions to flush contaminants out of the wound.

11. Prepping after cast or large dressing removal may necessitate soaking with sterile solutions to remove adherent dressings. Care must be taken in this situation because the skin may be sensitive and denuded.

12. Prepping for procedures involving grafts necessitates separate setups, or if it is a small area, one preparation setup may be used, cleansing the donor site first.

13. When preparing an area with a possible malignancy (e.g., a breast mass), omit scrubbing to avoid the possible spread of carcinoma, and only apply an antimicrobial paint or gel to the operative area.

14. After scrubbing, the lather should be either wiped off with a dry sponge or blotted dry with an absorbent towel. When removing the towel, grasp the edges farthest away and lift it up away from the skin, bringing the towel toward the person performing the preparation. Pay careful attention not to contaminate the prepared area with the edges of the towel.

15. Using a sponge stick and an outward circular motion, apply the antimicrobial solution starting at the incisional area and move to the periphery. A second

and third sponge stick may be necessary to completely cover the operative area.

16. If flammable solutions are used (alcohol, acetone, fat solvents), adequate time should elapse to allow the solution to dry and the fumes to evaporate before activating electrosurgical or laser equipment.

17. Remove the impervious preparation pad from under the extremities or remove the absorbent towels from each side of the patient; avoid bringing towels over the prepared area.

18. Remove the gloves and discard all preparation materials in a proper receptacle.

19. Document on the OR record the patient's skin condition and the effectiveness of hair removal before beginning the preparation; state the antimicrobial agent used, the area prepped, and the person performing the prep.

20. On completion of the surgical procedure, assess the patient's skin in and around the operative site and document on the OR record any redness, abrasions, or burns. Communicate the findings to the surgeon and the postanesthesia care nurse.

21. A surgical skin preparation procedure manual should specify the type of agent, the anatomical areas, and the procedure for each type of surgical procedure.

The following are surgical skin preparations designed for different anatomical areas of the body. These are not the only acceptable methods but are some of the most common procedures.

Scrub for Specific Anatomical Areas

Eye

1. Confine the patient's hair within a disposable surgical hat or towel.

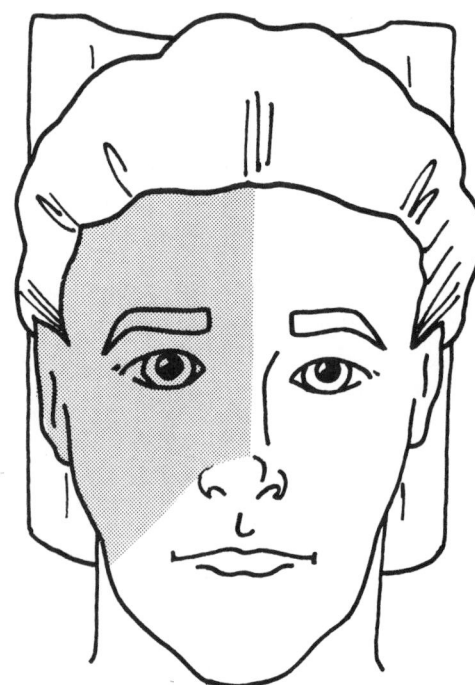

FIGURE 6–45. The shaded area is prepared for eye surgery.

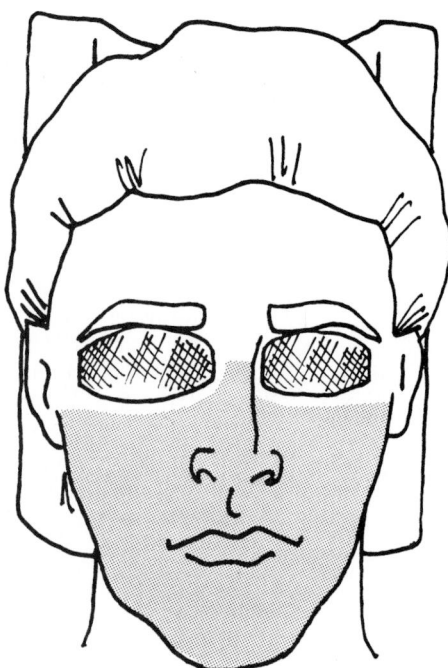

FIGURE 6–46. The shaded area is prepared for nose and lower face surgery.

2. Secure the head in a head support to prevent rolling or moving.

3. Trim the eyelashes (when ordered) with a fine scissors coated with sterile ophthalmic ointment to catch the lashes.

4. Squeeze sponges almost dry when cleansing, to prevent pooling of the solution in the eye.

5. Cleanse the periorbital area, the eyelid, the lashes, and at least a 1-inch-diameter area beyond the periphery of the eye using a nonirritating aqueous antimicrobial solution and sponges (Fig. 6–45).

6. Begin at the center of the eye and continue to the periphery using cotton-tipped applicators for difficult-to-reach areas.

7. Irrigate the periorbital area using a small bulb syringe and sterile water. Contain irrigating solution in a basin or with a towel at the side of the head.

8. Blot the area dry with a sterile sponge.

Lower Face and Nose

1. Confine the patient's hair within a disposable surgical hat or towel.

2. Secure the head in a head support to prevent rolling or moving.

3. Protect the patient's eyes with sponges or eye pads.

4. Squeeze the sponges almost dry when cleansing to prevent pooling of the solution in the patient's eyes or ears.

5. Begin cleansing at the bridge of the nose in a circular motion, moving out toward the hairline and down to the mandible (Fig. 6–46).

6. Use cotton-tipped applicators to cleanse the nostrils and hard-to-reach areas.

7. Squeeze excess antimicrobial solution from the sponge stick and paint from the nose to the periphery.

Ear

1. Confine the patient's hair within a disposable surgical hat or towel.
2. Turn the patient's head to the side, with the ear to be operated on up, and secure in head support to prevent rolling or moving.
3. When ordered, clip or wet shave the hair around the ear that may interfere with the procedure.
4. Secure the hair and define the operative area with tape or adhesive plastic towels.
5. Squeeze the sponges almost dry when cleansing to prevent pooling of the solution in the ear.
6. Prepare from the center of the ear using a nonirritating antimicrobial solution. Extend the prep onto the face and neck area (Fig. 6–47).
7. Use cotton-tipped applicators to cleanse the external ear canal.
8. A small piece of cotton ball may be placed in the external ear to absorb solution and prevent pooling of prepping solution.
9. Squeeze excessive antimicrobial solution from the sponge stick and paint from the center of the ear. Extend the prep into the face and neck area.

Neck and Combined Head and Neck

1. Expose the operative area to the nipple line.
2. Place an impervious pad at the table line beneath the head.
3. Begin cleansing in a circular motion from the incisional site to the periphery.
4. Prepare the neck anteriorly and laterally from the mandible to midsternum, including the tops of the shoulders (Fig. 6–48).
5. For combined head and neck procedure, also cleanse the lower portion of the face and the areas of the head around the ears.

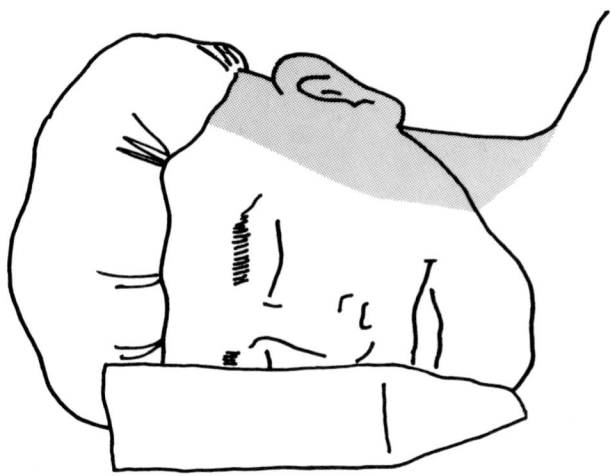

FIGURE 6–47. The shaded area is prepared for ear surgery.

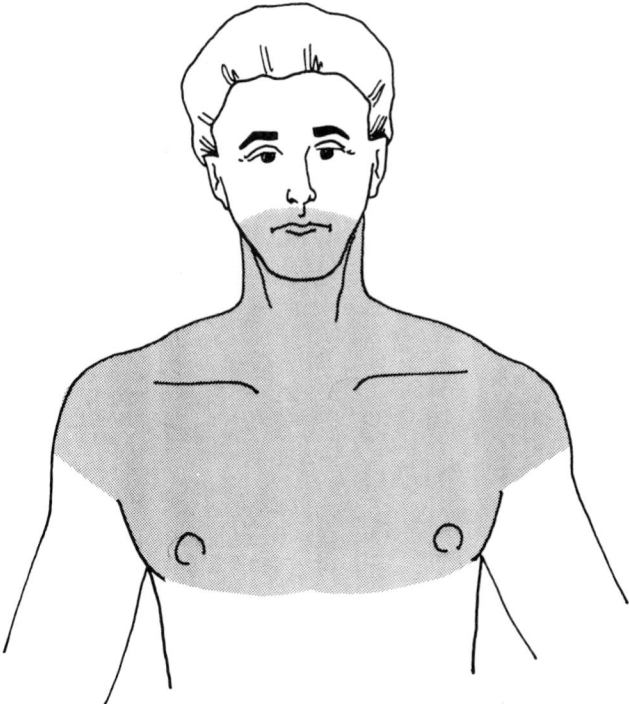

FIGURE 6–48. The shaded area is prepared for head and neck surgery.

6. Continue the scrubbing long enough to cleanse the area thoroughly.
7. Blot the area dry with absorbent sterile towels.
8. Paint with an antimicrobial solution.

Chest or Breast

1. Support the fingers in a hand-holder device, or obtain an assistant to elevate the patient's hand and arm.
2. Expose the operative area to the waistline.
3. Place an absorbent towel over the unoperative side and an impervious preparation pad on the table under the axilla and shoulder of the operative side.
4. Begin cleansing in a circular motion from the incisional site to the periphery.
5. Prepare from the top of the shoulder to below the diaphragm and from the edge of unoperative breast to the table line, including the upper arm to elbow circumferentially and the axilla (Fig. 6–49).
6. Cleanse the axillary area last or use a separate sponge and discard it because of the high bioburden in that area.
7. Prepare both sides of the chest for a bilateral procedure.
8. Paint with an antimicrobial solution.
9. For a breast biopsy, prepare the breast from the incisional area, to include an approximately 3-inch-diameter area beyond the breast.
10. When preparing a breast with a possible malignancy, omit scrubbing to avoid possible spread of carci-

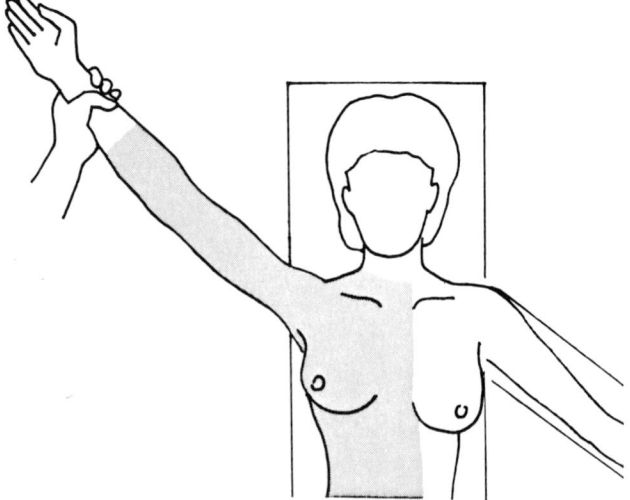

FIGURE 6–49. The shaded area is prepared for breast surgery.

noma; gently apply an antimicrobial paint or gel to the operative area only.

Abdomen, Supine Position

1. Expose the operative area from the nipple line to the pubis.
2. Place absorbent towels alongside the patient at the table line to absorb any solution and prevent pooling.
3. Begin cleansing in a circular motion from the incisional site to the periphery.
4. Prepare from the breast line to the groin area, and from table line to table line (Fig. 6–50).
5. Continue scrubbing long enough to cleanse the area thoroughly.
6. Blot the area dry with absorbent sterile towels.
7. Paint with an antimicrobial solution.

Back, Prone Position

1. Expose the operative area from the shoulders to the top of the buttocks.
2. Place absorbent towels alongside the patient at the table line to absorb any solution and prevent pooling.
3. Begin cleansing in a circular motion from the incisional site to the periphery.
4. Prepare from the shoulders to the top of the buttocks, and from table line to table line (Fig. 6–51).
5. Continue scrubbing long enough to cleanse the area thoroughly.
6. Blot the area dry with absorbent sterile towels.
7. Paint with an antimicrobial solution.

Chest and Kidney, Lateral Position

1. Expose the operative area to the ileum.
2. Place absorbent towels anteriorly and posteriorly under the chest at the table level.
3. Begin cleansing in a circular motion from the incisional site to the periphery.

4. Prepare the area from the shoulders to the ileum and the anterior and posterior chest wall for thoracic procedures (Fig. 6–52).
5. Prepare from midchest to the hip, anteriorly and posteriorly for kidney procedures.
6. Blot the area dry with absorbent sterile towels.
7. Paint with an antimicrobial solution.

Perineum or Vagina

1. Expose the perineal area.
2. Place an impervious pad under the buttocks and form a funnel into a kick bucket to collect fluids.
3. Prepare from the pubis to the anus, including the vulva, the labia, the perineum, the inner aspects of the thighs, and the vagina (Fig. 6–53).
4. Cleanse from the pubis area downward over the vulva and the perineum and past the anus; always discard the sponge after touching the anus because of the high bioburden in that area.
5. Scrub the inner aspects of the thighs beginning at the labia majora and moving outward.
6. Insert a narrow sponge stick saturated with an antimicrobial agent gently into the vagina and, using a rotating motion, cleanse the many folds of the vaginal

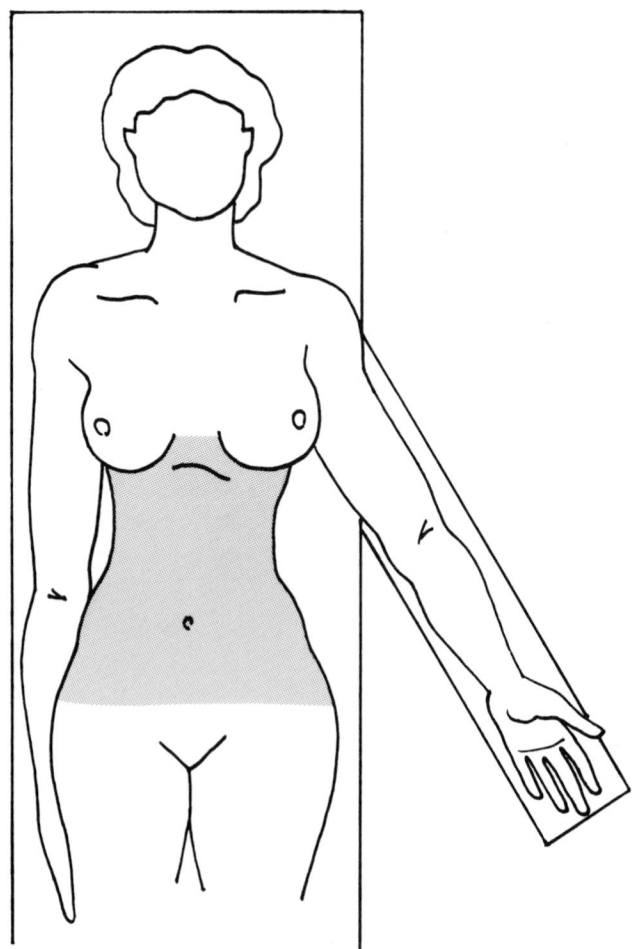

FIGURE 6–50. The shaded area is prepared for abdominal surgery.

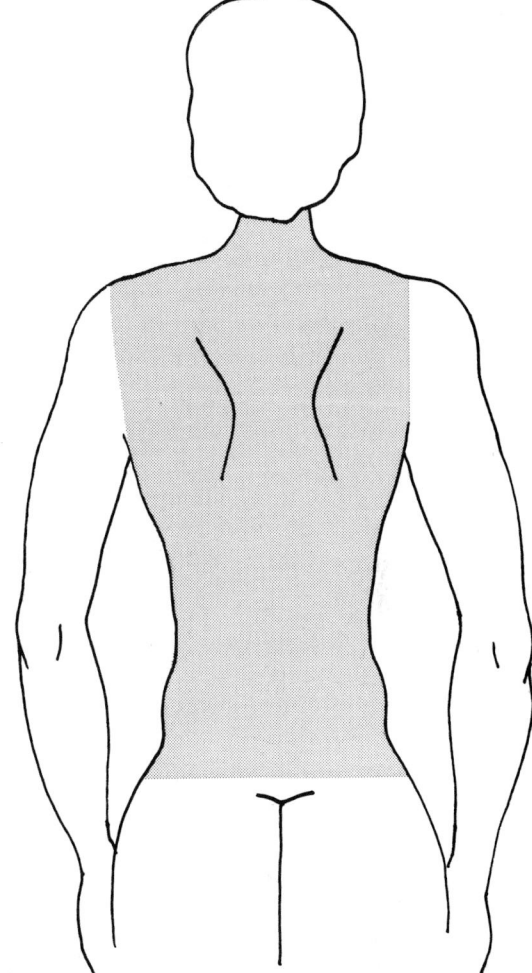

FIGURE 6–51. The shaded area is prepared for back surgery with the patient in the prone position.

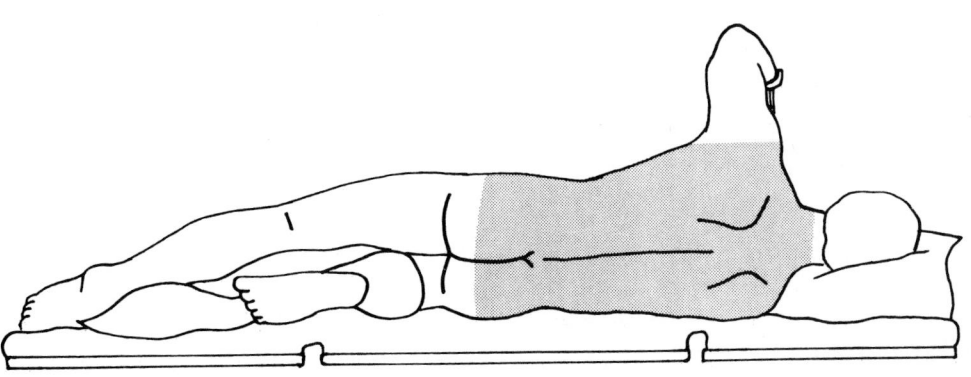

FIGURE 6–52. The shaded area is prepared for thoracic surgery with the patient in the lateral position.

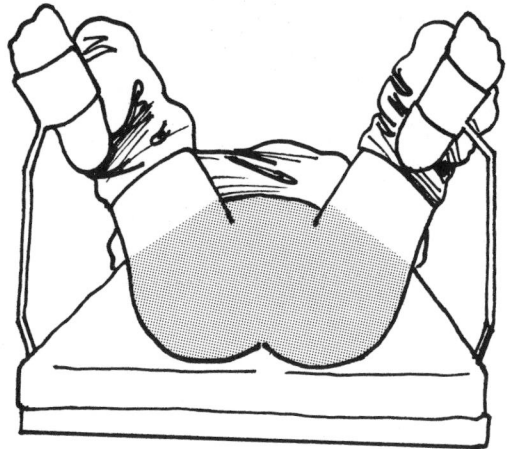

FIGURE 6–53. The shaded area is prepared for perineal or vaginal surgery.

mucosa. Repeat twice, discarding the sponge stick after each use.

7. Insert a dry narrow sponge gently into the vagina to absorb any pooling of antimicrobial agent.

Catheterization in Conjunction with Perineal-Vaginal Preparation

1. Remove the gloves; they are considered contaminated from the prep.
2. Don sterile gloves and insert a sterile catheter.

Hand or Forearm

1. Apply a tourniquet to the upper arm, when ordered (see Chapter 8).
2. Place the patient's arm on a hand table, which is protected with an impervious pad.
3. Elevate the forearm on an extremity support.
4. Begin cleansing at the fingertips and continue to the elbow circumferentially, paying close attention to areas under the nails and the cuticles (Fig. 6–54).

5. If the nail beds are dirty, soak a sudsy solution under the nails and clean with a nail cleaner and brush.
6. Blot the area dry with absorbent sterile towels.
7. Paint with an antimicrobial solution from the fingertips to the elbow.

Elbow and Upper Arm

1. Apply a tourniquet to the upper arm, when ordered (see Chapter 8).
2. Support the fingers in a hand-holder device, or obtain an assistant to elevate the patient's hand and arm.
3. Apply an impervious adhesive U-drape, sealing off a tourniquet to prevent the preparation solution from running or pooling under tourniquet.
4. Begin cleansing in a circular motion from the incisional site to the periphery.
5. Prepare from the wrist to the axilla, or to the tourniquet, if applied, circumferentially (Fig. 6–55).
6. Continue the scrubbing long enough to cleanse the area thoroughly.
7. Blot the area dry with absorbent sterile towels.
8. Paint with an antimicrobial solution from the incisional site to the periphery.

Shoulder

1. Support the fingers in a hand-holder device, or obtain an assistant to elevate the patient's shoulder from the table.
2. Place an impervious pad under the shoulder and axilla.
3. Begin cleansing in a circular motion from the incisional site to the periphery.
4. Prepare from midneck to the elbow circumferentially, including the shoulder, the scapula, the chest to the nipple, and the axilla (Fig. 6–56).
5. Cleanse the axillary area last, or use a separate sponge and discard because of the high bioburden in that area.

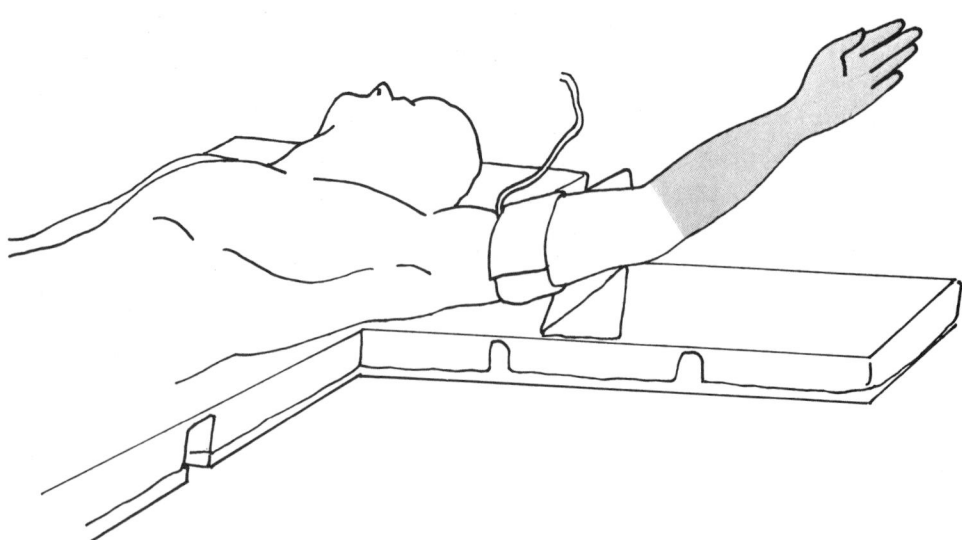

FIGURE 6–54. The shaded area is prepared for hand or forearm surgery.

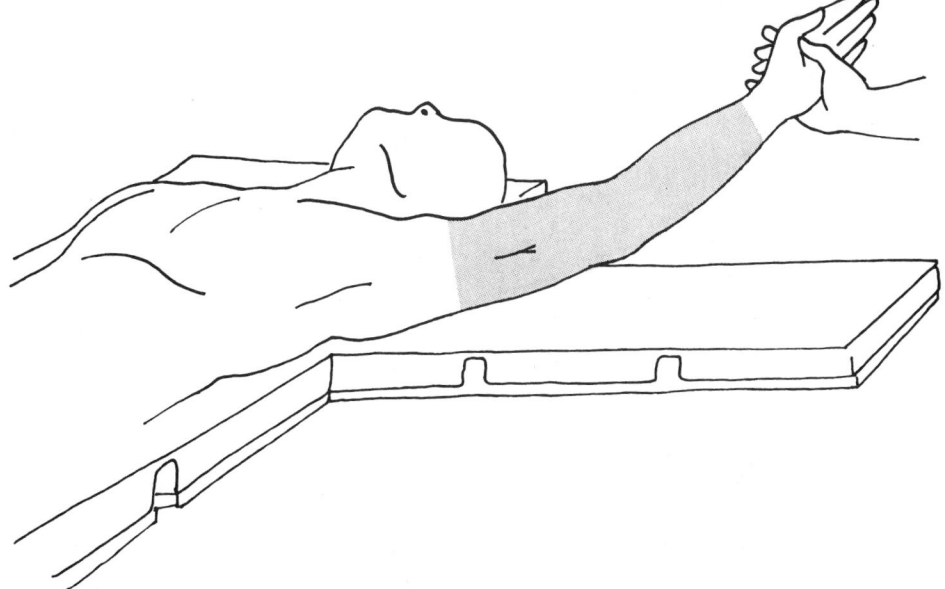

FIGURE 6–55. The shaded area is prepared for elbow and upper arm surgery.

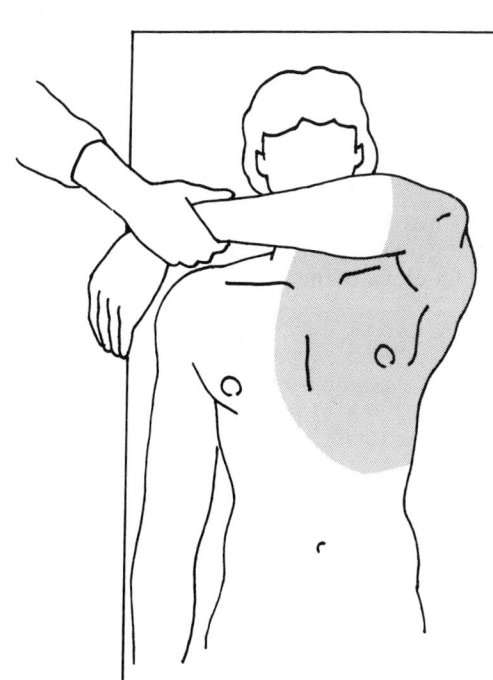

FIGURE 6–56. The shaded area is prepared for shoulder surgery.

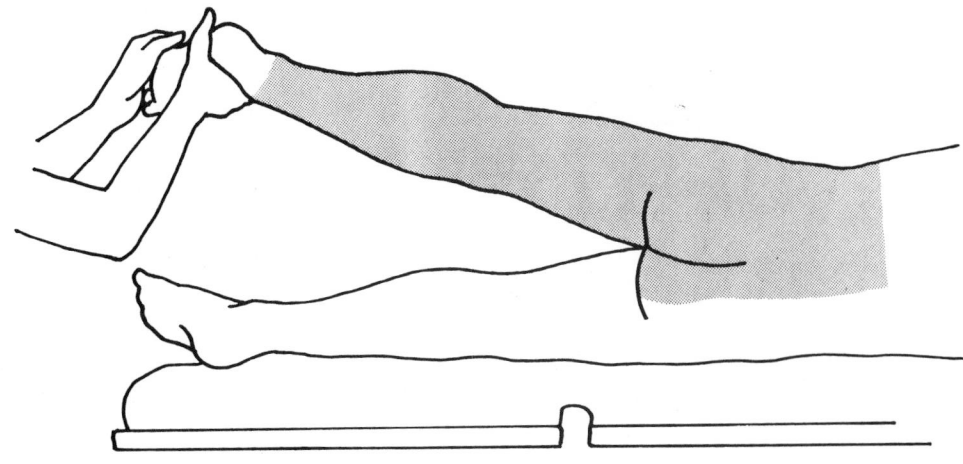

FIGURE 6–57. The shaded area is prepared for hip procedures with the patient in the semilateral position.

6. Continue scrubbing long enough to cleanse the area thoroughly.
7. Blot the area dry with absorbent sterile towels.
8. Paint with an antimicrobial solution from the incisional site to the periphery.

Hip, Semilateral Position

1. Support the foot in extremity-holder device, or obtain an assistant to elevate the patient's entire leg from the groin to the ankle.
2. Apply an impervious adhesive U-drape, isolating the perineal-rectal area.
3. Begin cleansing in a circular motion from the incisional site to the periphery.
4. Prepare from the waist to midbuttocks, and to the lower outer aspect of the abdomen, and include the leg circumferentially from the hip to the ankle (Fig. 6–57).
5. Blot the area dry with absorbent sterile towels.
6. Paint with an antimicrobial solution from the incisional site to the periphery.

Hip, Fracture Table

1. Position the patient on a fracture table with the affected leg in traction.
2. Apply an impervious adhesive U-drape, isolating the perineal/rectal area.
3. Place an impervious pad between the affected hip and the top of the fracture table.
4. Begin cleansing in a circular motion from the incisional site to the periphery.
5. Prepare from the waist to the abdominal midline, and to the table level, and include the leg circumferentially from the hip to the knee (Fig. 6–58).
6. Continue scrubbing long enough to cleanse the area thoroughly.
7. Blot the area dry with absorbent sterile towels.
8. Paint with an antimicrobial solution from the incisional site to the periphery.

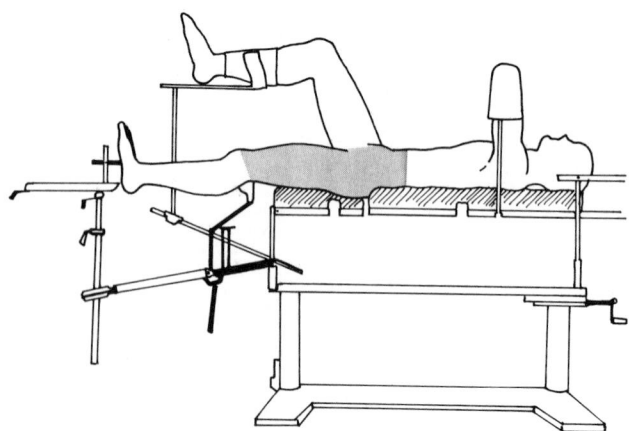

FIGURE 6–58. The shaded area is prepared for hip procedures with the patient on the fracture table.

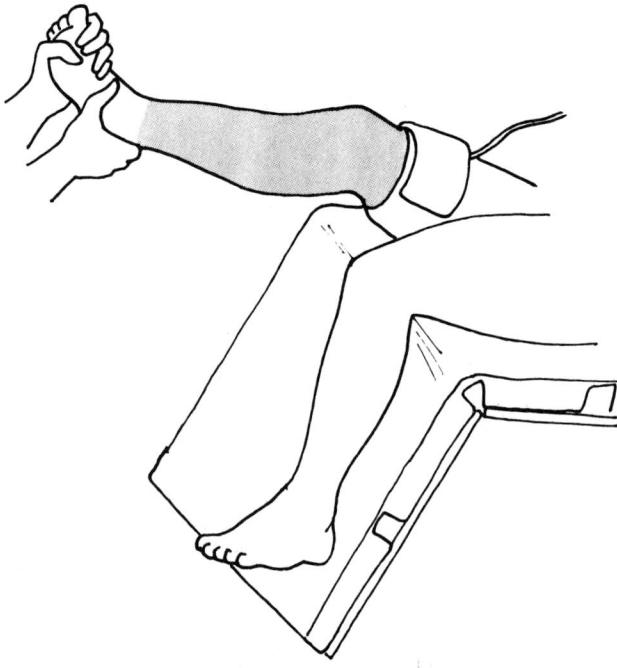

FIGURE 6–59. The shaded area is prepared for knee procedures.

Knee

1. Support the foot in extremity-holder device, or obtain an assistant to elevate the entire leg from the table.
2. Apply a tourniquet to the upper thigh, when ordered (see Chapter 8).
3. Apply an impervious U-drape, sealing off the tourniquet to prevent the solution from running or pooling under the tourniquet.
4. Prepare circumferentially from the ankle to the tourniquet (Fig. 6–59).
5. Begin cleansing at the knee in a circular motion, moving up toward the tourniquet, and discard sponges.
6. Begin cleansing again at the knee in a circular motion to the ankle and discard sponges.
7. Continue scrubbing long enough to cleanse the area thoroughly.
8. Blot the area dry with absorbent sterile towels.
9. Paint with an antimicrobial agent from the knee to the tourniquet, and discard the paint stick. With another paint stick, paint from the knee to the ankle.

Foot or Ankle

1. Apply a tourniquet to upper thigh, when ordered (see Chapter 8).
2. Elevate the lower leg on an extremity support.
3. Place an impervious pad under the foot.
4. Begin cleansing at the toes and move up toward the lower leg.
5. Prepare from the tip of the toes to the midcalf circumferentially, paying close attention to the area under and around the nails (Fig. 6–60).
6. Blot the area dry with absorbent sterile towels.

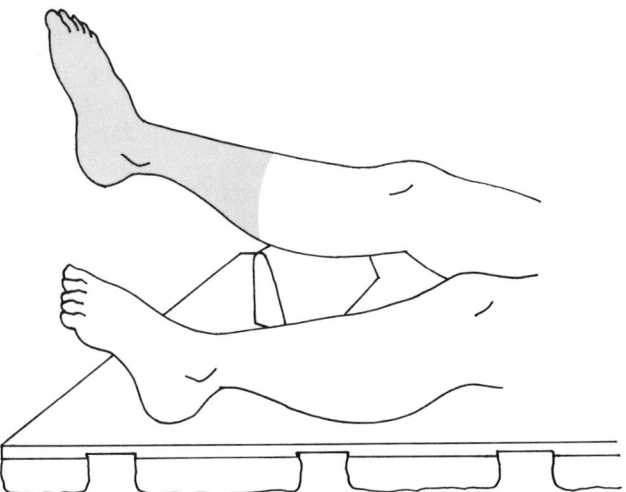

FIGURE 6–60. The shaded area is prepared for foot and ankle procedures.

7. Paint with an antimicrobial solution starting at the toes, and moving up toward the calf.

Open Heart

1. Expose the operative area from the neck to the toes.
2. Elevate the legs on an ankle support.
3. Place an impervious pad under the legs and towels alongside the patient at the table line to absorb excessive solution.
4. Prepare from the trachea to the toes, including both legs circumferentially (Fig. 6–61).
5. Begin cleansing in a circular motion at the sternum and move toward the periphery of the torso.
6. Prepare the leg circumferentially, beginning at the incision area, to the periphery of the legs.
7. Prepare the genital area separately and isolate the area with an impervious towel.
8. Continue scrubbing long enough to cleanse the area thoroughly.
9. Blot the area dry with absorbent sterile towels.
10. Paint with an antimicrobial solution from the incisional site to the periphery.
11. Separate preps may be done for the chest area and the leg areas.

Draping the Patient and Equipment
(AORN, 1992, *III*:2–1 and 6–1)

The primary functions of draping the surgical patient and equipment are to define and establish the sterile field during the surgical procedure by isolating the incisional site and to prevent microbial migration from nonsterile to sterile areas. The sterile field is the zone on the draped patient and the equipment considered to be free of microorganisms at the start of and throughout the surgical procedure. The area draped includes the patient; the area from the anesthesia screen and arm boards to the foot of the OR bed; the surgical team in sterile attire; and the Mayo stand, back table, ring stand, and any other equipment used during the surgical procedure.

Because of the possibility of direct contact with blood, tissues, and body fluids, universal precautions should be followed during surgical intervention for the prevention of transmission of the human immunodeficiency virus and hepatitis B virus. It is recommended that all patients be treated as though their blood and body fluids are infectious and that the precautions be practiced routinely and vigorously adhered to (OSHA Occupational exposure to bloodborne pathogens, 1991).

To prevent moist bacterial strike through and to contain and control body fluids, impervious barrier drapes are imperative. Strike through occurs when fluids penetrate sterile drapes from a sterile to a nonsterile area or vice versa, thus breaking the sterile barrier and allowing microbial transfer to and from the patient. Using an impervious fluid-proof fabric is the only way that strike through can be prevented.

Considerations

The importance of choosing the correct surgical drapes is increasing. The focus for preventing transmission of infectious microorganisms through barrier materials has grown to include both reducing postoperative wound infection and protecting the surgical team from contact with patients' body fluids.

The types of surgical draping material selected for each specific procedure depend on the degree of barrier

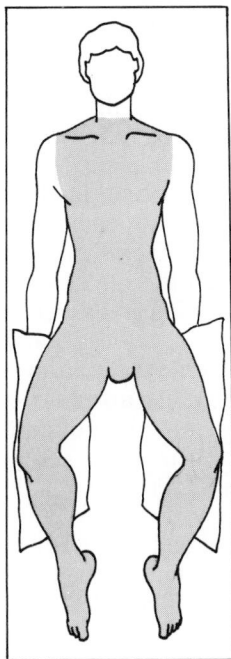

FIGURE 6–61. The shaded area is prepared for open heart surgery.

protection required for both the patient and the surgical team. Whether to choose a fluid-proof fabric with impervious barriers for areas where the soaking of blood and body fluids is a potential risk, or a fluid-resistant fabric for areas where the splashing or spraying of blood and body fluids is a potential risk depends on the anatomical area involved, the position required, and the amount of moisture inherent during the proposed surgery (OSHA Occupational Exposure to Bloodborne Pathogens, 1991).

When assessing the surgical patient to be draped, four areas of draping are taken into consideration:

1. The *patient critical area* is the draping area that immediately surrounds the operative site. Soaking of body fluids is a high risk in this area. To prevent strike through and maintain a sterile field for the duration of the procedure and to inhibit microbial transfer, it is essential that fluid-proof fabrics with impervious barriers are used in this area.
2. *Critical zones* are the draping areas where blood and irrigation fluids are increased and soaking of body fluids is a risk. The types of instruments or medical devices used have a tendency to cause tears, punctures, or abrasions of drapes, thus allowing strike through and causing a break in the sterile field; this permits microbial transfer to and from the patient. These areas include the back table, the Mayo stand, and the hand table; areas under or around extremities, areas of friction from retractors, and areas involved in a trauma procedure; and any other area where there is a potential risk of strike through. These draping areas require special attention where fluid-proof fabrics with impervious barriers and added strength or plastic pouches are necessary to contain and control body fluids.
3. The *patient peripheral area* is the draping area that covers the entire patient and surrounds the critical area. It includes both arm boards, the anesthesia screen, the area over the foot of the OR bed, and an adequate length beyond the OR bed level. In this area, splashing and spraying of body fluids is a risk and the chance of fluid strike through is less because of the small amount of moisture present. A fluid-resistant fabric can provide an effective sterile barrier in this area.
4. Equipment draping areas including surgical equipment and medical devices that will be used in and around the sterile field. Mayo stands and back tables where sterile instruments and supplies are placed require a fluid-proof fabric with impervious barriers to prevent strike through and to prevent microbial transfer and contamination. Equipment in the periphery of the sterile field, where splashing and spraying of body fluids is a risk, may be draped with a fluid-resistant fabric to provide an effective sterile barrier. Plastic, transparent impervious drapes are ideal for cameras, microscopes, laser arms, power equipment, and imaging equipment, and they provide an effective sterile barrier.

Most OR suites use a disposable nonwoven or a reusable linen draping system or a combination of both for surgical procedures. When selecting the correct surgical drapes for the proposed surgery, whether reusable or disposable, many qualities and characteristics need to be considered.

To be an effective sterile barrier, surgical drapes should be made of either fluid-proof fabrics with impervious barriers that avoid strike through, when soaking of blood and body fluids is a risk, or fluid-resistant fabrics, when splashing or spraying of blood and body fluids is a risk, thereby eliminating microorganism penetration. They should be lint free to minimize airborne contamination and the dissemination of particles into the wound. Drapes should be strong enough to resist abrasions, tears, or punctures yet porous enough to prevent heat build-up. This maintains an isothermic environment that is appropriate for the surgical patient's body temperature. Drapes should be made of fabrics that are easily drapeable, are memory free, have anti-slick surfaces, and do not allow light absorption or reflection. They should be nonabrasive, be free from toxic agents, inhibit the transfer of additives, and be permeable to sterilizing agents. All drapes should meet AORN's standards as described in Recommended Practices for Protective Barrier Materials for Surgical Gowns and Drapes (AORN, 1992, *III*:6–1—6–4) and the National Fire Prevention Association requirements for flammability.

All materials, both reusable woven linens and nonwoven disposables, can be hazardous in surgery in the presence of such ignition sources as electrosurgical pencils and units, unshielded grounding plates, laser beams, and endoscopic light sources. Wovens and nonwovens have the same ignition properties in that neither type is less susceptible to ignition with these sources.

Manufacturer's labels and instructions should be noted and their warnings must be heeded. Suppliers should be asked to document the degree of safety of their drapes, because all materials are capable of igniting and burning. It is essential that the members of the surgical team be apprised of the true flammability properties of the drape fabric so that they can take the necessary precautions.

Supplies and Equipment

Types of Fabric

Reusable Drapes

Reusable drapes are made of woven materials of various thread counts and are designed for multiple uses. Muslin of 140 to 160 thread count was the standard for many years in the construction of surgical drapes. It was an ineffective barrier to the migration of microorganisms because of the wicking action and therefore was not an acceptable sterile barrier (Beck, 1981, p. 241).

Tightly woven, polyester-cotton blends, treated with chemicals, were developed to improve barrier properties. This treatment renders them nonwicking and liquid resistant. Fabrics of polyester microfibers are durable, cool, and breathable and have a water-repellent finish.

In most cases, the barrier effectiveness achieved through waterproofing of reusable drapes deteriorates with multiple processings. The repeated processes of laundering and sterilization gradually disrupt the integrity of the fabrics. As they experience wear and then swell and shrink repeatedly in the laundering process, the threads begin to loosen, permanently altering their ability to protect the patient and the surgical team. Tests have shown that treated materials lose their barrier quality after being processed 75 times (Beck, 1981, p. 242).

The newest development in reusable fabrics is Gore-Tex, a barrier fabric laminate bonded between two layers of lightweight polyester. The fabric is liquid proof, durable, and breathable and prevents strike through.

When selecting a reusable woven system for surgical procedures, many factors should be considered. The most important consideration is the barrier quality of the fabric, which provides the best possible protection for the surgical patient and the surgical team. These drapes should provide that protection consistently, be cost effective, and not cause harm to the environment. To be cost effective, the entire reusable system needs to be analyzed.

The following should be considered:

- Initial purchase, inventory, and replacement costs
- Materials that meet AORN's standards as described in Recommended Practices for Protective Barrier Materials for Surgical Gowns and Drapes (AORN, 1992, III:6–1—6–4).
- Supplies to develop packs (tape, sterilizing indicators, wrappers, and so on)
- Inspection of drapes over a light table
- Use of a grid system to monitor the number of times that drapes are used and processed
- Space for delinting, folding, and assembling packs
- Adequate laundry facility and cost per pound
- Sterilization costs, labor, equipment, and utilities
- Storage area for sterile packs and gowns

When making a decision as to what type of fabric to purchase, the following questions should be asked:

- During the laundering process, do detergents cause a loss of barrier properties, and is there a special wash cycle and temperature?
- How is the loss of effective barrier and repellency measured? If the recommended use is 50 to 75 times, what happens between 50 and 75 uses? Can it fail after 25 times?
- Is the sterilization process for barrier drapes the same as for drapes without barriers? Is the sterilization time and drying time the same?
- What are the manufacturer's test methods and published clinical data for evaluating barrier effectiveness?
- What effect does the processing have on the environment? (The laundering and sterilizing of reusa-bles consumes water and chemicals, creates detergent waste water, uses a great deal of energy, and contributes to air pollution [Little, 1990, p. 3].)

Disposable Drapes

Disposable drapes made of nonwoven materials are designed for one-time use and may not be resterilized unless the manufacturer provides written instructions for reprocessing. Disposable nonwoven drapes are composed of both natural and synthetic fibers of various types. The most widely used are Sontara, a spun-laced, wet-laid wood pulp and polyester fiber blend, and SMS, a spun-bonded melt-blown polyethylene. Both of these fabrics have polyethylene film laminated beneath the nonwoven fabric in the critical areas of the drapes, thereby providing an effective fluid-proof sterile barrier. Areas that are not laminated with polyethylene provide an effective fluid-resistant sterile barrier.

Some nonwoven drapes are made with special reinforcement around the fenestrations to reduce instrument slippage. They also offer antimicrobial, absorbent reinforcements and attached plastic pouches in the critical area to contain and control body fluids. When these types of drapes are used, the handling of fluid-saturated linen is eliminated, thereby reducing the staff's exposure to fluid-borne contaminants. Nonwovens or disposable

---

TABLE 6–3. PRINCIPLES OF DRAPING

1. Aseptically prepare the operative site before applying sterile surgical drapes.
2. Impervious fluid-proof drapes provide an effective sterile barrier and must be used when soaking of blood and body fluids is a potential risk.
3. Fluid-resistant drapes provide an effective sterile barrier when splashing and spraying of body fluids is a potential risk.
4. Sterile drapes should be handled as little as possible; avoid shaking, fanning, or haphazard unfolding.
5. Drapes are carried folded to the operative site and are considered nonsterile if allowed to fall below the waist or table level.
6. The area around the incision is draped first and then the periphery.
7. When placing drapes, never reach across the nonsterile area to drape the other side, go around, all draping is done from the appropriate side.
8. Form a cuff with the sterile drape to protect the sterile gloved hands when draping the periphery or equipment.
9. Hold the drapes high enough to avoid touching the nonsterile areas of the OR bed.
10. After a drape is placed down, it is not moved or repositioned. Drapes that are incorrectly placed or become contaminated are removed by the circulating nurse, being careful not to contaminate the operative site or other drapes.
11. A towel clip that has been placed through a drape has its points contaminated and must not be repositioned or removed until completion of the procedure.
12. If the sterility of a drape is questionable, discard it.

Adapted from Atkinson, L. J., Kohn, M. L. (1986). *Berry and Kohn's Introduction to Operating Room Technique* (6th ed.) (pp. 317–318). New York: McGraw-Hill Book Co; Kneedler, J. A., Dodge, G. H. (1987). *Perioperative Patient Care* (2nd ed) (pp. 454–456). Boston: Blackwell Scientific Publications; Groah, L. (1983). *Operating Room Nursing: The Perioperative Role.* (pp. 274–279). Reston, VA: Reston Publishing Co.

drapes streamline the task of draping the patient. Many are designed for specific procedures and feature elastic fenestrations, built-in incise, and adhesives. Disposables reduce setup time and provide effective barriers with less material. The use of disposable nonwoven drapes significantly reduces postoperative wound infections (Moyland et al., 1987, p. 151).

Before selecting a disposable nonwoven draping system, a cost analysis should be completed. Ask each manufacturer to submit published clinical data to provide comparisons of impermeability on the various qualities and brands of their fabrics. Follow AORN's standards as described in Recommended Practices for Protective Barrier Materials for Surgical Gowns and Drapes (AORN, 1992, *III*:6–1—6–4). The following factors should be considered: the packaging and maintenance of sterility, cost effectiveness, storage space, delivery capabilities, and the cost of disposal. Take into consideration that some companies are beginning to recycle disposable drapes and gowns.

Types of Drapes

Barrier drapes use impervious material predominantly made of plastic. They are essential in providing fluid-proof barriers where soaking of blood and body fluids is a risk. They are usually used in conjunction with reusable drapes.

Fenestrated sheets are disposable or reusable with openings of a specific size for designated procedures (e.g., laparotomy, thyroid, hand, and extremity procedures). Disposable fenestrated sheets should have an impervious barrier of 8 to 10 inches surrounding the fenestration to prevent soaking of blood and body fluids.

Drape sheets are separate sheets that are disposable or reusable, are usually fan folded, and are predominantly used in free draping (squaring off the incision site with all separate sheets). They are also used for draping large areas (e.g., equipment, arm boards, the foot of the OR bed, and back table). They are also called three-quarter sheets, half sheet, medium sheet, and impervious table covers.

An *incise drape* is a self-adhering plastic film applied directly to the prepared dry skin (Fig. 6–62). It may be applied as a separate sheet or incorporated into a disposable fenestrated sheet. The surgical incision is made directly through the plastic film. It also helps stabilize other drapes, eliminates the need for towel clips, and isolates potential infection sources such as stomas, colostomies, and fistulas.

Specialty impervious drapes are also used. A U-drape is a plastic drape with adhesive strips used predominantly on extremities to seal off the perineal area, the tourniquet, and the axillary area to provide a totally impervious sterile barrier. Pouches are used to contain and control body fluids; they may be applied on top of disposable or reusable drapes or may be incorporated into disposable drapes.

A *towel drape* is a drape with a band of adhesive along one end of a towel, made of either disposable or clear plastic material.

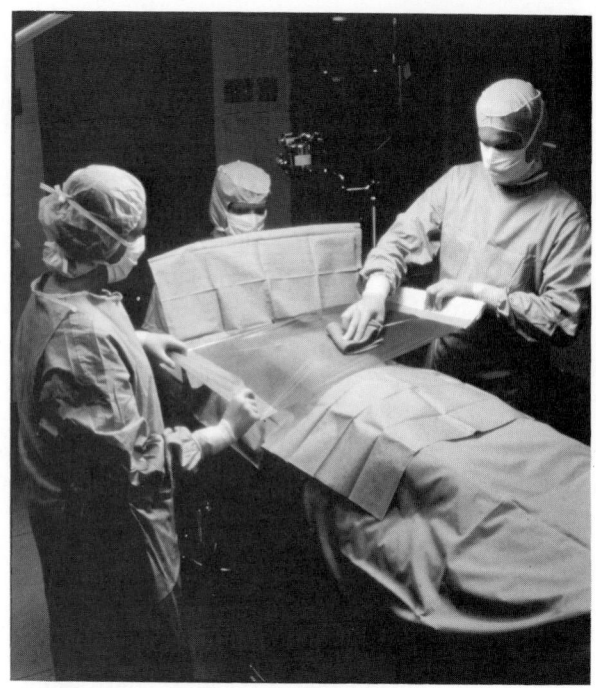

FIGURE 6–62. Application of an incise drape. (Courtesy of 3–M Health Care.)

An *aperture drape* is a small, clear plastic film drape with adhesive around the fenestration, which helps secure the drape to the skin around the incision site.

An *isolation drape* is a plastic transparent hanging drape used to isolate the C-arm, x-ray equipment, and other nonsterile equipment from the sterile operative field.

Stockinet is seamless tubing of stretchable impervious or woven material used to cover an extremity draped within the sterile operative field.

Equipment drapes are plastic transparent drapes to cover cameras, microscopes, the C-arm, x-ray equipment, and so on that are used within the sterile operative field.

No drapes presently withstand thermal laser beam impact. Wet towels should be applied around the area as a safety precaution where the laser will be used (American National Standards Institute, 1984). Fluid-proof drapes should be applied under the wet towels to prevent strike through and microbial migration. Research is presently being conducted to develop *laser-resistant drapes*.

The surgical team must determine how critical a given zone is and then use the proper type of fabrics and drapes to achieve the desired barrier protection.

Written policy and procedure should establish guidelines for the standardization of draping techniques and facilitate consistency of draping procedures. The following draping procedures elaborate the principles of draping (Table 6–3) for different anatomical areas of the body and equipment using nonwoven fluid-proof and fluid-resistant drapes.

Procedure

Draping the Patient and Equipment

1. Inspect the area in the OR where the sterile field will be set up.
   a. Assemble furniture and equipment to be draped within the sterile field.
   b. Check the surfaces of tables and equipment for cleanliness and dryness.
2. Gather all necessary draping supplies for the proposed surgery.
   a. Many ORs have a case cart system, in which all supplies and drapes for the procedure are assembled in advance and placed on a cart.
   b. Verify the correct surgical packs and drapes for the proposed surgery and anatomical area involved.
   c. Inspect the outer package for holes. If the integrity of the package has not been compromised, it is ready for use. If there are any defects, discard it.
3. Effective sterile barriers for back tables and Mayo stands are fluid-proof barrier drapes with impervious backings because these areas are considered critical zones.
4. Draping of the back table by a nonsterile team member:
   a. Remove the drape pack from the outer package.
   b. Place the drape pack on the center of the back table.
   c. Tear the seal and open toward the back of the table first and then open toward the front of the table. A nonsterile person should open the flap farthest away from her or him first, and the nearest flap last.
   d. Walk to either end of the table and grasp the cuff below table level and unfold the back table cover toward oneself (Fig. 6–63). Move to the other side of the table and repeat the same movements. The area touched falls below the nonsterile table level, leaving the surface of the table sterile while exposing the pack contents.
5. Draping of the back table by sterile team members:
   a. Open the table drape toward oneself to cover the nonsterile front edge of the table first to minimize the possibility of contaminating the front of the gown.
   b. Protect gloved hands in the folded cuffs and place a drape over the back of the table and then laterally to each side.
6. Draping of the Mayo stand is performed by a sterile team member.
   a. Place both hands under the cuff, palms down. A Mayo stand cover is a long tube (pillowcaselike) drape.
   b. Slide the cover over the Mayo stand, allowing it to unfold as it is being applied and taking precautions not to let it fall below waist level (Fig. 6–64).
   c. Stabilize the Mayo stand by placing the foot on its base while sliding the cover on.

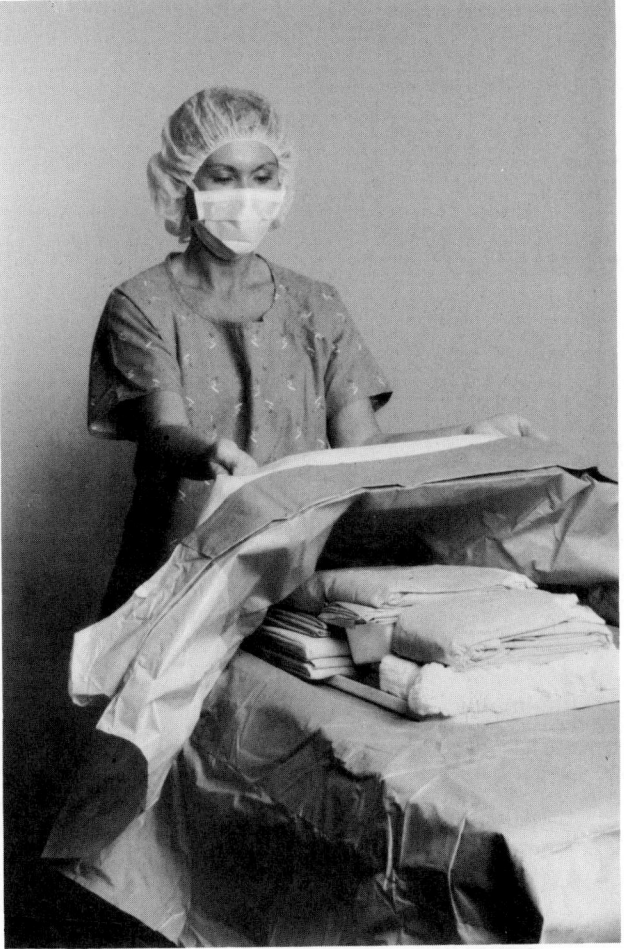

FIGURE 6–63. A back table drape pack is opened.

   d. Adjust the lower open end of the Mayo stand cover by pulling the cuff down the stand. This is performed by a nonsterile team member.
7. Arrange all drapes in sequence of their use and handle the drapes as little as possible.
8. Drapes must be correctly folded and have directional markings for ease in positioning and opening.

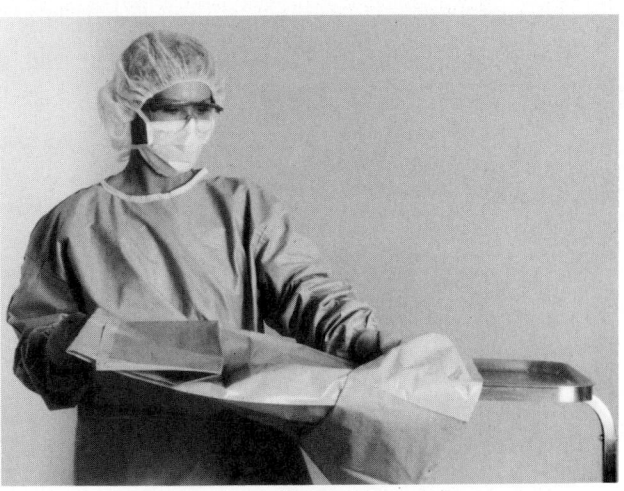

FIGURE 6–64. The Mayo stand is draped.

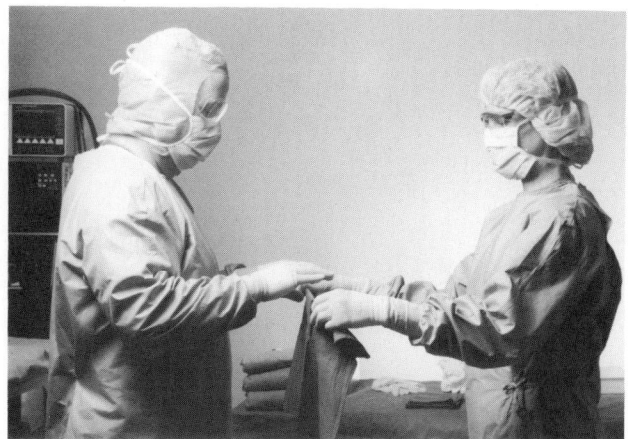

FIGURE 6–65. A folded towel is handed to the surgeon.

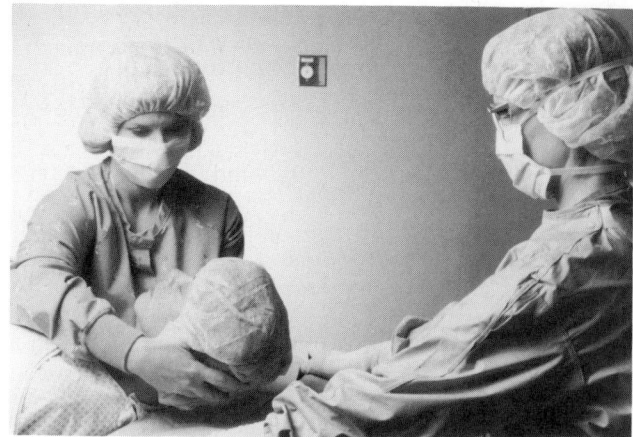

FIGURE 6–67. A drape is placed under the patient's head.

9. The surgeon may elect to drape the patient, assisted by other surgical team members, or the surgeon may indicate the proposed field of delineation and charge the nursing team with the responsibility for draping the patient.

10. It is the responsibility of the surgical team members to have all the appropriate drapes ready for the proposed procedure.

11. The circulating nurse should observe and direct the sterile surgical team members as necessary and watch carefully for breaks in aseptic technique when draping the surgical patient.

Draping for Specific Procedures and Anatomical Areas

Laparotomy or Any Flat Surface

1. Hand sterile adhesive drape towels with the folded adhesive edge toward oneself to the surgeon or place the adhesive towel, folded edge toward the patient, to outline the operative site.

2. If linen Huck towels are used, fold one third of the towel lengthwise with the folded side toward oneself

and hand it to the surgeon (Fig. 6–65) or place the folded edge toward the patient to outline the operative site.

3. Remove the release liners from the adhesive strips around the fenestration; place the folded laparotomy sheet, with the fenestration directly over the operative site (Fig. 6–66).

4. Unfold the drape to each side, keeping it at table level until it is unfolded toward the patient's head, including arm boards, and toward the patient's feet, including an adequate length over the OR bed.

Eye, Ear, Nose, and Face

1. Place the gloved hands, palms down, under the cuff of the head or bar drape.

2. Place the head or bar drape under the patient's head while a nonsterile team member lifts up the patient's head (Fig. 6–67).

3. Remove the release liner tabs from adhesive strips and draw the drape up separately on each side of the patient's face (turban style) and secure with adhesive.

4. Place a split sheet on the patient's chest with the tails toward the head, unfold to the sides and then to the

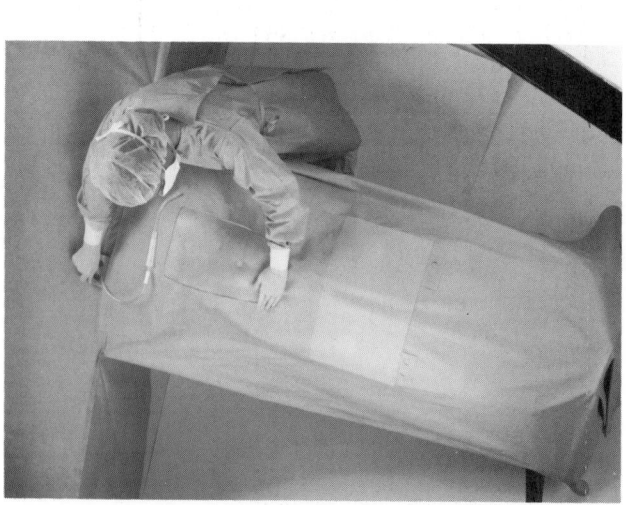

FIGURE 6–66. Laparotomy drape.

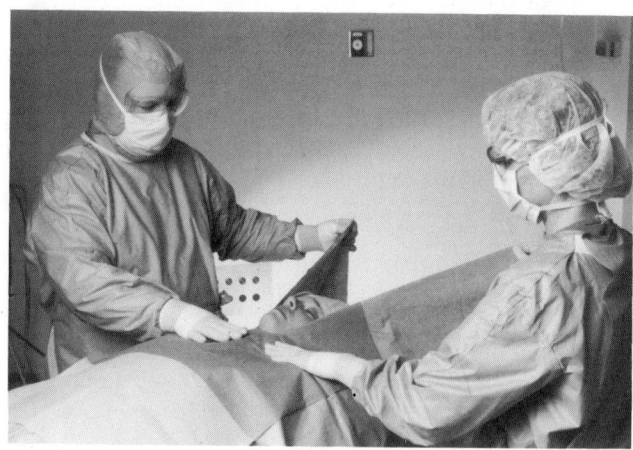

FIGURE 6–68. A split sheet is placed around the patient's head.

feet. Remove release liners from adhesive strips and simultaneously position the tails while adhering them around the operative site (Fig. 6–68).

5. Apply a small aperture drape by removing the release liner from the adhesive and then securing the edges to the skin around the operative site.

6. When applying drapes around the head and face of an awake patient, provide adequate breathing space and protect the patient from fear of claustrophobia.

Lithotomy

1. Separate leggings and sheet:
   a. Place the gloved hands, palms up, under the cuff of the under buttocks drape and position it under the patient's buttocks.
   b. Protect the gloved hands in the legging cuff and apply the legging over the leg and the stirrup. The telescope fold allows for ease of positioning. Repeat for the other leg.
   c. Place the sheet on the abdomen (firmly pressing the adhesive strip to stabilize the drape) and unfold laterally, then unfold to the head.

2. One-piece drape with attached leggings:
   a. Remove the release liner from the adhesive strip.
   b. Place the fenestration over the perineal area.
   c. Unfold the drape toward the patient's head while firmly pressing the adhesive strip to patient's abdomen to stabilize the drape.
   d. Grasp the legging marked toe with the right hand and pull it up over the patient's right leg and stirrup.
   e. Touching only the underside of the drape, the nonsterile team member assists in placing the drape over the patient's leg and stirrup.
   f. Repeat with the left hand for the left leg.
   g. Some drapes are designed with plastic pouches to help contain and control blood and body fluids (Fig. 6–69).

Hand

1. Drape the hand table with an impervious fluid-proof table cover.
2. Apply a rolled towel around the arm and secure it with a clip. If stockinet is preferred, the towel may be omitted.
3. Position the hand drape over the hand; grasp and pull the patient's hand through the elastic fenestration. Unfold the drape onto the hand table and across the patient's chest. Unfold toward the patient's feet, and unfold to the patient's head (Fig. 6–70).

Shoulder

1. With the patient's arm and shoulder elevated, apply a U-drape by removing the release liners from the adhesive strips and securing them to the skin below the arm, sealing off the axillary area.
2. Apply an impervious stockinet if the arm is draped

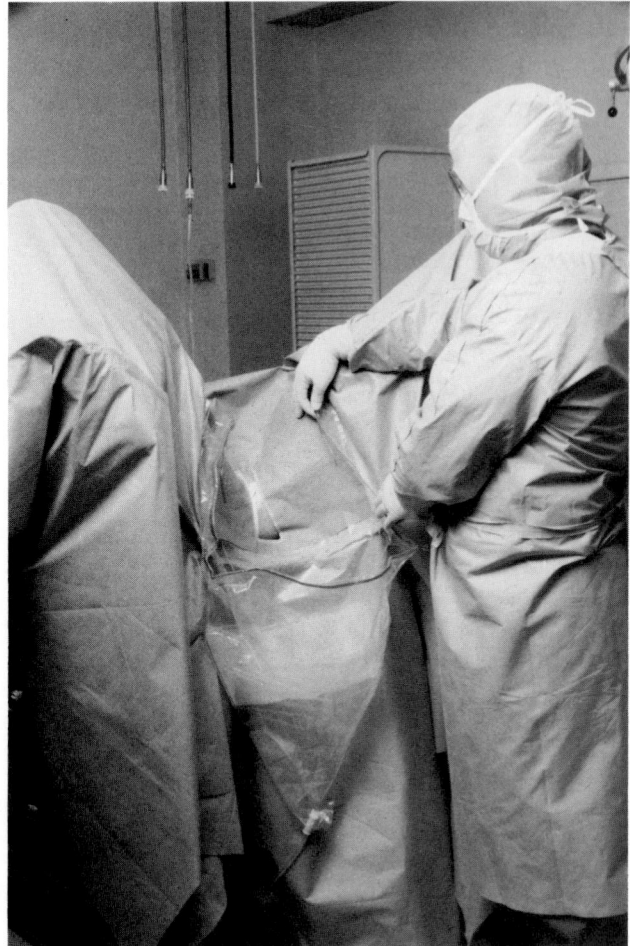

FIGURE 6–69. Plastic pouch on a drape for lithotomy.

within the sterile field. Twist it to achieve a better fit and to expel the air as it is rolled up the arm.

3. Apply an incise drape around the support apparatus if the arm is in traction.
4. Position the body split sheet below the arm at the axilla; unfold the sheet side to side, then toward the

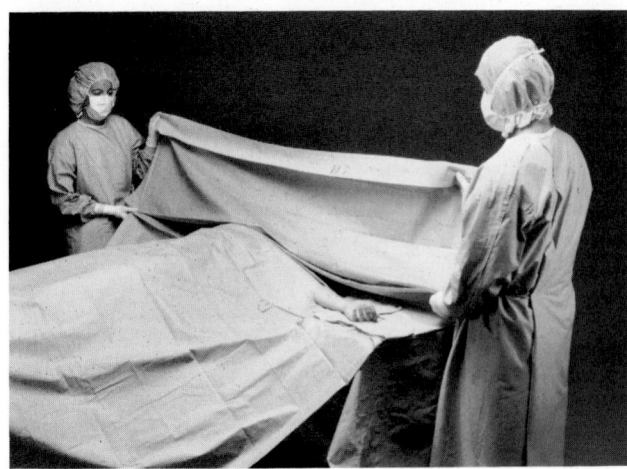

FIGURE 6–70. A drape is placed for hand procedures.

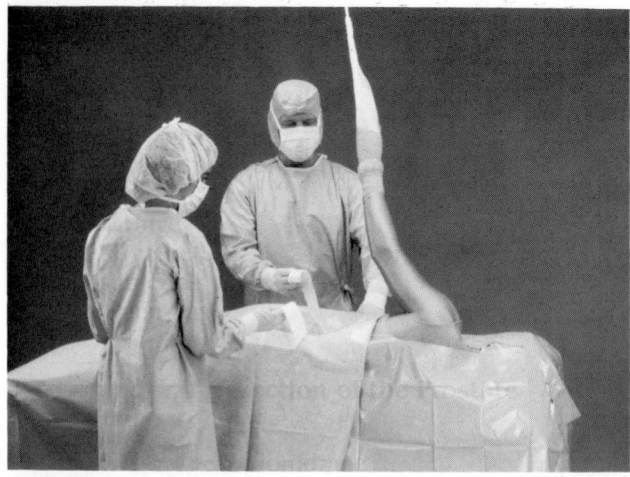

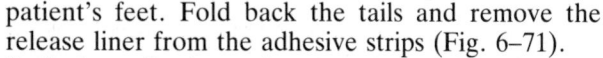

FIGURE 6–71. Release liners from adhesive strips are removed.

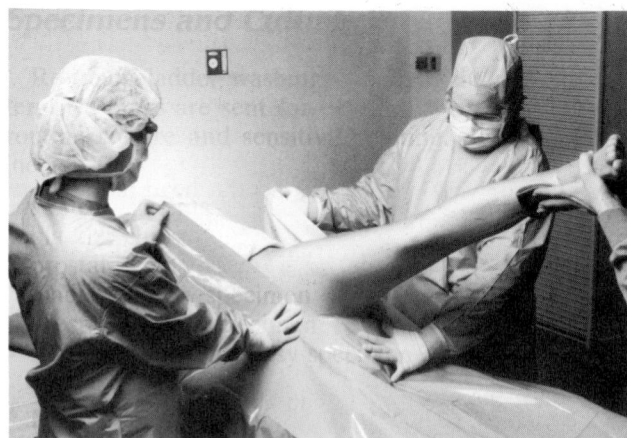

FIGURE 6–73. Application of U-drape to seal off the perineal area for hip procedures with the patient in the semilateral position.

patient's feet. Fold back the tails and remove the release liner from the adhesive strips (Fig. 6–71).

5. Seal the adhesive tails around the shoulder and toward the patient's head (Fig. 6–72).

6. Position the shoulder drape with the pouch above the shoulder. The arrow points toward the patient's feet. Unfold the drape from side to side and up to create the anesthesia screen.

7. Unfold the tails toward the anesthesia screen to expose the incise release liner, remove the release liner, bring both tails down around the shoulder simultaneously, and seal the adhesive to the bottom split sheet.

Hip, Semilateral Position

1. With the leg elevated, apply a U-drape by removing the release liner from the adhesive strips and securing

them to the skin, sealing off the perineal area and crossing the tails up over the iliac crest to complete the fenestration (Fig. 6–73).

2. Apply an impervious stockinet, twisting it to achieve a better fit and to expel the air as it is rolled up the leg.

3. Position the split sheet under the leg, with the tails toward the operative site. Unfold the drape to each side and then to the feet.

4. Fold back the tails and remove the release liners from the adhesive strips and simultaneously position the tails, adhering them around the operative site.

5. Position the top sheet with the arrow toward the incision, unfold to the side, remove the release liners from the adhesive strip, and seal to the split sheet, completing the fenestration around the operative site. Unfold up to create the anesthesia screen.

6. If an elastic fenestrated hip sheet is utilized, follow steps 1 and 2. Slip the fenestration over the patient's

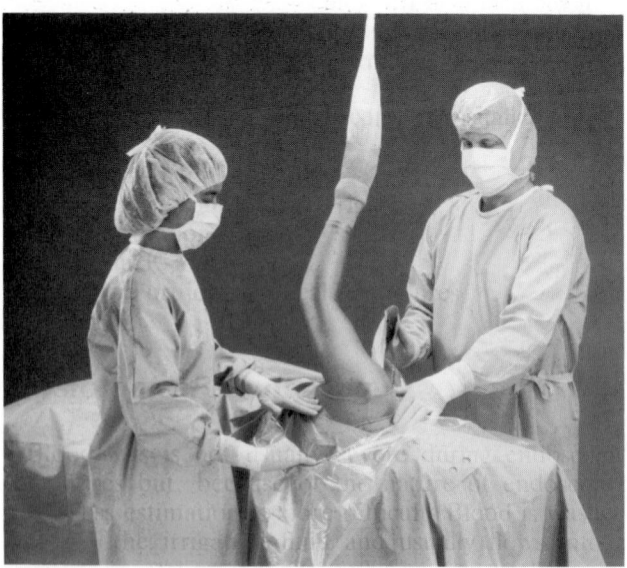

FIGURE 6–72. A split sheet with fluid control pouch is placed around the patient's shoulder.

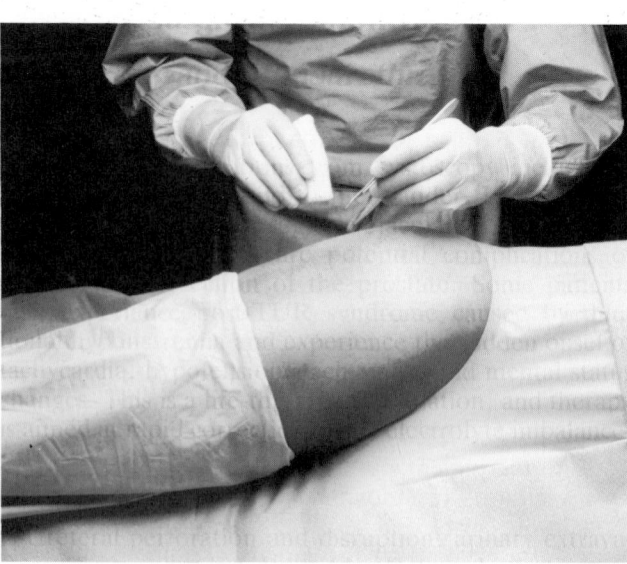

FIGURE 6–74. Hip drape.

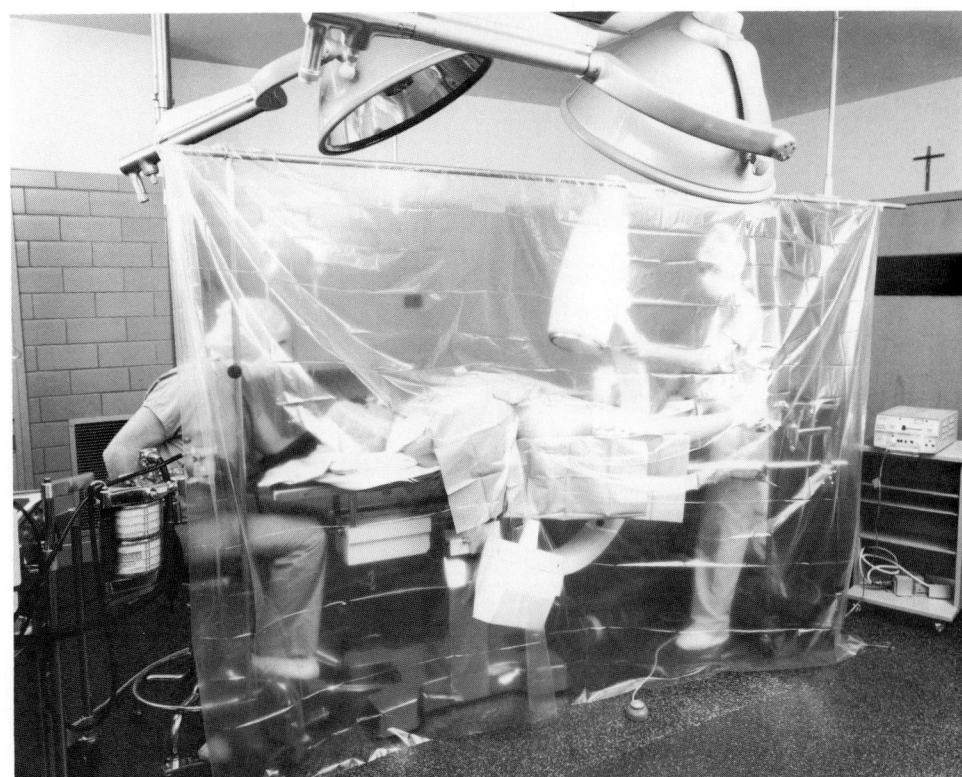

FIGURE 6–75. Isolation hanging drape. (Courtesy of 3–M Health Care.)

foot and unfold to each side and then toward the foot and up to create the anesthesia screen (Fig. 6–74).

7. If an incise drape is used, apply it over the operative site, securing the stockinet and all drapes in place.

Hip, Fracture Table

1. Square off the operative site with adhesive drape towels.
2. Apply an isolation hanging drape by removing the release liner from the incise area of the drape and firmly pressing the adhesive onto the operative site to stabilize the drape.
3. Unfold laterally to each side. Unfold to top toward the support bar.
4. Touching only the underside of the drape, the non-sterile team member assists in adhering the wall drape to the support bar (Fig. 6–75).
5. Unfold toward the floor.

Arthroscopy

1. With the patient's leg elevated, apply a U-drape by removing the release liner from the adhesive strips and securing them to the leg above the knee, sealing off the tourniquet and the leg-holder device.
2. Apply an impervious stockinet, twisting it to achieve a better fit and to expel the air as it is rolled up the leg.
3. Position the arthroscopy drape with the fluid control pouch at the knee. Grasp the foot and pull the

patient's leg through the double elastic fenestrations with the pouch.

4. Unfold the drape to each side, then to the head and to the feet.
5. To form a pouch, place one elastic fenestration above the knee and the other below the knee (Fig. 6–76).
6. If an elastic fenestrated arthroscopy drape is used without a pouch, follow steps 1 and 2.
7. Slip the fenestration over the patient's foot and unfold to each side and then to the head and to the feet.

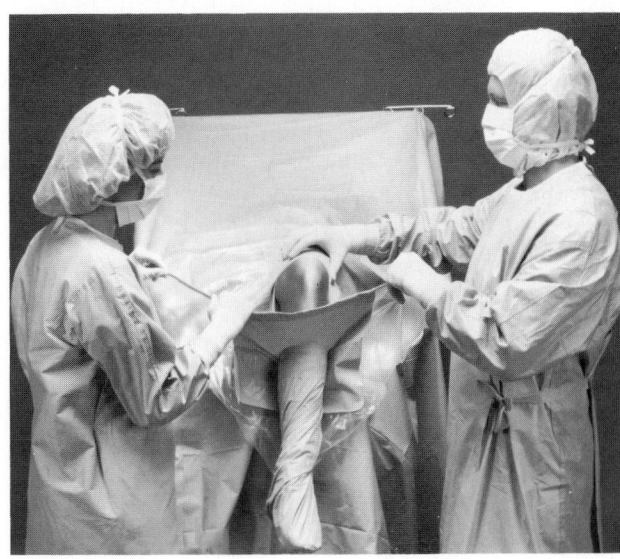

FIGURE 6–76. Drape (with fluid control pouch) for arthroscopy.

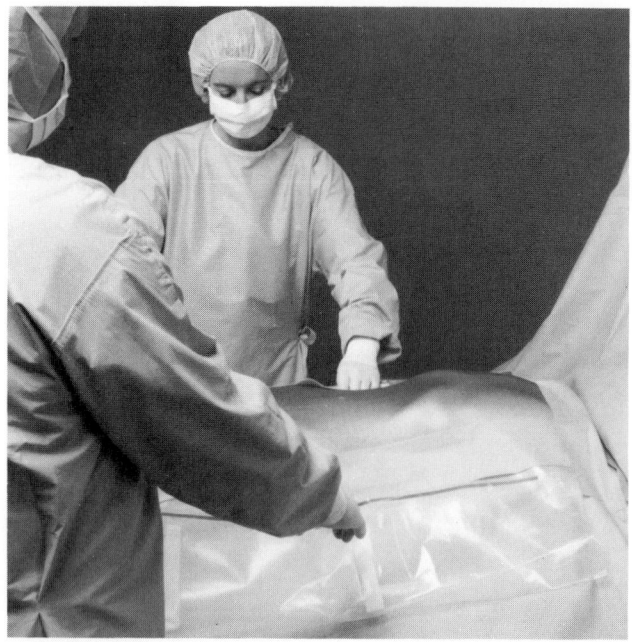

FIGURE 6–77. Drape (with pouch) for open heart surgery.

Ankle or Foot

1. With the patient's foot elevated, place an impervious fluid-proof barrier drape under the operative extremity.
2. Apply a rolled towel around the patient's thigh and secure it with a clip. If stockinet is preferred, the towel may be omitted.
3. Position the elastic fenestrated extremity sheet over the foot. Grasp and pull the patient's foot through the elastic fenestration.
4. Unfold the drape to each side, then to the head and to the foot.

Open Heart

1. With the patient's legs elevated, place an impervious fluid-proof barrier drape under the legs.
2. Place stockinet on each foot or drape the feet in a small drape. Lower the patient's legs onto the sterile barrier.
3. Seal off the perineal area with an impervious towel or drape.
4. Apply adhesive drape towels along the sides of the patient's chest and legs.
5. Apply a large incise sheet to cover the chest and the abdomen (Fig. 6–77).
6. Apply a large incise sheet over both legs and the groin area.
7. Position a cardiovascular split drape on the patient's chest; remove the release liners from adhesive and secure to the patient's chest.

ACKNOWLEDGEMENTS

Photographs are provided courtesy of Baxter Convertors/Custom Sterile, McGaw Park, Il. Photographer: Bob Morrison. Drawings are provided courtesy of Steve Brouwer.

Bibliography

American Hospital Association. (1979). *Infection control in the hospital* (4th ed.). Chicago: Visual Images.

American National Standards Institute. (1984). Laser safety in the health care environment. *Fire Hazards,* Z–136.3, section 7.5.

Association of the Nonwoven Fabrics Industry. (1991). *Facts about single-use and reusable drapes and gowns.* Cary, NC.

Association of Operating Room Nurses. (1992). *Standards and recommended practices for perioperative nursing.* Denver.

Atkinson, L. J., Kohn, M. L. (1986). *Berry and Kohn's introduction to operating room technique.* New York: McGraw-Hill.

Beck, W. C. (1981). Aseptic barriers in surgery. *Archives of Surgery, 116,* 240–244.

Beck, W. C. (1961). Justified faith in surgical drapes. *American Journal of Surgery, 105,* 560–562.

Belkin, L. B. (1988). Surgical gowns and drapes as aseptic barriers. *American Journal of Infection Control, 16,* 14–18.

Bloodborne pathogens. (1991, December 5). *Federal Register, 56*(235), 64176–64177.

Centers for Disease Control. (1988). Update: Universal precautions for prevention of transmission of HIV, HBV, and other blood borne pathogens in health-care settings. (1988). *AORN Journal, 48,* 586–594.

Centers for Disease Control. (1988). *Enforcement procedures for occupational exposure to hepatitis B virus (HBV) and human immuno-deficiency virus (HIV).* Atlanta.

Cruse, P. J. E., Foord, R. (1980). The epidemiology of wound infection, a 10-year study of 62,939 wounds. *Surgical Clinics of North America, 60,* 27–39.

Cruse, P. J. E., Foord, R. (1973). A five-year prospective study of 23,649 surgical wounds. *Archives of Surgery, 107,* 206–210.

Dineen, P. (1969). An evaluation of the duration of the surgical scrub. *Surgery, Gynecology and Obstetrics, 129,* 1181–1184.

Dinein, P. The role of impervious drapes and gowns in preventing surgical infection. *Clinical Orthopaedics and Related Research,* 210.

Fernsebner, B. (1986). Infection control survey. *AORN Journal, 43,* 891–897.

Garibaldi, R. (1988). Prevention of intraoperative wound contamination with chlorhexidine shower and scrub. *Journal of Hospital Infection, 11* (Suppl. B), 5.

Garner, J. (1985). *Guideline for prevention of surgical wound infections* (pp. 1–10). Atlanta: Centers for Disease Control, National Technical Information Service.

Garner, J., Favero, M. (1985). *Guidelines for handwashing and hospital environmental control* (pp. 1–20). Atlanta: Center for Disease Control, National Technical Information Service.

Gilbertson, W. (1972). *Progress report: The OTC drug review.* FDA's Bureau of Drugs.

Girard, N. J. (1990). *Aseptic technique: Stressing the fundamentals* (DG-1990). [Film]. Denver, CO: Association of Operating Room Nurses.

Gordon, M. (1979). The concept of nursing diagnosis. *Nursing Clinics of North America, 14,* 487–496.

Gordon, M. (1987). *Manual of Nursing Diagnosis: 1986–1987.* New York: McGraw-Hill.

Groah, L. K. (1983). *Operating room nursing: The perioperative role.* Reston, VA: Reston Publishing.

Gruendemann, B. J., Meeker, M. H. (1983). *Alexander's care of the patient in surgery.* St. Louis: C. V. Mosby.

Kneedler, J. A., Dodge, G. H. (1987). *Perioperative patient care: The nursing perspective.* Boston: Blackwell Scientific.

Larson, E. (1988). APIC guidelines for infection control practice, guideline for use of topical antimicrobial agents. *American Journal of Infection Control, 16,* 253–266.

Little, A. D. (1990). *Disposables versus reusable diapers: health, environmental and economic comparisons.* Report to Procter and Gamble. Cambridge, MA.

Moyland, J. A., Fitzpatrick, K. T., Davenport, K. E. (1987). Reducing wound infections—improved gown and drape barrier performance. *Archives of Surgery, 122,* 152–157.

Moyland, J., Kennedy, B. (1980). The importance of gown and drape barriers in the prevention of wound infection. *Surgery, Gynecology and Obstetrics, 151,* 465–470.

National Fire Prevention Association requirements for flammability. Patient preoperative skin preparation and surgical hand scrub. (1978). *Federal Register, 43,* 1229–1249.

Patterson, P. (1992). OSHA issues rules to protect workers from HIV, hepatitis B. *OR Manager,* 1–7.

Pfister, J. (1975). *Proper operating room attire.* (DG-1209) [Film]. Denver, CO: Association of Operating Room Nurses.

Price, S. A., Wilson, L. McC. (1986). *Pathophysiology, clinical concepts of disease processes* (3rd ed.). New York, NY: McGraw-Hill.

Recommendations for prevention of HIV transmission in health-care settings. (1988). *AORN Journal, 47,* 808–832.

Reed, E. A., Applegeet, C. J. (1986). Infection control. *AORN Journal, 43,* 1002–1005.

Rothrock, J. C. (1987). The RN First Assistant: an expanded perioperative nursing role. New York: J. B. Lippincott Company, 191–192.

Ryan, P. (1979). Reusables vs disposables? Defending your position. *AORN Journal, 30,* 415–424.

Schwartz, J. E., Saunders, D. E. (1980). Microbial penetration of surgical gown materials. *Surgery, Gynecology and Obstetrics, 150,* 507–512.

Spry, C. (1988). *Essentials of perioperative nursing.* Rockville, MD: Aspen Systems.

Tucci, V. J., Stone, A. M., Thompson, C., Isenberg, H. D. (1977). Studies of the surgical scrub. *Surgery, Gynecology and Obstetrics,* 145–416.

U.S. Department of Labor. (1991). OSHA Occupational exposure to bloodborne pathogens; final rule, federal register (29 CFR part 1910. 1030).

Wells, M. M. P. (1987). *Decision making in perioperative nursing.* Philadelphia: B. C. Decker.

Wells, P. (1976). *Fundamentals of aseptic technique* (DG-1223) [Film]. Denver, CO: Association of Operating Room Nurses.

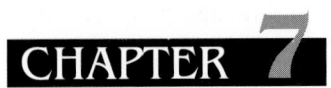
Performing Sponge, Sharps, and Instrument Counts

Rosemary Grandusky

DEFINITION

Performing counts of sponges, sharps, and instruments is the perioperative nursing activity of accounting for items to ensure that they are not retained in the surgical wound after closure. This crucial activity is an integral component of safe perioperative nursing practice. Because perioperative nurses have a grave responsibility to provide safe patient care, sponge, sharps, and instrument counts should be considered for every surgical procedure to ensure that the patient is not injured as a result of a retained foreign body.

MEASURABLE CRITERIA

The perioperative nurse demonstrates competency to perform sponge, sharps, and instrument counts by

- following operating room (OR) policy and procedure for counting
- initiating incorrect count procedures
- documenting the count results according to OR policy and procedure (Association of Operating Room Nurses [AORN], 1992)

ROLE OF THE PERIOPERATIVE NURSE

Members of the intraoperative nursing team are responsible for taking the measures necessary to provide safe patient care. The perioperative nurse, functioning as the circulator, ensures that the appropriate counting policies and procedures are implemented. The scrub person collaborates with the circulator in accounting for all sponges, sharps, and instruments.

CONSIDERATIONS

Recommended Practices

The AORN's Recommended Practices for Sponge, Sharp, and Instrument Counts (1992, *III*:19–1—19–6) provides guidelines for the development of institutional policies and procedures. These recommendations promote an optimal level of practice. They have no authority, however, to bind actual institutional practice. Each health care institution should use the recommended practices to develop policies and procedures specific to the needs of the institution. For example, recommended practice III states that "instruments should be counted on all procedures" (AORN, 1992). Many facilities do not count instruments for all procedures but choose to define for what procedures instruments are counted. These procedures usually include intraperitoneal and thoracic surgery.

Institutional Policies and Procedures

Policies and procedures for counts must be established by the institution. It is the perioperative nurse's legal responsibility to know and carry out these policies and procedures. Failure to do so places the patient at risk for injury and the nurse at risk for negligent practice.

According to AORN (1992, III:19–4) recommendations, institutional policies should address the following:

• Establish authority, responsibility, and accountability for sponge, sharps, and instrument counts.
• Provide direction for performing counts.
• Provide direction for discontinuing counts.
• Provide protocols for incorrect counts.

Legal Issues

Accountability for sponges, sharps, and instruments during a surgical procedure is a primary responsibility of the perioperative nurse. If a sponge, sharp, or instrument is left in a patient and the patient sues, and if the suit goes to trial, the jury will determine if the perioperative nurse did what any reasonable and prudent nurse would have done to account for the item prior to closure of the surgical wound. Jury members will be instructed to base their decision on the evidence presented at the trial, such as expert witness testimony, AORN's recommended practices, and the institution's policy. Retention of sponges, sharps, and instruments may result in a verdict of negligence against the perioperative nurse (Murphy, 1991, p. 878).

The case of *Northeast Alabama Regional Medical Center vs Robinson, 548 So 2d 439 (Ala 1989)*, clearly illustrates the importance of stringent count procedures. The patient had had a vaginal hysterectomy for an enlarged uterus and abnormal bleeding in September 1983. During follow-up care she complained of pain, nausea, vomiting, dizziness, and inability to sleep. In December, a sonogram revealed a large mass posterior to her vaginal cuff. The surgeon tentatively diagnosed this mass as an ovarian cyst. In January 1984, an exploratory laparotomy revealed a retained laparotomy sponge that had been cut in half. The patient sued the hospital, nurses, and physician for damages. In this case the jury returned a verdict that the surgeon was not liable for the retained sponge, even though a sponge had been cut in half and left in the wound. The nurses, however, who reported the count to be correct to the surgeon were held liable. The jury set damages at $250,000 (Murphy, 1990, pp. 1067–1068).

OUTCOME STANDARD

The patient is free from injury related to the retention of sponges, sharps, or instruments.

Criteria

There is an absence of

• unexplained pain, cramping, and fever
• formation of abscesses in the abdominal, retroperitoneal, and chest cavities
• retained sponges, sharps, or instruments seen on postoperative x-ray films

POTENTIAL ALTERATIONS IN FUNCTIONAL HEALTH PATTERNS

Health Perception–Health Management Pattern

Diagnosis

High risk for injury related to retained sponges, sharps, and instruments

Definition

Presence of risk factors for the patient to experience injury owing to sponges, sharps, or instruments inadvertently left in the surgical wound after closure

Risk Factors

• Emergency surgery that precludes counting sponges, sharps, and instruments
• Intraoperative hemorrhaging necessitating the immediate use of a great number of sponges
• Surgery entailing the packing of cavities with sponges
• Change of perioperative nursing staff during the procedure
• Lenient institutional count policies and procedures

Expected Outcome

The patient does not exhibit signs or symptoms indicating the retention of sponges, sharps, or instruments after surgery.

PERIOPERATIVE NURSING INTERVENTIONS

The following interventions serve as guidelines for counting sponges, sharps, and instruments. Institutional policies and procedures should be followed when implementing sponge, sharps, and instrument counts; initiating incorrect count procedures; and documenting counts (AORN, 1992, *III*:19–1—19–4).

Counting Sponges

- Count sponges before the beginning of the procedure, at the change of personnel, when sponges are added to the sterile field, before the closure of a deep or large incision or body cavity, and immediately before the completion of the procedure.
- The circulating nurse counts sponges out loud with the scrub nurse.
- The scrub nurse separates the sponges when counting. This enables the circulating nurse to verify that additional sponges, or pieces of sponge, are not concealed.
- Use only x-ray–detectable sponges during the procedure.
- Count sponges in units of 5 or 10, depending on how they are packaged.
- Remove packages of sponges that contain more or less than the packaged number from the operative field.
- Do not remove counted sponges from the OR during the procedure.
- The scrub nurse keeps sponges organized at all times on the operative field.
- Discard used sponges in an fluid-impervious, lined container. Count and bag sponges in groups of 5 or 10 as they are accumulated.

Counting Sharps

- Count sharps before the beginning of the procedure, at the change of personnel, when sharps are added to the sterile field, before the closure of a deep or large incision or body cavity, and immediately before the completion of the procedure.
- The circulating nurse counts sharps out loud with the scrub nurse.
- Count needles according to the number indicated on the package. When the package is opened, the circulating nurse verifies the number of needles with the scrub nurse.
- Do not remove counted sharps from the OR during the procedure.
- Use sharps-counting devices to assist in the counting procedure.
- The scrub nurse keeps sharps organized at all times on the operative field.
- The scrub nurse continually counts needles during the procedure and hands them to the surgeon on an exchange basis.
- Account for all pieces of broken sharps.

Counting Instruments

- Count instruments before the beginning of the procedure, at the change of personnel, when instruments are added to the sterile field, before the closure of a deep or large incision or body cavity, and immediately before the completion of the procedure.
- The circulating nurse counts instruments out loud with the scrub nurse.
- Use uniform instrument sets. This allows easy identification and counting.
- Use preprinted instrument work sheets. The work sheet should match each instrument set.
- Do not remove counted instruments from the OR during the procedure.
- The scrub nurse keeps the instruments organized at all times on the operative field.
- Account for all pieces of broken instruments.

Incorrect Counts

- In the event of an incorrect count, notify the surgeon and recount.
- If the problem is still not resolved after a recount, search for the missing item. Ask the surgeon to explore the wound. Look in areas where the item could be concealed such as under the OR bed, under the surgeon's or an assistant's feet, under instrument trays, and in trash containers.
- Request an x-ray film before the patient is taken from the OR.
- Implement documentation procedures according to policy and procedure.

DOCUMENTATION AND COMMUNICATION PROCEDURES

- The circulating nurse and the scrub nurse maintain communication about the status of sponge, sharps, and instrument counts throughout the procedure.
- Announce the results of the count to the surgeon. The surgeon should acknowledge the results of the count.
- Document the results of the count in the patient's record in compliance with facility policy and procedure. According to AORN's Recommended Practices for Sponge, Sharp, and Instrument Counts (1992), the perioperative nurse should document the types and number of counts taken, the names and titles of personnel taking the counts, the results of counts, the actions taken if discrepancies occur, the rationale if counts are not performed or completed, and the signature of the responsible party.

Bibliography

Association of Operating Room Nurses. (1992). *Standards and recommended practices for perioperative nursing.* Denver.

Murphy, E. K. (1990). OR Nursing Law: Nurses' liability for inaccurate counts. *AORN Journal, 51*(4), 1067–1068.

Murphy, E. K. (1991). OR Nursing Law: Counts, documentation revisited. *AORN Journal, 54*(4), 878.

CHAPTER 8

Providing Instruments, Equipment, and Supplies

Jean M. Allen and Mark L. Phippen

DEFINITION

Providing instruments, equipment, and supplies refers to the technical activities performed by the perioperative nurse functioning in the role of the circulating nurse or scrub nurse. These activities provide for safe patient care and enable the surgeon to effectively and efficiently perform surgery. This chapter gives an overview of some of the instruments, equipment, and supplies that the perioperative nurse may provide during a surgical procedure. See Chapter 16 for a more detailed discussion.

MEASURABLE CRITERIA

The perioperative nurse demonstrates competency to provide instruments, equipment, and supplies by safely and efficiently

- selecting instruments, equipment, supplies, and suture for a surgical procedure
- delivering instruments, supplies, and suture to the sterile field
- arranging instruments and supplies on the instrument table and the Mayo tray
- passing instruments and supplies to the surgeon
- preparing and passing sutures to the surgeon
- applying and removing a pneumatic tourniquet
- applying and removing the electrosurgical unit dispersive electrode
- operating the electrosurgical unit generator
- preparing electrical instruments for use
- preparing air-powered instruments for use
- preparing the hyperthermia or hypothermia unit for use
- applying dressings
- assisting with the application of casts and splints

ROLE OF THE PERIOPERATIVE NURSE

The perioperative nurse implements the measurable criteria described above as the circulating or scrub nurse. With appropriate supervision, delegation or assignment of these tasks to qualified assistive personnel is permissible. Accountability for the correct performance of the tasks rests with the perioperative nurse.

OUTCOME STANDARD

The patient is free from injury related to the provision of instruments, equipment, and supplies during surgery.

Criteria

The patient demonstrates no evidence of

- alterations in temperature
- electrical injury
- burns
- nosocomial infection

POTENTIAL ALTERATIONS IN FUNCTIONAL HEALTH PATTERNS

Health Perception–Health Management Pattern

Diagnosis

High risk for injury related to the use of electrical equipment

Definition

Presence of risk factors for the patient to experience impaired skin and tissue integrity, altered tissue perfusion and cardiac output, and impaired neurological function related to the use of electrical equipment during surgery

Risk Factors

- Excessive hair
- Scar tissue
- Internal or external metal prosthetic devices
- Impaired skin or tissue integrity, bony prominences, or impaired tissue perfusion at the site of the dispersive electrode or electrocardiographic lead placement
- Pacemakers
- Improper application of dispersive electrode
- Use of faulty equipment

Expected Outcome

The patient is free from electrical equipment–related injury during the perioperative period. There is no evidence of

- impaired skin and tissue integrity
- altered tissue perfusion
- altered cardiac output
- impaired neurological function

Diagnosis

High risk for injury related to the use of a pneumatic tourniquet

Definition

Presence of risk factors for the patient to experience impaired skin and tissue integrity, chemical skin burns, and nerve damage secondary to improper pneumatic tourniquet use

Risk Factors (Association of Operating Room Nurses [AORN], 1992, III:13–1—13–3)

- Improper cuff size
- Wrinkled padding
- Improper cuff positioning
- Cuff rotation after application
- Pooling of preparation solutions under the cuff
- Excessive cuff pressure
- Excessive cuff inflation time

Expected Outcome (AORN, 1992, III:13–1—13–3)

The patient is free from injury related to pneumatic tourniquet use. There is no evidence of

- bruising, blistering, pinching, or necrosis of skin
- skin abrasions or swelling
- chemical skin burns
- paralysis or other signs of nerve damage

Diagnosis

High risk for infection

Definition

Presence of risk factors for the patient to experience a nosocomial infection secondary to exposure to the surgical environment

Risk Factors (Gordon, 1987, p. 50)

- Surgical intervention that alters tissue and skin integrity
- Inadequate secondary defenses (e.g, decreased hemoglobin concentration, leukopenia, suppressed inflammatory response, and immunosuppression)

- Inadequate acquired immunity (e.g., acquired immunodeficiency syndrome)
- Chronic disease leading to suppressed immunity (e.g., lupus erythematosus)
- Invasive drains and monitors (intravenous catheters, hyperalimentation catheters, nasogastric tubes, Foley catheters, chest tubes)
- Malnutrition that interferes with tissue repair
- Blood abnormalities such as sickle cell anemia, thrombocytopenia, and thalassemia
- Impaired tissue perfusion
- High white blood cell count, low platelet count, and anemia
- Impaired skin integrity
- Impaired tissue integrity
- Failure of sterilization or disinfection processes
- Nonadherence to surgical suite traffic patterns
- Failure of environmental sanitation processes

Expected Outcome

The patient is free from nosocomial infection after surgery. There is no evidence of

- wound infection
- urinary tract infection
- upper respiratory tract infection

Nutritional-Metabolic Pattern

Diagnosis

High risk for altered body temperature during surgery

Definition

Presence of risk factors for the patient to experience hypothermia while in the surgical suite

Risk Factors (AORN, 1992, *III*:7–2)

- General or regional anesthesia
- Excessive sedation, especially in the patient receiving a local anesthetic
- Evaporative or conductive heat loss from prepared skin areas
- Use of unwarmed infusion or irrigating solutions
- Cold room temperature
- Surgical exposure of the abdominal or thoracic cavities
- Preexisting medical conditions (e.g., hypothyroid or hyperthyroid problems)
- Extremes in age, particularly infant, small child, and geriatric patients
- Decreased body fat for insulation
- Malnourishment
- Debilitated or chronically ill patients
- Anticipated long operative time
- Intracranial surgery

Expected Outcome

The patient's body temperature is maintained within normal limits during the perioperative period. There is no evidence of

- verbal complaint of feeling uncomfortably cold (for a conscious patient)
- shivering
- chattering of teeth
- cool skin
- decreased pulse and respiration rate (Gordon, 1987, p. 98)

PERIOPERATIVE NURSING INTERVENTIONS

Selecting Instruments, Equipment, Supplies, and Suture for a Surgical Procedure

Obtain the surgeon's preference card, pick list, and other forms used to select instruments, equipment, and supplies (Table 8–1). Select all items listed on the surgeon's preference card and other pertinent forms. Make a list of the items not available.

Check all sterile items for signs of moisture, lack of seal integrity, and compromise of packaging material, such as pinholes and tears (Fig. 8–1). Note the expiration dates. If a discrepancy is found, do not use the item.

Examine the autoclave tape on cloth-wrapped packages and the chemical sterilization indicators on or in paper or plastic packages for a color change to ensure that the item was subjected to a sterilization cycle. If a discrepancy is found, do not use the item.

If the setup is not immediately used, return the surgeon's preference card to the appropriate location. Close the case cart or cover the setup with a cloth sheet or other appropriate protective material and label with the surgeon's name, the date and time of the procedure, and the procedure name.

Accountability is established by initialing the label. Place the setup in the appropriate location. Attach the list of missing items to the setup. Communicate the list of missing items to the appropriate person.

Delivering Instruments, Supplies, and Suture to the Sterile Field

General Guidelines

Check all sterile items for signs of moisture, lack of seal integrity, compromise of packaging material, outdated expiration dates, and the absence of autoclave tape and chemical sterilization indicators of a color change before opening. If a discrepancy is found, do not use the item. Do not reach over the sterile field when delivering sterile items. Do not use cloth-wrapped

TABLE 8–1. **EXAMPLES OF SURGICAL INSTRUMENTS**

Grasping or holding clamps	Mosquito	Control superficial bleeders and handle delicate tissue
	Crile	Control bleeders in subcutaneous tissue
	Kelly	Control bleeders in muscle tissue; hold Kittner forceps; pass drains
	Allis	Retract tissue; grasp fascia, cysts, and knee cartilage
	Babcock	Grasp appendix, fallopian tubes, ureters, intestines, and stomach
	Right angle	Pull suture strands around or behind vessels; perform dissection; clamp deep bleeders in hard-to-reach places
	Kocher-Oschner	Grasp fascia on large patients when placing retention suture; grasp bone and cartilage; grasp uterine broad ligaments
	Rochester-Péan	Secure Kittner forceps; grasp broad ligaments of uterus; cross-clamp intestines
	Sponge forceps	Secure sponges; extract placenta from uterus; grasp tough tissue
	Tissue	Grasp and hold fascia and subcutaneous tissue
	Dressing	Hold gauze sponges and dressings; grasp and hold delicate tissue
	Adson	Perform skin closure
Needle holders	Hegar-Mayo	Hold medium- to heavy-gauge needles
	Collier	Hold medium-gauge needles
	Brown	Hold small-gauge needles
Retractors	Richardson (large and small)	Retract broad tissue such as subcutaneous tissue
	Army-Navy	Use for shallow incisions and tissue
	Vein	Use for shallow areas in arms and legs and veins
	Volkmann (sharp and dull)	Use for shallow incisions during orthopedic surgery
Suction devices	Poole	Abdominal cavity and obstetrical and gynecological surgery
	Yankauer tonsil	Use for a wide variety of surgical procedures
Scissors	Straight Mayo	Cut suture and other surgical materials such as dressings and drains
	Curved Mayo	Cut heavy, tough tissue such as muscle, fascia, and subcutaneous tissue; perform gross dissection
	Metzenbaum	Cut delicate tissue such as peritoneum, intestines, and stomach; perform delicate dissection
Scalpels	Knife handle No. 4	Fits blade No. 20; use for skin knife
	Knife handle No. 3	Fits blades Nos. 10, 11, 12, and 15; use for second knife
	Knife handle No. 7	Fits blades Nos. 10, 11, 12, and 15; use for eye, hand, and plastic surgery

Adapted from U.S. Army. (1988). 301–91D10 *Operating room specialist course competency based program of instruction student handbook.* Fort Sam Houston, TX: Academy of Health Sciences, U.S. Army.

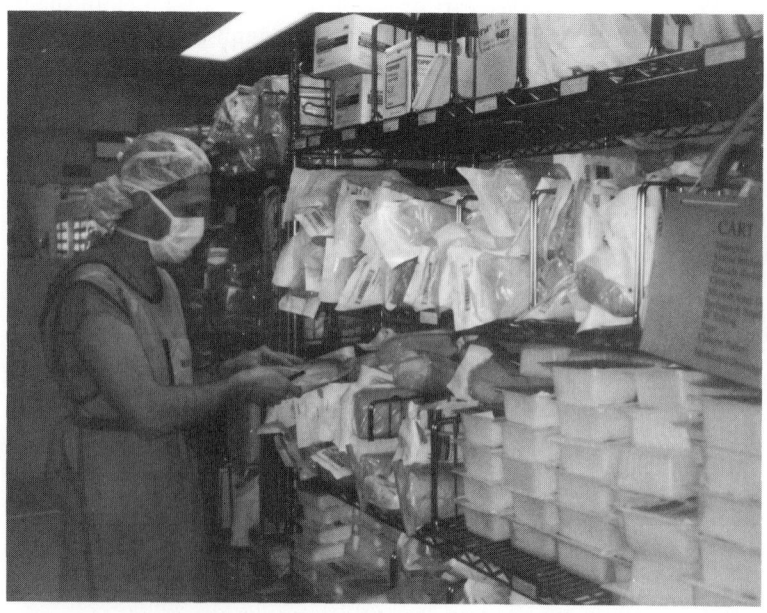

FIGURE 8–1. Checking the packaging of sterile items.

items that are dropped on the floor. The decision to open the inner wrappers or packages of double-wrapped or double-packaged items is determined by institutional policy (*AORN Journal*, 1990, p. 440; U.S. Army, 1988, p. 35).

Wrapped Items

Remove the autoclave tape and position the package so that it can be opened by lifting the top flap away from the body. Lift the top flap (first flap) away from the body, the second and third flaps to the left and the right, and the last flap toward the body. Gather the wrapper tails together with one hand when presenting the item to the sterile field. Open the wrappers for sharp, bulky, or heavy items on an appropriate-sized table or a Mayo stand (U.S. Army, 1988, pp. 47–48).

Items Sealed in Peel-Back Packages

Carefully peel the package apart. Present the item to the scrub person. The scrub nurse grasps the item and carefully lifts it from the package. The item must not touch the package's inner seal line during removal. If the scrub nurse cannot accept the sterile item, the circulating nurse flips the item onto the sterile field. The item must not touch the inner seal line while being passed to the sterile field (U.S. Army, 1988, pp. 47–48).

Arranging Instruments and Supplies on the Instrument Table and Mayo Tray

General Guidelines

Usually, the back table is divided into four sections. The scrub nurse stands next to the left and right lower sections. Depending on the number of instruments required, more than one back table and Mayo tray may be needed. To facilitate the continuity of care during staff changes, back tables and Mayo trays should be uniformly set up (Fig. 8–2). Before transferring an instrument set or other items to the back table, check the internal chemical sterilization indicator for a color change. If the color of the indicator has not changed or the indicator is missing, remove the item and regown and reglove. The following guidelines provide an example of organizing a back table and a Mayo tray (U.S. Army, 1988, p. 63).

Back Table

Place the instrument pan with instruments in the far upper right quadrant of the back table. Prepare towels for use on the Mayo tray and the back table by completely rolling two towels into cylinders. Place one towel lengthwise and next to the edge of the Mayo tray. Place the other towel in the far lower right quadrant of the back table. Lift the stringed instruments from the instrument pan, place them on the rolled towel, and remove the stringer. Arrange the retractors according to size in the upper right quadrant, to the left of the instrument pan (Fig. 8–3). If preferred, retractors may be left in the instrument pan and arranged according to size. Arrange tissue and dressing forceps in the lower right quadrant of the back table, to the left of the rolled towel. Scissors are placed in the left front quadrant of the back table, next to the tissue and dressing forceps. Place suture packages and free needles in the left front quadrant of the back table, to the left of the scissors. Place needle holders in the left front quadrant of the back table, to the left of the suture packages and free needles. Close the box-locks of the small and large towel clips and place them on the ring stand. Arrange sponges, special instruments, and supplies in the upper left quadrant of the back table (U.S. Army, 1988, pp. 63–65). The irrigation bowl or pitcher is placed in the upper left quadrant (Fig. 8–4).

Scalpels

Hold the scalpel handle in one hand. With the other hand, grasp the blade on the dull edge with a needle holder at the widest, strongest point without touching the cutting edge. Pointing the blade and handle down and away from the body, slide the blade into the groove of the scalpel handle until it is secured (U.S. Army, 1988, pp. 63–65). Place assembled scalpels ready for use on the back instrument table (Fig. 8–5).

Mayo Tray

Arrange suture ties on the covered Mayo tray and draped Mayo stand. Generally, silk and other nonabsorbable ties are placed to the rear, away from the scrub nurse, and absorbable ties are placed to the front. Drape a towel over the ties and tuck under the tray (Fig. 8–6). Arrange the clamps and hemostats needed for the first phase of the procedure on the rolled towel. Place the tissue forceps and scissors next to the instruments (Fig. 8–7). The scalpels are placed next to the tissue forceps and scissors. The blade should point away from the scrub nurse. Some scrub personnel tuck the blades under the rolled towel. Place four sponges, suction tubing, the electrosurgical unit active electrode, the electrode holster with attachment hardware, and light handles or gloves on the Mayo tray. If the suction or active electrode tubing is attached to the drapes with a nonpenetrating clamp, insert the tubing or the cord through the handle rings of the clamp. Attach the Yankauer tonsil suction tip to the tubing and electrode tip to the pencil (U.S. Army, 1988, pp. 63–65).

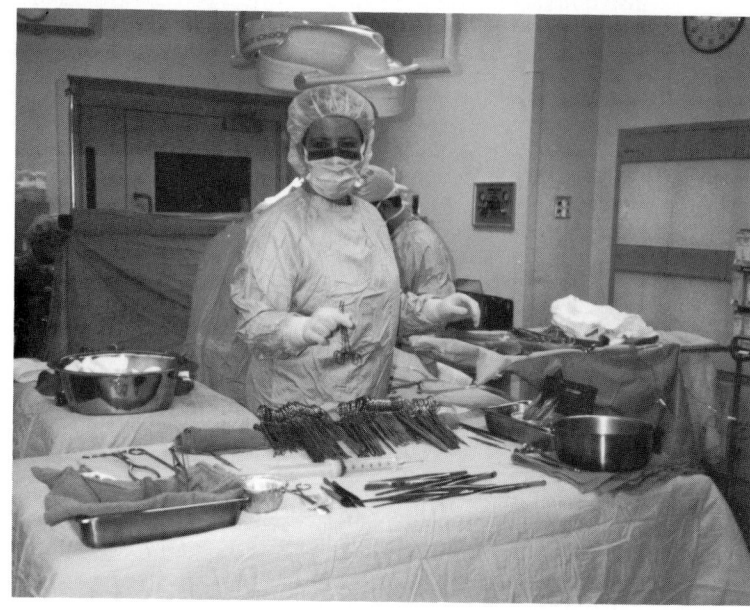

FIGURE 8–2. Setup of the back table.

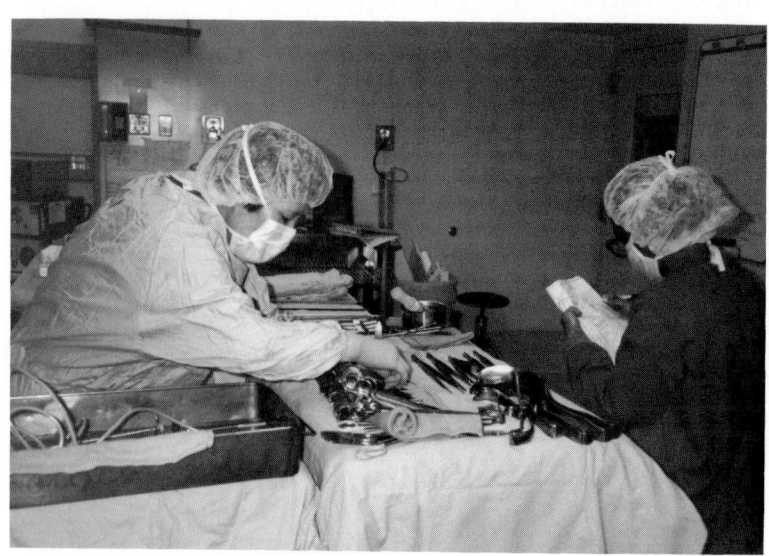

FIGURE 8–3. Arranging retractor, clamps, and forceps on the back table.

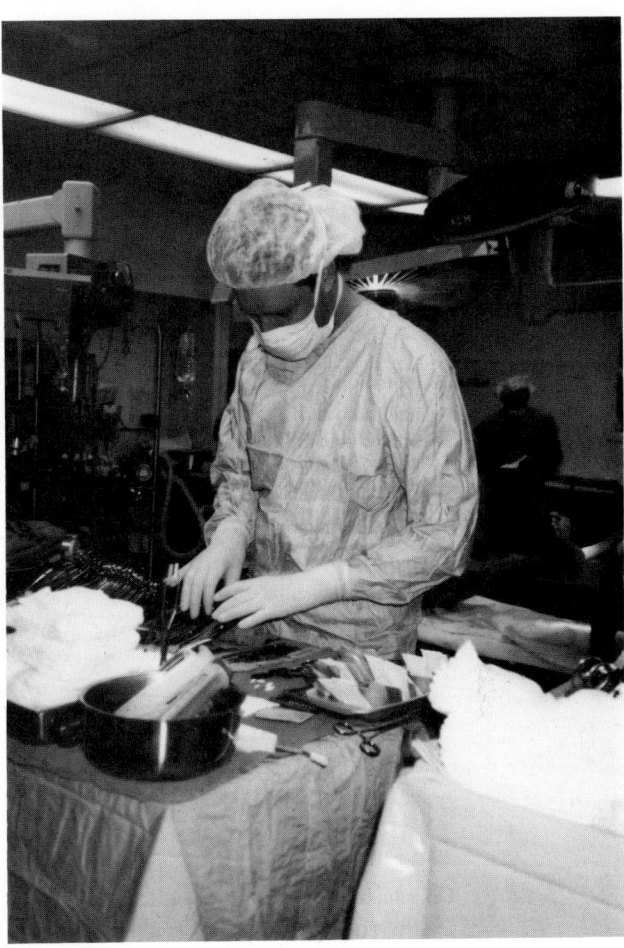

FIGURE 8–4. Sponges, suture, and irrigation bowl on the back table.

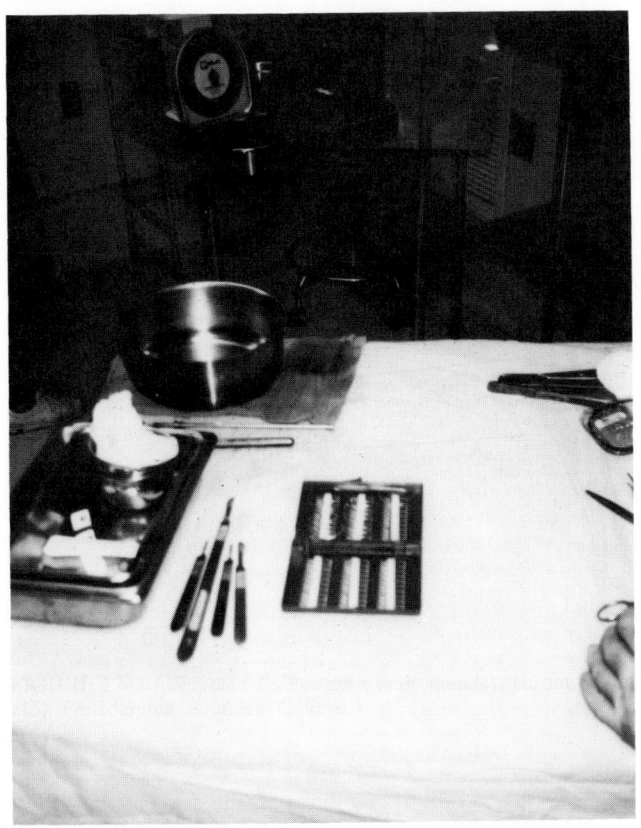

FIGURE 8–5. Scalpels on the back table.

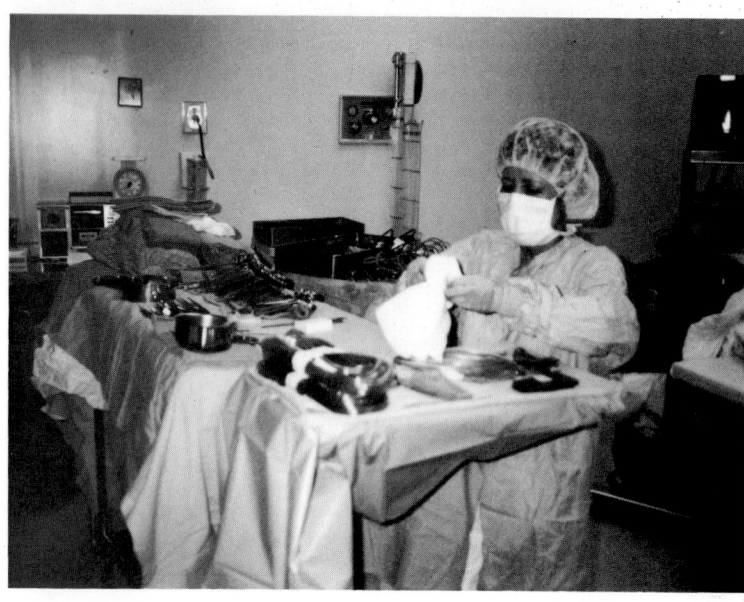

FIGURE 8–6. Preparation of the Mayo tray.

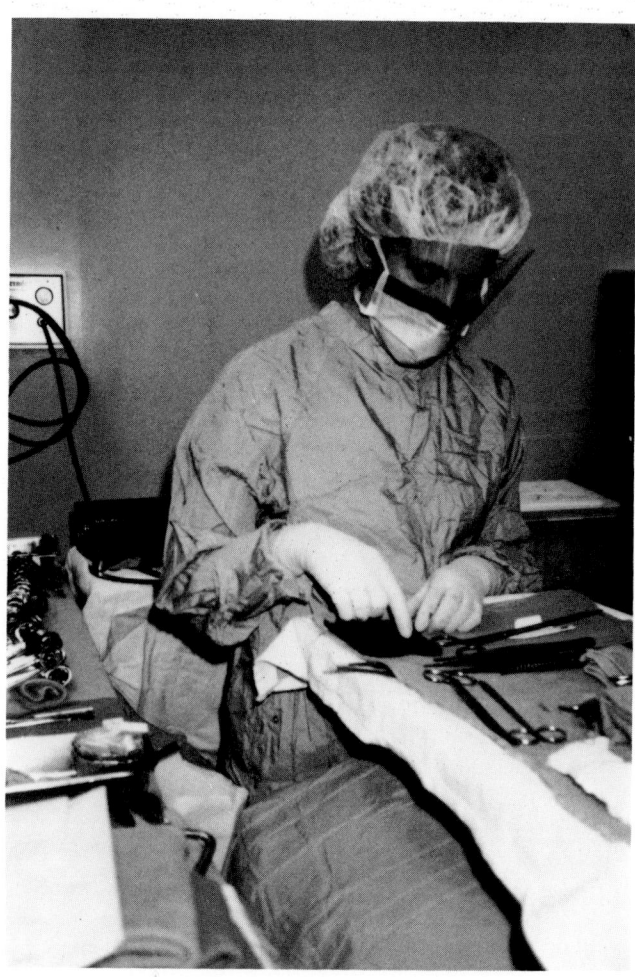

FIGURE 8–7. Instruments on the Mayo tray.

Passing Instruments and Supplies to the Surgeon

Pass the scalpel to the surgeon handle first with the cutting edge pointed downward. Tissue forceps and ringed or box-locked instruments are passed to the surgeon in the position of function. Multipiece retractors are assembled before being passed to the surgeon. Pass retractors handle first. Place sponges close to the operative site. Moisten and wring out sponges as requested by the surgeon. Sponges for the abdominal or thoracic cavity are usually moistened. Pass Kittner dissector sponges held in a Kelly clamp or Rochester-Péan forceps and stick sponges on a sponge forceps. Pass instruments by gently snapping them into the surgeon's hand. The instrument is released as soon as the surgeon has a firm grip (U.S. Army, 1988, pp. 97–98).

Preparing and Passing Suture to the Surgeon

Nonabsorbable Suture

Tear the foil pack at the notch and remove the suture strands from the package as a unit. Unfold the strands of suture to full length. Do not pull silk suture between gloved fingers. This prevents the build-up of static electricity in the suture. Place the strands under the towel on the Mayo tray according to type and size (U.S. Army, 1988, pp. 102–103).

Absorbable Suture

Tear the foil pack over a small basin to prevent fluid from dripping on the table drape. Remove the suture from the package. Place the center loop of the suture over two fingers of the nondominant hand and unwind the suture to half length. Gently pull to straighten the suture. Jerking the strand can lead to breakage. Fold and cut the suture into equal parts and cut with the suture scissors. Place the strands under the towel on the Mayo tray according to type and size (U.S. Army, 1988, p. 103).

Free Tie

Hold both ends of the suture securely with one end in each hand. Press the tie firmly into the palm of the surgeon's dominant hand. Release the suture as soon as the surgeon closes his or her hand (U.S. Army, 1988, p. 105).

Tie-to-Pass Ligature

Place the tip of the suture strand securely into the tip of a tonsil or right-angled clamp and lock the clamp.

Hold the box-lock of the clamp between the thumb and the index finger. The tip of the clamp should be positioned so it faces the back of the hand. Gently snap the rings of the clamp into the palm of the surgeon's hand so that the tip of the clamp points toward the center of the surgeon's body (U.S. Army, 1988, p. 105).

Stick-Tie Suture

Position the needle in the needle holder so that the point of the needle faces the midline and the suture end of the needle is on the right. Clamp the needle between one fourth and one third of the distance from the suture end of the needle to the point of the needle. The needle should be recessed approximately ⅛ inch into the jaws of the needle holder. Pass the needle holder so that the point of the needle is toward the center of the surgeon's body. Place the free end of the suture over the back of the surgeon's hand. Place used needles on the needle counter or in another appropriate container (U.S. Army, 1988, pp. 104–105).

Applying and Removing a Pneumatic Tourniquet

General Guidelines

Tourniquets are used to provide a bloodless field. Pneumatic tourniquet equipment includes a pressure source, a pressure gauge, a regulator, tubing, connectors, and an inflatable cuff. The entire system should be checked for discrepancies, such as cracks or holes in the tubing, before each use. Ensure that the inner tube of the cuff is completely encased (AORN, 1992, III:13–1). Check the pressure source for adequate gas. An inert nonflammable gas such as nitrogen is used to inflate the cuff. Pressure in the tank should read at least 500 pounds/square inch.

Selecting the Tourniquet Cuff

Inappropriate cuff size can injure the patient. The perioperative nurse should assess the size of the extremity and select a cuff that overlaps at the ends no more than 3 inches. Cuff width is important. The wider the cuff is, the larger the mass of tissue compressed, resulting in a lower pressure to provide hemostasis. Low pressure decreases the patient's risk of cuff-related nerve injury (AORN, 1992, III:13–1).

Applying the Tourniquet Cuff

Unless contraindicated by the manufacturer's instructions, before applying the tourniquet cuff, the perioperative nurse applies wrinkle-free padding. If applied correctly, the padding protects the skin under the cuff from mechanical injury. The nurse positions the cuff above the elbow or knee "at the point of maximum circumference of the limb" (AORN, 1992, *III*:13–2). Placement of the cuff below the elbow or the knee results in pressure that may cause nerve damage because of the thin layer of soft tissue between underlying bones and the cuff. Care must be taken to avoid an incomplete or overly aggressive seal of the cuff. An improper cuff seal may result in bruising, blistering, pinching, or necrosis of the skin. The perioperative nurse secures the tourniquet by tying the cuff strings in a bow. Do not tie a knot. This interferes with removal, especially in an emergency situation. After applying the tourniquet cuff, the perioperative nurse ensures that the cuff is *not* rotated to a new position. Rotating the cuff after application leads to shearing forces, which may damage the underlying tissue (AORN, 1992, *III*:13–2).

Preparing and Draping the Extremity After Tourniquet Application

The perioperative nurse applies an impervious barrier around the cuff during the skin preparation. Seepage of preparation solutions under the cuff and the subsequent pressure of the inflated cuff may result in chemical burns (AORN, 1992, *III*:13–2). If preparation solutions seep under the cuff during the preparation, the perioperative nurse should remove the cuff, dry the limb and the cuff, and then reapply the cuff.

While draping the extremity, especially around the tourniquet cuff, the scrub person must not puncture the cuff with the towel clip or other sharp object. Holes may not immediately affect cuff inflation. During the procedure, however, cuff effectiveness is diminished and hemostasis is compromised.

Preparing the Limb for Tourniquet Inflation

The surgeon may wrap the limb tightly before inflating the tourniquet cuff. This action compresses the veins and drains the blood from the limb. Depending on the size of the limb, use a 4- or 6-inch Esmarch or elastic (Ace) bandage. Starting with the hand or the foot, elevate and tightly wrap the limb toward the cuff. After wrapping, inflate the cuff. Unwrap the limb by reversing the procedure and rewind the bandage. Save the bandage for later use.

Inflating the Tourniquet

Because exact tourniquet inflation pressures have not been determined, the patient's age and systolic blood pressure, the width of the tourniquet, and the circumference of the limb should be considered when selecting a tourniquet inflation pressure. As a guideline, in the healthy adult patient, 50 to 75 mm Hg above the systolic

pressure for an arm and 100 to 150 mm Hg above the systolic pressure for a leg usually produce a bloodless field (AORN, 1992, *III*:13–2). Pressures are lower for children and patients with impaired tissue perfusion.

Monitoring the Tourniquet Intraoperatively

The perioperative nurse ensures that the pressure gauge is clearly visible. Do not cover it with drapes. Check the cuff periodically during inflation for pressure fluctuations. Excessive or insufficient tourniquet pressure may cause nerve damage. Hemorrhagic infiltration of the nerve secondary to passive venous congestion of the limb is another complication of insufficient tourniquet pressure.

Watch the tourniquet inflation time. Tourniquet paralysis may result from keeping the tourniquet in place too long. Exact tourniquet times have not been established. As a general guideline, however, the tourniquet should stay inflated no longer than 1 hour for an arm and 1½ hours for a leg in the healthy adult patient. As for inflation pressures, variables such as the patient's age, the condition of the limb, and the patient's health status affect the inflation time (AORN, 1992, *III*:13–2).

Removing the Tourniquet

Do not deflate the tourniquet cuff until instructed by the surgeon. After the cuff is deflated, remove the cuff and padding, and inspect the skin for signs of chemical burn, bruising, blistering, pinching, and necrosis.

Documenting Tourniquet Use

AORN's Recommended Practices for Use of the Pneumatic Tourniquet (1992, *III*:13–3) suggest that the perioperative nurse document the following information when using a pneumatic tourniquet:

- Location of the cuff
- Identification of the person who applied the cuff
- Cuff pressure and time of inflation and deflation
- Skin and tissue integrity under the cuff before and after the use of the pneumatic tourniquet
- Identification number of the specific tourniquet

Applying and Removing the Electrosurgical Unit Dispersive Electrode

General Guidelines

Electrosurgery is common to most surgical procedures. The perioperative nurse, therefore, should have the appropriate knowledge concerning the use of the electrosurgical unit to ensure patient and staff safety.

As for other electrical equipment, before use, inspect the electrosurgical unit by testing the alarm system and looking for frayed wires and loose connections. Place the generator close enough to the sterile field to ensure that the active electrode cord is connected without tension. This prevents inadvertent disconnection of the cord from the generator. Always use the electrosurgical unit at the lowest possible effective setting. Confirm orally with the operator the activation and settings. When higher than usual settings are requested, check for malfunction or loose connections. If no loose connections or malfunctions are found and high settings are still required, obtain another generator. Electrosurgical units are not usually used for patients with pacemakers owing to the potential for electrical interference with the pacemaker. To avoid possible fire, do not use electrosurgical units in the presence of flammable agents. Do not use extension cords on an electrosurgical unit generator (AORN, 1992, *III*:5–1—5–2).

Applying the Dispersive Electrode

Patient safety depends on a safe dispersive electrode (grounding pad). Ensure that the dispersive electrode has adequate gel for good conduction. Electrode size should provide adequate body contact and grounding. Place the grounding pad over a large muscle mass and as close to the wound site as possible. Do not apply the grounding pad over bony prominences, scar tissue, areas with large metal prosthetic implants (total hip replacements, internal rods, and plates), or excessively hairy areas. Shave hairy patients at the dispersive electrode site before applying the pad. This ensures good contact of the pad and gel with the skin. Apply the dispersive electrode with uniform contact with the skin. Do not place the dispersive electrode pad circumferentially on an extremity owing to the potential for a tourniquet effect and decreased tissue perfusion.

Protect the patient from a potential thermal injury by placing the grounding pad in areas where liquids do not accumulate. In addition, do not place the grounding pad near electrocardiographic electrodes or rectal probes. Before and during the procedure, check to ensure that the patient is not touching metal objects such as intravenous poles and stirrup holders. Contact with metal objects during electrosurgery provides the electrical current with an alternative exit pathway, which may lead to a patient burn. If contact with metal objects unavoidably occurs, insulate the object with a nonconductive material such as foam, rubber, or cloth. During the procedure, check the grounding pad for tenting and puckering, and reposition as necessary (AORN, 1992, *III*:5–2).

Removing the Dispersive Electrode

Do not remove the electrode until the dressing has been applied and the drapes taken off the patient. Carefully and slowly peel the dispersive electrode from the patient's skin. Assess the application site for signs of electrical burns. Check the patient for burns due to alternative exit pathway of electrical current, particularly at the application sites for electrocardiographic leads.

Monitoring the Active Electrode

The scrub nurse monitors the active electrode during surgery. Before use, inspect the active electrode for damage, especially if it is reusable. Look for frayed wires and check that the tip tightly fits in the pencil. Hand the active electrode cord from the sterile field without loops and twists. During the procedure, remove charred tissue from the blades and tips of the active electrode. When not using the active electrode, place it in a clean, dry, nonconductive, and highly visible area during procedures. Do not allow the active electrode to contact metal clamps or lie on exposed patient skin (AORN, 1992, *III*:5–2).

Documenting Electrosurgery

The perioperative nurse should document the following when using the electrosurgical unit:

- Patient's preoperative and postoperative skin condition at the dispersive electrode site
- Area of placement of the dispersive electrode
- Identification of the electrosurgical unit and its settings (AORN, 1992, *III*:4–1)

Preparing Electrical Instruments and Equipment for Use

Many types of electrical instruments and equipment are used during surgery (Fig. 8–8). The perioperative nurse should prepare and operate electrical instruments and equipment according to the manufacturer's instructions.

Inspect electrical instruments and equipment before use. Attachments should be affixed to the electrical instrument and the unit tested before use. To avoid accidental activation of the unit, triggers should be in the safety position and on-off switches should be in the off position when changing attachments and plugging in the instrument (AORN, 1992, *III*:9–5).

Check outlets and switch plates for damage. Examine cords and plugs for fraying or other damage. Damaged outlets and switch plates, as well as frayed cords and plugs, may result in excessive current leakage and cause patient or personnel injury (AORN, 1992, *III*:7–4).

Eliminate the potential for tripping or accidental unplugging of the equipment by laying cords flat on the floor (AORN, 1992, *III*:7–4). Watch for pooled fluids on the floor. Cords with undetected frays or damage that are lying in water or other fluid present an extreme electrical hazard to personnel.

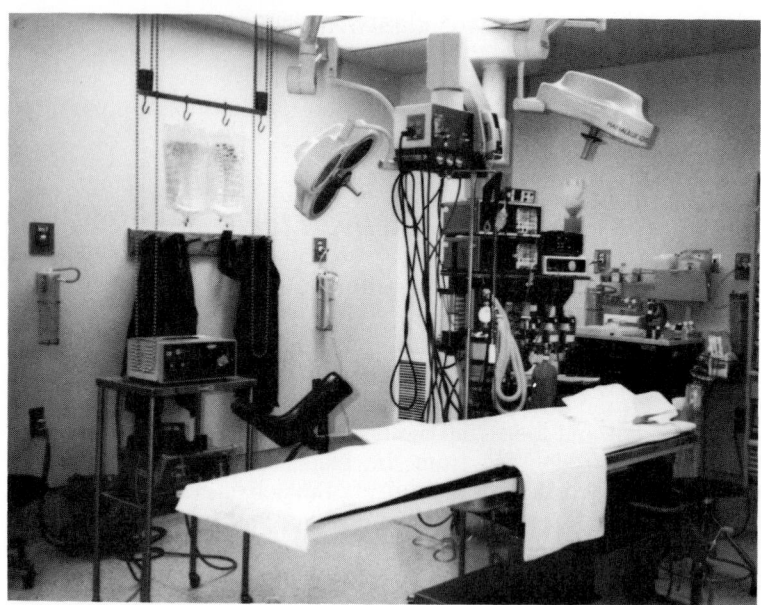

FIGURE 8–8. Electrical equipment in the operating room.

Preparing Air-Powered Instruments for Use

Inspect and test air-powered instruments before use. Ensure that the manufacturer's instructions are followed when an air-powered instrument is used. Because worn or damaged air hoses are a hazard to personnel and can cause delays in the surgical procedure, meticulously inspect hoses before using the air-powered instrument (AORN, 1992, III:9–5).

Prevent patient and personnel injury by connecting attachments and testing the unit before use. If not securely seated, improperly connected attachments may be thrown with great force when the unit is activated. Avoid accidental activation when changing attachments by placing the triggering mechanism in the safety position (AORN, 1992, III:9–5).

Use medical-grade compressed air or compressed dry nitrogen (99.97% pure) for air-powered instruments. Check the tank before use. At least 1000 pounds square inch should register on the tank pressure gauge. Do not set pounds per square inch unless the instrument is running. "Excessive ppsi can damage the air-powered surgical instrument and exert stress on the hose" (AORN, 1992, III:9–5). Use the manufacturer's recommended pounds per square inch when using an air-powered instrument. Do not automatically exceed the recommended pounds per square inch if the instrument operation is sluggish or erratic.

Many types of electrical instruments and equipment are used during surgery. The perioperative nurse should prepare and operate electrical instruments and equipment according to the manufacturer's instructions.

Preparing the Hyperthermia or Hypothermia Unit for Use

Hypothermia or hyperthermia units and blankets are used to maintain, increase, or decrease the patient's temperature. The perioperative nurse ensures that the hypothermia or hyperthermia unit and blanket is used in an effective and safe manner. Monitoring of the unit and blanket is essential during the surgical procedure (AORN, 1992, III:7–3).

Before using the hypothermia or hyperthermia unit, the perioperative nurse ensures that the fluid reservoir is filled according to the manufacturer's instructions. Controls are checked to ensure proper functioning. Lights should illuminate when the unit is on. Temperature-monitoring devices that connect to the unit should be available and in proper working order.

The perioperative nurse should inspect the blanket surfaces and tubing for holes and kinks before placing the blanket on the operating room (OR) bed. Attach the blanket tubing to the hypothermia or hyperthermia unit, set the controls to the desired heating or cooling temperature, and activate the unit. As the unit pumps fluid through the tubing and blanket, check for leaks.

After checking the blanket and tubing for leaks, place the blanket on the OR bed. Because patient thermal burns or pressure necrosis may occur with a hyperthermia or hypothermia blanket unless the blanket is designed for direct skin contact, cover the blanket with an absorbable pad or sheet. Prevent folds and creases in the blanket. These hinder the proper flow of fluid through the blanket and may cause hot or cold spots on the blanket's surface (AORN, 1992, III:7–3).

During unit use, the perioperative nurse should periodically assess its functioning. Feel for excessive heat or cold radiating from the tubing and the blanket. Check the temperature controls to ensure that they are set for the correct temperature.

Applying Dressings

Preparing the Incision

Before removing drapes, the scrub person should clean the incision site with a wet sterile sponge or towel to remove dried preparation solution, blood, other body fluid, and tissue. Tape applied over dried preparation solution may lead to skin irritation and possible chemical burn. Tape applied over blood, fluids, and tissue creates an environment conducive to microorganism growth. Dry the skin around the incision after cleaning.

Applying the Dressing

The scrub person applies the sterile dressing according to the surgeon's preference. Avoid using radiopaque sponges for dressings. Hold the dressing in place with one hand and remove the drapes from the incision site with the other hand.

Applying the Tape

The circulating nurse applies the tape. If the surgeon applies the tape, he or she should remove the gloves to prevent cross-contamination. Secure the dressing in place with tape. Do not stretch the skin while applying the tape.

Assisting with the Application of Casts and Splints

Preparing the Operating Room

Casting materials spilled or splattered during the application of casts or splints complicates room cleanup and increases turnover time. Protect the OR by spreading a disposable plastic or fabric sheet on the floor around the OR bed. The OR bed is protected by covering exposed areas with a suitable draping material.

Using Casting Materials

Plaster of Paris is made from hydrous calcium sulfate, also known as gypsum. During the manufacturing of plaster of Paris, the gypsum is ground to a fine powder and subjected to heat. The heat eliminates some of the water found in the compound. Plaster setting times are determined by adding chemicals to the dehydrated powder. Cast strength is determined by the formation of long cylindrical crystals. As the plaster of Paris sets, crystals form and interlock with each other to make a strong cast. If the cast is moved or manipulated before setting, the crystals break and do not interlock, and the cast becomes weak (U.S. Army, 1967, p. 93).

Plaster setting time can be slowed by leaving excessive amounts of water in the plaster roll and adding sugar or cold water to the water in the plaster bucket. Setting time can be accelerated by removing excessive water from the plaster roll, rubbing and working with the plaster as it is applied, and adding table salt or hot water to the water in the plaster bucket (U.S. Army, 1967, p. 93).

Preparing the Casting Materials and Equipment

Select the plaster rolls, cut the padding, and obtain other materials, such as stockinet and Webril, according to the physician's preference (Fig. 8–9) (Table 8–2). Place a plastic liner bag in the plaster bucket and fill with lukewarm water, about 70 to 80°F (U.S. Army, 1967, p. 94).

TABLE 8–2. BASIC CAST SUPPLIES AND EQUIPMENT	
Name	**Description**
Cotton bandages, plaster of Paris impregnated	Available in widths of 2, 3, 4, and 6 inches; used as the basic material to form casts
Splints, plaster of Paris impregnated for leg and arm	Lengths and width are short and narrow (3 × 15 inches), short and wide (4 × 15 inches), and long and wide (5 × 30 inches); used to reinforce casts and reduces the time for application
Stockinet	Tubular, seamless-ribbed knit material of natural color; available in widths of 3, 6, 10, and 12 inches; thin padding next to cast; helps to make close fitting, contoured cast
Cotton wadding	Available in widths of 5 inches × 6 yards; padding for casts
Webril bandage	Available in 2, 3, 4, and 6 inches × 4 yards; used as padding
Felt bandages	Available in large white rolls and can be split into the thickness and cut into the size and shape required; used for padding bony prominences
Electrical cutter	Available with 2- and 2½-inch blades; used for cutting casts; may have vacuum attached to confine plaster dust
Cast knives	Various sizes available; the compound dental knife with detachable No. 21 blade is commonly used
Spreaders, benders, scissors, and pliers	Spreaders used to spread the edges of casts; benders, for bending back the edges; bandage scissors, for cutting materials; ordinary pliers, for tightening blades on cast cutter
Plaster cart	Used for containing supplies and preparing casts
Metal splints, padded	Used for splinting finger fractures
Bucket, 8 quart	Used for dipping plaster products
Pillows, plastic covered	Used for elevating limbs after casting

Adapted from U.S. Army. (1967). *Orthopedic specialist: TM 8–231, AFM 160–6* (pp. 93–97). U.S. Departments of the Army and the Air Force. Baltimore: U.S. Army Publications Center.

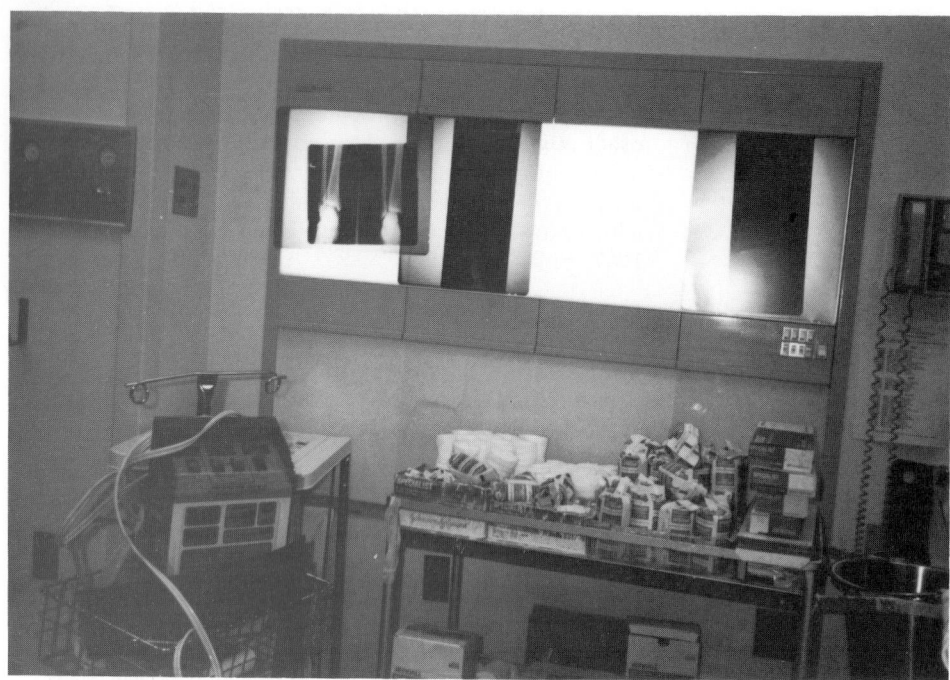

FIGURE 8–9. Casting materials and equipment under the light box.

Padding the Cast

Padding reduces the risk of pressure sore development over bony prominences, thereby making the cast more comfortable for the patient and facilitating removal of the cast.

For a close-fitting and well-contoured cast, use the stockinet for padding material. Because the stockinet tends to constrict, however, there is the potential for impaired circulation. Do not use it alone if the patient has an acute fracture or excessive swelling or immediately after an operation. If the stockinet is used without padding, document this fact on the cast using an indelible ink pen. This alerts the person who removes the cast to use caution when using the electrical cast cutter. The surgeon may elect to wrap sheet cotton or Webril bandage over the stockinet. If Webril is used, wrap it smoothly in one to three layers with the turns overlapping about one half the width of the bandage. Bony prominences must be padded to reduce the risk of skin breakdown after the cast has been applied. Heavy felt pieces can be placed over bony prominences (U.S. Army, 1967, p. 94).

Preparing the Plaster Bandage Roll

When dipping the plaster roll, hold it in a vertical position. This allows air to escape through the core of the roll. Dip the roll in the lukewarm water for approximately 5 seconds or until the water stops bubbling. Hold the roll at each end and squeeze. Do not wring the water out of the roll. Squeeze at the ends, while pushing toward the center. This forces the water out of the roll. Leave enough water in the roll to delay drying, thus ensuring proper application before the plaster sets.

Pass the plaster roll to the surgeon (U.S. Army, 1967, p. 94).

Preparing the Plaster Splint

The surgeon may apply splints to joint areas or to areas where additional strength is desired. Select the number and size of splint sheets according to the surgeon's preference, dip in the water and rapidly withdraw them. Place the splints on a work table and smooth out with the palm of the hand. Draw each side of the splint through the index and middle fingers and pass to the surgeon. Give the surgeon a plaster bandage to tie the splint (U.S. Army, 1967, p. 94).

Molding the Cast

The surgeon rubs and molds the cast over the contour of the body part. During this process, he or she may apply a few drops of water to make the surface smooth. If plaster crumbs develop, the surgeon should remove the crumbs with water, which prevents rough spots in the cast from forming. Molding continues until the plaster begins to set, or until the plaster is no longer glossy or creamy. Ventilating the cast is necessary because heat is generated as the plaster sets. Do not cover it (U.S. Army, 1967, p. 94).

Finishing the Cast

Finishing the cast involves trimming it with a cast knife. After trimming the cast, the edges of the stockinet are folded over, a plaster splint is applied over the folded edge, and the splint is smoothed over. Next, the patient's casted extremity is placed on a pillow. To prevent cast denting, the cast is protected from contacting rough surfaces (U.S. Army, 1967, p. 96).

Removing the Cast

Most casts are removed with an electrical cast cutter. The cast should be removed outside the restricted areas of the surgical suite to confine plaster dust. A cast cutter with an attached vacuum helps confine plaster dust that is generated during the removal process. When removing the cast, exercise care in cutting over bony prominences or areas where the bones are close to the surface of the skin, such as the shin. Look for notes on the cast that indicate areas of light padding (U.S. Army, 1967, pp. 96–97).

If an electrical cast cutter is not available, a cast can be removed by soaking it in water until it becomes soft. After the cast is softened, it is unraveled, starting with the end of the last roll applied. Another method is to use peroxide and a plaster knife. Grooves are made in the cast and peroxide is poured into the grooves. As the plaster softens, the knife is used to cut the layers of the cast (U.S. Army, 1967, pp. 96–97).

Precautions

When applying casts, the following precautions should be taken:

- Do not place circular dressing of cloth, adhesive, moleskin, elastic bandage, or any material other than acceptable padding under the cast.
- Use the palm of the hand, not the fingertips, to hold a wet cast.
- Because plaster generates heat while setting, expose the cast to air while it is drying (U.S. Army, 1967, p. 97).

Discharge Instructions for the Patient

The perioperative nurse may be in the position to provide discharge instructions to the patient. Instructions include cast care and complication prevention (U.S. Army, 1967, p. 97).

Cast Care

- Do not walk on new walking casts for 24 hours.
- Keep all casts dry.
- Do not alter casts.
- Do not remove casts.
- Do not put foreign objects inside of casts.

Prevention of Complications

- To prevent swelling when a cast is applied to a limb, elevate the limb for 2 days.
- Report pressure points.
- If a cast becomes soft or broken, return for repairs.
- If a cast becomes too loose, return for a new one.
- If in doubt, return to have the cast checked.
- Follow the physician's orders.

Bibliography

Association of Operating Room Nurses. (1992). *Standards and recommended practices for perioperative nursing.* Denver.

Fogg, D. M. (1990). Clinical issues. *AORN Journal, 51*(2), 440.

Gordon, M. (1987). *Manual of nursing diagnosis: 1986–1987.* New York: McGraw-Hill.

U.S. Army. (1988). *301–91D10 Operating room specialist course competency based program of instruction student handbook.* Fort Sam Houston, TX: Academy of Health Sciences, U.S. Army.

U.S. Army. (1967). *Orthopedic specialist: TM 8–231, AFM 160–6 (pp. 93–97).* U.S. Departments of the Army and the Air Force. Baltimore: U.S. Army Publications Center.

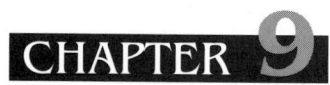

Administering Drugs and Solutions

Angela M. Martinelli

DEFINITION

Proper administration of drugs and solutions is essential for safe, quality patient care in the operating room (OR). The perioperative nurse ensures that the administration of drugs and solutions by the nursing team during the intraoperative period is performed correctly and does not result in harm to the patient. Although the perioperative nurse may administer medications and solutions orally or by inhalation, most medications and solutions given by the nurse during the intraoperative phase are administered by injection, topical application to the skin or mucous membranes, or irrigation of the operative site.

This chapter focuses on medications and solutions administered in the OR by the perioperative nurse. For a discussion of drugs and solutions usually administered by an anesthetist (e.g., anesthetic agents, intravenous, [IV] preparations, and blood products) refer to Chapter 19.

MEASURABLE CRITERIA

The perioperative nurse demonstrates competency to administer drugs and solutions by

- visiting the patient and the family before surgery to obtain a medication history (see Appendix A)
- verifying patient identification, the correct drug or solution, the correct dosage, the correct route, and the correct time for administration
- knowing potential drug reactions, complications, and contraindications
- having available specific antidotes and other emergency drugs and equipment
- gathering prescribed medications and necessary supplies and equipment (see Appendix B)
- using resources as needed (e.g., *AMA Drug Evaluations* [American Medical Association, 1984] FDA Drug Bulletin, *Physicians' Desk Reference* [1992], hospital formulary, manufacturer's product information, and other selected pharmacology texts and journal articles)
- communicating with the hospital pharmacist as needed
- preparing and administering drugs and solutions according to institutional policy, manufacturer's recommendations, and federal and state regulations
- verifying the drug, the doses, and the route of administration with the physician and the scrub nurse before transferring a drug to the sterile field
- performing procedures for charging the patient for drugs and solutions administered
- obtaining the patient's consent for the use of experimental drugs
- disposing of needles, syringes, glassware, and contaminated material according to accepted guidelines
- verifying verbal orders before administration
- questioning orders that appear to be erroneous
- documenting the drug or solution, its dosage, the time and route of administration, and the name of the individual who prepared and administered the substance

ROLE OF THE PERIOPERATIVE NURSE

The circulating nurse, first assistant, scrub person, and surgeon share in the responsibility for preparing and administering drugs and solutions during the intraoperative phase. Each team member is responsible for patient safety as it relates to identifying the patient and verifying the name of the medication, the dosage, the route by which it is to be administered, and the time and frequency of administration.

The circulating nurse receives a standing, written, or verbal order from the physician and is responsible for preparing the drug or solution. The circulating nurse then verifies this order with the surgeon before placing the medication on the operative field. The scrub person then labels the medication and identifies it each time it is administered.

CONSIDERATIONS

Potential for Adverse Drug Reactions

Pharmacological Toxicity

Toxicity is usually caused by drug overdose. When this occurs, it is an adverse effect of the drug's known pharmacological characteristics. If the dose is large enough, toxic effects can occur in any patient. Even with small doses, toxicity is possible if the patient is hypersusceptible to one or another of the drug's primary or secondary pharmacological effects (Rodman and Smith, 1984, p. 32).

The perioperative nurse must have knowledge of the type and the dose of drugs and solutions used during a surgical procedure. If excessive amounts are given, toxicity can result, even with commonly used drugs such as lidocaine (Xylocaine) for local anesthesia, a heparin solution for anticoagulation, and an antibacterial irrigation for the prevention of infection.

Drug Allergy and Idiosyncracy

Drug allergy and idiosyncracy are the result of a patient's sensitivity to a specific chemical. These conditions differ from toxicity in that they are not related to the drug's pharmacology. A reaction due to drug allergy does not occur at the first time of administration but only after the individual becomes sensitized. In an immediate, or anaphylactic, reaction, signs and symptoms develop within minutes after exposure. These reactions result from the release of active chemical mediators during the antigen-antibody reactions. The degree of severity does not depend on the drug but on how strongly sensitized the individual was when she or he received the drug at an earlier time.

In a delayed reaction, the appearance of signs and symptoms may not be evident until several hours or days after exposure to the chemical. These reactions often result in a variety of signs and symptoms such as contact dermatitis, hemolytic anemia, fever, swollen lymph nodes, and edema of the face and limbs. For example, the perioperative nurse who administers a penicillin compound or applies mafenide acetate cream (Sulfamylon) to treat burns may observe a delayed drug reaction during the postoperative visit to the patient.

Patients who are abnormally sensitive to small doses of a drug the first time it is administered may experience an idiosyncratic reaction. Malignant hyperthermia is an example. This uncommon response may occur in patients who receive inhalation anesthetics such as halothane or the skeletal muscle relaxant succinylcholine.

Potential Interaction of Drugs or Solutions with Other Substances

The presence of another chemical in the body may alter the desired effect of the drug or solution. Combinations of chemicals can result in a number of reactions. The most common reaction is a change in drug metabolism that can alter absorption, distribution, biotransformation, excretion, and concentration of one or more substances. The perioperative nurse must know the medications that the patient is taking, know the potential interactions, and take measures to prevent interactions.

Physical Factors That May Influence the Effect of Drugs

Each patient has a variety of unique physical characteristics that can influence his or her response to medications. For the most part, these characteristics cannot be altered.

Patient's Weight. The patient's body weight is usually the primary consideration when determining medication dosage. In general, weight affects the amount of administered dose that arrives at the reactive target tissues. In a low-weight patient, the reactive target tissue receives a greater portion of the dose. Consequently, the effect of the drug on the low-weight patient is greater than that on a heavier patient. Conversely, the reactive target tissue of a heavy patient receives a smaller portion of the dose, and the effect of the drug is less potent (Rodman and Smith, 1984, p. 21). The perioperative nurse notes the patient's weight, which is usually recorded in kilograms (2.2 pounds is equal to 1 kg). The kilogram weight is used when calculating dosage because dosage is often prescribed and administered on the basis of the ratio of milligrams of the drug to kilograms of body weight.

Patient's Age. A patient's age can influence the response to medication. In most cases, neonates, premature infants, and the elderly are more likely to experience intense effects produced by a drug because of an age-related inability to transform drugs to inactive metabolites or a decreased capability to excrete drugs and their remaining active metabolites.

Presence of Disease. Existing disease states can alter drug metabolism and excretion and cause an unexpected drug response. For example, the patient with severe liver disease is a poor candidate for general anesthesia with thiopental sodium (Pentothal) because the final elimination of this drug from the body requires enzymatic breakdown in the liver. In patients with renal dysfunction, administration of gentamicin can cause further renal damage. Diabetes, cardiac disease, cancer, and arthritis are common coexisting conditions that must be considered during the perioperative course.

Drug Tolerance. Drug tolerance to a particular substance can result in a decreased ability to break down the drug by means of hepatic or other enzymatic metabolism. Tolerance to a drug may also develop when a patient continues to take the drug for a long time.

Cross-tolerance can develop with different drugs that act at the same cellular site to produce similar effects. The drug- or alcohol-addicted patient, for example, may prove resistant to a general anesthetic that depresses the central nervous system (CNS) in much the same way that alcohol does.

Coexisting Drugs. Cumulative effects can occur when drugs are taken at a greater rate than the rate at which they can be eliminated by the patient. If several doses of a drug are taken at regular intervals, accumulation and overdose may result. The amount of drug that is then removed from the body in the time between doses also becomes greater. A point is then reached at which the amount of drug excreted is equal to the amount taken in the previous dose. As a result, the body harbors a steady state of the drug.

Human Response

Psychological factors influence the patient's willingness to take a medication and the degree of effectiveness of the drug. If a patient does not believe that the medication will be effective, chances are that the desired effect will not be achieved. In the case of the placebo effect, a patient who is unaware of the inactive properties of the placebo finds the substance effective for its intended use. There have been clinical studies in such therapies as guided imagery, hypnosis, therapeutic touch, and meditation for patient care. The perioperative nurse can use these techniques alone or in combination with medications administered during the intraoperative phase.

Religious beliefs and practices play an important role in the patient's perception of health, reaction to illness, and response to medications. By assessing the value-belief pattern, the perioperative nurse obtains data that can influence medication administration and patient compliance. For example, a Seventh-Day Adventist may refuse to ingest narcotics or stimulants because he or she believes that his or her body is a temple of the Holy Spirit and should be protected from such substances. Jehovah's Witnesses are generally opposed to blood transfusion, although individuals may be persuaded in emergencies to accept blood. Christian Scientists believe that their religion has a healing function and, although they may seek health care for childbirth and fracture, they generally refuse medications, vaccinations, and inoculations.

Like religious practices, culture and ethnicity may affect a patient's health beliefs. Many cultures employ folk beliefs and remedies in the treatment of illness. Some of these practices have a scientific basis. One common example is the use of the plant source *Digitalis lanata* (yellow foxglove) and *D. purpurea* (purple foxglove) to ameliorate the symptoms of congestive heart failure. Other folk practices and herbal treatments, although lacking in scientific basis, have significant value to those who use them. Understanding and respecting these beliefs fosters holistic care and promotes an awareness and use of many nontraditional resources.

Federal Drug Laws and Regulations

The Harrison Narcotic Act of 1914 was the first attempt in the prevention of drug abuse in the medical and nursing communities. Later regulations were enacted to control the use of marijuana and to make certain drugs available only by prescription (the Durham-Humphrey Amendment of 1951). Continued abuse of potentially dangerous drugs led to the passage of the Drug Abuse Amendments of 1965. With the continued spread of drug abuse in the 1960s, Congress enacted the Comprehensive Drug Abuse Prevention and Control Act of 1970, which identified five schedules of controlled substances. Drugs are listed in these categories according to the extent of their abuse potential and medical usefulness (Tables 9–1 and 9–2).

In addition to being aware of federal laws and regulations, the perioperative nurse is responsible for knowing the details of the nurse practice act for her or his particular state. This act, which is a collection of laws that regulate nursing, is included in the code of all 50 states, the District of Columbia, Puerto Rico, Guam, and the Virgin Islands.

OUTCOME STANDARD

The patient is free from injury related to the administration of medications and solutions.

Criteria

The patient is free from injury during the intraoperative phase and any sequela during the postoperative phase. There are no signs of

- drug overdose
- drug toxicity
- allergic reactions

ANTI-INFECTIVE AGENTS

Anti-infective agents are used to prevent an infection or control an existing infection (Table 9–3). The perioperative nurse is responsible for preparing and/or administering anti-infective agents during the intraoperative period.

Considerations

Drug Selection. Ideally, specimens for bacterial culture and sensitivity are obtained before beginning drug treatment. On occasion, when emergency surgery is indicated, it is unrealistic to wait for the results of bacterial analysis. With such cases, the patient's history and presenting signs and symptoms are used as indica-

TABLE 9–1. CONTROLLED SUBSTANCE CATEGORIES

Category	Interpretations
I	High potential for abuse and of no currently accepted medical use. Examples: heroin, LSD, mescaline, and peyote. Not obtainable by prescription, but may be legally procured for research, study, or instructional use.
II	High abuse potential and high liability for severe psychic or physical dependency. Prescription required and cannot be renewed. Examples: amphetamines, meperidine, morphine, and secobarbital.
III	Moderate to low physical dependence and high psychological dependency. Examples: codeine, paregoric, and preparations containing limited quantities of certain opiates.
IV	Lower potential for abuse than schedule III. Examples: certain psychotropic medications (tranquilizers), chloral hydrate, diazepam, and phenobarbital.
V	Composed of a mixture of limited quantities of narcotic drugs in combination with various nonnarcotic ingredients. Generally used for antitussive and antidiarrheal purposes.

tors of the treatment of choice until sensitivity testing is conducted (Table 9–4).

Dose and Route Selection. The dose and route of administration often depend on the severity of the infection. The most common intraoperative routes are IV administration, topical antibiotic irrigation, vaginal administration, and inunction (rubbing into the skin).

Length of Treatment. The length of treatment is important in avoiding relapse or the development of resistance or adverse reactions. After an anti-infective drug is selected and administered, its administration should be continued until signs of infection are absent for several days. Documentation of anti-infective drug administration started during the intraoperative phase

TABLE 9–2. U.S. FOOD AND DRUG ADMINISTRATION PREGNANCY CATEGORIES

Category	Interpretations
A	Controlled studies show no risk. Adequate, well-controlled studies in pregnant women have failed to demonstrate risk to the fetus.
B	No evidence of risk in humans. Either animal fndings show risk, but human findings do not, or if no adequate human studies have been done, animal findings are negative.
C	Fetal risk cannot be ruled out. Human studies are lacking, and animal studies are either positive for fetal risk, or lacking as well. Potential benefits, however, may justify the potential risks.
D	Positive evidence of risk. Investigational or postmarketing data show risk to the fetus. Nevertheless, potential benefits may outweigh the potential risk.
X	Contraindicated in pregnancy. Studies in animals or humans, or investigational or postmarketing reports, have shown fetal risks that clearly outweigh any possible benefit to the patient.

TABLE 9–3. KEY TERMS FOR ANTI-INFECTIVE DRUGS

Antibiotic	A chemical compound produced by microorganisms, which can inhibit the growth of, or kill, other organisms
Bactericial	A compound having direct action on bacteria that results in their destruction or death
Bacteriostatic	A compound that inhibits the growth or multiplication of bacteria
Gram stain	A method of staining bacteria that is used to identify various types of bacteria
Gram-negative	A characteristic of certain microorganisms whereby they lose their initial stain when treated with a decolorizing solution used in the Gram stain procedure
Gram-positive	A characteristic whereby certain microorganisms stained with crystal violet and iodine and retain their stain after decolorizing
Active immunity	Immunity that is attained by prior exposure to a pathogen or to its antigen, which stimulated production of specific antibodies; also known as acquired immunity
Passive immunity	Protection against a pathogen and its toxins by transfer of antibodies produced in the body of another individual or animal that has been actively immunized
Acquired resistance	A state in which an organism that was once sensitive to an anti-infective drug has developed the ability to remain unaffected by that drug
Congenital resistance	An inborn ability to remain unaffected by certain anti-infective drugs
Microbial resistance	The ability of a microorganism to withstand the effects of anti-infective drugs

must be accurate in case the surgeon decides to use the agent for postoperative anti-infective therapy.

Drug Combinations. Emergency treatment of infections before the causative agent is known is often begun with a combination of two broad-spectrum drugs. If culture and sensitivity testing indicate that the pathogenic strain is fully susceptible to one of the drugs, the other anti-infective agent may be withdrawn.

Adverse Reactions. Anti-infective agents may cause direct tissue damage when administered topically or in irrigation solutions. Although IV injection may result in phlebitis, some of the more serious forms of toxicity occur when absorbed antibiotics are poorly eliminated and accumulate in the tissue.

Allergic Reactions. Allergies have been reported with almost every kind of anti-infective drug. Reactions are most common with penicillin-type antibiotics.

Chemoprophylaxis. Anti-infective prophylaxis before and during surgery is common practice. Such therapy is successful when the goal is to prevent implantation and invasion by a specific pathogen that is known to be sensitive to the anti-infective agent. The use of anti-infectives to prevent or eliminate pathogens, however, should never take the place of strict adherence to aseptic technique in the operating field.

Use with Prosthetic Devices During Surgery. The perioperative nurse prepares and delivers anti-infective medications to the operative field to be used for soaking prosthetic devices. Prostheses, such as penile, testicular, breast, and orthopedic implants, are commonly soaked in an antibiotic solution before being implanted. One method is to dispense a solution of 500 to 1000 ml of 0.9% sodium chloride onto the field. To this, one or a combination of antibiotics is added. Commonly used antibiotics include bacitracin, polymyxin B, and gentamicin.

Specific Drug Groups

Penicillin G is frequently used as a prophylactic agent. The American Heart Association and the American Dental Association suggest the use of penicillin prophylaxis against bacterial endocarditis in patients with congenital heart disease or other valvular disease when they require oral or respiratory tract surgery.

Antipseudomonal penicillin, such as ticarcillin disodium (Ticar), is used to treat systemic infections such as septicemia, infected wounds, and acute respiratory tract infections.

The *cephalosporins*, such as cefamandole nafate (Mandol) and cefoxitin sodium (Mefoxin), are reactive against a wide range of gram-positive and gram-negative organisms. Third-generation products, such as cefoperazone sodium (Cefobid) and cefotaxime sodium (Cla-

TABLE 9–4. COMMON INTRAOPERATIVE ANTI-INFECTIVES

Generic Name	Trade Name	Adult Dosage
Polymyxin B sulfate	Aerosporin	1.5–2.5 mg/kg in divided doses
Amikacin sulfate	Amikin	IV; 15–30 mg/kg/d q 8–12 h
Ampicillin	—	IV; 150–200 mg/kg/d in divided doses
Cefazolin sodium	Ancef, Kefzol	2 g q 4 h
Azlocillin	Azlin	IV; 3 g q 4 h
Bacitracin	—	Irrigation; 50,000 U in 1000 ml of 0.9% sodium chloride
Cefoperazone sodium	Cefobid	IV; 2 g q 12 h
Cefotetan disodium	Cefotan	IV; 1–3 g q 12 h
Clindamycin	Cleocin hydrochloride	IV; 150–900 mg q 8 h
Chloramphenicol	Chloromycetin	IV; 50 mg/kg/d
Erythromycin gluceptate	Ilotycin gluceptate	IV; 250–500 mg q 4–6 h
Gentamicin	Garamycin	IV; 3–5 mg/kg/d in divided doses
Cefamandole nafate	Mandol	IV; 0.5–2 g q 4 h
Cefoxitin sodium	Mefoxin	IV; 2 g q 4 h
Mezlocillin sodium	Mezlin	IV; 3 mg q 4 h
Penicillin G	—	IV; usually greater than 20,000,000 U/d
Methicillin sodium	Staphcillin	IV; 1–2 g q 4 h
Ticarcillin disodium	Ticar	IV; 3 g q 4 h
Vancomycin	Vancocin	IV; 1 g q 12 h
Cefuroxime	Zinacef	IV; 1.5 g q 8 h

foran), possess a broader antibacterial spectrum than do second-generation drugs. The third-generation drugs also have a prolonged duration of action and better penetration into certain body parts. Cefonicid sodium (Monocid) is often administered before surgery to reduce the incidence of postoperative infections in patients undergoing surgical procedures classified as contaminated or potentially contaminated. It is also given when infections at the operative site present serious risk (e.g., for prosthetic arthroplasty and cardiothoracic and vascular procedures).

Erythromycin is similar to penicillin G in its effectiveness against the common gram-positive and gram-negative cocci. It is used in patients sensitive to penicillin for short-term prevention of streptococcal endocarditis during oral and respiratory tract surgery.

Clindamycin phosphate and lincomycin hydrochloride (Lincocin) are effective for treating infections resulting from anaerobic bacteria. They are used when anaerobic bacteria, which can cause abscess and peritonitis, spill into the abdominal cavity after a rupture of the appendix or other visceral organ.

Vancomycin has proved effective for penicillin-sensitive patients with severe infections who cannot receive or who have failed to respond to other drugs. Rapid bolus administration of this drug may be associated with exaggerated hypotension, nephrotoxicity, and cardiac arrest, although this last complication is rare.

Tetracyclines are rarely administered during the intraoperative period owing to potential enhancement of neuromuscular blockade and are contraindicated for concurrent use with methoxyflurane.

Chloramphenicol is effective against *Bacteroides fragilis* and other enteric anaerobes. It is used in treating peritonitis, postabortal sepsis, and septicemia.

Aminoglycoside antibiotics are used to treat life-threatening systemic infections such as gram-negative bacteremia, peritonitis, and meningitis. They can induce neuromuscular blockade. Aminoglycoside antibiotics are administered during 30 to 60 minutes to avoid nephrotoxicity and ototoxicity.

Polymyxins are active against a wide range of gram-negative bacilli but not against gram-negative or gram-positive cocci. Polymyxins are often used in combination with other antibiotics such as bacitracin and neomycin. These agents are mixed in 500 to 1000 ml of 0.9% sodium chloride and used as irrigating or soaking solutions during prosthetic arthroplasty or other procedures involving prosthetic implants.

Sulfonamides are active against a variety of both gram-positive and gram-negative species as well as yeast. Certain sulfonamide creams are used in the management of second- and third-degree burns to prevent local sepsis and subsequent septicemia.

Bacitracin is derived from culture of *Bacillus subtilis*. It is effective against a variety of gram-positive and a few gram-negative organisms. For antibiotic irrigation, 50,000 U of bacitracin is often mixed in a 1000-ml solution of 0.9% sodium chloride. The drug is assayed against a standard and its activity is expressed in units, 1 mg having a potency of not less than 50 U.

Supplies and Equipment

The selection of the size and type of syringe is determined by the type and amount of medication being prepared. For example, when administering a dose of less than 1 ml, the use of a tuberculin syringe reduces the risk of medication error. When diluting a powder with sterile water or normal saline, a 5- or 10-ml syringe can be used. After the antibiotic has been reconstituted and transferred onto the operative field, the scrub person hands it to the surgeon in an irrigation syringe (see Appendix B).

Needle selection is determined by the type of antibiotic being mixed and the route of administration. By using a 16- or 18-gauge, 2-inch needle, the nurse ensures a quick and easy injection, aspiration, and transfer of solution from the ampule or from one vial to another.

Whatever the size of the syringe and needle, strict aseptic technique must be maintained. The sterility of the syringe barrel, the part of the plunger that enters the barrel, the tip of the barrel, and the needle should not be compromised.

Potential Alterations in Functional Health Patterns

Health Perception–Health Management Pattern

Diagnosis

High risk for infection related to the administration of drugs and solutions

Definition

Presence of risk factors for the patient to experience a nosocomial infection secondary to the preparation and administration of drugs and solutions

Discussion. The surgical patient is at increased risk for postoperative infection if aseptic technique is breached during medication preparation and administration. Because the medication is often dispensed directly into the wound, strict measures must be taken to prevent the development of local, regional, and systemic infection.

Risk Factors

● Inadequate primary defense

Surgery, the administration of anesthesia, and invasive monitoring procedures involve loss of skin integrity, traumatization of the tissue, decrease in ciliary action, altered peristalsis, and stasis of body fluids. These stressors, either in isolation or in combination, put patients at increased risk for postoperative infection. The length of a procedure and the amount of time the surgical site is exposed to the environment also increase the risk of infection.

- Inadequate secondary defense

  The patient's immunological defenses may be deficient as a result of disease, drug therapy, radiation, or blood loss. Immunologically compromised patients often experience infection caused by endogenous microbial flora. Lack of integrity of the immune system, such as with leukopenia, acquired immunodeficiency syndrome, and defective immunoglobulin synthesis, can be life threatening.

- Chronic disease

  Chronic diseases such as diabetes, alcoholism, malignancies, arterial or vascular insufficiency, pulmonary disorders, and the presence of a chronic emotional disorder are stessors that may contribute to the development of infection.

- Malnutrition

  Whether primary or secondary to catabolic disease, malnutrition contributes to a patient's inability to fight infection. Protein deficiency is a major component of infection susceptibility in patients whose caloric requirements are raised owing to the presence of burns or multiple injuries. Gastrointestinal (GI) disorders that cause severe diarrhea and/or vomiting (e.g., ulcerative colitis or pyloric stenosis) may result in iron and vitamin loss. Obese patients with abundant poorly vascularized subcutaneous tissue are also at risk for the development of infection. The presence of excessive adipose tissue increases the length of the procedure, incisions are usually larger, and there is the potential for larger dead spaces after wound closure.

- Extremes of Age

  Premature and newborn infants and geriatric patients have a decreased ability to fight the stressor associated with the development of infection.

- Type of surgical procedure that predisposes to possible infection

  Surgical procedures of the GI and genitourinary tracts involve contamination. Patients who have injured or ischemic tissue, denuded bone, implanted foreign bodies, or prosthetic devices are at increased risk for microbial invasion. Patient acuity, the complexity and length of surgical procedure, and the length of hospital stay also play a major role in the development of postoperative infection.

Expected Outcome

The patient is free from infection related to the administration of drugs and solutions. There are no signs of localized or systemic infection 48 hours after surgery.

Diagnosis

High risk for injury related to hypersensitivity reaction because of improper identification of patient allergies

Definition

Presence of risk factors for the patient to experience a hypersensitivity reaction during drug administration owing to unidentified allergies

Discussion. Allergic reactions of the immediate or delayed type have been reported with almost every type of anti-infective drug. These are particularly common with penicillin-type antibiotics. Crossover reactions to cephalosporins occur in 10% of patients with allergies to penicillin.

Allergic response may range in intensity from mild rashes to fatal anaphylaxis or anaphylactoid reaction. The use of high concentrations of certain anti-infective agents can result in such toxic effects as neuropathy, ototoxicity, hepatotoxicity, nephrotoxicity, and electrolyte imbalance. Because the kidney is the major excretory pathway for most anti-infective drugs, impaired renal function frequently results in both prolonged and elevated drug levels.

Risk Factors

- History of a past reaction to specific or related anti-infective agents
- History of self-treatment with anti-infective drugs
- Inability of the patient or family members to provide an accurate drug history
- Use of anti-infective drugs for self-treatment of minor infections

Expected Outcome

The patient undergoes the surgical procedure without evidence or report of local or systemic drug reaction. There are no signs of

- patient uneasiness, apprehension, weakness, and feeling of impending doom
- generalized pruritus and urticaria
- erythema and angioedema of the eyes, lips, or tongue
- discrete cutaneous wheals or urticarial eruptions
- congestion, rhinorrhea, dyspnea, and increasing respiratory distress with audible wheezing
- rales, wheezing, and diminished breath sounds
- hypotension and a rapid, weak pulse
- abdominal cramping, diarrhea, or vomiting (Ignatavicius and Bayne, 1991, p. 654)

Perioperative Nursing Interventions

Preoperative

- Interview the patient and family members before surgery and obtain a medication history (see Appendix A).

- Check the patient identification or drug alert bracelet for allergies.

Intraoperative

- Prepare and administer drugs and solutions according to recommended methods (see Appendix C).
- Monitor physiological changes when administering anti-infective agents that are known to cause alterations in health patterns (e.g., vancomycin). Report changes in the patient's pulse, blood pressure, temperature, and respirations.
- Observe and report signs and symptoms of allergic response such as urticaria, itching, and wheezing.
- Apply ointments and dressing as indicated (see Appendix D).
- Document nursing actions in the patient's record.

Postoperative

- Communicate to the postanesthesia care unit (PACU) nurse the type, amount, and route of anti-infective drug given, along with the time of administration.
- Report known allergies to the PACU staff.
- Make a postoperative visit to evaluate the surgical outcome and assess the patient for signs of infection.
- If the patient is discharged while receiving anti-infective therapy, instruct the patient to take the drug for the entire length of time for which it is prescribed, even if symptoms subside.

ANTICOAGULANTS

The process of hemostasis involves the interplay of four phases. The first three, vascular response, platelet formation, and coagulation, promote blood clotting and prevent blood loss. The fourth, the fibrinolytic phase, helps maintain blood fluidity and prevents propagation of clotting beyond the site of injury. This phase is also involved in clot dissolution. For a thorough discussion on the process of hemostasis, see Chapter 17.

Considerations

Medications that prevent the coagulation of blood are classified into three groups: anticoagulant, antiplatelet, and fibrinolytic.

Anticoagulants prevent clot formation or, if they have already formed, keep clots from completely closing off a portion of the blood vessel (Table 9–5). Anticoagulant drugs used for this purpose are heparin and warfarin. Heparin exerts an effect on blood coagulation (clotting) by potentiating the action of antithrombin III, which subsequently acts on several kinds of circulating clotting factors to exert an immediate effect in preventing blood coagulation. Warfarin, an effective oral anticoagulant,

TABLE 9–5. KEY TERMS FOR ANTICOAGULANT THERAPY	
Ecchymosis	A small spot caused by bleeding in the skin or mucous membranes, forming a round or irregular purple patch
Embolus	A clot carried by the blood from a larger vessel to a smaller vessel, which becomes blocked
Hematoma	A localized collection of blood in a space, organ, or tissue
Petechia	A tiny red spot caused by the escape of a small amount of blood
Phlebothrombosis	The presence of blood clots in a vein without inflammation
Thrombophlebitis	Inflammation and clotting within a vein
Thrombus	A solid mass of clotted blood in a vessel or in the heart

acts in the liver to prevent the synthesis of vitamin K–dependent clotting factors. Subsequently, this prevents blood coagulation.

Antiplatelet drugs, such as aspirin, dipyridamole (Persantine), and dextran 40 injection (Rheomacrodex), interfere with the reaction that causes platelets to aggregate at arterial wall sites and in the veins.

Fibrinolytic agents, such as streptokinase, urokinase, and tissue plasminogen activator, speed the rate of the natural clot-resolving process. The proteolytic enzyme fibrinolysin, which is present in the blood as a precursor called plasminogen, breaks down the fibrin framework of blood clots. Plasminogen is activated by enzymes called kinins that split off certain amino acids from the inactive precursor. The plasmin produced in this way then digests fibrin. As the fibrin matrix dissolves, the clot is fragmented into soluble products and gradually resolves.

Specific Drugs

Heparin

- Heparin is measured in standard U.S. Pharmacopeia units and not in milligrams or International Units (IU), neither of which is equivalent to 1 U of heparin. One unit of heparin is defined as the amount of heparin required to anticoagulate 1 ml of blood.
- Strict adherence to heparin dosage and dilution instructions is essential in the prevention of excessive bleeding. Have an antidote available (protamine sulfate 1%).
- Coexisting drugs can interact with heparin (Table 9–6).

Dextran 40 Injection

- Use dextran 40 injection only if the seal is intact and the solution is absolutely clear. To dissolve crystals, place the unopened bottle in a warm water bath until the solution clears. Discard any unused portion because dextran 40 injection contains no preservatives.

TABLE 9–6. MEDICATIONS THAT INTERACT WITH HEPARIN*

Agent	Potential Effect
Anticoagulants, oral	Prolonged prothrombin time
Antihistamines	Partial antagonist of anticoagulant action of heparin
Aspirin and other salicylates	Inhibition of platelet adhesiveness and aggregation
Contraceptives, oral	Estrogen-containing contraceptives may reduce the concentration of antithrombin III and result in increased thrombotic activity
Digitalis glycosides	Partial antagonistic action of heparin
Dextran	Inhibition of platelet adhesiveness
Dipyridamole (Persantine)	
Indomethacin (Indocin)	
Ibuprofen (Motrin)	
Streptokinase	May partially antagonize anticoagulant action of heparin
Tetracyclines	
Urokinase	

*Heparin sodium is a common drug used in vascular and cardiac procedures and in selected cases involving injury or infection of limbs and pelvic organs. Frequently, patients requiring such surgical intervention are taking a variety of medications for one or more coexisting conditions or diseases (e.g., cardiac disease, arthritis, asthma, hay fever). Untoward effects can occur when heparin is administered in conjunction with other medications.

Adapted from Govoni, L. E., Hayes, J. E. (1985). *Drugs and nursing implications* (5th ed.) (p. 628). East Norwalk, CT: Appleton-Century-Crofts.

- Use vented IV tubing.
- Do not confuse dextran 40 injection with dextran 70 or other dextran solutions.
- A baseline hematocrit should be obtained before the initiation of dextran 40 injection and after administration. Notify the physician if the hematocrit is depressed below 30% by volume.

Potential Alterations in Functional Health Patterns

Nutritional-Metabolic Pattern

Diagnosis

High risk for fluid volume deficit related to the use of anticoagulants or antiplatelet agents

Definition

Presence of risk factors for the patient to experience excessive intraoperative blood loss owing to preoperative or intraoperative use of anticoagulant or antiplatelet agents

Discussion. Any intrinsic pathophysiological blood coagulation can alter the effect of anticoagulants and place the patient at increased risk for bleeding.

Risk Factors

- Surgical intervention

    The disruption of tissue and vascular integrity puts the patient at increased risk for bleeding.

Patients receiving prophylactic therapy to prevent postoperative deep venous thrombosis are also at risk for bleeding.

- CNS trauma

    Patients who have had recent surgery on the brain, spinal cord, or eyes; recent trauma to the CNS; or suspected intracranial bleeding are at increased risk.

- Pregnancy

    Pregnant women and the fetus in utero may experience bleeding when heparin is administered. Heparin may pass into the breast milk and reduce clotting factor levels in infants who are breast-feeding.

- Advanced age and female gender

    The risk of hemorrhage with heparin appears to be greatest in women and in patients 70 years and older.

- Renal insufficiency

    Renal insufficiency reduces the rate of heparin clearance from the blood, thereby prolonging the duration of its anticoagulant action.

- GI disorders

    Patients with ulcerations of the GI tract, or other GI disorders (e.g., visceral carcinoma, diverticulitis), or continuous drainage from the GI tract are at increased risk for bleeding.

- Alteration in vitamin K absorption

    Patients with severe liver or biliary tract disease may have interference in using vitamin K and a subsequent decrease in the production of vitamin K–dependent clotting factors, which in turn may lead to a bleeding tendency.

- Tobacco and alcohol use

    Smoking and alcohol consumption may alter the response to heparin therapy.

- Other medications

    The use of drugs such as aspirin, antihistamines, cough preparations containing guaifensin, and other over-the-counter medications may alter the effects of heparin.

Expected Outcome

The patient experiences minimal fluid deficit related to anticoagulant therapy. The hemodynamic status (blood pressure, pulse, and central pressures) is maintained within normal limits.

Health Perception–Health Management Pattern

Diagnosis

High risk for injury related to hypersensitivity or an adverse reaction to an anticoagulant

Definition

Presence of risk factors for the patient to experience an allergic reaction to the administration of anticoagulants

Discussion. Hypersensitivity to heparin is marked by chills, rash, urticaria, pruritus, fever, occasional respiratory allergic symptoms, and anaphylactic or anaphylactoid reactions. Similar signs and symptoms can occur with an allergic reaction to dextran 40 injection. Hypersensitivity is most likely to occur during the first few minutes of administration.

Risk Factors

- History of allergic hypersensitivity to heparin, dextran 40 injection, or other anticoagulant
- Heparin resistance resulting from large amounts of fibrin deposits in conditions such as early-stage thrombophlebitis, peritonitis, fever, pleurisy, cancer, myocardial infarction, and extensive surgery
- Dextran sensitivity

  A small percentage of individuals who never received dextran experience an allergic reaction because of previous sensitization by the dextrans present in commercial sugars and dextran-producing organisms found in the human GI tract.

Expected Outcome

The patient is free from an allergic reaction to anticoagulant therapy. There is an absence of chills, fever, rash, urticaria, and anaphylactic and anaphylactoid reactions.

Perioperative Nursing Interventions

Preoperative

- Interview the patient and/or family members before surgery and obtain a medication history. The patient may be taking medications such as aspirin, ibuprofen (Motrin), or other nonsteroidal anti-inflammatory drugs that can affect platelet function, thus resulting in a prolonged bleeding time. Such patients may have normal prothrombin time and partial thromboplastin time but still be at risk for intraoperative bleeding. Patients taking such preparations should have a bleeding time checked before surgery.
- Identify patient allergies and check the patient identification or drug alert bracelet for documentation of allergies.
- Note a patient or family history of blood dyscrasia or other bleeding disorders such as thrombocytic purpura, thrombocytopenia, hemophilia, and polycythemia.
- Assess the patient's need for transfusion and know the availability of whole blood, plasma, or other blood products for transfusion.
- Have laboratory tests results available (prothrombin time, partial thromboplastin time, and bleeding time).

Intraoperative

- Prepare requests for laboratory work (e.g., activated partial thromboplastin time, activated coagulation time, hematocrit, hemoglobin and red blood cell levels, and platelet count).
- Prepare and administer heparin.

  1. Heparin flush solution. Heparin flush solution is commonly used to maintain the patency of central venous, femoral or dialysis catheters. It is considered standard practice to flush a central catheter with 1 to 2 ml of normal saline before and after medication administration to avoid the possibility of drug interaction. Because heparin is strongly acidic, it is incompatible with many drugs. Avoid mixing any drug with heparin unless specifically advised by the physician or the pharmacist. Heparin is stable at room temperature of 15 to 30°C (59–86°F). Inspect all preparations for discoloration and particulate matter before administration. Heparin administration in bolus form can cause a significant transient decrease in blood pressure that may necessitate intervention.
  2. Diluting heparin solution for injection. When heparin is added to a solution of IV 0.9% sodium chloride for injection, the container should be inverted at least six times to ensure adequate mixing and to prevent pooling of the heparin. A common mix is 10,000 U of heparin in 1000 ml of 0.9% sodium chloride.

- Prepare and administer dextran.

  Monitor vital signs and observe the patient closely for at least the first few minutes of administration. Therapy should be terminated at the first sign of reaction. Other means of sustaining circulation should be available. Have on hand epinephrine, ephedrine, steroids, and antihistamines. Observe the patient for signs of circulatory overload: shortness of breath, wheezing, coughing, increased pulse and respiratory rate, and sensation of chest pressure. At the first indication of renal dysfunction, discontinue dextran administration. Monitor intake and output.

- Apply a pressure dressing to the IV and other puncture sites.
- Monitor vital signs for indications of hemorrhage or other adverse reactions. Report changes in the patient's pulse, blood pressure, temperature, and respirations. Observe and report indications of allergic response such as urticaria, itching, and wheezing.
- Pad and position the patient to avoid trauma to the skin and underlying tissue.
- Use electrical clippers or a depilatory cream for removal of body hair.
- Have an antidote available (protamine sulfate 1% solution).

  When administered alone, protamine has an anticoagulant effect. When it is given in the presence

208 ■ BASIC COMPETENCIES

of heparin (which is a strong acid), a stable salt is formed. The anticoagulant effect of both drugs is then lost.

- Administer protamine sulfate.

1. Dosage is guided by blood coagulation studies. Administer protamine sulfate slowly; too rapid administration of protamine can cause severe hypotension and anaphylactoid reactions. Do not exceed 50 mg in any 10-minute period. The antidote for protamine sulfate overdose is calcium chloride.
2. Do not use protamine sulfate with minor bleeding during heparin therapy because withdrawal of the heparin administration usually stops the bleeding.
3. Store protamine sulfate at 2 to 8°C (36–38°F). Protamine sulfate powder for injection and reconstitution solution are stable for 72 hours at 15 to 30°C (59–86°F).
4. Protamine sulfate may be contraindicated in patients with a history of seafood allergy because the drug is produced from a purified mixture of simple, low-molecular-weight proteins obtained from sperm or testes of suitable fish species. Patients taking neutral protamine Hagedorn (NPH) insulin may develop antibodies to protamine sulfate, resulting in an allergic reaction when the drug is administered.

- Record the amount, route, and time of anticoagulant and antidote given.

Postoperative

- Communicate with PACU unit nurses the type and dose of anticoagulant and the route and time of administration. Report the presence of allergies and reactions to medications and solutions.
- Assess the operative site, IV and intra-arterial sites, and other points of puncture, pressure, or potential injury.

LOCAL ANESTHETICS

Local anesthetics are used during minor surgical procedures and as an adjunct to general or regional anesthesia (Table 9–7). These drugs provide a loss of feeling without the loss of consciousness associated with general anesthesia. Local anesthetics act by temporarily interrupting the production and conduction of nerve impulses. This reversible block in conduction is brought about by a drug-induced reduction in the permeability of the nerve cell membrane to sodium and potassium ions. This then interferes with the ability of the neuronal membrane to depolarize in response to stimuli.

TABLE 9–7. KEY TERMS FOR LOCAL ANESTHETICS

Topical analgesia	Application of a cream, ointment, or fluid for the purpose of anesthetizing the skin or mucous membrane
Infiltration anesthesia	Injection of solutions of local anesthesia into tissue to bring the anesthetic into contact with nerve endings in the intracutaneous, subcutaneous, and deeper structure and keep these sensitive nerve terminals from transmitting pain impulses
Field block	A form of infiltration anesthesia in which the sensory nerve pathways from the operative field are blocked off by a circular ring of subcutaneously injected solution
Central nerve block	Block that affects the roots of nerves at various points close to their origin in the spinal cord
Peripheral nerve block	Block affecting the trunks of specific nerves such as the sciatic-femoral, ulnar, or intercostal nerves, or the brachial plexus
Intravenous regional block	Local anesthesia of an arm or a leg by injection of local anethetic into a vein after exsanguination and application of a pneumatic tourniquet

Considerations

Medication Administration

The perioperative nurse prepares local anesthetics used on the operative field. Precautions are taken to prevent rapid systemic absorption from the skin, subcutaneous tissue, fascia, and muscles, as well as accidental IV injection. Local anesthetics should not be injected into infected tissue or applied to traumatized mucous membranes.

Aspiration is performed in several planes to ensure that the needle has not entered a vessel. Injections are made systematically by first entering the cutaneous, then subcutaneous, and lastly interfascicular and intramuscular planes.

The surgeon allows enough time for the drug's action to take effect before the procedure is initiated or before administering additional anesthetic. Knowledge of the time it takes to achieve anesthesia is essential because there is great variation between local anesthetic actions.

Lidocaine injection and commercially prepared solutions containing the drug in 5% dextrose are stored preferably at 15 to 30°C (59–86°F) unless otherwise directed by the manufacturer. Inspect solutions for particulate matter and discoloration before administration and discard if either is present.

Drug Selection

Table 9–8 lists commonly used local anesthetics.

TABLE 9–8. FREQUENTLY USED LOCAL ANESTHETICS

Generic Name	Trade Name	Duration of Action*	Use and Maximal Dose
Benzocaine	Americaine, Anesthesin		Topical; used on broken and mucous membrane
Mepivacaine hydrochloride	Carbocaine	60–120 min	Infiltration and conduction; plain, 300 mg; with epinephrine, 500 mg
Prilocaine hydrochloride	Citanest hydrochloride	30–120 min	Infiltration and conduction; plain, 600 mg; with epinephrine, 600 mg
Cocaine hydrochloride topical solution	—		Topical, 200 mg
Bupivacaine hydrochloride	Marcaine hydrochloride, Sensorcaine	120–240 min	Infiltration and conduction; plain, 175 mg; with epinephrine, 225 mg
Chloroprocaine hydrochloride	Nesacaine, Nesacaine CE	15–30 min	Infiltration and conduction; plain, 800 mg; with epinephrine, 1000 mg
Procaine hydrochloride	Novocain	15–30 min	Infiltration and conduction; plain, 1000 mg; with epinephrine, 600 mg
Tetracaine	Pontocaine hydrochloride, Anacel	120–240 min	Infiltration and conduction; plain, 100 mg; with epinephrine, 200 mg
Lidocaine	Xylocaine	30–120 min	Infiltration and conduction; plain, 300 mg; with epinephrine, 500 mg

*Epinephrine-containing solutions have a duration of 1½ to 2 times as long as plain solutions.

Dose and Route Selection

Only the minimal amount of medication effective for producing anesthesia should be injected. A record is kept of the total amount of solution injected, and the actual number of milligrams administered is calculated. The method for calculation of a dose of injected anesthetic agent is as follows:

$$\text{Percentage of concentration} \times 10 = \text{mg/ml}$$

For example, a 2% solution contains 20 mg/ml.

For solutions containing epinephrine, a 1:1000 concentration has 1 mg of epinephrine per 1 ml. All variations of concentration are proportions of this equation. For example, a solution containing epinephrine 1:100,000 has 1 mg of epinephrine per 100 ml of solution.

Specific Drugs

Vasoconstrictors. Epinephrine and phenylephrine are often added to local anesthetic solutions to slow down the absorption of the drug and to keep the anesthetic at the desired site. This prolongs its blocking effect. In addition, epinephrine diminishes blood loss because of its vasoconstrictive action. High concentrations of epinephrine (1:100,000) are used in vascular areas such as the scalp and face. Lower concentrations (1:200,000) are used for areas such as the skin of the back or the extremities. Vasoconstrictors are not added to anesthetic solutions that are used in areas of restricted circulation such as the fingers, the toes, the tip of the nose, the ears, or the penis.

Cocaine. Cocaine produces local anesthesia of mucous membranes such as the nose, the throat, and the tracheobronchial tree. Cocaine hydrochloride topical solution (4% per 4 ml and 10% per 4 ml) is commonly applied to the nares with cotton pledgets before septorhinoplasty or sprayed into the throat before endotra-

cheal intubation. Ophthalmological application produces surface anesthesia, vasoconstriction, and mydriasis.

Cocaine is not administered by injection. Systemic absorption can result in tachycardia, increased blood pressure, tremors, convulsive seizures, and respiratory failure. The use of cocaine can cause physical and psychological dependence.

Care of the Awake Patient

The perioperative team should avoid conversation that may be upsetting to the patient. Post patient awake signs at each entry and alert personnel who may use the intercom system that the patient is awake. This is of particular importance when conveying information that may be upsetting to the patient.

Position the patient to provide comfort and maintain body alignment. Diversional techniques such as conversing using audio headphones or a radio, and reading can help lessen the patient's anxiety and decrease the amount of anesthetic needed.

Physiological Monitoring of the Patient

Patient monitoring during procedures involving the use of local anesthesia is often the responsibility of the perioperative nurse. For additional information about local anesthesia and patient monitoring, see Chapter 10.

Supplies and Equipment

Syringes. The size and type of syringe is determined by the amount of local anesthetic to be delivered. Ring syringes are preferred because they provide added control over the injection and allow for aspiration and injection with one hand.

Needles. A short ½-inch, 25-gauge needle is often used for the initial infiltration. For deeper injection, a longer 23- or 25-gauge needle or 2½-inch spinal needle is used.

Topical Application Supplies. Cotton pledgets, usually ½ × 3 inches, a bayonet forceps, and 30-ml cup for cocaine solution are used.

Emergency Drugs, Supplies, and Equipment. Whenever local anesthetics are used, oxygen, rapid-acting barbiturates, and vasopressor agents should be available.

Potential Alterations in Functional Health Patterns

Health Perception–Health Management Pattern

Diagnosis

High risk for injury related to an allergic reaction

Definition

Presence of risk factors for the patient's experiencing an allergic reaction to a local anesthetic agent

Risk Factors

- Sensitivity to local anesthetic, methylparaben, or p-aminobenzoic acid (PABA)

   Allergic reaction may occur as a result of sensitivity to the local anesthetic or sensitivity to the methylparaben used as a preservative in multiple-dose vials. The amino esters (procaine, chloroprocaine, tetracaine) are metabolized by pseudocholinesterase. An end product of this metabolism is PABA. Approximately 1% of the patients receiving local anesthesia are allergic to PABA (Covoni and Vassallo, 1976, pp. 9–10).

- Patients with hepatic dysfunction, congestive heart failure, and cardiogenic shock

   These patients tends to metabolize local anesthetic drugs at a slower rate than usual.

- Patients at risk for malignant hyperthermia

   It is unclear whether lidocaine triggers a malignant hyperthermia episode in patients genetically prone to this disorder. Unexplained signs of tachycardia, rapid respirations, changes in blood pressure, metabolic acidosis, and muscle rigidity may precede temperature elevation and should be noted.

Expected Outcome

The patient is free from allergic reaction related to the administration local anesthetic agents. There is an absence of allergic responses such as

- redness
- rash
- urticaria
- bronchoconstriction

Diagnosis

High risk for injury related to toxicity

Definition

Presence of risk factors for the patient to experience a toxic reaction to a local anesthetic agent

Toxicity can occur when blood concentration of the local anesthetic reaches a level that affects the CNS. This level varies from 1.6 µg/ml with bupivacaine to 6 µg/ml with lidocaine. Clinical manifestations may include excitement marked by nervousness, apprehension, disorientation, dizziness, confusion, vertigo, nausea, and vomiting. These reactions may be followed by tremors and tonic-clonic convulsions. Convulsions may be followed by a loss of reflexes, coma, respiratory depression, and respiratory arrest.

Risk Factors

- Systemic diseases that slow the metabolism of the local anesthetic agent

   A pseudocholinesterase deficiency increases the chance of toxic responses with an amino ester agent.

Projected Outcome

The patient is free from allergic or toxic reaction related to the administration of local anesthetic agents. There is an absence of toxic response such as

- apprehension
- blurred vision
- tinnitus
- dizziness
- loss of consciousness
- convulsions
- central nervous system depression
- respiratory depression

Activity-Exercise Pattern

Diagnosis

High risk for decreased cardiac output related to toxicity

Definition

Presence of risk factors for the patient to experience a gradual or abrupt fall in blood pressure caused by a toxic response to the local anesthetic

Discussion. The patient with cardiodepression may appear pale and complain of feeling weak, dizzy, or faint. Tachycardia may occur as the heart tries to compensate for the hypotension. The patient may become sleepy and then unconscious as the blood pressure falls to shock levels. If the condition progresses, the heart rate may decrease with a coexisting reduction in pulse pressure. Cardiac arrest or ventricular fibrillation may suddenly develop.

Risk Factors

- The presence of cardiac depressants can increase the effect of local anesthetics.
- Local anesthetics containing epinephrine can precipitate arrhythmias.

Expected Outcome

The patient does not experience cardiodepression associated with the administration of local anesthesia. The patient is free from

- local anesthetic–induced hypotension
- tachycardia
- cardiac arrhythmias

Perioperative Nursing Interventions

Preoperative

- Interview the patient before surgery and obtain a medication history. Note the presence of allergy to local anesthetic, past reaction to local anesthesia, a family or personal history of malignant hyperthermia, and the presence of hepatic or cardiac disease.
- Assess for the presence of cardiac disease.
- Note the patient's weight and calculate the maximal dose of anesthetic that can be safely administered.

Intraoperative

- Warn the patient before injection with local anesthetic. The anesthetic may sting and burn before taking effect.
- Provide emotional support by reassuring the patient with conversation and touch.
- Assess for local and systemic signs of adverse reactions.

  1. Monitor the patient at scheduled intervals for allergic or toxic effects of the local anesthetic. Note the patient's blood pressure, oxygen saturation, skin condition, mental status, and emotional response.
  2. The application of topical medication may cause itching, burning, redness, or other local skin reaction. The use of topical eye anesthetics may cause corneal ulcerations. Local reactions are characterized by redness, cutaneous lesions, urticaria, and edema.
  3. Systemic reactions include bronchoconstriction, hypotension, syncope, and ultimately respiratory arrest.

- Record and report the total amount of solution injected and the actual numbers of milligrams administered. If an adverse reaction is suspected, communicate this to the physician at once. Document the signs and symptoms of local or systemic reactions as they occur.

Postoperative

- Communicate to the PACU or ward nurse, the type, dose, and route of administration of the local anesthetic. Alert the staff of the need for special medications or treatments.
- Explain to the patient that the anesthetized area may feel numb until the effects of the medication wear off. Instruct the patient to avoid using the anesthetized area (hand, arm, throat, and so on) until the effect of the agent has worn off. Use of the affected area may result in injury such as burns, abrasions, and aspiration. Instruct the patient to avoid extended use of over-the-counter local anesthetics for the relief of chronic irritations (cutaneous, anal, and vaginal). Extended use may result in the patient's developing a sensitivity to the agent.

OPHTHALMIC AGENTS

The perioperative nurse prepares and administers a variety of ophthalmic medications for use during eye examinations and ophthalmological procedures (Table 9–9). Ophthalmic medications and solutions are used during procedures such as cataract extraction, intraocular lens implantation, glaucoma filtration, correction of muscle disorders, corneal transplant, and retinal attachment surgery.

Considerations

Specific Drugs

Topical anesthetic agents, such as such as proparacaine hydrochloride (Ophthain) and tetracaine hydrochloride (Pontocaine), act by stabilizing the neuronal membrane and preventing the initiation and transmission of nerve impulses. The onset of anesthesia begins within 20 seconds and lasts up to 15 minutes. Topical anesthetics are used in conjunction with retrobulbar infiltration anesthesia for surgical procedures. Topical anesthetics are used before the removal of foreign bodies and sutures and during tonometry and gonioscopy to promote comfort. Topical anesthetics can also retard wound healing. Subsequent corneal infection and/or corneal opacity with accompanying permanent visual loss or corneal perforation may occur. The recommended dose for proparacaine hydrochloride is 1 to 2 drops of a 0.5% solution. The dose for tetracaine hydrochloride is also 1 to 2 drops of a 0.5% solution.

Hyperosmotic agents, such as mannitol (Osmitrol) and

TABLE 9–9. KEY TERMS FOR OPHTHALMIC AGENTS

Aphakia	Absence of the lens of the eye, may be congenital or occur after injury or surgery.
Adrenergic agents	Medications that constrict the vessels of the eye, thereby reducing the rate at which aqueous fluid is formed within the eye. In addition, the outflow of fluid may be increased. This mechanism, which is not clearly understood, helps to lower the intraocular pressure.
Cholinergic agents	Medications that directly or indirectly cause the sphincter muscles of the iris and of the ciliary body to contract.
Cycloplegic agent	Medication that causes paralysis of accommodation by relaxing the ciliary muscles of the eye.
Gonioscopy	Examination of the filtration angle of the anterior eye chamber with an optical instrument designed to visualize the area and determine anterior chamber width.
Hyperosmotic agents	Medications that increase the osmotic pressure of the blood plasma to a point above that of the aqueous humor and the vitreous body of the eye. Intraocular fluid then follows the osmotic gradient into the hyperosmotic plasma. The loss of fluid leads to a reduction in intraocular pressure.
Inner canthus	The angle at the nasal end of the opening between the eyelids.
Miotic agent	Medication that causes constriction of the pupil.
Mydriatic agent	Medication that causes dilatation of the pupil of the eye.
Tonometry	The process of using a tonometer to measure intraocular pressure.
Trabecula	Supporting fibers of connecting tissue.

glycerin (Osmoglyn, Glyrol), act by increasing the osmotic pressure of the blood plasma to a point above that of the aqueous humor and the vitreous body of the eye. Fluid within the eye then follows the osmotic gradient into the hyperosmotic plasma. This loss of pressure leads to a reduction of intraocular pressure so that surgery can safely be performed on a softened eye. The recommended dose of mannitol is 2 g/kg of a 20% solution given IV during a 30-minute period. The dose of glycerin is 1 to 1.5 mg/kg of a 50% solution mixed in a chilled fruit juice or cola.

Miotic agents, such as acetylcholine chloride (Miochol), pilocarpine hydrochloride, and physostigmine (Eserine), cause the sphincter muscles of the iris and the ciliary body to contract. Constriction of the pupil tends to thin the iris and pull its folds and roots out of the anterior chamber angle. This leads to a reduction of intraocular pressure in acute angle-closure glaucoma, also known as closed-angle and narrow-angle glaucoma. In open-angle glaucoma, these drugs act by opening the closed or narrowed trabecular channel and allowing fluid to escape. Store miotic solutions in a cool place and protect them from light to reduce the rate of deterioration. Check the solution before use. Discolored or cloudy solutions should be discarded. Physostigmine

tends to turn pink or red. Epinephrine turns brown. Phenylephrine becomes cloudy.

To administer acetylcholine chloride, the rubber stopper of the vial is pressed down sufficiently to dislodge the center rubber plug seal. This releases the solvent (sterile water) from the upper chamber. Shake the vial gently to dissolve and mix the drug in the lower chamber. If the center rubber plug seal does not move down, or is in the down position, do not use the medication. After mixing, clean the stopper with 70% alcohol and aspirate the desired dose into a dry sterile syringe with a sterile 18- to 22-gauge needle. Because acetylcholine chloride is an unstable solution, it must be reconstituted immediately before use. Discard unused portion.

Mydriatic or cycloplegic agents include atropine sulfate, cyclopentolate hydrochloride, homatropine hydrobromide (Homatrocel), and tropicamide (Mydriacyl). The parasympatholytic action of cycloplegic agents causes the smooth muscle of the ciliary body and iris to relax, resulting in pupillary dilatation and paralysis of the ciliary muscles. Cycloplegic agents are contraindicated in persons with primary glaucoma or a tendency toward glaucoma.

Cycloplegic agents are administered at least 1 hour before refraction and/or surgery. When instilling drops, apply pressure to the inner canthus to lessen systemic absorption of the drug. The solution may otherwise run into the respiratory tract via the lacrimal duct and be absorbed into the blood stream. Keep the lids open for several seconds after application to retain the solution on the surface of the eye. This prolongs ocular action. After administration, the nurse should wash his or her hands and instruct the patient to do so because these drugs may be absorbed from the mucosa of the nose and mouth if fingers contaminated with the drug come in contact with these areas.

Cycloplegic Agent	Recommended Doses
Atropine sulfate	1 to 2 drops of a 1% solution
Cyclopentolate hydrochloride	2 drops of 0.5% solution or 1 drop of a 1% solution
Homatropine	1 to 2 drops of a 1 to 2% solution
Tropicamide	1 to 2 drops of a 0.5 to 1% solution

Sympathomimetic drugs (adrenergics), such as phenylephrine hydrochloride (Neo-Synephrine), 0.5% to 2% solution, and epinephrine hydrochloride (Adrenalin) 1:1000, are used to produce pupillary dilatation and vasoconstriction without muscle relaxation. Vasoconstriction decreases the production rate of aqueous humor and may increase the outflow of aqueous fluid, thus reducing intraocular pressure. Although used to treat some types of glaucoma, these agents are contraindicated in acute angle-closure glaucoma.

A note concerning *miotics and mydriatics*: Accidental administration of a mydriatic instead of a miotic to a patient with angle-closure glaucoma may precipitate an acute attack, which could lead to blindness. Never administer mydriatics routinely for eye examinations. Ask the physician for specific instructions for each patient.

Chymotrypsin (Zolyse) is a proteolytic enzyme that is instilled into the posterior chamber of the eye to cause dissolution of zonular fibers attached to the lens, thereby facilitating the removal of the lens during cataract extraction. Reconstitute this drug immediately before surgery. Do not use the reconstituted solution if it is cloudy or if it contains a precipitate. Do not resterilize the drug. Excessive heat, alcohol, and other chemicals inactivate the enzyme. Store chymotrypsin at 8 to 24°C (46–75°F).

Sodium hyaluronate (Healon) is used as a surgical aid in cataract extraction, intraocular lens implantation, corneal transplant, glaucoma filtration, and retinal attachment surgery. Instillation of sodium hyaluronate maintains a deep anterior chamber during surgery and allows for effective manipulation with less trauma to the cornea and surrounding tissue.

The surgeon should express a small amount of sodium hyaluronate from the syringe before use and carefully examine the remainder as it is injected. The literature reports an occasional release of minute rubber particles, presumably formed when the diaphragm is punctured. Avoid the reuse of cannulas. If reuse becomes necessary, rinse the cannula with sterile distilled water. Store sodium hyaluronate at 2 to 8°C (36–46°F) and protect it from freezing and light. Allow refrigerated sodium hyaluronate to attain room temperature for approximately 30 minutes before use.

Anti-infective–steroid combination agents, such as dexamethasone 0.1%, neomycin sulfate, and polymyxin B sulfate, are used for steroid-responsive inflammatory ocular conditions for which a corticosteroid is indicated and when bacterial infection or risk of bacterial ocular infection exists.

Glucocorticoids, such as sterile methylprednisolone acetate suspension (Depo-Medrol) and sterile betamethasone sodium phosphate and betamethasone acetate suspension (Celestone Soluspan), are used for their potent anti-inflammatory effects. Glucocorticoids are injected during or immediately after ocular surgery to prevent the inflammatory process. They are also used to treat severe acute and chronic allergic and inflammatory processes involving the eye such as herpes zoster ophthalmicus, iritis, diffuse posterior uveitis and choroiditis, sympathetic ophthalmia, anterior segment inflammation, and keratitis.

Hyaluronidase, 150 U (Wydase), is a *mucolytic enzyme* that is added to the retrobulbar injection of local anesthetic to promote diffusion and absorption of the anesthetic agent. Injection of hyaluronidase is contraindicated in or around inflamed, infected, or cancerous areas. Because absorption of accompanying drug is enhanced, watch for adverse reactions and expect a shortened duration of drug action. Hyaluronidase for injection is reported to be stable for up to 3 months when stored at 2 to 8°C (36–46°F).

Supplies and Equipment

In addition to the medication to be administered, the perioperative nurse needs cotton balls, gauze, and cotton-tipped applicators to roll the upper eyelid. A sterile dropper should come with the vial of medication. All equipment for administration of ophthalmic medications, including droppers, tubes, and plastic containers, must be sterile and never allowed to touch the eye. This helps prevent nosocomial infection in the eye and surrounding structures.

Potential Alterations in Functional Health Patterns

Health Perception–Health Management Pattern

Diagnosis

High risk for injury related to mydriatic agent administration causing an acute angle-closure glaucoma episode

Definition

Presence of risk factors for the patient to experience an acute glaucoma episode owing to the inadvertent administration of a mydriatic agent

Discussion. Acute angle-closure glaucoma is a medical emergency that can result from the administration of a mydriatic such as atropine to a patient with a history of angle-closure glaucoma. Unlike the case with an asymptomatic patient with open-angle glaucoma, when an acute episode of angle-closure glaucoma occurs, definite symptoms are present. Clinical signs include a moderately dilated pupil that does not react to light, complaints of blurred vision, halos around lights or a rapid loss of vision, excruciating eye and facial pain, nausea, and vomiting.

Risk Factors

- History of angle-closure glaucoma
- Age 40 years or older

Expected Outcome

The patient undergoes an eye examination or ophthalmological surgery without experiencing an episode of acute angle-closure glaucoma.

Nutrition-Metabolic Pattern

Diagnosis

High risk for fluid volume deficit related to the administration of hyperosmotic agents

Definition

Presence of risk factors for the patient to experience a decrease in circulating volume

Discussion. IV administration of hyperosmotic agents, such as mannitol and glycerin, may reduce intraocular pressure by increasing the osmotic pressure of glomerular filtration, thereby inhibiting tubular reabsorption of water and solutes. Elevated intraocular pressure is lowered within 30 to 60 minutes for a period of 4 to 6 hours. High oral doses of glycerin raise plasma osmotic pressure by withdrawing fluid from the extravascular spaces. Ocular pressure is then decreased by the reduction in volume of intraocular fluid.

Risk Factors

- Extremes in age and weight
- Presence of other diuretics in the system
- Nausea and vomiting related to the pain of acute angle-closure glaucoma

Expected Outcome

The patient does not experience fluid deficit secondary to the administration of hyperosmotic agents. There is an absence of unintentional increase in intraocular pressure. Intraoperative fluid volume is maintained.

Perioperative Nursing Interventions

Preoperative

- Interview the patient and family members to obtain a medication history. Pay close attention to patients who report past responses to eye medications. Check the patient or family history for glaucoma.
- Review the chart for additional information about medication and past ocular procedures.

Intraoperative

- Position the patient to ensure the proper administration of ophthalmic medications. Many patients undergo ocular procedures under local anesthesia. A pillow under the knees may increase patient comfort by relieving strain in the lower back.
- Provide emotional support during the administration of medications. A hand on the shoulder, brow, arm, or hand can decrease anxiety and ensure proper instillation of the medication.
- Alert the patient before instillation of drops, ointments, and injections. Some medications can cause temporary burning and/or irritation.
- Prepare and administer eye medications as needed (see Appendix E).
- Monitor the patient's pulse, blood pressure, and respirations because systemic absorption of medications can occur.
- Report changes in physiologic status and take necessary actions.
- Record the type and dose of all ocular medications and the time and route of administration.

Postoperative

- Communicate to the PACU or ward nurse the type of procedure performed and the type, dose, and time of administration of medications used during the procedure.
- Determine the patient's immediate response to medications (e.g., blurred vision, headache, and signs of systemic absorption).
- Provide patient education. Instruct patients with eye disorders to
  1. visit their physician and obtain eye examinations as needed according to their specific eye disorder
  2. avoid the use of nonprescription ophthalmic medications without medical advice
  3. properly instill eyedrops and ointments
  4. wear dark glasses when outdoors to avoid discomfort caused by sunlight that enters the dilated pupil, because the pupil cannot dilate reflexively after a refractory examination or surgery

OTIC AGENTS

The perioperative nurse prepares and administers a variety of otic medications for use during ear examinations and otolaryngological procedures (Table 9–10).

Considerations

Observe strict asepsis when the ear has been opened surgically, or opened because of trauma. Infection is especially hazardous because of the ear's close proximity to the brain.

Straighten the ear canal for optimal visualization and so medication flows into the canal. In adults, the auricle is pulled upward and backward and the tragus is pulled forward. In infants and children, the auricle is pulled downward.

TABLE 9–10. KEY TERMS FOR OTIC MEDICATIONS	
Auricle or pinna	External part of the ear composed of cartilage and covered by skin.
Cochlea	Winding cone-shaped tube forming a portion of the inner ear.
Eustachian tube	Tube that brings air to the middle ear, thus equalizing pressure on both sides of the tympanic membrane.
External auditory canal	Includes the outer portion of the ear, the canal, and the tympanic membrane.
Inner ear or labyrinth	A system of tubes and spaces within a hollowed-out temporal bone, collectively called the bony labyrinth.
Mastoid air cells	Air-filled spaces in the temporal bone. The middle ear communicates posteriorly with the mastoid ear cells.
Ossicles	Three bones of the ear: malleolus, incus, and stapes.
Tragus	Cartilaginous projection in front of the exterior meatus of the ear.
Tympanic membrane	The eardrum, which divides the meatus and the middle ear cavity.

Warm medications. Solutions and/or suspensions used for irrigation and eardrops should be warmed to body temperature before they are instilled. Hot or cold solutions can cause vertigo, nausea, and vomiting.

Never obstruct the ear canal when instilling drops. Obstruction may result in a pressure increase against the tympanic membrane.

Examine glass-tipped medication droppers to ensure that the tip of the dropper is not chipped.

Clean and dry the ear canal before the instillation of medication.

Know medication contraindications. Preparations of polymyxin B, neomycin, and hydrocortisone used for the prevention and treatment of inflammation and superficial bacterial infections of the external auditory canal are contraindicated in patients who have shown hypersensitivity to any of their components, and in herpes simplex, vaccinia, and varicella.

Supplies and Equipment

Medication with a sterile dropper
Cotton ball or ear wick
Gauze or tissue to remove excessive solution from the skin

Potential Alterations in Functional Health Patterns

Health Perception–Health Management Pattern

Diagnosis

High risk for injury related to an allergic or adverse reaction because of patient sensitivity to medication

Definition

Presence of risk factors for the patient to experience injury as a result of the allergic response or other adverse reaction to the administration of an otic preparation

Discussion. Allergic cross-reactions may occur, which could prevent the use of any or all of the following antibiotics: kanamycin, paromomycin, streptomycin, and possibly gentamicin. Neomycin is a common cutaneous sensitizer. When using neomycin-containing products to control secondary skin infections, such as chronic otitis externa, note that the skin in these conditions is more liable than normal skin to become sensitized to many substances, including neomycin.

Risk Factors

- Hypersensitivity to any of the components of antibiotics
- Presence of secondary infections in chronic dermatoses

Expected Outcome

The patient receives otic suspensions or solutions without allergic or adverse reaction. There is an absence of

- pruritus
- swelling
- inflammation
- other clinical manifestation of allergic reaction or secondary infection

Perioperative Nursing Interventions

Preoperative

- Interview the patient and family members and obtain a medication history. Note the presence of allergy to neomycin.
- Review the patient record for a past history of ear surgery and the use of otic medication.

Intraoperative

- Position the patient on her or his side with the affected ear up. A pillow under the head and between the knees may promote comfort.
- Instill otic solution or suspension as ordered (see Appendix F).
- Insert and remove ear wicks.

  Wicks of small pieces of cotton or commercially made wicks may be used as drains in the ear to remove exudate or excessive eardrops. Gently insert the wick into the canal only as far as it is possible to see. Leave the end of the wick extending out of the canal. Keep the wick moist by adding solution if the patient is in the OR for an extended period. Change the wick as needed to prevent hardening and/or obstruction of drainage flow.

- Provide emotional support during the procedure. A hand to the face or brow can offer support and remind the patient to remain in the proper position.
- Record the type, amount, and time of administration of medications.

Postoperative

- Communicate to the PACU or ward nurse the type of procedure and the type, amount, and time of administration of medications.
- Determine the immediate response to the medication. Note stinging, burning, redness, swelling, vertigo, nausea, and vomiting.
- Instruct the patient or parent in the proper method of cleaning the ear and instilling otic medications.

SKIN MEDICATIONS

The perioperative nurse selects, prepares, and administers a variety of topical skin preparations (Table 9–

TABLE 9–11. KEY TERMS FOR SKIN MEDICATIONS

Antihistaminic	Antagonizes the effects of free histamine on the skin and its blood vessels and thus relieves the cutaneous signs and symptoms of allergy
Anti-infective	Used to treat or prevent skin or mucous membrane infection by pathogenic microbes (e.g., antimicrobials, antifungals, antiseptics, antibacterials)
Anti-inflammatory	Used to reduce skin inflammation and relieve its signs and symptoms
Antiseptic	Chemical substance that kills microorganisms and prevents their growth
Demulcent	Used to coat the skin and mucous membranes, thereby providing mechanical protection against irritation of these surfaces
Depilatory	Chemical used to remove hair
Detergent	Used to clean the skin; usually has some antiseptic properties
Dusting powder	Inert substance applied to the skin to protect the irritated surface or to absorb excessive moisture
Emollient	Oily or fatty substance used to prevent the evaporation of water and drying of the skin
Proteolytic enzymes	Chemical substance applied to the skin to speed the breakdown of necrotic tissue in ulcerated or burned skin areas (e.g., for chemical débridement of dead tissue)

11). Each preparation, whether ointment, solution, cream, lotion, or impregnated dressing, should be applied to ensure desired penetration and absorption so that the intended result is achieved.

Considerations

Avoid applying ointments, creams, and lotions in copious amounts. Not only is this practice messy, it may result in excessive absorption of the product, especially when using corticosteroids. Apply liquids and other fluids sparingly to the scalp area to prevent fluids from running into the patient's eyes. Remove blood, pus, cellular debris, or other drainage because some topical applications are inactivated by these substances.

Specific Drugs

- Benzoin compound tincture

  The skin should be cleaned thoroughly before benzoin is applied because it forms an occlusive coating and may promote the retention of moisture and bacterial growth.

- Collodion, flexible

  Clean and dry the skin before application.

- Glycerin

  Undiluted glycerin (95–99%) absorbs moisture and therefore may result in dehydration and irritation when applied to mucous membranes.

- Petrolatum, hydrophilic

  Avoid the use of excessive amounts. As petrolatum warms from contact with the skin, the product may liquefy and run from the desired application location. This may cause discomfort to the patient.

- Starch

  Ensure that powdered substances such as starch do not come in contact with open stomas or wounds.

- Talc

  Dry skin surfaces before applying powder because caking of powder can lead to further irritation.

- Xeroform petroleum dressing

  Do not use on patients with hypersensitivity to bismuth tribromphenate.

- Zinc oxide

  Zinc, like other metals, may cause an alteration of x-ray films or x-ray therapy.

Chemicals That Cause Local Irritation

- Alcohol (ethyl and isopropyl)

  Avoid contact with open wounds, mucous membranes, and the eyes.

- Acetone

  Avoid contact with open wounds and mucous membranes, especially the eyes.

- Silver nitrate

  Use for wound cauterization. Before use, clean the area to remove organic material that may inhibit drug action. If a silver nitrate pencil is used, it should be dipped in water and applied to the areas for the time that promotes the desired action. If healthy tissue is accidentally treated, it may be washed with a saline solution because the chloride in the saline forms insoluble precipitates with silver nitrate and thus inhibits its action.

Occlusive Dressings for Topical Corticosteroids

Penetration of a steroid can be increased about 10-fold by covering the areas of application with an impermeable plastic. The plastic covering is kept in place for several hours and then removed to prevent prickly heat lesions and maceration. Systemic toxicity, such as cushingoid signs or suppression of adrenal function, is possible but is rarely associated with topical application. The risk of adrenal suppression is increased, however, when a large occlusive dressing is used.

Topical Anti-infective Agents

- Antibiotics

  Topical antibiotic therapy most commonly makes use of combinations of several antibiotics such as bacitracin, polymyxin B, neomycin, and sometimes trythricin and gramicidin.

- Antibacterial sulfonamides

  When sulfonamides are applied to extensive areas, serum sulfa concentrations, urinalysis, and kidney function tests should be monitored because significant quantities of the drug may be absorbed. Sulfonamides are incompatible with silver preparations.

- Topical dyes (gentian violet)

  Wear protective gloves to avoid staining the hands. Avoid accidental spilling onto the patient's skin.

- Oxidizing agents (hydrogen peroxide)

  Never instill oxidizing agents into closed body cavities or into abscesses that do not allow the free oxygen to escape. Deep wound irrigation can result in systemic oxygen microemboli by passage of oxygen into the vascular system.

Supplies and Equipment

- Varies depending on the type of application
- Sterile gloves
- Dry sterile dressings
- Occlusive dressing
- Sterile elastic (Ace) wrap, bandage (Kling), or other roll of gauze to secure the dressing
- Cotton-tipped applicators or tongue blades

Potential Alterations in Functional Health Patterns

Nutritional-Metabolic Pattern

Diagnosis

High risk for impaired skin integrity related to the administration of skin medications

Definition

Presence of risk factors for the patient to experience altered skin integrity owing to an allergic response to or contact dermatitis from skin medications

Discussion. Allergic contact dermatitis may result from exposure of the skin to a product that causes an inflammatory reaction. Contact dermatitis is caused by sensitizers and can result from the application of almost any skin product. Irritant contact dermatitis can be caused by any skin irritant. If body secretions are not properly removed before application of a skin product, the secretions, alone or in combination with the product, can cause skin breakdown. Local allergic reaction is the most common adverse effect associated with topical preparations. Skin sensitivity may develop after brief or prolonged exposure. The clinical picture may appear hours or weeks after the sensitized skin has been exposed. Symptoms may include itching, burning, erythema, vesiculation, and edema and swelling, followed by weeping, crusting, and drying and peeling of the skin.

Risk Factors

- Presence of irritating secretions, blood, pus, or infected drainage
- History of sensitivity to the specific agent or a related compound
- Existing impaired skin integrity

Expected Outcome

The patient's skin remains intact after the application of skin medications. There is an absence of

- redness
- swelling
- drainage
- other signs of local irritation

Perioperative Nursing Interventions

Preoperative

- Conduct a patient or family interview and obtain a medication history. Include any local systemic reactions to over-the-counter or prescribed medications or skin products.
- Review the patient's record and collect additional data regarding past and present skin conditions and reactions to skin products or medications.
- Inspect the skin for scars, abrasions, healing incisions, open wounds, and areas of skin breakdown.
- Identify infected skin lesions and take appropriate precautions.

Intraoperative

- Note the reaction of the skin to locally applied medications.
- Report signs of irritation.
- Apply lotions and ointments with a firm touch. Light dabbing can increase the sensation of itching.
- Apply skin preparations as needed (see Appendix D).
- Record the type, amount, time, and location of skin medication application.

Postoperative

- Communicate to the PACU or ward nurse the type, amount, time, and location of skin medication application during the procedure.
- Determine the immediate response or allergic reaction to the medication. Report the reaction and take appropriate measures.
- Teach patients with a history of allergy to skin medications to avoid trying a variety of skin products. They should stick to a few products that they know cause no adverse reaction.

CONTRAST MEDIA

Contrast media are administered to highlight a body structure during radiographic examination (Table 9–12). Media intended for intravascular and intrathecal use include metrizamide (Amipaque) and iohexol (Omnipaque). Agents used for intravascular injection alone include diatrizoate meglumine and diatrizoate sodium injection (Angiovist), iothalamate meglumine (Conray), and diatrizoate sodium (Hypaque). Diatrizoate meglumine (Renografin) can be used for intraureteral studies as well as IV studies.

The dosage, concentration, and route of administration vary depending on the patient and the procedure being performed. The perioperative nurse should always refer to the manufacturer's recommendations and consult with the physician before preparing contrast media for administration.

Considerations

Contrast media may interfere with some chemical determinations made on urine specimens. Urine needed for study should be collected before the administration of the contrast media or 2 days or more after the radiographic study.

A *scout film* is recommended before administration of the contrast media. This helps set the limits for the study and reduces the patient's exposure to contrast media.

Protect vials from direct exposure to sunlight. Do not freeze contrast media. Store it at 15 to 30°C (59–86°F).

Urography and nephrotomography are contraindicated in patients with anuria.

Visually inspect parental products for particulate matter and discoloration before administration.

Supplies and Equipment

- Syringes
- Needles
- IV tubing with a three-way adapter (for intraoperative cholangiogram)
- 0.9% sodium chloride for injection to dilute the media if needed

Potential Alterations in Functional Health Patterns

Health Perception–Health Management Pattern

Diagnosis

High risk for injury related to an allergic reaction to contrast media

Definition

Presence of risk factors for the patient to experience an allergic reaction to contrast media during a radiographic examination

Discussion. Many minor reactions to the opaque media require no treatment. Patients may complain of a flush and warm feeling. Other symptoms include urticaria, pain at the injection site, nausea, and excessive salivation. Major reactions, however, can occur in almost any system. Respiratory reactions include respiratory arrest, severe asthmatic attacks, laryngospasm, and laryngeal edema. CNS reactions include syncope, convulsion, aphasia, paraplegia, and coma. Cardiovascular reactions include shock, cardiac arrest, congestive heart failure, and arrhythmias. Renal reactions include flank pain, oliguria or anuria, hematuria, and renal failure.

Risk Factors

- History of allergy to contrast media or a related compound
- Hypersensitivity to iodine
- Bronchial asthma

TABLE 9–12. **KEY TERMS FOR CONTRAST MEDIA**	
Arteriogram	Radiographic study of an artery to determine arterial perfusion, size, and shape.
Arthrogram	Radiographic study of a joint cavity to outline the contour of the joint.
Cholangiogram	Radiographic study of the bile ducts.
Cystogram	Radiographic study of the bladder.
Cystourethrogram	Radiographic study of the bladder and ureters.
Diskogram	Radiographic study of intervertebral disks.
Hysterosalpingogram	Study of the uterus and fallopian tubes after injection of radiopaque material into those structures.
Pyelogram	Radiographic study of the ureter and renal pelvis. For an IV pyelogram, the contrast medium is given intravenously and an x-ray film of the urinary tract is taken while the material is excreted. This provides important information about the structure and function of the kidney, ureter, and bladder.

- Hay fever
- Food allergies such as shellfish allergy

Expected Outcome

The patient does not experience injury (allergic reaction) related to the administration of contrast media. There is an absence of respiratory, CNS, cardiovascular, renal, and local reactions to contrast media.

Perioperative Nursing Interventions

Preoperative

- Interview the patient and family members and obtain a medication history. Pay special attention to past reactions to contrast media or a history of asthma, hay fever, or food allergies.
- Note a history of multiple myeloma or other paraproteinemia. Using radiopaque agents with such conditions may cause anuria, resulting in progressive uremia, renal failure, and eventually death.
- Note the presence of sickle cell disease. Contrast media promote the phenomenon of sickling in individuals who are homozygous for sickle cell disease when the material is injected intravenously or intra-arterially.

Intraoperative

- Aseptically withdraw contrast media from the vial using a sterile syringe and needle. Contrast media should be at body temperature when injected.
- Avoid contaminating catheters, syringes, needles, and contrast media with glove powder or draping material fibers.
- If nondisposable equipment is used, care should be taken to prevent residual contamination with traces of cleansing agents.
- Monitor the patient for a reaction to the contrast media. Report physiological or psychological changes and take appropriate actions if necessary.
- Have emergency equipment available:

  100% oxygen
  Adrenalin chloride
  Aminophylline
  Aromatic ammonia
  Atropine sulfate
  Cortisone
  Metaraminol (Aramine)
  Succinylcholine chloride (Anectine)

- Provide emotional support during the procedure. Patients are sometimes awake during radiographic procedures. Use conversation and touch to offer support and reassurance. Diversional techniques such as listening to the radio, using audio headphones, or reading may help decrease anxiety and facilitate the patient's cooperation.

- Record the type, amount, route, and time of administration of media.

Postoperative

- Communicate to the PACU or unit staff the type, amount, route, and time of administration of contrast media. Alert the staff if dyes that stain the patient's urine were administered.
- Determine immediate response to the contrast media.
- Inform the patient to contact the physician or return to the health care facility if he or she suspects a reaction to the media. Most adverse reactions occur within 1 to 3 minutes after the start of injection. Delayed reactions, however, can occur at a later time.

IRRIGATING FLUIDS FOR TRANSURETHRAL PROCEDURES

The perioperative nurse administers glycine (1.5% glycine irrigation) or other suitable nonelectrolyte solutions for transurethral surgical procedures. Glycine is an amino acid. Because it does not contain electrolytes, it is nonconductive and suitable for urological irrigation during electrosurgical procedures.

A 1.5% concentration of glycine in water is sufficient to minimize the risk of intravascular hemolysis, which can occur from absorption of plain water through open prostatic veins during transurethral resection. Glycine is hypotonic in relation to extracellular fluid. Any solution absorbed intravascularly during transurethral resection or bladder surgery is excreted by the kidneys.

Considerations

Discard any unused portion. Glycine contains no bacteriostatic, anti-infective agent, or acid buffer. It is intended for use as a single-dose irrigation.

Do *not* inject by parenteral routes.

Do *not* administer in patients who have a history of anuria.

Warm the solution to prevent hypothermia. Do not warm, however, over 150°F (66°C).

Administer the solution only if it is clear, the seal is intact, and the container is undamaged.

Supplies and Equipment

- At least 10 3000-ml 1.5% glycine irrigation containers
- Sterile irrigation set

Potential Alterations in Functional Health Patterns

Nutritional-Metabolic Pattern

Diagnosis

High risk for fluid volume excess related to the absorption of large amounts of irrigating fluid into the systemic circulation

Definition

Presence of risk factors for the patient to experience excessive circulation volume owing to absorption of irrigating fluid into the vascular system

Discussion. Fluid absorbed into the systemic circulation via open prostatic veins may increase the volume of extracellular fluid and lead to congestive heart failure.

Risk Factors

- History of cardiopulmonary disease
- History of renal dysfunction

Expected Outcome

The patient's hemodynamic status is maintained within normal limits. There is an absence of

- edema
- hypotension
- tachycardia
- anginalike pains
- pulmonary congestion

Perioperative Nursing Interventions

Preoperative

- Interview the patient and family members to obtain a medication history. Note a prior history of transurethral procedures.
- Warm the solution to prevent hypothermia. Do not heat the container to more than 150°F (66°C).

Intraoperative

- Aseptically prepare the solution for administration. Use the appropriate administration set and attach the tubing promptly after protective seals are removed.
- Do not elevate the container more than 60 cm (about 2 feet) above the OR bed. Excessive elevation can increase intravascular absorption of the irrigating fluid.
- Monitor the physiological status and note and re-

port adverse reactions. In the event of adverse reaction, alert the physician, and as directed by the physician, discontinue the irrigation and institute appropriate treatment. Save the remainder of the fluid for examination.

- Patients are often awake for transurethral procedures. Use conversation and therapeutic touch to provide reassurance and decrease anxiety.
- Record intake and output, noting the amount of irrigation fluid used and the amount of fluid removed from the bladder.
- Record the amount, type, and time of administration of fluid.

Postoperative

- Communicate to the PACU nurse the type, amount, and time of administration of irrigation fluid.
- Note an immediate response to irrigation (e.g., chills, vertigo, backache, and nausea)

SUMMARY

The perioperative nurse is responsible for the preparation and administration of many medications and solutions in the surgical setting. Most importantly, the nurse must remember the "rights" involved in medication administration: right patient, right drug, right dose, route, and time. The nurse should always read accompanying drug literature and refer to the package insert, the *Physicians' Desk Reference* (1992), or other suitable reference before administering an unfamiliar product.

Bibliography

American Medical Association. (1984). *AMA drug evaluations* (5th ed.). Chicago: Author.
Association of Operating Room Nurses. (1992). *Standards and recommended practices for perioperative nursing.* Denver.
Centers for Disease Control. (1985). *Guidelines for handwashing and hospital environmental control.* Atlanta.
Covoni, B., Vassallo, H. (1976). *Local anesthetics: Mechanisms of action and clinical use* pp. 9–10). New York: Grune & Stratton.
Gordon, M. (1991). *Manual of nursing diagnoses: 1986–1987.* New York: McGraw-Hill.
Ignatavicius, D., Bayne, M. V. (1991). *Medical-surgical nursing: A nursing process approach.* Philadelphia: W. B. Saunders.
Perry, A. G., Potter, P. A. (1986). *Clinical nursing skills and techniques.* St. Louis: C. V. Mosby.
Physicians' desk reference (46th ed.). (1992). Montvale, NJ: Medical Economics Company.
Rodman, M. J., Smith, D. W. (1984). *Clinical pharmacology in nursing* (2nd ed.) (pp. 21 and 32). Philadelphia: J. B. Lippincott.
Wolff, L., Weitzel, M. H., Zsohar, H. (1983). *Fundamentals of nursing* (7th ed.). Philadelphia: J. B. Lippincott.

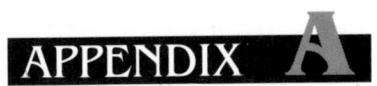

Preoperative Medication History

Health Perception—Health Management Pattern

What medications are you presently taking?
What do these medications do for you?
Do they seem to work?
What medications have you taken in the past?
Did they seem to work for you?
Do you have any allergies to drugs, foods, chemicals, or other materials such as tape or iodine?
Do you use alcohol, tobacco, or recreational drugs?
On a scale of 1 to 10, rate your compliance with (how well you stick to) your medication regimen (10 being 100% compliance).

Nutritional-Metabolic Pattern

Age _____
Weight _____
Height _____

Abnormal laboratory values or test results

_____
_____
_____

Do you take any special foods with, before, or after your medications?
Do you have any problems associated with your medications? Skin problems? Dental or gum problems? Difficulty healing?

Elimination Pattern

Have your medications caused any problems with elimination (constipation, polyuria, diarrhea)?
Do you use over-the-counter laxatives?

Activity-Exercise Pattern

Have you had a change in energy related to your medications?

Are you able to take your medications or do you need assistance?
Functional level related to the ability to self-medicate:

Level 0: Full self-care
Level I: Requires use of equipment or devices
Level II: Requires assistance or supervision from another person
Level III: Requires assistance or supervision from another person and equipment or devices
Level IV: Is dependent and does not participate

Sleep-Rest Pattern

Have your medications changed your sleep habits?
Do you have any nightmares or dreams associated with your medications?
Do you use any aids to sleep (alcohol, medications, foods)?

Cognitive-Perceptual Pattern

Have you experienced any changes related to your medications? Changes in vision, hearing, memory, decision making, and associated pain or discomfort?

Self-perception—Self-concept Pattern

Have you noticed any changes in how you feel about yourself since you have been taking _____?
Have you had any changes in your body such as weight gain or loss, enlarged breasts, and fluid retention?
Have you had a change in your attitude such as anger, depression, and fear?

Role-Relationship Pattern

If need be, is there someone at home who can help you with your medications?
Has taking _____ interfered with your

ability to perform your life roles (wife/husband, parent, jobholder, and so on)?

Sexuality-Reproductive Pattern

Has your medication altered your sexual drive or changed your sexual relationship?

If appropriate: Do you use contraception? When was your last menstrual period? Are there any menstrual problems related to medications?

Coping–Stress Tolerance Pattern

Do you use any medications, herbs, folk remedies, or alcohol to help you cope with stress?

Are these methods effective?

Do you presently use or have a history of using recreational drugs?

Values-Beliefs Pattern

Does taking your medication interfere with your religious beliefs or values? If so, how? Is there interference with your cultural or ethnic beliefs or values? If so, how?

Supplies and Equipment for Medication Administration

Syringes

Syringes with needles are commonly used in the process of reconstituting powders with a diluent and for aspirating a solution or suspension from a vial or an ampule. Syringe selection (size and type) is usually dependent on the medication being prepared and dispensed.

Because the amount of medication varies depending on its type and function, the perioperative nurse must use judgment in selecting syringe size. Generally, a 10-ml syringe is used for injection of local anesthetics and for reconstituting powders with diluent. Larger syringes are usually more difficult to control than smaller ones because greater force is needed for aspiration and injection.

When preparing small doses of potentially dangerous medications such as heparin or epinephrine, it is best to use a 1-ml insulin or tuberculin syringe to ensure accurate dosage.

Types

Luer-Lok tip

This syringe has a tip that locks over the needle hub. It is used whenever pressure is exerted to inject or aspirate fluid. Sizes range from 2 to 60 ml.

Luer-slip tip

This syringe has a plain tip that may not provide a secure connection on a needle hub. It is not recommended for preparing medications but may be needed when administering medications through catheters and ports. Sizes range from 1 to 60 ml.

Ring control

This syringe has a Luer-Lok tip with a finger hold and thumb hold. It is ideal for injection of local anesthetics. The syringe allows firm control when injecting with only one hand. Sizes range from 3 to 10 ml.

For Irrigation

Bulb syringe with barrel

This syringe has a rubber or plastic bulb attached to the neck of the barrel. It is used for irrigation in many types of procedures. Sizes have a solution capacity ranging from ¼ to 4 ounces.

Bulb syringe without barrel

This syringe is also known as the ear syringe. It is a one-piece bulb that tapers to a blunt end. It is used for irrigating the ear, the eye, or other small structures.

Needles

The size of a needle is designated by length and gauge. Gauge is the outside diameter of the needle. The bevel of a needle is its sloped edge. Commonly used sizes include

½ inch × 30 gauge	for local anesthesia in plastic surgery
¾ inch × 25 gauge	for local anesthesia or conjunctival injection
1½ inches × 22 gauge	for subcutaneous or intramuscular injection
2 inches × 16 or 18 gauge	for preparation of medications and solutions
4 inches × 20 or 22 gauge	spinal needles used for deep injection of local anesthetic

Diluent

0.9% sodium chloride

This preparation is designed for parenteral use only after the addition of drugs that require dilution or must be dissolved in an aqueous vehicle before injection. Do not use unless the solution is clear and the container is undamaged. When diluting or dissolving drugs, mix thoroughly and use promptly.

Bacteriostatic water for injection

Used as a diluting or dissolving agent according to the drug manufacturer's recommendation.

Preparing Medications and Solutions from Ampules and Vials

Task Standard

The perioperative nurse prepares medications and solutions from ampules and vials in a manner that

- prevents contamination of the ampule or vial contents
- maintains sterility of the needle and syringe parts
- ensures accurate dosage of medication or solution

Considerations

- Knowledge of the principles of medical and surgical asepsis
- Knowledge of sterile technique in placing solution onto a sterile field
- Knowledge of how to calculate medication and solution dosage

Supplies and Equipment

Appropriate-sized syringe and needle
Protective pad for opening ampule
Sharps container
Diluent
    0.9% sodium chloride injection
    Bacteriostatic water for injection

Removing Medication or Solution from an Ampule

- Identify the type, dose, and expiration date of the medication.
- Tap the ampule lightly and quickly until the fluid leaves the neck of the ampule and flows to the lower chamber.
- Place a gauze or alcohol pad around the neck of the ampule. This helps protect the fingers when breaking the ampule. Do not remove the alcohol pad from its wrapper. Alcohol may lead into the ampule.
- Snap the neck of the ampule along the prescored line. The snapping motion should be directed away from the body. While snapping the top off, avoid shattering the glass. If it is suspected that glass has entered the ampule, discard it and start again.
- Hold the ampule upside down or place it on a flat surface. The ampule may be held upside down without danger of spillage as long as the needle tip or shaft does not touch the ampule. After the needle touches the ampule, surface tension breaks down and fluid leaks out.
- Insert the needle into the ampule without touching the rim.
- Keep the needle tip below the surface of the liquid and quickly draw up the medication without injecting air into the ampule. Injection of air forces the fluid out of the ampule. Because the fluid in the ampule is immediately displaced by air, there is no resistance to its withdrawal.
- Confirm the type, dose, and expiration date of the medication with the scrub person.
- Dispense the medication onto the sterile field. The scrub person should position the medication receptacle at the edge of the field or hold it so that the solution can be released without contamination.
- Dispose of the needle, syringe, and gauze or alcohol pad. This protects other personnel from inadvertent injury from the needle or glass slivers. Discard unused medication.

Removing Medication or Solution from a Vial

- Identify the type, dose, and expiration date of the medication.
- Remove the plastic or metal cap covering the top of the unused vial. If the vial is a multiple-dose vial and has been previously used, wipe the rubber seal with alcohol before and after each use. This removes surface bacteria, dust, and dried solution from the stopper.
- Prepare the syringe with as much air as solution to be removed from the vial. As medication is removed, replacement with air is required to prevent a build-up of negative pressure.
- Insert the needle, with the bevel pointing up, through the center of the vial. The center of the vial is thinner and is designed for penetration. Keep the bevel up to prevent cutting a rubber core from the seal.
- Inject air into the vial. While injecting air, hold onto the plunger. The plunger may be forced backward by air pressure within the vial. For vials with dry medication, diluent is used to replace air, thereby creating positive pressure in the vial.
- Invert the vial with the nondominant hand while grasping the syringe barrel and plunger with the thumb and forefinger of the dominant hand. Inverting the vial allows fluid to settle in the lower section of the vial.
- Allow air pressure to fill the syringe; pull back slightly on the plunger if necessary. Positive pressure in the vial causes the syringe to fill.
- After the correct volume is obtained, withdraw the needle from the vial.
- For multiple-dose vials, prepare a label that includes the date and time of mixing and concentration per milliliter.
- Confirm the type, dose, and expiration date of the medication with the scrub person.
- Dispense the medication onto the sterile field. The scrub person should position the medication receptacle at the edge of the field or hold it so that the solution can be released without contamination.
- Dispose of the needle and syringe in an appropriate container.

Applying Skin Medications

Task Standard

The perioperative nurse applies topical medications to ensure proper penetration and absorption.

Considerations

- Knowledge of how to assess the skin and mucous membranes
- Knowledge of the purpose of skin application
  1. Prevention or treatment of inflammation, discomfort, or infection
  2. Protection of the suture line or other skin surface
  3. Provision of local anesthesia over the skin surface
- Knowledge of the anatomy and physiology of the skin and mucous membrane
- Knowledge of dosage calculation
  Apply the least amount of medication to obtain the desired effect. Excessive application of creams, ointments, or powders can result in skin irritation.

Supplies and Equipment

Desired cream, ointment, or solution
Sterile gloves
Tongue blade or cotton-tipped applicators
Dry sterile dressing
Tape (paper or plastic)

Assessing the Patient

Inspect the site of application for lesions, reddened areas, signs of infection, and breaks in skin or membranes.

Applying the Topical Ointment or Cream

- Don sterile gloves.
- Wash the application site to remove microorganisms, blood, debris, and fluids.
- Dry the application site. Moisture can interfere with application of the medication and hinder absorption of the medication.
- Apply the medication.
  1. Place the desired amount of medication on the sterile gauze.
  2. Apply the medication with a sterile tongue blade onto the suture line or desired skin surface. If a gloved finger is used for application, a fresh sterile glove should be donned. Glove powder should be removed.
  3. Avoid rubbing the skin, which may cause irritation, disruption of the suture line, or bleeding.
- Apply a dry sterile gauze or dressing as desired and secure with paper or plastic tape.

Applying an Aerosol Spray

- Shake the can vigorously, which mixes the contents and propellant to ensure a fine and even spray.
- Protect the patient's eyes and face from the spray by having the patient turn his or her head or by covering the face with a towel.
- Hold the can the recommended distance from the skin, usually 6 to 12 inches.
- Spray the desired area and allow it to dry before applying dressing or tape. This prevents the product from being removed by the dressing or tape.
- Cover the area with dressing as desired by the physician. Covering may help maintain the application on the skin.

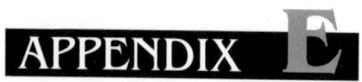

Administering Ophthalmic Medications

Task Standard

The perioperative nurse administers ocular solutions and ointments in a manner that

- prevents injury to the eye
- maintains the sterility of droppers, tubes, or medication containers

Considerations

- Knowledge of the principles of medical and surgical asepsis
- Knowledge of the anatomy and physiology of the eye
- Knowledge of dosage calculations
- Knowledge of the purpose of ophthalmic applications
  1. Dilatation of the pupil for remeasurement of lens refraction or visualization of internal eye structures
  2. Paralysis of lens muscles for measurement of lens refraction
  3. Prevention or relief of local irritation or infection of the eye
  4. Local treatment of an increase in intraocular pressure
  5. Maintenance of lubrication of the cornea or the conjunctiva

Supplies and Equipment

Desired ointment, eyedrop, or insert
Gloves to protect the hands from purulent drainage or blood
Cotton ball, gauze, or tissue
Eye pad and tape for dressing if needed

Assessing the Patient

Inspect the site of application for drainage, reddened areas, and encrusted areas.

Preparing the Patient

- Position the patient in a supine or a semi-Fowler position. These positions provide access to the eye and minimize drainage of medication through the lacrimal duct.
- If the eyelids are covered with crust or drainage, clean with sterile water or saline solution. Soak crust with warm solution if it is dry and difficult to remove. Soaking allows easy removal of crust and drainage that may harbor microorganisms. Always wipe from the inner to the outer canthus. This prevents carrying debris to the lacrimal duct.
- Place the thumb and index finger near the margin of the lower eyelid immediately below the eyelashes, and exert downward pressure over the bony prominence of the cheek. Ask the patient to look upward while this is being done. This maneuver provides exposure of the lower conjunctival sac while retraction against the bony orbit prevents pressure and trauma to the eyeball. Upward eye motion retracts the cornea up and away from the conjunctival sac and reduces stimulation of the blink reflex.

Instilling Eyedrops

- Hold the dropper in the dominant hand about 1 to 2 cm above the conjunctival sac. This prevents dropper contact with the eyeball.
- Instill the prescribed number of drops into the eye.

If the patient blinks and drops do not enter the eye, repeat the procedure. The conjunctival sac normally holds 1 to 2 drops.

- When administering drops that cause a systemic effect, protect the fingers with gloves or a tissue and apply gentle pressure to the patient's nasolacrimal duct for 30 to 60 seconds. This prevents absorption of the medication into the systemic circulation and prevents overflow of the drops into the nasopharyngeal passage.

Instilling Eye Ointment

- Have the patient look down to reduce the blinking reflex during ointment instillation.

- Hold the applicator above the lid margin and apply a thin stream of ointment evenly along the inside of the lower lid on the conjunctiva. Evenly distribute the ointment.
- Have the patient close the eye and gently rub the lid in a circular motion with a cotton ball. This helps distribute the ointment without causing injury to the eye.
- Remove excessive solution or ointment from the lids or face. This promotes comfort and prevents undesired absorption of the medication.
- If ordered by the physician, apply a clean eye patch.

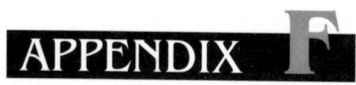

Administering Otic Medications

Task Standard

The perioperative nurse administers otic medications in a manner that

- prevents injury to the ear
- maintains the sterility of the medicine dropper
- prevents the transmission of infection

Considerations

- Knowledge of the principles of medical and surgical asepsis
- Knowledge of the anatomy and physiology of the ear
- Knowledge of dosage calculations
- Knowledge of the purpose of otic instillation
  1. Prevention or treatment of inflammation, discomfort, or infection
  2. Softening of cerumen for removal

Supplies and Equipment

Desired otic solution or suspension
Cotton ball or wick
Cotton-tipped applicator

Assessing the Patient

Inspect the site of application for reddened areas, signs of infection, breaks in the skin, and cerumen build-up.

Preparing the Patient

- Position the patient in a comfortable sitting or side-lying position so that the affected ear is facing up. An infant or child can be held by the parent or another adult.
- If cerumen or drainage occludes the outer ear canal, clean the canal with a cotton-tipped applicator. Do not force the cerumen inward or occlude the canal in any way.
- Straighten the patient's ear by pulling the pinna upward and outward for adults. For children, pull the pinna down and back. Straightening the canal provides direct access to deeper ear structures.

Instilling the Medication

- Instill the medication by holding the dropper 1 cm above the ear canal. Do not force the drops into the canal under pressure.
- Have the patient maintain the body position for 2 to 3 minutes while applying gentle pressure to the tragus. This allows complete distribution of the solution. Gentle pressure moves the medication inward.
- Insert a cotton ball or wick into the ear (optional). This prevents the solution from running out of the ear when the patient moves the head. Remember to remove the cotton ball.

CHAPTER 10

Physiologically Monitoring the Patient

Angela M. Martinelli

DEFINITION

Safe monitoring of the surgical patient is essential if quality care is to be delivered in the operating room. The perioperative nurse monitors the physical, psychological, sociocultural, and spiritual stressors that can affect the surgical patient. This chapter focuses on physical stressors that can have an impact during the intraoperative period (Table 10–1).

MEASURABLE CRITERIA

The perioperative nurse demonstrates competency to perform physiological monitoring of the patient by evaluating

- the airway
- intake
- output
- body temperature
- the effects of local anesthesia

ROLE OF THE PERIOPERATIVE NURSE

The perioperative nurse assists the anesthetist in monitoring the patient during surgery. When assigned as the monitoring nurse during procedures using intravenous (IV) conscious sedation or local anesthesia, the perioperative nurse assumes total responsibility for monitoring duties.

CONSIDERATIONS

The perioperative nurse is responsible for knowing the standards of care cited in the state nurse practice act and for complying with the standards that are used

TABLE 10–1. ROUTINE METHODS OF MONITORING

Airway Patency, Gas Exchange, and Tissue Perfusion

Use pulse oximetry
Inspect the skin and nails for color and capillary refill
Inspect the surgical field for the color of tissue and blood
Listen to lung sounds and ventilatory rate
Monitor arterial blood gas values as needed

Hemodynamic Status

Assess blood pressure and pulse (rate, rhythm, and quality)
Note the amount and rate of blood loss

Fluid Intake

Inspect mucous membranes and conjunctiva for color, moisture, and edema
Monitor intravenous fluids and blood products
Note the amount and type of surgical irrigation used

Output and Fluid Loss

Assess blood loss, urine output, and other drainage
Assess for third-space fluid loss and insensible fluid loss

Body Temperature

Assess skin temperature and core temperature as needed

Effects of Local Anesthesia

Inspect the skin for rash, edema, or pruritus
Note changes in hemodynamic status, respiratory function, and mental and neurologic status (seizure activity)

---

in the local community. Additionally, it is a professional responsibility to have knowledge of the recommendations put forth by the Joint Commission on Accreditation of Healthcare Organizations and the *Standards and Recommended Practices for Perioperative Nursing* (Association of Operating Room Nurses [AORN], 1992).

OUTCOME STANDARD

Standard I

The patient's breathing patterns are maintained during surgery.

Criteria

Depending on the physical and psychological status, the patient exhibits no signs of

- ineffective airway clearance and obstruction
- respiratory depression related to IV sedation

Standard II

The patient is free from injuries associated with IV fluid intake.

Criteria

Depending on the physical and psychological status, the patient exhibits no signs of

- alteration in cardiac output related to air embolism associated with fluid administration
- alteration in tissue integrity related to infiltration of IV fluid
- alteration in fluid volume related to the administration of excessive fluid

Standard III

The patient maintains a balanced circulating blood volume.

Criteria

Depending on the physical and psychological status, the patient exhibits no signs of fluid deficit associated with intraoperative blood loss.

Standard IV

The patient maintains normal body temperature.

Criteria

Depending on the physical and psychological status, the patient exhibits no signs of hypothermia or hyperthermia.

Standard V

The patient is free from complications associated with the administration of local anesthesia.

Criteria

Depending on the physical and psychological status, the patient exhibits no signs of

- impaired tissue integrity related to extravasation of medication
- allergic reaction to the local anesthetic
- toxic effects of the local anesthetic

MONITORING THE AIRWAY

The perioperative nurse is responsible for monitoring the airway of a patient who is not monitored by the anesthetist. Upper airway obstruction may occur in patients who are receiving IV conscious sedation, who have an impaired airway, or who are comatose. During the procedure, sedated patients may be unable, reluctant, or forget to breathe deeply and cough, if necessary. In addition, unconscious or comatose patients lose their protective reflexes as well as the tone of pharyngeal muscles with the result that the tongue falls back and obstructs the airway.

Considerations

Factors That Affect Airway Clearance

- Excessive secretions
- Coexisting respiratory disease
- Tracheostomy
- Obesity
- Fatigue
- Weight of drapes
- Noxious odors
- Flow of blood or secretions into the airway
- Use of medications that produce sedation
- Body position

  Mechanical restriction or reduced ability of the diaphragm to push down against the abdominal contents can impair lung expansion. Lung compliance is then decreased, reducing the amount of alveolar volume available for gas exchange and the functional residual capacity.

Supplies and Equipment

Nasal cannula or face mask
Oropharyngeal or nasopharyngeal airway
Pulse oximeter
Oxygen
Endotracheal tube, laryngoscope, self-inflating bag, and pressure-controlled ventilator
Suction equipment

Potential Alterations in Functional Health Patterns

Activity-Exercise Pattern

Diagnosis

High risk for ineffective airway clearance

Definition

Presence of risk factors for the patient to experience an inability to clear the airway during the surgical procedure

Discussion. The surgical patient is at particular risk for obstruction owing to a variety of irritants that can partially or completely obstruct the movement of air through the upper airway. Common irritants that may enter the trachea or the larynx include saliva, blood, vomitus, and other dry particulate matter.

Risk Factors

- Alteration in level of consciousness caused by sedation
- History of sleep apnea or obstruction because of the position of the tongue
- Excessive salivation or the presence of viscous secretions

- Ineffective coughing or an inability to cough due to the nature of the procedure (cataract or other ocular procedure) or lack of understanding of how and when to deep breathe and cough
- Pain or fear of pain that may discourage coughing
- Fatigue, weakness, or drowsiness

Expected Outcome

The patient is free from airway obstruction during the perioperative period.

Perioperative Nursing Interventions

Preoperative

- Interview the patient and the family to assess for a history of airway obstruction or respiratory disease.
- Conduct an assessment and note the presence of a cough, dyspnea, rales, clubbing of the fingers, abnormal breath sounds, a change in the rate or depth of respiration, and cyanosis.
- Review related laboratory studies:

  X-ray film of chest
  Sputum studies
  Pulmonary function tests
  Arterial blood gas studies

Intraoperative

- Administer oxygen as needed via nasal prongs or a face mask
- Use a pulse oximeter to determine the blood oxygen saturation
- Position the patient with the head slightly elevated or in a semisitting position if permitted by the surgical procedure
- Provide emotional support by maintaining contact through touch and communication
- Monitor the respiratory rate and the quality of chest excursion. Note stridor, a skin color change, or a change in mental alertness or personality
- Observe for signs of airway obstruction:
  1. Inspiration will cause drawing in of parts of the upper chest, the sternum, and the intercostal spaces.
  2. Exhalation is characterized by jerky protrusion and prolonged contractions of abdominal muscles.
  3. Seesaw movement of the chest and abdomen may occur.
  4. Tracheal tug or indrawing of the suprasternal notch may occur.
- Initiate corrective action if airway obstruction occurs.
  1. Open and inspect the mouth for displacement of the tongue and the presence of secretions, blood, or other substances.
  2. Extend the head by lifting the jaw. This increases the distance between the chin and the cervical spine, which puts the muscles that support the chin under tension and pulls the tongue forward. This maneuver puts further tension on the musculature that supports the tongue. The mandible

is lifted upward by exerting pressure on the ascending ramus of the mandible and at the same time tilting the head backward. The fingers and palm of each hand are applied on each side of the face to maintain head extension.

- If the head tilt or extension is not effective, an oral airway may need to be inserted or endotracheal intubation may have to be performed. The perioperative nurse should call for assistance from an anesthetist while administering supplemental oxygen and assisting with ventilation using a self-inflating bag.
- Record findings and report as needed.

Postoperative

- Report intraoperative events to the postanesthesia care unit (PACU) or unit nurse.
- Determine the immediate response to therapeutic measures.
- If needed, consult with a respiratory therapist for assistance.

MONITORING INTAKE

The administration of IV fluids is sometimes managed by the perioperative nurse. Usually, patients undergoing surgical intervention are provided with IV access to administer fluids and to establish a route for drug administration. Perioperative fluid alterations can range from minimal blood loss to massive loss and severe alteration of electrolyte levels. In addition, because most surgical patients have fluid intake restrictions before surgery, IV therapy provides water, electrolytes, and nutrients to meet body requirements; to replace water and electrolyte deficiencies; and to provide a means for IV drug administration.

Body fluid (water and electrolytes) accounts for 60% of adult male and 50% of adult female body weight. The difference is attributed to more body fat in females. Intracellular fluid in the adult exceeds extracellular water and approximates 40% of the body weight. Total extracellular fluid in an adult is half that of intracellular water, accounting for 20% of body weight (Masiak et al., 1985, p. 6).

Extracellular water can further be divided into a number of types: plasma (intravascular fluid), interstitial fluid, lymph, inaccessible bone water, transcellular fluids, and fluid of the potential spaces (Masiak et al., 1985, p. 6).

Considerations

Factors That Affect Fluid and Electrolyte Balance

- Fluid and food intake

  During assessment, note the last time the patient ate or drank and the type of diet.

- Excessive thirst
- Sources of fluid loss such as diarrhea, draining wounds, excessive urine output, and excessive perspiration
- Use of prescribed medications, such as diuretics and adrenocorticosteroids, that may cause fluid and electrolyte imbalances
- Use of over-the-counter agents to induce urinary and bowel elimination
- Excessive ingestion of alcohol or the use of illegal drugs that may interfere with a proper nutrition
- Preexisting conditions or disease states that can result in fluid and electrolyte imbalances such as diabetes, renal failure, cancer, burns or trauma, and exposure to toxic agents.
- Inadequate IV fluid flow.

  The flow of IV fluid is directly proportional to the height of the liquid column. Raising the height of the infusion container sometimes improves the flow. Fluid flow is directly proportional to the diameter of the tubing. The clamp on the IV tubing regulates the flow by changing the tubing diameter. The flow will be faster through large-gauge cannulas (14, 16, or 18 gauge). Fluid flow is inversely proportional to the length of the tubing. Adding tubing to provide more length decreases the flow rate. Fluid flow is inversely proportional to the viscosity of the fluid. Solutions such as blood products and hyperalimentation fluids require a larger cannula than do normal solutions.

Calculating Fluid Need and Flow Rate

Fluid needs can be calculated in several ways. A common guide is to use a combination of weight and age. Using the patient's weight to estimate body surface area can also be effective. Charts that list estimates of surface area in relation to weight are available, although calculations are necessary when the patient's body fluid deviates from the average for her or his age.

Regardless of the method used to select the type and amount of fluid, the perioperative nurse must consider the patient's clinical condition. Patients in need of preventive therapy or IV infusions for drug administration have varied needs from those patients experiencing a severe depletion of fluid.

Monitor IV solutions frequently to ensure that they are flowing at the desired rate. The IV container should be marked with a tape indicating how much fluid should be infused per hour. To calculate the flow rate, the number of drops per milliliter must be determined. This number varies with the type of tubing and drip chamber and is usually included with the product information.

The following formulas can be used to calculate drip rates:

$$\frac{\text{Amount of solution to infuse}}{\text{Hours to infuse the solution}} = \text{amount to infuse each hour}$$

or

$$\frac{\text{Amount of solution/hour} \times \text{drops/ml}}{60 \text{ (minutes/hour)}} = \text{drops to infuse/minute}$$

Types of Intravenous Solutions

IV solutions are classified as isotonic, hypotonic, or hypertonic according to whether their osmolality is, respectively, the same as, less than, or greater than that of blood.

Isotonic fluids have a total osmolality close to that of intravascular fluid and do not cause red blood cells to shrink or swell. Commonly used isotonic fluids include 5% dextrose in water, normal saline (0.9% sodium chloride), and lactated Ringer solution.

Hypotonic fluids replace transcellular fluid because they are hypotonic as compared with plasma. Commonly used hypotonic fluids include half-normal saline (0.45% sodium chloride) and fructose-electrolyte solution (Normosol-M).

Hypertonic fluids have a total osmolality that exceeds that of extracellular fluid. Commonly used hypertonic solutions include 5% dextrose in normal saline (0.9% sodium chloride), dextrose-electrolyte solution (Ionosol MB with 5% dextrose), and hypertonic saline (3% sodium chloride).

Infusion Pumps

A variety of infusion pumps are available to assist in the delivery of fluids and medications. Although these devices are helpful for delivering solutions at a controlled rate and volume, they do not eliminate the need for frequent monitoring of the infusion.

The *syringe infusion pump* is a small pump that may be worn by the patient and used to deliver a small volume of solution during a 24-hour period. This device monitors actual volume infused.

The *peristaltic infusion pump* is a large infusion pump with a sensor that attaches to any standard IV drip chamber. It regulates the rate of solution by exerting pressure on the IV tubing and monitors drops per minute infused.

The *piston infusion pump* is a large pump that controls solution flow rate by piston action. It monitors actual volume of fluid infused.

Supplies and Equipment

IV fluid as ordered by the physician
Venipuncture cannulas

The major types of cannulas used for IV infusion are the steel scalp vein needle (butterfly), indwelling plastic catheters inserted over a steel needle, and indwelling plastic catheters inserted through a sterile needle.

Tubing
Infusion pump

Potential Alterations in Functional Health Patterns

Nutritional-Metabolic Pattern

Diagnosis

High risk for impaired tissue integrity related to local infiltration of IV fluid

Definition

Presence of risk factors for the patient to experience infiltration of IV fluid into the interstitial spaces

Risk Factors

● Fragile venous condition due to age or coexisting disease.
● Disoriented or confused patient who may inadvertently dislodge the catheter

Expected Outcome

The patient's tissue integrity is maintained at the site of the IV infusion.

Perioperative Nursing Interventions

Preoperative

● Interview the patient or family members and assess for a history of infiltration or problems associated with IV infusion.
● Assess for disease that may alter vascular integrity.
● Select an optimal site for IV entry.

> Upper extremity veins are commonly used. Avoid the antecubital fossa, however, because flexion of the arm can impede the flow of the infusion. Select a site that does not impede mobility. Use of the patient's nondominant hand is preferred. Palpate the vein for elasticity and the absence of hard knots that may indicate thromboses.

Intraoperative

● Frequently inspect the infusion site for infiltration, swelling, redness, or coolness.
● If infiltration occurs, alert the physician. The infusion should be discontinued and restarted.
● Apply a warm, moist compress to the affected area.
● Explain to the patient what has occurred and provide support as needed.
● Record and report care and the patient's response to therapy.

Postoperative

● Report intraoperative events to the PACU or unit nurse.

- Determine the immediate response to interventions.

Diagnosis

High risk for fluid volume excess

Definition

Presence of risk factors for the patient to experience an increase in body fluid volume from the administration of IV fluids during the perioperative period.

Discussion. An increase in fluid volume can result when the patient is receiving IV fluid in the operating room. Fluid volume excess can occur and result in generalized fluid volume overload.

Hypervolemia occurs when the intravascular volume receives an excessive amount of IV fluid. If not corrected, hypervolemia can lead to congestive heart failure, which is manifested by dyspnea, neck vein distention, tachycardia, hypertension or hypotension, and cardiac ischemia. Hypervolemia can also lead to dependent edema. Laboratory findings may include a low hematocrit and low total protein count owing to dilution. The serum sodium level may be low or normal (Masiak et al., 1985, p. 48).

Risk Factors

- Rapid intake of excessive fluid or sodium

  The serum sodium level is a reflection of the osmolality of the blood. Homeostasis of osmolality is regulated by the relative proportions of water and salt in the extracellular fluid.

- Presence of congestive heart failure, chronic renal failure, or liver disease, resulting in sodium retention
- Stress of surgical intervention

  The endocrine response to stress includes the release of antidiuretic hormone and aldosterone. Antidiuretic hormone results in renal water reabsorption, thus decreasing osmolality of the blood. Aldosterone increases tubular reabsorption of sodium, thus expanding the extracellular volume.

- Cushing syndrome or corticosteroid therapy

  Cushing syndrome and corticosteroid therapy can cause extracellular volume excess and resultant edema. This may be due to the disease process or to the drugs used to treat the disease.

Expected Outcome

The patient's fluid volume is maintained. There are no signs of

- edema or effusion
- changes in mental status
- intake greater than output, oliguria, and specific gravity changes
- shortness of breath, dyspnea, and orthopnea
- abnormal breath sounds
- blood pressure, venous pressure, or pulmonary arterial pressure changes
- jugular venous distention
- hemoglobin and hematocrit decrease
- alteration in electrolytes (Gordon, 1987, p. 82)

Perioperative Nursing Interventions

Preoperative

- Conduct a nursing history and assess the patient for the presence of disease conditions that may put him or her at risk for volume overload.
- Assess baseline laboratory values.
- If the patient is at high risk for hypervolemia, use microdrip tubing and an infusion pump to assist in monitoring intake.
- Note the presence of edema, bounding pulse, distended neck veins, rales, dyspnea, orthopnea, elevated central venous pressure, and recent unexplained weight gain.

Intraoperative

- If symptoms of fluid excess develop, slow the rate of the infusion at once and alert the physician.
- Continue to monitor vital signs and report findings to the physician.
- Document findings on the intraoperative record.
- Measure and document urine and blood loss.
- Record and report patient care and response to therapy.

Postoperative

- Report intraoperative events to the PACU or unit nurse.
- Determine the immediate response to interventions.

Activity-Exercise Pattern

Diagnosis

High risk for decreased cardiac output related to air embolus from IV catheters

Definition

Presence of risk factors for the patient to experience alterations in cardiac output secondary to an air embolus from the IV catheter

Discussion. Air, when introduced into the circulation in large quantity, impedes the flow of blood and thus acts as an embolus. As a result of decreased blood flow, the patient becomes cyanotic, hypotensive, and unresponsive. Infusions given under pressure are far more likely to be associated with air embolism than are peripheral infusions delivered by gravity. In addition, infusions delivered by central catheters are more prone to air embolus formation.

Although small amounts of air are not hazardous, a volume of 50 ml can be lethal when delivered as a bolus.

A large air embolus in the right atrium or the right ventricle can cause an air lock that prevents returning blood from filling the right side of the heart. The result is a significant decrease in cardiac output, which can lead to hypotension and cardiac arrest.

Risk Factors

- Delivery of fluid under pressure
- Presence of a central IV catheter

Expected Outcome

The patient's cardiac output is maintained.

Perioperative Nursing Interventions

Preoperative

- Inspect the tubing for the presence of air.
- Flush air from the tubing before connecting it to the patient. Discontinue or replace the infusion before the container is empty.
- Ensure that all connections are tight.

Intraoperative

- Allow a loop of tubing to drop below the extremity as an added precaution against air embolus.
- If an air embolus is suspected, clamp the tubing, turn the patient onto the left side, and place the patient in the Trendelenburg position.

   These interventions keep the air in the right atrium, where it can be absorbed or removed through a central venous catheter.

- Administer oxygen if an air embolus is suspected and support the circulation with emergency medications as ordered by the physician.
- Record and report intraoperative events, patient care, and the patient's response to care.

Postoperative

- Report intraoperative events to the PACU or unit nurse.
- Determine the immediate response to interventions.

MONITORING OUTPUT

During surgery, the perioperative nurse monitors blood loss and urine output for patients at risk for fluid deficit. Monitoring activities include measuring blood loss and urine output from receptacles and weighing sponges.

Considerations

Factors That Affect Output

- Coexisting disease such as renal failure, neurogenic bladder, urinary retention or diabetes, which can alter normal urine output
- Clotting disorders or the presence of medications in the system that alter normal blood coagulation
- Extremes of age and weight
- Diarrhea
- Artificial urinary drainage system (cystostomy, peritoneal or renal dialysis, ureteral stents)
- Type of surgical procedure, its length and location, and the size of the incision
- Trauma
- Use of blood, blood products, IV fluids, and volume expanders

Supplies and Equipment

Suction tubing and containers
Sponges
Graduated measuring devices
Sterile skin marker and paper for recording the amount of irrigation used

Potential Alterations in Functional Health Patterns

Nutritional-Metabolic Pattern

Diagnosis

High risk for fluid volume deficit related to intraoperative bleeding

Definition

Presence of risk factors for the patient to experience significant fluid loss during the intraoperative period owing to hemorrhaging

Discussion. Intraoperative bleeding, if not controlled, can have dire consequences for the patient. The perioperative nurse remains alert for the possibility of bleeding and is prepared to take actions necessary to determine the extent of blood and other fluid loss.

The type and amount of bleeding depends on the type of vessels involved. Capillary hemorrhage is characterized by a slow, general ooze. Venous hemorrhage bubbles out quickly and is dark in color. Arterial hemorrhage is bright red in color and spurts out with each heart beat.

Hypovolemic shock results in a decreased fluid volume owing to loss of blood, plasma, or water. Hypovolemia is characterized by a fall in venous pressure, a rise in peripheral resistance, and tachycardia. Classic signs of shock include pallor; cool, moist skin; restlessness; rapid breathing; cyanosis of the lips, eyelids, and gums; weak, thready pulse; small pulse pressure; lowering of blood pressure and oliguria; concentrated urine; and anuria.

Patients undergoing procedures with local anesthesia monitored solely by the perioperative nurse are not immune from experiencing excessive intraoperative bleeding. Procedures such as hair transplants, facial reconstruction, and excision of scalp lesions are prone to result in bleeding owing to the vascularity of the operative site. Additionally, blood may be lost when excisions of lesions thought to be small or superficial become more extensive than anticipated or involve the dissection of major blood vessels.

Risk Factors

- Type of surgery, the location of the incision, and the duration of the procedure predisposing to bleeding
- Preexisting bleeding disorders and coexisting disease
- Trauma
- Presence of anticoagulant medications in the patient's system (e.g., aspirin, heparin, or warfarin sodium)

Expected Outcome

The patient's fluid volume is maintained during the intraoperative period.

Perioperative Nursing Interventions

Preoperative

- Conduct an assessment and evaluate for the presence of disease, bleeding or clotting disorders, or medications that may influence blood loss during surgery.
- Assess for the presence of fluid deficit by evaluation of the nutritional status and skin turgor and auscultation of lung field for abnormal breath sounds. Note the presence of medications that may alter fluid balance (IV fluids, bowel preparations, and diuretics).
- Note a family history of bleeding or clotting disorders.
- Start an IV infusion to provide access to the circulatory system.
- Monitor vital signs.

Intraoperative

- Prepare and administer IV fluids as needed.
- Insert an indwelling urinary catheter, depending on the patient's fluid status, the anticipated length of the procedure, and the anticipated amount of blood loss.

  Urine output is one of the most valuable indexes of adequacy of renal perfusion. A drop in renal arterial pressure and flow produces renal arterial vasoconstriction and results in decreased glomerular filtration and decreased urine output. Normal urine flow is 50 ml/hour. An output of 0.5 ml/kg/hour is suggestive of inadequate volume replacement or cardiac failure.

- Monitor blood loss and the amount of irrigation solution used. Use warm, moistened sponges to prevent tissue from becoming dry and from losing heat via evaporation and convection.
- If the patient is awake, provide psychosocial support during the procedure by using touch, conver-

sation, and measures to distract the patient. Keep blood-soaked sponges and soiled instruments and supplies out of the patient's visual field.

- If hypotension occurs, place the patient in the Trendelenburg position.
- Administer oxygen, fluids, and medications as needed.
- Call for emergency assistance if needed.
- Inspect the wound for a bleeding site if it has not already been located.
- Continue to monitor vital signs.
- Monitor blood loss via suction and saturation of sponges. Weigh sponges as needed.
- Record the type and amount of irrigation fluid used during the procedure.
- Record and report intraoperative care and response to therapy.

Postoperative

- Report intraoperative events to the PACU or unit nurse. Communicate estimated blood loss, amount of IV fluid infused, the number or units of blood or blood products transfused, and the presence of drains and catheters.
- Determine the immediate response to interventions.

MONITORING BODY TEMPERATURE

The perioperative nurse monitors body temperature to determine the extent of heat production and heat loss.

Considerations

Factors That Affect Body Temperature

- Hypothalamus

  Body temperature is controlled by the hypothalamus, which acts as the body's thermostat. The anterior hypothalamus controls heat dissipation, and the posterior hypothalamus controls heat conservation. Illness or trauma to these centers can alter temperature control.

- Age and weight
- Activity level

  Inactivity decreases the temperature, whereas vigorous activity may cause an increase.

- Metabolic rate

  Increases in metabolic rate, as seen with malignant hyperthermia, thyroid disease, or imbalances of hormonal production, may alter temperature. Heat production is increased by the body's secretions of epinephrine, norepinephrine, and thyroxine. Production of these hormones can be influenced by the stressors associated with surgery.

- Radiation, convection, evaporation, and conduction

  As much as 95% of the body's heat is lost through radiation, convection, and evaporation of water through the lungs and the skin. *Radiation* is the dissemination of heat through electromagnetic waves. *Convection* is the dissemination of heat by motion between areas of unequal density, such as from the body to cool water in a swimming pool. *Evaporation* is the conversion of liquid to vapor, as in the evaporation of perspiration. *Conduction* is the transfer of heat to another object by direct contract as occurs with the use of a cooling blanket. Heat is lost in small amounts through the feces and urine (Wolff et al., 1983, p. 323).

A decrease in body temperature triggers a series of responses, including sympathetic activation, catecholamine release, vasoconstriction, shivering, and thermogenesis (Miller, 1986, p. 1995). Piloerection, the contracture of smooth muscles, and shivering, the involuntary movement of skeletal muscles, produce body heat by increasing metabolism and conserving heat by constricting superficial vessels in the skin. Exposure to cold environments results in heat loss through convection and conduction. Sedation decreases the metabolic rate, causing a drop in temperature. Medications causing vasoconstriction or vasodilation influence heat loss and conservation. When blood vessels are dilated, heat is lost through the skin. When vessels are contracted, heat is conserved.

Supplies and Equipment

Thermometer (conventional, electronic, or temperature-sensitive patch or tape)
Warm blankets
Fluid warmer
Hyperthermia or hypothermia blanket and machine

Potential Alterations in Functional Health Patterns

Nutritional-Metabolic Pattern

Diagnosis

High risk for hypothermia

Definition

Presence of risk factors for the patient to experience a decrease in body temperature during the intraoperative period

Discussion. The surgical patient is at risk for the development of hypothermia. The cool ambient temperature of the operating room, the use of cool fluids for irrigation or IV infusion, a prolonged duration of surgery, and the exposure of internal organs or body cavities can precipitate a drop in core temperature. Other causes include loss of temperature-sensing and temperature-regulating mechanisms (hypothalamic anesthesia), loss of shivering ability, decreased metabolism and free heat production, ventilation with dry gases (evaporation loss), skin vasodilation, and losses due to evaporation, convection, and radiation from the wound.

The awake patient may respond with apathy, confusion, or drowsiness. The patient with hypothermia may also exhibit arrhythmias, ventricular irritability, increased bleeding tendency and changes in arterial blood gas values, alteration in acid-base balance, and increase in heart rate, stroke volume, arterial blood pressure, cardiac output, and oxygen consumption (Luckmann and Sorenson, 1987, p. 550).

Risk Factors

- Trauma
- Exposure of internal organs and body cavities
- Extreme in age

  Children less than 3 months of age are at particular risk because hypothermia can induce reopening of fetal circulation, with resultant acidosis and hypoxemia, which becomes a circular pattern of events that is difficult to reverse.

- Malnutrition
- Inactivity
- Sedation
- Decreased metabolism
- Use of cool fluids for irrigation and infusion

Expected Outcome

The patient maintains a normal body temperature during the perioperative period.

Perioperative Nursing Interventions

Preoperative

- Interview the patient and family members to assess for factors that may put the patient at risk for hypothermia.
- Wrap the patient in warm sheets or blankets, if needed, while he or she is in the surgical suite holding area.
- Note the preoperative temperature.

Intraoperative

- Monitor the patient's temperature and assess physiological changes.

  Body metabolism is reduced by almost 50% when body temperature is reduced to 86°F (60°C), and is reduced to 25% of normal if temperature reaches 68°F (20°C). Endocrine, liver, and kidney functions decrease as the rate of metabolism decreases (Luckmann and Sorenson, 1987, p. 550).

- Use measures to maintain comfort and warmth.
  1. Increase the ambient temperature of the room.
  2. Provide surface warming with a heating blanket.
  3. Wrap the patient in warm blankets.
  4. Wrap limbs in stockinet, elastic (Ace) wraps, or webril.
  5. Use warm IV fluids or blood products.
  6. Humidify inspired gases and oxygen.
- Monitor vital signs and note changes in the electrocardiogram, blood pressure, arterial blood gas values, and blood chemistry values.

  The critical level below which arrhythmias result from altered myocardial irritability varies with the degree of hypothermia and the patient's age and condition. The volume of circulating blood is reduced as plasma pools in peripheral capillary beds. Cardiac rate decreases as the heart's neuromuscular tissue is affected by the reduced temperature. Oxygen consumption is reduced and respiratory rate and blood pressure also fall.

- Monitor a change in the behavior in the awake patient.

  Hypothermia may result in a decrease in venous and intracranial pressure. In addition, for every degree centigrade reduction in temperature, cerebral blood flow is reduced about 6% and cerebral function is diminished.

- If body temperature drops below the desired level, rewarm the patient as needed. If the temperature is greater than 35°C, passive rewarming is preferred to active rewarming, because the latter method may result in hyperthermia. Warming methods include
  1. internal surface warming with warm saline, moist sponges, and warm IV fluids
  2. external surface warming using a warming blanket, warm sheets, and external packs
- Be prepared for emergency measures, which may include
  1. cardiac massage (external or internal)
  2. mechanical ventilation
  3. infusion of IV fluids and blood products
  4. cardioversion for ventricular fibrillation
  5. use of antiarrhythmic drugs
  6. insertion of an indwelling catheter to monitor fluid status
- Record and report intraoperative findings and care activities.

Postoperative

- Report intraoperative events to the PACU or unit nurse.
- Determine the immediate response to interventions.
- Alert the PACU or unit staff to the need for special warming equipment and medications. A number of

medications may be used to suppress shivering, including nondepolarizing muscle relaxants in the intubated patient, chlorpromazine, droperidol, magnesium sulfate, and methylphenidate (Miller, 1986, p. 2014).

Diagnosis

High risk for hyperthermia

Definition

Presence of risk factors for the patient to experience an increase in body temperature during the intraoperative period

Discussion. The patient's ability to maintain normal body temperature may be influenced by the use of copious amounts of warm irrigating solutions, the application of impervious surgical drapes, the use of internal or external warming techniques, the use of medications such as vasoconstrictors, and the stress associated with surgery. Malignant hyperthermia that is associated with general anesthesia is discussed in Chapter 19.

Damage to the hypothalamus or severe intracranial infection may result in hyperthermia in the patient with neurological disease or the patient undergoing neurosurgery. Such temperature elevations must be controlled, because the increased metabolic demands by the brain stress the circulation and oxygenation of the brain. Persistent hyperthermia is indicative of brain stem damage. Intraventricular blood can also cause temperature elevations.

The patient with hyperthermia may complain of headache, thirst, general malaise, and palpitations. Overt signs can include increased body temperature, flushed skin, warm skin, increased respirations, tachycardia, seizures, and convulsion.

Risk Factors

- Dehydration
- Illness resulting in fever
- Use of warm fluids for irrigation and infusion
- Use of medication causing vasoconstriction
- Endocrine disorders such as thyroid disease
- Intracranial infection or injury to the hypothalamus

Expected Outcome

The patient maintains a normal body temperature during the perioperative period.

Perioperative Nursing Interventions

Preoperative

- Interview the patient and family members and assess for factors that may put the patient at risk for hyperthermia.
- Note the presence of fever, infection, or diseases associated with hyperthermia.

Intraoperative

- Use a thermometer to monitor the patient's temperature and assess changes as needed.
- Maintain the patient's comfort and normal body temperature by removing excessive drapes as needed.
- Cool the patient's skin with alcohol or cool water as needed.
- Monitor vital signs and note changes in the electrocardiogram, blood pressure, arterial blood gas values, and blood chemistry values.
- If body temperature increases, use a cooling blanket as needed. Be prepared for emergency measures, including the use of oxygen, the infusion of cool IV fluids, the use of emergency medications, the use of antiarrhythmic drugs, and the insertion of indwelling urinary catheter to monitor fluid status.
- Record and report intraoperative findings and care activities.

Postoperative

- Report intraoperative events to the PACU or unit nurse.
- Determine the immediate response to interventions.
- Alert the staff of the need for special equipment or medications (e.g., antibiotics and antipyretics).

MONITORING THE EFFECTS OF LOCAL ANESTHESIA

Monitoring the patient who is receiving local anesthesia, analgesia, and sedation consists of constant vigilance for patient reactions to external and internal stressors.

Considerations

Factors That Affect the Patient Receiving a Local Anesthetic

- Local anesthetic agents, analgesics, and sedatives may cause hypersensitivity reactions, cardiovascular depression, respiratory depression, central nervous system depression, and toxicity.
- Before monitoring a patient receiving local anesthesia, the perioperative nurse must understand the mechanism of action of the agents that are being used. Depending on their chemical structure, local anesthetic agents are placed into two categories: amino esters and amino amides. Both groups block depolarization of the nerve cell membrane by inhibiting sodium conduction across the membrane. The amino esters are broken down by the enzyme pseudocholinesterase. A product of this breakdown is *p*-aminobenzoic acid. About 1% of patients have

an allergic reaction to this metabolite. Amino amides are metabolized by hepatic enzymes. Patients with hepatic disease may have ineffective metabolism, which may result in toxic responses, even with normal doses. For further information, refer to Chapter 9.
- Surgery itself may result in stress by combining fear and anxiety with factors such as pain and blood loss. In addition, the anesthetic agent itself, surgical manipulation, conversation of the perioperative staff, or attitudes and values conveyed by the body language and expressions of the surgical team can lead to patient stress. Some patients, because of age or certain physiological and psychological factors, are not candidates for local anesthesia with monitoring by the perioperative nurse.

Standards of Care

The perioperative nursing department in conjunction with the departments of surgery and anesthesia is responsible for the development of standards of care for the patient receiving local anesthesia. Essential considerations include recommended practices set by the Association of Operating Room Nurses, the American Society of Anesthesiologists, and the Joint Commission on the Accreditation of Healthcare Organizations. Other considerations include the level of patient function, the presence of preexisting diseases, the type and duration of the procedure, the amount of sedation required, and the extent of monitoring required.

Supplies and Equipment

Local anesthetic agents
Marker and labels to identify the anesthetic agent on the sterile field
IV therapy supplies and equipment
Blood pressure monitor
Electrocardiographic monitor
Pulse oximeter
Emergency supplies
    Oxygen with self-inflating bag and mask
    Endotracheal tube and laryngoscope
    Medications such as diazepam or ultrashort-acting barbiturates such as sodium thiopental, methohexital (Brevital) sodium
    Resuscitative agents

Potential Alterations in Functional Health Patterns

Allergic and toxic reactions, although not common, are nevertheless serious complications that a patient might experience when receiving a local anesthetic. For a discussion concerning the patient's risk of allergic and toxic reactions to local anesthetics, see Chapter 9.

Nutritional-Metabolic Pattern

Diagnosis

High risk for impaired tissue integrity related to extravasation of IV medication

Definition

Presence of risk factors for the patient to experience injury to subcutaneous tissue owing to extravasation of the medications and IV solutions

Discussion. Tissue can be impaired by infiltration and/or extravasation of IV medications into the subcutaneous tissue. Local reaction can include burning, tissue irritation, tissue necrosis, skin discoloration, hives, hive-like elevations, swelling, burning, warmth or coldness at the injection site, rash, and pruritus.

Risk Factors

- Elderly patients or debilitated individuals with poor venous access

Expected Outcome

The patient is free from tissue damage related to subcutaneous infiltration of medications and IV fluids.

Perioperative Nursing Interventions

Preoperative

- Assess the patient for a history of a local reaction to IV medication.
- Ensure that the IV catheter is patent and flowing before the administration of medication.

Intraoperative

- Consult accompanying drug information and related literature before the administration of medication.
- Administer diazepam (Valium).
  1. Do not mix or dilute with other drugs or solutions in the same syringe or container.
  2. Inject slowly taking at least 1 minute for each 5 mg (1 ml) given to adults, and taking 3 minutes to inject 0.25 mg/kg of body weight for children.
  3. Avoid using small veins for diazepam administration.
- Administer midazolam hydrochloride (Versed).
  1. Midazolam injection is compatible with 5% dextrose in water, 0.9% sodium chloride, and lactated Ringer solution.
  2. When used for sedation, the perioperative nurse must individualize and titrate the dose. Do not administer midazolam hydrochloride by rapid or single-bolus IV administration. The patient's response varies with age, physical status, and concomitant medication.
- Communicate and record the type of medication administered, the dose, the route, the time of administration, and any local reaction to IV medication.

Postoperative

- Report intraoperative events to the PACU or unit nurse.
- Determine the immediate response to interventions.
- Assess postoperative response to local anesthetic agent.

Activity-Exercise Pattern

Diagnosis

High risk for decreased cardiac output (cardiodepression) related to the administration of local anesthetics

Definition

Presence of risk factors for the patient to experience cardiodepression during the administration of a local anesthetic

Discussion. A hypotensive reaction may occur as a toxic response to a local anesthetic. Blood pressure may fall gradually or abruptly. The patient may show pallor and report feeling faint and dizzy. Tachycardia may occur, followed by bradycardia, cardiovascular collapse, and cardiac arrest.

Risk Factors

- Patient receiving cardiodepressant medications

  Local anesthetics can increase the effect of these medications. When given in conjunction with tricyclic antidepressants, monoamine oxidase inhibitors, and pressor medications, local anesthetics can increase blood pressure.

- Local anesthetics with epinephrine
- Heart block or other cardiac disease

Expected Outcome

The patient's cardiac output is maintained during the surgical procedure. There are no signs or reports of

- gradual or abrupt hypotension
- pallor
- feeling faint or dizzy
- tachycardia
- bradycardia

Perioperative Nursing Interventions

Preoperative

- Assess the patient for cardiac disease or the presence of risk factors for cardiac disease. Note drug allergies.
- Establish physiological baseline values to assess cardiac function during the procedure.

Intraoperative

- Monitor the patient. Evaluate

  blood pressure
  heart rate and rhythm
  respiratory rate
  oxygen saturation
  skin condition
  mental status
  emotional response to surgery and anesthesia

- Record and report findings.
- Document at 5-minute intervals and at any significant event.
- Document the dosage, the route and time of administration, and the effect of medications administered, oxygen therapy, and IV therapy and the patient's response to the surgery and anesthesia.

Postoperative

- Report intraoperative events to the PACU or unit nurse.
- Determine the immediate response to interventions.

Diagnosis

High risk for ineffective breathing pattern related to IV sedation

Definition

Presence of risk factors for the patient to experience sedative-induced breathing difficulty

Discussion. The patient may be provided with sedation, analgesia, relaxation, and amnesia through the use of a combination of medications from a variety of chemical classes. Commonly used agents include tranquilizers, such as diazepam and midazolam; neuroleptics, such as droperidol; narcotic analgesics, such as fentanyl, morphine, and meperidine; and dissociative anesthetics, such as ketamine.

The use of IV medications in combination with local anesthesia is preferred for many minor surgical procedures. Central nervous system depression caused by the depressant drugs may lead to hypoxia, hypercapnia, and respiratory failure resulting from diminished sensitivity of the respiratory center to carbon dioxide. Careful calculation and administration, as well as vigilant monitoring, are necessary. Overdose can result in laryngospasm, bronchospasm, dyspnea, hyperventilation, wheezing, shallow respirations, airway obstruction, tachypnea, or respiratory arrest.

Risk Factors

- Respiratory disorders such as emphysema, asthma, pneumonia, pulmonary tumor, and chronic obstructive pulmonary disease
- Conditions that interfere with normal breathing patterns such as obesity, third trimester of pregnancy, and neuromuscular disorders
- Liver disease that interferes with the metabolism of sedatives and narcotics

Expected Outcome

The patient's breathing patterns are maintained during the surgical procedure. There are no signs of

- wheezing
- shallow respirations
- dyspnea
- hyperventilation
- tachypnea
- airway obstruction
- laryngospasm
- bronchospasm

Perioperative Nursing Interventions

Preoperative

- Assess the patient for a history of sensitivity to sedatives and narcotics.
- Assess for signs of pulmonary dysfunction: dyspnea, tachypnea, orthopnea, skin color changes, absence or diminished breath sounds, rhonchi, wheezing, or rales.
- Establish physiological baseline values to assess respiratory function during the procedure.
- Note the patient's weight and calculate the maximal dosage.
- Note reports of respiratory status tests (chest x-ray films, pulmonary function tests).

Intraoperative

- Position the patient to facilitate breathing. Elevate the head and ensure that drapes and equipment are kept off the chest, if possible.
- As ordered by the physician, provide humidified oxygen at the desired rate (liters per minute).
- Monitor the patient. Evaluate

  blood pressure
  heart rate and rhythm
  respiratory rate
  oxygen saturation
  skin condition
  mental status
  emotional response to surgery and anesthesia

- Record and report findings.
- Document at 5-minute intervals and at any significant event.
- Document the dosage, the route and time of administration, and the effect of medications administered, oxygen therapy, and IV therapy and the patient's response to the surgery and anesthesia.

Postoperative

- Report intraoperative events to the PACU or unit nurse.
- Determine the immediate response to interventions.

SUMMARY

The perioperative nurse is constantly challenged to meet the physiological monitoring needs of the patient during all surgical procedures. Depending on the type of anesthesia administered, the perioperative nurse may assist the anesthetist in monitoring, or become the caregiver responsible for total monitoring of the patient. Potential problems associated with airway maintenance, bleeding, fluid balance, body temperature, and the use of anesthetic agents can develop into life-threatening events. The perioperative nurse must be constantly aware of stressors that may alter the patient's health status during surgery. Prompt action must be taken to prevent or correct problems as they occur. The patient's responses must be documented in the patient's record and communicated to appropriate caregivers.

Bibliography

Covoni, B., Vassallo, H. (1976). *Local anesthetics: Mechanisms of action and clinical use*. New York: Grune & Stratton.

Cousins, M., Bridenbaugh, P. (1980). *Neural blockade in clinical anesthesia and management of pain*. Philadelphia: J. B. Lippincott.

Gordon, M. (1987). *Manual of nursing diagnosis, 1986–1987*. New York: McGraw-Hill.

Luckmann, J., Sorenson, K. C. (1987). *Medical-surgical nursing: A psychophysiologic approach*. (3rd ed.). Philadelphia: W. B. Saunders.

Masiak, M. J., Naylor, M. D., Hayman, L. L. (1985). *Fluid and electrolytes throughout the life cycle*. East Norwalt, CT: Appleton-Century-Crofts.

Miller, R. D. (1986). *Anesthesia* (2nd ed.). New York: Churchill Livingstone.

Wolff, L., Weitzel, M. H., Zornow, R. A., Zsohar, H. (1983). *Fundamentals of nursing* (7th ed.). Philadelphia: J. B. Lippincott.

CHAPTER 11

Monitoring and Controlling the Environment

Leana Revell

DEFINITION

Monitoring and controlling the environment refers to those activities performed by the perioperative nurse that promote the safety and well-being of the patient during surgery. The perioperative nurse protects the patient from hazards within the environment and provides an environment that promotes infection control.

MEASURABLE CRITERIA

The perioperative nurse demonstrates competency to monitor and control the environment by

- regulating temperature and humidity
- ensuring electrical safety
- monitoring the sensory environment
- ensuring radiation safety
- maintaining surgical suite traffic patterns
- performing operating room (OR) sanitation
- sterilizing instruments, supplies, and equipment (AORN, 1992)

ROLE OF THE PERIOPERATIVE NURSE

The perioperative nurse implements the measurable criteria. With appropriate supervision, assignment of these tasks to qualified assistive personnel is permissible. If an assistive person helps the perioperative nurse accomplish the measurable criteria, however, the nurse remains accountable.

OUTCOME STANDARD

The patient is free from injury related to environmental hazards.

Criteria

The patient demonstrates no evidence of

- alterations in temperature
- electrical injury

245

- radiation injury
- nosocomial infection
- fear

POTENTIAL ALTERATIONS IN FUNCTIONAL HEALTH PATTERNS

Health Perception–Health Management Pattern

Diagnosis

High risk for injury related to the use of electrical equipment

Definition

Presence of risk factors for the patient to experience shock, cardiac fibrillation, or burns from electrical current flowing through the patient's body to the ground, related to the use of electrical equipment during surgery

Risk Factors (Association of Operating Room Nurses [AORN], 1992, *III*:5–2, 7–4)

- Excessive hair
- Scar tissue
- Internal or external metal prosthetic devices
- Impaired skin or tissue integrity, bony prominences, or impaired tissue perfusion at site of dispersive electrode or electrocardiographic lead placement
- Pacemakers
- Frayed or damaged power cords
- Damaged outlets
- Malfunctioning isolated power system

Expected Outcome

The patient is free from electrical equipment–related injury during the perioperative period. There is no evidence of

- impaired skin and tissue integrity
- altered tissue perfusion
- altered cardiac output
- impaired neurological function

Diagnosis

High risk for injury related to ionizing radiation exposure

Definition

Presence of risk factors for the patient to experience injury from exposure to ionizing radiation

Risk Factors

- Fluoroscopy
- Multiple x-ray films during surgery
- Pregnancy

Expected Outcome

The patient is free from injury related to ionizing radiation. There is no evidence of

- fetal exposure
- tissue trauma (burns)
- anemia
- sterility

Diagnosis

High risk for injury related to nonionizing radiation exposure

Definition

Presence of risk factors for the patient to experience impaired skin and tissue integrity from exposure to laser beams

Risk Factors

- Unprotected eyes during laser use
- Aberrant and reflected laser beams
- Plume and noxious fumes
- Use of flammable or combustible anesthetics, preparation solutions, drying agents, ointments, plastic resins, or plastics

Expected Outcome

The patient is free from injury related to nonionizing radiation. There is no evidence of

- retinal trauma
- impaired tissue integrity
- impaired skin integrity
- respiratory difficulty related to breathing laser plume or noxious odors

Diagnosis

High risk for infection

Definition

Presence of risk factors for the patient to experience a nosocomial infection secondary to exposure to the surgical environment

Risk Factors (Gordon, 1987, p. 50)

- Surgical intervention that alters tissue and skin integrity

- Inadequate secondary defenses (e.g., decreased hemoglobin concentration, leukopenia, suppressed inflammatory response, and immunosuppression)
- Inadequate acquired immunity (e.g., acquired immunodeficiency syndrome)
- Chronic disease leading to suppressed immunity (e.g., lupus erythematosus)
- Invasive drains and monitors (intravenous catheters, hyperalimentation catheters, nasogastric tubes, Foley catheters, chest tubes)
- Malnutrition that interferes with tissue repair
- Blood abnormalities such as sickle cell anemia, thrombocytopenia, and thalassemia
- Impaired tissue perfusion
- High white blood cell count, low platelet count, and anemia
- Impaired skin integrity
- Impaired tissue integrity
- Failure of sterilization or disinfection processes
- Nonadherence to surgical suite traffic patterns
- Failure of environmental sanitation processes

Expected Outcome

The patient is free from nosocomial infection after surgery. There is no evidence of

- wound infection
- urinary tract infection
- upper respiratory tract infection

Nutritional-Metabolic Pattern

Diagnosis

High risk for altered body temperature

Definition

Presence of risk factors for the patient to experience environment-induced hyperthermia or hypothermia while in the surgical suite

Risk Factors (AORN, 1992, III:7–23)

- General or regional anesthesia
- Excessive sedation, especially in the patient receiving local anesthetia
- Evaporative or conductive heat loss from prepared skin areas
- Use of unwarmed infusion or irrigating solutions
- Ambient room temperature and humidity
- Surgical exposure of the abdominal or thoracic cavities
- Preexisting medical conditions (e.g., hypothyroid or hyperthyroid problems)
- Extremes in age, particularly infant, small child, and geriatric patients

- Decreased body fat for insulation
- Malnourishment
- Debilitated or chronically ill patients
- Anticipated long operative time
- Intracranial surgery

Expected Outcome

Depending on anesthetic technique and level of consciousness, the patient is free from environment-related alterations in body temperature during the perioperative period. There is no evidence of

- hyperthermia: verbal complaint of feeling uncomfortably warm (for a conscious patient), elevated body temperature, perspiration, tachycardia, warm skin, flushed skin, increased respiratory rate, and seizures or convulsions
- hypothermia: verbal complaint of feeling uncomfortably cold (for a conscious patient), shivering, chattering of teeth, cool skin, and decreased pulse and respiration rate (Gordon, 1987, pp. 98–100)

Self-perception–Self-concept Pattern

Diagnosis

Fear

Definition

Presence of risk factors for the patient to experience a feeling of dread related to the impending surgery
The patient perceives surgery as a threat or danger to the self (Gordon, 1987, p. 198).

Risk Factors

- Knowledge deficit concerning the anticipated surgical environment
- Perceived powerlessness to control events
- History of a previous difficult surgical experience

Expected Outcome

The patient is free from fear related to impending surgery. There is no evidence of

- restlessness
- voice tremors or pitch changes
- increased verbalization (quantity and rate)
- hand tremor
- increased muscle tension
- narrowing focus of attention progressing to a fixed focus
- diaphoresis
- increased heart rate
- increased respiratory rate (Gordon, 1987, p. 198)

PERIOPERATIVE NURSING INTERVENTIONS

Regulating Temperature and Humidity

The perioperative nurse is responsible for monitoring room temperature and humidity levels. A relative humidity of 50 to 60% inhibits bacterial growth and decreases the potential for static electricity. Room temperatures of 68 to 76°F also inhibit bacterial growth. Although comfortable for staff dressed in sterile attire, these temperatures are potentially hazardous for the compromised patient, particularly geriatric and pediatric patients. Consequently, it is necessary for the perioperative nurse to monitor and control not only the environmental temperature and humidity, but also the temperature of the patient. The supplies and equipment needed for regulating temperature and humidity are room temperature– and humidity-monitoring devices, overhead warming units, heat conduction lamps, cooling or warming blankets, blood warmers, thermal body drapes, cloth blankets, warming cabinets for solutions and blankets, and patient temperature–monitoring devices, which may be esophageal, urinary bladder, axillary, rectal, or tympanic.

Monitoring the Temperature and Humidity of the Operating Room

Before starting the first case of the day, the perioperative nurse should take a baseline reading of the OR temperature and humidity level. The temperature should range between 68 and 76°F. The humidity level should range between 50 and 60%. Report variations of these ranges to the OR manager. Except in extenuating circumstances, such as an emergency situation or when the room temperature is raised to accommodate a patient at risk for alteration in body temperature, avoid using ORs that do not adhere to these ranges. A room temperature and humidity level that varies from the norm may contribute to alterations in patient body temperature. Likewise, an elevated room temperature or humidity level is uncomfortable, as well as stressful, for the surgical team, especially those who are gowned and gloved. Exceptionally low temperature and humidity ranges may also cause discomfort and stress to the surgical team.

Assessing the Need for Devices to Monitor and/or Control the Patient's Temperature

The perioperative nurse should consider the following factors when assessing the patient for temperature monitoring and/or control devices:

- the patient's age
- the patient's physical status
- type of anesthesia planned
- ambient room temperature
- length and type of surgical procedure (AORN, 1992, III:7–2)

Monitoring the Temperature of the Patient

A thermometer with an appropriate esophageal, urinary bladder, tympanic, axillary, or rectal probe is used to monitor patients at risk for experiencing intraoperative alterations in body temperature. Before using the thermometer, test it to ensure that it is in working order. Testing procedures are usually found in the manufacturer's instructions. After obtaining the desired probe, carefully insert it into the appropriate orifice. Probes are best inserted after the patient is anesthetized because insertion is usually easier, the patient's dignity and comfort are not compromised, and adverse affects, such as vagal stimulation with the rectal probe, are avoided. When placing the rectal probe in the adult patient, insert it 1 to 2 inches within the rectum. For the infant, insert the probe no more than 1 inch. Gently insert tympanic membrane probes. Aggressive insertion can cause perforation of the tympanic membrane. After inserting a probe, tape it into place to avoid inadvertent removal during the procedure.

Conserving the Patient's Body Heat

Preventing heat loss through evaporation, radiation, convection, and conduction is essential when protecting the patient's body temperature. When the skin becomes wet, the body loses heat through evaporation. Radiation heat loss occurs when heat is transferred from the body surface to another surface. Air currents passing over the exposed skin cause heat loss by convection. Conduction heat loss occurs when the patient is in contact with cold or damp materials such as a wet sheet (Atkinson and Kohn, 1986, p. 592). Conserve the patient's body heat by covering the patient with warm blankets; exposing only the operative area; decreasing air currents by keeping the OR doors closed and limiting movement within the OR; warming preparation solutions, intravenous infusions, blood, and irrigating solutions; moistening sponges with warm saline before handing them to the surgeon; keeping OR bed linens dry; and blotting the patient's skin dry after the skin preparation.

Alternative Methods of Temperature Regulation

Thermoregulation devices such as warming or cooling blankets and heat lamps provide an external source of heat. Provide these devices for patients identified as at high risk for alterations in body temperature. Chapter 8 describes the use of thermoregulation devices.

Neonates

Because of an incompletely developed thermoregulatory mechanism and a thin layer of insulating subcutaneous fat, neonates, particularly the premature, have a wider average range of body temperature (97–100°F). Temperature begins to stabilize, however, during the first 12 to 24 hours after birth, if the environment is controlled (Atkinson and Kohn, 1986, p. 592). Consequently, the neonate, especially during the first 24 hours of life, is at risk for experiencing an intraoperative alteration in body temperature. Conserve the neonate's body heat by covering the head with a stockinet cap, encasing the extremities in stockinet, or wrapping the extremities with webril or plastic wrap. Warming blankets and heat lamps are good sources of external heat. The perioperative nurse, however, should exercise caution when employing these devices because the thin layer of subcutaneous fat places the neonate at risk for experiencing a thermal injury. Keeping the neonate in an isolette and dressed before and immediately after the procedure also helps to conserve the patient's body heat.

Documenting Procedures

Document the use of thermoregulation devices (e.g., the use of hyperthermia or hypothermia blankets, the wrapping of extremities, and the application of blankets) and skin conditions before and after the procedure. Record a baseline patient temperature. This helps in the detection of malignant hyperthermia and overheating from auxiliary heating equipment.

Ensuring Electrical Safety

The expanding inventory of electrical equipment within the surgical environment increases the possibility that the patient and staff experience an injury related to electrical hazard. Implementation of appropriate nursing interventions and continuous observation for potential electrical hazards by the perioperative nurse, however, ensure electrical safety within the OR.

Monitoring Isolated Power Systems for Effectiveness

An OR, as a hazardous area, has an isolated power system that prevents accidental grounding of persons in contact with a hot wire (Fig. 11–1). The isolated power system continually monitors for current leaks and grounding and thus reduces the hazard of shock, cardiac fibrillation, or burns from electrical current flowing through the patient's body to ground (AORN, 1992, III:7–4).

The system uses an isolation transformer to isolate OR electrical circuits from the grounded circuits in the

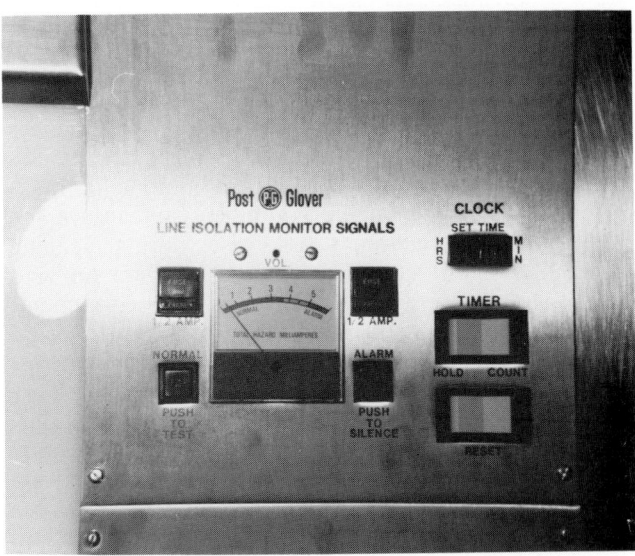

FIGURE 11–1. Isolated power system used for the OR.

power mains. Consequently, the electrical current seeks to flow only from one isolated line to the other, thus preventing accidental grounding.

A line isolation monitor measures resistance and capacitance between the two isolated lines and ground. If an inadvertent grounding of the isolated circuits occurs, the monitor sounds an alarm. If the isolated power system is functional, the alarm sounds only when faulty equipment is plugged into ungrounded circuits. In such a case, the perioperative nurse should shut off and unplug the last electrical device plugged into the electrical system. If the warning system alarm light remains lit, unplug electrical equipment until the defective device is identified. After it is found, send the defective device to the bioengineering department for repair.

Providing Safe Electrical Equipment

All electrical equipment, including the surgeon's personal equipment, must meet hospital performance and safety standards. Responsibility for ensuring that electrical equipment is safe rests with the OR manager. Routine inspections at least every 6 months to check for defects and scheduled preventive maintenance in accordance with manufacturer's recommendations prolong equipment life and enhance patient safety.

Before using electrical equipment for patient care, inspect the equipment for frayed cords, loose wires, and lack of secure connections. Test the electrical units before use for functioning audio alarms and lights. Check outlets and switch plates for damage (AORN, 1992, III:7–4). Do not use equipment that requires unusually high power settings to function. Turn this equipment in for repair. Test electrical adapters for tightness to ensure a secure connection. If necessary, replace the adapter.

Implementing Electrical Safety Practices

Electrical equipment is only as safe as the practices employed by the operator. Do not place receptacles containing liquid on top of electrical equipment. Inadvertent spills may ruin the equipment and injure the patient and staff members. Likewise, during cleaning procedures, avoid saturating electrical equipment with liquid. Do not spray liquid directly onto equipment; clean with a damp cloth. During the procedure, ensure that foot pedals that activate electrical equipment remain dry. Do not roll heavy equipment (beds, x-ray machines) over electrical cords. Position equipment during procedures to decrease stress on electrical cords and connections. When possible, avoid using extension cords. However, if extension cords are necessary, use only those that are designed for heavy-duty use and approved by the hospital biomedical engineering department. Replace short cords of high-use equipment with long cords. Maintain a safe traffic pattern by taping electrical cords securely to the floor. When removing cords from sockets, do not pull on the wire; remove by the plug.

Monitoring the Sensory Environment

Surgical patients frequently experience psychological stress. The sights, sounds, smells, and cold temperatures of an OR may further increase the patient's anxiety and fear. The perioperative nurse has the ability to control and monitor the sensory environment and thus minimize the patient's anxiety or fear. The supplies and equipment needed to monitor the sensory environment include audio equipment, air freshener devices, air filtration devices, and screens.

Providing Preoperative Teaching

Fear and anxiety, common reactions in many surgical patients, are often related to knowledge deficit. Preoperative teaching can put the surgical experience into perspective for the patient by confirming expectations and clarifying misconceptions. Begin the preoperative teaching by assessing the patient's knowledge level about the surgical environment. Clarify misconceptions and explain what to expect in the surgical suite. Tell the patient about environmental sights, sounds, and smells.

Eliminating, Attenuating, or Modifying Sensory Stimuli

Sometimes, the sight, sound, or smell of a particular item or area within the surgical suite causes undue stress for the patient. Witnessing an intubation or extubation, smelling laser plume, or hearing the whine of a craniotome can turn a calm patient into a fearful and anxious patient. Establish traffic patterns so that the patient avoids areas where noxious sights, sounds, or smells occur. Place the patient in an area that shields him or her from distressing stimuli. If the patient has a local, regional, or spinal anesthetic, arrange the drapes and screen to prevent visualization of the procedure, blood, specimens, instruments, and equipment.

Keep loud talking to a minimum. Monitor conversations and exercise caution when using the intercom. Conscious patients may think that a conversation applies to them and draw inaccurate conclusions about their condition.

Do not talk during the induction of general anesthesia. Quietly handle instruments in the presence of the patient. When testing or using noisy instruments and equipment (drills, saws, alarms, laminar air flow equipment), warn the patient and explain what to expect. If surgery generates noxious odors, explain these to the conscious patient.

Use music to distract the conscious patient during surgery. A headset playing a favorite selection of music helps the patient to focus on something other than the surgery and its assorted sights, sounds, and smells. Music may also decrease the patient's fear or anxiety level during the procedure. Provide diversionary activities when appropriate. Like music, coached breathing exercises and guided imagery may distract the patient. Touch and verbal reassurance usually comfort the patient and may reduce anxiety and fear.

Ensuring Radiation Safety

Excessive radiation modifies the molecular structure of body cells. The use of ionizing radiation, such as x-rays, fluoroscopy, and implantation of radioactive substances require special handling and precautions. As with any potential hazard associated with the OR, the implementation of safe radiation practices by the perioperative nurse protects staff members and patients against the dangerous effects of radiation exposure. Supplies and equipment needed for ensuring radiation safety include radiation exposure badges or monitoring devices, lead aprons, lead gloves, lead collars and shields, x-ray cassette holding devices, and portable or stationary x-ray equipment.

Monitoring the Amount of Radiation Exposure

The OR manager should provide radiation-monitoring badges for personnel frequently exposed to ionizing radiation. Table 11–1 outlines the maximal permissible dose of x-rays per year. Personnel should wear badges outside lead aprons at the neckline and ring dosimeters when the hands are exposed to radiation. Pregnant personnel should avoid radiation exposure.

TABLE 11–1. MAXIMAL PERMISSIBLE YEARLY X-RAY EXPOSURE	
Whole body, eye, blood-forming organs	5 REM
Skin	15 REM
Hands	75 REM
Other organs (thyroid)	15 REM
Pregnant women (total during gestation)	0 REM

Providing Protective Devices

Protective devices decrease radiographic exposure of the patient and staff members. Before use, leaded protective devices should be inspected for cracks. Biannually, the OR manager should have leaded protective devices radiographically inspected for cracks and structural integrity. Provide lead gloves to personnel who must hold the x-ray cassette while x-ray films are taken; this protects their hands. Wear lead aprons to protect the torso and gonads. Likewise, wear lead collars to protect the thyroid. During upper torso exposure of the male patient, place a lead collar over the testicles. During x-ray exposures, the surgical team should move as far away from the radiation source as possible. Protect the staff who cannot leave the room by placing a portable lead shield on a movable stand in a convenient

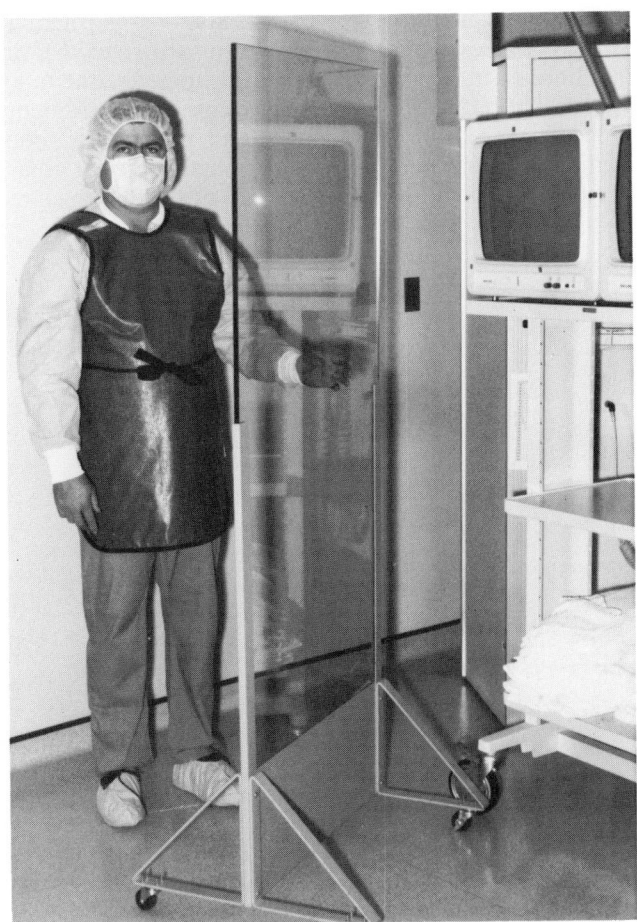

FIGURE 11–2. Portable lead shield on a movable stand to protect staff from x-ray exposure.

location in the OR (Fig. 11–2). Drape shields adjacent to the sterile field with sterile sheets. After use, leaded protective devices are stored flat or hanging, never folded.

Implementing Radioactive Material Safety Precautions

The perioperative nurse coordinates the intraoperative insertion of radioactive materials (seeds, needles, capsules). Careful coordination facilitates rapid insertion and decreases the exposure time of personnel. Nuclear medicine personnel transport radioactive material to the OR. Store the carrier for radioactive implants away from personnel and patient care areas. Identify and document the number of radioactive items when they are delivered to the OR. During insertion, stay as far away from the source of radiation as possible. Do not touch radioactive material with bare or gloved hands. Use the instruments provided for insertion and handling when moving or touching radioactive material. Handle radiation material as quickly as possible to limit exposure. Before the patient leaves the OR, establish accountability by counting the radioactive material. Account for each item implanted and retained in the container. This procedure prevents inadvertent loss of radioactive material in the OR. After implantation of radioactive materials, notify recovery or floor personnel that they will receive a patient with radioactive implants.

Documenting Procedures

Include in the operative record the type of ionizing radiation used. Monitor and record the monthly radiation exposures for personnel. Document the time, number, location, and types of radioactive material inserted. Place a sign indicating that radiation is in use on the door of the OR while the procedure is in progress. Inform postanesthesia care unit or floor personnel before receiving the patient so that they can make arrangements for care of the patient. A radiation safety officer should maintain written records of radioactive materials.

Ensuring Laser Safety

Lasers have dramatically increased the range of surgery. Yet, as with much sophisticated surgical equipment, lasers are hazardous if not used correctly. The perioperative nurse ensures that only qualified personnel operate the laser, provides a safe laser unit, monitors the use of protective devices during laser procedures, and protects the patient and staff from injury.

Selecting Qualified Personnel for Laser Use

Physicians, nurses, technicians, and others required to work with lasers must demonstrate competency in laser techniques and have knowledge concerning the hazards of and safety measures for laser surgery. As the patient advocate, the perioperative nurse limits the use of laser units to qualified personnel. Use of laser equipment by unqualified personnel is reported to the OR manager.

Providing Safe Laser Units

When laser equipment is not in use, the OR manager is responsible for securing (locking) it. Access to the laser key is limited to personnel qualified in laser use. Before each use, and before bringing the patient into the room, check and test the laser equipment. Immediately report equipment malfunction, and do not use the unit until it is repaired. Closely follow the manufacturer's recommendations and instructions when operating laser equipment. Rooms for laser use should not have windows, or the windows should have blinds. Evacuate the laser plume through filtered hospital lines or specific equipment designed for this purpose. When not in immediate use, place the laser on standby to avoid accidental discharge.

Providing Laser Protective Devices

When using the laser, place on the door a warning sign that a laser is in use and protective eyewear is required. Ensure that personnel wear approved protective glasses with side shields. Each laser light has a specific wavelength. Eye protection should have the appropriate wavelength and optical density. Cover the eyes of the awake patient with appropriate protective glasses. Cover the eyes of anesthetized patients with wet gauze and tape it securely in place. Patients and health care workers should be protected from inhaling laser fumes. Special smoke evacuators and surgical masks should be used. Use special nonreflective, ebonized instruments during laser surgery. Laser safety devices include protective eyewear specific for laser beam, wet gauze or cloth towels, special anesthesia endotracheal equipment for head and neck surgery, nonreflective instruments, and signs identifying that laser surgery is in progress (AORN, 1992, *III*:10–1—10–3).

Implementing Fire Safety Precautions

Laser beams may ignite flammable supplies such as drapes, gowns, and clothing. Do not allow the use of flammable anesthetics. For head and neck procedures, provide anesthesia endotracheal tubes designed for laser use. Ensure that skin preparation solutions do not have an alcohol base. Drape moistened towels around the incision area before laser use. Laser-retardant drapes should be used to drape the operative site. Keep the towels and sponges surrounding the target tissue wet at all times. Have a bucket of water in the room in case flammable materials are ignited. A halon fire extinguisher should be readily available.

Documenting Procedures

Documentation on the operative record should include the name of the surgeon, the support staff, the procedure, the type of laser used, the lens used, the length of laser use, and wattage. Additional laser logs may be required by the institution or the U.S. Food and Drug Administration if equipment is listed as investigational. Document orientation and ongoing education programs for nursing personnel performing laser procedures. Post warning signs indicating laser use.

Maintaining Traffic Patterns

Maintaining strict control of traffic patterns within the surgical suite decreases the potential for cross-contamination, regulates access to the suite, and facilitates efficiency. The surgical suite is divided into three zones: unrestricted, semirestricted, and restricted. The unrestricted zone usually includes the areas where OR personnel interface with outside departments, the patient reception and holding areas, and areas where supplies are received. In some surgical suites, the unrestricted zone also includes communication stations and administrative offices. Personnel may wear street clothes in the unrestricted zone. The semirestricted zone may include, but is not restricted to, storage and instrument-processing areas and, depending on design, corridors leading to restricted areas and peripheral support areas. Personnel must don appropriate scrub attire to enter

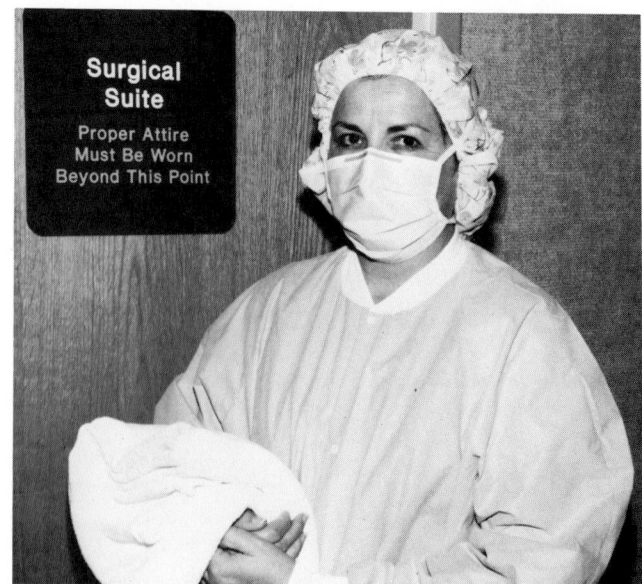

FIGURE 11–3. Appropriate attire for personnel entering the restricted zone.

the semirestricted zone. In the restricted zone, personnel must wear appropriate scrub attire and surgical masks. This area includes the ORs, substerile areas, and the sterile core areas (Fig. 11–3).

Established traffic patterns reduce the potential for cross-contamination. This is accomplished by correlating an area within the surgical suite according to the level of contamination found in the area. At a minimum, the surgical suite should have sterile, clean, and contaminated areas designated. Sterile and clean supplies and equipment are separated from soiled equipment and waste by space, time, or traffic patterns. Where architectural design permits, clean and contaminated items are moved using separate traffic patterns.

The supplies and equipment needed for maintaining traffic patterns are scrub attire, masks, hair covering, shoe covers, germicidal solutions for cleaning, personal protective attire (eyewear, gloves, aprons), and enclosed transport carts for contaminated items.

Decreasing Potential Airborne Contamination

Keep traffic flow into and out of the room to a minimum. When the number of personnel increases, the environmental microbial count also increases. Because corridor air may contain a higher bacterial count than OR air, keep doors closed. Open doors only when transporting patients, supplies, or equipment (AORN, 1992, III:22–2). Sick personnel, or those with skin infections, should not work in restricted areas.

Decreasing Potential Contamination from Outside Environmental Sources

Before use, damp dust or wipe down with a germicidal solution all equipment brought into the surgical suite. Transport clean and sterile items to the OR in an enclosed container or on a covered cart. Before bringing supply carts into the OR, remove protective coverings. Clean patient transport gurneys after each use (AORN, 1992, III:17–3).

Confining Contamination Within Established Traffic Patterns

Contain contamination by transporting trash, soiled linen, soiled instruments, and nonsterile equipment and supplies in an enclosed cart or an impervious system. Ensure that contaminated objects and waste disposal operations are separate from patient care areas. Contaminated items should never enter clean or sterile areas. Contain contaminated items at the source or origin to decrease airborne contamination (AORN, 1992, III:17–2).

Providing Clear Pathways for Traffic Flow

To facilitate retrieval and traffic patterns, store supplies as close as possible to their point of use. Keep hallways free of clutter to decrease potential injury and ease the flow of traffic. When hallways must have carts and equipment in them, keep them isolated to one side of the hallway so there is an aisle for traffic flow.

Performing Operating Room Sanitation

An OR environment that ensures cleanliness and minimal bacterial growth is essential to the well-being of the patient. Unless properly cleaned and disinfected, the OR can become heavily contaminated by pathogenic microorganisms. Every surgical procedure is considered potentially contaminated. Therefore, consistently implement the same environmental sanitation protocols for every surgical procedure (AORN, 1992, III:17–1). Universal precautions, as designated by the Centers for Disease Control (CDC), should be closely followed during all environmental sanitation procedures.

Sanitation measures are required before, during, and after each procedure. OR sanitation is a team effort by nursing and housekeeping personnel. No matter who performs OR sanitation, however, the ultimate responsibility for a clean OR rests with the perioperative nurse. The perioperative nurse should not allow patient care in a dirty OR.

The supplies and equipment needed to perform OR sanitation are lint-free cloths for cleaning, germicidal solutions, a wet vacuum (preferred) or a mop and clean mop heads, a mechanical floor scrubber, plastic liners, gloves, a pistol grip sprayer, laundry bags, disposable suction tubing, suction containers, utility carts, and covered carts for linens and trash disposal (Fig. 11–4).

Personnel with exudative lesions or weeping dermatitis should not perform environmental sanitation duties. Use protective devices such as gloves, gowns, masks, protective eyewear, and instruments when handling contaminated articles.

Preoperative Sanitation

Before the first scheduled surgery, damp dust all horizontal surfaces, including furniture, surgical lights, and equipment, with a clean, lint-free cloth moistened in a hospital-grade disinfectant. This procedure removes dust that might have settled on horizontal surfaces after terminal cleaning. Use friction while damp dusting. For subsequent procedures, perform preoperative sanitation by inspecting the room for cleanliness. If discrepancies are found, make corrections before preparing the room for the next procedure. If additional equipment is needed for the next procedure, damp dust the equip-

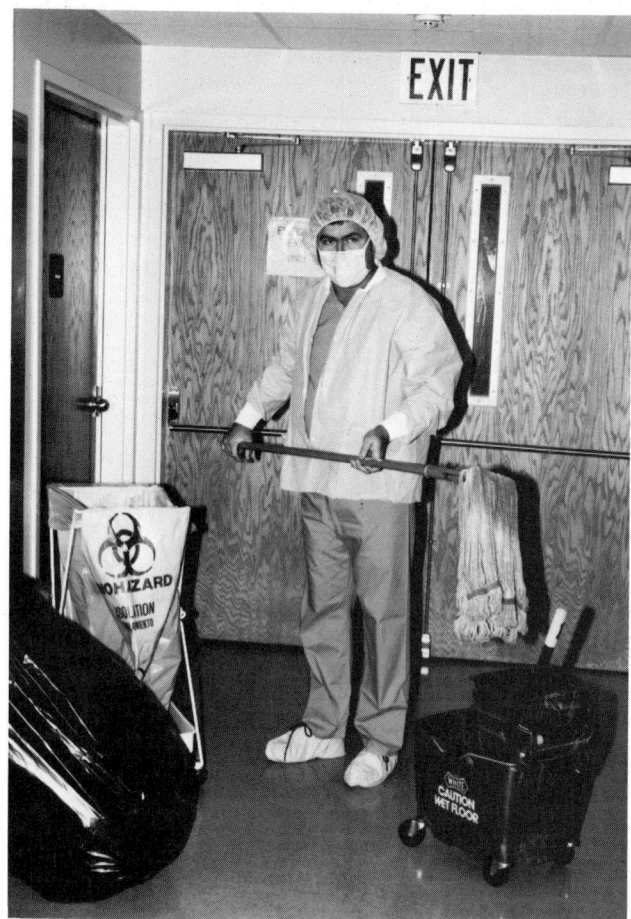

FIGURE 11–4. Equipment used to sanitize the OR.

vious container, such as a plastic bag or case cart. If contaminated instruments are required for immediate use, before sterilization, wash in a germicidal detergent and rinse. Clean the exterior surfaces of impervious specimen containers received from the operative field with a disinfectant before attaching a label and removing from the OR. Ensure that documents submitted with specimens are free from contamination. Identify and label specimens as contaminated (AORN, 1992, *III*:17–2).

Postoperative Sanitation

At the end of the procedure, clean all horizontal surfaces, and surfaces that have come in immediate contact with a patient or patient secretions, with germicidal solution. Carefully disconnect disposable suction units, seal, and discard. If hospital policy dictates disposal of suction container fluids, empty contents of the suction container into a flushing hopper. Use protective eyewear, masks or face shield, apron or gown, and gloves when disposing of suction container fluids. If a reusable suction container is used, disinfect after each use (AORN, 1992, *III*:17–2).

Confine all disposable items used during the procedure in impervious containers. Use gloves when handling contaminated linens or trash and handle as little as possible. Place all linens, used and unused, in a designated laundry bag. Place wet linen in the center of the bag to prevent inadvertent seepage. This is particularly important if laundry bag liners are not available. Trash, linen, and hazardous wastes are sealed and removed to a designated area (AORN, 1992, *III*:17–2).

Wear gloves when handling items that were on the sterile field or came in contact with the patient. Many items from the sterile field that look clean, however, are nonetheless contaminated. Instruments and supplies that were not on the sterile field or in contact with the patient are separated from contaminated items. Irrigate suction tips with clean water before disconnecting. Remove all visible debris from contaminated instruments and open the jaws of locking instruments. Separate delicate instruments for special handling and disassemble instruments that can reasonably be handled without losing parts. Carefully place sharps into puncture-proof containers. Do not recap needles or disassemble disposable syringes when disposing of sharps. Using caution, carefully remove blades from knife handles with a needle holder. Separate sharp instruments (skin hooks, scissors, rakes, osteotome, towel clips) and place in an appropriate container such as an emesis basin. Deposit reusable needles and sharp instruments in a puncture-proof container for transport to a processing area. If the substerile area adjacent to the OR contains the washer-sterilizer, place instruments in a wire mesh tray for processing. If the processing area is not adjacent to the OR, place contaminated instruments in a plastic bag or enclosed cart for transport. Remove gown and gloves before leaving the OR (AORN, 1992, *III*:17–2).

After removing trash, linen, and instruments, flood the floors with a germicidal detergent and wet vacuum.

ment before bringing it into the room (AORN, 1992, *III*:17–3).

Intraoperative Sanitation

During the surgical procedure, as much as possible, confine and contain contamination to a small area. Use appropriate protective devices (gloves, instruments, eyewear, gowns) when handling contaminated articles. When organic debris falls from the sterile field, remove with a disposable cloth and promptly disinfect the area. Saturate the area with a germicidal solution and wipe with a clean cloth. Discard the contaminated cloth into an impervious container. Deposit soiled sponges in a plastic-lined bucket. Do not place soiled sponges on a draped table or spread on an impervious barrier on the floor. If the anesthetist must see the sponges, ask her or him to stand up and look or take the bucket to the anesthetist. When necessary, count sponges and seal them in an impervious bag (AORN, 1992, *III*:19–2).

While wearing gloves, pick up surgical instruments that fall on the floor and submerge them in a pan containing germicidal detergent. This prevents drying of debris, which would become airborne contamination. Enclose nonsubmersible instruments in a clean imper-

If a wet vacuum is not available, mop the floor with a clean mop head soaked in fresh germicidal detergent solution. After mopping, discard the mop head (AORN, 1992, *III*:17–3).

When cleaning the OR bed, wipe all surfaces and mattress pads with a lint-free cloth soaked in germicidal detergent. Pay particular attention to the sides of the OR bed. Blood and other fluids may have spilled from the patient. If the OR bed was modified for the lithotomy position, inspect and clean the underside of the foot section. After thoroughly cleaning the OR bed, move it to the periphery of the OR, thus allowing easy access to the center of the room for wet vacuuming or mopping. When moving the OR bed, move casters of the table through the cleaning solution.

Carefully inspect the overhead lights for contamination and spot clean as needed. After cleaning, wipe the surgical light reflector shields with 70% isopropyl alcohol to remove detergent film. Return the lights to the center of the room for optimum lighting exposure.

Remove reusable anesthesia tubing, masks, and equipment and deposit for terminal cleaning. Discard disposable tubing, masks, endotracheal tubes, and other equipment into trash containers. Disinfect horizontal surfaces of the anesthesia machine (AORN, 1992, *III*:1–1).

Inspect OR walls for contamination and spot clean as necessary (AORN, 1992, *III*:17–3).

Clean transportation gurneys after each use with germicidal solution. Pay attention to cleaning side rails, mattress, pillows, and any other area that may have been contaminated with blood or body fluids (AORN, 1992, *III*:17–3).

After the room is cleaned, remove gloves, wash the hands, and prepare the room for the next case by placing new liners and bags in the appropriate receptacles for trash and linen. Reassemble the suction canisters and attach clean tubing. Prepare the OR bed with fresh linen and a clean safety strap.

Sanitation at the Conclusion of the Scheduled Day

At the end of each day, all ORs, substerile areas, scrub sinks, scrub or utility areas, hallways, furniture, and equipment are terminally cleaned. In sterile storage areas, care must be taken not to contaminate any sterile supplies with cleaning solutions. Remove all portable equipment from the room, such as kick buckets, linen hamper frames, suction canisters, and other waste receptacles, and clean with a germicidal detergent. If feasible, autoclave items such as kick buckets that contained body fluids. Wipe down overhead lights, doors, handles on cabinets, waste receptacles, and remaining furniture or room equipment. Wheels and casters on equipment need special attention, as these tend to pick up sutures and other debris readily. Flood the floor with a germicidal detergent for 5 minutes and thoroughly scrub with a floor scrubber. Remove the solution with a wet vacuum or a sterilized, single-use mop head. If baseboards are present, use a baseboard brush for cleaning before removing the floor cleaning solution. Disassemble, clean, and if possible, autoclave reusable soap dispensers before refilling. Remove and autoclave spray heads of faucets. Inspect walls, particularly around scrub sink areas, for cleanliness. Clean transportation and storage carts. After performing OR sanitation, clean the housekeeping equipment. Before storing the equipment, ensure that it is dry because moisture tends to enhance bacterial growth (AORN, 1992, *III*:17–3).

Periodic Sanitation for the Surgical Suite

Usually, cabinets and shelves, walls, the ceiling, air conditioning and heating grills, ducts and filters, sterilizers, warming cabinets, refrigerator, offices, lounges, and locker rooms are cleaned routinely (AORN, 1992, *III*:17–3).

Sterilizing Instruments, Supplies, and Equipment

Sterilization renders instruments, supplies, and equipment free from all forms of microorganisms, including spores. Several methods of sterilization are available; the use of each sterilization method is dictated by the nature of the instrument, supply, or piece of equipment. Steam under pressure and ethylene oxide are two of the primary methods used in most health care agencies. Specific knowledge of each method is needed by the perioperative nurse for the daily delivery of patient care.

The supplies and equipment needed for sterilizing instruments, supplies, and equipment are a gravity displacement autoclave, a prevacuum autoclave, autoclave recording graphs, biological and chemical sterilization indicators, an ethylene oxide sterilizer, and an ethylene oxide aerator.

Decontaminating Instruments

All instrument trays and/or instruments opened during the procedure should be decontaminated. Instrument care varies depending on the type of cleaning process required. Most general instruments can withstand washer-sterilizer decontamination (Fig. 11–5) and ultrasonic cleaning. Specialty instruments, however, frequently require special handling. Usually, these instruments are not placed in washer-sterilizers. Because some should not be immersed in liquid, ultrasonic cleaning is also inappropriate for these instruments. Examples of special instruments include endoscopes, pneumatic drills, saws and hoses, dermatomes, dermabraders, cords and cable, electronic devices, Silastic tubing, reusable plastic equipment, and delicate instruments. Each of these categories necessitates special decontamination

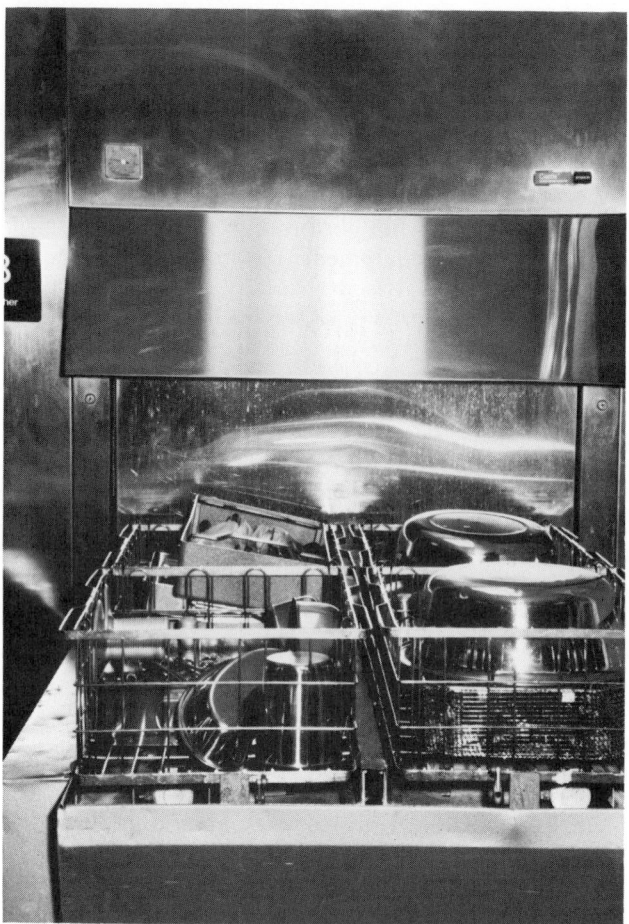

FIGURE 11–5. General instruments placed in a washer-sterilizer for decontamination.

and cleaning procedures. When available, the manufacturer's protocols for decontamination and processing for sterilization should be followed.

Cleaning

During the surgical procedure, instruments should be kept free from gross blood and other debris by wiping or prerinsing with distilled water. After the procedure is completed, the used instruments should be opened and placed in water or a germicidal solution. Equipment should be covered in impervious containers, closed carts, or plastic bags. Used supplies and equipment are collected and taken to the decontamination section of the instrument-processing area in a way that avoids contamination of personnel or any area of the hospital.

Personnel in the decontamination area should wear protective clothing, which includes a scrub uniform, a plastic apron or jump suit, hair covering, rubber or plastic gloves, and safety glasses.

Delicate instruments are usually hand washed using a germicidal detergent, which will not damage the instrument. After being washed, they are placed in a wire mesh pan, put in a sterilizer, and sterilized for 3 minutes at 270°F. Some institutions use liquid disinfectants for the processing of the hand-washed instruments. The disinfecting solution should be in sufficient concentration and must remain in contact with instrument surfaces for the manufacturer's recommended time. Disinfectants should not be mixed with other disinfectants or combined with detergents. Instruments should be thoroughly washed and dried before being placed in the disinfectant. Drying prevents dilution of the disinfectant. Personnel should take precautions to avoid contact with these chemicals. After the disinfection process is complete, the items are rinsed in distilled water, dried, and stored or sent to the packaging area for further processing.

For general instruments, automated cleaners or washer-sterilizers should be used for decontamination. The instruments are carefully taken from the fluid-filled basins, placed in wire mesh trays, and put into the washer-sterilizer for washing, rinsing, and sterilizing. If washer-sterilizers are not available, the instruments should be washed manually. When manual cleaning of instruments is used, instruments are submerged in the appropriate germicidal detergent and cleaned while submerged. Cleaning the instruments while they are under water decreases the occurrence of aerosolization.

After the initial washing of general instruments, the instruments are placed in an ultrasonic cleaner, which removes debris that may have been missed. Dissimilar metal such as copper, stainless steel, and brass should not be combined in the ultrasonic cleaner. Make sure that all instruments in the ultrasonic baskets are covered by solution. After the ultrasonic cycle, drain and rinse instruments. Instruments that have been in the ultrasonic cleaner should be lubricated with a water-soluble solution, which protects the instruments from corrosion and rust and improves the movement of joints. These water-soluble solutions are usually allowed to dry on the instrument, thereby providing a protective coating.

After the decontamination process is completed, instruments should be inspected for cleanliness and proper functioning. Instrument trays are then assembled, inventoried, packaged, and readied for the sterilization process.

Preparing Instruments, Equipment, and Supplies for Sterilization

Open the box-locks of instruments for the sterilization cycle. Stringers or racks ensure that box locks remain open. If possible, disassemble instruments with multiple parts before sterilization. Instruments that will be sterilized together are placed in perforated container systems or wire-mesh trays. Place heavy instruments in the bottom of the tray. Wrap delicate instruments separately and place on the top of the heavy instruments. To ensure that all surfaces are exposed to the sterilizing agent, place absorbent towels between nested articles. Tightly packed and large instrument sets decrease the penetration of the sterilizing agent; therefore, the weight of these sets should not exceed approximately 16 pounds (AORN, 1992, *III*:20–1). Before wrapping the instruments, place chemical sterilization indicators in the center of the each pack. When steam sterilizing items with lumina, such as tubes, needles, and drains, flush with distilled water before placing in the tray. This prevents the trapping of air, thus facilitating the steam sterilization process. If ethylene oxide or chemical sterilization processes are used, lumina must be dry.

Wrapping Items

Materials used for wrapping items for sterilization must permit the penetration of the sterilizing agent to all items in the package. The material must also allow the evacuation or release of the sterilizing agent and drying. These may be woven (cloth) or nonwoven fabrics. If they are cloth, use only freshly laundered fabric outerwraps. The fabric must have no holes, or a minimal number of heat-sealed patches. Whether using single-use disposable or reusable fabric wrappers, sequentially double wrap the items for sterilization. Peel-pack pouches should have as much air as possible removed before sealing. Like materials of peel-pack pouches should touch when double wrapping (paper to paper, see-through plastic to plastic). To provide an impermeable barrier to microorganisms, moisture, and dust, packaging must completely cover the item. Packaging materials must allow sealing that is tamper proof; the package cannot be opened and resealed without evidence that sterility has been broken. When selecting packaging material, choose a material that is durable and that withstands tearing, puncturing, and the pressures of normal handling. In addition, packaging materials should adapt to the size, shape, and nature of the item to be packaged (AORN, 1992, *III*:12–1—12–2).

A containerized packaging system (metal or plastic) (Fig. 11–6) should have the following characteristics: a removable top that facilitates aseptic presentation of the contents, perforations or valves that allow for sterilant penetration and removal, a filter or valve system that maintains the sterility of contents, a means to identify processed or sterile containers from unprocessed or unsterile containers, and a way of securing the top of the container to the bottom. Prevacuum steam sterilizing is the only acceptable method of sterilizing containerized packaging systems.

Performing Steam Sterilization

Loading Items for Steam Sterilization

Place each item on the autoclave racks to ensure free circulation of steam. If an item capable of holding water, such as basins and solid-bottomed trays, is sterilized, place it on its side during the sterilization cycle. Likewise, flat packages are placed on the shelf vertically. Large packages are placed so that they do not touch. Linen packages go on the top level of the sterilizer and metal on the bottom when running a mixed load. To keep them upright, place heat-sealed plastic-paper peel-down packages on end. Instrument container systems

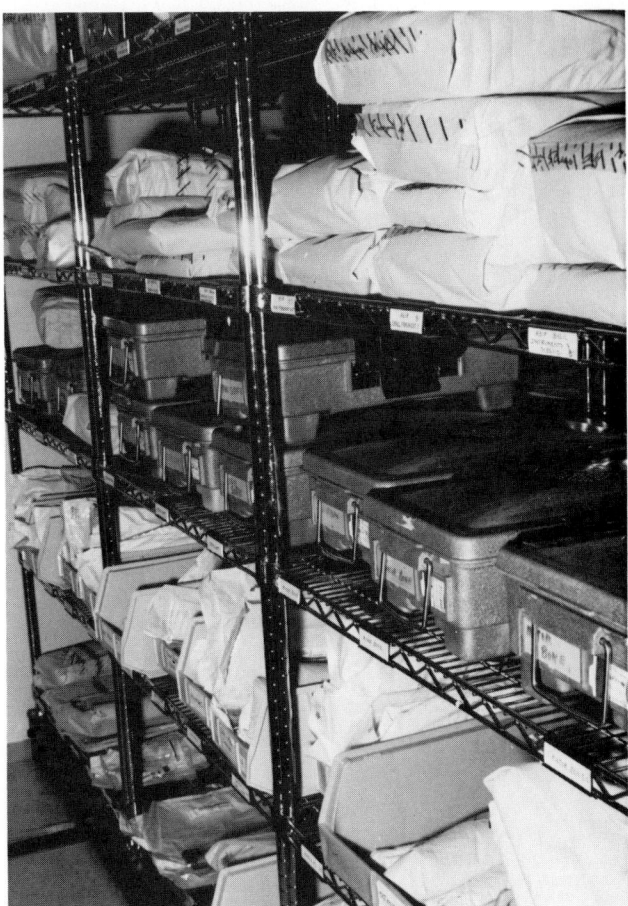

FIGURE 11–6. A containerized packaging system.

and sets with perforated trays may be placed flat during the sterilization cycle.

Operating a Steam Sterilizer

Follow the manufacturer's written instructions when operating the steam sterilizer. Before removing the contents, check the sterilizer graph or printed read-out to verify that sterilization objectives were met (Fig. 11–7). When ready to remove the sterilizer contents, before opening the door, verify that the exhaust valve reading is zero to ensure complete dissipation of steam. Stand behind the door and open it slowly to avoid the steam escaping from around the door (Fig. 11–8). Do not touch the interior surfaces of the sterilizer owing to the potential for burn. Keep the doors of sterilizers closed when not in use. Sterilize supplies requiring the same exposure cycle in the same load (Table 11–2). After removing the cart from the sterilizer, do not place it near air vents or fans owing to the possibility of condensation. Items removed from the sterilizer after processing should remain on the cart until adequately cooled. In addition, do not touch sterile items while cooling. Wet packages are considered unsterile. Apply dust covers to designated items after they are completely cooled.

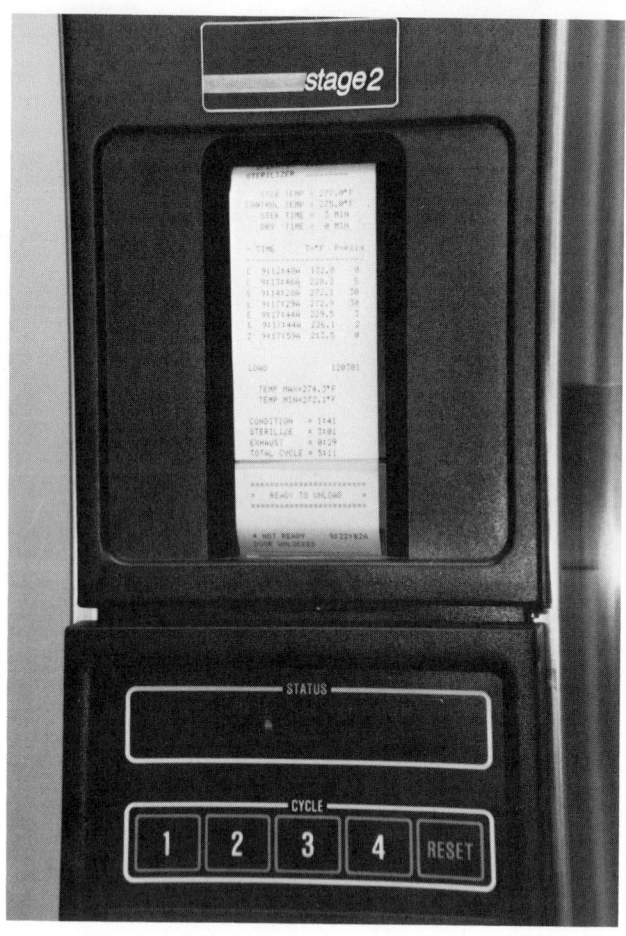

FIGURE 11–7. Printed read-out on steam sterilizer.

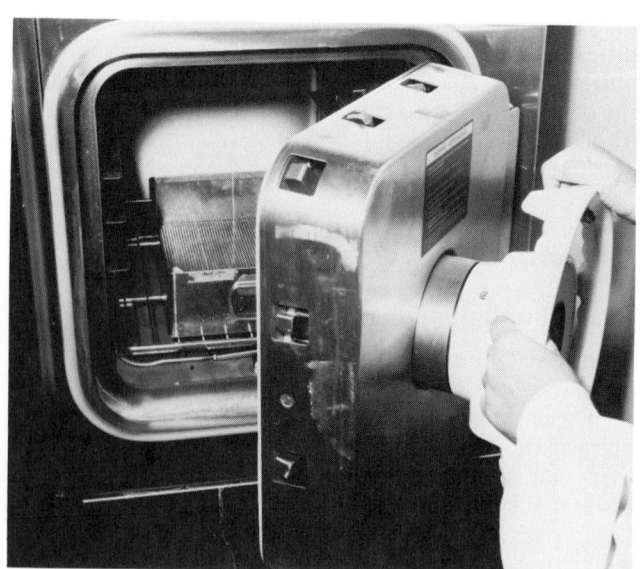

FIGURE 11–8. One should avoid the steam that escapes around the door when opening the steam sterilizer.

TABLE 11–2. MINIMUM STERILIZATION EXPOSURE PERIOD FOR WRAPPED AND UNWRAPPED GOODS: GRAVITY CYCLE ONLY

Items	Sterilize Times at 250°F (121°C) (Minutes)	Sterilize Times at 270°F (132°C) (Minutes)	Dry Times (Minutes)
Dressings, wrapped in muslin or an equivalent	30	25	30*
Glassware, empty, inverted	15	3	0**
Instruments, metal combined with suture, tubing, or other porous materials, unwrapped	20	10	0**
Instruments, metal only, in mesh-bottomed tray, unwrapped	15	3	0**
Instruments, wrapped in double-thickness muslin or an equivalent	30	15	30*
Textile packs (maximum size: 12 × 12 × 20 inches; maximum weight: 12 pounds)	30	25	30*
Treatment trays, wrapped in muslin or an equivalent	30	15	30*
Utensils, wrapped in muslin or an equivalent	30	15	30*
Utensils, unwrapped	15	3	0**
Flasked solutions ■ 75 ml ■ 250 ml ■ 500 ml ■ 1000 ml ■ 1500 ml ■ 2000 ml	25 30 40 45 50 55	N/A	N/A

*Dry time for wrapped goods can vary depending on pack density, instrument tray weight, pack preparation technique including type of wrapping material used, and sterilizer loading procedures.

**Dry time is not required for unwrapped goods; however, on older sterilizers a dry time of 1 or 2 minutes will help reduce excess steam when opening chamber door at end of cycle.

Adapted with permission from American Sterilizer Company (AMSCO), *Eagle series 3000 equipment manual*, AMSCO publication number P-129362-451 (pp. 12–13) Erie, PA.

Operating a High-Speed Pressure (Flash) Sterilizer

Place unwrapped items in a perforated or mesh-bottomed tray (Fig. 11–9). Position instruments with concave surfaces with the open side down and open all hinged instruments. Use racks or stringers to ensure that instruments stay open during sterilization. Disassemble items with easily removable parts. Separate heavy items from delicate instruments to decrease potential damage. Sterilize metal instruments for 3 minutes at or above 270°F. Sterilize porous items (towels, rubber or plastic), or mixed porous-nonporous items for 10 minutes at or above 270°F. Specialty instruments may require different exposure times based on the manufacturers' recommendations. Additionally, some specialty instruments should not be flash sterilized—heat-sensitive items would be destroyed. Do not flash sterilize implants; these require sterilization in conjunction with biological monitoring. Use a sterile device (towels, handles, mittens) for removing instruments from the autoclave. Remove instruments utilizing aseptic technique (AORN, 1992, *III*:20–6).

Sterilizing with Ethylene Oxide

Implementing Safety Procedures

Operate ethylene oxide sterilizers according to the manufacturer's recommendation and equipment speci-

fications. Ethylene oxide vapor is extremely hazardous and should be avoided. Therefore, isolate all ethylene oxide sterilizers and aerators to minimize human exposure to toxic vapors. Additionally, do not smoke near ethylene oxide because it is highly flammable and explosive. Post signs identifying where ethylene oxide is in

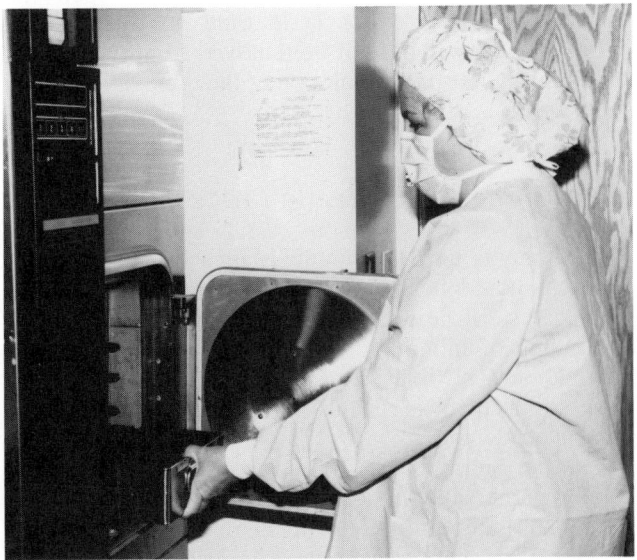

FIGURE 11–9. Placement of items into a high-speed pressure sterilizer.

use. Individuals operating ethylene oxide sterilizers should be thoroughly knowledgeable of chemical hazards and emergency procedures. All personnel who may be potentially exposed to ethylene oxide must be monitored. An annual physical examination for those working in areas containing ethylene oxide vapor is recommended.

Loading Ethylene Oxide Sterilizers

Sterilize items having common aeration times together. Thoroughly clean and dry items before sterilization. Unlike the case for steam sterilization, dry the lumina of tubing and needles. The combination of water and ethylene oxide forms ethylene glycol, a toxic substance. After packaging the items, place on metal carts or in wire baskets. Avoid overloading the sterilizer. This allows circulation of sterilant to all surfaces. Arrange items so that they do not touch the walls of the sterilizing chamber during the sterilizing cycle. Do not stack heavy packages on top of one another and place pouches on edge in a wire basket (AORN, 1992, *III*:20–4—20–5).

Transferring Items from Sterilizer to Aerator

Open the sterilizer door as soon as possible after completion of the sterilization cycle to decrease ethylene oxide vapor build-up. If sterilizer carts are used when moving equipment from the sterilizer to the aerator, pull the carts, do not push, to avoid inhaling ethylene oxide. Avoid touching sterilized items when transferring sterilized items to the aerator because ethylene oxide can burn the skin. Use gloves when removing the biological indicator test pack from the sterilized load and wash the hands to remove any possible gas residue.

Aerating Items

Leave approximately 1 inch between all items. Overloading the aerator decreases air circulation, which in turn prolongs the aeration cycle. Do not open the aerators until the entire cycle time has elapsed. In addition, items should not be removed from the aerator prematurely. At the completion of the cycle, allow items to cool before storage.

Liquid Chemical Sterile Processing

Instruments used in minimally invasive surgical procedures should be sterilized. Low-temperature, liquid chemical sterilization methods are an option for the processing of minimally invasive instrumentation such as rigid and flexible scopes and cameras. The Steris Process is a chemical sterilization method that has gained clinical acceptance.

Use the Steris Process only for instruments that are totally immersible in a liquid and able to withstand processing temperatures of up to 56°C for 12 minutes. Preclean and mechanically prepare instruments accord-

ing to the instruments' manufacturers' recommendations for liquid immersion or according to current department practices. It is not necessary to dry instruments prior to placing them into the Steris System 1 Processor. Place unwrapped instruments into the appropriate tray or container. For flexible endoscopes, the scopes' lumen(a) must be properly connected according to Steris' instructions to permit the liquid sterilant to reach internal and external surfaces. Insert a sealed container of sterilant (Steris 20 Sterilant Concentrate) into the Processor. The Processor automatically prepares the working concentration of sterilant and controls the exposure time (12 minutes) and temperature (50–56°C). Following sterilization, the Processor rinses the instruments with sterile water to remove chemical residues without recontaminating the instruments. Upon completion of the 30-minute cycle, the instruments are immediately available for use. Before removing the instruments from the Processor, observe the control panel lights and printout to verify that a successful cycle was achieved. Initial and save the cycle printout for quality assurance records. Report a failed cycle to the appropriate person for corrective action. Do not use instruments from a failed cycle.

Instruments should be distributed and used promptly following sterilization in System 1 because the instrument containers are not intended for storage. Do not sterilize implants in System 1; these require sterilization in conjunction with biological monitoring.

Safety Procedures

When direct physical contact with the sterilant is a possibility, as in case of an incomplete cycle, protective eyewear (chemical goggles) and waterproof gloves should be worn. The diluted sterilant is nontoxic and safe for direct disposal into a sanitary sewer. No environmental or personal exposure monitoring is required; however, ensuring adequate ventilation in the work area is desirable to minimize the vinegar-like chemical odor.

Monitoring the Cycle

Chemical and biological indicators provide the same level of Steris cycle quality assurance as apply to steam and ethylene oxide sterilization processes. A chemical indicator may be run with each instrument load as a secondary check of the Processor's ability to monitor sterilant potency. A biological indicator should be run weekly. Use the indicator systems available from Steris and interpret results according to the manufacturer's criteria.

Monitoring the Sterilization Process

Mechanical Control Measures

Mechanical control monitors such as time-temperature recording devices, temperature gauges, and pressure gauges should be monitored at the beginning and ending of each cycle to verify that adequate parameters have been achieved. Before removing any materials from the sterilizer, verify that adequate temperature and duration have been achieved. Report sterilizer malfunction or suspicious operation to the appropriate person. If automated mechanical control measures are used, evaluate and initial the recording at the end of each cycle.

Chemical Indicators

External or internal chemical indicators may include sterilization indicating tape, labels, cards, or strips that visually identify that the package has been exposed to sterilizing conditions. It does not validate that sterilization has been achieved. Use the manufacturer's criteria to interpret chemical indicator results. Use an external chemical indicator with every package. Place an internal chemical indicator in the most inaccessible area of every pack.

Efficacy of Vacuum System on Prevacuum Sterilizers

The Bowie-Dick test is carried out to determine the efficacy of the vacuum system of a pre-vacuum sterilizer and does not indicate sterilization. A Bowie-Dick–type test sheet is placed in the center of a pack consisting of folded towels, 9 × 12 inches, with a height of 10 to 11 inches. The pack is loosely single wrapped. Place the test pack horizontally on the bottom front rack of the sterilizer, near the door and over the drain of an otherwise empty chamber. Run this test each day before the first sterilization cycle. Do not perform this test on gravity displacement sterilizers.

Biological Testing of Sterilizers

Perform biological testing for routine monitoring and as a challenge test after any major sterilizer redesign or relocation, suspected malfunction, and major repair. Perform biological testing at least weekly or as needed for steam autoclaves.

Procedure

Label the biological indicator with sterilizer load information. Place the indicator in the area of the sterilizer chamber that is least favorable to sterilization. Remove it from the sterilizer after exposure to sterilization cycle. Incubate the biological indicator according to the manufacturer's recommendations. Schedule biological testing according to institutional policies. At a minimum, biologically test a sterilizer at least weekly. Record the results of biological indicator tests. Notify appropriate personnel immediately if abnormal results occur. Biological indicators are placed in any load that includes implants. Do not use the implants until the return of a normal biological indicator at 48 hours. Use *Bacillus stearothermophilus* to test steam sterilization and *B.*

subtilis for ethylene oxide sterilizers. If the test is positive for growth, immediately rechallenge the sterilizer. If there is a subsequent abnormal result of biological indicators, take the sterilizer out of service until the problem is corrected and a normal reading is obtained. Recall and reprocess suspected load items if a sterilizer malfunction in found (AORN, 1992, *III*:20–2—20–3).

Test Packs for Biological Challenge Steam Sterilization Monitoring

A routine test pack consists of three muslin gowns, 12 towels, 30 4 × 4 inch gauze sponges, five laparotomy sponges, and one muslin drape sheet. Place two biological indicators in the center of the pack. Place a chemical indicator one towel above or below the biological indicators. Place the test pack on edge at the front bottom, near the door, in a routinely loaded gravity displacement sterilizer. Place the test pack on edge at the front bottom, near the door, by itself in a prevacuum steam sterilizer (AORN, 1992, *III*:20–3).

Biological Challenge Test for Ethylene Oxide Sterilizers

A general purpose ethylene oxide sterilizer is a chamber-type sterilizer that provides humidity adjustment during the sterilization cycle. Make a general test pack of four clean surgical towels, each folded in thirds and then halved to create six layers per towel. Place these on top of one another. Add one adult plastic airway, a 10-inch section of latex tubing with internal diameter of 3/16 inch, and two plastic or glass syringes with biological indicators placed in the barrels of the syringes to the center of the towels. Insert the plungers into the barrels of the syringes. The plunger diaphragm should not touch the biological indicator. Sequentially wrap the pack with two 24 × 24 inch wrappers and secure with tape. Chemical indicators and a biological indicator may be used in the same sterilization cycle as the general test pack (AORN, 1992, *III*:20–3).

Special Purpose. A special purpose ethylene oxide sterilization system requires prehumidification of items to be sterilized and usually operates at atmospheric pressure. Special test packs include one 10-inch length of latex tubing of ³⁄₁₆ inch diameter and two syringes with biological indicators enclosed in the syringe barrel and the syringe tip open. Wrap in single-thickness wrapper and tape closed.

For challenge test pack placement in an 80 to 100 cubic foot chamber, five test packs are used, one placed in the center front and the others in diagonally opposite corners in the upper and lower levels. For a 40 to 79 cubic foot chamber, three test packs are used, one each placed in the center, front section, rear upper section. For a 16 to 39 cubic foot chamber, two test packs are used, one in the rear corner and one in the front corner. For a chamber less than 16 cubic foot, one pack is placed in the front of the chamber near the door.

In a routine test pack, one biological indicator is

placed in a plastic syringe of sufficient size that the indicator does not touch the plunger. This syringe has an open tip and is placed inside of a folded, clean, 100% cotton towel. These articles are placed in a single-peel pouch wrapper and placed in the center of the load. After the sterilization cycle, biological test pack indicators and controls are removed and incubated according to the manufacturer's recommendations (AORN, 1992, III:20–3).

Sterilizers Performance Records

Each package to be sterilized is labeled with a lot control number, which designates the sterilizer used, the date of sterilization, the cycle number, and an expiration date. Sterilizer performance records for each sterilizer are kept. These should include the contents of each load as to general category, the duration and temperature of the sterilization phase, the identification of the operator, the results of biological testing, a time and temperature recording chart for the sterilizer, and a record of repairs and preventive maintenance (AORN, 1992, III:20–6).

Preventive Maintenance

Preventive maintenance procedures are outlined by the manufacturer of the sterilizer. In general, areas that need attention are air filters, steam traps, drain pipes, and door gaskets.

Daily Inspection and Cleaning

Daily care of sterilizer is done while sterilizer is cool. Remove the chamber drain strainer and eliminate debris and sediment. Wash and rinse all internal surfaces of the sterilizer, using only the recommended cleaning agent. Clean door gaskets. Observe for evidence of gasket failure leaks, blowing of steam, water on the interior of the autoclave, and low pressures. Check for proper functioning of the recording chart and pen. Weekly inspection and cleaning should include discharge system and accessories. Routine maintenance is done at least every 6 months. This includes inspection, servicing, and calibration (AORN, 1992, III:20–6).

Documenting Procedures

Permanent records are kept regarding the results of biological monitoring, autoclave graphs and recording charts, load contents, and load control numbers. Maintenance records are kept for each sterilizer. Include a date of service, the model and serial number, a description of the service performed, the name of the individual performing the service, a description and quantity of the parts replaced, the results of biological indicator and/or a Bowie-Dick test after the repair, the name of the authorized individual requesting service, and the signature of the person acknowledging completed work.

Each item or pack intended for use as a sterile product is labeled with a lot control number, which designates the sterilizer identification number, the date of sterilization, and the cycle number. Specific policies and procedures must provide for checking items that may be outdated, damaged, or contaminated (AORN, 1992, III:20–5).

ACKNOWLEDGEMENT

Special thanks to Pamela C. Tanner, V.P. Regulatory Affairs, Steris Corp., Painesville, OH, for contributing the discussion about liquid chemical sterile processing.

Bibliography

Association of Operating Room Nurses. (1992). Recommended practices for safe care through identification of potential hazards in the surgical environment. *Standards and recommended practices for perioperative nursing.* III(7), 1–6. Denver.

Association of Operating Room Nurses. (1992). Recommended practices for electrosurgery. *Standards and recommended practices for perioperative nursing.* III(5), 1–4. Denver.

Association of Operating Room Nurses. (1992). Recommended practices for safe care through identification of potential hazards in the surgical environment. *Standards and recommended practices for perioperative nursing.* III(7), 1–6. Denver.

Association of Operating Room Nurses. (1992). Recommended practices for radiological safety in the practice setting. *Standards and recommended practices for perioperative nursing.* III(16), 1–7. Denver.

Association of Operating Room Nurses. (1992). Recommended practices for laser safety in the practice setting. *Standards and recommended practices for perioperative nursing.* III(10), 1–5. Denver.

Association of Operating Room Nurses. (1992). Recommended practices for traffic patterns in the surgical suite. *Standards and recommended practices for perioperative nursing.* III(22), 1–4. Denver.

Association of Operating Room Nurses. (1992). Recommended practices for operating room environmental sanitation. *Standards and recommended practices for perioperative nursing.* III(17), 1–6. Denver.

Association of Operating Room Nurses. (1992). Recommended practices for aseptic technique. *Standards and recommended practices for perioperative nursing.* III(2), 1–6. Denver.

Association of Operating Room Nurses. (1992). Recommended practices for care of instruments, scopes and powered surgical instruments. *Standards and recommended practices for perioperative nursing.* III(9), 1–9. Denver.

Association of Operating Room Nurses. (1992). Recommended practices for selection and use of packaging materials. *Standards and recommended practices for perioperative nursing.* III(12), 1–4. Denver.

Association of Operating Room Nurses. (1992). Recommended practices for sterilization and disinfection. *Standards and recommended practices for perioperative nursing.* III(20), 1–11. Denver.

Association for the Advancement of Medical Instrumentation. (1985, February). Good hospital practice: Performance evaluation of ethylene oxide—ethylene oxide test packs. Arlington, Va: Association for the Advancement of Medical Instrumentation.

Association for the Advancement of Medical Instrumentation. (1981, March). Good hospital practice: Ethylene oxide gas—Ventilation recommendations and safe use. Arlington, Va: Association for the Advancement of Medical Instrumentation.

Association for the Advancement of Medical Instrumentation. (June, 1986). Good hospital practice: Steam sterilization using the unwrapped method (Flash sterilization). Arlington, VA.

Association for the Advancement of Medical Instrumentation. (1980, January). Good hospital practice: Steam sterilization and sterility assurance. Arlington, VA.

Atkinson, L., Kohn, M. (1986). *Berry and Kohn's introduction to operating room technique* (6th ed.). New York: McGraw-Hill Book Co., 200–207.

Beare, P., Myers, J. (1990). *Principles and practice of adult health nursing.* St. Louis: C. V. Mosby Co., 308–312.

Bennett, J., Brachman, P. (1986). *Hospital infections.* (2nd ed.). Boston: Little, Brown and Company.

Buczko, G. B., McKay, W. P. S. (1987). Electrical safety in the operating room. *Canadian Journal of Anesthesia, 34,* 315–322.

Carmody, S., Hickey, P., Bookbinder, M. (1991, July). Perioperative needs of families: Results of a survey. *AORN Journal, 54,* 561–567.

Centers for Disease Control. (1987, August). Recommendations for preventions of HIV transmission in health-care settings. *Morbidity and Mortality Weekly Report, 36*(25),

Council on Scientific Affairs. (1986, August). Lasers in medicine and surgery. *Journal of American Medical Association, 256*(7), 900–907.

England, E. (1985). Lasers: Issues, problems, and implications for practice. *Perioperative Nursing Quarterly, 1*(2), 29–38.

Fay, M., Beck, W., Fay, J., et al. (1990, June). Medical waste: The growing issues of management and disposal. *AORN, 51,* 1493–1508.

Filston, H., Izant, R. (1985). *The surgical neonate: Evaluation and care.* New York: Appleton-Century-Crofts.

Fitzpatrick, B., Reich, R. (1989, October). Sterilization monitoring in vacuum steam sterilizers. *Healthcare Material Management,* 82–85.

Fogg, D. (1989, October). Criteria for flash sterilization. *AORN Journal, 50,* 888–892.

Gillette, M., Caruso, G. (1989, July). Intraoperative tissue injury: major causes and preventative measures. *AORN Journal, 50,* 66–78.

Gorman, N. (1988). Non-woven material: Manufacturing process for sterilization wraps. *Hospital Material Management Quarterly, 9*(3), 1–8.

Haney, P., Raymond, B., Lewis, L. (1990, February). Ethylene oxide: An occupational health hazard for hospital workers. *AORN Journal, 52,* 480–485.

Johnston, C., et al. (1988, January). Parental presence during anesthesia induction: A research study. *AORN Journal, 47,* 187–194.

Kalapes, A., Greene, V., Langholz, A., et al. (1987). Effect of long-term storage on sterile status of devices in surgical packs. *Infection Control, 8*(7), 289–293.

Kneedler, J., Dodge, G. (1986). *Perioperative patient care.* Boston: Blackwell Scientific Publications, pp. 117–126, 289–294.

Loving, T., Allen, R. (1985, March/April). EtO personnel monitoring devices: The state of the art. *Journal of Hospital Supply, Processing and Distribution,* pp. 38–42.

Meeker, M., Rothrock, J. (1991). *Alexander's care of the patient in surgery* (9th ed.). St. Louis: C. V. Mosby Co., pp. 33–39.

Mock, E. (1991, March). Electrosurgical unit safety: The role of the perioperative nurse. *AORN Journal 53,* 744–752.

Moddeman, G. (1991, May). The elderly surgical patient: A high risk for hypothermia. *AORN Journal, 53,* 1270–1272.

Moss, R. (1986, May). Overcoming fear: A review of research on patient, family instruction. *AORN Journal, 43,* 1107–1114.

Moss, V. (1988, July). Music and the surgical patient: The effect of music on anxiety. *AORN Journal, 48,* 64–69.

National Institute for Occupational Safety and Health. (1989, July). Ethylene oxide sterilizers in health care facilities, engineering controls and work practices. Cincinnati, OH: *Current Intelligence Bulletin,* 52, 1989.

Nyamathi, A., Kashiwabara, A. (1988, January). Preoperative anxiety: Its affect on cognitive thinking. *AORN Journal, 47,* 164–170.

Ryan, P. (1987, November/December). Concepts of cleaning technologies and processes. *Journal of Healthcare Material Management,* 20–27.

Smith, R. (1986, July/August). Sterile: The ten parameters of steam sterilization. *Journal of Healthcare Material Management,* 34–39.

Spry, C. (1988). *Essentials of perioperative nursing: A self-learning guide.* Rockville, MD: Aspen Publishers.

Vidor, K. (1990, September). Anxiety related to impending surgery. *Today's OR Nurse, 12*(9), 36.

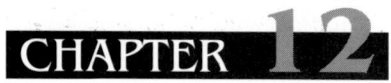

CHAPTER 12

Positioning the Patient

Steven L. Perry

DEFINITION

Positioning the patient for surgery is a crucial element of perioperative nursing care. Careless positioning can potentially jeopardize the patient's well-being and possibly hinder the surgeon. The perioperative nurse must be proficient in safely positioning the patient while providing the optimal operative exposure.

MEASURABLE CRITERIA

The perioperative nurse demonstrates competency to position by placing the patient in the

- supine position
- Trendelenburg position
- reverse Trendelenburg position
- low lithotomy position
- high lithotomy position
- lateral decubitus position
- prone position
- jackknife position
- sitting position

The views expressed in this chapter are those of the author and do not reflect the official position or policy of the Department of the Army, the Department of Defense, or the U.S. Government.

264

ROLE OF THE PERIOPERATIVE NURSE

The perioperative nurse's responsibility toward the patient encompasses all phases of perioperative patient care: preoperative, intraoperative, and postoperative. The nurse must possess the knowledge, proficiency, and problem-solving and communication skills necessary competently to position the surgical patient. The nurse must be knowledgeable about the physiological effects of surgery and positioning. The nurse should have a thorough understanding of and be able to apply the nursing process. She or he should be proficient in the correct operation of the operating room (OR) bed and the various accessories and positioning devices. The nurse must possess the problem-solving skills necessary to develop a plan of care that meets the needs of the patient. She or he should exhibit the communication skills necessary to document and inform others about the individual plan of care. Most of all, the nurse must assess each patient and provide care that meets the patient's needs.

As the circulating nurse, the perioperative nurse usually positions the patient for surgery. Assignment of positioning activities to assistive personnel is permissible. If positioning is assigned to assistive personnel, the perioperative nurse maintains accountability.

OUTCOME STANDARD

Surgical positioning does not physiologically compromise or cause injury to the patient.

Criteria

There are no signs or symptoms of

- physical injury reported by the patient or significant others
- impaired skin integrity or breakdown
- ineffective breathing
- altered tissue perfusion
- postoperative pain
- uncompensated sensory deficit (touch or kinesthesia)

POTENTIAL ALTERATIONS IN FUNCTIONAL HEALTH PATTERNS

Health Perception–Health Management Pattern

Diagnosis

High risk for injury

Definition

Presence of risk factors for the patient to experience bodily injury owing to surgical positioning

Risk Factors

- Disorientation
- Impaired judgment
- Muscle weakness
- Paralysis
- Incoordination
- Sensory/perceptual deterioration due to disease, medication, or anesthesia
- Existing or previous trauma or accidental injury
- Lack of safety precautions attributed to inadequate, untrained, or inattentive staff; a shortage of equipment; and a hazardous environment

Expected Outcome

The patient does not show evidence of injury related to positioning. There are no signs of the following:

- inability to resume preoperative patterns of ambulation
- tingling, numbness, cramping, pain, or aches in the joints

- weakness and stiffness in the upper and lower extremities
- inability to abduct, adduct, flex, and extend the upper and lower extremities without experiencing pain or discomfort (Rothrock, 1987, p. 271)

Nutritional-Metabolic Pattern

Diagnosis

High risk for impaired skin integrity

Definition

Presence of risk factors for the patient to experience skin disruption over bony prominences owing to surgical positioning (Gordon, 1987, p. 84)

Risk Factors

- Prolonged pressure on the bony prominences
- Shearing force
- Pressure on the peripheral nervous or vascular systems
- Physical immobilization, lack of position change for more than 1½ hours
- Inattentive staff leaning on the patient
- Obesity or emaciation
- Change in skin turgor
- Edema
- Pooling of preparation solutions

Expected Outcome

The patient does not show evidence of skin breakdown related to positioning. There are no signs of disruption of skin surfaces or destruction of skin layers, especially over bony prominences (Gordon, 1987, p. 88).

Activity-Exercise Pattern

Diagnosis

High risk for ineffective breathing pattern

Definition

Presence of risk factors for the patient to experience respirations inadequate to maintain sufficient oxygen supply for cellular requirements because of surgical positioning (Gordon, 1987, p. 154)

Risk Factors

- Obesity
- Inattentive staff leaning on the patient

- Existing neuromuscular or musculoskeletal impairment
- Pregnancy

Expected Outcome

The patient shows no evidence of ineffective breathing patterns during the intraoperative period. There are no signs of labored breathing in the conscious patient, abnormal arterial blood gas values because of ineffective respirations, and cyanosis (Gordon, 1987, p. 154).

Diagnosis

High risk for altered tissue perfusion

Definition

Presence of risk factors for the patient to experience a blood supply deficit to a body part owing to surgical positioning (Gordon, 1987, p. 160)

Risk Factors

- Compression of the extremities against positioning devices or OR bed accessories
- Excessive abduction of the arm boards
- Inattentive staff leaning on the patient

Expected Outcome

The patient shows no evidence of altered tissue perfusion related to surgical positioning during the intraoperative period. There are no signs of the following:

- cold extremities
- diminished arterial pulsations
- blood pressure changes in the extremities
- edema
- discoloration in the extremities (Rothrock, 1987, p. 272)

PERIOPERATIVE NURSING INTERVENTIONS

All Surgical Positions

Communication. Communication with the patient and members of the operative team is essential. The perioperative nurse should inform the patient of the positioning procedure during the patient teaching session. Specific intraoperative patient requirements should be communicated with other members of the operative team (AORN, 1992, *III*:14–1).

Preparing the Operating Room Bed. Before transferring the patient, modify the OR bed. Ensure that the OR bed is functioning properly, clean, free from hazards, and padded (AORN, 1992, *III*:14–1). The pads should be of equal height. Lock the OR bed in place.

Ensure that all required positioning devices and attachments are immediately available for use, functional, clean, and free from hazards. Attach a padded table extension if the patient's body will extend beyond the end of the OR bed. Transfer the patient to the OR bed, as described in Chapter 4.

Centering the Patient on the Operating Room Bed. Ensure that the head, spine, and legs are aligned. The patient's legs should not be crossed. Apply the safety strap at least 2 inches above the knees without excessive pressure. Insert a hand between the strap and the thighs to check for excessive pressure.

Placing the Patient's Arms on the Arm Boards. The arm boards should be at less than a 90-degree angle to the body. Ensure that the arm boards and bed pad are of the same height. Secure each arm with a safety strap. If the palms are placed at the sides, they should be turned toward the patient's sides with the fingers extended. Pad the arms and tuck them with the draw sheet. Check the elbows to ensure that they are not flexed or resting on the metal edge of the OR bed. Ensure that the fingers are clear of the OR bed breaks and other possible hazards.

Padding Bony Prominences. Bony prominences should be padded and free of excessive pressure.

Moving the Anesthetized Patient. Check with the anesthetist before positioning or repositioning the anesthetized patient. Do not move the patient without adequate assistance available. Move the patient slowly, as a coordinated team. Reassess the patient for body alignment and tissue integrity (AORN, 1992, *III*:14–3) before draping. Examine the safety strap to ensure that it is secure and not constrictive.

Documenting Interventions. Document all intraoperative nursing interventions. Continually monitor the patient's position during the procedure. After the operative procedure, assess the patient and document the findings. Transfer the patient to the recovery bed, as described in Chapter 4. Document and communicate the postoperative evaluation with other members of the perioperative team (AORN, 1992, *III*:4–1—4–3).

Supine Position

The supine position, also known as the dorsal recumbent position, is the most frequently used position for patients undergoing a surgical procedure. The patient is placed on his or her back with the legs extended and the arms resting on arm boards (Fig. 12–1) or at the sides (Fig. 12–2). This position is routinely used in abdominal, thoracic, vascular, and orthopedic procedures.

Considerations

Staffing Requirements. The perioperative nurse is the minimal nursing staff needed to position the patient.

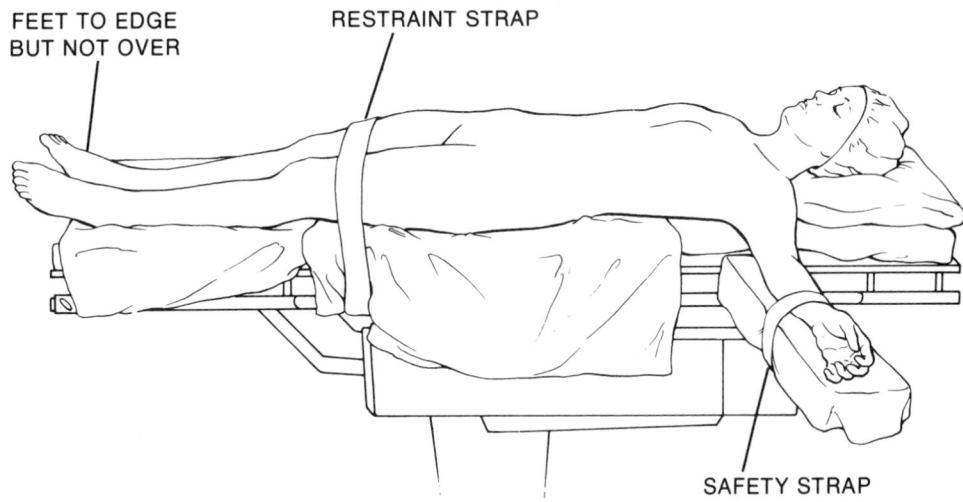

FEET TO EDGE
BUT NOT OVER

RESTRAINT STRAP

SAFETY STRAP

FIGURE 12–1. Supine position, arms extended. (From Fuller, J. R. [1986]. *Surgical technology: Principles and practice* [2nd ed.]. Philadelphia: W. B. Saunders.)

However, the staffing requirement should be based on the need to provide safe patient care without jeopardizing the safety of the operative team.

Body Structures at Risk. (Table 12–1)

Potential Adverse Effects. (Rothrock, 1987, pp. 253–254)

- Position-induced hypotension
- Venous pooling in the legs resulting from a reduction of venous pressure
- Decreased diaphragmatic excursion due to abdominal organs' resting against the upper abdominal wall
- Restriction of posterolateral chest movement, causing a reduction in vital capacity
- Decreased mean arterial pressure, heart rate, and peripheral resistance, particularly during the induction of anesthesia

Supplies and Equipment

The routine supplies and equipment needed for placing the patient in the supine position are arm boards, arm restraints, a pillow or headrest, padding for bony prominences (foam, sheepskin, blankets, pillows), and a safety strap. Supplementary supplies and equipment such as a padded footboard, a pelvic wedge, a table

extension, and toboggans are identified in the perioperative nursing care plan.

Procedure

Inform the conscious patient before performing any interventions. After the transfer, ensure that the patient's head, neck, spine, and legs are in proper alignment, the legs are not crossed and are slightly apart, the safety belt is secured above the knees, the patient is not resting on any unpadded surfaces, and the extremities are secured away from the OR bed joints (breaks) and attachments.

If arm boards are to be used, the patient's arms must not be abducted beyond 90 degrees; if the patient's range of motion is restricted (e.g., in thoracic outlet syndrome and arthritis), the arms should be abducted less than 90 degrees (Dornette, 1986, p. 210) and secured to the arm boards. If the arms are to be placed at the patient's sides, the palms should be turned toward

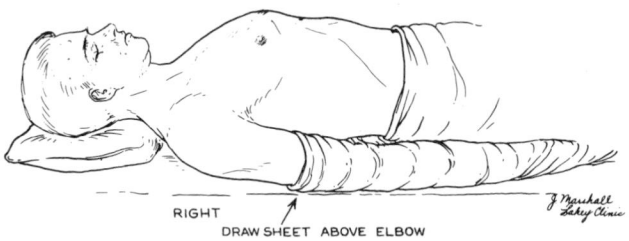

RIGHT

DRAW SHEET ABOVE ELBOW

FIGURE 12–2. Supine position, arms tucked. (From Ginsberg, F. [1966]. *A Manual of operating room technology*. Philadelphia: J. B. Lippincott.)

TABLE 12–1. **BODY STRUCTURES AT RISK FOR INJURY IN SUPINE POSITION**
Integumentary system
Scalp and all skin layers, particularly over bony prominences
Nervous system
Brachial plexus; radial, ulnar, median, common peroneal, and tibial nerves
Musculoskeletal system
Bony prominences: occiput, spinous processes, scapulae, medial and lateral epicondyles of humerus, olecranon process, styloid process of ulna and radius, sacrum, and calcaneus
Joints: supine, shoulders, elbows, wrists, knees, and hips
Muscles: calf and strap
Respiratory system
Diaphragm
Vascular system
Aorta, inferior vena cava, popliteal artery, and saphenous vein

Data from Aldrete, 1987; Dornette, 1986; Gruendemann, 1987; Schmaus et al., 1987; Smith, 1987.

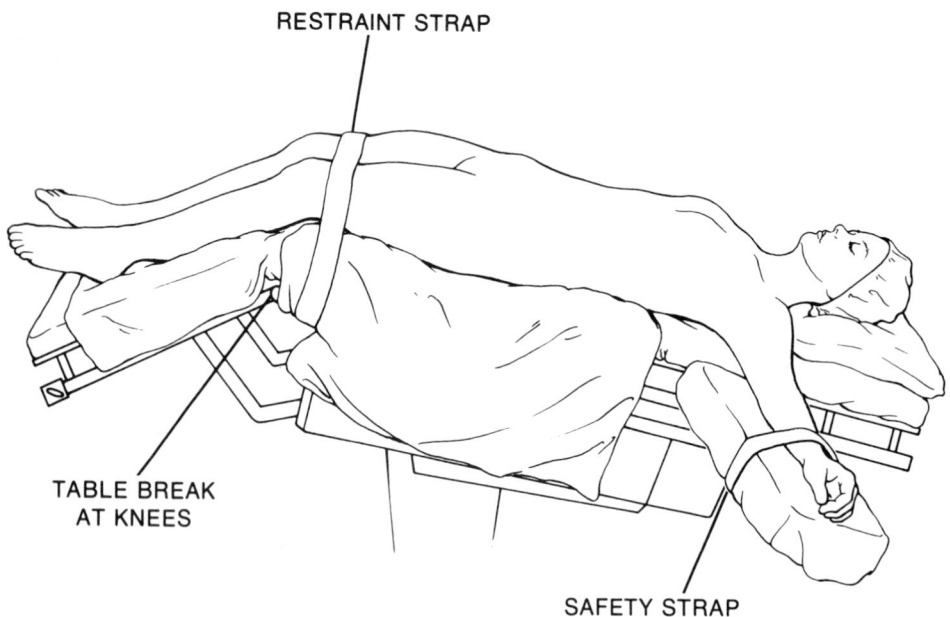

RESTRAINT STRAP

TABLE BREAK
AT KNEES

SAFETY STRAP

FIGURE 12–3. Trendelenburg position. (From Fuller, J. R. [1986]. *Surgical technology: Principles and practice* [2nd ed.]. Philadelphia: W. B. Saunders.)

the body or the bed, and the full length of the arms should be secured by a draw sheet or a padded toboggan (McAlpine and Sechel, 1987, pp. 317, 319).

Apply protective padding to all areas susceptible to injury, as identified in the nursing care plan. Place a small pad under the patient's head, lower lumbar area, and heels and avoid hyperextending the knees (Smith, 1987, p. 34). For pregnant or obese patients, place a small pelvic wedge under the right side of the patient to relieve pressure on the vena cava (Smith, 1987, p. 35). Attach a padded footboard to the bed if the need has been identified in the nursing care plan.

Trendelenburg Position

The Trendelenburg position is a modification of the supine (dorsal recumbent) position. The patient is placed in the supine position and the OR bed is modified to a head-down tilt; the lower section of the bed may be altered to lower the knees (Fig. 12–3). This position causes the abdominal organs to move out of the pelvis, improving the visualization of the pelvic organs (Schiller, 1987, p. 117).

Considerations

Staffing Requirements. The perioperative nurse is the minimal nursing staff needed to position the patient.

Body Structures at Risk. (Table 12–2)

Potential Adverse Effects. (Rothrock, 1987, p. 262)

- Hypotension related to reflex-induced vasodilation, unrecognized blood loss, and reduced cardiac output
- Air embolism

- Retinal detachment or cerebral edema due to increased venous pressure
- Venous thrombosis related to congestion of the cerebral vessels
- Occlusion of superficial veins by positioning and restraining devices and lower extremity phlebothrombosis, especially when the knees are bent
- Atelectasis caused by drug-induced hypoventilation or lung compression by the abdominal contents
- Nerve injury

Supplies and Equipment

The routine supplies needed for placing the patient in the Trendelenburg position are arm boards, arm re-

TABLE 12–2. **BODY STRUCTURES AT RISK FOR INJURY IN TRENDELENBURG POSITION**
Cerebrovascular system
Integumentary system
Scalp and all skin layers, particularly over bony prominences
Nervous system
Brachial plexus; radial, ulnar, median, common peroneal, and tibial nerves
Musculoskeletal system
Bony prominences: occiput, spinous processes, scapulae, medial and lateral epicondyles of humerus, olecranon process, styloid process of ulna and radius, sacrum, and calcaneus
Joints: spine, shoulders, elbows, wrists, knees, and hips
Muscles: calf and strap
Respiratory system
Diaphragm
Vascular system
Aorta, heart, inferior vena cava, carotid artery, popliteal artery, and jugular and saphenous veins

Data from Aldrete, 1987; Dornette, 1986; Gruendemann, 1987; Prentice and Martin, 1987; Schmaus et al., 1987; Smith, 1987.

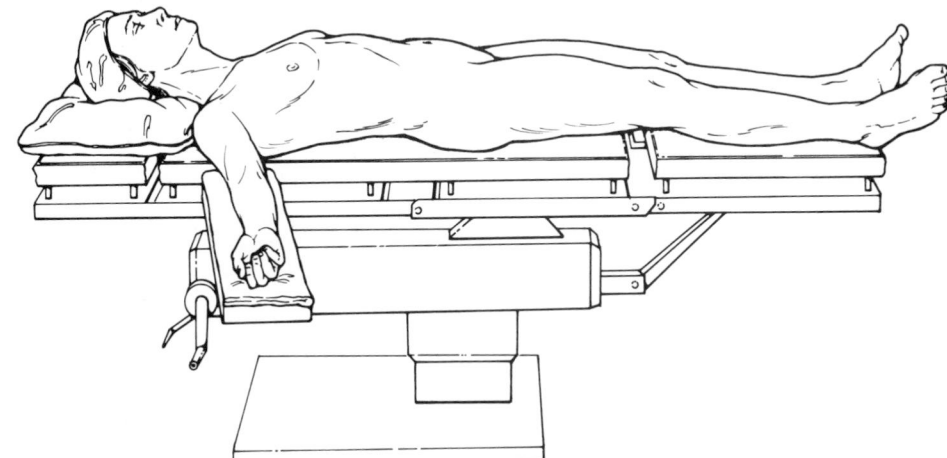

FIGURE 12–4. Preparation for substantial Trendelenburg tilt. (Modified from Martin, J. T. [Ed.]. [1987]. *Positioning in anesthesia and surgery* [2nd ed.]. Philadelphia: W. B. Saunders.)

straints, a pillow or headrest, padding for bony prominences (foam, sheepskin, blankets, pillows), and a safety strap. Supplementary supplies and equipment such as a padded footboard, a pelvic wedge, a table extension, and toboggans are identified in the perioperative nursing care plan. The use of shoulder braces is not recommended (Prentice and Martin, 1987, p. 143; Schmaus et al., 1987, p. 40).

Procedure

Position the patient as described for the supine position. If the knee section of the OR bed is to be lowered to minimize pressure on the calves and knee joints, position the top edge of the patient's knees below the hinge, at a distance approximately equal to the thickness of the OR bed pad and x-ray tunnel (Prentice and Martin, 1987, pp. 130–131; Rothrock, 1987, p. 266) (Fig. 12–4). Tilt the bed, feet up and head down, to the desired angle.

Reverse Trendelenburg Position

The reverse Trendelenburg position is a modification of the supine position. The patient is placed in the supine position and the OR bed is adjusted to a head-up tilt (Fig. 12–5). This position is used for procedures of the head and neck.

Considerations

Staffing Requirement. The perioperative nurse is the minimal nursing staff needed to position the patient.

Body Structures at Risk. (Table 12–3)

Potential Adverse Effects. (Rothrock, 1987, p. 259)

- Venous pooling in the legs
- If arms are placed at the sides, misalignment or compression of the arms against the OR bed resulting in radial, median, or ulnar nerve damage
- Impaired tissue integrity from shearing forces if the patient slides toward the foot of the bed

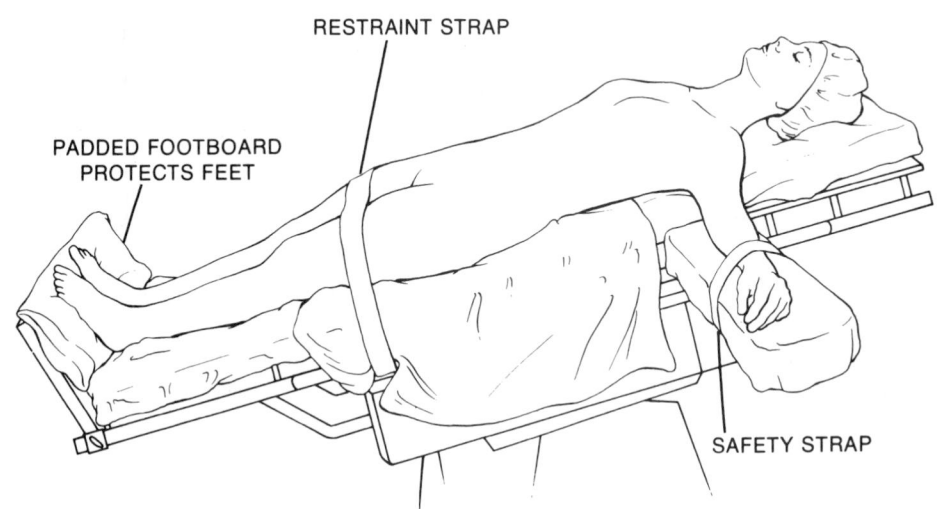

FIGURE 12–5. Reverse Trendelenburg position. (From Fuller, J. R. [1986]. *Surgical technology: Principles and practice* [2nd ed.]. Philadelphia: W. B. Saunders.)

TABLE 12–3. **BODY STRUCTURES AT RISK FOR INJURY IN REVERSE TRENDELENBURG POSITION**
Integumentary system
Scalp and all skin layers, particularly over bony prominences
Nervous system
Brachial plexus; radial, ulnar, median, common peroneal, and tibial nerves
Musculoskeletal system
Bony prominences: occiput, spinous processes, scapulae, medial and lateral epicondyles of humerus, olecranon process, styloid process of ulna and radius, sacrum, and calcaneus
Joints: spine, shoulders, elbows, wrists, knees, and hips
Muscles: calf and strap
Vascular system
Aorta, inferior vena cava, popliteal artery, and saphenous vein

Data from Aldrete, 1987; Dornette, 1986; Gruendemann, 1987; Schmaus et al., 1987; Smith, 1987.

Supplies and Equipment

The routine supplies and equipment need to place the patient in reverse Trendelenburg position are arm boards, arm restraints, a padded footboard, a pillow or headrest, padding for bony prominences (foam, sheepskin, blankets, pillows), and a safety strap. Supplementary supplies and equipment such as a pelvic wedge, a table extension, and toboggans are listed in the perioperative nursing care plan.

Procedure

Position the patient as described for the supine position. Attach a padded footboard to the foot of the bed to keep the patient from sliding toward the foot of the OR bed. Tilt the bed, feet down and head up, to the desired angle.

High Lithotomy Position

The high lithotomy position is frequently used for procedures requiring a vaginal or perineal approach. The patient is supine with the legs raised and abducted by positioning stirrups (Fig. 12–6). The bottom section of the OR bed is lowered out of the surgeon's way.

Considerations

Staffing Requirements. The perioperative nurse and an assistant are the minimal nursing staff needed to position the patient.

Body Structures at Risk. (Table 12–4)

Potential Adverse Effects. (Rothrock, 1987, pp. 267–268)

- Venous pooling in the lumbar region
- Vein compression in the groin due to thigh flexion

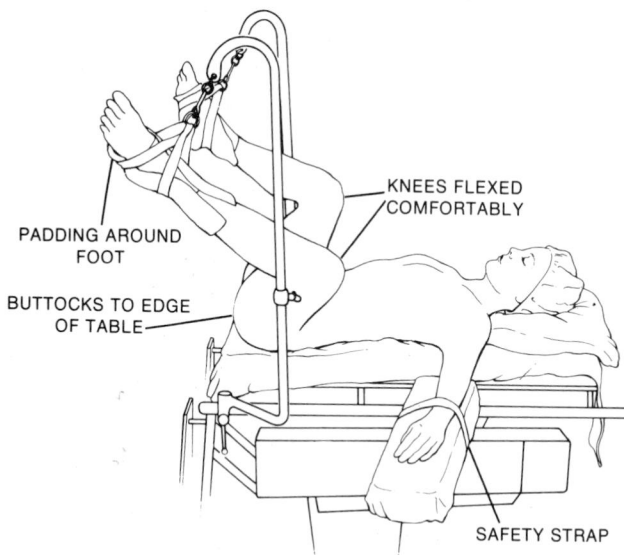

FIGURE 12–6. High lithotomy position. (From Fuller, J. R. [1986]. *Surgical technology: Principles and practice* [2nd ed.]. Philadelphia: W. B. Saunders.)

- Vein compression in the legs due to positioning equipment
- Increased intraabdominal pressure with a subsequent reduction in diaphragmatic movement due to the thighs' pressing against the abdomen, especially in obese patients
- Severe hypotension due to blood's draining from the torso into the legs when the legs are lowered from the lithotomy position
- Injury to the obturator and femoral nerves due to acute flexion of the thighs
- Injury to the saphenous and common peroneal nerves due to misplaced or unpadded stirrups
- Hip injury due to excessive abduction of the legs during positioning

TABLE 12–4. **BODY STRUCTURES AT RISK FOR INJURY IN HIGH LITHOTOMY POSITION**
Integumentary system
Scalp and all skin layers, particularly over bony prominences
Nervous system
Brachial plexus; radial, ulnar, median, common peroneal, tibial, sciatic, saphenous, femoral, and obturator nerves
Musculoskeletal system
Bony prominences: occiput, spinous processes, scapulae, medial and lateral epicondyles of humerus, olecranon process, styloid process of ulna and radius, sacrum, femoral epicondyle, tibial condyles, and lateral malleolus
Joints: spine, shoulders, elbows, wrists, knees, and hips
Muscles: calf and strap
Respiratory system
Diaphragm
Vascular system
Inferior vena cava, external iliac artery, femoral artery, and saphenous vein

Data from Aldrete, 1987; Dornette, 1986; Goldstein, 1987; Gruendemann, 1987; Schmaus et al., 1987; Smith, 1987; Welborn, 1987.

- Brachial plexus injury due to hyperextension of the arms when moving the patient toward the break in the OR bed after positioning

Supplies and Equipment

The routine supplies and equipment needed for placing the patient in the high lithotomy position are arm boards, arm restraints, a pillow or headrest, padding for bony prominences (foam, sheepskin, blankets, pillows), a safety strap, protective leg coverings (foam boots, towels), stirrups, and stirrup holders.

Procedure

Adjust the Operating Room Bed and Transfer the Patient. Before transferring the patient, adjust the OR bed. Begin by releasing the head section of the mattress pad. Pull the headpiece and mattress pad out. Attach the headpiece and mattress to the foot of the OR bed. Refit the bed sheet to the OR bed. Transfer and prepare the patient for anesthesia administration in the supine position as described for interventions for all surgical positions. Apply protective padding to the patient's feet and lower legs. Other protective padding is used as described for interventions for all surgical positions.

Attach the Stirrups. Attach the stirrup holders to the OR bed above the knee break hinge. Insert the stirrups into the holders and tighten. Adjust the stirrups to the appropriate height; ensure that they are level and secure.

Place the Patient in the High Lithotomy Position. After the patient is anesthetized, remove the safety strap from the legs. Grasp the sole of one foot in one hand, supporting the leg at the knee with the other hand. Instruct the assistant to perform the same maneuver for the other leg. Together with the assistant, *slowly* flex the legs toward the abdomen, then slightly externally rotate the hips and secure the feet to the stirrups (Fuller, 1986, p. 73). Cover the patient's genitalia and perineum with a towel or sheet.

Complete Modification of the Operating Room Bed. Remove the headrest and the leg section of the OR bed. Place the headrest and the leg section on a clean surface outside the surgeon's work area. Ensure that the patient's fingers are not in the hinges of the bed. Lower the leg section of the OR bed.

Reposition if Necessary. Remove the arm board straps and fold the patient's arms across the abdomen. Have the assistant stand by the patient to protect the arms. Stand between the patient's legs and move the patient to the edge of the OR bed break by placing the hands and arms under the patient's buttocks and gently lifting using proper body mechanics, or with another team member lift the patient using the draw sheet. Move the arm boards and resecure the patient's arms.

Reposition After Surgery. Check to ensure that the patient's hands and fingers are not extending beyond the OR bed break. Elevate the leg section to the horizontal position. Replace the mattress pad on the leg section. Put the head section and mattress pad back on the foot of the bed. Have the assistant stand on the opposite side of the OR bed and perform the same maneuvers for the other leg. When given clearance by the anesthetist, grasp the patient's legs and remove the stirrup strap. With one hand under the patient's heel and the other under the knee, *slowly* extend the legs and lower them together. Reapply the safety strap securely across the thighs. Cover the patient with a warm sheet or blanket. Remove the positioning equipment from the OR bed.

Low Lithotomy Position

The low lithotomy position is a modification of the high lithotomy position. The patient is placed in the supine position with the legs raised and abducted, exposing the perineum (Fig. 12–7). The angle between the patient's thighs and the trunk is not as acute as for the high lithotomy position. This position is used for surgical procedures entailing a vaginal or perineal approach and laparoscopic examinations.

Considerations

Staffing Requirements. The perioperative nurse and an assistant are the minimal nursing staff needed to position the patient.

Body Structures at Risk. (Table 12–5)

Potential Adverse Effects. See under discussion of the high lithotomy position.

Supplies and Equipment

The routine supplies and equipment needed for placing the patient in low lithotomy position are arm boards, arm restraints, a pillow or headrest, padding for bony prominences (foam, sheepskin, blankets, pillows), a safety strap, protective leg coverings (foam boots, towels), leg holders, and a rail socket.

Procedure

Adjust the Operating Room Bed and Transfer the Patient. Adjust the OR bed as described for the high lithotomy position. Transfer and prepare the patient for anesthesia administration in the supine position as described under interventions for all surgical positions.

Apply Protective Devices. Apply protective padding to the patient's feet and lower legs. Additional protective padding should be applied as described under interventions for all surgical positions.

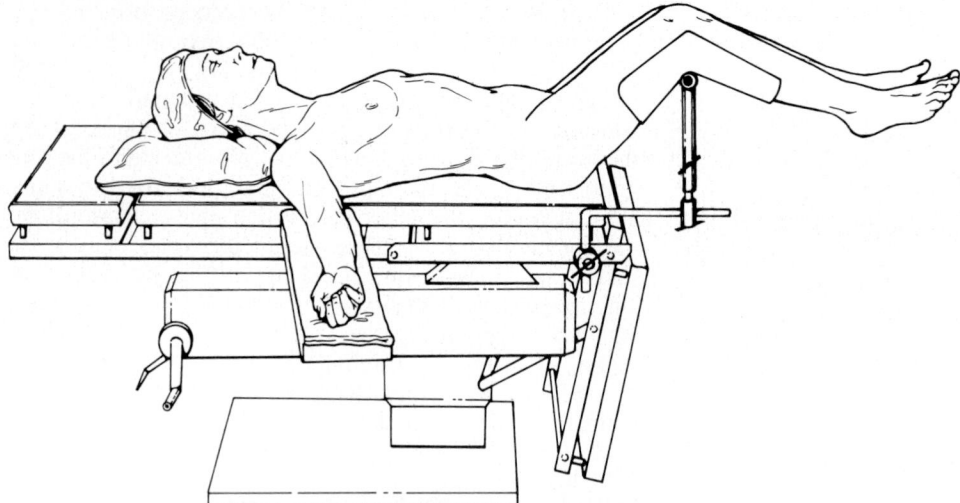

FIGURE 12–7. Low lithotomy position. (Modified from Martin, J. T. [Ed.]. [1987]. *Positioning in anesthesia and surgery* [2nd ed.]. Philadelphia: W. B. Saunders.)

Attach the Leg Holders. Attach the rail socket to the OR bed above the knee break hinge. Insert the leg holders into the rail socket and tighten. Adjust the leg holders to the appropriate height; ensure that they are level and secure.

Place the Patient in the Low Lithotomy Position. After the patient is anesthetized, remove the safety strap from the legs. Grasp the sole of one foot in one hand, supporting the leg at the knee with the other hand. Instruct the assistant to perform the same maneuver with the other leg. Together with the assistant, *slowly* flex the legs toward the abdomen, then slightly externally rotate the hips and secure the legs to the leg holders (Fuller, 1986, p. 73; Kropp, 1987, p. 54). As seen in Figure 12–7, the thighs should be at an obtuse angle to the trunk. Cover the patient's genitalia and perineum with a towel or a sheet. Complete modification of the OR bed as described for the high lithotomy position. Reposition the patient if necessary as described for the high lithotomy position.

TABLE 12–5. **BODY STRUCTURES AT RISK FOR INJURY IN LOW LITHOTOMY POSITION**

Integumentary system
  Scalp and all skin layers, particularly over bony prominences
Nervous system
  Brachial plexus; radial, ulnar, median, common peroneal, tibial, sciatic, saphenous, femoral, and obturator nerves
Musculoskeletal system
  Bony prominences: occiput, spinous processes, scapulae, medial and lateral epicondyles of humerus, olecranon process, styloid process of ulna and radius, sacrum, femoral epicondyle, tibial condyles, and lateral malleolus
  Joints: spine, shoulders, elbows, wrists, knees, and hips
  Muscles: calf and strap
Respiratory system
  Diaphragm
Vascular system
  Inferior vena cava, external iliac artery, femoral artery, and saphenous vein

Data from Aldrete, 1987; Dornette, 1986; Goldstein, 1987; Gruendemann, 1987; Schmaus et al., 1987; Smith, 1987; Welborn, 1987.

Reposition After Surgery. Check to ensure that the patient's hands and fingers are not extending beyond the OR bed break. Elevate the leg section to the horizontal position. Replace the mattress pad on the leg section. Put the head section and mattress pad back on the foot of the bed. Have the assistant stand on the opposite side of the OR bed and perform the same maneuvers for the other leg. When given clearance by the anesthetist, place one hand under the patient's heel and the other under the knee, *slowly* lift the legs off the leg holder, extend the legs, and lower them together. Reapply the safety strap. Cover the patient with a warm sheet or blanket. Remove the positioning equipment from the OR bed.

Lateral Decubitus Position

For the lateral decubitus position, the patient is placed in a stabilized position resting on his or her side (Fig. 12–8). This position can be modified to place the patient in the Sims, kidney, or semiprone position. The lateral position and its variations are employed for thoracic, renal, or orthopedic (hip) procedures.

Considerations

Staffing Requirements. The perioperative nurse and three assistants are the minimum nursing staff needed to position the patient.

Body Structures at Risk. (Table 12–6)

Potential Adverse Effects. (Rothrock, 1987, pp. 281–282)

- Injury to the dependent brachial plexus
- Injury to the median, radial, ulnar, and peroneal nerves
- Pressure sore development over the dependent greater trochanter of the femur
- Potential interference with cardiac action because of a possible shift in heart position

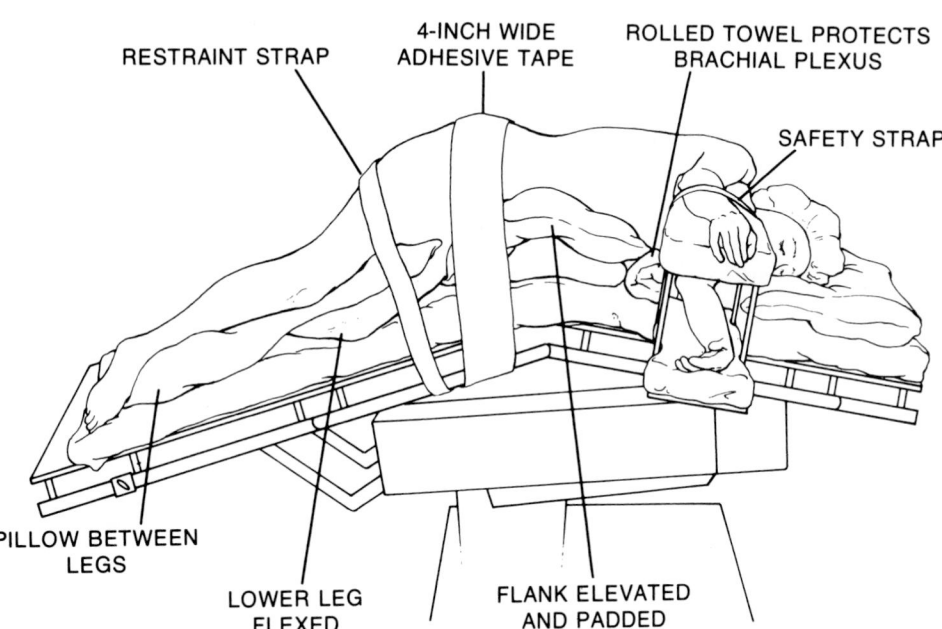

RESTRAINT STRAP

4-INCH WIDE
ADHESIVE TAPE

ROLLED TOWEL PROTECTS
BRACHIAL PLEXUS

SAFETY STRAP

PILLOW BETWEEN
LEGS

LOWER LEG
FLEXED

FLANK ELEVATED
AND PADDED

FIGURE 12–8. Lateral position. (From Fuller, J. R. [1986]. *Surgical technology: Principles and practice* [2nd ed.]. Philadelphia: W. B. Saunders.)

- Potential drop in arterial pressure of up to 24 mm Hg with the left lateral position
- Potential drop in arterial pressure of up to 33 mm Hg with the right lateral position

Supplies and Equipment

The routine supplies and equipment needed for placing the position in the lateral decubitus position are pillows, a headrest, padding for bony prominences (foam, sheepskin, blankets, pillows), arm boards, a

TABLE 12–6. BODY STRUCTURES AT RISK FOR INJURY IN LATERAL DECUBITUS POSITION

Integumentary system
  Eyelids, ear, scalp, and all skin layers, particularly over bony prominences
Nervous system
  Brachial plexus; suprascapular, radial, ulnar, median, sciatic, lateral femoral cutaneous, and common peroneal nerves
Musculoskeletal system
  Bony prominences: temporal area, zygomatic arch, acromion process, greater tubercle of humerus, lateral and medial epicondyles of humerus, olecranon process, styloid process of ulna and radius, iliac crest, greater trochanter of femur, lateral and medial femoral epicondyles, lateral tibial condyles, and lateral and medial malleoli
  Joints: spine, shoulders, elbows, hips, and knees
  Muscles: neck
Respiratory system
  Chest wall and diaphragm
Vascular system
  Carotid artery, axillary artery, brachial artery, abdominal aorta, inferior vena cava, and saphenous vein
Breast and genitalia

Data from Aldrete, 1987; Biddle and Cannady, 1990; Dornette, 1986; Goldstein, 1987; Gruendemann, 1987; Lawson, 1987; Schmaus et al., 1987; Smith, 1987; Welborn, 1987.

safety strap, a beanbag, and other special positioning equipment.

Procedure

Transfer the Patient to the Operating Room Bed. Transfer and prepare the patient for anesthesia administration in the supine position as described for interventions for all surgical positions.

Prepare the Assistants. Ensure that the assistants understand their individual roles. The circulating nurse and one assistant stand on the right side of the OR bed if the patient's left side will be facing down. If the patient's right side will be facing down, the circulating nurse and assistant stand on the left side of the OR bed. The other two assistants stand on the opposite side of the OR bed, one across from the circulating nurse and the other near the foot of the OR bed.

Turn and Position the Patient. The anesthetist controls the head and neck and initiates the movement. After the patient's arms are placed at his or her sides, the circulating nurse and assistant reach under the patient's shoulders and hips, lift slightly, and draw the patient's far shoulder and hip toward the middle of the OR bed. Next they concurrently rotate the patient to the lateral position. The assistant across from the circulating nurse helps rotate the patient. The assistant near the foot of the OR bed controls the patient's legs. Support the patient until after the anesthetist has reestablished ventilation. Place a rolled towel or other type of padding (axillary roll) under the patient below the axilla, not in the axilla (Thomas, 1987, p. 151). Secure the patient with tape, beanbags, rolls, or other type of support. Flex the down-side leg at the knee to add stability. Place a pillow or padding between the patient's legs. After positioning the patient, ensure that

- the patient's head, neck, and spine are in proper alignment and the axillary roll is in the proper position, below the axilla
- the genitals and breast are free from pressure
- the legs and knees are padded
- no part of the patient's anatomy is resting on an unpadded surface
- the extremities are secured away from the OR bed joints (breaks) and attachments

Stabilize and secure the patient's body to the OR bed.

Prone Position

For the prone position (also known as the ventral recumbent or ventral decubitus position), the patient is placed face down, resting on his or her abdomen and chest (Fig. 12–9). This position and modifications of this position, such as the Kraske position, are used for procedures of the cervical spine, back, rectal area, and lower extremities.

Typically, the patient is placed under general anesthesia on the gurney before being transferred to the OR bed. However, the patient may be anesthetized on the OR bed and then rotated into the prone position.

Considerations

Staffing Requirements. The perioperative nurse and three assistants are the minimal nursing staff needed to position the patient.

Body Structures at Risk. (Table 12–7)

Potential Adverse Effects. (Rothrock, 1987, p. 275)

- Pressure on the inferior vena cava and femoral veins, resulting in hypotension, "causing blood to seek another pathway, such as the perineal venous plexus and the veins of the vertebral column"
- Excessive intraoperative blood loss due to increased blood flow through the veins of the vertebral column
- Injury to the brachial plexuses due to improperly placed support devices
- Injury to the lateral femoral cutaneous nerves due to compression against the pelvic support device
- Injury to the facial nerves in the intraparotic areas
- Injury to the ulnar nerves due to incorrect positioning
- Injury to nerves and tendons of the dorsa of the feet due to incorrect positioning, especially if the feet rest on the edge of the OR bed
- Injury to the genitalia and breasts

Supplies and Equipment

The routine supplies and equipment needed to place the patient in the prone position are pillows, a headrest,

---

TABLE 12–7. BODY STRUCTURES AT RISK FOR INJURY IN PRONE POSITION

Cerebrovascular system
Integumentary system
  Cornea, eyelids, ear, and all skin layers, particularly over bony prominences and pendulous abdomen
Nervous system
  Brachial plexus; optic, facial, radial, ulnar, and median nerves
Musculoskeletal system
  Bony prominences: temporal area, zygomatic arch, acromion process, clavicle, lateral chest wall, olecranon process, anterior superior iliac spine, pubic tubercle, patella, tibial tuberosity, and dorsal area of feet
  Joints: spine, shoulders, elbows, wrists, knees, hips, and toes
  Muscles: neck
Respiratory system
  Diaphragm
Vascular system
  Carotid artery, abdominal aorta, inferior vena cava, and saphenous vein
Breast and genitalia

Data from Aldrete, 1987; Dornette, 1986; Martin, 1987c; Schmaus et al., 1987; Smith, 1987; Winter and Munro, 1989.

chest rolls or a supporting frame (Relton, Wilson, and so on), padding for bony prominences and the dorsa of the feet (foam, sheepskin, blankets, pillows), arm boards, arm restraints, and a safety strap. Other supplementary equipment includes a face rest (horseshoe, Mayfield, and so on), a padded knee rest, and a table extension.

Procedure

Transfer the Patient to the Operating Room Bed. Transfer and prepare the patient for anesthesia administration in the supine position as described for interventions for all surgical positions.

Turn the Patient on the Operating Room Bed. Prepare the assistants by ensuring that the assistants understand their individual roles. The circulating nurse and one assistant stand on one side of the OR bed and the other two assistants stand on the opposite side of the OR bed. The anesthetist controls the head and neck and initiates the movement. After the patient's arms are placed at his or her sides, the circulating nurse and assistant reach under the patient's shoulders and hips, lift slightly, and draw the patient's far shoulder and hip toward the middle of the OR bed. The nurse and assistant concurrently rotate the patient to the lateral position. The assistant across from the circulating nurse helps rotate the patient. The assistant near the foot of the bed should control the legs. Continue rotating the patient while centering the trunk on the OR bed. Support the patient until after the anesthetist has reestablished ventilation. Place the positioning devices under the patient (Martin, 1987, p. 199).

Place the Patient in Position. After turning the patient, ensure that the chest rolls extend from the acromioclavicular joint to the iliac crest and do not impinge on the chest expansion (Gruendemann, 1987, p. 62). Ensure that the breasts are displaced medially on the

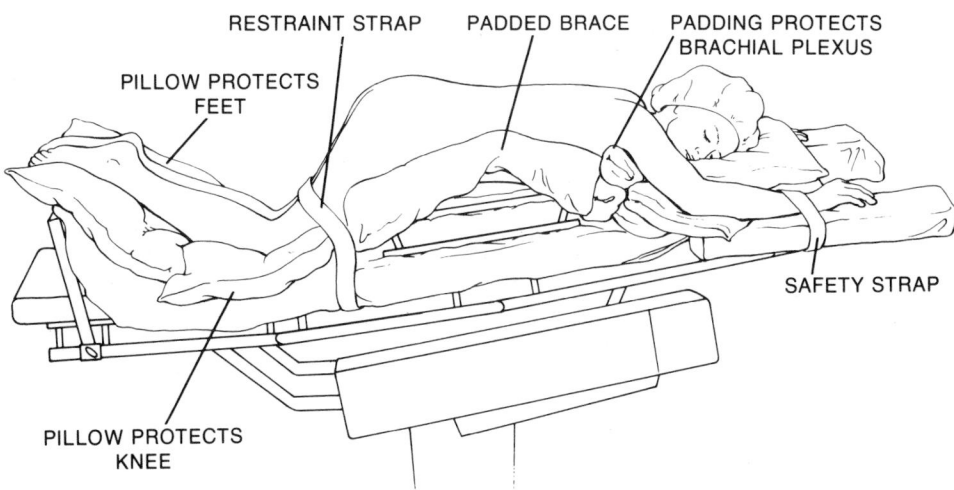

RESTRAINT STRAP PADDED BRACE PADDING PROTECTS
BRACHIAL PLEXUS
PILLOW PROTECTS
FEET

SAFETY STRAP

PILLOW PROTECTS
KNEE

FIGURE 12–9. Prone position with the OR bed modified for laminectomy. (From Fuller, J. R. [1986]. *Surgical technology: Principles and practice* [2nd ed.]. Philadelphia: W. B. Saunders.)

chest rolls (Martin, 1987, pp. 216–217). Check that the head, neck, spine, and legs are in proper alignment. Ensure that the legs are uncrossed and slightly apart. Check and free genitals from pressure. Pad iliac crests and knees. Support the dorsum of the foot with a pillow to prevent pressure on the toes. Ensure that no part of the patient's anatomy is resting on an unpadded surface. Ensure that the extremities are secured away from the OR bed joints (breaks) and attachments. Secure the body to the bed.

Position the Arms. If arm boards are used, the patient's arms "should be rotated cephalad in a plane roughly parallel to the sagittal plane of the body" (Martin, 1987, p. 202); the arms are positioned above the patient's head with the elbows flexed as seen in Figure 12–9 and secured to the arm boards. If the arms are placed at the patient's side, the palms should be turned toward the body or the bed and the full length of the arms needs to be secured by a draw sheet or padded toboggan.

Reassess the Patient. Reassess the patient before draping. Ensure that the chest rolls extend from the clavicle to the iliac crest and do not impinge on the

chest expansion. Check that the female breasts are displaced medially on the chest rolls. The body should be properly aligned and the safety strap in place. The arms should be properly secured and placed on the arm boards or at the patient's side. Check that there is no pressure on the genitals. The dorsum of the foot should be supported to prevent pressure on the toes.

Jackknife (Kraske) Position

The jackknife, or Kraske, position is a modification of the prone position. The patient is placed in the prone position and the bed is adjusted, placing the patient in an inverted V position (Fig. 12–10). This position is frequently used in gluteal and anorectal surgeries.

Considerations

Staffing Requirements. The perioperative nurse and three assistants are the minimal nursing staff needed to position the patient.

Body Structures at Risk. (Table 12–8)

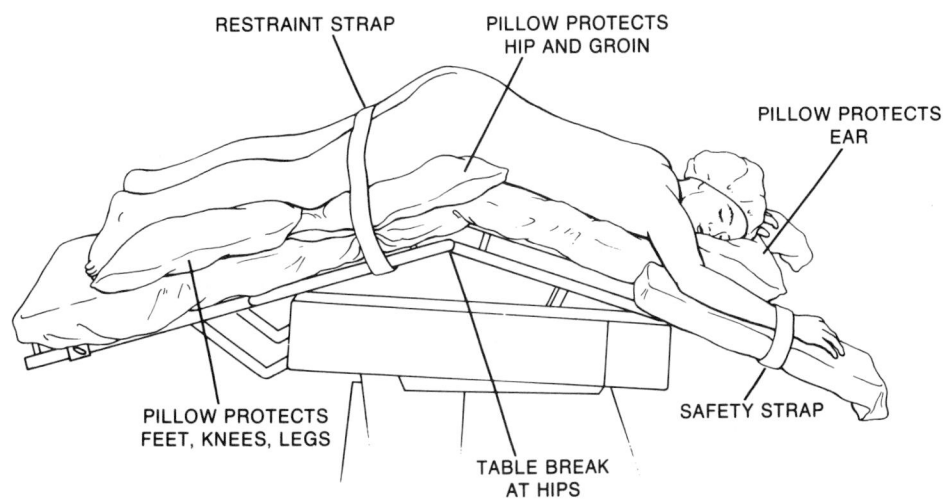

RESTRAINT STRAP PILLOW PROTECTS
HIP AND GROIN

PILLOW PROTECTS
EAR

PILLOW PROTECTS
FEET, KNEES, LEGS

TABLE BREAK
AT HIPS

SAFETY STRAP

FIGURE 12–10. Jackknife (Kraske) position. (From Fuller, J. R. [1986]. *Surgical technology: Principles and practice* [2nd ed.]. Philadelphia: W. B. Saunders.)

TABLE 12–8. **BODY STRUCTURES AT RISK FOR INJURY IN JACKKNIFE (KRASKE) POSITION**

Cerebrovascular system
Integumentary system
  Cornea, eyelids, ear, and all skin layers, particularly over bony
    prominences and pendulous abdomen
Nervous system
  Brachial plexus; optic, facial, radial, ulnar, and median nerves
Musculoskeletal system
  Bony prominences: temporal area, zygomatic arch, acromion
    process, clavicle, lateral chest wall, olecranon process, anterior
    superior iliac spine, pubic tubercle, patella, tibial tuberosity,
    and the dorsal area of the feet
  Joints: spine, shoulders, elbows, wrists, knees, hips, and toes
  Muscles: neck
Respiratory system
  Diaphragm
Vascular system
  Carotid artery, abdominal aorta, inferior vena cava, and
    saphenous vein
Breast and genitalia

Data from Aldrete, 1987; Dornette, 1986; Martin, 1987c; Schmaus et al., 1987; Smith, 1987; Winter and Munro, 1989.

Potential Adverse Effects. See under discussion of the prone position.

Supplies and Equipment

The routine supplies and equipment needed for placing the patient in the jackknife position are pillows, a headrest, chest rolls or a supporting frame (Relton, Wilson, and so on), padding for bony prominences and the dorsa of the feet (foam, sheepskin, blankets, pil-

lows), arm boards, arm restraints, and a safety strap. A face rest (horseshoe, Mayfield, and so on), a padded knee rest, and a table extension might also be needed.

Procedure

Transfer the Patient to the Operating Room Bed. Transfer and prepare the patient for anesthesia administration in the supine position as described for interventions for all surgical positions.

Turn and Position the Patient. Ensure that the assistants understand their individual roles. The circulating nurse and one assistant stand on one side of the OR bed and the other two assistants stand on the opposite side of the OR bed. Position the patient as described for the prone position.

Adjust the Operating Room Bed. Ensure that the patient's hips are positioned over the OR bed break. Check that there is no pressure on the patient's genitalia. Reverse flex the OR bed until the patient is in an inverted V position.

Reassess the Patient. Reassess the patient before draping for any potential discrepancies as described for the prone position.

Sitting Position

The sitting position is common for neurosurgery. The patient's back is raised with the thighs and legs flexed (Fig. 12–11).

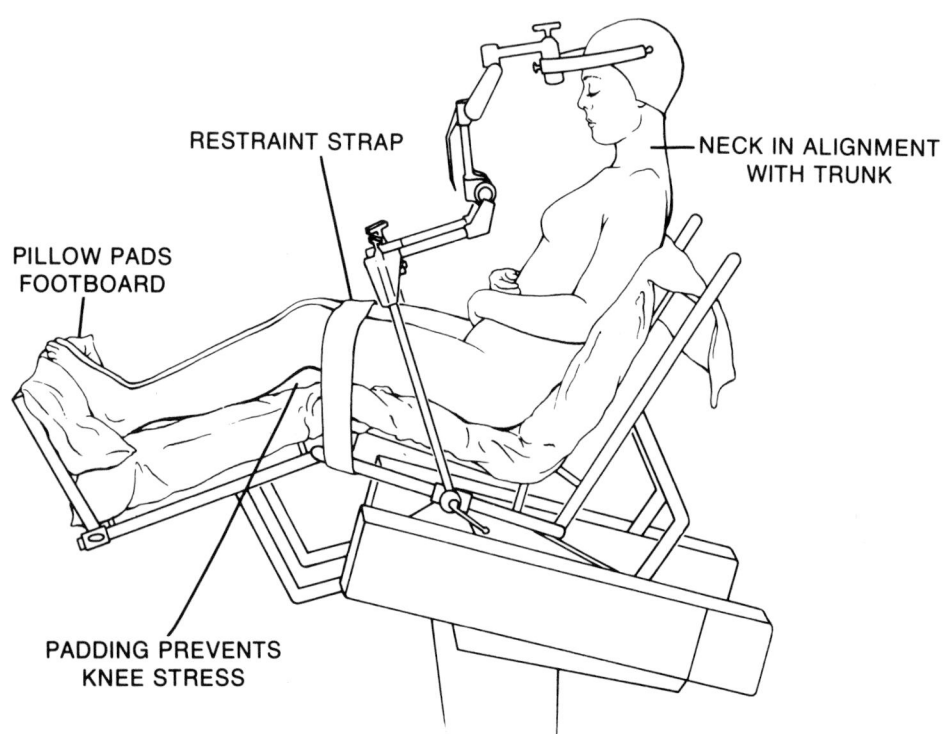

RESTRAINT STRAP

NECK IN ALIGNMENT WITH TRUNK

PILLOW PADS FOOTBOARD

PADDING PREVENTS KNEE STRESS

FIGURE 12–11. Sitting position. (From Fuller, J. R. [1986]. *Surgical technology: Principles and practice* [2nd ed.]. Philadelphia: W. B. Saunders.)

TABLE 12–9. BODY STRUCTURES AT RISK FOR INJURY IN SITTING POSITION

Integumentary system
 Scalp and all skin layers, particularly over bony prominences
Nervous system
 Cervical portion of the spinal cord; brachial plexus; and radial, ulnar, median, and sciatic nerves
Musculoskeletal system
 Bony prominences: spine, scapulae, olecranon process, sacrum, ischial tuberosities, and calcaneus
 Joints: spine, shoulders, elbows, knees, and hips
Vascular system
 Superficial temporal, occipital, and popliteal arteries and saphenous vein

Data from Aldrete, 1987; Dornette, 1986; Goldstein, 1987; Gruendemann, 1987; Martin, 1987a; Poppi et al., 1989; Reid and Grundy, 1987; Schmaus et al., 1987; Smith, 1987; Welborn, 1987.

Considerations

Staffing Requirement. The perioperative nurse is the minimal staff needed. Additional staffing requirements need to be noted on the perioperative nursing care plan.

Body Structures at Risk. (Table 12–9)

Potential Adverse Effects. (Rothrock, 1987, pp. 286–287)

- Intraoperative hypotension leading to cerebral hypoperfusion and hypoxia
- Venous pooling in the legs
- Venous air embolism
- Pressure sore development on the ischial tuberosities
- Injury to the sciatic nerves due to prolonged extension of the knees
- Footdrop due to pressure on the Achilles tendons

Supplies and Equipment

The routine supplies and equipment needed to place the patient in the sitting position are arm boards, arm restraints, a head holder (e.g., skull clamp, Mayfield, Gardner, with sterile skull pins), padding for bony prominences (foam, sheepskin, blankets, pillows), a padded footboard, and a safety strap. Additional supplies and equipment may include an antigravity suit, medical antishock trousers, elastic bandages, a table extension, and toboggans.

Procedure

Transfer the Patient to the Operating Room Bed. Transfer and prepare the patient for anesthesia administration in the supine position as described for interventions for all surgical positions.

Prepare the Patient. Before placing the patient in the sitting position, wrap both legs of the patient to the groin with elastic bandages or compression stockings.

The surgeon may request that an antigravity suit or medical antishock trousers be applied. Generously pad the patient under the buttocks and place padding under each heel. A padded footboard should be attached to the end of the OR bed (Rothrock, 1987, p. 290).

Modify the Operating Room Bed to the Sitting Position. Elevate the patient's back, flex the bed, and lower the footpiece. After the patient is in position, place the patient's arms on a pillow that has been set on her or his lap and secure with 3-inch adhesive tape attached to the OR bed frame. Pad each elbow with rubber. If available, place the patient's arms in arm holders. Attach the accessories for the skull clamp (Rothrock, 1987, p. 290).

Reassessing the Patient. Check the patient for alignment. If the patient is male, check to ensure that the scrotum and penis are not twisted or compressed between the legs (Rothrock, 1987, p. 290).

DOCUMENTATION AND COMMUNICATION PROCEDURES

Documenting surgical positioning and the nursing interventions associated with positioning is a professional responsibility. Perioperative nursing documentation should include a preoperative nursing history, assessment, and care plan. At a minimum, the assessment should include

- physical limitations
- weight
- height
- nutritional status
- skin condition
- preexisting disease
- type and length of procedure (Association of Operating Room Nurses [AORN], 1992, *III*:14–7)

The nurses' notes should contain information about the interventions used to eliminate, diminish, or alter the patient risk factors identified in the care plan. The intraoperative nursing record should include the following:

- position
- safety and security measures
- the use and the location of positioning devices (AORN, 1992, *III*:14–3)

Postoperatively, the nurse should assess and document the patient's physical condition.

SUMMARY

Positioning the patient for surgery takes skill. The perioperative nurse ensures that the surgical position does not compromise access to the patient's airway, intravenous lines, and monitoring devices. Injury to the patient's integumentary, circulatory, respiratory, musculoskeletal, and neurological structures can be prevented by identifying patients at risk for injury prior to initiating positioning activities. Careful planning and cooperation among surgical team members help avoid intraoperative and postoperative complications related to positioning (AORN, 1992, *III*:14–1).

Bibliography

Aldrete, J. A. (1987). Complications of positioning. In J. T. Martin (Ed.), *Positioning in anesthesia and surgery* (2nd ed.) (pp. 329–335). Philadelphia: W. B. Saunders.

Association of Operating Room Nurses. (1992). *Standards and recommended practices for perioperative nursing.* Denver.

Biddle, C., Cannady, M. J. (1990). Surgical positions: Their effects on cardiovascular, respiratory systems. *AORN Journal, 52*(2), 350–359.

Dornette, W. H. L. (1986). Compression neuropathies: Medical aspects and legal implications. *International Anesthesiology Clinics, 24*(4), 201–299.

Fuller, J. R. (1986). *Surgical technology: Principles and practice* (2nd ed.). Philadelphia: W. B. Saunders.

Goldstein, P. J. (1987). Surgical aspects: Obstetrics and gynecology. In J. T. Martin (Ed.), *Positioning in anesthesia and surgery* (2nd ed.) (pp. 41–51). Philadelphia: W. B. Saunders.

Gordon, M. (1987). *Nursing diagnosis: Process and application* (2nd ed.). New York: McGraw-Hill.

Gordon, M. (1989). Manual of Nursing Diagnosis: 1988–1989. St. Louis: C. V. Mosby.

Gruendemann, B. J. (1987). *Positioning plus.* Chatsworth, CA: Devon Industries.

Kropp, K. A. (1987). Urology: Surgical aspects. In J. T. Martin (Ed.), *Positioning in anesthesia and surgery* (2nd ed.) (pp. 241–254). Philadelphia: W. B. Saunders.

Lawson, N. W. (1987). The lateral decubitus position: Anesthesiologic considerations. In J. T. Martin (Ed.), *Positioning in anesthesia and surgery* (2nd ed.) (pp. 155–179). Philadelphia: W. B. Saunders.

Martin, J. T. (1987). *Positioning in anesthesia and surgery* (2nd ed.). Philadelphia: W. B. Saunders.

McAlpine, F. S., Seckel, B. R. (1987). Complications of positioning: The peripheral nervous system. In J. T. Martin (Ed.), *Positioning in anesthesia and surgery* (2nd ed.) (pp. 303–328). Philadelphia: W. B. Saunders.

Poppi, M., Giuliani, G., Gambari, P. I., et al. (1989). Hazard of craniotomy in the sitting position: The posterior compartment syndrome of the thigh. *Journal of Neurosurgery, 71*(4), 618–619.

Prentice, J. A., Martin, J. T. (1987). The Trendelenburg position: Anesthesiologic considerations. In J. T. Martin (Ed.), *Positioning in anesthesia and surgery* (2nd ed.) (pp. 127–145). Philadelphia: W. B. Saunders.

Reid, S. A., Grundy, B. L. (1987). The head-elevated positions. Surgical aspects: The neurosurgical skull clamp. In J. T. Martin (Ed.), *Positioning in anesthesia and surgery* (2nd ed.) (pp. 71–77). Philadelphia: W. B. Saunders.

Rothrock, J. C. (1987). *The RN first assistant: An expanded perioperative nursing role.* New York: J. B. Lippincott.

Schiller, W. R. (1987). The Trendelenburg position: Surgical aspects. In J. T. Martin (Ed.), *Positioning in anesthesia and surgery* (2nd ed.) (pp. 117–126). Philadelphia: W. B. Saunders.

Schmaus, D. C., Nelson, S. L., Davis, D. L. (1987). *Positioning the surgical patient.* Denver, CO: Association of Operating Room Nurses.

Smith, B. L. (1987). The traditional supine position. In J. T. Martin (Ed.), *Positioning in anesthesia and surgery* (2nd ed.) (pp. 33–35). Philadelphia: W. B. Saunders.

Thomas, A. N. (1987). The lateral decubitus position: Surgical aspects. In J. T. Martin (Ed.), *Positioning in anesthesia and surgery* (2nd ed.) (pp. 147–154). Philadelphia: W. B. Saunders.

Welborn, S. G. (1987). The lithotomy position: Anesthesiologic considerations. In J. T. Martin (Ed.), *Positioning in anesthesia and surgery* (2nd ed.) (pp. 57–62). Philadelphia: W. B. Saunders.

Winter, R., Munro, M. (1989). Lingual and buccal nerve neuropathy in a patient in the prone position: A case report. *Anesthesiology, 71*(3), 452–454.

CHAPTER 13

Handling Cultures and Specimens

Sharon Hendricks

DEFINITION

Handling cultures and specimens refers to the nursing activities performed or supervised by the perioperative nurse to collect, process, store, preserve, and transport surgical cultures and tissue specimens.

MEASURABLE CRITERIA

The perioperative nurse demonstrates competency to handle cultures and specimens by correctly

- providing supplies and equipment needed for the collection of cultures and specimens
- labeling culture and tissue specimen containers
- completing laboratory slips
- documenting the collection of cultures and specimens on the patient's operative record
- establishing chain of custody for cultures and tissue specimens

- obtaining and processing cultures for examination
- obtaining and processing tissue for examination
- storing, preserving, and maintaining tissue
- directing the transfer of cultures and specimens to the laboratory
- communicating intraoperative pathology reports to the surgeon

ROLE OF THE PERIOPERATIVE NURSE

The perioperative nurse, as the circulator, implements the measurable criteria described above. With appropriate supervision, assignment of these tasks to qualified assistive personnel is permissible. If an assistive person helps the perioperative nurse accomplish the measurable criteria, however, the nurse remains accountable. If the handling of cultures and specimens is assigned to assistive personnel, the perioperative nurse must ensure that identification and documentation procedures are accurately implemented.

CONSIDERATIONS

Legal Implications

Proper labeling of cultures and specimens ensures continuity of care for the patient. With proper documentation, the specimen can be tracked from its source to its disposition. In addition, "documentation provides a comprehensive method of retrieving information in the event of legal action and for the measuring of the quality of care delivered in quality assurance programs" (Groah, 1983, p. 128).

Infection Control

All cultures and specimens are potentially infectious. Thus, personnel must use universal precautions while collecting and preparing cultures and specimens for examination. Gloves are essential and must be worn at all times. After the gloves are removed, the hands must be washed. The perioperative nurse must avoid contaminating the exterior surface of culture tubes or specimen containers with blood or other body fluids. If contamination occurs, the exterior surfaces of tubes or containers "should be cleaned with a tuberculocidal hospital-grade disinfectant or a 1:10 dilution of household bleach before they are removed from the operating room" (Association of Operating Room Nurses [AORN], 1992, III:17–2) (Fig. 13–1). If tubes or containers cannot be disinfected, they should be placed in an impervious clear bag for transportation to the laboratory and labeled that the exterior surface of the tube or container is contam-

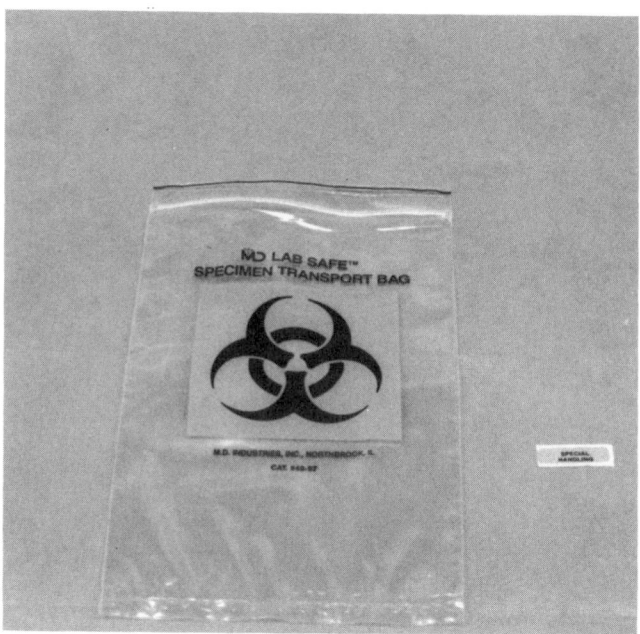

FIGURE 13–2. A contaminated culture tube is placed in an impervious clear bag for transport to the laboratory. (Courtesy of Santa Rosa Hospital, San Antonio, TX.)

inated (Fig. 13–2). This alerts the person receiving the culture or specimen to use caution when handling the tube or container.

The perioperative nurse should also prevent contamination of documents such as labels and laboratory slips (AORN, 1992, III:1–2). If they become contaminated, fresh documents should be prepared.

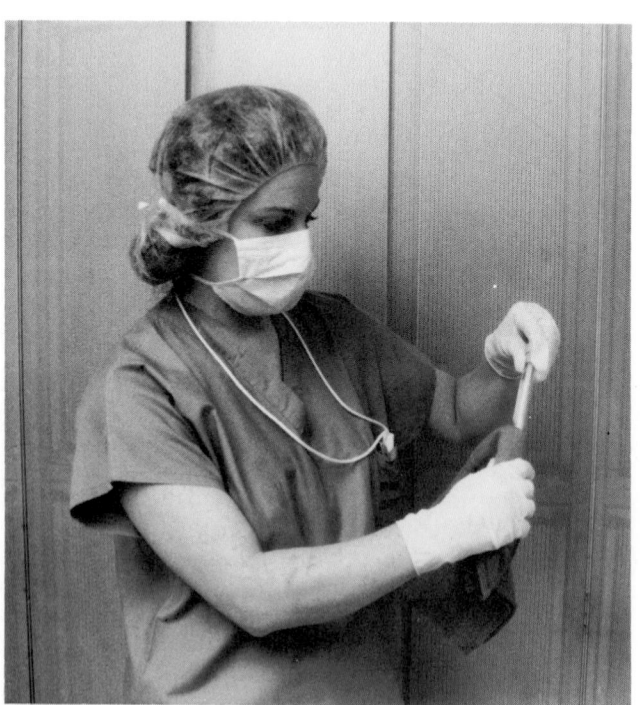

FIGURE 13–1. The nurse disinfects the exterior surface of the culture tube. (Courtesy of Santa Rosa Hospital, San Antonio, TX.)

Supplies and Equipment

Addressograph
Labels and laboratory slips (histology, cytology, aerobic, anaerobic, and acid fast)

Culture Tubes

Anaerobic (Fig. 13–3, right), aerobic (Fig. 13–3, left), and test tube with cap (Fig. 13–4, left); blood culture bottles (Fig. 13–5); and Petri dishes (Fig. 13–4, right) are used.

Tissue Specimen Containers

Tissue containers are designed to hold permanent specimens. They should be rigid, impermeable, unbreakable, and nonreactive to fixative solutions such as formalin and alcohol. Lids should be tight fitting, prevent fluids from spilling from the container, and suppress odors. A variety of container sizes should be available for use (Fig. 13–6).

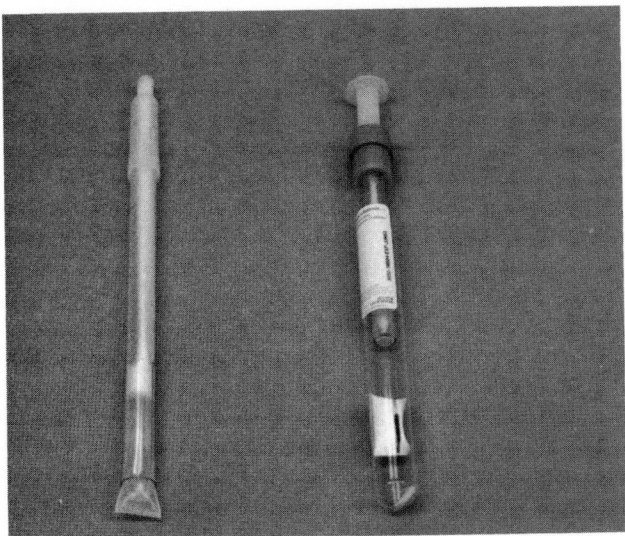

FIGURE 13–3. Aerobic and anaerobic culture tubes. (Courtesy of Santa Rosa Hospital, San Antonio, TX.)

Formalin

Formalin is a clear aqueous solution of formaldehyde with a small amount of methanol. The solution is commonly used as a preservative for permanent specimens. Formalin is usually prepared as a 10% solution by laboratory personnel.

When used in the surgical suite, formalin may be poured directly over a specimen that has been placed in a specimen container or poured into a container before specimen collection. When pouring formalin over a specimen or into a container, extreme caution must be exercised to avoid splashing, contact with body surfaces, and breathing of the vapors. Whenever containers are prepared, the employee should wear protective eyewear and gloves (Fig. 13–7). A hazard label should be affixed to receptacles containing formalin (Fig. 13–8).

Because formalin is designated a hazardous material by federal law, a material safety data sheet (MSDS) is distributed to the purchaser of the chemical. The formalin MSDS should be maintained on file with MSDSs of other hazardous chemicals. According to the formalin

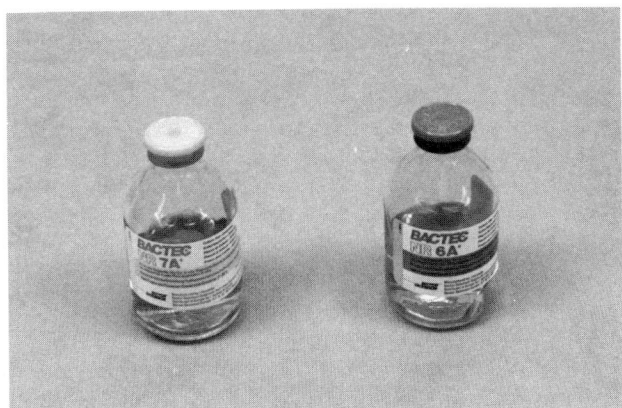

FIGURE 13–5. Blood culture bottles. (Courtesy of Santa Rosa Hospital, San Antonio, TX.)

MSDS, the following precautions should be used when handling the chemical:

- Formalin is flammable. Keep it away from heat, sparks, and flames. If needed, use a water fire extinguisher.
- Formalin vapors are toxic. The chemical should be used only with adequate ventilation. When filling specimen containers or preparing specimens, employees must avoid breathing the vapors. Formalin may cause sore throat, coughing, shortness of breath, and irritation of the respiratory tract. In high concentration, formalin may be fatal. If formalin is inhaled, move the person to fresh air. Oxygen therapy is appropriate if breathing is difficult. If the person is not breathing, give artificial respiration.
- Formalin is toxic to the skin. Redness, pain, and possibly burns may result from skin exposure. When formalin is absorbed by the skin, symptoms paralleling those of ingestion may occur. Exposed skin surfaces should be flushed with water for 15 minutes. As a precaution, after handling formalin, thoroughly wash the hands with soap and water.
- In the event of eye contact, immediately flush the eyes with plenty of water for at least 15 minutes.

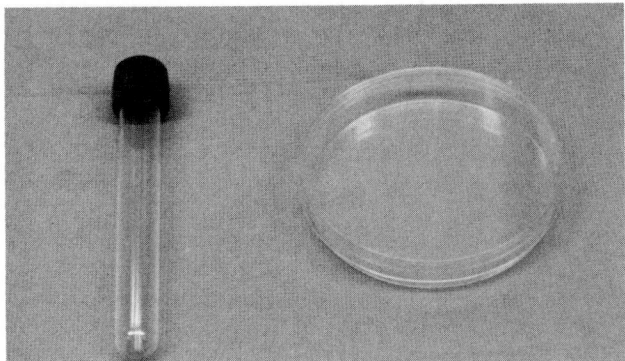

FIGURE 13–4. Test tube with cap and Petri dish. (Courtesy of Santa Rosa Hospital, San Antonio, TX.)

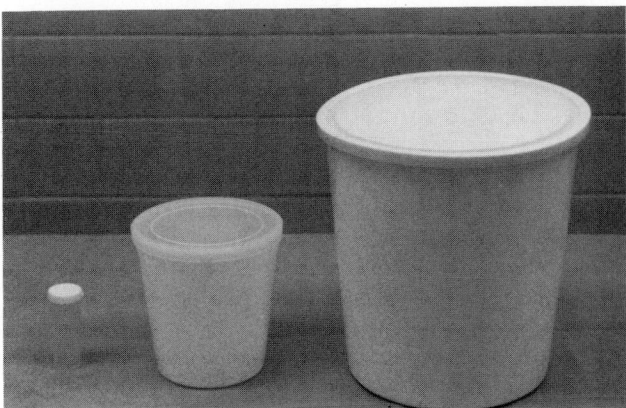

FIGURE 13–6. Specimen containers. (Courtesy of Santa Rosa Hospital, San Antonio, TX.)

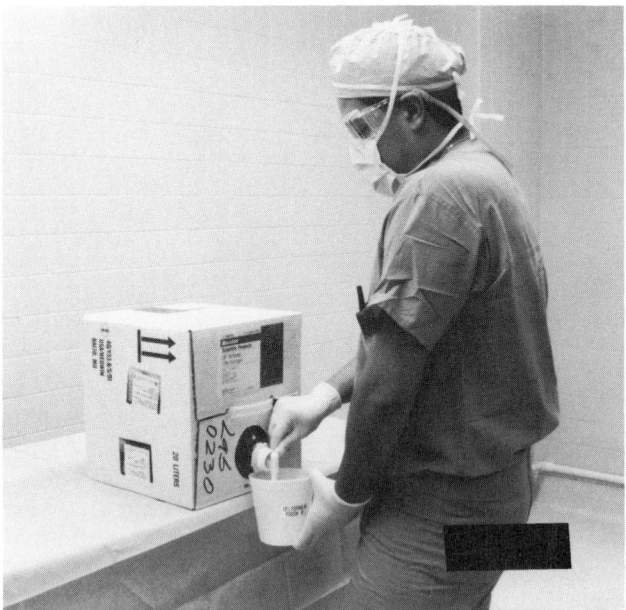

FIGURE 13–7. An employee wears protective eyewear, gloves, and a mask while dispensing hazardous fluid. (Courtesy of Santa Rosa Hospital, San Antonio, TX.)

Vapors may cause irritation of the eyes, with redness, pain, and possibly burns.

- The ingestion of formalin may cause severe abdominal pain, violent vomiting, headache, and diarrhea. Larger doses may lead to decreased body temperature, pain in the digestive tract, shallow respirations, weak irregular pulse, unconsciousness, and death. The methanol component of formalin affects the optic nerve and may cause blindness.
- In the event of a formalin spill, ventilate the area and remove sources of ignition. The area should be cleaned according to the hospital policy and procedure.

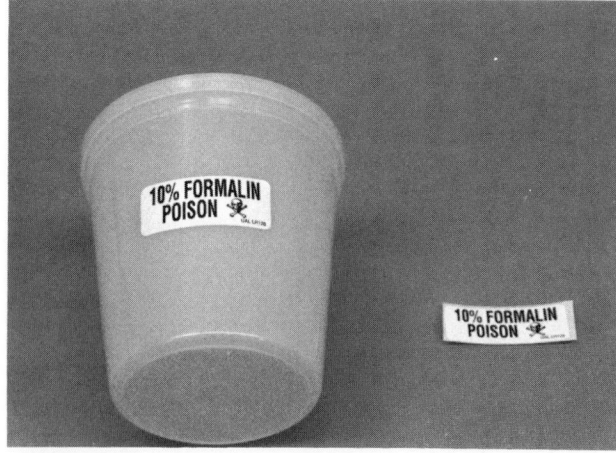

FIGURE 13–8. Specimen container with warning labels. (Courtesy of Santa Rosa Hospital, San Antonio, TX.)

OUTCOME STANDARD

The patient is free from injury related to the handling of cultures and specimens during the perioperative period.

Criteria

The patient does not experience a compromised diagnosis because of inappropriate handling of cultures and specimens.

POTENTIAL ALTERATIONS IN FUNCTIONAL HEALTH PATTERNS

Health Perception–Health Management Pattern

Diagnosis

High risk for injury related to improper handling of cultures and specimens obtained during surgery

Definition

Presence of risk factors for the patient to experience a wrong diagnosis, no diagnosis, or the prevention of definitive therapy because of improper handling of cultures and specimens by the perioperative nursing team

Risk Factors

- Failure to provide the correct supplies and equipment for culture and specimen collection
- Incorrect labeling of culture and tissue specimen containers
- Incorrect completion of laboratory slips
- Incorrect documentation of cultures and specimens on the patient's operative record
- Failure to establish chain of custody for cultures and tissue specimens
- Improper intraoperative processing of cultures and tissue for examination
- Improper storage, preservation, and maintenance of tissue
- Failure to direct properly the transfer of cultures and specimens to the laboratory
- Incorrect communication of intraoperative pathology reports to the surgeon

Expected Outcome

The patient does not experience injury related to the handling of specimens and cultures. There is no evidence of incorrect medical diagnosis or treatment due to improper handling of cultures and specimens by the perioperative nursing team.

PERIOPERATIVE NURSING INTERVENTIONS

Providing Supplies and Equipment

To ensure continuity of care, facilitate the surgical procedure, and prevent delays, the perioperative nurse gathers supplies and equipment needed for cultures and specimens before the patient is transferred to the operating room (OR) bed. The perioperative nurse determines the types of supplies and equipment needed by assessing the patient, reviewing the patient's record, checking the surgeon's preference card, and questioning the surgeon concerning specific culture and specimen needs. If appropriate, the nurse contacts laboratory personnel or pathologists to make arrangements for special tests or procedures.

Labeling Culture and Specimen Containers

Correct labeling of culture and specimen containers is essential for the prevention of patient injury. Proper labeling ensures that the patient receives the appropriate diagnosis (Atkinson and Kohn, 1986, p. 217). By affixing a label to the container, the culture or specimen can still be identified if the laboratory slip is lost. A stamped label, using the addressograph card, or a hand written label is appropriate. The label should contain at least the following information:

- patient's name
- patient's identification number
- physician's name
- source of the culture or type of tissue specimen
- date and time of collection

Completing Laboratory Slips

All cultures and specimens must be dispatched to the laboratory or pathology department with an appropriate laboratory slip (Fig. 13–9). The number and the format of laboratory slips vary from hospital to hospital. All slips, however, have the same purposes: to identify the type of study requested, to communicate pertinent patient information to the laboratory technologist or pathologist, and to serve as a reporting document for the attending physician. Like the container label, the laboratory slip must be correctly completed. Information must be legible and accurate. The addressograph card is used to stamp identifying information on the slip. If an addressograph card is not available, the information should be carefully written in the space provided on the slip. The following information should be recorded on the laboratory slip:

- patient's name
- patient's identification number

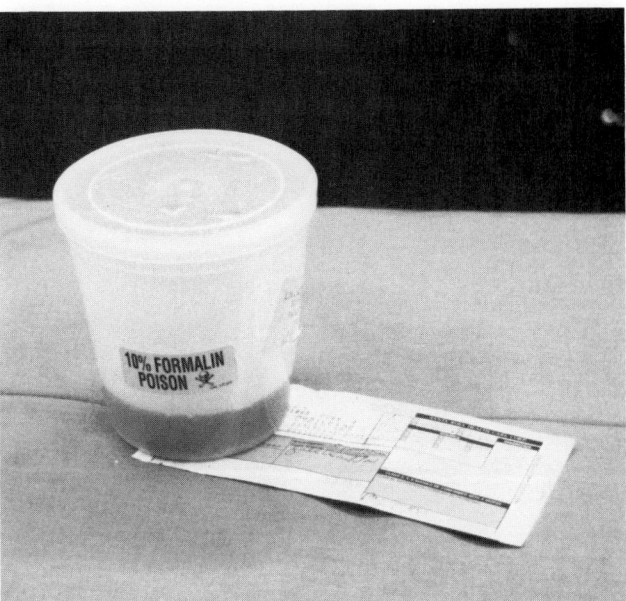

FIGURE 13–9. A laboratory slip is completed for each specimen. (Courtesy of Santa Rosa Hospital, San Antonio, TX.)

- physician's name
- culture or tissue source (specific)
- date and time of collection
- patient's medical diagnosis
- patient's unit room number
- identification of the study requested
- other pertinent information such as antibiotics being administered

Documenting the Collection of Cultures and Specimens

Accurate documentation of the collection, identification, and disposition of cultures and specimens on the patient's operative record is essential. The operative record should reflect the source of the culture or the type of specimen, the time of collection, and the studies requested (Table 13–1). Noting the final disposition of the culture and specimen is also important. If a specimen is not obtained, this too should be reflected on the operative record. Although not part of the operative record, laboratory slips, if returned to the OR during the intraoperative period with study results, should be placed in the patient's chart.

Establishing Chain of Custody

Chain of custody is a mechanism to ensure accountability for culture and tissue specimens. Log books are used to track the specimen from the surgical suite to the laboratory or pathology department (Fig. 13–10). Various systems are used. The dual–log book system, however, is recommended. One log book is used to register

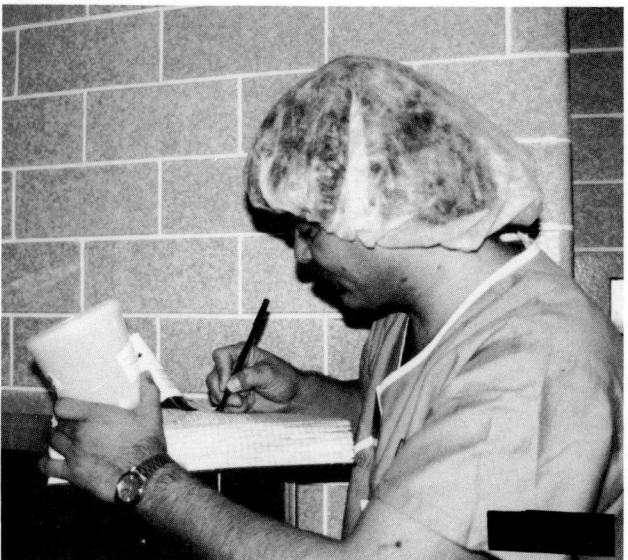

FIGURE 13–10. Careful documentation ensures that cultures, tissue specimens, and other objects removed from the patient are not lost. (Courtesy of Santa Rosa Hospital, San Antonio, TX.)

specimens for culture, and the other log book is used to register tissue permanent specimens and frozen sections, as well as other objects removed from the patient. The following information should be recorded in the log book:

- patient's name
- patient's identification number
- physician's name
- source of culture or type of tissue specimen or object
- person logging the specimen
- date and time of log in
- person receiving the specimen
- date and time of disposition

Maintaining accountability can be a tedious process. Diligence in the task, however, ensures that cultures, tissue specimens, and other objects removed from the patient are not lost.

TABLE 13–1. **TYPES OF SPECIMENS**
Tissue
Permanent
Frozen section
Biopsy: tissue or fluid
Hormonal receptor site
Papanicolaou smears (in alcohol)
Skin sent for storage
Fluid
Aerobic cultures
Anaerobic cultures
Gram stain
Spinal fluid
Acid fast: culture or smear
Fungus: culture or smear
Miscellaneous
Foreign bodies (e.g., bullets)
Orthopedic hardware

Collecting and Preparing Cultures for Examination

If the surgeon identifies or suspects an infectious process during the surgical procedure, a specimen for culture or other bacteriological study is obtained. Types of studies include aerobic, anaerobic, Gram stain, acid-fast, and mycological examinations. Whatever the type of study, the purpose of the culture is to identify the pathogen causing the infection. The surgeon uses this information to order appropriate antibiotics and start a treatment regimen.

Four types of microorganisms cause most nosocomial infections: aerobic bacteria, microaerophilic bacteria, anaerobic bacteria, and nonbacterial microorganisms, such as viruses and fungi (Table 13–2). Aerobic bacteria require the presence of oxygen for survival. Microaerophilic bacteria require oxygen but can survive with amounts less than are found in the atmosphere, and anaerobic bacteria grow in the absence of oxygen.

General Guidelines

When obtaining fluid, tissue, or other material for culture, enough should be obtained to permit all tests requested by the physician to be performed. Sterile equipment and receptacles must be used so as not to contaminate the specimen with exogenous microorganisms. Integrity of the culture specimen must be maintained. Specimen contact with chemicals, germicides, or disinfectants may compromise laboratory processing and invalidate study results. If multiple studies are ordered,

TABLE 13–2. **COMMON PATHOGENS OF NOSOCOMIAL INFECTIONS**	
Aerobic bacteria	Microaerophilic bacteria
Gram-positive cocci	Gram-positive cocci
Staphylococcus aureus	Hemolytic streptococci
S. epidermidis	Nonhemolytic streptococci
Streptococcus group B	Anaerobic bacteria
Streptococcus group D	Gram-positive cocci
Gram-negative cocci	*Peptostreptococcus*
Neisseria gonorrhoeae	*Peptococcus*
Gram-positive bacilli	Gram-positive bacilli
Bacillus subtilis	*Clostridium tetani*
Mycobacterium tuberculosis	*C. welchii*
Gram-negative bacilli	Gram-negative bacilli
Escherichia coli	*Bacteroides* species
Klebsiella pneumoniae	*B. fragilis*
Pseudomonas aeruginosa	Nonbacterial microorganisms
P. cepacia	Viruses
Proteus vulgaris	Herpesvirus
Serratia marcescens	Hepatitis virus
Salmonella species	Human immunodeficiency
Alcaligenes faecalis	virus
Haemophilus influenzae	Fungi
Enterobacter species	*Candida albicans*
	Histoplasma capsulatum
	Phycomycosis species

Adapted from Atkinson, L. J., Kohn, M. L. (1986). *Berry and Kohn's introduction to operating room technique* (6th ed.) (p. 103). New York: McGraw-Hill. Reproduced by permission of Mosby-Year Book, St. Louis, MO.

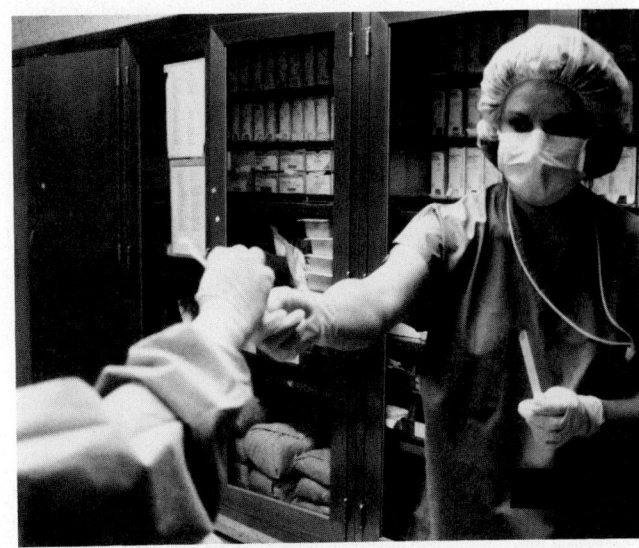

FIGURE 13–11. The circulating nurse presents the culture swab to the scrub person. (Courtesy of Santa Rosa Hospital, San Antonio, TX.)

one culture should be obtained for each test (Santa Rosa Hospital, 1988, #161, p. 0003).

Aerobic Cultures

The surgeon uses a sterile culture tube with a cotton swab to obtain an aerobic culture during the operative procedure. After the surgeon notifies the nursing team that she or he wants aerobic cultures taken, the circulator prepares the culture system. Two methods of obtaining the culture are acceptable.

With the first method, the circulating nurse removes the sterile tube from the package. The bottom of the tube is held with one hand, while the other hand carefully removes the top of the tube and exposes the distal end of the cotton swab. The scrub nurse grasps the end of the swab attached to the top and pulls it from the culture tube (Fig. 13–11). Avoid touching or contaminating the cotton swabs. If the culture is to be taken immediately, the circulating nurse should stand adjacent to the sterile field, tube and cap in hand, ready to accept the swab. If the culture will be taken later, the circulating nurse should recap the tube.

After the culture is taken, the scrub nurse carefully inserts the swab into the tube, which is held by the circulating nurse (Fig. 13–12). The circulating nurse then recaps the tube (Fig. 13–13) and crushes the media ampule at the midpoint of the bottom tube by gently squeezing the tube over the ampule (Fig. 13–14). Next, the circulating nurse pushes on the cap to ensure that the swab tip contacts the moistened pledgets (Fig. 13–15). The tube is labeled and sent to the laboratory with

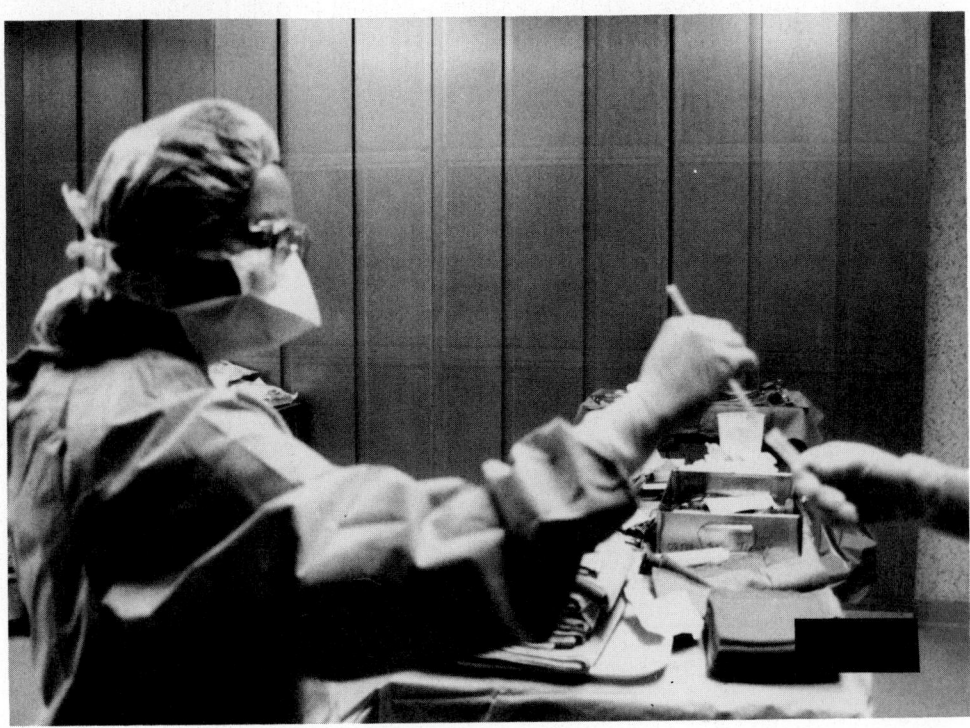

FIGURE 13–12. The scrub nurse returns the aerobic culture tube to the culture container. (Courtesy of Santa Rosa Hospital, San Antonio, TX.)

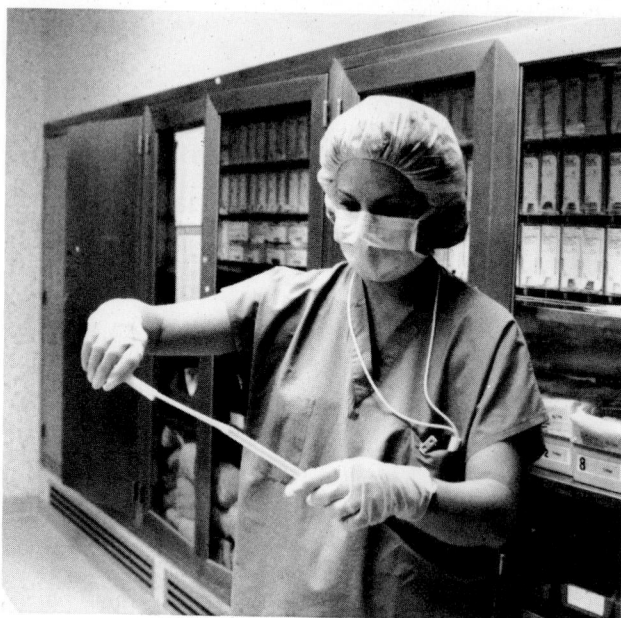

FIGURE 13–13. The circulating nurse inserts the culture swab into the aerobic culture tube. (Courtesy of Santa Rosa Hospital, San Antonio, TX.)

FIGURE 13–14. The circulating nurse activates the medium in the culture tube by crushing the bottom of the tube. (Courtesy of Santa Rosa Hospital, San Antonio, TX.)

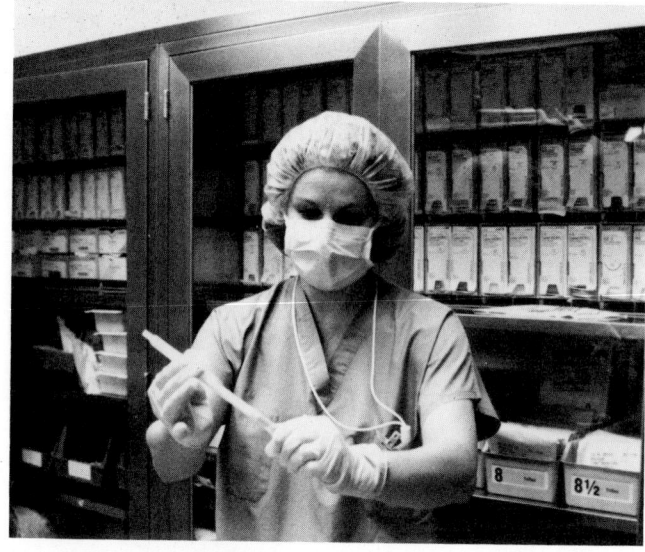

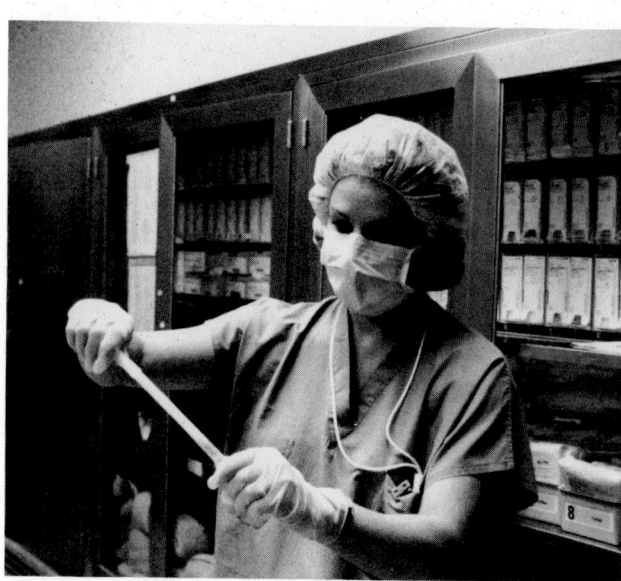

FIGURE 13–15. The circulating nurse pushes on the aerobic culture tube cap to ensure that the swab tip enters the culture medium. (Courtesy of Santa Rosa Hospital, San Antonio, TX.)

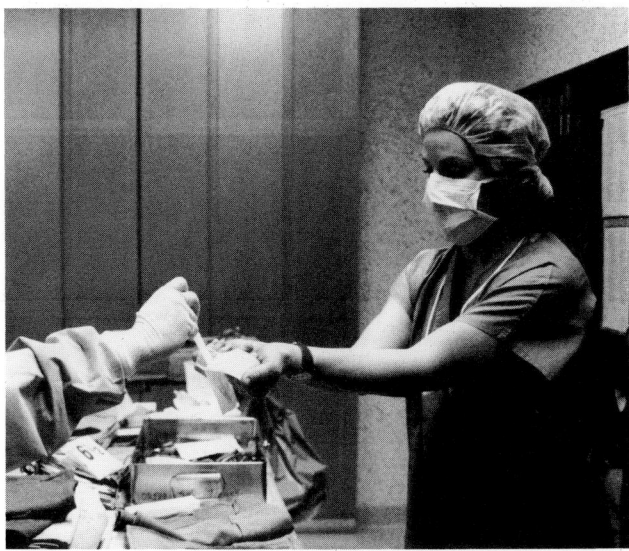

FIGURE 13-16. The circulating nurse aseptically delivers the aerobic culture tube and swab to the sterile field. (Courtesy of Santa Rosa Hospital, San Antonio, TX.)

the appropriate laboratory slip. If done correctly, this method is preferable because it ensures that the exterior of the culture tube is not contaminated.

With the second method, the circulating nurse aseptically delivers the culture tube and swab to the sterile field (Fig. 13-16). The scrub nurse removes the cotton swab and passes it to the surgeon (Fig. 13-17). After the culture is taken, the surgeon or the scrub nurse inserts the swab into the tube. The scrub nurse recaps the tube (Fig. 13-18) and passes it off the sterile field to the circulating nurse (Fig. 13-19). Wearing gloves, the circulating nurse receives the tube, decontaminates it with a tuberculocidal hospital-grade disinfectant or a 1:10 dilution of household bleach (Fig. 13-20), breaks

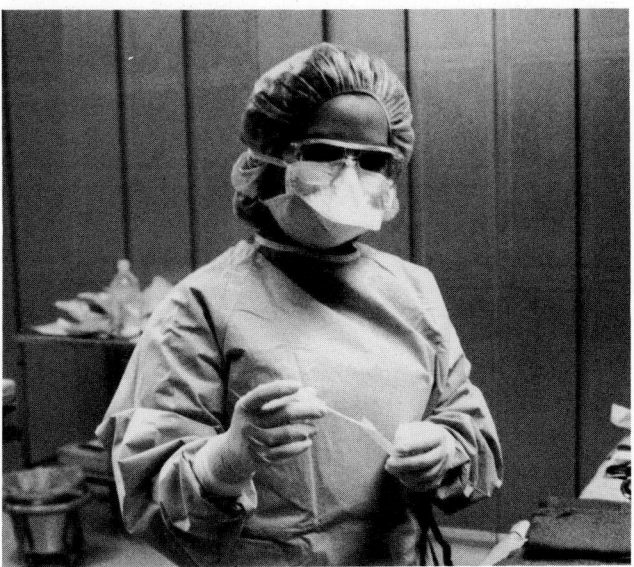

FIGURE 13-17. The scrub nurse removes the culture swab and passes it to the surgeon. (Courtesy of Santa Rosa Hospital, San Antonio, TX.)

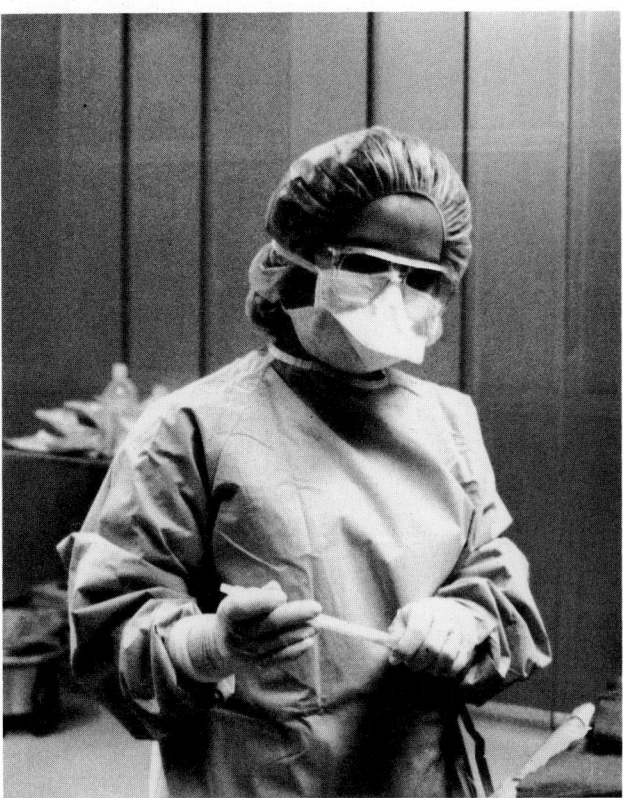

FIGURE 13-18. The scrub nurse recaps the aerobic culture tube. (Courtesy of Santa Rosa Hospital, San Antonio, TX.)

the media ampule, pushes the swab into the media, attaches a label, and sends the tube to the laboratory with the appropriate laboratory slip.

Anaerobic Cultures

Anaerobic cultures must be obtained in such a manner that the specimen is not in contact with air for a long period of time. If a swab is used to obtain the specimen, care should be taken to ensure that it is not aerated. Fluid for anaerobic cultures may be sent to the laboratory in an anaerobic culture transport system or a syringe with all air removed. A sterile plastic tube may be used for tissue obtained for anaerobic study. In such cases, however, the specimen must be immediately sent to the laboratory. Even though anaerobic bacteria survive longer in tissue, delay in dispatching the specimen can hinder the culturing process (Santa Rosa Hospital, 1988, #166, p. 0002).

The circulating nurse aseptically delivers the anaerobic culture system to the sterile field (Fig. 13-21). The scrub nurse pulls the cap with the swab attached out of the tube and passes it to the surgeon (Fig. 13-22). After obtaining the culture, the surgeon or the scrub nurse inserts the swab into the tube (Fig. 13-23). While recapping the tube, the scrub nurse pushes the cap firmly onto the tube with a downward motion (Fig. 13-24).

The gloved circulating nurse receives the anaerobic

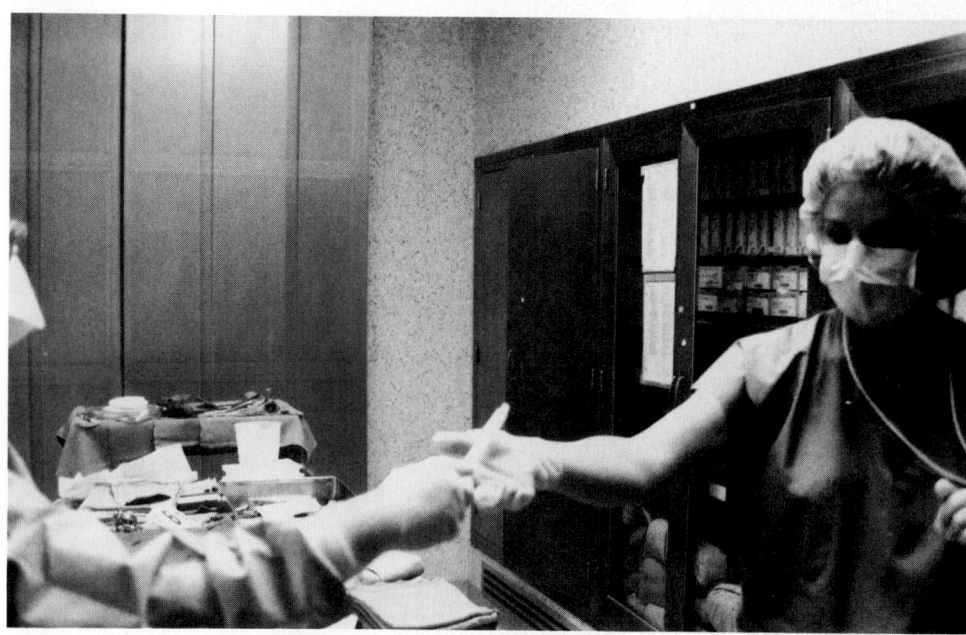

FIGURE 13–19. The scrub nurse passes the aerobic culture tube to the gloved circulating nurse. (Courtesy of Santa Rosa Hospital, San Antonio, TX.)

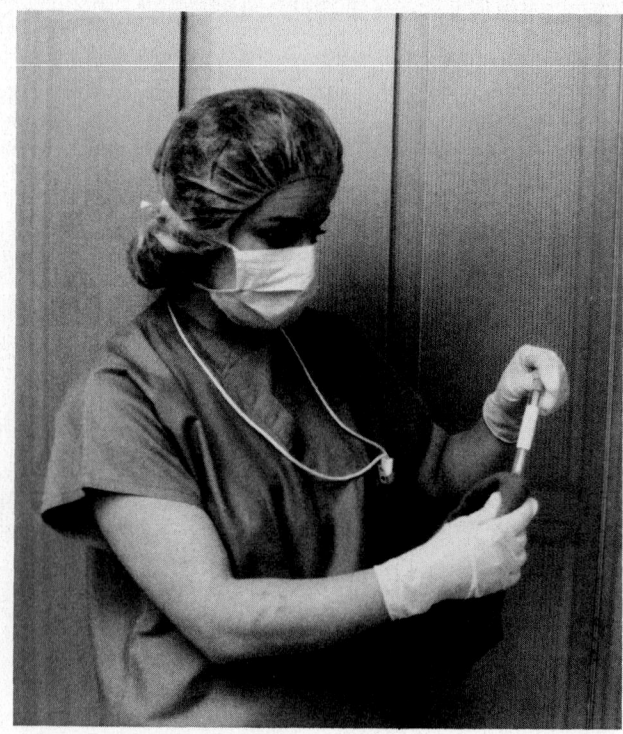

FIGURE 13–20. The circulating nurse disinfects the aerobic culture tube. (Courtesy of Santa Rosa Hospital, San Antonio, TX.)

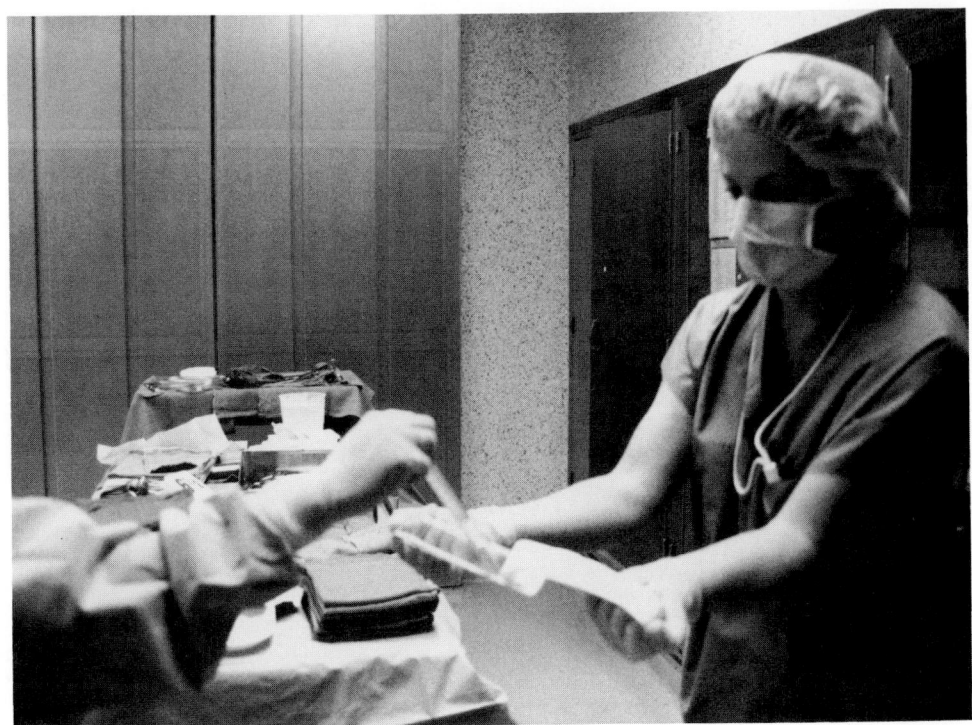

FIGURE 13–21. The circulating nurse passes the anaerobic culture tube to the sterile field. (Courtesy of Santa Rosa Hospital, San Antonio, TX.)

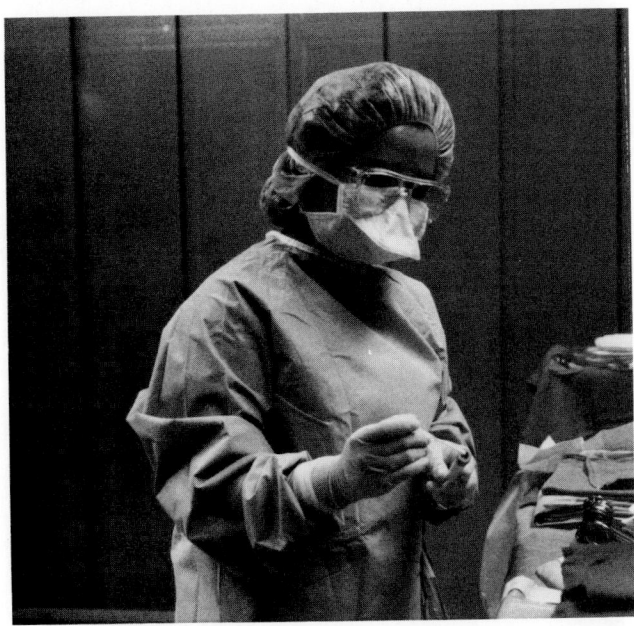

FIGURE 13–22. The scrub nurse takes the cap of the anaerobic culture tube and gives the swab to the surgeon. (Courtesy of Santa Rosa Hospital, San Antonio, TX.)

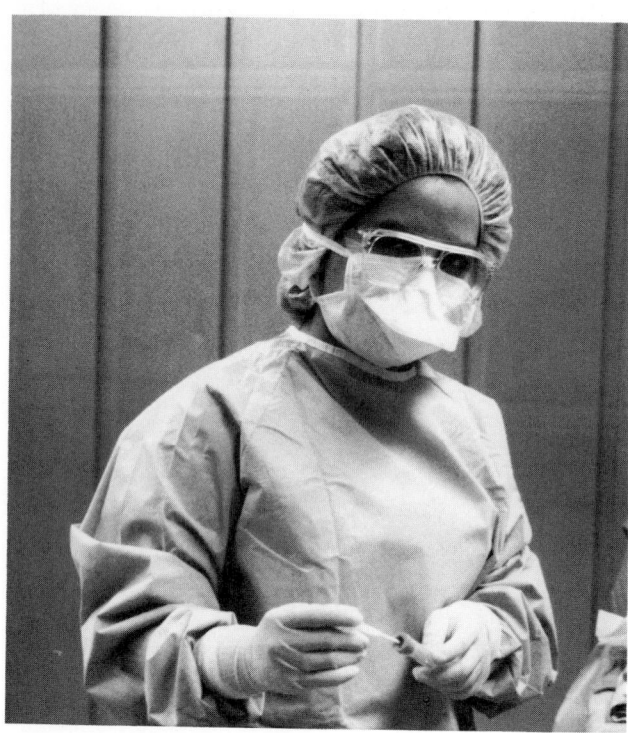

FIGURE 13–23. The scrub nurse inserts the swab back into the anaerobic culture tube. (Courtesy of Santa Rosa Hospital, San Antonio, TX.)

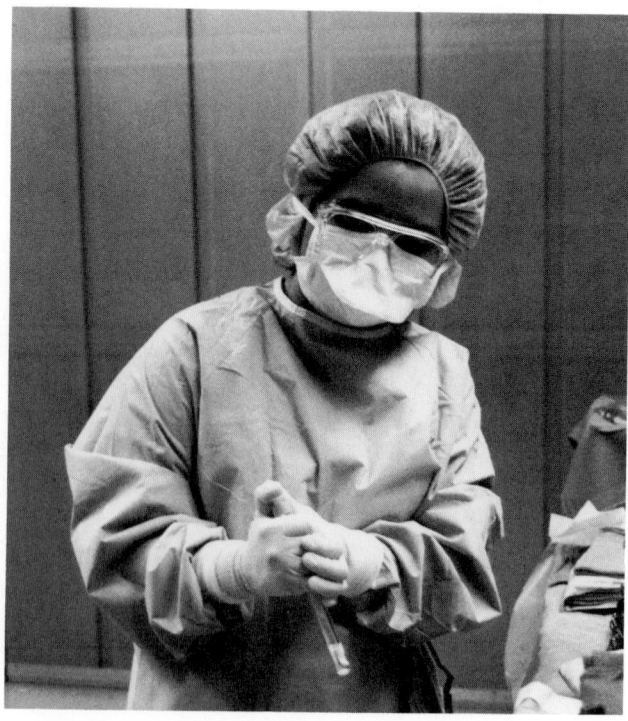

FIGURE 13–24. The scrub nurse pushes the cap on the anaerobic culture tube and activates the medium. (Courtesy of Santa Rosa Hospital, San Antonio, TX.)

culture tube from the sterile field, decontaminates it as described for aerobic culture tubes, attaches a label, and immediately sends it to the laboratory with the appropriate laboratory slip.

When the surgeon asks for a syringe to collect fluid for an anaerobic or aerobic culture, the circulating nurse aseptically delivers an appropriate-sized syringe to the sterile field. If a needle is needed for collection, a large-gauge needle should be used.

If the surgeon aspirates the fluid without a needle, the scrub nurse recaps the syringe and passes it to the gloved circulating nurse. Preferably, the scrub nurse drops the syringe into an impervious container, such as a plastic bag, held by the circulating nurse. Decontamination of a fluid-filled syringe by the circulating nurse should be avoided. During decontamination, ejection or leakage of syringe contents is possible by inadvertent pushing or pulling of the plunger by the circulating nurse.

The circulating nurse labels the container with patient and specimen data, marks it to alert laboratory personnel that the syringe is contaminated, and sends the container to the laboratory with the appropriate laboratory slip.

If the surgeon uses a needle to aspirate fluid for culture, extreme caution must be exercised by the scrub nurse. *The syringe should not be recapped.* After the surgeon passes the syringe and needle to the scrub nurse, the needle should be carefully removed with a clamp and placed in a sharps container on the sterile field. Next, the syringe is recapped and passed to the circulating nurse as described above.

Gram Stains

A Gram stain is done to classify species of bacteria. Test results guide the surgeon in initiating appropriate antibiotic therapy. Cultures for Gram stains are collected using an aerobic culture tube and immediately sent to the laboratory for smear and fixation. An appropriate laboratory slip is forwarded with the culture.

After receiving a culture, the laboratory technician prepares a film of the culture specimen on a slide. After drying and fixing the film with heat, a stain of aniline gentian violet or ammonium oxalate crystal violet is applied. The stain is rinsed in water and immersed in Gram iodine solution. The iodine solution is rinsed off with water and decolorized in ethyl alcohol or acetone. A counterstain of dilute carbolfuchsin or safranine is applied. After being rinsed with water, the slide is blotted dry. Gram-negative bacteria lose the stain and take the color of the counterstain (pink); gram-positive bacteria retain the color of the gentian violet stain (blue) (Thomas, 1976, p. G-32).

Spinal Fluid

Fluid removed during a spinal tap may be sent to the laboratory in sterile tubes (Fig. 13–25). The perioperative nurse must ensure that sufficient fluid is collected for the requested study. Guidelines for minimal amounts include

- aerobic culture and smear: 1.5 to 2 ml
- fungus culture: 1 ml
- acid-fast culture and smear: 2 ml

If cell count, cell differentiation, glucose, or protein studies are requested, separate tubes must be sent. Label the tubes and send with the appropriate laboratory requisition slips immediately to the laboratory.

Acid-fast Cultures and Smears

Acid-fast cultures and smears are done to diagnose tuberculosis. These cultures and smears are sent in the aerobic transport system. One swab is needed for each test. The specimen is labeled and sent immediately to

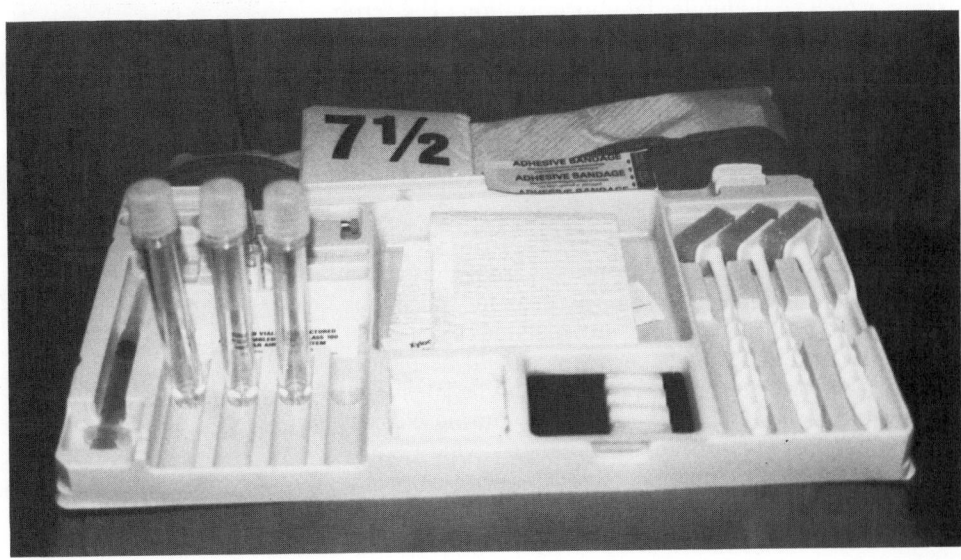

FIGURE 13–25. A spinal tray set-up. (Courtesy of Santa Rosa Hospital, San Antonio, TX.)

the laboratory with the proper laboratory requisition slip (Santa Rosa Hospital, 1988, #171, p. 0002).

Fungus Cultures

Mycological studies include direct microscopic examination of a smear and culturing. Fluid or pus should be collected in a syringe. A dry, sterile Petri dish may also be used. The perioperative nurse should collect as much of the specimen as possible. Like other specimens, the specimen for mycological studies is labeled and immediately sent to the laboratory with the appropriate laboratory slip.

Collecting and Preparing Tissue for Examination

Tissue may be taken during the intraoperative period for a number of studies. Examples are permanent surgical, frozen section, excisional biopsy, bone marrow biopsy, percutaneous needle biopsy, estrogen receptor site study, and Papanicolaou smear specimens.

General Guidelines

The perioperative nurse should handle all specimens carefully and as little as possible. Fluid specimens should not be shaken. This may rupture the cells. In addition, specimens should not be crushed or torn. Crushing or tearing may damage cells and hinder the pathologist in making a conclusive diagnosis. When transferring a specimen with an instrument, care should be taken to protect the specimen from tearing or damage (Atkinson and Kohn, 1986, p. 174).

Tissue should remain in a near-natural state, particularly tissues sent for frozen section examination. The work of the pathologist is facilitated if the specimen is received in the same condition as when removed. Consequently, care must be taken to prevent specimen drying, which could hinder later examination. The scrub should place the specimen in a container, such as an emesis basin. While the specimen is on the sterile field, the scrub nurse should keep the specimen damp by frequently wetting it with normal saline.

Permanent Specimens

All tissue or other objects removed from the patient are sent to the laboratory as permanent specimens. Exceptions to this guideline are dictated by hospital policy. After removal, all specimens should be handed off the sterile field as soon as possible. This helps prevent inadvertent discarding of the specimen during cleanup after the end of the procedure. After receiving permission from the surgeon, the scrub nurse passes the specimen to the gloved circulating nurse. The specimen

is transferred to an appropriate-sized container by tipping the emesis basin, thus causing the specimen to slide from the basin into the container (Fig. 13–26). The circulating nurse may also use an instrument to transfer the specimen to the container. Care should be taken to avoid splashing if the container is already filled with formalin. Likewise, if the circulating nurse pours formalin over the specimen, care must be taken to avoid splashing. The specimen should be completely covered by formalin. An exception is bladder or gallstones. These are sent dry to prevent decomposition.

When the size of a specimen makes it difficult to see, the scrub nurse should place the specimen on a piece of material that provides contrast. Telfa is suitable and may be submerged in formalin and sent to the laboratory.

Each container should contain only one specimen. If specimens are bilateral, such as fallopian tubes, each specimen should be labeled as left or right. Medial and lateral designations are also made.

Specimens too large for standard containers should be placed in an appropriate-sized basin and transported immediately to the laboratory with the appropriate paperwork. Care must be taken to avoid contamination

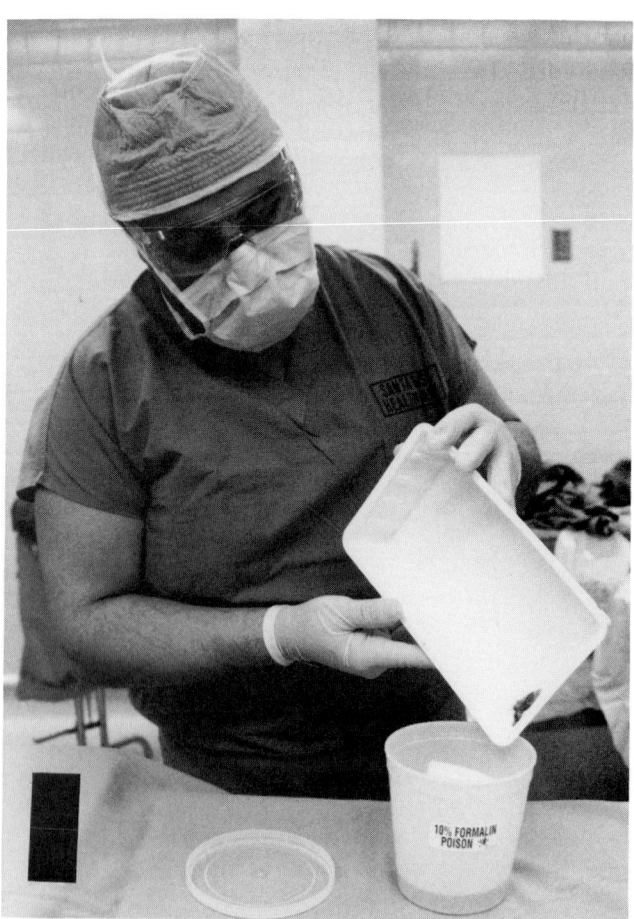

FIGURE 13–26. After donning protective eyewear, gloves, and a mask, the circulating nurse transfers the specimen to the container. (Courtesy of Santa Rosa Hospital, San Antonio, TX.)

of the transporter and laboratory personnel. Placing the basin containing the specimen in a clear impervious bag protects personnel and enables the circulating nurse to attach an identification label. The impervious bag should be covered with a towel during transport. Pathology department personnel should be alerted concerning such specimens.

In most hospitals, permanent specimens are collected by laboratory personnel or carried to the laboratory by OR personnel at designated times during the day. Care must be taken to ensure that all permanent specimens are appropriately labeled. The laboratory slip should be attached to the container with a rubber band or placed in a readily accessible place near the specimen container.

Specimens for Frozen Section

Some specimens are sent from the OR directly to the pathologist for a frozen section examination. The frozen section examination provides the surgeon with a quick preliminary diagnosis. Frozen sections are analyzed to determine the presence of malignancy and identify tissue during surgery, such as parathyroid tissue and lymph nodes. When a frozen section examination is anticipated, the pathologist should be notified before the surgical procedure begins. This ensures that the pathologist is available and able to prepare for the specimen before it arrives in the pathology department.

After the specimen is obtained from the patient, it is passed off the sterile field on a section of dampened telfa, on a towel, or in a container such as an emesis basin. Specimens should not be passed off the field on a counted sponge. The gloved circulating nurse receives the specimen and transfers it to an appropriate-sized dry container. The specimen is *not* placed in fluid such as formalin or saline. During the freezing process, moisture forms ice crystals and interferes with the examination. A label is attached and the specimen is immediately taken to the pathology department. A report of the frozen section examination may be called to the OR via telephone or intercom, or the pathologist may come directly to the OR to give the report in person. The pathologist is told if the patient is conscious.

Depending on hospital policy, the specimen may be retained by the pathologist or returned to the OR. If it is returned, the circulating nurse should place it in formalin and handle it as a permanent specimen.

Tissue and Fluid for Biopsy

Biopsy refers to a procedure in which tissue or fluid is removed for diagnosis. The surgeon does a biopsy to have a definitive diagnosis before scheduling further surgical intervention or medical treatment. Types of biopsies include excisional biopsy, bone marrow biopsy, and percutaneous needle biopsy.

An excisional biopsy is done to remove tissue from the body through an incision in the skin or mucous membranes. It may also be done using endoscopic instruments (Atkinson and Kohn, 1986, p. 384). Unless the tissue is obtained for frozen section examination, it is sent to the laboratory as described for permanent specimens.

A bone marrow biopsy or aspiration is done by a physician and a technologist from the hematology department. The specimen is obtained using a trocar puncture needle or an aspiration needle. A skin incision or percutaneous puncture is made; the needle is inserted into the bone, usually the sternum or the iliac crest; and the bone marrow is aspirated (Atkinson and Kohn, 1986, p. 384). The syringe containing the marrow is mixed with a fixative and the specimen is labeled and sent to the laboratory with the proper requisitions (Santa Rosa Hospital, 1988, p. 0010).

Percutaneous needle biopsy is done to obtain tissue from internal organs, such as the liver or the prostate gland. A hollow needle is inserted through the body wall and the tissue is removed (Atkinson and Kohn, 1986, p. 384). Unless instructed otherwise by the surgeon, the circulating nurse prepares the specimen as described for permanent specimens.

Tissue for Hormonal Receptor Site Studies

The surgeon may choose hormonal receptor site studies as a way to select patients who will benefit from postoperative endocrine manipulation. "Endocrine manipulation does not cure, but it can control dissemination of disease if the tumor progresses beyond the limits of effective operative resection or radiation therapy" (Atkinson and Kohn, 1986, p. 620).

This study identifies hormonal dependence of primary tumors. Breast and uterine tumors in a female patient may be stimulated by estrogen and/or progesterone. Prostate tumors in a male patient may be stimulated by androgens. Because these hormones affect the cellular metabolism of specific hormone receptors in tumor cells of some breast, endometrial, and prostate cancers, the tumors cells depend on these hormones for growth and maintenance (Atkinson and Kohn, 1986, p. 620).

After a positive diagnosis of malignancy is made by frozen section or routine tissue examination studies, the surgeon obtains a specimen from the primary breast, uterine, or prostate tumor site. The scrub nurse passes the tissue to the gloved circulating nurse. The tissue is *not* placed in formalin because this alters receptor sites and negates the hormonal study results (Atkinson and Kohn, 1986, p. 620). The specimen is labeled and sent to the laboratory with the appropriate paperwork.

Papanicolaou Test Specimen

The Papanicolaou test, commonly called a Pap smear, is a uterine smear to detect cancer cells in the mucus of the uterus. The following items are needed for this test:

- bottle of fixative (95% alcohol)
- cystospatula
- two glass slides (Fig. 13–27)

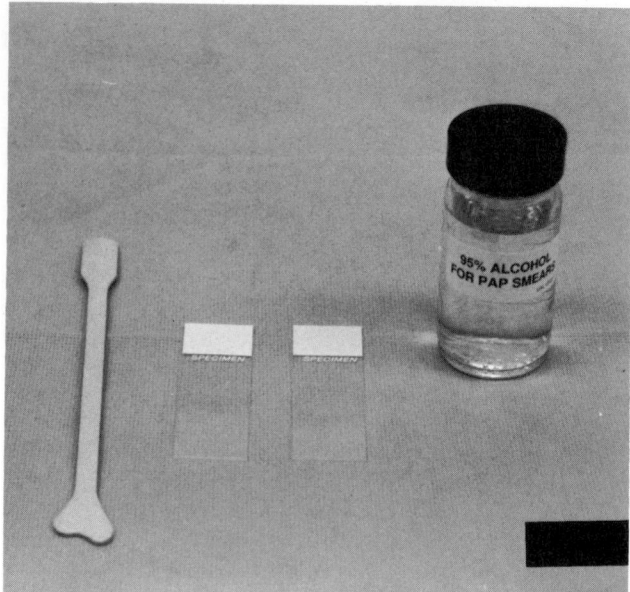

FIGURE 13–27. Set-up for a Papanicolaou test. (Courtesy of Santa Rosa Hospital, San Antonio, TX.)

The surgeon obtains the specimen from the vaginal pool and the cervical os with the cystospatula and spreads the material on one side of each of the glass slides. The slides are immediately placed in the fixative solution, back to back, with the smeared sides exposed to the fixative. The circulating nurse recaps the bottle, attaches a label, and sends it to the laboratory with the appropriate laboratory slip (Santa Rosa Hospital, 1988, #301, p. 0001).

Other Types of Surgical Specimens

Examples of other types of surgical specimens are missiles (bullets), intrauterine devices, heart valves, screws, and other foreign objects. These specimens are processed according to hospital policy and are usually sent to the pathologist for cataloging. These objects are sent to the laboratory in a dry container.

In the case of a foreign object that may be used as evidence in a court case, care must be taken to preserve the integrity of the specimen. A bullet should be removed, wrapped in gauze sponge, and placed in a dry container. If there is more than one bullet, separate containers should be used for each bullet. The bullet should not touch metal and care should be taken to avoid scratching it. This could interfere with the police ballistics test. The patient's clothes may be used as evidence in the case. Do not cut through the hole made by the bullet when removing the clothing.

Storing, Preserving, and Maintaining Tissue

Human tissue removed for banking may include cartilage, bone, and skin. Potential donors should be as-

sessed and be free from transmissible infection, malignancy, autoimmune disease, neurologic disease of unknown cause, and human-derived growth hormone. Policies regarding donor and recipient tissue banking vary from hospital to hospital.

Tissue should be removed under strict aseptic conditions and be stored in a controlled environment. Several methods are acceptable:

- For short-term storage, "place skin in an isotonic solution (eg, normal saline or balanced salt solution) or tissue medium and refrigerate at 1 degree C (33.8 degrees F) to 10 degrees C (50 degrees F) for up to 14 days."
- For long-term storage, "skin should be maintained in a cryoprotectant under controlled cooling and freezing conditions. Freeze by cooling skin to at least −70 degrees C (−94 degrees F) at a rate of decline between 1 degree C (1.8 degrees F) to 5 degrees C (9 degrees F) per minute. The skin can then be stored in a liquid nitrogen freezer." (AORN, 1992, III:21–3)

Label the tissue with the following information:

- donor's name
- donor's identification number
- donor's pertinent medical information
- donor's history
- pathology report
- culture and serological testing reports
- type and anatomical site of tissue
- date and time of collection
- method of collection
- preservation solution and composition
- recipient of the graft
- recipient's identification number
- date and time of transplantation
- anatomical site of transplantation
- informed consents from donor or donor's responsible party (AORN, 1992, III:21–1—21–2)

Directing the Transfer of Cultures and Specimens to the Laboratory

Correctly transporting cultures and specimens to the laboratory is essential for continuity of care. The transporter must understand where and to whom the culture or specimen is to be delivered. Assistive personnel responsible for transportation duties should receive specific training on handling cultures and specimens during transportation. Training should include log book completion, precautions to take if the specimen container is contaminated, and recognition and identification of laboratory slips.

Communicating Intraoperative Laboratory or Pathology Reports to the Surgeon

The circulating nurse facilitates the communication of intraoperative laboratory or pathology reports between the surgeon and the laboratory or the pathology department. Direct communication between the surgeon and the laboratory technician or the pathologist is preferred. The technician or pathologist should be notified if the patient is awake for the procedure. If this method is not possible, however, a written report should be presented to the surgeon. If the circulating nurse must serve as a conduit of oral communication, the information should be written by the nurse, verified for accuracy with the pathologist or the laboratory technician, and then given to the surgeon. Written reports received intraoperatively should be attached to the patient's record.

Bibliography

Association of Operating Room Nurses. (1992). *Standards and recommended practices for perioperative nursing.* Denver.

Atkinson, L. J., Kohn, M. L. (1986). *Berry and Kohn's introduction to operating room technique* (6th ed.). New York: McGraw-Hill.

Groah, L. (1983). *Operating room nursing: The perioperative role.* Reston, VA: Reston Publishing Co.

Santa Rosa Hospital. (1988). *Laboratory policy and procedure book.* San Antonio, TX: Santa Rosa Hospital.

Santa Rosa Hospital. (1989). *Hazardous communication book.* San Antonio, TX: Santa Rosa Hospital.

Thomas, C. L. (Ed.). (1976). *Taber's cyclopedic medical dictionary.* Philadelphia: F. A. Davis.

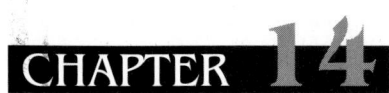

Evaluating Patient Care: A Functional Health Patterns Approach

Cynthia A. Abbott

Evaluation is the fourth component of the nursing process after assessment, planning, and implementation. Evaluation compares the expected outcomes and patient goals established in the planning phase with patient's current health status to determine which future nursing actions will benefit the patient. By evaluating patient care, perioperative nurses can determine which nursing actions are necessary to provide quality care. By applying the nursing process, using evaluation data, and communicating with the patient and others the status of health problem resolution, perioperative nurses build a foundation for nursing research and a body of knowledge for the management of surgical patients.

DEFINITION

Evaluation is an appraisal of the changes in the patient's condition that result from perioperative nursing actions (Yura and Walsh, 1983, p. 192). This appraisal indicates the degree of goal achievement and health problem resolution experienced by the patient (Yura and Walsh, 1983, p. 192). Evaluation is the review of the patient's responses to the perioperative nursing actions contained in the nursing care plan (Yura and Walsh, 1983, p. 193). The nursing care plan contains the nursing diagnosis (health problem), the goal for

health problem resolution, and projected patient outcomes, which are the framework for the evaluation process (Yura and Walsh, 1983, p. 193).

MEASURABLE CRITERIA

The perioperative nurse demonstrates competency to evaluate patient care by

- evaluating patient outcomes according to identified criteria
- measuring patient outcomes
- conducting a postoperative assessment
- measuring the degree of goal achievement
- reassessing patient care
- documenting and communicating the evaluation process (AORN, 1992)

THE EVALUATION PROCESS

Evaluating Patient Outcomes According to Criteria

The development of measurable criteria, expected outcomes, and patient goals was discussed in Chapter 3. The evaluation phase of the nursing process reviews

The views expressed in this chapter are those of the author and do not reflect the official position or policy of the Department of the Army, the Department of Defense, or the U.S. Government.

the criteria and expected outcomes identified in the planning phase. The perioperative nurse compares the expected outcomes with the patient's postoperative response. By comparing the results of nursing actions (a patient's response) with the desired patient outcome, the perioperative nurse identifies the extent of goal achievement. Criteria written in the planning phase enable objective measurement of expected patient outcomes during the evaluation phase of the patient's surgical experience.

Measuring Patient Outcomes

Measurement of expected patient outcomes assists the perioperative nurse in determining the degree of goal achievement experienced by the patient. To measure actual patient outcomes, the perioperative nurse collects data about the patient's postoperative condition and compares the data with expected outcomes and criteria identified in the planning phase of care plan development.

The perioperative nurse collects three types of data about the patient's condition during evaluation: physiological data, observable patient behavior, and subjective patient responses (Yura and Walsh, 1983, p. 194). After data collection of postoperative results, the perioperative nurse compares this information with preoperative and intraoperative findings to accurately interpret the patient's postoperative status. Physiological measurements such as temperature, pulse rate, blood pressure, weight, diagnostic test results, and laboratory test results objectively reflect the patient's status during the perioperative experience. Observable behaviors such as posture, appearance, skin color, and level of orientation, as well as subjective responses of the patient and family members, also provide data to the perioperative nurse in determining whether patient outcomes were achieved as expected. The perioperative nurse identifies perceptual and physiological disparities between outcome criteria and postoperative status and uses these cues to initiate the process of care reassessment (see later).

Conducting a Postoperative Assessment

The postoperative phase begins when the patient is admitted to the postanesthesia care unit and ends with the resolution of surgical health problems (Association of Operating Room Nurses [AORN], 1992, *I*:3–1). *Assessment* is a continuous process of data collection to identify the patient's actual and potential health problems (AORN, 1992, *I*:3–1).

The perioperative nurse performs postoperative assessment in a variety of settings. The nurse in the ambulatory surgical setting may be able only to evaluate the patient's immediate goals before discharge of the patient from the health care facility but may use the discharge plan to communicate the patient's intermediate and long-term needs to other health care team members in the community (e.g., community health nurse and visiting nurse). In addition, the perioperative nurse in the ambulatory surgical setting may choose to schedule an additional evaluation via telephone with the patient to complete a postoperative assessment of the patient's condition. The perioperative nurse in an inpatient setting may choose postoperative assessment strategies similar to those for the ambulatory surgical setting. The perioperative nurse can perform the postoperative assessment in the hospital, the patient's home, or a specialty term care facility (e.g., long-term care and rehabilitation).

The perioperative nurse needs several skills to collect data about the patient's condition and compare these data with expected patient outcomes. Astute observation enables the perioperative nurse to identify subtle differences in a patient's condition (e.g., in appearance, posture, and skin color) during the preoperative, intraoperative, and postoperative phases of the patient's surgical experience. The nurse uses communication techniques to assist the patient in identifying and clarifying expected outcomes and differences between anticipated and actual results postoperatively. The perioperative nurse employs sophisticated analytical and perceptual skills to compare the patient's postoperative status with the criteria and expected outcomes identified in the planning phase.

During the postoperative assessment, the perioperative nurse uses reasoning skills to determine the cause of not meeting expected outcomes for the patient. The initial step in postoperative assessment is to review expected outcomes to determine if statements written in the planning phase were realistic and achievable. Next, the perioperative nurse reviews the criteria to identify if they were appropriate to measure the expected outcomes postoperatively. Lastly, the nurse reviews the nursing actions used to meet the expected patient outcomes. A review of the nursing actions reveals omissions and ineffectiveness of nursing intervention in resolving patient health problems (nursing diagnoses).

The perioperative nurse analyzes the assessment, planning, and implementation phases of care plan design to determine the accuracy of identified nursing diagnoses and the efficacy of nursing actions. A systematic examination of the care plan postoperatively prevents inappropriate or unsuccessful nursing actions, outcomes, and goals from being continued for the patient and family. This review demonstrates accountability for patient- and family-centered care. The perioperative nurse determines the suitability of expected patient outcomes and criteria for measuring the attainment of actual outcomes used to measure goals.

Measuring the Degree of Goal Achievement

Goal attainment is measured according to the extent of achieving patient outcomes. Expected patient outcomes determine the degree to which health problems (nursing diagnoses) are resolved (Yura and Walsh, 1983, pp. 193–194). As noted in Chapter 3, not all patient goals must be met at the time of postoperative evaluation. The perioperative nurse categorizes goal achievement and evaluation according to immediate, intermediate, and long-term goal priorities.

The perioperative nurse expects that many of the immediate goals related to the surgical experience can be evaluated postoperatively. However, nursing actions necessary to meet intermediate and long-term goals may not be completed until after the patient's discharge from the hospital. Continuity of information is important for the health care team members working with the patient and the family in the community. The perioperative nurse needs to evaluate objectively the completion of goals and communicate the partial completion or failure to address remaining goals for follow-up by others.

Evaluation of goals may result in one of the following outcomes:

1. The patient responds as expected and the *health problem* (nursing diagnosis) *is resolved*. Further nursing actions are not needed because those implemented were effective in resolving the health problem. An appointment with the patient may be made for a future date to confirm the patient's problem-free status.
2. The patient's objective and subjective responses indicate that the *problem has not been resolved*. Immediate goals have been achieved, but intermediate and long-term goals have not been met. If goal attainment is possible, resolution of the health problem will be slow or will be achieved with alterations in the care plan. Nursing actions are geared to meet unresolved goals and prevent potential problems. Reevaluation of the patient's expected outcomes is needed at a later time.
3. The patient's objective and subjective *responses are similar to those present in the assessment phase*. Few or no changes in the patient's condition indicate that the patient's health problem has not been resolved. Immediate goals have not been achieved and the attainment of intermediate and long-term goals is doubtful. Resolving the patient's health problem necessitates reassessing the patient's health status, refining nursing diagnoses, establishing different goals, revising the care plan, and instituting nursing actions.
4. The patient's responses indicate that *new problems have developed as a result of unmet needs*. The entire nursing process must be repeated to identify the entire spectrum of patient health problems. The perioperative nurse reviews decisions of the planning phase and the effectiveness of nursing actions in resolving health problems before identifying new health problems in the nursing care plan. Evaluation follows implementation of new nursing actions to resolve the additional health problems (Yura and Walsh, 1983, pp. 194–195).

When patient goals and expected outcomes fall into the second, third, or fourth categories, the perioperative nurse reviews the possible reasons for failure to resolve the health problems. Factors that affect patient responses, patient outcomes, and goal achievement include internal and external variables involving the patient, the family, significant others, the nursing team, and health care team members.

Personal values, religious beliefs, and internalized cultural attitudes are examples of internal variables that influence the patient's response to nursing actions and the achievement of patient outcomes. The perioperative nurse or other health care providers may employ values in their care delivery that threaten the patient's values, attitudes, or beliefs. This threat may cause the patient to withdraw his or her support of goal achievement if the unconscious threat is not identified and resolved. Financial resources, support systems, and communication barriers exemplify potential sources of conflict for goal achievement. The family of a comatose patient with a poor prognosis may not believe that invasive surgery and prolonged suffering are justified at the expense of exhausting limited financial resources. The perioperative nurse reviews internal and external factors in health care team members as well as the patient to identify possible obstacles to the achievement of patient goals.

The quality and quantity of information shared with the perioperative nurse has a significant impact on care plan design and evaluation. Inaccurate or insufficient information offered by the patient owing to religious, cultural, or psychosocial beliefs results in difficulties with problem identification, prioritization, resolution, and evaluation. An increase in the patient's health problem may occur intraoperatively or postoperatively. This increase may change the expected patient outcome and goal identified as appropriate in the preoperative planning phase. In addition, the patient may experience a decrease in energy and coping mechanisms resulting from multiple stressors from the environment (e.g., loss of job, loss of self-esteem, low income, and absence of significant others). The perioperative nurse must ensure that the patient participates in prioritizing health problems and planning for their resolution. If the patient wishes to participate in her or his plan of care, attainment of patient outcomes is enhanced. The patient who participates in prioritizing and resolving health problems is interested in meeting expected outcomes and goals (Yura and Walsh, 1983, p. 200).

Actions by the perioperative nurse can lead to problems in goal attainment and health problem resolution. The nurse may overlook important data or fail to perform nursing actions appropriately because of intellectual, interpersonal, or technical limitations (e.g., an inability to perform nursing actions confidently) (Yura & Walsh, 1983, p. 201). An inadequate understanding about gas exchange is an example of an intellectual limitation. The perioperative nurse must be familiar with the implications of abnormal oxygen and carbon dioxide values for the patient undergoing anesthesia. Depersonalizing the patient is an example of interpersonal limitations that perioperative nurses may not recognize in themselves. Depersonalizing the patient may decrease the patient's desire to participate in goal attainment. A nurse's lack of familiarity with a procedure with complex and unfamiliar instruments that interferes with the nurse's ability to assess, plan, and implement nursing actions is an example of a technical limitation. These limitations unintentionally affect the achievement of expected outcomes and goals.

If the perioperative nurse does not recognize intellectual, interpersonal, or technical limitations and strengths, several problems that affect the evaluation process could arise. First, the perioperative nurse may assign high or low priorities to health problems inappropriately. Second, the nurse may fail to validate a perception or inference with the patient. Third, inadequate or inaccurate collection of data regarding the patient's socioeconomic, cultural, religious, physical, and psychological variables may occur. Lastly, the perioperative nurse may fail to (1) involve the patient in planning, (2) identify realistic goals and achievable patient outcomes, and (3) recognize patient strengths and the need for independence within the limits of wellness or illness (Yura and Walsh, 1983, pp. 201–202).

Goal achievement and expected outcome attainment may fail to occur because of the patient's significant others. The patient's support system may not be available or interested in the resolution of health problems. Significant others may not understand the health problem or resolution and may be unable to assist the patient in goal achievement. In addition, significant others may perceive that resolving the health problem will further drain limited financial, physical, emotional, and intellectual resources. Moral, cultural, and religious influences may interfere with a significant other's ability to aid in resolving health problems and support the patient in goal achievement (Yura and Walsh, 1983, p. 202).

After comparing the evaluation data with the expected patient outcomes and analyzing the possible causes of altered patient outcomes, the perioperative nurse reassesses the nursing care plan.

Reassessing Patient Care

Reassessment is the mechanism perioperative nurses may use to analyze the nursing care planned for and delivered to the patient (AORN, 1992, I:2–12, 3–2). After perioperative nursing care has been delivered, the nurse reviews the evaluation data to determine which health problems have not been resolved. The perioperative nurse then reassesses the patient's health status to ensure that new and existing problems have been identified. The nursing diagnoses from the previous planning phase are reviewed and modified as needed. New nursing diagnoses arising from the reassessment are developed. All nursing diagnoses are classified according to immediate, intermediate, and long-term priorities.

The care plan includes nursing actions appropriate for existing, revised, and new nursing diagnoses. The pa-

tient's attainment of expected outcomes demonstrated by meeting criteria and the degree of goal achievement is reevaluated. Repeating the steps of the nursing process allows the perioperative nurse to implement, modify, and communicate nursing strategies for goal achievement as the status of the patient changes according to internal factors and external influences from the environment. Reassessment of patient care involves reexamining the patient's health status, refining nursing diagnoses, reestablishing patient goals, revising the nursing care plan, implementing nursing actions, and reevaluating the achievement of expected patient outcomes (AORN, 1992, I:2–12).

DOCUMENTATION AND COMMUNICATION PROCEDURES

Written records should reflect the review or revision of the care plan, and the status of the care plan should be communicated to others as appropriate (AORN, 1992, III:4–2). Written communication of the patient's health status in the preoperative, intraoperative, and postoperative phases of the surgical experience is ensured when a nursing care plan is developed, updated, and revised. The care plan provides continuity of information regarding the patient's health problems. This information is vital to ensure that quality perioperative nursing care is delivered to the patient. Several nurses may participate in the assessment, planning, implementation, and evaluation phases of perioperative nursing care.

A written care plan reflecting the nursing process ensures that the attainment of outcomes and goals for patient care can be ascertained by the nursing team. A documented care plan with evaluation data demonstrates accountability for nursing care delivered to the surgical patient. Following the nursing process, evaluating patient outcomes according to criteria, measuring the degree of goal achievement, and reassessing patient care according to evaluation data place the patient at the center of nursing care. This patient-oriented approach ensures a high degree of success for goal achievement and resolution of patient health problems.

Bibliography

Association of Operating Room Nurses. (1992). *Standards and recommended practices for perioperative nursing.* Denver.
Yura, H., Walsh, M. (1983). *The nursing process: Assessing, planning, implementing, evaluation* (4th ed.). East Norwalk, CT: Appleton-Century-Crofts.

COMPETENCIES FOR THE REGISTERED NURSE FIRST ASSISTANT

CHAPTER 15

Preparing the Patient for Surgery

Lori Ominsky and Mark L. Phippen

DEFINITION

Preparing the patient for surgery refers to the activities performed by the registered nurse first assistant (RNFA) during the preoperative period to make the patient physically and psychologically ready for surgical intervention.

MEASURABLE CRITERIA

The RNFA demonstrates competency to prepare the patient for surgery by

- facilitating patient admission to the health care facility
- obtaining informed consent
- performing a preoperative assessment
- facilitating preoperative care

ROLE OF THE REGISTERED NURSE FIRST ASSISTANT

The role that the RNFA plays in preparing the patient for surgery depends on the extent of collaboration with the surgeon and the health care facility policies and procedures. The RNFA who has a collaborative relationship with the surgeon may admit the patient to the health care facility, obtain the consent, do the initial preoperative work-up, and oversee the patient's preoperative regimen.

The extent to which the perioperative nurse prepares the patient for surgery depends on the practice setting. Perioperative nurses practicing in ambulatory surgery facilities may admit the patient, collect laboratory specimens, obtain the consent, and provide any ordered preoperative treatments or care. However, nurses practicing in a setting that is predominantly inpatient may find the extent of involvement in the preoperative care of the patient limited to activities performed immediately before surgery in the holding area.

CONSIDERATIONS

Categories of Surgery

Table 15–1 shows categories of surgery.

The Patient Self-Determination Act
(American Nurses Association, 1992)

As more and more outpatient surgical procedures are performed and perioperative nurses expand their prac-

303

TABLE 15–1. CLASSIFICATION OF SURGICAL PROCEDURES

Classification	Characteristics	Condition or Procedure
Emergency	Requires immediate interventions because of life-threatening consequences	Abdominal aortic aneurysm Gunshot or stab wound Severe bleeding Major open bone fracture Appendectomy
Urgent	Requires prompt interventions; is potentially life-threatening if treatment is delayed more than 24–48 h	Intestinal obstruction Eye injury Bladder obstruction Kidney or ureteral stones Cholecystectomy with acute inflammation Bone fracture
Diagnostic	Requires intervention to determine origin, cause, and cell type	Cancer Endoscopy Colonoscopy Bronchoscopy Biopsy Exploratory laparotomy
Elective	Is planned for correction of nonacute problem	Cataracts Hernia repair Hemorrhoidectomy Total joint arthroplasty
Cosmetic	Is intervention primarily for alteration of personal appearance	Suction lipectomy Revision of scars Rhinoplasty Blepharoplasty
Palliative	Is performed to relieve symptoms of a disease process but is not curative	Colostomy Nerve root resection Tumor debulking

From Ignatavicius, D., Bayne, M. V. (1991). *Medical-surgical nursing: A nursing process approach* (p. 428). Philadelphia: W. B. Saunders.

tice domain, the RNFA and the perioperative nurse play an important role in ensuring that surgical and invasive procedure patients know and understand their choices regarding end-of-life decisions and that these decisions are implemented in compliance with the Patient Self-Determination Act (Fig. 15–1).

The Patient Self-Determination Act requires that individuals receiving medical care receive *written* information about their rights under state law to make decisions about medical care, including the right to

- accept or refuse medical or surgical treatment
- initiate advance directives such as living wills and durable power of attorney

There are the two types of advance medical directives: treatment directives (living wills) and appointment directives (power of attorney or health proxies). The intent of an advance directive is to help others make decisions for the patient should it become necessary. The treatment directive delineates what treatments to omit or refuse if a patient is unable to make treatment decisions and is terminally ill. The appointment directive designates a proxy to make medical decisions if the patient can no longer make the decisions concerning appropriate medical treatment. This directive has broader applications than the treatment directive because it applies to any incapacitating illness or injury.

An advance directive is a legal document. It may be as simple or as complex as necessary and does not necessitate the services of an attorney for initiation or implementation. Two witnesses, however, must sign an advance directive. State laws delineate who can sign as a witness. In some states, heirs, relatives, or physicians are prohibited from signing. An advance directive applies only if the incapacitated patient cannot make decisions concerning treatment. Two physicians may activate the advance directive, however, if they are of the opinion that the patient is unable to make decisions. The patient may change or cancel an advance directive at any time. After the patient signs an advance directive, a family member, the physician, and the person designated as the proxy should receive a copy. If the patient initiated an advance directive before admission to the health care facility, a copy should be given to the health care facility.

The Patient Self-Determination Act does not require that an advance directive be written. It merely requires hospitals and other health care facilities to tell patients that they have a right to do so.

The American Nurses Association (1992) recommends that nurses question the patient about advance care directives during the assessment (Fig. 15–1).

OUTCOME STANDARD

The patient receives care that reflects an ongoing process of management of his or her health status during

AMERICAN NURSES ASSOCIATION

BOARD OF DIRECTORS TASK FORCE ON THE NURSE'S ROLE IN END OF LIFE DECISIONS

NURSING AND THE PATIENT SELF-DETERMINATION ACT

The Patient Self-Determination Act, passed as part of the Omnibus Budget Reconciliation Act of 1990, becomes effective December 1, 1991. The federal law applies to all health care institutions receiving Medicare or Medicaid funds and requires that all individuals receiving medical care must be given written information about their rights under state law to make decisions about medical care, including the right to accept or refuse medical or surgical treatment. Individuals must also be given information about their rights to formulate advance directives such as living wills and durable powers of attorney for health care. Patients must be made aware of their rights to make decisions about these issues upon admission (in the case of hospitals or skilled nursing facilities), enrollment (in the case of health maintenance organizations), on first receipt of care (in the case of hospices) or before the patient comes under an agency's care (in the case of home health personal care agencies).

We support the patient's right to self-determination and believe that nurses will and must play a primary role in implementation of the law. Ideally, decisions about advance directives should be made by the patient with the family and the primary care provider prior to admission. The formation of advance directives is an important decision and will inevitably involve nurses who are the most omnipresent professionals in health care facilities. It is imperative that the decision making that will fall to patients and their families as they make choices about end of life care be facilitated by nurses.

- Each nurse should know the laws of the state in which she/he is practicing pertaining to advance directives, and should be familiar with the strengths and limitations of the various forms of advance directive.

- The nurse is one of several health care professionals who has a responsibility for ensuring that the advance care directives initiated by the patient are current and reflective of the patient's choices. Facilitating self-determination of patients with respect to end of life decisions is a process that includes evaluating changes in the patient's perspective and health state.

- The nurse has a responsibility to facilitate informed decision making, including but not limited to advance directives.

- We recommend that these questions about advance directives be part of the nursing admission assessment: Do you have basic information about advance care directives including living wills and durable power of attorney? Do you wish to initiate an advance care directive? If you have already prepared an advance care directive, can you provide it now? Have you discussed your end of life choices with your family and/or designated surrogate and health care team workers?

- The role of the nurse is critical in implementation of the Patient Self-Determination Act and includes public education, research, patient care, advocacy, education of the profession and inservice education of other health care providers.

IN END-OF-LIFE DECISIONS

FIGURE 15–1. Statement of the American Nurses Association Board of Directors Task Force on the Nurse's Role in End-of-Life Decisions. (From American Nurses Association. [1992, January]. What is an advanced medical directive? *The American Nurse*, p. 9.)

the perioperative period. Care is planned on the basis of nursing diagnoses identified during the assessment.

Criteria

Depending on the patient's physical, psychological, sociocultural, and spiritual status, the patient or the significant other (if applicable) can expect a plan of care that ensures that the patient

- complies with the prescribed therapeutic regimen before and after surgery
- is free from nosocomial infection after surgery
- is free from injury related to electrical and radiation hazards, chemicals, extraneous objectives, positioning, the administration of drugs and solutions, the improper handling of cultures and specimens, and the handling of tissue with instruments during surgery
- maintains fluid volume
- maintains skin and tissue integrity
- maintains body temperature within normal limits
- is free from prolonged adynamic ileus following surgery
- demonstrates self-care activities after surgery
- demonstrates effective airway clearance
- demonstrates an effective postoperative breathing pattern
- maintains cardiac output
- has adequate postoperative tissue perfusion
- experiences minimal postoperative pain
- is knowledgeable about the perioperative experience
- copes with feelings of fear before surgery
- recognizes the presence of anticipatory grief
- copes with changes in body image after surgery
- demonstrates functional grieving
- demonstrates effective coping in response to the stress of impending surgery

POTENTIAL ALTERATIONS IN FUNCTIONAL HEALTH PATTERNS

Response to surgical intervention varies from patient to patient. The goal of surgery is to improve, or at least maintain, the patient's health status. Some patients, however, have complications that if not dealt with can ultimately affect their health status during and after surgery. Throughout the text, potential alterations in functional health patterns that have an impact on the patient's status as it relates to surgery are discussed. Because the discussion in other chapters is primarily concerned with physiological factors, this chapter focuses on the psychological and sociocultural factors affecting the patient during the perioperative period. The actual and potential diagnoses cited are not meant to be all inclusive, rather they highlight some of the alterations in functional health patterns that surgical patients may experience.

Health Perception–Health Management Pattern

Diagnosis

High risk for noncompliance with the prescribed therapeutic regimen after surgery

Definition

Presence of risk factors for the patient's or family members' nonadherence to the prescribed postoperative treatment regimen

Discussion. The success of an operative procedure often depends on the type of care the patient receives after surgery not only in the hospital, but also after discharge. The physician may order a specific diet, give instructions for wound care, prescribe medications, and arrange for further treatments. The success of the postoperative treatment regimen depends on the patient's or the family's physical, mental, and emotional ability to cooperate with the health care team. Identification of a patient or families at risk for noncompliance provides the RNFA or the perioperative nurse with the opportunity to implement interventions designed to ensure successful rehabilitation after discharge from the hospital.

Risk Factors (Gordon, 1987, p. 48)

- Patient history of noncompliance with prescribed therapeutic regimens
- For patients unable to provide self-care, a family history of noncompliance with prescribed therapeutic regimens
- Lack of patient support systems (family, friends)
- Denial of illness by the patient or the family (if the patient is unable to provide self-care)
- Perceived ineffectiveness of the recommended therapeutic regimens by the patient or the family
- Perceived lack of seriousness by the patient or the family of the health problems or risk factors
- Perceived lack of susceptibility to the potential complications secondary to noncompliance by the patient or the family
- Insufficient knowledge or skills of the patient or the family to implement the recommended therapeutic regimens
- Lack of a plan by the patient or the family for integrating therapeutic recommendations into daily routines

Expected Outcome

The patient complies with the prescribed therapeutic regimen after surgery.

Perioperative Nursing Interventions

A thorough preoperative assessment is the key to planning interventions to eliminate the risk of noncompliance. During the preoperative assessment, ask open-ended questions to determine if the patient or family members have had difficulty complying with prescribed therapeutic regimens in the past. Questions should determine if the patient or the family

- failed to understand postoperative instructions given by the nurse and the physician during the past hospitalization
- lacked support systems (family, friends) for encouragement or care
- denied the presence of the illness
- perceived the recommended treatment modalities as ineffective
- failed to understand the seriousness of the health problem or risk factors associated with the health problem
- believed that the patient was not susceptible to complications that might result if the postoperative instructions and the treatment regimen were not followed
- had insufficient knowledge or skills to comply with the postoperative instructions and treatment regimen
- lacked a plan for integrating therapeutic recommendations into daily routines

Assessment questions should also identify the presence of family members or significant others in the patient's support system. If family or friends are present during the assessment, determine their willingness to participate in the patient's care after surgery.

If the patient denies the illness, the nurse should explore strategies to help him or her accept the current health status. Close collaboration of the nurse with the physician and the family is crucial if the patient is to move to a stage of acceptance.

Perceived ineffectiveness of recommended practices, perceived lack of seriousness of problems or risk factors, and perceived lack of susceptibility to postoperative complications often stem from insufficient knowledge or skills on the part of the patient or family members. The nurse should implement patient and family teaching strategies, especially concerning postoperative care routines. Chapter 5 provides examples of home instructions for the postoperative patient. Helping the patient and the family plan for the integration of the therapeutic recommendations into daily routines may also prove effective in ensuring compliance. Postoperative home visits or telephone calls enable the nurse to verify compliance, provide motivation when needed, and identify problems.

Diagnoses

High risk for infection (see Chapters 6, 8, 9, 11, 16, 17, and 18)

High risk for injury (see Chapters 4, 6, 7, 8, 9, 11, 12, 13, 16, and 17)

Nutritional-Metabolic Pattern

Diagnoses

High risk for fluid volume deficit (see Chapters 9, 10, and 17)

High risk for fluid volume excess (see Chapters 9 and 10)

High risk for impaired skin integrity (see Chapters 9 and 12)

High risk for impaired tissue integrity (see Chapters 6, 9, 10, 12, 16, 17, and 18)

High risk for hyperthermia (see Chapters 10, 11, and 18)

High risk for hypothermia (see Chapters 4, 6, 8, 10, and 11)

High risk for alteration in bowel function (see Chapter 18)

Activity-Exercise Pattern

Diagnosis

High risk for self-care deficit following surgery

Definition

Presence of risk factors for the patient to experience a temporary or permanent inability to complete one or more the following activities of daily living as a result of surgery: feeding, bathing, toileting, dressing, and grooming

Discussion. Some surgical procedures may temporarily or permanently leave the patient incapacitated and unable to manage self-care. For example, consider the elderly diabetic patient who is scheduled for a below-knee amputation. Most likely, because of age and probable alteration in mobility related to the disease process, the patient is already experiencing difficulty with toileting and bathing. Clearly, managing toileting and bathing will become more difficult after surgery. Another example is the orthopedic trauma patient who has casts applied to both arms. This patient will experience temporary difficulty with feeding, toileting, bathing, dressing, and grooming. These are clear examples of patients at risk for self-care deficit.

Other cases, however, may be more subtle. Patients experiencing psychosocial problems, such as severe anxiety or depression, may lack the motivation to participate in self-care activities after surgery, even though the surgery was a success and did not compromise the patient's physical ability to perform the activities of daily living.

The RNFA and the perioperative nurse play an important role in identifying patients at risk for self-care deficit after surgery. As more surgeries are performed in the outpatient setting, identification of patients at risk for self-care deficit becomes imperative. Assumptions that all patients have the support systems to deal with temporary or permanent disability cannot be made.

Risk Factors (Gordon, 1987, p. 132)

- Activity intolerance: decreased strength and endurance related to age, the presence of disease, or the effect of surgery
- Chronic pain or discomfort
- Acute pain or discomfort after surgery
- Uncompensated perceptual-cognitive impairment
- Uncompensated neuromuscular or musculoskeletal impairment
- Severe anxiety
- Depression
- Restrictive treatment modalities after surgery such as immobilization (casts and traction)
- Surgery resulting in loss of limb, sight, hearing, or bowel or bladder control
- Lack of functional support systems in the home

Expected Outcome

The patient demonstrates the ability to manage self-care after discharge from the health care facility.

Perioperative Nursing Interventions

The role that perioperative nurses play in identifying and managing patients at risk for self-care deficit varies with the nurse's practice focus. Nurses engaged in outpatient surgery practice have the opportunity to identify high-risk patients and follow up to ensure that a self-care deficit risk has not become a reality. RNFAs in practice with surgeons can extend their contact with a patient identified at risk by evaluating the patient during office visits after surgery and visiting the patient in the home. The perioperative nurse with a practice primarily focused on the intraoperative setting plays an important role by participating in the surgical procedure. This nurse is in the position to document in the patient's record and communicate to appropriate health care personnel surgical events that have an impact on the patient's ability for self-care after discharge from the health care facility. During the perioperative period, the nurse should

- identify patients at risk for self-care deficit after surgery
- determine the quality of home support systems available to the patient
- document and communicate to appropriate health care workers that a patient is at risk for self-care deficit after discharge from the hospital

Diagnoses

High risk for ineffective airway clearance (see Chapters 10 and 18)

High risk for ineffective breathing pattern (see Chapters 6, 10, 12, and 18)

High risk for decreased cardiac output (see Chapters 9, 10, and 18)

High risk for altered tissue perfusion (see Chapters 4, 12, and 18)

Cognitive-Perceptual Pattern

Diagnoses

High risk for postoperative discomfort: acute pain (see Chapters 4 and 18)

High risk for postoperative discomfort: nausea and vomiting (see Chapter 18)

Knowledge deficit (see Chapter 5)

Self-perception—Self-concept Pattern

Diagnosis

Fear related to the perioperative experience

Definition

A feeling of dread by the patient because he or she perceives surgery as a threat or danger to the self (Gordon, 1987, p. 198)

Discussion. Unlike the case with anticipatory anxiety, the patient experiencing fear knows the reason for the fear; he or she is afraid of the impending surgery. Fear is a common reaction to surgery, even though patients are becoming more knowledgeable about their health care alternatives. The patient may be able to discuss the rationale for the surgery and accept the event as inevitable, but the fact that his or her body will be cut, explored, manipulated, and sewn up again instills a feeling of dread.

Defining Characteristics

- Surgery as the focus of threat or danger
- Feelings of dread, nervousness, or concern about the surgical event
- Verbalized expectation of danger to self
- Increased questioning or information-seeking
- Voice tremors, pitch changes
- Increase in quantity of verbalization
- Increased rate of verbalization
- Hand tremor
- Increased muscle tension
- Narrowing focus of attention progressing to fixed
- Diaphoresis
- Increased heart rate
- Increased respiratory rate (Gordon, 1987, p. 198)

Related Factors (Gordon, 1987, p. 198)

- Knowledge deficit about the impending surgical event or health status

- Perceived inability to control the surgical event or the outcome of surgery

Expected Outcome

The patient recognizes and manages fear during the perioperative period.

Perioperative Nursing Interventions

The perioperative nurse can help the patient recognize that he or she is experiencing fear and then assist him or her to manage the feeling of fear. Elimination of fear is an unrealistic expectation because it is a human response to threat and impending danger. The RNFA can start this process in the surgeon's office when the patient consents to surgery. At this time, the patient's knowledge level about the surgery should be determined and appropriate teaching about the surgical event begun. Perioperative nurses providing outpatient and inpatient care should also look for the defining characteristics of fear. Interventions aimed at calming the patient should be implemented during the preoperative period (see the interventions described for managing anticipatory anxiety during the immediate preoperative period).

Diagnosis

Anticipatory anxiety (mild, moderate, or severe) related to the perioperative experience

Definition

Patients experiencing anticipatory anxiety have an "increased level of arousal associated with a perceived future threat (unfocused) to the self or significant relationships" (Gordon, 1987, p. 200)

Discussion. Surgery often causes the patient to experience a mild, moderate, or even severe anticipatory anxiety reaction. Perioperative events such as the disclosure of possible complications, anesthesia, intraoperative diagnosis, postoperative pain, and therapeutic treatment regimens such as chemotherapy and radiation may trigger an anticipatory anxiety reaction.

Defining Characteristics

- Verbalization of apprehension, uncertainty, fear, distress, or worry
- Verbalization of painful and persistent feelings of increased helplessness, inadequacy, regret
- Expressions of concern (change in life events)
- Fear of unspecified consequences
- Overexcited, rattled, jittery, scared state
- Restlessness, focus on self, insomnia, increased perspiration
- Increased wariness, glancing about, poor eye contact, facial tension, voice quivering
- Increased tension, foot shuffling, hand/arm movements, trembling, hand tremor, shakiness (Gordon, 1987, pp. 200, 202)

Related Factors

- Perceived threat of death related to the surgical experience
- Unconscious conflict (essential values, life goals) triggered by surgical intervention
- Surgical intervention perceived by the patient "as a threat to self concept, health status, socioeconomic status, role functioning, interaction patterns, or environment" (Gordon, 1987, p. 202)

Discussion. A person submitting to sterilization provides an example of unconscious conflict associated with essential values. Religious norms or values may prohibit sterilization, whereas the economic reality of controlling the size of the family may necessitate the procedure. An example of unconscious conflict associated with life goals can be seen in a patient facing a permanent surgical outcome that limits mobility. If a patient has a life goal that focuses on a career entailing the use of the legs, such as a career in professional sports, the fact that the person will have to rely on career skills that do not entail the use of the legs may precipitate unconscious conflict.

Expected Outcome

The patient identifies and manages anticipatory anxiety.

Perioperative Nursing Interventions

Because most patients experience some form of anticipatory anxiety when confronted with surgical intervention, the perioperative nurse can help the patient identify the source of his or her anxiety and suggest strategies for managing the anxiety. The RNFA in practice with a surgeon should start the intervention process early in the patient's perioperative experience. Assessment that focuses on the identification of anticipatory anxiety as soon as the patient consents to surgical intervention provides an opportunity to work with the patient and family members in developing a plan of care that addresses anxiety management. Interventions should focus on providing information about the impending surgery, clarifying misinformation the patient may have, teaching the patient relaxation techniques, helping the patient explore the source of anxiety, and communicating the patient's psychosocial status to the outpatient and/or inpatient perioperative nursing staff.

Perioperative nurses with practices limited to the outpatient or the inpatient setting are also able to identify defining characteristics that indicate when a patient is experiencing anticipatory anxiety. For these nurses, anticipatory anxiety may be easier to identify because the patient is more likely to exhibit signs of anxiety when surgery is imminent. However, developing a plan of care with interventions to manage the anxiety may be more difficult because of the immediacy of the situation. Interventions should focus on providing support, particularly during the immediate preoperative period. Gentle physical contact, a quiet and unhurried surgical environment, soothing words, and provision of amenities such as a warm blanket, a pillow, and headphones for listening to music help the patient deal with anxiety.

Diagnosis

High risk for body image disturbance related to anticipated changes in body appearance or function secondary to surgical intervention

Definition

Presence of risk factors for the patient to experience negative feelings or perceptions about characteristics, functions, or limits of the body or a body part as a result of surgical intervention (Gordon, 1987, p. 220)

Discussion. Surgery may result in the removal of a body part, a change in body functioning, or limits on the extent to which a patient is able to use his or her body. When this occurs, the patient may experience a body image disturbance. Identifying the risk of body image disturbance before surgery provides an opportunity for the perioperative nurse and the patient to develop a plan of care that assists the patient in accepting forthcoming body changes.

Risk Factors

- Surgery for removal of a body part significant to sexual identity
- Surgery resulting in a change in the appearance of body parts visible to others (face, neck, hands)
- Amputation
- Verbalization by the patient that he or she will experience difficulty in integrating the impending body change
- Verbalization by the patient that the body will be imperfect after surgery

Expected Outcome

The patient acknowledges the presence of body image disturbance after surgery and engages in functional coping behaviors.

Perioperative Nursing Interventions

Society focuses on beauty, vitality, strength of body, and independence. Consequently, surgery that changes one of these characteristics may negatively affect the patient, even though surgery is done to eradicate disease or even extend life. Identification of patients at risk for body image disturbance early in the perioperative period enables the perioperative nurse to assist the patient in preventing a body image disturbance.

The RNFA in practice with a surgeon should look for risk factors as soon as the patient agrees to surgery. Interventions should focus on helping the patient begin integration of the impending change into his or her body image. Depending on the severity of the surgical result,

the patient may need the assistance of an experienced counselor. Exposure to a person who experienced a similar surgical result often proves useful. This intervention, however, should only be done if the other person has successfully integrated the body change into his or her body image. Other interventions include asking the patient to verbalize feelings about changes in body image and self-esteem, providing realistic information about potential life style changes, working with the patient to set realistic goals, and helping the patient to recognize personal strengths to cope with changes in body image (Ignatavicius et al., 1992, p. 23).

Body image disturbance is a profound life event and a significant amount of time is needed to implement quality intervention. Most perioperative nurses in outpatient and inpatient settings are limited because of time and the episodic nature of their practice environment. Consequently, interventions designed to resolve body image disturbance, should it occur, are difficult to plan and implement. These nurses, however, play a crucial role by identifying patients at risk for body image disturbance. Documentation and communication of the risk to appropriate health care personnel activates the resources necessary to help the patient avoid or resolve a body image disturbance. Resources for patients with potential or actual body image disturbance include social workers, pastoral care personnel, psychologists, marriage counselors, and organizations with a mission to assist in the rehabilitation of patients with specific disease entities.

Role-Relationship Pattern

Diagnosis

Anticipatory grieving related to the effect of surgery

Definition

Expectation by the patient that he or she will experience a disruption in familiar patterns or significant relationships concerning other people, possessions, job, status, home, ideals, and parts and processes of the body after surgery (Gordon, 1987, p. 228)

Discussion. In their zeal to care and cure, perioperative nurses and surgeons sometimes forget that surgery is a disrupting event in the life of a patient, which may lead to an anticipatory grief response. Patients consenting to surgery for removal of a body part often grieve before surgery because of the anticipated loss. As an example, it is not uncommon for a patient to grieve before hysterectomy for the expected loss of her uterus, even though the patient is past childbearing years. For some, the loss of the uterus signifies the loss of femininity.

Defining Characteristics

- Verbal expression of distress at potential (anticipated) loss

- Anger
- Sadness, sorrow, crying
- Crying at frequent intervals, choked feeling
- Change in eating habits
- Alteration in sleep or dream patterns
- Alteration in activity level
- Altered libido
- Idealization of anticipated loss
- Developmental regression
- Alterations in concentration or pursuit of tasks (Gordon, 1987, p. 228)

Related Factors (Gordon, 1987, p. 228)

- Expected loss or change related to anticipated surgical result
- Surgery for removal of a body part significant to sexual identity
- Surgery resulting in a change in the appearance of body parts visible to others (face, neck, hands)
- Amputation

Expected Outcome

The patient recognizes the presence of anticipatory grief and engages in a functional grieving process.

Perioperative Nursing Interventions

Grieving is part of the human experience. When one is confronted with a precipitating event, functional grieving is necessary for good physical, psychological, sociocultural, and spiritual health. Dysfunctional grieving, on the other hand, has a negative impact on the holistic well-being of the individual. Such grief can lead to physical, psychological, and sociocultural imbalances and damage the human spirit.

The RNFA who has extensive patient interaction before surgery has the opportunity to identify the presence of anticipatory grieving. Helping the patient move along the grief continuum to the point of acceptance places the patient in a position in which he or she is better able to deal with the physiological and psychosocial stressors of surgery. If the patient exhibits signs of anticipatory grieving, help him or her to get in touch with the grief and understand that the experience is not uncommon. Discuss the stages of grieving with the patient and encourage him or her to set goals in response to the expected loss.

Perioperative nurses in the inpatient and outpatient setting should look for the defining characteristics of anticipatory grieving. If these are present, document and communicate the findings to the appropriate members of the health care team such as pastoral care personnel, social workers, and psychologists. If the patient exhibits behaviors such as crying or expresses anger, sorrow, or sadness, respond appropriately by listening and showing empathy. If not contraindicated because of the patient's cultural practices or preference, establish body contact with the patient by touching the hand, the shoulder, or the side of the face. Prepare the patient for the sensations that she or he will experience during the intraoperative and postoperative period. Explain that feelings of loss and grieving are normal (Ignatavicius et al., 1992, pp. 23–24).

Coping–Stress Tolerance Pattern

Diagnosis

Ineffective individual coping related to the stress of impending surgery

Definition

Impairment of a patient's abilities to use adaptive behaviors and problem-solving techniques for meeting life's demands and roles during the perioperative period. The patient's usual patterns of coping with stressful life situations are insufficient to control the anxiety, fear, or anger related to surgery (Gordon, 1987, p. 284)

Discussion. Effective individual coping, although not a guarantee for successful rehabilitation and recuperation, is nonetheless an important contributing factor. Ineffective coping on the part of the patient affects the control of anxiety and fear. Inability to cope may also interfere with the patient's compliance with the postoperative treatment regimen.

Defining Characteristics (Gordon, 1987, p. 284)

- Verbalization of inability to cope
- Inability to ask for help
- Inability to effectively solve problems
- Anxiety, fear, anger, irritability, tension
- Presence of life stress [such as a major surgical experience or disease process]
- Inability to meet role expectations [such as a permanent or temporary loss of employment as a consequence of surgery]
- Inability to meet basic needs
- Alteration in societal participation
- Destructive behavior toward self and others
- Inappropriate or ineffective use of defense mechanisms
- Change in usual communication patterns
- Excess food intake, alcohol consumption; smoking
- Digestive, bowel, appetite disturbance; chronic fatigue or sleep pattern disturbance

Related Factors (Gordon, 1987, p. 284)

- Situational crises such as surgery
- Personal vulnerability
- Knowledge deficit concerning surgery
- Problem-solving skills deficit, particularly in relation to dealing with the consequences of the surgical experience

Expected Outcome

The patient demonstrates the ability to cope with the stresses associated with surgical intervention.

Perioperative Nursing Interventions

For many people, surgery is a significant crisis in their lives. Suddenly, they are personally vulnerable in that they must submit, even though willingly, to therapeutic interventions. They lose control over their senses and sometimes their normal body functions. Interventions that focus on eliminating knowledge deficit and strengthening problem-solving skills as they relate to the surgical experience help enable the patient to be better able to cope with surgery. Possible intervention strategies include

- identification of the patient's past experiences and coping strategies as they relate to surgery or illness and then encouragement that they be implemented
- facilitation of open communication
- encouragement of the patient to participate in the decision-making process concerning surgery
- promotion of the acknowledgment of the possible outcomes of surgery
- encouragement to share the fears and anxieties related to the act of surgery and the outcome of surgery
- facilitation of the implementation of relaxation and meditation techniques (Ignatavicius et al., 1992, p. 100)

Diagnosis

Ineffective family coping: disabling related to surgery and the surgical outcome for a loved one

Definition

Behavior demonstrated by a significant other that disables the significant other's or the patient's ability to perform the tasks essential to either person's adaptation to the process or outcome of the surgical experience (Gordon, 1987, p. 300)

Discussion. Effective family coping benefits the patient throughout the perioperative period, especially during rehabilitation and recuperation. Occasionally, however, patients have family members who worry and fuss to such an extent that the ability to concentrate on the task at hand, coping with the surgery or the rehabilitation and recuperation process, is impaired.

Defining Characteristics (Gordon, 1987, p. 300)

- Neglectful care of the patient in regard to basic human needs or illness treatment
- Distortion of reality concerning the patient's health problem or denial of the existence or the severity of the disease process
- Intolerance toward the patient
- Rejection, abandonment, or desertion of the patient
- Carrying on usual routines while disregarding the patient's needs
- Taking on illness signs of the patient
- Implementation of decisions and actions by the family that are detrimental to the economic or social well-being of the patient
- Demonstration of agitation, aggression, or hostility toward the patient
- Family member's depression
- Demonstration of neglectful relationship with other family members
- Patient's helpless or inactive dependence behaviors

Related Factors (Gordon, 1987, p. 302)

- Persistent unexpressed guilt, anxiety, or hostility by family members
- Incongruity of coping styles for dealing with adaptive tasks between the significant person and the patient or among significant people
- Ambivalent family relationships

Expected Outcome

Ineffective family coping does not disable the patient's or significant other's ability to address the tasks essential to the process or outcome of the surgical experience. The patient or the significant other

- complies with preoperative and postoperative instructions
- complies with the treatment regimen after surgery

Perioperative Nursing Interventions

Usually, unless the perioperative nurse has had lengthy exposure to the patient's family dynamics, the presence of ineffective family coping may be difficult to diagnose. When it is diagnosed, however, the nurse should refer the patient and the family to appropriate family counseling. During the perioperative period, the nurse

- assists the patient and the family in identifying mechanisms to assist in coping with the surgical procedure
- plans with the patient and the family all aspects of care to ensure functional rehabilitation and recuperation
- identifies problem-solving skills of the patient and family members
- encourages family members to increase communication with the patient (Ignatavicius et al., 1992, p. 186)

CRITICAL CRITERIA FOR PATIENT PREPARATION

Facilitating Admission to the Health Care Facility

The surgeon, RNFA, office nurse, or surgeon's secretary usually schedules the surgery or invasive procedure. When scheduling surgery, the following information should be provided to the clerk or secretary posting the case:

- patient's full name
- patient's age and birth date
- patient's sex
- surgeon's name
- date and time of surgery
- planned procedure
- special instrument, supply, and equipment requests
- preoperative diagnosis
- preauthorization number for Medicare patients
- insurance information

Surgical case posting varies by institution. In some institutions, all the information listed above is obtained by the surgery posting clerk. In others, admitting personnel obtain information about insurance and preauthorization numbers.

After posting the case, the RNFA or nurse instructs the patient to

- report to the facility at a specified time
- wear comfortable, loose-fitting clothing
- bring all home prescription medications to the hospital when admitted
- leave valuables at home

If outpatient surgery is scheduled, the nurse also instructs the patient to

- maintain nothing by mouth status after midnight
- plan for child care the day of surgery
- have transportation home after the procedure
- have a responsible person stay with the patient at home after the procedure

Obtaining Informed Consent (Fay, 1986, pp. 6–10)

Informed consent implies that the patient has a right to know. A patient's right to give consent before medical care stems from the common law right of an individual to be free from unwanted, offensive, or harmful touching by another person. A valid consent implies that the patient knows about the planned procedure, its anticipated effects and possible complications, and alternative treatments. A valid consent must also be voluntary and given by a competent person. Normally, the patient gives consent verbally and in writing. Occasionally, however, consent may be inferred or legally implied. A patient may infer consent by his or her actions. For example, a patient being admitted for a cardiopulmonary bypass and coronary arterial grafting who experiences a cardiac arrest before actually signing the consent infers consent because of taking action to be admitted for the purpose of undergoing cardiac surgery. An emergency situation is an example of a consent that is legally implied because it is assumed that the patient, if he or she were able, would give consent for the procedure.

Consent may also be delegated or assisted. An example of a delegated or assisted consent is the one obtained for a minor or incompetent patient.

In general, one should always get a valid consent. Circumstances, however, may warrant the performance of surgery or other invasive procedures without a valid consent. Examples of these circumstances are emergencies, situations of therapeutic privilege, and occasions of patient waiver. Emergency situations include those in which the patient is unconscious or unable to give consent because of an extenuating circumstance or in which life or limb is at stake. If the physician believes that disclosure would have a significant negative impact on the patient and constitute unsound medical practice, therapeutic privilege may be invoked. Finally, some patients choose to be uninformed and thus waive consent.

Three parties have a responsibility for obtaining an informed consent: the health care facility, the physician, and the nurse. The health care facility is responsible for adopting and enforcing policies governing informed consent.

The physician is responsible for providing sufficient information so that the patient can make an informed consent. RNFAs in collaborative practice with surgeons should not assume this responsibility unless they have credentials to do so from the health care facility and it is allowed by the state. Information should include the medical diagnosis and the purpose of surgery, as well as the expected outcome. The patient should be told who will perform or supervise the surgery. Potential risks and reasonable alternatives to the proposed surgery should be explained. The patient should also understand the possible effects of refusing surgery, other pertinent facts that might affect the course of treatment, and the products that might be used, such as prostheses and orthopedic implants.

Nurses have the responsibility of knowing and following health care facility policies and procedures concerning informed consent. During the preoperative assessment, the perioperative nurse should determine if the patient and the physician have discussed surgery. If the consent has not been signed, the nurse should determine if the patient is ready to sign and is competent to give consent. Giving consent for an invasive or surgical procedure can cause anxiety and fear in the patient. The nurse should help put the patient at ease. While obtaining consent, the nurse should avoid providing information detailing surgical risks, benefits, alternatives, or adverse reactions. If the patient asks such questions, the surgeon or RNFA should be notified. Validity of an informed consent remains intact until the risks, benefits, or alternatives to surgery change, or until the consent is withdrawn.

The decision of who should determine if consent has been obtained is made by the health care facility. In most cases, however, the health care facility assumes this responsibility. Obtaining witnesses for the patient's signature is up to health care facility policy. In addition, depending on state regulations, a physician's signature may be required.

In the past, a consent could not be changed if premedication was given to a patient. Now, if allowed by institution policy, a consent may be changed after premedication is administered. In such cases, the patient should sign the change and the nurse should document that a change was made after premedication was administered. If at the last minute, the surgeon determines that additional procedures should be performed, notation by the surgeon should be made in the record that the patient gave prior consent to the change. The nurse should also document this change in the record.

When a consent is incomplete, the surgeon decides if the procedure should be done as planned. In such cases, the nurse should follow institutional policy and document in the record that the surgeon was notified that the consent was incomplete.

Illiterate patients or patients unable to sign owing to a physical disability should mark the consent in the presence of two witnesses. The witnesses in turn should also sign the consent.

On occasion, a telephone consent must be obtained. This type of consent should be witnessed by another person listening to the conversation. The person obtaining the consent should specify the date, note the time, and sign the record. The witness should also sign to verify that consent was given. The person giving the consent should be instructed to send confirmation of the consent via facsimile or telegram.

Figures 15–2 and 15–3 provide examples of consent forms in English and Spanish. These consents list procedures that require mandatory disclosure according to the Texas State Board of Health.

Performing the Preoperative Assessment

The purpose of the preoperative assessment is to collect sufficient data to enable

- the RNFA or the perioperative nurse to diagnose actual or potential alterations in health patterns that may affect the patient during the perioperative period
- the physician to diagnose acute or chronic medical conditions that may affect the performance of surgery and establish the patient's risk of postoperative complications

Careful evaluation and examination of major systems gives the RNFA a good idea of the physical status of the patient. The RNFA should be familiar with major symptom patterns and the probable organ pathological changes causing the symptoms.

Baseline Vital Data

The RNFA begins the assessment by introducing himself or herself to the patient and explaining the purpose of the assessment. Establish contact with the patient by touching or shaking the patient's hand during the introduction. This helps to establish rapport and puts the patient at ease. Continue contact by taking vital signs: pulse, temperature, blood pressure, and respirations. Table 2–2 lists abnormal findings for vital signs, possible indications, and possible postoperative complications. Communicate abnormal vital signs to the surgeon and the anesthetist. Postponement of surgery may be necessary to treat the underlying problem associated with the abnormal vital sign.

Determine the patient's weight and height. If measurements are recorded in pounds and inches, also note the metric equivalents. Record the patient's chronological age. If the patient is younger than 2 years of age, record the age in months. An accurate weight is critical when calculating medication dosage, especially for pediatric patients. Both weight and height help determine the patient's risk of some potential alterations in health patterns during the perioperative period.

Surgical or Invasive Procedure History

Ask the patient about prior hospitalizations. Obtain the date and reason for the hospitalization. If available, old medical records are included in the chart. As for hospitalization, ask about prior surgical and invasive procedures. Obtain the date of the past procedures and have the patient explain why the procedure was done. Also ask the patient to describe the outcome of past procedures. If the patient had a surgical or invasive procedure in the past, ask about the type of anesthesia that was used and if there was a reaction to the anesthetic.

Laboratory and Diagnostic Studies

The extent and type of laboratory and diagnostic studies depends on a multitude of factors such as the patient's condition and medical diagnosis, the type of surgery or invasive procedure planned, the physician's preference, and facility policy. Common laboratory and diagnostic studies include complete blood count, fasting blood glucose levels, urinalysis, blood electrolyte determination, electrocardiographic studies, and chest x-ray films.

White Blood Cell Count. During any acute infection, the white blood cell count (WBC) is liable to be ele-

Text continued on page 327

SANTA ROSA
HEALTH CARE CORPORATION
Conducted by Sisters of Charity of the Incarnate Word

(ADDRESSOGRAPH)

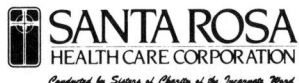

DISCLOSURE AND CONSENT

Medical, Surgical and Diagnostic Procedures

TO THE PATIENT: *You have the right, as a patient, to be informed about your condition and the recommended surgical, medical, or diagnostic procedure to be used so that you may make the decision whether or not to undergo the procedure after knowing the risks and hazards involved. This disclosure is not meant to scare or alarm you; it is simply an effort to make you better informed so you may give or withhold your consent to the procedure.*

I (we) voluntarily request Dr.________________________ as my physician, and such associates, technical assistants and other health care providers as they may deem necessary, to treat my condition which has been explained to me as:________________________

____

____

I (we) understand that the following surgical, medical, and/or diagnostic procedures are planned for me and I (we) voluntarily consent and authorize these procedures:________________________

____

____

I (we) understand that my physician may discover other or different conditions which require additional or different procedures than those planned. I (we) authorize my physician, and such associates, technical assistants and other health care providers to perform such other procedures which are advisable in their professional judgement.

I (we) do (do not) consent to the use of blood and blood products as deemed necessary.

I (we) understand that no warranty or guarantee has been made to me as to result or cure.

I (we) consent to the disposal by hospital authorities of any tissues or parts which may be removed.

*Exception:*____

Just as there may be risks and hazards in continuing my present condition without treatment, there are also risks and hazards related to the performance of the surgical, medical, and/or diagnostic procedures planned for me. I (we) realize that common to surgical, medical, and/or diagnostic procedures is the potential for infection, blood clots in veins and lungs, hemorrhage, allergic reactions, and even death. I (we) also realize that the following risks and hazards may occur in connection with this particular procedure:

____

____

____

____

____

____

____

____

____

____

FIGURE 15–2. Disclosure and consent. (Courtesy of Santa Rosa Hospital, San Antonio, TX. Santa Rosa Health Care Corporation, 519 West Houston Street, San Antonio, TX 78207. All rights reserved.)

Illustration continued on following page

I (we) do (do not) consent to the photographing of the operations or procedures to be performed, including appropriate portions of my body, for medical, scientific or educational purposes, providing my identity is not revealed by descriptive texts accompanying the pictures.

I (we) do (do not) agree to the possible presence of a scientific observer in the operating room during my surgical care should my surgeon make such a request, I (we) understand that said observer is not in any way associated with the Santa Rosa Medical Center. I (we) hereby release the Santa Rosa Medical Center, its agents, assigns and successors from any and all liability which may result from the presence of a scientific observer in the operating room.

I (we) understand that anesthesia involves additional risks and hazards but I (we) request the use of anesthetics for the relief and protection from pain during the planned and additional procedures. I (we) realize the anesthesia may have to be changed possibly without explanation to me (us).
I (we) understand that certain complications may result from the use of any anesthetic including respiratory problems, drug reaction, paralysis, brain damage or even death. Other risks and hazards which may result from the use of general anesthetics range from minor discomfort to injury to vocal cords, teeth or eyes. I (we) understand that other risks and hazards resulting from spinal and epidural anesthetics include headache and chronic pain.

I (we) have been given an opportunity to ask questions about my condition, alternative forms of anesthesia and treatment, risks of nontreatment, the procedures to be used, and the risks and hazards involved, and I (we) believe that I (we) have sufficient information to give this informed consent.

I (we) certify this form has been fully explained to me, that I (we) have read it or have had it read to me (us), that the blank spaces have been filled in, and that I (we) understand its contents.

AM
DATE: _____   TIME: _____ PM

PATIENT: _____   WITNESS: _____
                                                            N A M E
                                              ADDRESS: _____

                                              CITY, STATE, ZIP CODE _____

_____
OTHER LEGALLY RESPONSIBLE PARTY
SIGNATURE

_____
Relationship to Patient

Verification of Informed Consent   Verification of Patient Signature:

_____   Witness: _____
Physician   Hospital Employee

_____
Surgeon

_____
Anesthesiologist

FIGURE 15–2 *Continued*

List A INFORMED CONSENT
(EFFECTIVE: JULY 8, 1988)

Procedures requiring full disclosure (List A). The following treatments and procedures require full disclosure by the physician or health care provider to the patient or person authorized to consent for the patient.

1. Anesthesia
☐   1. Epidural
        1. Risks are enumerated in the informed consent form.
☐   2. General
        1. Risks are enumerated in the informed consent form.
☐   3. Spinal
        1. Risks are enumerated in the informed consent form.

2. Cardiovascular system.
(No procedures assigned at this time.)

3. Digestive system treatments and procedures
   1. Cholecystectomy with or without common bile duct exploration.
☐   1. Pancreatitis.
      2. Injury to the tube between the liver and the bowel.
      3. Retained stones in the tube between the liver and the bowel.
      4. Narrowing or obstruction of the tube between the liver and the bowel.
      5. Injury to the bowel and/or intestinal obstruction.

4. Ear treatments and procedures
   1. Stapedectomy
☐   1. Diminished or bad taste.
      2. Total or partial loss of hearing in the operated ear.
      3. Brief or long-standing dizziness.
      4. Eardrum hole requiring more surgery.
      5. Ringing in the ear.
   2. Reconstruction of auricle of ear for congenital deformity or trauma.
☐   1. Less satisfactory appearance compared to possible alternative artificial ear.
      2. Exposure of implanted material.
   3. Tympanoplasty with mastoidectomy
☐   1. Facial nerve paralysis.
      2. Altered or loss of taste.
      3. Recurrence of original disease process.
      4. Total loss of hearing in operated ear.
      5. Dizziness
      6. Ringing in the ear.

5. Endocrine system treatments and procedures
   1. Thyroidectomy
      1. Injury to nerves resulting in hoarseness or impairment of speech.
☐   2. Injury to parathyroid glands resulting in low blood calcium levels that require extensive medication to avoid serious degenerative conditions such as cataracts, brittle bones, muscle weakness and muscle irritability.
      3. Lifelong requirement of thyroid medication.

6. Eye treatments and procedures
   1. Eye muscle surgery
☐   1. Additional treatment and/or surgery.
      2. Double vision.
      3. Partial or total loss of vision.
   2. Surgery for cataract with or without implantation of intraocular lens.
      1. Complications requiring additional treatment and/or surgery.
☐   2. Need for glasses or contact lenses.
      3. Complications requiring the removal of implanted lens.
      4. Partial or total loss of vision.
   3. Retinal or vitreous surgery
      1. Complications requiring additional treatment and/or surgery.
☐   2. Recurrence or spread of disease.
      3. Partial or total loss of vision.

   4. Reconstructive and/or plastic surgical procedures of the eye and eye region, such as blepharoplasty, tumor, fracture, lacrimal surgery, foreign body, abscess, or trauma.
☐   1. Worsening or unsatisfactory appearance.
      2. Creation of additional problems such as:
        1. Poor healing or skin loss.
        2. Nerve damage
        3. Painful or unattractive scarring.
        4. Impairment of regional organs, such as eye or lip function.
      3. Recurrence of the original condition
   5. Photocoagulation and/or cryotherapy.
      1. Complications requiring additional treatment and/or surgery.
☐   2. Pain.
      3. Partial or total loss of vision.
   6. Corneal surgery, such as corneal transplant, refractive surgery and pterygium.
      1. Complications requiring additional treatment and/or surgery.
☐   2. Possible pain.
      3. Need for glasses or contact lenses.
      4. Partial or total loss of vision.
   7. Glaucoma surgery by any method.
      1. Complications requiring addtional treatment and/or surgery.
☐   2. Worsening of the glaucoma.
      3. Pain.
      4. Partial or total loss of vision.
   8. Removal of the eye or its contents (enucleation or evisceration).
      1. Complications requiring additional treatment and/or surgery.
☐   2. Worsening or unsatisfactory appearance.
      3. Recurrence or spread of disease.
   9. Surgery for penetrating ocular injury, including intraocular foreign body.
      1. Complications requiring additional treatment and/or surgery, including removal of the eye.
☐   2. Chronic pain.
      3. Partial or total loss of vision.

7. Female genital system treatments and procedures
   1. Abdominal hysterectomy (total).
      1. Uncontrollable leakage of urine.
☐   2. Injury to bladder.
      3. Sterility.
      4. Injury to the tube (ureter) between the kidney and the bladder.
      5. Injury to the bowel and/or intestinal obstruction.
   2. Vaginal hysterectomy.
      1. Uncontrollable leakage of urine.
☐   2. Injury to bladder.
      3. Sterility.
      4. Injury to the tube (ureter) between the kidney and the bladder.
      5. Injury to the bowel and/or intestinal obstruction.
      6. Completion of operation by abdominal incision.

   3. All fallopian tube and ovarian surgery with or without hysterectomy, including removal and lysis of adhesions.
      1. Injury to the bowel and/or bladder.
☐   2. Sterility.
      3. Failure to obtain fertility(if applicable).
      4. Failure to obtain sterility(if applicable).
      5. Loss of ovarian functions or hormone production from ovary(ies).
   4. Abdominal endoscopy (peritoneoscopy, laparoscopy).
      1. Puncture of the bowel or blood vessel.
☐   2. Abdominal injection and complications of infection.
      3. Abdominal incision and operation to correct injury.
   5. Removing fibroids (uterine myomectomy).
      1. Uncontrolled leakage of urine.
☐   2. Injury to bladder.
      3. Sterility.
      4. Injury to the tube (ureter) between the kidney and the bladder.

FIGURE 15–2 *Continued*

Illustration continued on following page

5. Injury to the bowel and/or intestinal ob—struction.
6. Uterine suspension.
  ☐ 1. Uncontrollable leakage of urine.
  2. Injury to bladder.
  3. Sterility.
  4. Injury to the tube (ureter) between the kidney and the bladder.
  5. Injury to the bowel and/or intestinal ob—struction.
7. Removal of the nerves to the uterus (presacral neurectomy).
  1. Uncontrolled leakage of urine.
  2. Injury to bladder.
  ☐ 3. Sterility.
  4. Injury to the tube (ureter) between the kidney and the bladder.
  5. Injury to the bowel and/or intestinal ob—struction.
  6. Hemorrhage, complications of hemorr—hage, with additional operation.
8. Removal of the cervix.
  1. Uncontrolled leakage of urine.
  2. Injury to bladder.
  3. Sterility.
  ☐ 4. Injury to the tube (ureter) between the kidney and the bladder.
  5. Injury to the bowel and/or intestinal ob—struction.
  6. Completion of operation by abdominal incision.
9. Repair of vaginal hernia (anterior and/or posterior colporrhaphy and/or enterocele repair).
  1. Uncontrollable leakage of urine.
  2. Injury to bladder.
  ☐ 3. Sterility.
  4. Injury to the tube (ureter) between the kidney and the bladder.
  5. Injury to the bowel and/or intestinal ob—struction.
10. Abdominal suspension of the bladder (retropubic urethropexy).
  1. Uncontrolled leakage of urine.
  2. Injury to bladder.
  ☐ 3. Injury to the tube (ureter) between the kidney and the bladder.
  4. Injury to the bowel and/or intestinal ob—struction.
11. Conization of cervix.
  1. Hemorrhage with possible hysterectomy to control.
  2. Sterility.
  ☐ 3. Injury to bladder.
  4. Injury to rectum.
  5. Failure of procedure to remove all of cer—vical abnormality.
12. Dilation and curettage of uterus (diagnostic).
  1. Hemorrhage with possible hysterectomy
  2. Perforation of the uterus.
  ☐ 3. Sterilty.
  4. Injury to bowel and/or bladder.
  5. Abdominal incision and operation to cor—rect injury.
13. Dilation and curettage of uterus (obstetrical).
  1. Hemorrhage with possible hysterectomy to control.
  2. Perforation of the uterus.
  ☐ 3. Sterility.
  4. Injury to the bowel and/or bladder.
  5. Abdominal incision and operation to cor—rect injury.
  6. Failure to remove all products of concep—tion.

8. Hematic and lymphatic system.
1. Transfusion of blood and blood components.
  1. Fever.
  ☐ 2. Transfusion reaction which may include kidney failure or anemia.
  3. Heart failure.

4. Hepatitis.
5. A.I.D.S. (acquired immune deficiency syndrome).
6. Other infections.

9. Integumentary system treatments and procedures
1. Radical or modified radical mastectomy. (Simple mastectomy excluded.)
  ☐ 1. Limitation of movement of shoulder and arm.
  2. Swelling of the arm.
  3. Loss of the skin of the chest requiring skin graft.
  4. Recurrence of malignancy, if present.
  5. Decreased sensation or numbness of the inner aspect of the arm and chest wall.
2. Reconstruction and/or plastic surgical operations of the face and neck.
  ☐ 1. Worsening or unsatisfactory appearance.
  2. Creation of several additional problems, such as:
    1. Poor healing or skin loss.
    2. Nerve damage.
    3. Painful or unattractive scarring.
    4. Impairment of regional organs, such as eye or lip function.
  3. Recurrence of the original condition.

10. Male genital system
1. Orchidopexy [reposition of testis(es)]
  ☐ 1. Removal of testicle.
  2. Atrophy (shriveling) of the testicle with loss of function.
2. Orchiectomy [removal of the testis(es)].
  ☐ 1. Decreased sexual desire.
  2. Difficulties with penile erection.
3. Vasectomy.
  ☐ 1. Loss of testicle.
  2. Failure to produce permanent sterility.

11. Maternity and related cases.
1. Delivery (vaginal).
  ☐ 1. Injury to bladder and/or rectum, including a hole (fistula) between bladder and vagina and/or rectum and vagina.
  2. Hemorrhage possible requiring blood ad—ministration and/or hysterectomy and/or artery ligation to control.
  3. Sterility.
  4. Brain damage, injury or even death occur—ing to the fetus before or during labor and/or vaginal delivery whether or not the cause is known.
2. Delivery (cesarean section).
  ☐ 1. Injury to bowel and/or bladder.
  2. Sterility.
  3. Injury to tube (ureter) between kidney and bladder.
  4. Brain damage, injury or even death oc—curring to the fetus before or during labor and/or cesarean delivery whether or not the cause is known.
  5. Uterine disease or injury requiring hys—terectomy.

12. Musculoskeletal system treatments and procedures
1. Arthroplasty of all joints with mechanical device.
  ☐ 1. Impaired function such as shortening or deformity of an arm or leg, limp or foot drop.
  2. Blood vessel or nerve injury.
  3. Pain or discomfort.
  4. Fat escaping from bone with possible damage to a vital organ.
  5. Failure of bone to heal.
  6. Bone infection.
  7. Removal or replacement of any implanted device or material.
2. Mechanical internal prosthetic device.
  ☐ 1. Impaired function such as shortening or deformity of an arm or leg, limp or foot drop.
  2. Blood vessel or nerve injury.
  3. Pain or discomfort.
  4. Fat escaping from bone with possible damage to a vital organ.

FIGURE 15–2 *Continued*

5. Failure of bone to heal.
6. Bone infection.
7. Removal or replacement of any implanted device or material.

3. Open reduction with internal fixation.
   1. Impaired function such as shortening or deformity of an arm or leg, limp or foot drop.
   2. Blood vessel or nerve injury.
   3. Pain or discomfort.
   4. Fat escaping from bone with possible damage to a vital organ.
   5. Failure of bone to heal.
   6. Bone infection.
   7. Removal or replacement of any implanted device or material.

4. Osteotomy.
   1. Impaired function such as shortening or deformity of an arm or leg, limp or foot drop.
   2. Blood vessel or nerve injury.
   3. Pain or discomfort.
   4. Fat escaping from bone with possible damage to a vital organ.
   5. Failure of bone to heal.
   6. Bone infection.
   7. Removal or replacement of any implanted device or material.

5. Ligamentous reconstruction of joints.
   1. Failure of reconstruction to work.
   2. Continued loosening of the joint.
   3. Degenerative arthritis.
   4. Continued pain.
   5. Increased stiffening.
   6. Blood vessel or nerve injury.
   7. Cosmetic and/or functional deformity.

6. Children's orthopedics (bone, joint, ligament, or muscle).
   1. Growth deformity.
   2. Additional surgery.

13. **Nervous system treatments and procedures**
1. Craniotomy (craniectomy) for excision of brain tissue, tumor, vascular malformation and cerebral revascularization.
   1. Additional loss of brain function including memory.
   2. Recurrence or continuation of the condition that required this operation.
   3. Stroke.
   4. Blindness, deafness, inability to smell, double vision, coordination loss, seizures, pain, numbness and paralysis.

2. Craniotomy (craniectomy) for cranial nerve operation including neurectomy, avulsion, rhizotomy or neurolysis.
   1. Numbness, impaired muscle function or paralysis.
   2. Recurrence or continuation of the condition that required this operation.
   3. Seizures.

3. Spine operation. Including: laminectomy, decompression, fusion, internal fixation or procedures for nerve root or spinal cord compression; diagnosis; pain; deformity; mechanical instability; injury; removal of tumor, abscess or hematoma. (Excluding coccygeal operations.)
   1. Pain, numbness or clumsiness.
   2. Impaired muscle function.
   3. Incontinence or impotence.
   4. Unstable spine.
   5. Recurrence or continuation of the condition that required the operation.
   6. Injury to major blood vessels.

4. Peripheral nerve operation; nerve grafts, decompression, transposition or tumor removal; neurorrhaphy, neurectomy or neurolysis.
   1. Numbness
   2. Impaired muscle function.
   3. Recurrence or persistence of the condition that required the operation.
   4. Continued, increased or different pain.

5. Correction of cranial deformity.
   1. Loss of brain function.
   2. Seizures.
   3. Recurrence or continuation of the condition that required this operation.

6. Transphenoidal hypophysectomy or other pituitary gland operation.
   1. Spinal fluid leak.
   2. Necessity for hormone replacement
   3. Recurrence or continuation of the condition that re-

quired this operation.
4. Nasal septal deformity or perforation.
7. Cerebral spinal fluid shunting procedure or revision.
   1. Shunt obstruction or infection.
   2. Seizure disorder.
   3. Recurrence or continuation of brain dysfunction.

14. **Radiology**
1. Angiography, aortography, arteriography (arterial injection of contrast media-diagnostic).
   1. Injury to artery.
   2. Damage to parts of the body supplied by the artery with resulting loss of function or amputation.
   3. Swelling, pain, tenderness or bleeding at the site of the blood vessel perforation.
   4. Aggravation of the condition that necessitated the procedure.
   5. Allergic sensitivity reaction to injected contrast media.

2. Myelography.
   1. Chronic pain.
   2. Transient headache, nausea, vomiting.
   3. Numbness.
   4. Impaired muscle function.

3. Angiography with occlusion techniques-therapeutic.
   1. Injury to artery.
   2. Loss or injury to body parts.
   3. Swelling, pain, tenderness or bleeding at the site of the blood vessel perforation.
   4. Aggravation of the condition that necessitated the procedure.
   5. Allergic sensitivity reaction to injected contrast media.

4. Angioplasty (intravascular dilatation technique).
   1. Swelling, pain, tenderness, or bleeding at the site of vessel puncture.
   2. Damage to parts of the body supplied by the artery with resulting loss of function or amputation.
   3. Injury to the vessel that may require immediate surgical intervention.
   4. Recurrence or continuation of the original condition.
   5. Allergic sensitivity reaction to injected contrast media.

5. Splenoportography (needle injection of contrast media into the spleen).
   1. Injury to the spleen requiring blood transfusion and/or removal of the spleen.

15. **Respiratory system treatments and procedures**
1. Excision of lesion of larynx, vocal cords, trachea.
   (No risks or hazards assigned at this time).
2. Rhinoplasty or nasal reconstruction with or without septoplasty.
   1. Deformity of skin, bone or cartilage.
   2. Creation of new problems, such as septal perforation or breathing difficulty.
3. Submucus resection of nasal septum or nasal septoplasty.
   1. Persistence, recurrence or worsening of the obstruction.
   2. Perforation of nasal septum with dryness and crusting.
   3. External deformity of the nose.

16. **Urinary system**
1. Partial nephrectomy (removal of part of the kidney).
   1. Incomplete removal of stone(s) or tumor, if present.
   2. Obstruction of urinary flow.
   3. Leakage of urine at surgical site.
   4. Injury to or loss of the kidney.
   5. Damage to adjacent organs.
2. Radical nephrectomy (removal of kidney and adrenal gland for cancer).
   1. Loss of the adrenal gland.
   2. Incomplete removal of tumor.
   3. Damage to adjacent organs.
3. Nephrectomy (removal of kidney).
   1. Incomplete removal of tumor if present.
   2. Damage to adjacent organs.
   3. Injury to or loss of the kidney
4. Nephrolithotomy and pyelolithotomy [removal of kidney stone(s)].
   1. Incomplete removal of stone(s).
   2. Obstruction of urinary flow.
   3. Leakage of urine at surgical site.
   4. Injury to or loss of the kidney.
   5. Damage to adjacent organs.
5. Pyeloureteroplasty (pyeloplasty or reconstruction of the kidney drainage system).
   1. Obstruction of urinary flow.
   2. Leakage of urine at surgical site.

FIGURE 15–2 Continued

Illustration continued on following page

3. Injury to or loss of the kidney.
4. Damage to adjacent organs.

6. Exploration of kidney or perinephric mass.

☐
1. Incomplete removal of stone(s) or tumor, if present.
2. Leakage of urine at surgical site.
3. Injury to or loss of the kidney.
4. Damage to adjacent organs.

7. Ureteroplasty [reconstruction of ureter (tube between kidney and bladder)].

☐
1. Leakage of urine at surgical site.
2. Incomplete removal of the stone or tumor (when applicable).
3. Obstruction of urine flow.
4. Damage to other adjacent organs.
5. Damage to or loss of the ureter.

8. Ureterolithotomy [surgical removal of stone(s) from ureter (tube between kidney and bladder)].

☐
1. Leakage of urine at surgical site.
2. Incomplete removal of stone.
3. Obstruction of urine flow.
4. Damage to other adjacent organs.
5. Damage to or loss of ureter.

9. Ureterectomy [partial/complete removal of ureter (tube between kidney and bladder)].

☐
1. Leakage of urine at surgical site.
2. Incomplete removal of tumor (when applicable).
3. Obstruction of urine flow.
4. Damage to other adjacent organs.

10. Ureterolysis [freeing of ureter (tube between kidney and bladder) from adjacent tissue].

☐
1. Leakage of urine at surgical site.
2. Obstruction to urine flow.
3. Damage to other adjacent organs.
4. Damage to or loss of ureter.

11. Ureteral reimplantation [reinserting ureter (tube between kidney and bladder) into the bladder].

☐
1. Leakage of urine at surgical site.
2. Obstruction to urine flow.
3. Damage to or loss of ureter.
4. Backward flow of urine from bladder into ureter.
5. Damage to other adjacent organs.

12. Prostatectomy (partial or total removal of prostate).

☐
1. Leakage of urine at surgical site.
2. Obstruction to urine flow.
3. Incontinence (difficulty with urinary control.)
4. Semen passing backward into bladder.
5. Difficulty with penile erection (possible with partial and probable with total prostatectomy).

13. Total cystectomy (removal of urinary bladder).

☐
1. Probable loss of penile erection and ejaculation in the male.
2. Damage to other adjacent organs.
3. This procedure will require an alternate method of urinary drainage.

14. Partial cystectomy (partial removal of urinary bladder).

☐
1. Leakage of urine at surgical site.
2. Incontinence (difficulty with urinary control).
3. Backward flow of urine from bladder into ureter (tube between kidney and bladder).
4. Obstruction of urine flow.
5. Damage to other adjacent organs.

15. Urinary diversion (ileal conduit, colon conduit).

☐
1. Blood chemistry abnormalities requiring medication.
2. Development of stones, strictures or infection.
3. Routine lifelong medical evaluation.
4. Leakage of urine at surgical site.
5. Requires wearing a bag for urine collection.

16. Ureterosigmoidostomy (placement of kidney drainage tubes into the large bowel).

☐
1. Blood chemistry abnormalities requiring medication.
2. Development of stones. strictures or infection.
3. Routine lifelong medical evaluation.
4. Leakage of urine at surgical site.
5. Difficulty in holding urine in the rectum.

17. Urethroplasty (construction/reconstruction of drainage tube from bladder).

☐
1. Leakage of urine at surgical site.
2. Stricture formation.
3. Additional operation(s).

FIGURE 15–2 *Continued*

Santa Rosa
CORPORACION DE ESMERO DE SALUD
Conducted by Sisters of Charity of the Incarnate Word

DECLARACION
Y CONSENTIMIENTO

(ADDRESSOGRAPH)

Procedimientos Medicos Y Quirurgicos

PARA EL PACIENTE: *Usted tiene el derecho, como paciente, de ser informodo acerca de su condición; y las recomendaciones quirúrgicas (operación), médicas, o procedimientos diagnósticos que van a ser usados; para que usted decida si va a someterse al procedimiento o nó; despues de conocer los riesgos y peligros relacionados. Esta explicación no tiene como intención asustarlo o alarmarlo; simplemente es un esfuerzo para darle mejor información; de tal manera que usted pueda otorgar o rehusar su consentimiento para el procedimiento.*

Yo (Nosotros) voluntariamente, pido al Doctor _____
como mi médico, y sus asociados, asistentes tecnicos y otros proveedores de servicios de salud como sean necesarios, para tratar mi condición médica, explicada a mí como _____

_____

Yo (Nosotros), comprendo que los siguientes procedimientos quirúrgicos (Operación) médicos, o exámenes de diagnóstico estan planeados para mi y Yo (Nosotros) voluntariamente doy consentimiento y autorizo estos procedimientos. _____

_____

Yo (Nosotros) comprendo que mi Doctor puede encontrar otra condición; o condiciones diferentes, que requieran procedimentos adiciónales o diferentes de lo planeado. Yo (Nosotros) autorizo mi Doctor, los asociados, asistentes técnicos y otros proveedores de servicios de salud; para que lleven a cabo aquellos otros procedimientos que sean aconsejables de acuerdo con su jucio profesional.

Yo (Nosotros) (Doy) (No Doy) consentimiento para el uso de sangre o derivados de sangre como sea necesario.

Yo (Nosotros) comprendo que no hay garantía y que ninguna garantía se me ha hecho acerca de resultados o curación.

Yo (Nosotros) consiento a la disposición, por las autoridades del hospital, de cualquier tejido o partes que hayan sido removidas.

Excepción: _____

De la misma manera que existen riesgos y peligros de continuar en mi condición presente, sin tratamiento, existen tambien riesgos y peligros relacionados con los procedimientos operatorios, médicos o de diagnóstico, planeados para mi. Yo (Nosotros) entiendo que relacionado a estos procedimientos operatorios, médicos, o de diagnostico, existen riesgos de infección, coágulos en las venas y en los pulmones, hemorragia, reacciones alérgicas y posible fallecimiento.
Yo (Nosotros) comprendo que los siguientes riesgos y peligros pueden ocurrir con este procedimiento en particular.

_____

_____

_____

_____

_____

_____

_____

FIGURE 15–3. Declaracion y consentimiento. (Courtesy of Santa Rosa Hospital, San Antonio, TX. Santa Rosa Health Care Corporation, 519 West Houston Street, San Antonio, TX 78207. All rights reserved.)

Illustration continued on following page

Yo (nosotros) doy (no doy) consentimiento para que tomen fotografias durante la operación o procedimiento, incluyendo partes apropiadas de mi cuerpo, para propositos cientificos, médicos o educacionales, con la condición que mi identidad no sea revelada con textos discriptivos acompañando las fotografias.

Yo (nosotros) estoy (no estoy) de acuerdo con la posible presencia de observadores cientificos durante mi operación en caso que mi cirujano lo requiera. Yo (nosotros) entiendo (entendemos) que este observador no está asociado en ninguna forma con el Centro Medico Santa Rosa. Yo (nosotros) libero (liberamos) al Centro Medico Santa Rosa, sus agentes, asignos y sucesores de cualquier causa legal que pueda resultar por la presencia de un observador cientifico en la sala de operaciones.

Yo (Nosotros) comprendo que la anestesia, agrega riesgos y peligros adicionales pero Yo (Nosotros) pido el uso de anesteticos para el alivio y protección de dolar durante el procedimiento a procedimientos adicionales planeados.

Yo (Nosotros) comprendo que algunas complicaciones pueden resultar por el uso de cualquier anestetico, como problemas respiratorios, reacciones a la drogas, parálisis, daño al cerebro o posible fallecimiento.

Otros riesgos y peligros que pueden resultar por el uso de anesteticos generales varian; de molestias menores a lesiones de las cuerdas vocales, los dientes; o los ojos; Yo (Nosotros) comprendo que otros riesgos y peligros relacionados con anesteticos espinales o epidurales, incluyen dolores de cabeza y dolor crónico.

Yo (Nosotros) he tenido la oportunidad de preguntar acerca de mi condición, otras formas de anestesia y tratamiento, riesgos por no ser tratado, los procedimientos que se van a usar y los riesgos y peligros consiguientes, y Yo (Nosotros) creo (creemos) que Yo (Nosotros) tenemos la información suficiente para dar este consentimiento informado.

Yo (Nosotros) certifíco que ésta forma me ha sido completamente explicada y que yo (Nosotros) la he leído, o me ha sido leída; que los espacios en blanco han sido llenadas por escrito, y que Yo (Nosotros) comprendo su contenido.

FECHA: _____

PACIENTE: _____
　　　　　　　　(Firma)

OTRA PERSONA LEGALMENTE RESPONSABLE (firma)

Relación al Paciente

HORA: _____ AM/PM

TESTIGO: _____
　　　　　　　(Firma)

DIRECCION

CIUDAD,　　　ESTADO,　　　ZONA POSTAL

Verificación de Informe:

MEDICO

MEDICO (Cirujano)　　FIRMA

MEDICO (Anestesista)　　FIRMA

Verificación de Firma del Paciente:

TESTIGO (firma)　　　(Empleado del Hospital)

FIGURE 15–3 *Continued*

Lista A CONSENTIMIENTO INFORMADO
(EFFECTIVO: 1 de Julio de 1988)

Procedimientos que exigen declaracion amplia (Lista A). Los tratamientos y prodecimientos a continuación, exigen declaraciones amplias por parte del médico o del proveedor de cuidado de la salud al paciente o a la persona autorizada a dar el consentimiento o permiso del paciente.

1. Anestesia
- 1. Epidural
  - 1. Los riesgos estan incluidos en la forma de consentimiento.
- 2. General
  - 1. Los riesgos estan incluidos en la forma de consentimiento.
- 3. Espinal
  - 1. Los riegos estan incluidos en la forma de consentimiento.

2. Sistema Cardiovascular
(No hay procedimientos fijados a la fecha.)

3. Tratamientos y prodecimientos del sistema digestivo
1. Colecistectomía con o sin exploración del conducto biliar comun.
   1. Pancreatitis.
   2. Daño al tubo entre el hígado y el intestino.
   3. Piedras retenidas entre el hígado y el intestino.
   4. Estrechamiento u obstrucción del tubo entre el hígado y el intestino.
   5. Daño al intestino y/u obstrucción intestinal.

4. Tratamientos y procedimientos del oido
1. Estapedectomía
   1. Sabor disminuido o mal sabor.
   2. Pérdida total o parcial del oir en el oído operado.
   3. Mareo breve o de larga duración
   4. Perforación del tímpano requeriendo otra cirugía
   5. Zumbido en el oído.
2. Reconstrucción de la aurícula del oído por causa de deformidad congenital o por trauma.
   1. Aspecto menos favorable comparado a un oído alternativo artificial.
   2. Exposición del material implantado.
3. Timpanoplastía con mastoidectomía
   1. Parálisis del nervio facial.
   2. Gusto alterado o perdido.
   3. Reaparición del progreso de la enfermedad original.
   4. Pérdida total del oir en el oído operado.
   5. Mareo
   6. Zumbido en el oído.

5. Tratamientos y procedimientos del sistema endocrino
1. Tiroidectomía
   1. Daño a los nervios resultando en ronquera o deterioramiento del habla.
   2. Daño a las glándulas paratiroideas resultando en niveles bajos de calcio en la sangre que requieran medicación extensiva para evitar condiciones degenerativas serias como cataratas, huesos quebradizos, debilidad de los músculos e irritabilidad de los músculos.
   3. Requerimiento de por vida de medicina para la tiroidea.

6. Tratamientos y procedimientos para los ojos.
1. Cirugía de los músculos de los ojos.
   1. Tratamientos adicionales y/o cirugía adicional.
   2. Visión doble.
   3. Pérdida parcial o total de la vista.
2. Cirugía para catarata con o sin la implantación de un lente intraocular.
   1. Complicaciones que requieren tratamientos adicionales y/o cirugía adicional.
   2. La necesidad de usar pupilentes (lentes de contacto) o anteojos.
   3. Complicaciones que requieren la extracción del lente intracular.
   4. Pérdida parcial o total de la vista.
3. Cirugía retinal o vítrea.
   1. Complicaciones que requieren tratamientos adicionales y/o cirugía adicional.
   2. Repetición o desparramiento de la enfermedad.
   3. Pérdida parcial o total de la vista.
4. Procedimientos reconstructivos y/o cirugía plastica del ojo y de la región del ojo, como blefaroplastía, tumor, fractura, cirugía lacrimal, objeto extraño en el ojo, abceso, o trauma.
   1. Semblante peor o insatisfactorio.
   2. Problemas adicionales que pueden resultarse como:
      1. Cicatrización pobre o la perdida de la piel.
      2. Daño a los nervios
      3. Cicatrización dolorosa o inatractiva.
      4. Perjuico a órganos regionales, como la función del ojo o el labio.
   3. Repetición de la condición original.
5. Fotocoagulación y/o crioterapia.
   1. Complicaciones que requieren tratamientos adicionales y/o cirugía adicional.
   2. Dolor.
   3. Pérdida parcial o total de la vista.
6. Cirugia de la córnea, como transplante de la córnea, cirugía refractiva y pterigión.
   1. Complicaciones que requieren tratamientos adicionales y/o cirugía adicional.
   2. Posible dolor.
   3. La necesidad de usar pupilentes (lentes de contacto) o anteojos.
   4. Perdida parcial o total de la vista.
7. Cirugía sobre cualquier metodo para glaucoma.
   1. Complicaciones que requieren tratamientos adicionales y/o cirugía adicional.
   2. Empeoramiento de la glaucoma.
   3. Dolor.
   4. Pérdida parcial o total de la vista.
8. Remoción del ojo o de su contenido (enucleación o evisceración)
   1. Complicaciones que requieren tratamientos adicionales y/o cirugía adicional.
   2. Semblante peor o no satisfactorio.
   3. Repetición o desparramiento de la enfermedad.
9. Cirugía para daño penetrante ocular, incluyendo objeto extraño intraocular.
   1. Complicaciones que requieren tratamientos adicionales y/o cirugía adicional.
   2. Dolor crónico.
   3. Pérdida parcial o total de la vista.

7. Tratamientos y procedimientos del sistema genital de la mujer
1. Histerectomía abdominal (total).
   1. Goteo incontrolable de orina.
   2. Daño a la vejiga.
   3. Esterilidad.
   4. Daño al tubo (ureter) entre el riñon y vejiga.
   5. Daño al intestino y/u obstrucción intestinal.
2. Histerectomía vaginal.
   1. Goteo incontrolable de orina.
   2. Daño a la vejiga.
   3. Esterilidad.
   4. Daño al tubo (ureter) entre el riñon y vejiga.
   5. Daño al intestino y/u obstrucción intestinal.
   6. Necesidad de terminar la cirugía por incisión abdominal.
3. Toda cirugía del tubo de Falopio y ovario, con o sin histerectomía, removiendo aderencias.
   1. Daño al intestino y /o vejiga.
   2. Esterilidad.
   3. Falla de obtener fertilidad (si aplica).
   4. Falla de obtener esterilidad (si aplica).
   5. Pérdida de función del ovario y producción de hormonas ováricas.
4. Endoscopía abdominal (peritoneoscopía, laparoscopía).
   1. Perforación del intestino o vaso sanguíneo.
   2. Infección abdominal y complicaciones de infección.
   3. Incisión abdominal y cirugía para correguir daño.
5. Eliminación de fibromas (miomectomía uterina).
   1. Goteo o escape de orina sin control.

FIGURE 15-3 *Continued*

Illustration continued on following page

2. Daño a la vejiga.
3. Esterilidad.
4. Daño al tubo (ureter) entre el riñón y vejiga.
5. Daño al intestino y/o obstrucción intestinal.
6. Suspensión uterina.
  1. Incontrolable goteo o escape de orina.
  2. Daño a la vejiga.
  3. Esterilidad.
  4. Daño al tubo (ureter) entre el riñón y vejiga.
  5. Daño al intestino y/o obstrucción intestinal.
7. Eliminación de los nervios del útero (neurectomía presacral).
  1. Goteo o escape de orina incontrolables.
  2. Daño a la vejiga.
  3. Esterilidad.
  4. Daño al tubo (ureter) entre el riñón y vejiga.
  5. Daño al intestino y/o obstrucción intestinal.
  6. Hemorragia, complicaciones de hemorragia, con cirugía adicional.
8. Eliminación del cuello uterino (cervix)
  1. Goteo o escape de orina incontrolable.
  2. Daño a la vejiga.
  3. Esterilidad.
  4. Daño al tubo (ureter) entre el riñón y vejiga.
  5. Daño al intestino y/o obstrucción intestinal.
  6. Operación con terminación a base de incisión abdominal.
9. Reparación de hernia vaginal (colporrafia anterior y/o posterior y/o reparación de enterocele).
  1. Goteo o escape de orina, incontrolable.
  2. Daño a la vejiga.
  3. Esterilidad.
  4. Daño al tubo (ureter entre el riñón y vejiga.
  5. Daño al intestino y/o obstrucción intestinal.
10. Suspensión abdominal de la vejiga (uteropexia retropúbica).
  1. Incontrolable goteo o escape de orina.
  2. Daño a la vejiga.
  3. Daño al tubo (ureter) entre el riñón y vejiga.
  4. Daño al intestino y/o obstruccion intestinal.
11. Conización del cervix.
  1. Hemorragia con necesidad de histerotomía.
  2. Esterilidad.
  3. Daño a la vejiga.
  4. Daño al recto.
  5. Imposibilidad de remover todo el tejido anormal del cervix.
12. Dilatación y curetaje del útero (para diagnosis).
  1. Hemorragia con necesidad de histerotomia.
  2. Perforación del útero.
  3. Esterilidad.
  4. Daño al intestino y/o vejiga.
  5. Incisión abdominal y cirugía para corregir daño.
13. Dilatación y curetaje del útero con fimes obstétricos.
  1. Hemorragia con posible histerectomía.
  2. Perforación del útero.
  3. Esterilidad.
  4. Daño al intestino y/o vejiga.
  5. Incisión abdominal y cirugía para corregir daño.
  6 Falla en sacar todos los productos de concepción.

8. Sistema hemático y linfático.
  1. Transfusión de sangre y componentes de sangre.
    1. Calentura (fiebre).
    2. Reacción de transfusión que puede incluir falla de riñón o anemia.
    3. Falla de corazón.
    4. Hepatitis.
    5. S.I.D.A. (síndrome de inmuno deficiencia adquirida).
    6. Otras infecciones.

9. Tratamientos y procedimientos del sistema integumentario
  1. Mastectomía radical o radical modificada (mastectomía simple excluida)
    1. Movimiento limitado del hombro o brazo.
    2. Hinchazón del brazo.
    3. Pérdida de la piel del pecho requeriendo injerto de piel.
    4. Recurrencia de malignidad, si estuvo presente.

5. Disminución de sensacion o adormecimiento de la superficie interior del brazo y la pared del pecho.
  2. Reconstrucción y/o cirugía plastica de la cara y cuello
    1. Insatisfacción o empeoramiento de la apariencia.
    2. Cración de varios problemas adicionales tales como:
      a. curación deficiente o pérdida de la piel.
      b. daño a los nervios
      c. cicatrización dolorosa o inatractiva
      d. deterioramiento de los órganos regionales tales como el funcionamiento del ojo o labio
    3. Reaparición de la condición original.
10. Sistema genital del hombre
  1. Orquidopexia [reposición del testículo(s)]
    1. Extirpación del testículo.
    2. Atrofia (encogimiento) del testículo con pérdida de función.
  2. Orquidectomía [extirpción del testículo(s)]
    1. Disminución del deseo sexual.
    2. Dificultad con la erección del pene.
  3. Vasectomía.
    1. Pérdida del testículo.
    2. Falla de producir esterilidad permanente.
11. Maternidad y casos relacionados
  1. Parto vaginal.
    1. Daño a la vejiga y/o recto, incluyendo un agujero (fístula) entre la vejiga y la vagina y/o recto y vagina.
    2. Posible hemorragia necesitando administración de sangre y/o histerotomía y/o ligadura de arteria.
    3. Esterilidad.
    4. Daño cerebral, daño o aún muerte del feto antes o durante el parto y/o parto vaginal sea o no conocida la causa.
  2. Operación cesárea.
    1. Daño al intestino y/o vejiga.
    2. Esterilidad.
    3. Daño al tubo (ureter) entre el riñón y vejiga.
    4. Daño cerebral daño o aún muerte del feto antes o durante el parto y/o parto vaginal sea o no conocida la causa.
    5. Enfermedad uterina o daño que requiera histerectomía.
12. Tratamientos y procedimientos del sistema musculoesqueleto
  1. Artroplastia de todas las articulaciones con aparato mecanico.
    1. Función deteriorada como acortamiento o deformidad de un brazo o pierna, cojera o pie caído.
    2. Daño a vasos sanguíneos o a nervios.
    3. Dolor o incomodidad.
    4. Escape de grasa del hueso con daño posible a un órgano vital.
    5. Insuficiencia del hueso para curarse.
    6. Infección en el hueso.
    7. Quitar o reemplazar algún aparato o material injertado.
  2. Aparato interno prostético mecánico
    1. Función deteriorada como acortamiento o deformidad de un brazo o pierna, cojera o pie caído.
    2. Daño a vasos sanguíneos o a nervios.
    3. Dolor o incomodidad.
    4. Escape de grasa del hueso con daño posible a un órgano vital.
    5. Insuficiencia del hueso para curarse.
    6. Infección en el hueso.
    7. Quitar o reemplazar algún aparato o material injertado.
  3. Reducción abierta con fijación interna
    1. Función deteriorada como acortamiento o deformidad de un brazo o pierna, cojera o pie caído.
    2. Daño a vasos sanguíneos o a nervios.
    3. Dolor o incomodidad.
    4. Escape de grasa del hueso con daño posible a un órgano vital.
    5. Insuficiencia del hueso para curarse.
    6. Infección del hueso.
    7. Quitar o reemplazar algún aparato o material injertado.
  4. Osteotomia
    1. Función deteriorada como acortamiento o deformidad de un brazo o una pierna, cojera, o pie caído.
    2. Daño a vasos sanguíneos o a nervios.
    3. Dolor o incomodidad.

FIGURE 15–3 *Continued*

4. Escape de grasa del hueso con daño posible a un órgano vital.
5. Insuficiencia del hueso para curarse.
6. Infección del hueso.
7. Quitar o reemplazar algún aparato o material injertado.
5. Reconstrucción ligamentosa de articulaciones.
    1. Insuficiencia de la reconstrucción en su funcionamiento.
    2. Aflojamiento continuado de la articulación.
    3. Artritis degenerativa.
    4. Continuación del dolor.
    5. Rigidez aumentada.
    6. Daño a vasos sanguíneos o a nervios.
    7. Deformidad cosmética o functional.
6. Ortopédico para niños (hueso, articulaciones, ligamento o músculo.)
    1. Deformidad en el crecimiento.
    2. Cirugía adicional.

13. Tratamientos y procedimientos del sistema nervioso
1. Craniotomía (craniectomía) para excision de tijido cerebral, tumor, malformación vascular y revascularización cerebral.
    1. Pérdida adicional de función cerebral incluyendo la memoria.
    2. Reaparición o continuación de la condición que demandó esta operación.
    3. Embolia (accidente cerebrovascular).
    4. Ceguera, sordera, inhabilidad de oler, doble visión, pérdida de la coordinación, convulsiones, dolor, adormecimiento y parálisis.
2. Craniotomía (craniectomía para cirugía del nervio cranial incluyendo neurectomía, avulsión, rizotomía o neurólisis.)
    1. Adormecimiento, función deteriorada del músculo o parálisis.
    2. Reaparición o continuación de la condición que demando esta operación.
    3. Convulsiones.
3. Cirugía de la espina, incluyendo: laminectomía, descompresión, fusión, fijación interna o procedimientos para la compresión de raiz del nervio o cordón espinal; diagnosis; dolor; deformidad; inestabilidad mecánica; daño; extirpación de tumor; abceso o hematoma (excluyendo cirugías de coccígeo.)
    1. Dolor, adormecimiento o torpeza.
    2. Función deteriorada del músculo.
    3. Incontinencia o impotencia.
    4. Espina inestable.
    5. Reaparición o continuación de la condición que demando esta operación.
    6. Daño a los pricipales vasos sanguíneos.
4. Cirugía del nervio periférico; injertos de nervio, descompresión, transposición o extirpación de tumor; neurorrafía, neurectomía o neurólisis.
    1. Adormecimiento.
    2. Empeoramiento de la función del músculo.
    3. Reaparición o continuación de la condición que demando esta operación.
    4. Dolor persistente, aumentado o diferente.
5. Corrección de deformidad cranial.
    1. Perdida de función cerebral.
    2. Convulsiones.
    3. Reaparición o continuación de la condición que demando esta operación.
6. Hipofisectomía transesfenoidal o otra cirugia de la glándula pituitaria.
    1. Goteo o escape de fluido espinal.
    2. Necesidad de reemplazo de hormonas.
    3. Reaparición o continuación de la condición que demando esta operación.
    4. Deformidad o perforación del tabique nasal.
7. Procedimiento o revisión de la desviación del flúido espinal cerebral.
    1. Obstrucción o infección de la desviación (shunt).
    2. Desorden de convulsiones.
    3. Reaparición o continuación de la disfunción cerebral.

14. Radiología
1. Angiografía, aortagrafía, arteriografía (inyección arterial de media de contrastre diagnóstica).
    1. Daño a la arteria.
    2. Daño a partes del cuerpo abastecidas por la arteria resultando en una pérdida de función o amputación.
    3. Hinchazón, dolor, dolorimiento o sangría en el lugar del la perforación del vaso sanguineo.
    4. Agravacion de la condición que demandó el procedimiento.

5. Reacción de sensibilidad alérgica a la media de contraste inyectada.
2. Mielografía
    1. Dolor crónico.
    2. Dolor de cabeza, náusea, vómito transitorio.
    3. Adormecimiento.
    4. Función del músculo deteriorada.
3. Angiografía con oclusiones técnicas-terapéuticas.
    1. Daño a la arteria.
    2. Pérdida o daño a partes del cuerpo.
    3. Hinchazón, dolor, dolorimiento o sangría en el lugar de la perforación del vaso sanguíneo.
    4. Agravación de la condición que demandó el procedimiento.
    5. Reacción de sensibilidad alérgica a la media de contraste inyectada.
4. Angioplastia (técnica intravascular de dilatación).
    1. Hinchazón, dolor, dolorimiento o sangría en el sitio de la perforación del vaso sanguíneo.
    2. Daño a partes del cuerpo abastecidas por la arteria resultando en una pérdida de función o amputación.
    3. Daño al vaso que pueda resultar en intervención quirúrgica inmediata.
    4. Reaparición o continuación de la condición original.
    5. Reacción de sensibilidad alérgica a la media de contraste inyectada.
5. Esplinoportografía (injección de media de contrastre al esplín)
    1. Daño al esplín requiriendo transfusion de sangre y/o estirpación del esplín.

15. Tratamientos y procedimientos del sistema respiratorio.
1. Excision de lesión de laringe, cuerdas vocales, tráquea. (No hay riesgos ni peligros fijados a la fecha.)
2. Rhinoplastia o reconstrucción nasal con o sin septoplastía.
    1. Deformidad de la piel, hueso, o cartílago.
    2. Creacion de nuevos problemas, tales como, perforación del tabique o dificultad al respirar.
3. Resección submucosa del tabique nasal o septoplastia nasal.
    1. Persistencia, reaparición o empeoramiento de la obstrucción.
    2. Perforacion del tabique nasal con resequedad y formacion de costra.
    3. Deformidad externa de la nariz.

16. Sistema urinario
1. Nefrectomía parcial (extirpación de parte del riñón).
    1. Extirpación incompleta de piedra(s) o tumor, si estuvo presente.
    2. Obstrucción del flujo urinario.
    3. Goteo o escape de orina en el lugar quirúrgico.
    4. Daño o pérdida del riñón.
    5. Daño a órganos adyacentes.
2. Nefrectomía radical (extirpación del riñón y glándula adrenal por cancer).
    1. Perdida de la glándula adrenal.
    2. Extirpación incompleta del tumor.
    3. Daño a los órganos adyacentes.
3. Nefrectomía (extirpación del riñón).
    1. Extirpación incompleta del tumor.
    2. Daño a los órganos adyacentes.
    3. Daño o pérdida del riñón.
4. Nefrolitotomía and pielolitotomía [extirpación de piedra(s) del riñón].
    1. Extirpación imcompleta de la piedras(s).
    2. Obstrucción del flujo de la orina.
    3. Goteo o escape de orina en el lugar quirúrgico.
    4. Daño o pérdida del riñón.
    5. Daño a los órganos adyacentes.
5. Pieloureteroplastía (pieloplastía o reconstrucción del sistema de drenaje del riñón).
    1. Obstrucción del flujo de orina.
    2. Goteo de orina en el lugar quirúrgico.
    3. Daño o pérdida del riñón.
    4. Daño a órganos adyacentes.
6. Exploración del riñón o masa perinéfrica.
    1. Extirpación incompleta de piedra(s) o tumor, si estuvo presente.
    2. Goteo o escape de orina en el lugar quirúrgico.
    3. Daño o pérdida del riñón.
    4. Daño a órganos adyacentes.
7. Ureteroplastía [reconstrucción del uréter (tubo entre el riñón y vejiga)].
    1. Goteo o escape de orina en el lugar quirúrgico..
    2. Extirpación incompleta de piedra o tumor (cuando sea pertinente.)
    3. Obstrucción del flujo urinario.

FIGURE 15-3 *Continued*

Illustration continued on following page

4. Daño a otros órganos adyacentes.

8. Ureterlitotomía [extirpación quirúrgica de piedra(s) del uréter (tubo entre el riñón y vejiga)].

☐
    1. Goteo o escape de orina en el lugar quirúrgico.
    2. Extirpación incompleta de la piedra(s).
    3. Obstrucción del flujo urinario.
    4. Daño a otros órganos adyacentes.
    5. Daño o pérdida del uretér.

9. Ureterectomía [extirpación parcial o completa del uréter (tubo entre el riñón y vejiga)].

☐
    1. Goteo o escape de orina en el lugar quirúrgico.
    2. Extirpación incompleta del tumor (cuando sea pertinente).
    3. Obstrucción del tubo urinario.
    4. Daño a otros órganos adyacentes.

10. Ureterólisis [libración del uréter (tubo entre el riñon y vejiga) del tejido adyacente]

☐
    1. Goteo o escape de orina en el lugar quirúrgico.
    2. Obstrucción del flujo urinario.
    3. Daño a otros órganos adyacentes.
    4. Daño o pérdida del uréter.

11. Reimplantación ureteral [reintroducción del ureter (tubo entre el riñón y vejiga) en la vejiga].

☐
    1. Goteo o escape de orina en el lugar quirúrgico.
    2. Obstrucción del flujo urinario.
    3. Daño o pérdida del uréter.
    4. Regreso del flujo de la vejiga al uréter.
    5. Dãno a otros órganos adyacentes.

12. Prostatectomía (extirpación parcial o total de la próstrata).

☐
    1. Goteo o excape de orina en el lugar quirúrgico.
    2. Obstrucción del flujo urinario.
    3. Incontinencia (dificultad con el control urinario.)
    4. Paseo de semen hacia atrás dentro de la vejiga.
    5. Dificultad con erección del pene (posible con parcial y probable con prostatectomía total).

13. Cistectomía (extirpación de vejiga urinaria).

☐
    1. Perdida probable de erección del pene y eyaculación en el hombre.
    2. Daño a otros órganos adyacentes.
    3. Este procedimiento requerirá un método alternativo para el drenaje de la orina.

14. Cistectomía parcial (estirpación parcial de la vejiga urinaria).

☐
    1. Goteo o escape de orina en el lugar quirúrgico.
    2. Incontinencia (dificultad con el control urinario).
    3. Flujo de orina hacia atras de la vejiga al uréter (tubo entre el riñón y la vejiga).
    4. Obstrucción del flujo urinario.
    5. Daño a los órganos adyacentes.

15. Desviación urinaria (conducto del ilíaco, conducto del colon).

☐
    1. Abnormalidades en la química de la sangre que requieran medicación.
    2. Desarrollo de piedras, estricturas o infección.
    3. Evaluación médica de rutina de por vida.
    4. Goteo o escape de orina en el lugar quirúrgico.
    5. Requiere el uso de una bolsa para la colección de orina.

16. Ureterosigmoidostomía (Colocar tubos para drenaje del riñón en el intestino grueso).

☐
    1. Abnormalidades en la química de la sangre que requieran medicación.
    2. Desarrollo de piedras, estricturas o infección.
    3. Evaluación médica de rutina de por vida.
    4. Goteo o escape de orina en el lugar quirúrgico.
    5. Dificultad en retener orina en el recto.

17. Urethroplastía (construcción/reconstrucción del tubo de drenaje de la vejiga).

☐
    1. Goteo o escape de orina en el lugar quirúrgico.
    2. Formación de estricturas.
    3. Cirugía adicional.

FIGURE 15–3 *Continued*

vated. If surgery is planned to treat an infectious condition (e.g., acute appendicitis), an elevated WBC is not a contraindication to surgery. On the other hand, high WBCs in patients undergoing elective procedures may be indicative of an unsuspected inflammatory process that could contraindicate surgery. For example, an acute pneumonitis suspected by an elevated WBC and confirmed by chest x-ray film necessitates cancellation of elective surgery. Extremely high WBCs are rarely due to infection alone and may suggest a leukemia condition. Unusually low WBCs might suggest bone marrow depression, which contraindicates elective surgery.

Red Blood Cell Count. The state of the patient's blood volume may be approximately determined by a red blood cell count, hematocrit, or hemoglobin determination. An abnormal hematocrit reading, for example, may reveal an unsuspected anemia and force delay of surgery. If an anemic state is suspected, as in gastrointestinal bleeding, the hematocrit level aids in determining the need for blood preoperatively.

Fasting Blood Glucose. A fasting blood glucose study is routine for patients 50 years of age or older and those suspected of having diabetes or with a family history of diabetes. A high fasting blood glucose level is suggestive of diabetes mellitus and requires further study.

Urinalysis. Urinalysis is an extremely important clearance test before any surgical procedure. Much can be learned concerning the status of the kidneys, which infrequently remain asymptomatic in serious renal disease. The nurse is responsible for seeing that a clean and freshly voided urine specimen is sent to the laboratory for each surgical patient. Specimens decrease in diagnostic value with the passage of time. Several important things can be determined by the urine study.

- Red or white blood cells in the urine may suggest renal or bladder tumors as well as chronic or acute infections of the urinary system.
- Casts, which develop from cast-off debris from various sites in the urinary tract, may, depending on their type and number, indicate severe chronic renal disease.
- An excessive spillage of protein into the urine is frequently associated with poor renal function secondary to chronic or acute renal disease.
- Spillage of glucose into the urine may be the first clue to the presence of diabetic state.
- A low specific gravity (less that 1.01) may indicate poor renal function, with the kidney unable to concentrate its urine; a high specific gravity (greater that 1.025) may indicate a dehydrated state. Often, this test has to be repeated several times to validate the concentrating ability of the kidney.

Blood Urea Nitrogen and Creatinine. Elevated blood urea nitrogen and creatinine levels may suggest poor renal function and may lead one to anticipate renal failure postoperatively.

Chest Radiography. Chest x-ray films should be a routine study for all surgical patients. Unsuspected acute and chronic pulmonary problems may manifest themselves only by chest x-ray film. The nurse should read the written x-ray report and report abnormalities to the physician.

Electrocardiogram. Electrocardiography is frequently a routine test for patients older than the age of 40 years and those suspected of having cardiac disease, diabetes, and hypertension. The nurse should note the cardiologist's interpretation and discuss any obscure points with the physician.

Other Studies

- Radiological studies such as angiography and cholangiography
- Intravenous pyelography
- Myelography
- Computed tomography
- Magnetic-resonance imaging
- Ultrasonography
- Biopsies and aspirations such as liver biopsy and bone marrow aspiration
- Endoscopic procedure such as colonoscopy, esophagoscopy, and duodenoscopy

The RNFA should determine what laboratory and diagnostic studies the physician wants ordered, ensure that they are ordered, and ascertain that the results are on the chart. Results of studies should be reviewed to determine if they are within normal ranges. If abnormal findings are reported, notify the surgeon and the anesthetist.

Table 2–1 lists common preoperative blood test values. Table 15–2 lists common preoperative urine chemistry values. Both tables list normal findings and possible alterations in health status associated with abnormal findings.

Patient Allergies and Hypersensitivity Reactions

Ask the patient about allergies or hypersensitivity reactions to tape, iodine products, narcotics, antibiotics, local anesthetics, and other drugs. If the patient reports allergies or hypersensitivity reactions to food or chemical substances, determine what type of foods or substances and the type of reaction experienced. A history of anaphylaxis, asthma, or other respiratory difficulties related to the presence of allergens, toxins, or antigens should be noted and communicated to the anesthetist. Table 15–3 lists the most common agents that cause anaphylaxis.

Nutritional Status

Proper assessment of the nutritional status of the patient is an important aspect of preoperative care.

TABLE 15–2. COMMON PREOPERATIVE URINE CHEMISTRY VALUES

Characteristic/ Component	Normal Finding	Significance of Abnormal Finding
Color	Pale yellow	Dark amber indicates concentrated urine. Pale yellow indicates dilute urine. Dark red or brown indicates blood in the urine; brown also may indicate increased urinary bilirubin level. Other color changes may result from diet or medications.
Odor	Specific aromatic odor, similar to that of ammonia	Foul smell indicates possible infection and/or dehydration.
Turbidity	Clear	Cloudy urine indicates infection or sediment.
Specific gravity	Usually 1.015–1.025; possible range 1.01–1.03	Changes reflect a disturbance in the concentrating and diluting function of the tubules. Specific gravity may become fixed in renal insufficiency.
pH	6; possible range 4.6–8	Changes are caused by diet, medications, infection, acid-base imbalance, and altered renal function.
Glucose	None or <15 mg/dl	Presence may indicate decreased tubular reabsorption capacity or hyperglycemia that exceeds this capacity.
Ketones	None	Presence reflects incomplete metabolism of fatty acids, as in diabetes mellitus.
Protein	2–8 mg/100 ml	Increased levels may indicate stress, infection, strenuous exercise, or glomerular disorders.
Red blood cells	1 or 2 per high-power field	Increased levels are normal with indwelling or intermittent catheterization or menses, but may reflect tumor, stones, or glomerular disorders.
White blood cells	1 to 3 per high-power field	Increased levels may indicate infectious or inflammatory processes.
Bilirubin	None	Presence suggests hepatic or biliary disease or obstruction.
Casts	A few or none, composed of red or white blood cells, protein, or tubular cell casts	Increased levels indicate presence of bacteria or protein, which is seen in severe renal disease.
Crystals	None	Presence of normal and/or abnormal crystals may indicate that the specimen has been allowed to stand.
Bacteria	<1000 colonies/ml	Increased levels indicate need for urine culture to determine the presence of urinary tract infection.
Creatinine (clearance)	0.8–2 g/24 h Males: 1–2 g/24 h Females: 0.6–1.8 g/24 h	Increased levels indicate glomerular dysfunction caused by renal disease, shock, or hypovolemia.
Urea nitrogen	6–17 g/24 h	Increased levels commonly result from high-protein diet, dehydration, trauma, or sepsis.
Sodium	40–180 mEq/24 h	Decreased levels are seen in hemorrhage, shock, and hyperaldosteronism. Increased levels are common with diuretic therapy, excessive salt intake, and hypokalemia.
Chloride	110–254 mEq/24 h	Decreased levels are seen in certain renal diseases.
Calcium	50–300 mg/24 h	Increased levels are commonly seen with calcium renal stones and hypercalcemia. Decreased levels indicate hypocalcemia.
Total catecholamines	110–254 mEq/24 h	Increased levels occur with hypertension, pheochromocytoma, neuroblastomas, stress, or strenuous exercise.

From Ignatavicius, D., Bayne, M. V. (1991). *Medical-surgical nursing: A nursing process approach* (pp. 1816, 1819). Philadelphia: W. B. Saunders.

TABLE 15–3. MOST COMMON AGENTS THAT CAUSE ANAPHYLAXIS

Drugs/Foreign Proteins

■ Antibiotics: penicillin, cephalosporins, tetracycline, sulfonamides, streptomycin, vancomycin, chloramphenicol, amphotericin B, and others
■ Adrenocorticotropic hormone, insulin, vasopressin, protamine
■ Allergen extracts, muscle relaxants, hydrocortisone, vaccines
■ Local anesthetics: lidocaine, procaine
■ Whole blood, cryoprecipitate, immune serum globulin
■ Radiocontrast media
■ Opiates

Foods

■ Shellfish
■ Eggs
■ Legumes, nuts
■ Grains
■ Berries
■ Preservatives

Insects/Animals

■ Hymenoptera: bees, wasps, hornets
■ Fire ants
■ Snake venom

Other Agents

■ Pollens
■ Exercise
■ Heat/cold
■ Other agents

From Ignatavicius, D., Bayne, M. V. (1991). *Medical-surgical nursing: A nursing process approach* (p. 654). Philadelphia: W. B. Saunders.

Nutritional defects may be acute or chronic. The signs of depletion may be obvious or concealed. They may result from inadequate intake, absorption, or utilization. Absence of teeth should alert the nurse to nutritional defects. Any patient with a malignancy, chronic infection, or chronic gastrointestinal disease may enter the hospital in a poor state of nutrition. Under this condition, surgery is extremely hazardous, as wounds do not heal properly, anesthesia is poorly tolerated by the liver, the kidneys fail to excrete toxins adequately, and blood-clotting mechanisms fail. Restoration of adequate nutritional status is frequently required to reduce the operative risk. High-protein, high-carbohydrate diets are sometimes supplemented by enteral nutrition. If oral intake is impossible, such as in obstructing carcinoma of the esophagus, a feeding via jejunostomy may be necessary before the major surgical procedure (Le Maitre and Finnegan, 1980, p. 56).

During the nutritional assessment, look at the patient's fluid and electrolyte status. Determine the presence of acute gastrointestinal disorders, such as vomiting and diarrhea, which may result in a serious imbalance of fluids and electrolytes. A fluid and electrolyte imbalance must be corrected before surgery. Accurate measurements of fluid intake and output must be assessed and recorded to help the physician decide on future allowances for fluids as well as the patient's response to those already administered.

Integumentary System

History (Ignatavicius and Bayne, 1991, p. 1139)

● Determine if the patient's family has a chronic tendency toward skin disorders. Ask if there have been recent complaints with skin problems.
● When assessing the patient for allergies or reactions to toxic substances, determine if there have been skin reactions.
● Ask the patient his or her occupation and if he or she is exposed to irritants.
● Review the nutritional assessment data.
● If the patient has existing skin problems, determine when the problem began.
● If a skin problem exists, determine if it is associated with itching, burning, stinging, numbness, pain, fever, nausea and vomiting, diarrhea, sore throat, cold, stiff neck, exposure to new foods, new soaps or cosmetics, new clothing or bed linens, or stressful situations.
● Describe what makes the skin problem worse and what makes it better.

Physical Examination (Ignatavicius and Bayne, 1991, pp. 1140–1151)

● Perform the skin inspection in a well-lighted room. During the skin examination, inspect each skin surface to include the scalp, the hair, the nails, and the mucous membranes.
● Observe the patient's skin color, temperature, and texture (Table 15–4).
● Check the patient's skin for lesions. The initial skin reaction to a problem is called a *primary lesion* and consists of an alteration in one of the structural components of the skin. A *secondary lesion* results with the normal progression of the disease causing the primary lesion or the therapeutic intervention. For example, a primary lesion may consist of a contact dermatitis with vesicles. As the vesicles are disrupted because of scratching, the serous exudate dries and crust forms, resulting in the secondary lesion.
● Check the patient's nails (Table 15–5).
● Look for signs of edema (see Table 15–4). Edematous tissue appears shiny, taut, and paler in color than uninvolved skin. While looking for edema, check skin elasticity. Using moderate pressure, press the tip of the index finger against edematous tissue to determine the degree of indentation or pitting. Localized edema may be caused by an inflammatory response and is usually confined to an area of injury. Dependent or pitting edema, however, may be caused by fluid and electrolyte imbalance and venous and cardiac insufficiency. Common sites of dependent or pitting edema are found on the dorsum of the foot and medial aspect of the ankle in ambulatory patients and on the

TABLE 15-4. ASSESSING THE INTEGUMENT

Alteration	Cause	Location	Significance
White skin color (pallor)	Decreased hemoglobin level	Conjunctivae	Anemia
	Decreased blood flow to the skin (vasoconstriction)	Mucous membranes	Shock or blood loss
		Nail beds	Chronic vascular compromise
		Palms and soles	Sudden emotional upset
		Lips	Edema
	Genetically determined defect of the melanocyte (decreased pigmentation)	Generalized	Albinism
	Acquired patchy loss of pigmentation	Localized	Vitiligo; tinea versicolor
Yellow-orange skin color	Increased total serum bilirubin level (jaundice)	Generalized	Increased hemolysis of red blood cells
		Mucous membranes	
		Sclera	Liver disorders
	Increased serum carotene level (carotenemia)	Perioral	Increased ingestion of carotene-containing foods
		Palms and soles	
		Absent in sclera and mucous membranes	Pregnancy
			Thyroid deficiency
			Diabetes
	Increased urochrome level	Generalized	Chronic renal failure (uremia)
		Absent in sclera and mucous membranes	
Red skin color (erythema)	Increased blood flow to the skin (vasodilation)	Generalized	Generalized inflammation
		Localized	Localized inflammation (sunburn, cellulitis, trauma, and rashes)
		Face, cheeks, nose, and upper chest	Fever; increased alcohol intake
		Area of exposure	Exposure to cold
Blue skin color	Increase in deoxygenated blood (cyanosis)	Nail beds	Cardiopulmonary disease
		Mucous membranes	Methemoglobinemia
		Generalized	
	Bleeding from vessels in tissue:		
	Petechiae (1–3 mm)	Localized	Thrombocytopenia
	Ecchymosis (>3 mm)		Increased blood vessel fragility
Reddish blue skin color	Increased overall amount of hemoglobin	Generalized	Polycythemia vera
	Decreased peripheral circulation		
Brown skin color	Increased melanin production	Localized (to area of involvement)	Chronic inflammation
			Exposure to sunlight
		Pressure points, areolae, palmar creases, and genitalia	Addison disease
		Face, areolae, vulva, and linea nigra	Pregnancy; oral contraceptives (melasma)
	Café au lait spots (tan-brown patches)		
	<6 spots	Localized	Nonpathogenic
	>6 spots	Generalized	Neurofibromatosis
	Melanin and hemosiderin deposits (bronze or grayish tan color)	Distal lower extremities	Chronic venous stasis
		Exposed areas or generalized	Hemochromatosis
Localized edema	Inflammatory response	Area of injury or involvement	Trauma
Dependent or pitting edema	Fluid and electrolyte imbalance	Ambulatory: dorsum of foot and medial ankle	Congestive heart failure
	Venous and cardiac insufficiency		Renal disease
		Bedridden: buttocks, sacrum, and lower back	Hepatic cirrhosis
			Venous thrombosis or stasis
Nonpitting edema	Endocrine imbalance	Generalized, but more easily seen over the tibia	Hypothyroidism (myxedema)
Increased moisture	Autonomic nervous system stimulation	Face, axillae, skin folds, palms, and soles	Fever, anxiety, activity
			Hyperthyroidism
Decreased moisture	Dehydration	Buccal mucous membranes with progressive involvement of other skin surfaces	Postmenopause
	Endocrine imbalance		Hypothyroidism
			Normal aging
Increased temperature	Increased blood flow to skin	Generalized	Fever, hypermetabolic states
		Localized	Inflammation
Decreased temperature	Decreased blood flow to skin	Generalized	Impending shock, sepsis, anxiety
			Hypothyroidism
		Localized	Interference with vascular flow

TABLE 15-4. ASSESSING THE INTEGUMENT *Continued*

Alteration	Cause	Location	Significance
Decreased turgor	Decreased elasticity of dermis (tenting when pinched)	Abdomen, forehead, or radial aspect of wrist	Severe dehydration Sudden severe weight loss Normal aging
Rough or thick skin	Irritation, friction	Pressure points (soles, palms, and elbows)	Calluses Chronic eczema Atopic skin diseases
	Sun damage Excessive collagen production	Areas of sun exposure Localized or generalized	Normal aging Scleroderma Keloids
Soft or smooth skin	Endocrine disturbances	Generalized	Hyperthyroidism

From Ignatavicius, D., Bayne, M. V. (1991). *Medical-surgical nursing: A nursing process approach* (pp. 1142, 1147). Philadelphia: W. B. Saunders.

buttocks, sacrum, and lower back of bedridden patients. An endocrine imbalance may cause non-pitting edema, which is generalized but more easily seen over the tibia.

- Examine the patient's skin for moisture content (see Table 15–4). Autonomic nervous system stimulation may cause an increase in moisture. Look for increased moisture on the face, in the axillae and skin folds, and on the palms and the soles of the feet. Fever, anxiety, activity, and hyperthyroidism are other conditions that may cause an increase in moisture. Fluid loss with subsequent dehydration, normal aging, and endocrine imbalance secondary to hypothyroidism may result in decreased skin moisture. Areas of decreased moisture include the buccal mucous membranes, with progressive involvement of other skin surfaces.

Nursing Diagnoses

Integumentary assessment data provide clues for identifying alterations in the nutritional-metabolic pattern. Potential nursing diagnoses include the following:

- high risk for impaired skin integrity
- impaired skin integrity
- impaired tissue integrity

Cardiovascular System

History (Melonakos, 1990, p. 26)

- Ask the patient if she or he has experienced progressive weakness, shortness of breath, syncope, diaphoresis, nausea, or vomiting. If the patient has had these symptoms, ask under what circumstances they occurred.

TABLE 15-5. ASSESSING NAIL COLOR

Alteration	Clinical Findings	Significance
White	Horizontal white banding or areas of opacity Generalized pallor of nail bed	Chronic hepatic or renal disease (hypoalbuminemia) Shock Anemia Early arteriosclerotic changes (toenails) Myocardial infarction
Yellow-brown	Diffuse yellow to brown discoloration	Jaundice Peripheral lymphedema Bacterial or fungal infection of the nail Psoriasis Diabetes Cardiac failure Staining from tobacco, nail polish, or dyes Chronic tetracycline therapy Normal aging (yellow-gray color)
	Vertical brown banding extending from the proximal nail fold distally	Normal finding in black patients Nevus or melanoma of nail matrix in Caucasian patients
Red	Thin, dark red vertical lines 1–3 mm in length (splinter hemorrhages)	Bacterial endocarditis Trichinosis Trauma to nail bed Normal finding in some patients
	Red discoloration of lunula Dark red nail beds	Cardiac insufficiency Polycythemia vera
Blue	Diffuse blue discoloration that blanches with pressure	Respiratory failure Methemoglobinuria Venous stasis disease (toenails)

From Ignatavicius, D., Bayne, M. V. (1991). *Medical-surgical nursing: A nursing process approach* (p. 1149). Philadelphia: W. B. Saunders.

- Determine if the patient has a history of heart disease. If so, ask what type of heart disease.
- Ask the patient if family members have experienced heart disease, diabetes, stroke, and thromboembolism.
- Explore the type of medications the patient takes for existing cardiovascular disease such as nitroglycerin, digitalis, diuretics, antihypertensives, and potassium supplements.
- Assess the patient's social history. Look for occupation-related stress, type A behavior patterns, stress related to marital or family status, and recent stressful life events.
- Determine the patient's smoking and alcohol habits and the amount of caffeine intake.
- Assess the patient's nutritional status to include typical eating patterns and salt intake.
- Assess the patient's activity level. Ask about exercise patterns and participation in cardiac rehabilitation activities.

Physical Examination (Melonakos, 1990, pp. 26–28)

- Thoroughly assess the patient's pulse, including rate, amplitude, deficits, and peripheral pulses (Tables 15–6 and 15–7).
- Assess the cardiac area for pulsations or other abnormalities.
- Look for distended neck veins. The veins should distend only if the patient lowers the head to assume the supine position. They should not distend if the patient remains in the sitting position.
- Check the patient for cardiomegaly. It is present if the apex of the heart is percussed past the midclavicular line.
- Palpate for thrills or murmurs over heart valve areas (aortic, pulmonic, tricuspid, and mitral).
- Check the patient for pitting edema. Use the 1+, 2+, 3+, or 4+ scale to describe the severity of edema.
- Assess the patient for cold or pale feet, absent or diminished peripheral pulses, cyanosis or flushing of the extremities, and leg cramps on walking. Pay particular attention to leg and foot care in the postoperative period in any patient demonstrating one or more of these symptoms.

TABLE 15–6. ASSESSING PULSE

Measurement

Place first, second, and third fingers on the patient's radial artery to determine the radial pulse.
Evaluate rate, rhythm, and amplitude.
Count the radial pulse for 30 s and multiply by 2.
If irregularities are noted, take an apical pulse for 1 min.
Normal pulse rate is 60–80 beats/min for an average adult.

Pulse Rhythm

Normal dysrhythmias
   The pulse rate speeds up at the end of inspiration and slows down with expiration in young adults and children.
   Occasional premature beats are normal.
Abnormal dysrhythmias
   See Figures 2–3 through 2–9.
   Pulse deficit exists if the apical rate differs from the radial rate.

Pulse Amplitude

Pulse amplitude refers to the measurement of pulse force or strength.
Amplitude
   3+ = bounding pulse
   2+ = normal pulse
   1+ = weak, thready pulse
   0 = absent pulse
Bounding pulse implies a widened pulse pressure, which is the difference between the systolic and diastolic pressures.
Weak, thready pulse implies a narrowed pulse pressure.

Pulse Points

Obtain peripheral pulses for patients undergoing angiography or cardiac or vascular surgery.
Peripheral pulses include radial, ulnar, brachial, femoral, popliteal, dorsalis pedis, and posterior tibialis.

Data from Melonakos, K. (1990). *Saunders pocket reference for nurses* (pp. 10–12). Philadelphia: W. B. Saunders.

- Review laboratory values (Table 15–8).
- If indicated, obtain electrocardiographic readings.
- Evaluate the outcomes of angiography, scans, stress testing, pulmonary function tests, x-ray studies, fluoroscopy, and other diagnostic tests.

Nursing Diagnoses

Cardiovascular assessment data provide clues for identifying alterations in the activity-exercise pattern. Potential nursing diagnoses include the following:

TABLE 15–7. ABNORMAL HEART SOUNDS

Sound	Description	Cause
Quiet or muffled heart sounds		Thick chest wall, severe overload, cardiac tamponade
Gallops	Extra heart sounds best heard over apex	Cardinal sign of congestive heart failure
Snaps and clicks	High-pitched sounds usually associated with murmurs	Caused by rapid displacement of a valve from high pressure due to stenosis
Murmurs	High- or low-pitched sounds	Caused by turbulent blood flow through a valve due to congenital or acquired defects
Friction rub	A sound like two pieces of leather rubbing together	Associated with pericarditis

Adapted from Melonakos, K. (1990). *Saunders pocket reference for nurses* (p. 11). Philadelphia: W. B. Saunders.

TABLE 15–8. USING LABORATORY VALUES TO ASSESS CARDIOVASCULAR STATUS

Parameter	Assessment
Complete blood count	Check WBC, hemoglobin level, and hematocrit to identify infectious or anemic trends.
Electrolytes	Check potassium to determine if the patient is receiving diuretics or potassium supplements.
Blood gases	Check pH, oxygen pressure, and bicarbonate level for normal limits.
Cardiac enzymes	Check for trends in elevation of creatine kinase, lactate dehydrogenase, aspartate aminotransferase (formerly known as serum glutamic-oxaloacetic transaminase), and isoenzyme studies.
Coagulation studies	Check prothrombin time for oral coagulants, partial thromboplastin time for heparin therapy.
Urinalysis	Check specific gravity and look for presence of protein.
Blood urea nitrogen	Check kidney function.
Serum drug levels	Check for presence of digitalis, lidocaine, procainamide, and quinidine.

Data from Melonakos, K. (1990). *Saunders pocket reference for nurses* (pp. 28–29, 726). Philadelphia: W. B. Saunders.

- high risk for activity intolerance
- activity intolerance
- decreased cardiac output
- altered tissue perfusion

Respiratory System

History (Melonakos, 1990, pp. 20–22)

- If the patient reports episodes of shortness of breath, ask when they occur.
- Evaluate the patient for the presence of a cough. If a cough is present, determine if it is productive, hacking, paroxysmal, brassy, habitual, or nervous.
- Explore the patient's medical history for episodes of respiratory disease. If present, determine the type of therapy prescribed and the effectiveness of treatment.

- If the patient engages in an exercise program, determine if breathing exercises are part of the program.

Physical Examination (Melonakos, 1990, pp. 21–23)

- Check the patient's chest symmetry on inspiration.
- Look for abnormalities such as barrel-, funnel-, or pigeon-shaped chest and spinal deformities.
- Evaluate the patient's skin for mottling, scars, irregularities, and odor.
- Assess the patient's respiratory pattern, including rate and rhythm. Watch the patient breathe to determine the presence of pursed-lip breathing, nasal flaring, chest breathing versus abdominal breathing, retractions, or splinting because of pain. See Tables 15–9 through 15–13 for more information about assessing the respiratory system.
- Review laboratory results, especially complete blood count, electrolyte values, hematocrit, and hemoglobin concentration.
- If indicated, carefully evaluate blood gas results for abnormalities (Table 15–14).
- Review diagnostic studies and note and communicate to the physician abnormal results, especially abnormal findings of radiography, electrocardiography, biopsies, fluid aspirations, lung scans, pulmonary function studies, and bronchoscopy.

Nursing Diagnoses

Respiratory assessment data provide clues for identifying alterations in the activity-exercise pattern. Potential nursing diagnoses include the following:

- ineffective airway clearance
- ineffective breathing pattern
- impaired gas exchange

Gastrointestinal System

History (Melonakos, 1990, pp. 29–31)

TABLE 15–9. TYPES OF SPUTUM

Type of Sputum	Characteristics	Indications
Mucoid	Thin, clear	Early bronchitis
Mucopurulent	Thick, viscous, greenish color, frothy	Pneumonia, late bronchitis, tuberculosis
Purulent	Thick, viscous, yellowish, offensive smell	Lung abscess, advanced tuberculosis, bronchiectasis, pneumonia
Nummular	Mucopurulent with small semisolid masses that sink in water	Advanced tuberculosis
Rusty	Mucopurulent, rust tinged, viscous	Pneumonia
Prune juice	Dark brown, offensive smelling	Late pneumonia or gangrene of lung
Hemoptysis	Bright red and frothy	Cancer, tuberculosis, pneumonia, pulmonary embolism, mitral stenosis, or aneurysm rupturing into bronchial tubes

Adapted from Melonakos, K. (1990). *Saunders pocket reference for nurses* (p. 22). Philadelphia: W. B. Saunders.

TABLE 15–10. EXAMINING THE LUNGS

Palpation

Gently palpate the patient all over the thorax for any tender areas.

Check the patient's chest expansion by placing the hands on either side of the chest at the lung bases and ask the patient to inhale deeply. Look for equal expansion. The hands should move equally upward and slightly outward.

Assess the patient for tactile fremitus by palpating for vibrations on the chest wall when the patient says "ninety-nine." A decreased fremitus may indicate pneumothorax or pleural effusion. Increased fremitus may indicate consolidation secondary to atelectasis or pneumonia.

Percussion

Dullness on percussion may indicate consolidation, atelectasis, or effusion.

Hyperresonance on percussion may indicate pneumothorax or chronic obstructive pulmonary disease.

Auscultation

Instruct the patient to cough and clear the upper airway. Next, have the patient breathe deeply through the mouth.

Start at the trachea and move in a zigzag pattern, auscultating the anterior, posterior, and lateral parts of the patient's thorax.

Listen for resonance, breath and voice sounds, rales and rhonchi, and friction rub.

Adapted from Melonakos, K. (1990). *Saunders pocket reference for nurses* (pp. 7, 22–23). Philadelphia: W. B. Saunders.

TABLE 15–11. ABNORMAL BREATH SOUNDS

Breath Sounds	Characteristics	Indications
Rales	Sounds like fizzing seltzer; may be fine, medium, or coarse; wet or crackling	"Wet," pulmonary edema; "dry," pulmonary fibrosis
Rhonchi	Bubbling or rumbling sounds	Chronic bronchitis or any disorder with retained pulmonary secretions
Wheezing	Musical sounds, varied pitch	Asthma, chronic bronchitis, or any disorder reducing the caliber of airways
Pleural friction rub	Like a squeaky, groaning leather shoe	Pleurisy, pulmonary embolus

Adapted from Melonakos, K. (1990). *Saunders pocket reference for nurses* (p. 23). Philadelphia: W. B. Saunders.

TABLE 15–12. ASSESSING RESPIRATIONS

Assess the patient's respirations for rate and quality.

Count the rate for 30 s and multiply by 2. If respiratory or cardiac problems are identified, evaluate the respiratory rate for 60 s.

For the average adult, the normal respiratory rate is 16–20 breaths/min. A patient's rate varies depending on age, exercise, and environmental conditions. Normally, a patient takes 3 deep breaths/min.

Adapted from Melonakos, K. (1990). *Saunders pocket reference for nurses* (p. 12). Philadelphia: W. B. Saunders.

TABLE 15–13. ABNORMAL RESPIRATORY PATTERNS

Pattern	Characteristics	Indications
Tachypnea	Rapid and shallow breathing	Associated with fever, pneumonia, respiratory alkalosis, and salicylate poisoning
Bradypnea	Slowed but regular breathing	Associated with the use of opiates and alcohol, tumors, metabolic disorders, and conditions affecting the medulla oblongata
Hyperventilation or Kussmaul breathing	Increased rate and depth of breathing	Associated with renal failure and diabetic ketoacidosis
Apnea	Periodic absence of breathing	Caused by mechanical obstruction or conditions affecting the respiratory center
Cheyne-Stokes	Periods of apnea followed by breath of increasing depth	Caused by increased intracranial pressure, severe congestive heart failure, renal failure, meningitis, drug overdose, and cerebral anoxia
Biot fast	Uniformly deep respirations marked by abrupt pauses	Associated with head injury
Ataxic breathing	Completely chaotic and irregular breathing	Associated with severe brain stem damage

Adapted from Melonakos, K. (1990). *Saunders pocket reference for nurses* (pp. 12–13). Philadelphia: W. B. Saunders.

- The major symptoms indicating alterations in the gastrointestinal system include belching, heartburn, bowel habit changes, weight loss, past history of ulcers, gastrointestinal bleeding, and jaundice. Postoperative gastrointestinal complications include bleeding ulcers, liver failure, and intestinal obstruction.
- Assess the patient for gastrointestinal pain (Table 15–15).
- Assess for the presence of nausea, vomiting, and diarrhea. Determine when episodes of gastrointestinal distress occur, such as before or after meals. Search for precipitating factors such as emotional stress, medications, specific foods, treatments, and exercise.
- If the patient reports vomiting or diarrhea, describe the frequency, amount, color, odor, and consistency.
- Assess the patient for constipation. Determine the time of the last bowel movement. Ask if laxatives or enemas were used.
- Assess the patient for episodes of belching, gas, and flatulence. Determine their frequency.

- Determine if the patient has episodes of gastrointestinal bleeding. If so, describe the type of bleeding (Table 15–16).
- Ask the patient about recent weight gain or loss.
- Determine if the patient has a history of gastrointestinal problems. If so, inquire about the type of therapy used and if it was effective.
- Ask if the patient has experienced gastrointestinal problems related to allergies.
- Determine and list all medications the patient uses for gastrointestinal problems such as over-the-counter antacids, laxatives, and sodium bicarbonate.
- Determine bowel and bladder habits and if there has been a recent change in habits.

Physical Examination (Melonakos, 1990, pp. 31–33)

- Before the examination, instruct the patient to empty the bladder.
- Position the patient in the supine position, expose

TABLE 15–14. EVALUATING BLOOD GASES

Test	Value	Abnormal Findings	
		Increased	*Decreased*
pH	7.35–7.45	Alkalosis	Acidosis
Arterial carbon dioxide pressure (pCO_2)	35–45 mm Hg	Compensated metabolic alkalosis Respiratory acidosis Administration of high concentration of oxygen	Compensated metabolic acidosis Respiratory alkalosis Decreased cardiac output Chronic lung disease
Oxygen pressure (pO_2)	75–100 mm Hg (dependent on age and altitude); above 500 mg while receiving 100% oxygen	Polycythemia	Decreased efficiency of the lungs
Oxygen (O_2) saturation	95% or greater	Oxygen administration	High altitude Lung diseases
Bicarbonate (HCO_3)	24–28 mEq/L	Compensated respiratory acidosis Metabolic alkalosis	Compensated respiratory alkalosis Metabolic acidosis

Adapted from Melonakos, K. (1990). *Saunders pocket reference for nurses* (p. 106). Philadelphia: W. B. Saunders.

TABLE 15–15. PRIMARY CAUSES OF ABDOMINAL PAIN

Obstruction
Peritoneal irritation
Vascular insufficiency
Ulceration
Altered bowel motility
Nerve injury
Referred pain from an extraabdominal site
Emotional stress

Adapted from Melonakos, K. (1990). *Saunders pocket reference for nurses* (p. 29). Philadelphia: W. B. Saunders.

the abdomen, and cover the breast and pubic areas with a gown and bed sheet.

* Observe the patient's skin color and hair distribution.
* Look for jaundice.
* Inspect the skin for rashes, striae, pigmentations, or surgical wounds.
* Assess the patient for asymmetry, masses, herniations, visible peristalsis, or pulsations.
* Look at the contour of the patient's abdomen and describe in terms of obesity, flatness, distention, hollowness, and cachexia.
* Auscultate, percuss, and palpate the abdomen (Table 15–17).
* Examine the rectum and anus (Table 15–18).
* Review laboratory results, especially complete blood count, electrolyte values, and blood urea nitrogen level.
* Review diagnostic studies and note and communicate to the physician abnormal reports, especially reports of common gastrointestinal studies such as barium enema and barium swallow examinations, endoscopy, nuclear scans, sigmoidoscopy, ultrasonography, and radiography.

Nursing Diagnoses

Gastrointestinal assessment data provide clues for identifying alterations in the elimination pattern. Potential nursing diagnoses include the following:

* constipation
* diarrhea
* bowel incontinence

TABLE 15–16. CHARACTERISTICS OF GASTROINTESTINAL BLEEDING

Vomitus	Stool
Bright red	Bright red
Brown	Blood tinged
Coffee grounds	Dark and tarry
Blood tinged	Positive for occult blood
Positive for occult blood	

Adapted from Melonakos, K. (1990). *Saunders pocket reference for nurses* (p. 31). Philadelphia: W. B. Saunders.

TABLE 15–17. EXAMINING THE ABDOMEN

Auscultation

Perform auscultation before percussion or palpation to avoid stimulating peristalsis.
Because bowel sounds are high pitched, use the diaphragm of the stethoscope.
Normal bowel sounds should be heard in all four quadrants every 5–20 s.
Evaluate abnormal findings.
   Hypoactive bowel sounds (less than one per minute) indicate paralytic ileus, peritonitis, obstruction, hemorrhage, post abdominal surgery, mesenteric infarct, or no food in the bowel.
   Hyperactive bowel sounds (continuous sounds) may occur with vomiting or diarrhea, above bowel obstruction, or after eating.
   Vascular sounds may indicate aneurysm, vascular disease, heart murmur, or liver disease.

Percussion

Percuss all four quadrants.
Listen for areas of dullness and tympany.
   Tympanic areas: large and small intestines
   Dull areas: liver, spleen, bladder, and gravid uterus

Palpation

Palpate lightly for areas of tenderness, masses, and involuntary guarding.
Palpate deeply for normal anatomy, enlarged structures, masses, and pain.
   Liver, spleen, pancreas, and urinary bladder are not normally palpable.
   The lower pole of the right kidney may be palpated. The left kidney, however, is not normally palpable, except occasionally in thin individuals.
   Aorta is often palpable at the epigastrium slightly left of the midline. Aorta feels like a long thin, consistent, pulsatile mass. An enlarged area may indicate aneurysm.
Do not mistake normal structures (such as feces-filled colon, distended bladder, gravid uterus, aorta, and sacral promontory for masses).
Techniques for assessment of abdominal fluid include flank bulging and fluid shift.

Adapted from Melonakos, K. (1990). *Saunders pocket reference for nurses* (pp. 32–33). Philadelphia: W. B. Saunders.

Musculoskeletal System

History (Ignatavicius and Bayne, 1991, pp. 721–722)

* Obtain information about the patient's previous illnesses and accidents related to the musculoskeletal system. Ask about traumatic incidents such as sprains and fractures. Note the date of traumatic incidents, even if they occurred years in the past.
* Explore the patient's family history because osteoporosis is often seen in several family generations and bone cancer tends to be genetically linked.
* Determine if the patient receives regular exposure to sunlight. Inadequate exposure predisposes the patient to bone and muscle tone loss.
* Ask the patient or a significant other to describe the patient's eating patterns. Calcium or protein deficiency predisposes the patient to bone and muscle tone loss.

TABLE 15–18. EXAMINING THE RECTUM AND ANUS

Don protective gloves.
Place the patient in the lateral Sims' position.
Observe the skin and surface characteristics of the perianal area.
The perianal area should be smooth and clear with no tenderness, fissures, hemorrhoids, scars, ulcers, skin irritation, or rectal prolapse.
Palpate the perianal area for tenderness and masses.
With gloved, lubricated index finger, perform digital examination.
Sphincter muscle should tighten evenly around the finger with minimal discomfort for the patient.
The rectal wall should be a continuous, smooth surface with no areas of tenderness, tumors, lumps, or masses.

Data from Melonakos, K. (1990). *Saunders pocket reference for nurses* (p. 33). Philadelphia: W. B. Saunders.

- Determine if the patient has adequate vitamin C intake. Inadequate intake inhibits bone and tissue healing.
- Note the patient's weight. Obese patients with musculoskeletal problems are at risk for respiratory and circulatory complications. Obesity also places excessive strain and stress on joints and bones, which may lead to fractures and cartilage degeneration.
- Determine the patient's occupation, which may place the patient at risk for musculoskeletal injury or health problems.

Physical Examination (Ignatavicius and Bayne, 1991, pp. 722–724)

- Look for gross deformities or impairment by observing the patient's posture, gait, and mobility (Table 15–19).

TABLE 15–19. ASSESSING POSTURE, GAIT, AND MOBILITY

Posture

Evaluate the patient's body build and alignment when standing and walking.
Look for curvature of the spine.
  Lordosis
  Scoliosis
  Kyphosis
Inspect the extremities for length, shape, and symmetry.

Gait

Evaluate the patient's balance and steadiness.
Determine the patient's ease and length of stride.
Look for limp or other asymmetrical leg movements or deformities.
Determine the patient's need for ambulatory assistive devices.

Mobility

Assess the patient's ability to perform activities of daily living.
Determine the extent of range of motion by having the patient demonstrate active movement of major joints.

From Ignatavicius, D., Bayne, M. V. (1991). *Medical-surgical nursing: A nursing process approach* (p. 723). Philadelphia: W. B. Saunders.

TABLE 15–20. ASSESSING THE SKELETAL SYSTEM

Head and Neck

Inspect and palpate the skull for shape, symmetry, tenderness, and masses.
Evaluate the temporomandibular joints by palpating while the patient opens his or her mouth. Common abnormal findings are tenderness or pain, crepitus, and a spongy swelling caused by excessive synovium and fluid, which can be palpated.
Observe and palpate each vertebra in the neck.

Vertebral Spine

Observe and palpate the thoracic, lumbar, and sacral spine. Look for malalignment, tenderness, and inability to flex, extend, and rotate.
Check for discomfort in the lower back by placing both hands over the lumbosacral area and applying pressure with the thumbs to elicit tenderness.

Upper Extremities

Assess both extremities concurrently.
Starting with the shoulders and moving to the elbows and then the wrists, check for size, swelling, deformity, malalignment, tenderness or pain, and mobility.
Assess hand function by palpating the metacarpophalangeal, proximal interphalangeal, and distal interphalangeal joints. Compare the same digits on the right and left hands.
Determine range of motion for each joint.

Lower Extremities

Evaluate the hip joints by determining the degree of mobility.
Assess the knee joints with the patient in a sitting position with the knees flexed. Look for fluid accumulation, or effusion, and limitations in movement with accompanying pain.
Inspect the ankles and feet. Observe, palpate, and test each joint for range of motion.

Data from Ignatavicius, D., Bayne, M. V. (1991). *Medical-surgical nursing: A nursing process approach* (p. 723). Philadelphia: W. B. Saunders.

- Inspect the patient's muscle mass for size and symmetry. Look at tone, shape, and strength. Determine the grip strength by having the patient squeeze a sphygmomanometer bulb and record the level of pressure achieved.
- Assess the head and neck, the vertebral spine, and the upper and lower extremities (Table 15–20).
- Review laboratory studies, especially serum calcium, phosphorus, and phosphate levels; erythrocyte sedimentation rate; and serum muscle enzyme levels (Table 15–21).
- Review diagnostic studies such as radiography, tomography and xeroradiography, myelography, diskography, arthrography, computed tomography, and bone or muscle biopsies (Table 15–22).

Nursing Diagnoses

Musculoskeletal assessment data provide clues for identifying alterations in the activity-exercise pattern. Potential nursing diagnoses include the following:

- high risk for injury related to musculoskeletal impairment

TABLE 15–21. USING LABORATORY STUDIES FOR MUSCULOSKELETAL ASSESSMENT

Test	Normal Range (Adults)	Interpreting Abnormal Ranges

Serum calcium level	8–10.5 mg/dl or 4.5–5.5 mEq/L	Hypercalcemia
		  Metastatic cancers of the bone
		  Paget disease
		  Bone fractures in healing stage
		Hypocalcemia
		  Osteoporosis
		  Osteomalacia

Serum phosphorus level	2.5–4 mg/dl	Hyperphosphatemia
		  Bone fractures in healing stage
		  Bone tumors
		  Acromegaly
		Hypophosphatemia
		  Osteomalacia

Alkaline phosphatase level	30–90 IU/L (slightly higher in elderly)	Elevations
		  Metastatic cancers of the bone
		  Paget disease
		  Osteomalacia

Erythrocyte sedimentation rate	Westergren method
	  Males: 0–15 mm/h
	  Females: 0–20 mm/h
	Wintrobe method
	  Males: 0–9 mm/h
	  Females: 0–15 mm/h
		Elevations
		  Infection
		  Inflammation
		  Carcinoma
		  Cell or tissue destruction

Serum muscle enzyme level
  Creatine kinase (CK_3)
	15–150 IU/L	Elevations
		  Muscle trauma
		  Progressive muscular dystrophy
		  Effects of electromyography

Lactate dehydrogenase (LDH_4 and LDH_5)	60–150 IU/L	Elevations
		  Skeletal muscle necrosis
		  Extensive cancer
		  Progressive muscular dystrophy

Aspartate aminotransferase (serum glutamic-oxaloacetic transaminase)	10–50 mU/mL (slightly lower in women)	Elevations
		  Skeletal muscle trauma
		  Progressive muscular dystrophy

Aldolase A	1.3–8.2 U/dl	Elevations
		  Polymyositis and dermatomyositis
		  Muscular dystrophy

From Ignatavicius, D., Bayne, M. V. (1991). *Medical-surgical nursing: A nursing process approach* (p. 725). Philadelphia: W. B. Saunders.

- impaired physical mobility
- self-care deficit

Urinary System

History (Ignatavicius and Bayne, 1991, pp. 1808–1810)

- Note the patient's age and sex. Some urinary tract disorders are related to the age or sex of the patient. For example, sudden hypertension in a patient older than the age of 50 years may indicate the presence of renovascular disease. Another example is polycystic disease, which typically occurs in patients in their 40s or 50s. Men older than the age of 50 years may experience dysfunctional urinary patterns as a result of prostatic disease. Women, because of their short urethra, may experience cystitis.
- Assess the patient's personal and family history. Ask the patient about a history of urinary tract infections or urological surgery. Note any history of arthritis, hypertension, and diabetes mellitus. Arthritis medication may result in injury to renal tissue. Hypertension, especially if untreated or uncontrolled, may result in nephrosclerosis, leading to renal failure. Diabetes mellitus may lead to renal failure. Determine if the patient's family has a history of renal disease.
- Review nutritional assessment data. Symptoms such as changes in appetite and taste acuity or an inability to discriminate tastes are associated with the accumulation of nitrogenous waste products from renal failure. High protein intake can result in transient renal problems. Some patients are prone to renal calculi formation secondary to excessive calcium intake.
- Review the patient's medication history. Determine if the patient has taken medications for chronic health problems such as diabetes mellitus, hypertension, cardiac disorders, hormone deficiencies, and arthritis. Medications used to treat these disorders may lead to renal dysfunction. Antibiotics such as gentamicin, are also associated with sudden

TABLE 15–22. DIAGNOSTIC STUDIES OF THE MUSCULOSKELETAL SYSTEM

Examination or Test	Purpose	Method
Standard radiography	Visualize the skeleton and supporting structures Observe bone density, alignment, swelling, and intactness Determine condition of joints, including the size of the joint space, the smoothness of articular cartilage, and synovial swelling Determine soft tissue involvement	Standard x-ray imaging
Tomography and xeroradiography	Tomography is helpful in musculoskeletal assessment because it produces planes, or slices, for focus and blurs the images of other structures Xeroradiography highlights the contrast between structures, allowing margins and edges to be clearly seen	X-ray imaging with higher doses of radiation
Myelography	Visualize the vertebral column, intervertebral disks, spinal nerve roots, and blood vessels	Injection of a contrast medium into the subarachnoid space of the spine
Diskography	Visualize an intervertebral disk	Injection of a contrast medium directly into the target disk
Arthrography	Visualize a joint	X-ray imaging of a joint after injection of a contrast medium (air or solution) to enhance visualization
Computed tomography	Detect musculoskeletal problems (used with or without contrast medium)	Scanner produces a narrow x-ray beam that examines body sections from many different angles A computer produces a three-dimensional picture of the structure being studied Small tumors may not be detected without the use of oral or intravenous contrast medium
Bone biopsy	Confirm the presence of infection or neoplasm	Collection of a bone specimen for microscopic examination via needle or open extraction
Muscle biopsy	Diagnose muscle atrophy (as in muscular dystrophy) and inflammation (as in polymyositis)	Collection of a muscle specimen for microscopic examination via needle or open extraction
Electromyography	Determine the electrical potential generated in an individual muscle Usually accompanied by nerve conduction studies Helpful in the diagnosis of neuromuscular, lower motor neuron, and peripheral nerve disorders	Multiple needle electrodes, varying from 1.3 to 7.5 cm (½ to 3 inches), are inserted The patient performs activities to measure muscle potential during minimal and maximal contractions Nerve and muscle activity is recorded on an oscilloscope When done in conjunction with nerve conduction studies, flat electrodes are placed along the nerve to be evaluated, and small doses of electrical current are passed via the electrodes to the nerve and muscle innervated. If the muscle contracts, nerve conduction is confirmed
Bone scan	Radionuclide test used to detect tumors, arthritis, osteomyelitis, osteoporosis, vertebral compression fractures, and unexplained bone pain	The radioactive isotope technetium (^{99m}Tc) is injected intravenously for visualization of the entire skeleton
Gallium scan	This test is similar to the bone scan, but is more specific and sensitive in detecting bone problems	Radioactive medium used is gallium citrate (^{67}Ga), which is administered 3 d before the test owing to the slow absorption rate of the material
Indium imaging	Used primarily to detect bone infection	The patient's leukocytes are separated from a blood sample, tagged with indium (^{111}In), and injected intravenously. In acute bone infections (osteomyelitis), the tagged leukocytes accumulate and can be seen on scanning
Magnetic resonance imaging	Identify problems with muscle, tendons and ligaments	The image is produced through the interaction of magnetic fields, radiowaves, and atomic nuclei showing hydrogen density. The lack of hydrogen ions in cortical bone makes it easily distinguishable from soft tissues
Ultrasonography	Detect soft tissue disorders such as masses and fluid accumulation	Use of sound waves to produce an image of the tissue being studied

Adapted from Ignatavicius, D., Bayne, M. V. (1991). *Medical-surgical nursing: A nursing process approach* (pp. 726–731). Philadelphia: W. B. Saunders; and Melonakos, K. (1990). *Saunders pocket reference for nurses* (p. 154). Philadelphia: W. B. Saunders.

TABLE 15–23. **TERMS FOR URINARY DYSFUNCTION**	
Oliguria	Decrease in urine output, specifically an output of 100–400 ml/24 h
Anuria	Absence of urine output, specifically less than 100 ml/24 h
Polyuria	Increase in urine output, usually greater than 1500 ml/24 h
Dysuria	Any discomfort associated with urination
Hesitancy	Difficulties in initiating the flow of urine
Urgency	Sensations experienced when there is a sudden need to urinate; may be associated with urinary incontinence
Renal colic	Severe or spasmodic pain associated with renal or ureteral irritation that radiates into the perineal area, groin, scrotum, or labia

Adapted from Ignatavicius, D., Bayne, M. V. (1991). *Medical-surgical nursing: A nursing process approach* (p. 1810). Philadelphia: W. B. Saunders.

renal dysfunction. Determine if the patient takes over-the-counter medications. Some (e.g., analgesics), especially when combined with other agents, can affect renal function.

● Assess the patient's urinary patterns. Ask if the patient has experienced changes in the color of the urine, the pattern of urination, and the ability to start or control urination. Determine if the patient has experienced alterations in the appearance of the urine (see Table 15–2). Ask if the patient has experienced oliguria, anuria, polyuria, hesitancy, dysuria, or urgency (Table 15–23). Determine if the patient has episodes of urinary incontinence. If so, describe the situations that result in incontinence.

Physical Examination (Ignatavicius and Bayne, 1991, pp. 1810–1811)

● Assess the general condition of the patient. Look at the skin. Determine if there is a yellow tinge, rashes, ecchymoses, and other discoloration. Check the pedal, pretibial, presacral, and periorbital tissues, which are common sites for edema in renal disorders. Assess the patient's level of consciousness. Deficits in concentration, impaired thought processes or memory, dysarthria (the inability to speak clearly and distinctly), and an altered level of alertness may indicate the presence of renal disease. Check the patient's gait and hand coordination, which may also be affected by the presence of renal disease.

● Assess the kidneys, ureters, and bladder in conjunction with the abdominal assessment (Table 15–24).

● Inspect the urethra by checking the meatus for discharge such as blood, mucus, or purulent drainage. Check the surrounding tissues for the presence of lesions, rashes, or other abnormalities of the penis or scrotum or of the labia or vagina. Suspect urethral irritation if the patient reports discomfort when initiating urination.

Nursing Diagnoses

Urinary system assessment data provide clues for identifying alterations in the nutritional-metabolic and elimination patterns. Potential nursing diagnoses include the following:

● high risk for fluid volume deficit
● fluid volume deficit
● fluid volume excess
● altered patterns of urinary elimination
● functional incontinence
● stress incontinence
● total incontinence

Facilitating Preoperative Care

Before surgery, patients require special preparation. This is done so that the patient will experience surgery with the least amount of risk, discomfort, and fear and will recover from it with a minimum of pain and other complications. The patient should also have an understanding of how he or she can assist in speeding recovery

TABLE 15–24. **ASSESSING THE KIDNEYS, URETERS, AND BLADDER**

Auscultation

Listen to the aorta and renal arteries for the presence of a *bruit* (an audible sound produced when the volume of blood or the diameter of the blood vessel is changed).
If a bruit is detected, listen for a *thrill* (a palpable sensation of blood that is similar to a rippling pulse).

Palpation

Lightly palpate all quadrants of the abdomen. Note areas of tenderness or discomfort. If severe bladder distention is present, the outline of the bladder may be identified as high as the umbilicus.
The ureters are not palpable, however, a spasm of the ureteral musculature results in flank or low abdominal pain that is severe, excruciating, and similar to colic.
Do not palpate the kidneys unless appropriately trained. The ability to palpate the kidneys requires special training and practice under the guidance of a qualified practitioner and is usually reserved for nurses in advanced practice.

Percussion

Gently palpate the outline of the distended bladder, then place the fingertips of one hand on the lower abdomen. Use the fingertips of the other hand to thump over the top of the fingers of the hand resting on the abdomen. A distended bladder sounds dull when percussed. Move the hand resting on the bladder toward the umbilicus until the dull sounds are no longer heard.
Usually, the patient complains of discomfort or a constant, dull ache with inflammation or infection of the kidney, the renal capsule, or the adjacent fascia. If the patient has not identified flank pain, percuss the nontender costovertebral angle, which is the lower portion of the rib cage and the vertebral column. Have the patient assume the sitting, lateral, or supine position for this percussion. Clench the examining hand into a fist. With the heel of the hand and the little finger, quickly and firmly thump the costovertebral area. The elicitation of costovertebral tenderness is highly suggestive of kidney infection or inflammation.

Adapted from Ignatavicius, D., Bayne, M. V. (1991). *Medical-surgical nursing: A nursing process approach* (pp. 1811–1812). Philadelphia: W. B. Saunders.

TABLE 15–25. GASTROINTESTINAL PREPARATION

Surgical Site	Preparation	Complications
Stomach, duodenum, and proximal jejunum	Oral laxative (e.g., castor oil preparation or bisacodyl [Dulcolax]) Clear liquid diet the evening before surgery NPO after midnight	Abdominal cramping Dehydration Electrolyte imbalance Fatigue
Small intestine	Oral laxative (e.g., magnesium citrate) Clear liquid the evening before surgery NPO after midnight	Dehydration Electrolyte imbalance Fatigue
Large intestine to rectum	Multiple or combination of oral laxatives 12–24 h before surgery Multiple-position tap water or antibiotic (neomycin) enemas (3 times) or until return flow is clear the evening and morning before surgery Oral antibiotics to sterilize bowel (e.g., neomycin and erythromycin 24 h before surgery) Clear liquid diet the day before surgery NPO after midnight	Fatigue and weakness Fluid excess or deficit Potassium and/or sodium deficit Decreased cardiac output from vagal stimulation Irritation of bowel and rectal mucosa from enemas

Adapted from Ignatavicius, D., Bayne, M. V. (1991). *Medical-surgical nursing: A nursing process approach* (p. 441). Philadelphia: W. B. Saunders.

and convalescence. Before the patient's admission to the health care facility, or soon after, the surgeon or the RNFA writes orders specifying the type of preparation the surgeon desires for the patient. These orders may vary and are designed to meet the specific needs of each patient relating to the planned surgical procedure. The orders may include all or some of the following:

Skin Preparation. Skin preparation includes a complete bath and removal of hair from the operative site, if preferred by the surgeon. The bath is usually done with a special cleansing agent, such as povidone-iodine (betadine) or Hibiclens. Chapter 6 discusses preparing the patient's skin for surgery.

Diet. By withholding food and fluids before the operation, the patient accepts the induction of anesthesia more easily, and the surgeon is able to perform better

surgery. All patients should have nothing by mouth (NPO) after midnight of the night before surgery. This means not only no food and fluids, including water, but also no candy, nuts, gum, or smoking.

Gastrointestinal Tract Preparation. Enemas are not needed routinely, but may be required for abdominal operations likely to be followed by paralytic ileus and delayed bowel function and for operations on the colon, rectum, and anus. Table 15–25 describes common gastrointestinal tract preparation regimens.

In certain types of abdominal operations, particularly those on the intestinal tract, it is necessary to have a nasogastric tube inserted through the nose to the esophagus and into the stomach. The tube is fastened in place and aids in removing fluid and gas, which can cause distention and postoperative discomfort. If a patient has gastrointestinal obstruction, a nasogastric tube is passed

TABLE 15–26. COMMON PREOPERATIVE MEDICATIONS

Drug	Usual Preoperative Dose*	Precautions
Sedatives and Hypnotics		
Pentobarbital sodium (Nembutal)	50–200 mg PO	Monitor respiratory status.
Secobarbital sodium (Seconal)	200–300 mg PO	Monitor level of anxiety; encourage verbalization and
Chloral hydrate	0.5–1 g PO	relaxation
Tranquilizers		
Chlorpromazine hydrochloride (Thorazine)	25–50 mg PO, 12.5–25 mg IM	Maintain NPO status and assess for gastrointestinal upset
Hydroxyzine hydrochloride (Vistaril)	50–100 mg PO, 25–100 mg IM	or nausea.
Diazepam (Valium)	5–10 mg PO or IM	Promote relaxation by dimming lights and instructing the
Promethazine hydrochloride (Phenergan)	50 mg PO, 25–50 mg IM	patient on the importance of relaxation.
Narcotics (Opiates)		
Meperidine hydrochloride (Demerol)	50–100 mg IM or SC	Give deep intramuscular injection with 1- or 1½-inch
Morphine sulfate	5–15 mg IM or SC	needle.
Hydromorphone hydrochloride (Dilaudid)	2–4 mg PO or IM	Monitor blood pressure and respiratory status.
Anticholinergics		
Atropine sulfate	0.4–0.6 mg PO, SC, IM, or IV	Monitor blood pressure and heart rate.
Glycopyrrolate (Robinul)	0.002 mg/pound (0.004 mg/kg) of body weight IM	Monitor hydration and maintain NPO status.
Scopolamine (hyoscine)	0.3–0.6 mg IM or SC	

*PO, orally; IM, intramuscularly; SC, subcutaneously; IV, intravenously.
From Ignatavicius, D., Bayne, M. V. (1991). *Medical-surgical nursing: A nursing process approach* (p. 451). Philadelphia: W. B. Saunders.

preoperatively and the stomach is aspirated or placed on continuous suction to reduce the possibility of regurgitation and aspiration during the induction of anesthesia. If an emergency operation is to be performed on a patient who has eaten within 12 hours of surgery, insertion of a nasogastric tube is mandatory. When there is no indication for a nasogastric tube before surgery and one is needed during surgery, the anesthetist can pass the tube into the stomach after the patient is asleep.

Preoperative Medications. To alleviate anxiety and to ensure a restful sleep, a barbiturate or sleeping pill generally is prescribed the night before surgery for inpatients. About 1 or 2 hours before the operation, preoperative medications may be given to the patient (Table 15–26).

Blood Transfusion. If the use of blood or blood products is anticipated during surgery or after the operation, the patient's blood must be typed and arrangements need to be made for a sufficient number of units of blood to be cross-matched and available before surgery.

Urinary Bladder Preparation. If urinary retention is anticipated or if there is a need for hourly monitoring of urine output before, during, or after surgery, a Foley catheter can be inserted for constant bladder drainage. If bladder distention interferes with exposure in the pelvis, a catheter should be placed preoperatively. Catheterization can be done in the patient's room before leaving for the operation, although it may preferably be done after the patient has been anesthetized.

Intravenous Therapy. For operations associated with marked blood loss, a 14- or 16-gauge intravenous catheter is used for the rapid administration of blood, fluid, or medication. Intravenous therapy may be needed preoperatively for providing hydration as well as for maintaining adequate fluid and electrolyte balances.

Instructions for Postoperative Exercises. Depending on the operation, it may be helpful to teach the patient before the operation how to perform certain exercises that she or he will be expected to perform postoperatively. These may include coughing, turning, performing leg exercises, deep breathing, and practicing the use of special respiratory equipment (see Figs. 5–1 through 5–3).

SUMMARY

The RNFA plays a crucial role in preparing patients for surgery. Central to this role is facilitating the patient's admission to the health care facility, obtaining informed consent, performing a preoperative assessment, and facilitating preoperative care.

Bibliography

American Nurses Association (1992, January). What is an advanced medical directive? *The American Nurse*, p. 9.

Fay, M. F. (1986). Informed consent: A confusing concept. *Today's OR Nurse, 8*(7), 6–10.

Gordon, M. (1987). *Manual of Nursing Diagnosis: 1968–1987*. New York: McGraw-Hill.

Ignatavicius, D., Bayne, M. V. (1991). *Medical-surgical nursing: A nursing process approach*. Philadelphia: W. B. Saunders.

Ignatavicius, D., Batterden, R. A., Hausman, K. A. (1992). *Pocket companion for medical-surgical nursing*. Philadelphia: W. B. Saunders.

Le Maitre, G. D., Finnegan, J. A. (1980). *The patient in surgery: A guide for nurses* (4th ed.). Philadelphia: W. B. Saunders.

Melonakos, K. (1990). *Pocket reference for nurses*. Philadelphia: W. B. Saunders.

CHAPTER 16

Handling Tissues with Instruments

Rosalie Stewart and Joseph A. Kinnaman

DEFINITION

Handling tissues with instruments refers to those skills that the registered nurse first assistant (RNFA) uses to provide exposure of the operative site and clamp, grasp, suture, and cut tissue.

MEASURABLE CRITERIA

The RNFA demonstrates competency to handle tissues with instruments by

- providing exposure during surgery
- clamping tissue
- grasping tissue
- suturing
- cutting tissue

ROLE OF THE PERIOPERATIVE NURSE

Every operation, by the mere fact that tissue is cut, causes injury to the patient. The role of the perioperative nurse practicing as an RNFA is to minimize this injury by carefully and gently handling tissues. Careful, gentle, correct handling of tissues and instruments improves the result of any operation, thus minimizing damage and accelerating healing.

CONSIDERATIONS

Historical Perspectives

As early as 10,000 BC, sharpened flint knives were used to perform surgery. Egyptian writings dating back to 3000 BC tell of tourniquets. From these early writings, and from mummies found with wounds sutured with linen, we learn of the use of suture ligatures. Early Hindu surgeons were even more skillful than the Egyptians. They treated fractures and also practiced a crude form of plastic surgery. Early Greek carvings depict the use of scalpels. Early Arabian surgeons used cautery to control hemorrhage. Hippocrates (460–377 BC) recommended hot irons to control bleeding.

Ammonius (c. 247 BC) wrote of an instrument used to impale a bladder stone. Albucasis (d. AD 1013) illustrated a large number of instruments, including a trochar for paracentesis, a scissors, and a syringe. He also described the use of animal gut for sutures. Galen

(AD 130) depicted a method of grasping a vein with a hook and twisting it to stop bleeding, and he also recommended the use of a linen ligature for an artery.

In the 14th century, instruments remained relatively crude, even though modifications were being seen. During this century, the bullet extractor was introduced. Riveted handles were designed in the 16th century. Ambrose Pare (1510–1590) used a forceps shaped like a "crow's bill." Instruments remained crude, however, because they were being made by blacksmiths, armorers, and cutlers. It was not uncommon for a surgeon to use carpenter's tools, as well as kitchen knives and forks.

Hospitals began to provide appointments for surgeons in the 18th century. More surgery was being attempted and it was evolving into a scientific discipline. Coppersmiths, silversmiths, woodcutters, and steelworkers began to produce instruments. These instruments were limited in scope, however, as only operations of dire need such as amputations were regularly performed. Surgeon's instruments were often works of art with intricately carved handles made of wood or ivory and were stored in velvet-lined boxes.

The 19th century produced great changes in the design of instruments. Two important discoveries were responsible. The first was the introduction of anesthesia in 1846. This enabled the surgeon to work more cautiously because the surgeon no longer had to operate speedily on a struggling patient. As surgical techniques were refined, a larger array of instruments was needed. The second development, in 1867, was Lister's antiseptic method for the prevention of infection. Instruments needed to be sterilized and so the ornate, hand-carved instrument handles were replaced with metal ones. This was the beginning of modern surgery.

In 1900, stainless steel was introduced and became the preferred metal for making instruments. The pivot forceps and ratchet were also developed. As surgical specialties evolved, the number of different instruments increased vastly. Today, thousands of instruments are available for every purpose and preference to fulfill the needs of all surgeons.

Gentle Handling of Tissue

William Stewart Halsted (1852–1922) established the first school of surgery in the late 19th century at Johns Hopkins Hospital in Baltimore. He emphasized the concept of complete hemostasis, absolute asepsis, gentleness in the manipulation of tissues, sharp dissection, and accurate reapproximation of divided tissues. He also introduced the wearing of rubber gloves during an operation. When Halsted's principles of operative technique were abused, complications such as hematoma, infection, wound disruption, and contracture often occurred. Over the years, Halsted's principles have remained intact and surgeons have learned that there is no substitute for careful, gentle handling of tissue and accurate surgical technique.

Instrument Terminology

Thousands of surgical instruments of varying sizes and shapes are available for use by the surgeon. Most of these instruments are categorized as sharps, clamps, graspers, and retractors (Table 16–1).

OUTCOME STANDARD

Handling tissue with instruments does not compromise or cause injury to the patient.

Criteria

The patient is free from evidence of

- postoperative hematoma
- serous discharge or local infection
- wound dehiscence
- excessive scar formation
- postoperative neuromuscular impairment
- postoperative impaired tissue integrity

TABLE 16–1. CATEGORIES OF SURGICAL INSTRUMENTS

Category	Examples	Uses
Sharps	Scalpels Scissors Bone cutters Rongeurs Chisels Osteotomes Saws Curets Dermatomes	Designed to incise and dissect tissue and bone
Clamps	Hemostats (artery forceps) Vascular clamps Intestinal clamps	Designed to control bleeding and maintain hemostasis; may be used to grasp or retract tissue
Graspers	Tissue forceps Tenacula Rib approximators Sponge forceps Towel clips Needle holders	Used to grasp and hold tissue or bone for dissection or retraction or to assist in suturing
Retractors	Self-retaining Hand-held	Designed to provide the best exposure with minimal trauma to surrounding tissue
Other	Suction tubes Dilators	Designed to clear the operative field of fluids and open or clear anatomical passages

Adapted from Groah, L. K. (1983). *Operating room nursing: The perioperative role* (pp. 283–287). Reston, VA: Reston Publishing.

POTENTIAL ALTERATIONS IN FUNCTIONAL HEALTH PATTERNS

Health Perception–Health Management Pattern

Diagnosis

High risk for infection related to the handling of tissue with instruments during surgery

Definition

Presence of risk factors for the patient to experience a postoperative wound infection related to the exposure, clamping, grasping, suturing, and cutting of tissue during surgery

Risk Factors (Gordon, 1987, p. 50)

- Nutritional deficiencies: proteins, carbohydrates, zinc, and vitamins A, B, C, and K
- Obesity
- Fluid volume deficit or excess secondary to trauma or illness
- Impaired tissue integrity secondary to trauma
- Impaired tissue perfusion secondary to trauma
- Decreased hemoglobin concentration, leukopenia, and suppressed inflammatory response
- Immunosuppression
- Inadequate acquired immunity
- Existing infection
- Inadequate hemostasis
- Poor approximation of tissues, resulting in the formation of dead space
- Excessive handling of tissue
- Use of contaminated instruments

Expected Outcome

The patient is free from wound infection 72 hours postoperatively. Depending on the patient's health status and wound classification designation at the time of surgery, the patient shows no evidence of

- cellulitis
- abscess
- lymphangitis
- gas gangrene
- Meleney ulcer
- dehiscence (Rothrock, 1987, pp. 191–192)

Diagnosis

High risk for injury related to handling of tissue with instruments during surgery

Definition

Presence of risk factors for the patient to experience postoperative impaired physical mobility, impaired tissue integrity, altered tissue perfusion, and discomfort related to the exposure, clamping, grasping, suturing, and cutting of tissue during surgery

Risk Factors (Rothrock, 1987, pp. 124–125; Ethicon, 1988, p. 5)

- Altered circulation
- Obesity
- Emaciation
- Extremes in age, height, and body build
- Presence of physical deformities or limitations
- Failure to evaluate the type of tissue, location of vascular or nerve structures, and the presence of organs in relation to the method used to provide exposure
- Inadequate hemostasis
- Extended surgical procedure
- Excessive intraoperative abduction or adduction of extremities
- Direct pressure on body surface from members of the surgical team
- Exposure of the operative site with a retractor intended for use only on selected surgical procedures or on a specific type of tissue
- Use of an intestinal bag
- Excessive or improper retraction of tissue
- Improper clamping or grasping of tissue

Expected Outcome

The patient is free from injury related to the handling of tissue with instruments. Postoperatively, the patient shows no evidence of

- impaired physical mobility (inability to move, decreased active joint range of motion, and decreased muscle strength or control)
- impaired tissue integrity (excessive swelling at the surgical site, skin discoloration on body surfaces)
- altered tissue perfusion (cold extremities, diminished arterial pulses, blood pressure changes in extremities, discoloration of an extremity) (Gordon, 1987, p. 160)
- discomfort (excluding incisional pain)

Nutritional-Metabolic Pattern

Diagnosis

High risk for impaired tissue integrity related to the handling of tissue with instruments during surgery

Definition

Presence of risk factors for the patient to experience damage to muscle, fascia, subcutaneous tissue, and skin after surgery related to the approximation of tissue and the ligation of blood vessels with suture material

Risk Factors (Ethicon, 1988, pp. 5, 13)

- Obesity
- Wound infection
- Bleeding disorders
- Nutritional deficiencies
- Poor intraoperative hemostasis
- Inadequate approximation of tissue, resulting in the formation of dead space
- Poor knot tying technique; use of an inappropriate knot

Expected Outcome

The patient is free from signs of impaired tissue integrity at the wound site. The patient shows no evidence of

- swelling at the wound site
- excessive discoloration, swelling, or serosanguineous discharge at the wound site
- excessive pain at the wound site

PERIOPERATIVE NURSING INTERVENTIONS

Providing Exposure

Achieving exposure of the operative site requires adequate traction. A poorly exposed operative site, because of inadequate retraction, impedes the surgeon. Likewise, overly aggressive traction, although achieving good exposure, may cause injury to the patient.

The RNFA should approach the task of providing exposure from a nursing perspective. This means considering the provision of exposure during the preoperative assessment, while planning and implementing patient care, and during the postoperative evaluation.

The RNFA assesses the patient preoperatively and develops a plan of care that provides balanced traction to meet the exposure needs of the surgeon and protect the patient from injury. The assessment focuses on patient variables that affect the ability to provide exposure age, height, weight, body build, and physical deformities or limitations. The RNFA also reviews the planned procedure. This review includes the stages of the procedure that require exposure, the type of tissue and the location of vascular or nerve structures, the presence of organs, and the type of instruments available for exposure (Rothrock, 1987, pp. 124–125).

Intraoperatively, the RNFA implements the plan and continually assesses the operative site to determine the effectiveness of providing exposure. If variables change during the procedure, the RNFA modifies the plan. After surgery, the RNFA assesses the patient to determine the presence of injury related to the provision of exposure.

Stabilization of Anatomical Structures

Sponges

The RNFA uses laparotomy and 4 × 4 or 4 × 8 inch radiopaque sponges to stabilize and hold anatomical structures. Used either wet or dry, sponges enable the RNFA to hold back tissue or push it out of the way, thus providing better exposure for the surgeon. Radiopaque sponges, 4 × 4 or 4 × 8 inches, enable the RNFA to grasp and hold tissue such as muscle, fasciae, subcutaneous tissue, and skin. Because of the small size of radiopaque sponges, however, they should not be used in the abdominal cavity. Laparotomy sponges provide an excellent means for grasping and holding internal organs such as the large and small intestines. When using sponges to move or hold anatomical structures, handle the tissue gently, but with a firm touch. A gentle touch prevents bruising, tearing, and puncturing of the tissue, whereas a firm touch prevents slipping of the tissue from the assistant's hand. Figure 16–1 shows the surgeon holding skin and subcutaneous tissue with a laparotomy sponge during a total mastectomy. When packing the bowel, use laparotomy sponges. Before packing, ensure that the scrub nurse moistens the sponges in warm normal saline. Keep track of the number of sponges used and thoroughly examine the cavity for retained sponges before closure.

Intestinal Bag

An intestinal bag keeps the bowel moist, aids in retaining body heat, and protects the bowel from inadvertent abrasion during an extended procedure. The RNFA must monitor the moisture content of the intestinal bag and the tissue integrity of the bowel. Maintain

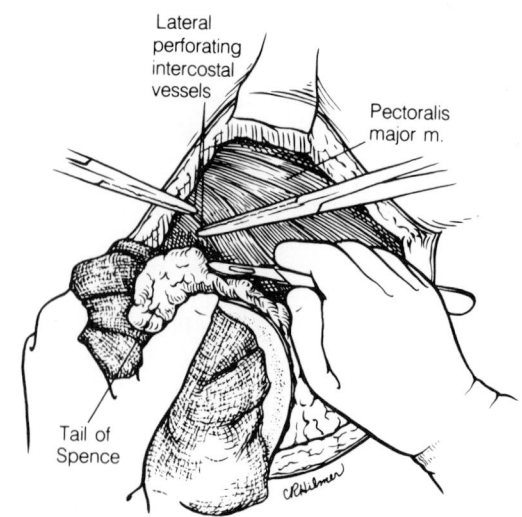

FIGURE 16–1. Holding tissue with a sponge during a mastectomy. (From Nora, P. F. [1991]. *Operative surgery: Principles and techniques* [3rd ed.] [p. 246]. Philadelphia: W. B. Saunders.)

moisture content with a wet towel or a large laparotomy sponge. Prevent inadvertent strangulation of the bowel by supporting the bag. A stack of towels placed between the assistant and the patient aids in this process.

Impervious Stockinet

When isolating an extremity, use an impervious stockinet. The stockinet enables the RNFA to hold, reposition, or provide traction on the extremity during the procedure.

Tapes and Other Devices

Use tapes, such as cotton cord ties, vessel loops, and Penrose drains to move or hold anatomical structures during surgery and better view the operative field. When using tapes, the surgeon exposes the tissue and then passes the tape around the tissue. After the tape is in place, the surgeon can gently move the structure from the operative field. Exercise care when moving or holding a structure with a tape. Too much traction may tear the tissue. Likewise, insufficient traction does not hold the structure steady and moves it from the operative field. A gentle, steady pull usually provides adequate traction. With experience, the RNFA learns to apply the correct amount of traction in varying situations. Figure 16–2 shows a Penrose drain placed around the spermatic cord.

Suture Stitch

The surgeon or RNFA may use a suture stitch to roll or hold tissue out of the way. After the surgeon places the stitch, the RNFA uses it to apply the necessary

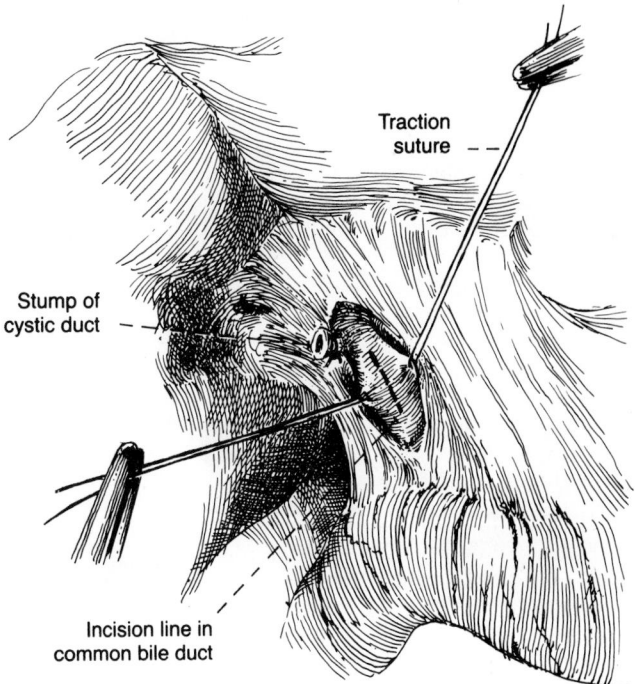

FIGURE 16–3. Traction sutures. (From Nora, P. F. [1991]. *Operative surgery: Principles and techniques* [3rd ed.] [p. 718]. Philadelphia: W. B. Saunders.)

traction. The surgeon may also attach the stitch to an instrument and use the weight of the instrument to apply the traction. The RNFA can also use this stitch to lift or hold tissue out of the operative field. Figure 16–3 shows two traction sutures placed in the common duct before incision.

Use of Retractors, Grasping Instruments, and Other Devices

All members of the surgical team use retractors, grasping instruments, and other devices to expose the operative field. Hand-held or self-retaining retractors move and hold tissue and organs out of the operative field. Other instruments such as clamps, stick sponges, and suction cannulas push tissue and organs away from or pull them toward the surgeon, thus providing exposure of the operative field.

Before using a retractor, or any other device, the RNFA must assess the operative site. A misplaced retractor can compress, tear, or stretch blood vessels, nerves, and organs. The wrong type of grasping instrument can puncture delicate tissue, thus causing intraoperative and postoperative complications. Intraoperative assessment factors include the size and depth of the operative site, the physiological status of the tissue, and the operative time. After placing retractors or using exposure devices, the RNFA must evaluate the tissue. If signs such as tissue blanching, cessation of pulse, or leaking of fluid appear, the RNFA should evaluate exposure methods. Excessive musculoskeletal pain, neu-

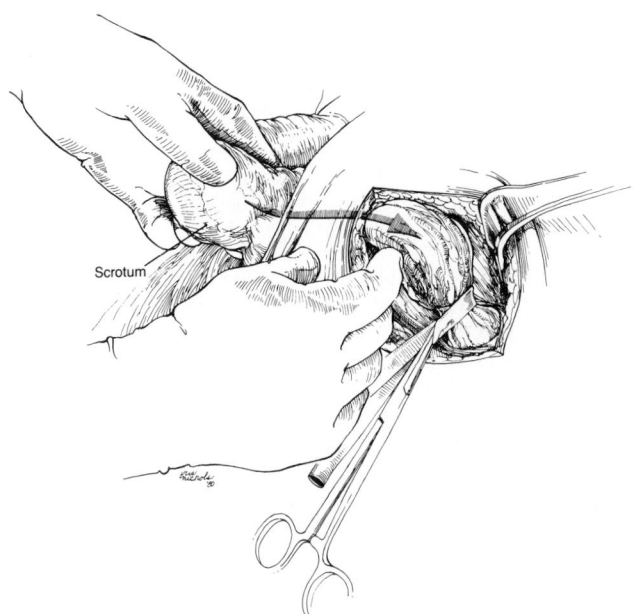

FIGURE 16–2. A Penrose drain is placed around the spermatic cord during radical inguinal orchiectomy. (From Gottesman, J. E. Radical inguinal orchiectomy. In Crawford, E. D., Bordon, T. A. [1982]. *Genitourinary cancer surgery*. Philadelphia: Lea & Febiger.)

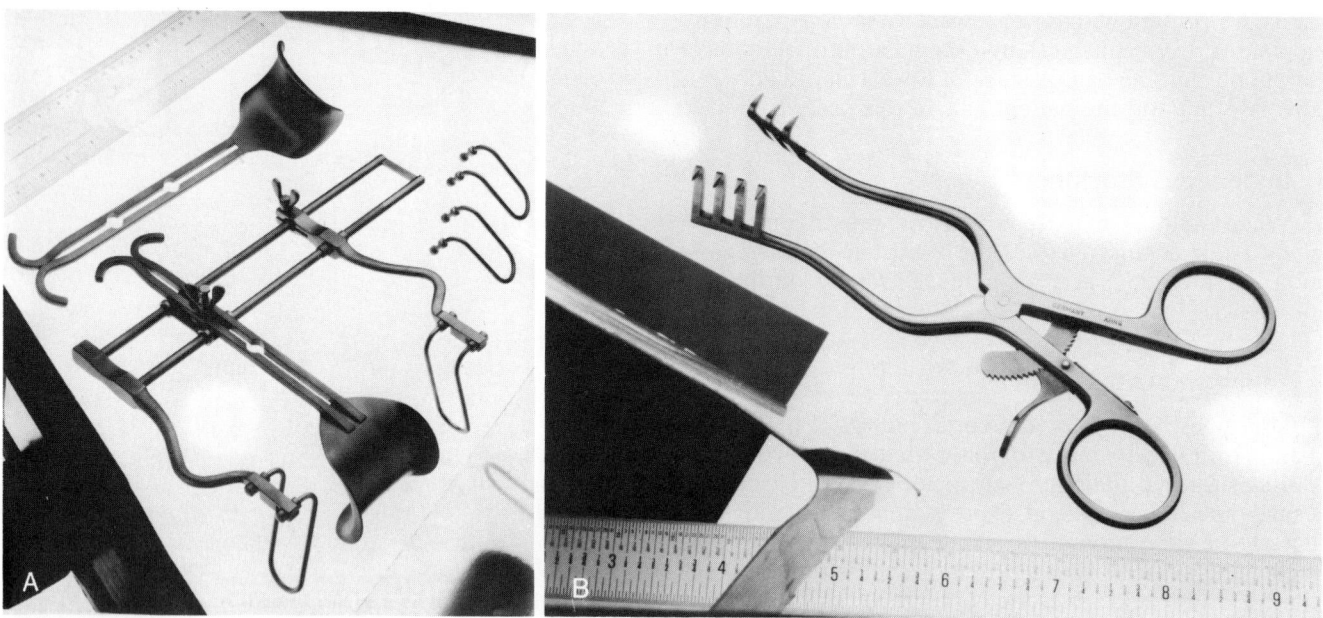

FIGURE 16–4. Self-retaining retractors. *A,* V. Mueller-Balfour abdominal retractor. *B,* Weitlaner retractor. (Courtesy of Baxter Healthcare Corporation, McGaw Park, IL.)

romuscular impairment, or unexplained fever after surgery should prompt the RNFA to determine whether exposure techniques were too aggressive or whether an organ was inadvertently punctured.

Self-retaining Retractors. Available in all sizes, shapes, and forms, self-retaining retractors isolate and hold all types of tissue, from the most superficial to the deepest. Figure 16–4*A* shows a V. Mueller-Balfour abdominal retractor. Figure 16–4*B* shows a Weitlaner retractor. Normally used on muscle, smooth self-retaining retractor blades prevent tearing. Blades with sharp or dull teeth hold fascia, subcutaneous tissue, and skin. Figure 16–5 shows the Gomez self-retaining retractor in place for abdominal aortic surgery.

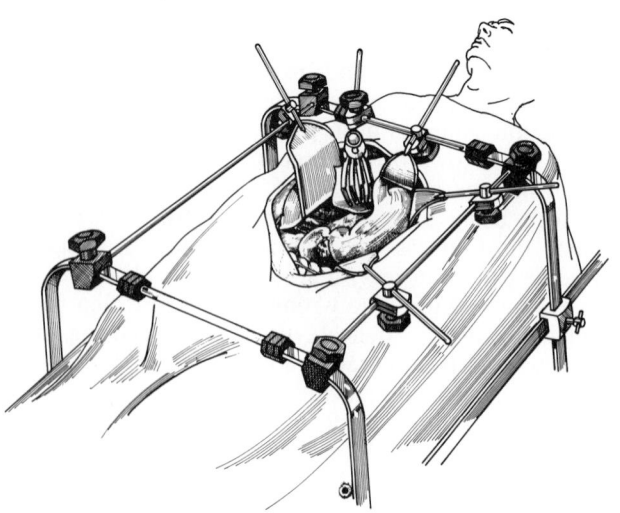

FIGURE 16–5. Gomez self-retaining retractor in place for abdominal aortic surgery.

Hand-held Retractors. Hand-held retractors, such as Lahey goiter, Green goiter, Senn, U.S. Army, Mayo-Davis, and Volkmann retractors, allow the assistant to fine tune exposure (Fig. 16–6). In Figure 16–7, three types of hand-held retractors are used during a portacaval shunt.

Stick and Peanut Sponges. Tissue can be pushed aside using stick sponges and peanut sponges (Kittner dissector sponges). Stick sponges are used on straight or curved Foerster sponge forceps (Fig. 16–8) and peanut sponges on a Rochester-Péan clamp. The peanut sponge is frequently used as a tissue dissector. Blunt dissection of the proximal duct from the hilus of the liver with a Kittner sponge is shown in Figure 16–9.

Suction Devices. Suction cannulas such as the Poole abdominal and Yankauer tonsil suction tubes may be used as exposure devices. When used in such a way, they clear fluids from the field as well as push tissue out of the way. Figure 16–10 shows blunt suction technique.

Hand. The hands enable the RNFA to provide exposure by manually cupping, compressing, and pulling tissue and organs out of the way or into the line of sight. Manual retraction reduces the risk of tearing or puncturing the tissue or organ because the RNFA controls the amount of pressure applied. Many times, hands provide better exposure than instruments. In Figure 16–11, the assistant uses two hands to retract the stomach and greater omentum, thus exposing the pancreas during gastrectomy.

Traction and Countertraction Techniques

When a surgeon requests exposure, the RNFA applies the principles of traction and countertraction. Counter-

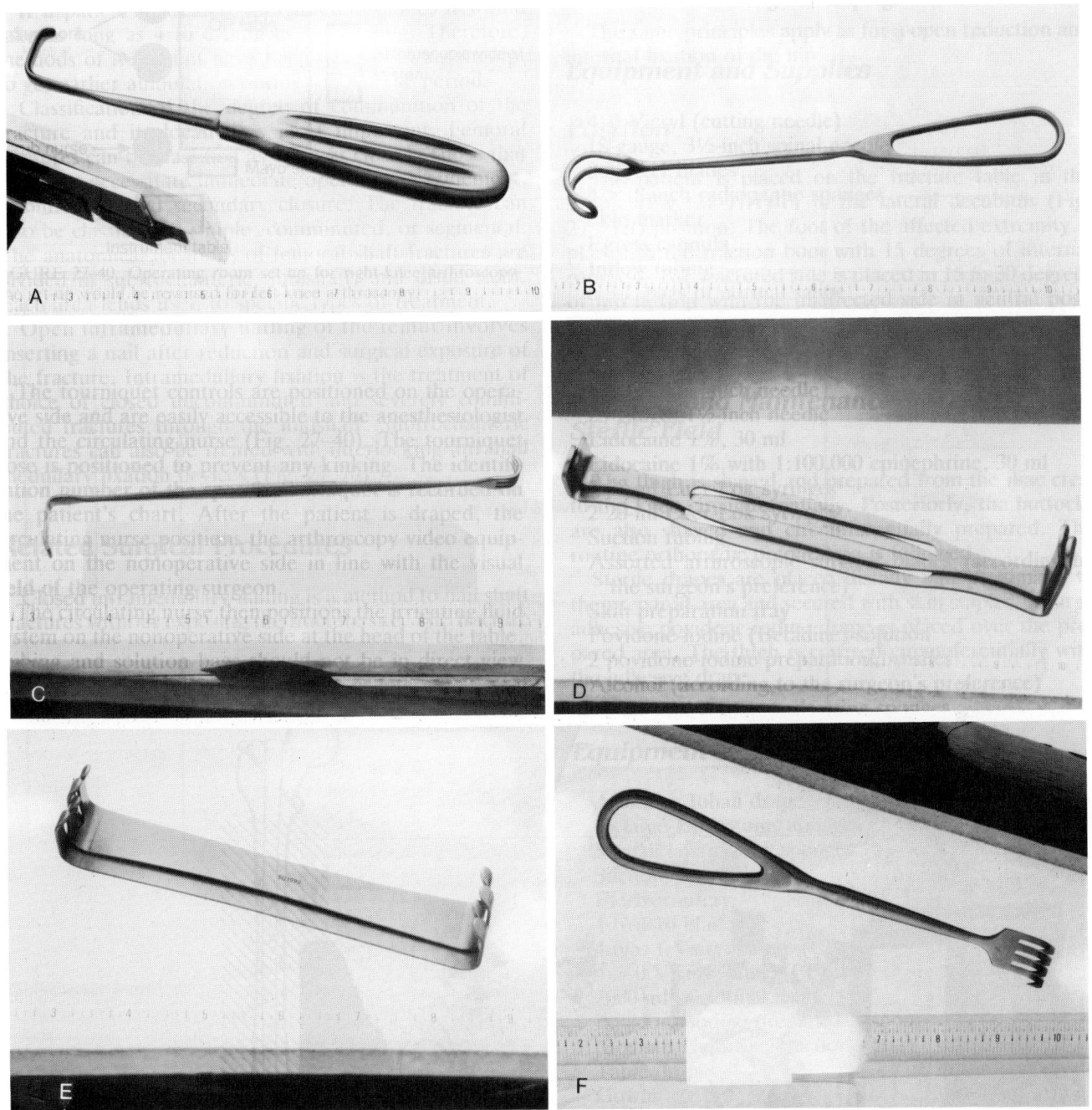

FIGURE 16–6. Hand-held retractors. *A*, Lahey goiter retractor. *B*, Green goiter retractor. *C*, Senn retractor. *D*, U.S. Army retractor. *E*, Mayo-Davis retractor. *F*, Volkmann retractor. (Courtesy of Baxter Healthcare Corporation, McGaw Park, IL.)

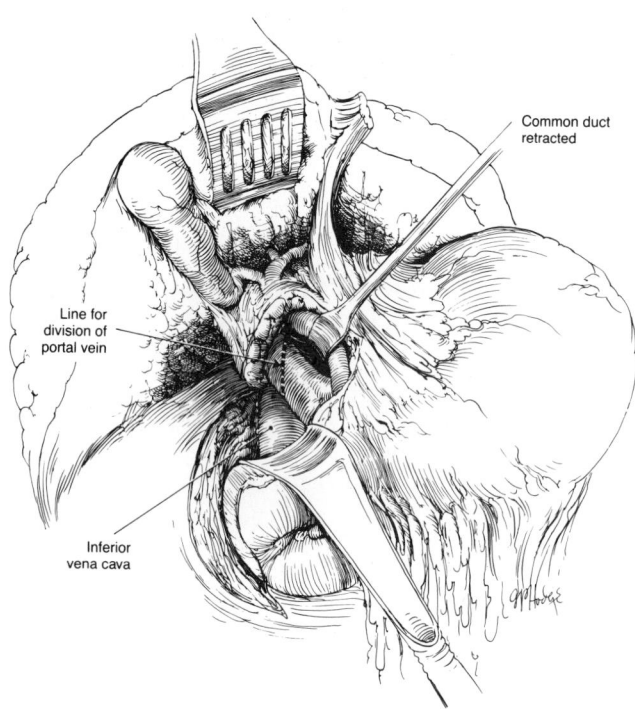

Common duct
retracted

Line for
division of
portal vein

Inferior
vena cava

FIGURE 16–7. Hand-held retractors in use during a portacaval shunt. (From Nora, P. F. [1991]. *Operative surgery: Principles and techniques* [3rd ed.] [p. 812]. Philadelphia: W. B. Saunders.)

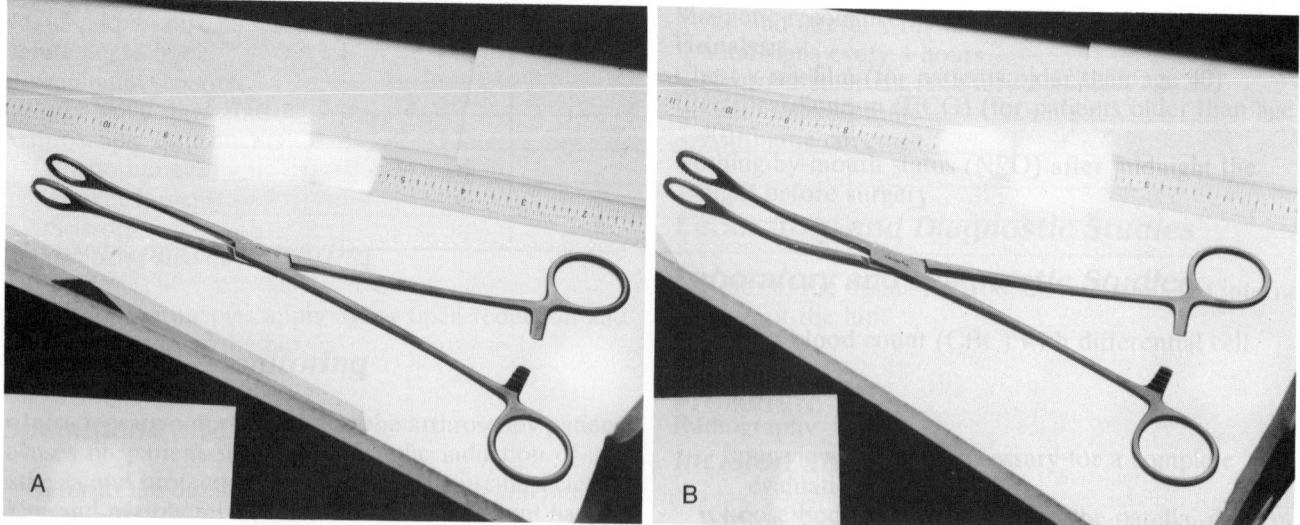

FIGURE 16–8. Sponge forceps. *A,* Straight Foerster sponge forceps. *B,* Curved Foerster sponge forceps. (Courtesy of Baxter Healthcare Corporation, McGaw Park, IL.)

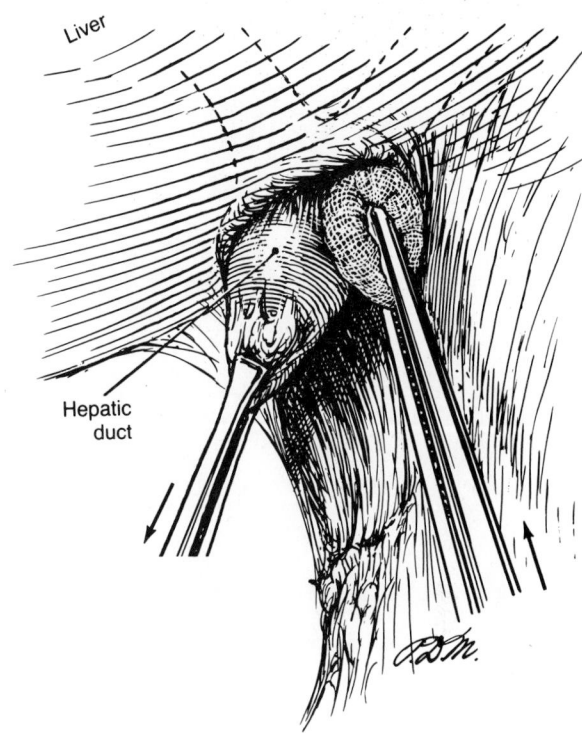

FIGURE 16–9. Blunt dissection with a Kittner sponge. (From Nora, P. F. [1991]. *Operative Surgery: Principles and techniques* [3rd ed.] [p. 732]. Philadelphia: W. B. Saunders.)

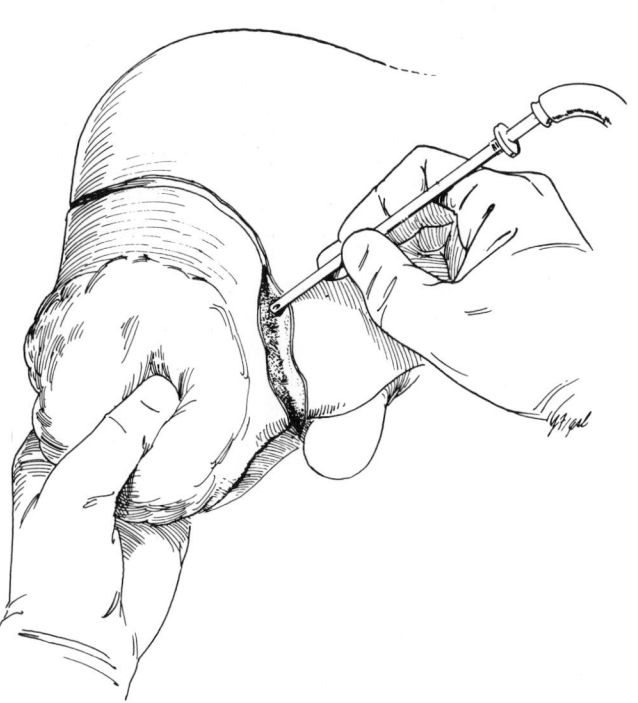

FIGURE 16–10. Blunt suction technique during liver resection. (From Foster, J. H. and Bermam, M. H. [1977]. *Solid liver tumors*. Philadelphia: W. B. Saunders.)

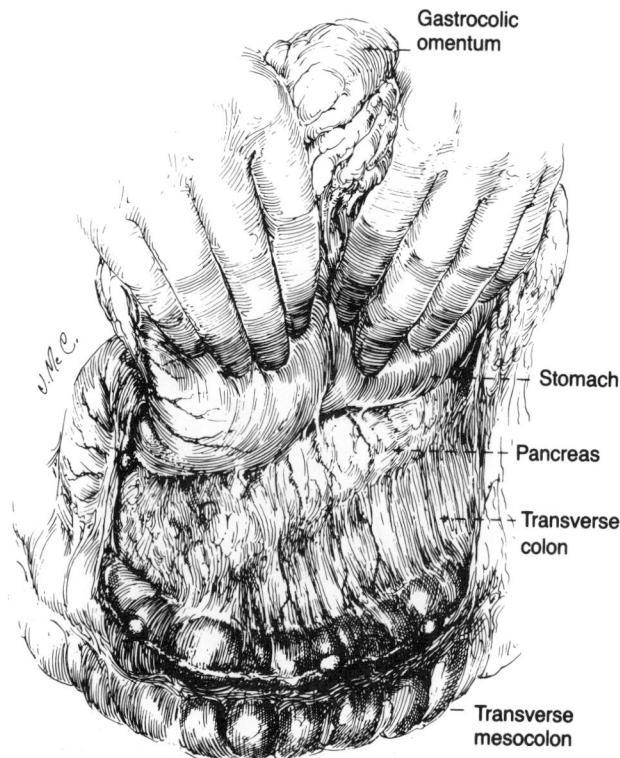

FIGURE 16–11. Using the hands to expose tissue during exploratory laparotomy. (From Nora, P. F. [1991]. *Operative surgery: Principles and techniques* [3rd ed.] [p. 548]. Philadelphia: W. B. Saunders.)

traction creates a plane of dissection that opens the connective tissue and provides exposure. It also gives the surgeon the necessary resistance during dissection of the organ or structure.

Clamping Tissue

Clamps are used to hold tissue in place. They are available in many sizes and shapes to accommodate the purposes of use and varieties of tissue in the body. They can be small and delicate such as those used in eye surgery or large and heavy for use on bone. Clamps also vary in length and type of serration. Tips may be straight, curved, or angled, or they may have unusual configurations such as oval, triangular, or barrel shaped.

The most widely used instrument in surgery is the *hemostatic artery forceps*. Figure 16–12 shows examples of artery forceps. Also called a hemostat, this instrument is commonly used to grasp superficial vessels. When using a hemostat, the thumb and second long finger are placed inside the rings and the index finger is held against the hand for stabilization. The hemostat is applied so that the tip is as close as possible to the divided end of the vessel. The fingers are then removed from inside the rings and the thumb and middle finger grasp the closed ring. When this position is obtained, the assistant gently and slightly lifts and tilts the tip toward the surgeon. The index finger is then free to open the ratchet by applying pressure against the ring just as the

surgeon increases the tension on the first knot. The hemostat is carefully released and fully opened with a gradual, smooth motion. In Figure 16–13, the cystic duct is doubly clamped with a Mixter forceps.

Vascular clamps provide hemostasis or partial occlusion until the vessel can be sutured. These, too, are available in many sizes and shapes. Some jaws have many rows of fine teeth; others are designed to receive cushioned insets. After it is placed, the clamp is held gently by the shank to avoid twisting or pulling. As with any hemostat, it is important to open the clamp widely before removing it to prevent drag on or accidental tears of the vessel. Vascular clamps are shown occluding the vena cava and portal vein in Figure 16–14. Bulldog clamps occlude the popliteal, anterior tibial, posterior tibial, and peroneal arteries during popliteal artery thromboembolectomy (Fig. 16–15).

Noncrushing clamps are used in general surgery for intestinal operations. Figure 16–16 shows examples. During transection of the small bowel, shodded intestinal clamps are placed on a segment of the bowel to prevent spillage of enteric contents during the procedure (Fig. 16–17). Clamps are designed to be used on every organ of the body. Examples of commonly used clamps designed for specific tissue are Heaney uterine clamp (hysterectomy forceps), Herrick kidney pedicle clamp, Best common duct stone forceps, and Judd-DeMartel gallbladder forceps (Fig. 16–18).

Grasping Tissue

When possible, the lifting of tissue should be done with the gentlest of all instruments—the fingers. Because good exposure is necessary and tissue is slippery, however, forceps are used as an extension of the surgeon's or assistant's fingers. The forceps are grasped like a pencil and squeezed together by applying pressure with the thumb and index finger.

Forceps should have light springs so that the surgeon or the assistant may apply the least possible pressure to hold the tissue. Crushed tissue can result if the grip is too tight. Forceps should be checked before surgery to see that they close precisely. Many varieties are available: smooth-jawed or single or multiple-toothed and fine or bulky forceps. Most forceps are straight. The bayonet forceps, often used in small deep areas, is shaped so that the fingers do not block visibility.

Smooth-jawed forceps are applied to tissue that would likely bleed or easily perforate, such as bowel and liver. Toothed forceps are used on skin, dense tissue, or scar tissue. Forceps are used throughout the surgery to lift tissue and provide countertraction and stabilization. When selecting forceps, the RNFA considers tissue sensitivity and its susceptibility to crushing. Figure 16–19 shows examples of Cushing and Brophy dressing forceps and Cushing, Adson, and Singley tissue forceps. In Figure 16–20, smooth tissue forceps and scissors are used to open the peritoneum. Figures 16–21 and 16–22 show examples of other types of instruments used to grasp and hold tissue. Lahey forceps are used to grasp the thyroid gland during thyroidectomy (Fig. 16–23).

Text continued on page 361

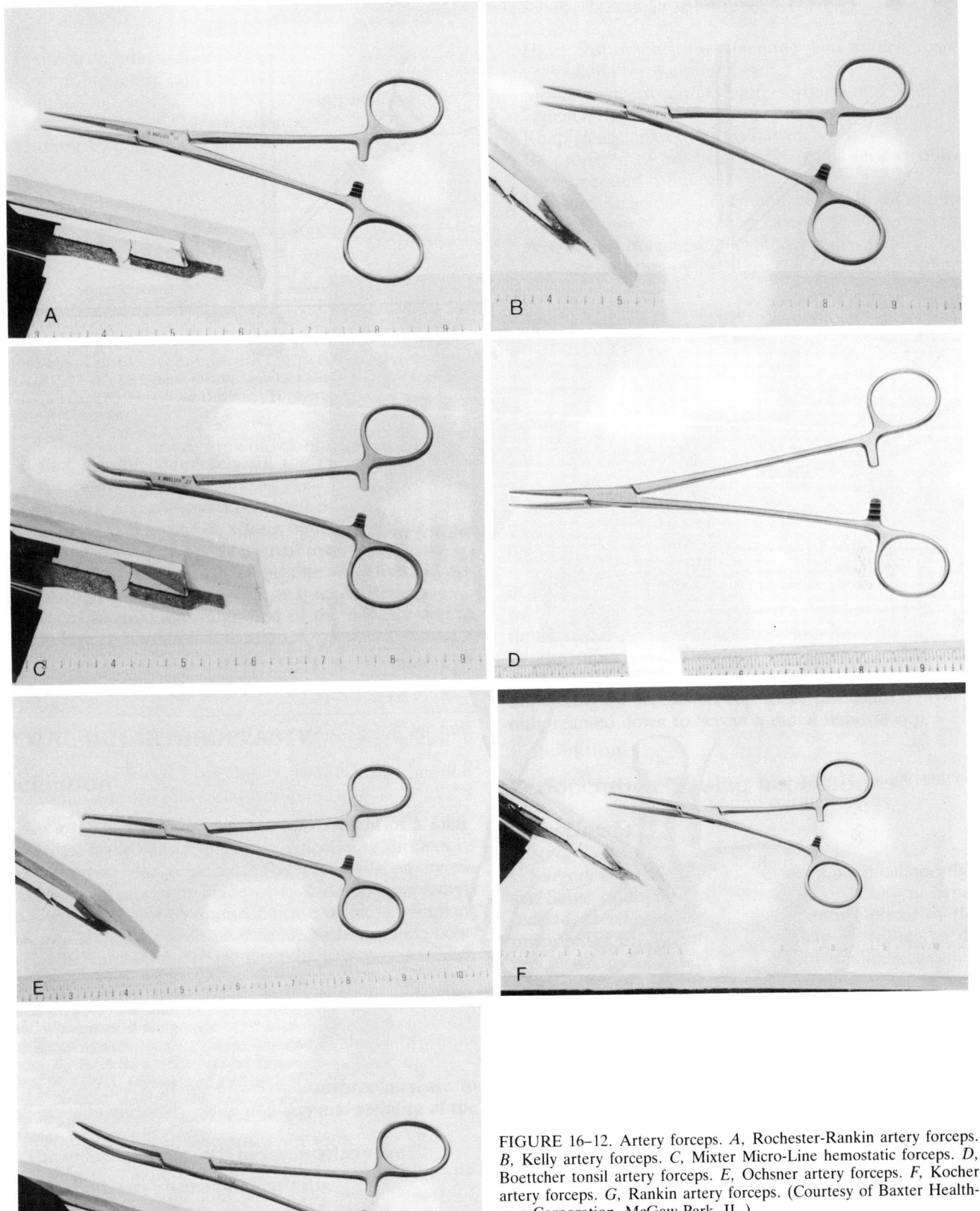

FIGURE 16–12. Artery forceps. *A*, Rochester-Rankin artery forceps. *B*, Kelly artery forceps. *C*, Mixter Micro-Line hemostatic forceps. *D*, Boettcher tonsil artery forceps. *E*, Ochsner artery forceps. *F*, Kocher artery forceps. *G*, Rankin artery forceps. (Courtesy of Baxter Health-care Corporation, McGaw Park, IL.)

353

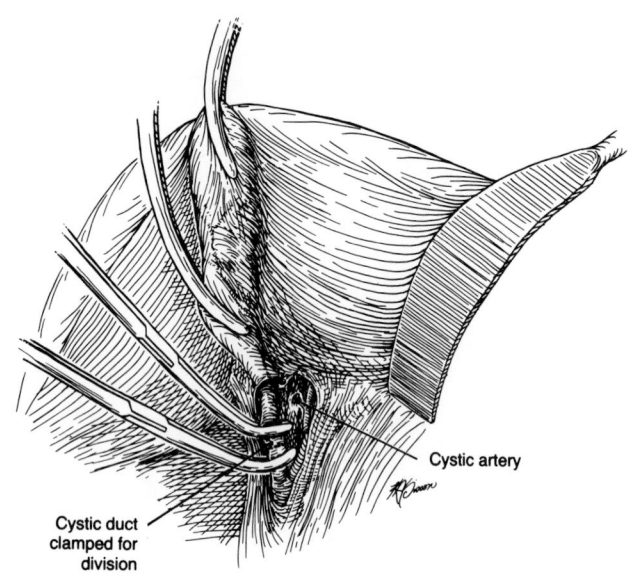

Cystic artery

Cystic duct
clamped for
division

FIGURE 16–13. Clamping the cystic duct during cholecystectomy. (From Nora, P. F. [1991]. *Operative surgery: Principles and techniques* [3rd ed.]. [p. 713]. Philadelphia: W. B. Saunders.)

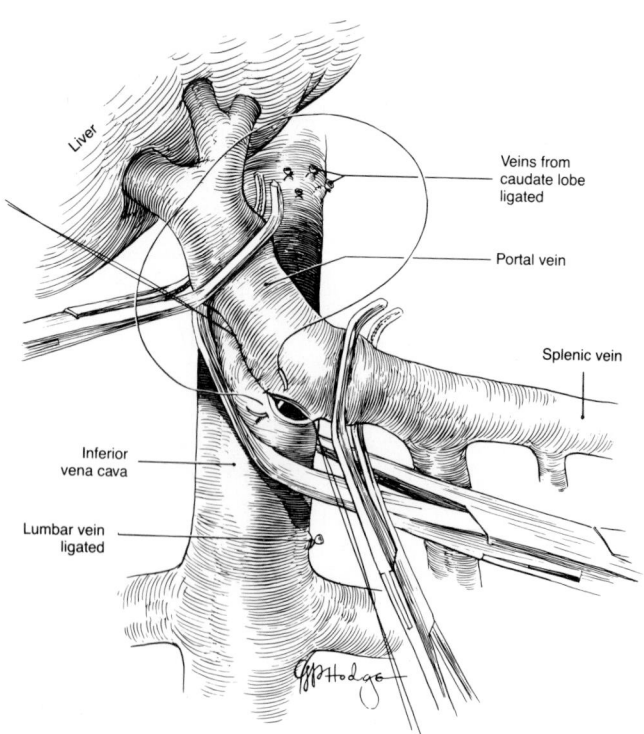

Liver

Veins from
caudate lobe
ligated

Portal vein

Splenic vein

Inferior
vena cava

Lumbar vein
ligated

FIGURE 16–14. Vascular clamps are used to occlude the inferior vena cava and portal vein during side-to-side portacaval anastomosis. (From Nora, P. F. [1991]. *Operative surgery: Principles and techniques* [3rd ed.]. [p. 814]. Philadelphia: W. B. Saunders.)

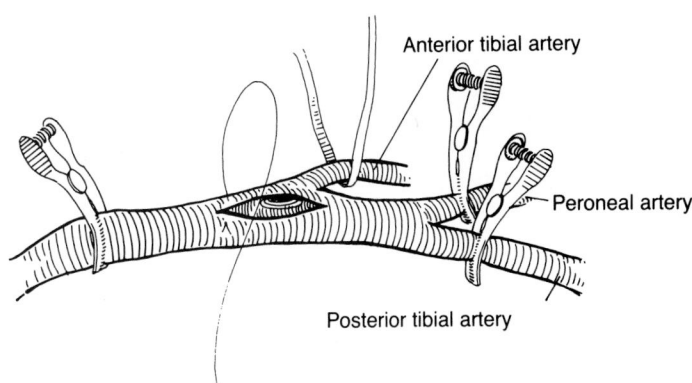

FIGURE 16–15. Bulldog clamps are used during popliteal artery thromboembolectomy. (From Nora, P. F. [1991]. *Operative surgery: Principles and techniques* [3rd ed.] [p. 976]. Philadelphia: W. B. Saunders.)

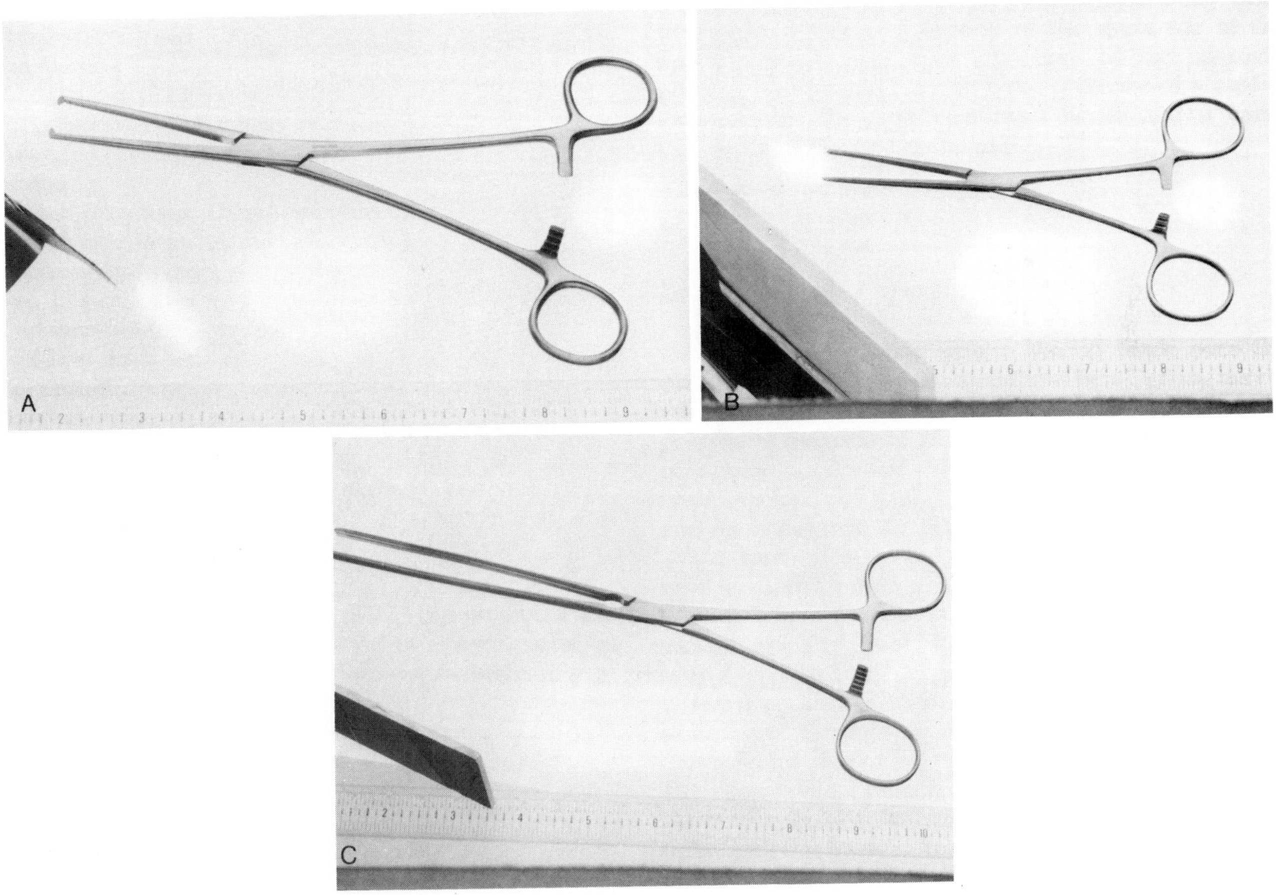

FIGURE 16–16. Intestinal clamps and forceps. *A,* Allen intestinal clamp. *B,* Bainbridge intestinal forceps. *C,* Kocher intestinal forceps.

Illustration continued on following page

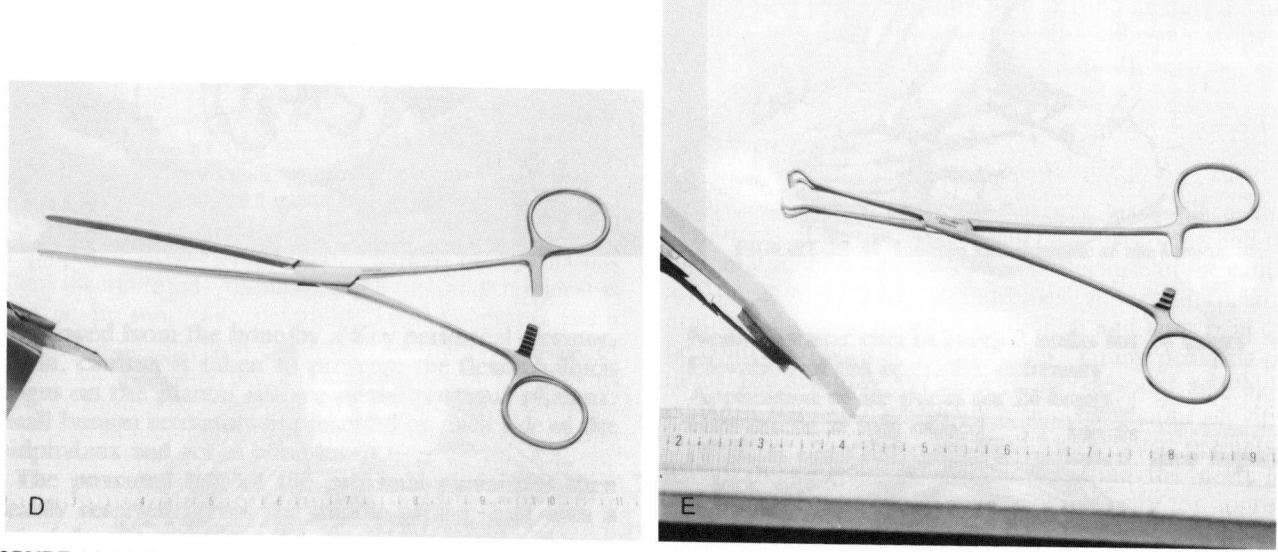

FIGURE 16–16 *Continued D*, Doyen intestinal forceps. *E*, Babcock tissue forceps. (Courtesy of Baxter Healthcare Corporation, McGaw Park, IL.)

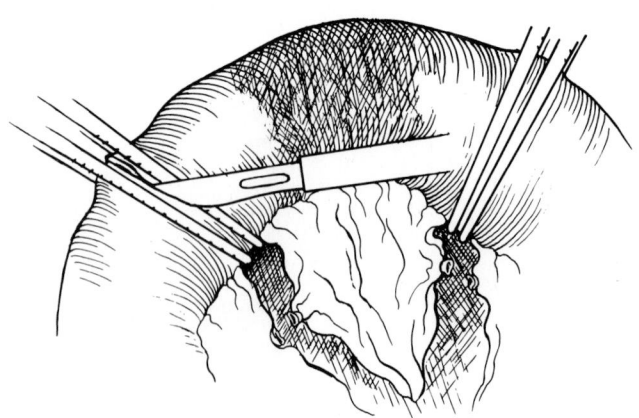

FIGURE 16–17. Intestinal clamps placed for transection of the small bowel. (From Nora, P. F. [1991]. *Operative surgery: Principles and techniques* [3rd ed.] [p. 587]. Philadelphia: W. B. Saunders.)

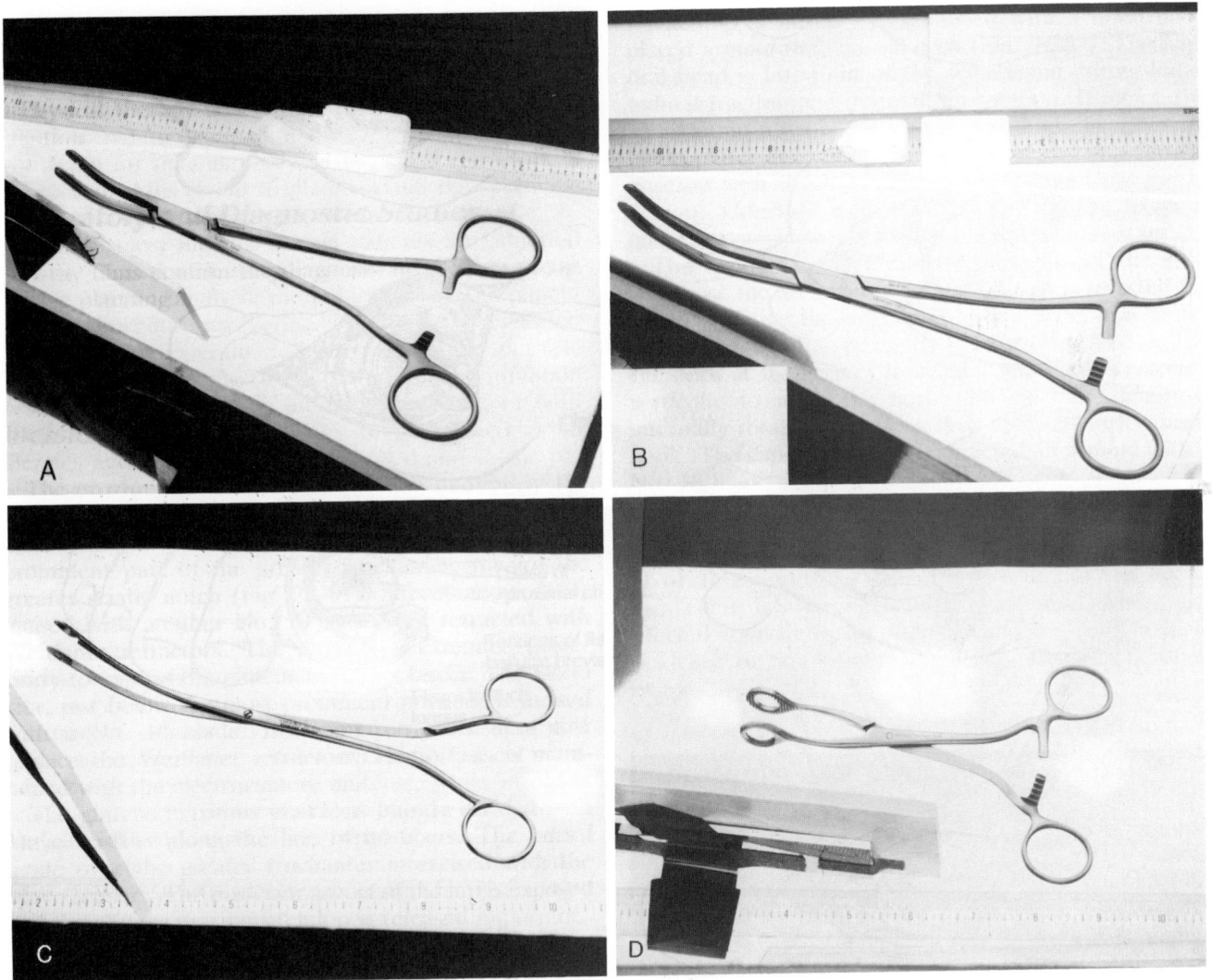

FIGURE 16–18. Specific body organ clamps. *A,* Heaney hysterectomy forceps. *B,* Herrick kidney pedicle clamp. *C,* Best common duct stone forceps. *D,* Judd-DeMartel gallbladder forceps. (Courtesy of Baxter Healthcare Corporation, McGaw Park, IL.)

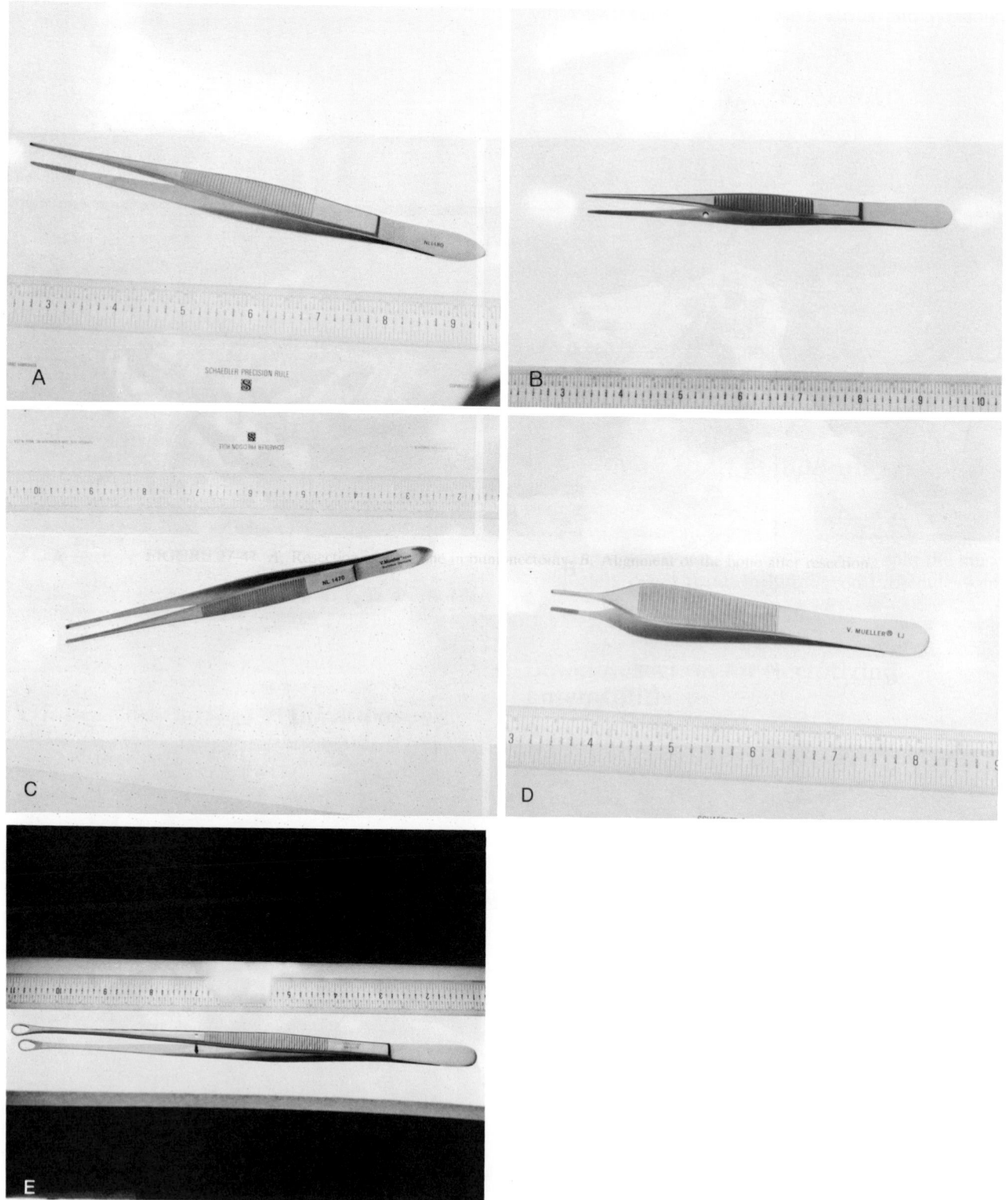

FIGURE 16–19. Dressing and tissue forceps. *A*, Cushing dressing forceps. *B*, Brophy dressing forceps. *C*, Cushing tissue forceps. *D*, Adson tissue forceps. *E*, Singley tissue forceps. (Courtesy of Baxter Healthcare Corporation, McGaw Park, IL.)

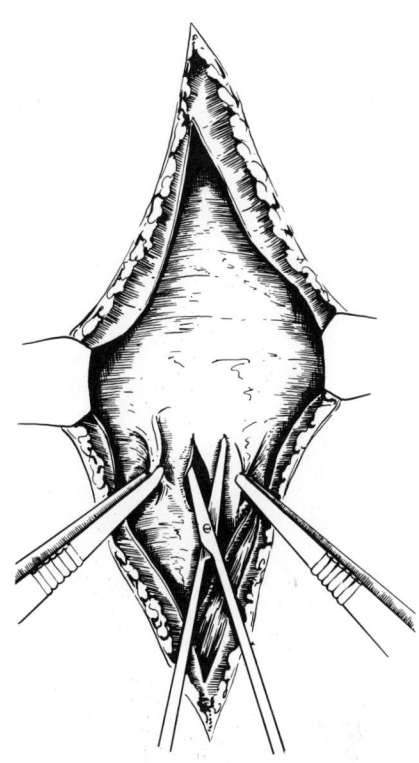

FIGURE 16–20. Smooth tissue forceps and scissors are used to open the peritoneum. (From Nora, P. F. [1991]. *Operative surgery: Principles and techniques* [3rd ed.] [p. 447]. Philadelphia: W. B. Saunders.)

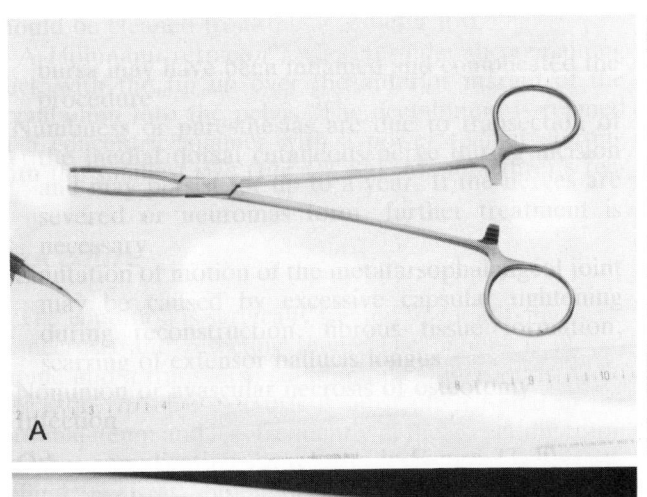

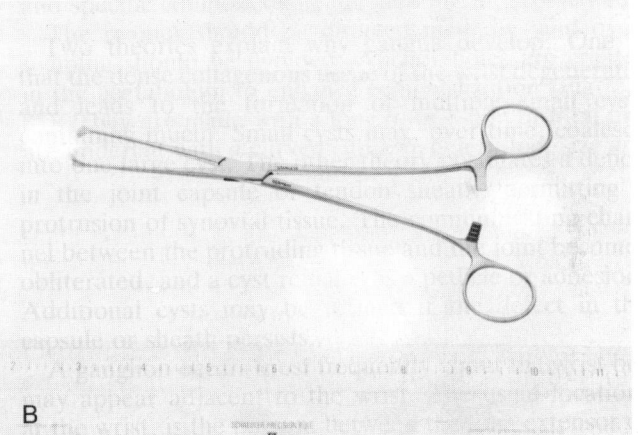

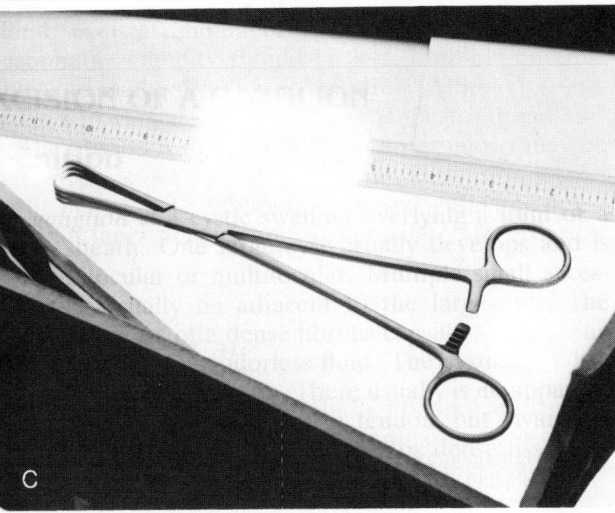

FIGURE 16–21. Tissue forceps. *A,* Judd-Allis tissue forceps. *B,* Allis tissue forceps. *C,* Gordon uterine vulsellum forceps. (Courtesy of Baxter Healthcare Corporation, McGaw Park, IL.)

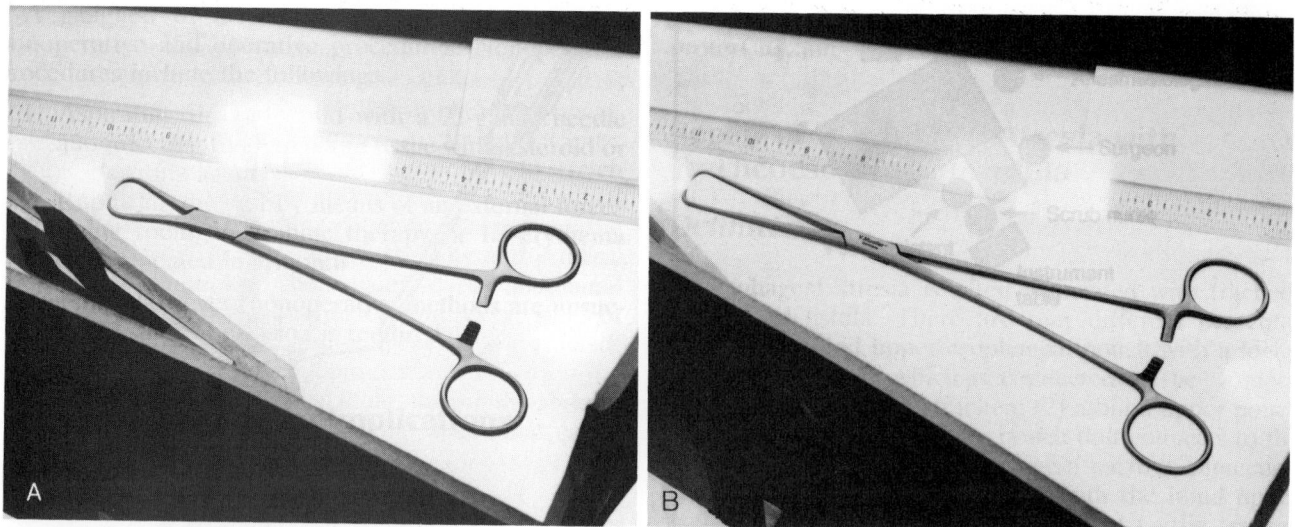

FIGURE 16–22. Tenaculum forceps. *A,* Adair uterine tenaculum forceps. *B,* Braun uterine tenaculum forceps. (Courtesy of Baxter Healthcare Corporation, McGaw Park, IL.)

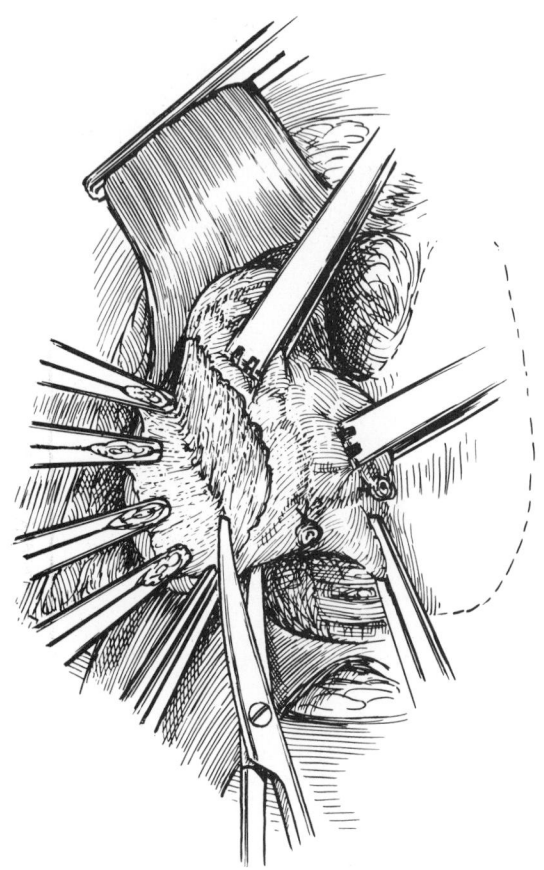

FIGURE 16–23. Lahey forceps are used to grasp the thyroid gland during thyroidectomy. (From Nora, P. F. [1991]. *Operative surgery: principles and techniques* [3rd ed.] [p. 198]. Philadelphia: W. B. Saunders.)

Suturing

Injured body tissues, whether from trauma or surgery, respond immediately and begin to heal. The healing process is facilitated if the surgical team controls infection by (1) maintaining sterile and aseptic technique and (2) properly ligating and approximating tissues with sutures to control bleeding, bring tissues together, and hold them in place while healing. Table 16–2 lists principles that the surgeon and the RNFA should keep in mind to ensure optimal wound healing.

Wound Healing

Wound healing occurs by first, second, or third intention (Fig. 16–24). The RNFA must understand these processes because each has useful applications when closing surgical incisions or traumatic wounds.

First-Intention Wound Healing. First-intention healing occurs by primary union of the incised tissues. Most surgical patients heal by first intention if

- tissue damage was minimal during the operation
- aseptic conditions were maintained
- tissue was gently handled
- dead space was eliminated

- hemostasis was achieved
- tissues were accurately approximated

Second-Intention Wound Healing. Postoperative complications such as wound dehiscence, infection, excessive drainage, and excessive scar formation impede healing by first intention. Infection, trauma resulting in excessive tissue destruction or loss, and poor approximation of tissues set the stage for healing by second-intention.

When a wound heals by second intention, rather than primary union with sutures, the wound is often left open and allowed to heal from the bottom up. This is called *contraction*. During this process, granulation tissue forms in the wound defect. As the defect fills with granulation tissue, contraction begins with the secondary growth of epithelium and the wound begins to close. Because this type of healing takes longer than first-intention healing, excessive scar tissue forms. The possibility of postoperative incisional herniation is also greater because of poor wound union.

Third-Intention Wound Healing. When the wound heals by third intention, two surfaces of granulation tissue join. A deeper and wider scar usually forms. The surgeon relies on third-intention healing in an area of gross infection, after extensive tissue loss from injury, or after aggressive débridement of infected or damaged

---

TABLE 16–2. PRINCIPLES OF SURGICAL TECHNIQUE

Plan the incision.	Planning and designing the location, length, and depth of the incision achieves optimal exposure. Making the incision just long enough affords sufficient operating space while reducing the amount of tissue trauma. The direction of the incision may be a factor in wound healing. Wounds heal side to side, not end to end.
Make the skin incision with one stroke of evenly applied pressure on the scalpel.	Making the skin incision with one stroke of evenly applied pressure on the scalpel aids in tissue approximation during wound closure. Sharp dissection cuts through other tissues. While cutting, watch for underlying nerves, blood vessels, and muscles to preserve as many as possible.
Handle tissue carefully and as little as possible.	Carefully placed and handled retractors prevent undue pressure on tissues. Excessive pressure and tension on tissues impairs circulation of blood, slows lymph flow, alters the local physiological state of the wound, and predisposes to microbial colonization. Reducing tissue trauma to a minimum aids the healing mechanisms of the body.
Provide hemostasis.	Hemostasis not only prevents loss of the patient's blood, but also provides a field as bloodless as possible for accurate dissection. Bleeding may occur from transected or penetrated vessels or a diffuse oozing from large denuded surfaces. Mass ligation of large areas of tissue may produce necrosis and prolong healing time. Complete hemostasis before closing the wound reduces the chance of hematoma formation. A hematoma or seroma in the incision prevents the direct apposition essential to the union of wound surfaces. These can act as a culture medium for microbial growth, leading to wound infection.
Preserve blood supply.	Preservation of the blood supply to the wound promotes optimal healing.
Débride necrotic and devitalized tissue.	Adequate débridement of all necrotic and devitalized tissue and removal of inflicted foreign bodies promote healing, especially of traumatic wounds. Foreign bodies, such as dirt, metal, and glass, increase the probability of wound infection.
Keep tissues moist.	Periodic irrigation of the wound with warm normal saline solution or covering exposed surfaces with saline-moistened sponges or laparotomy tapes prevents drying of tissues during long procedures.
Carefully and accurately approximate tissues.	Approximation of tissues as nontraumatically as possible and with precision eliminates dead space and minimizes the potential for wound disruption. Evaluation of each patient and selection of the proper wound closure materials for the particular surgical circumstance provides maximal opportunity for healing. Accurate approximation of tissue without tension or strangulation promotes healing.
Immobilize the wound.	Adequate immobilization of the approximated wound, but not necessarily the entire anatomical part, promotes efficient healing and minimal scar formation.

Adapted from *Ethicon wound closure manual* (1988). (p. 5). Somerville, NJ: Ethicon, Inc.

HEALING BY FIRST INTENTION

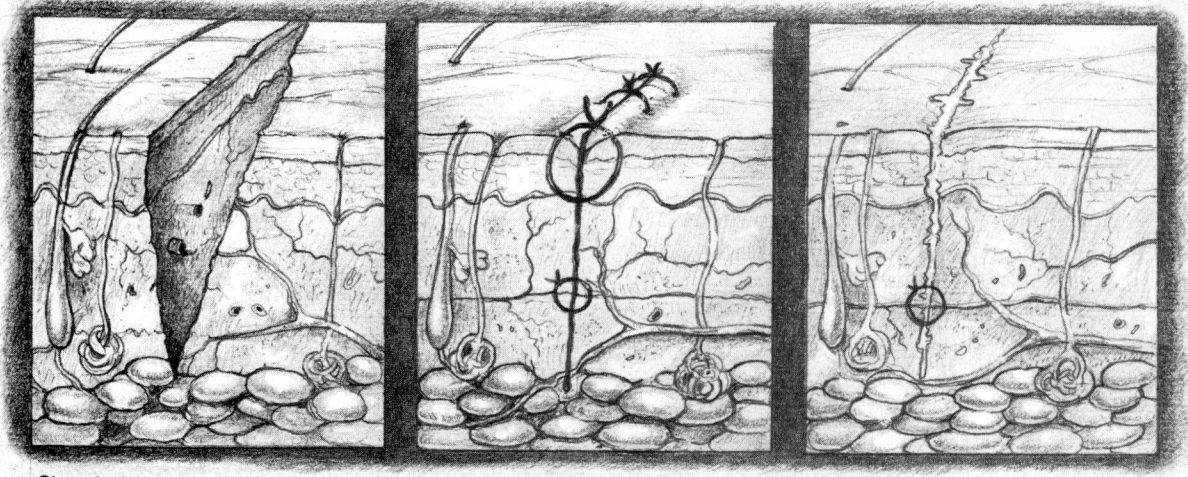

Clean incision   Early suture   "Hairline" scar

An aseptically made wound with minimal tissue destruction and minimal tissue reaction begins to heal as the edges are approximated by close sutures or staples. No open areas or dead spaces are left to serve as potential sites of infection.

HEALING BY SECOND INTENTION (GRANULATION)

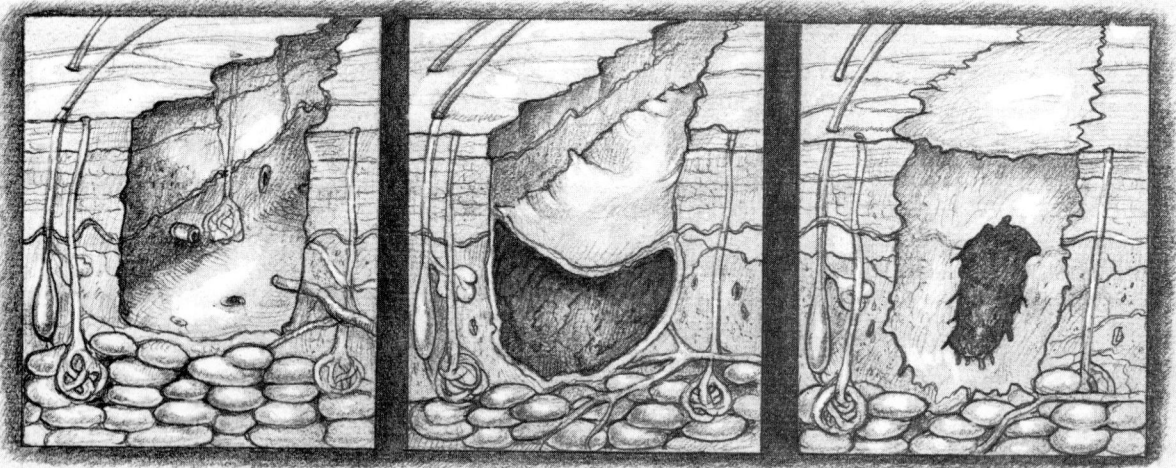

Gaping, irregular wound   Granulation   Growth of epithelium over scar

An infected wound or one with tissue damage so extensive that the edges cannot be smoothly approximated is usually left open and allowed to heal from the inside out. The nurse periodically cleans and assesses the infected wound for healthy tissue production. Scar tissue is extensive, and healing is prolonged.

HEALING BY THIRD INTENTION (DELAYED CLOSURE)

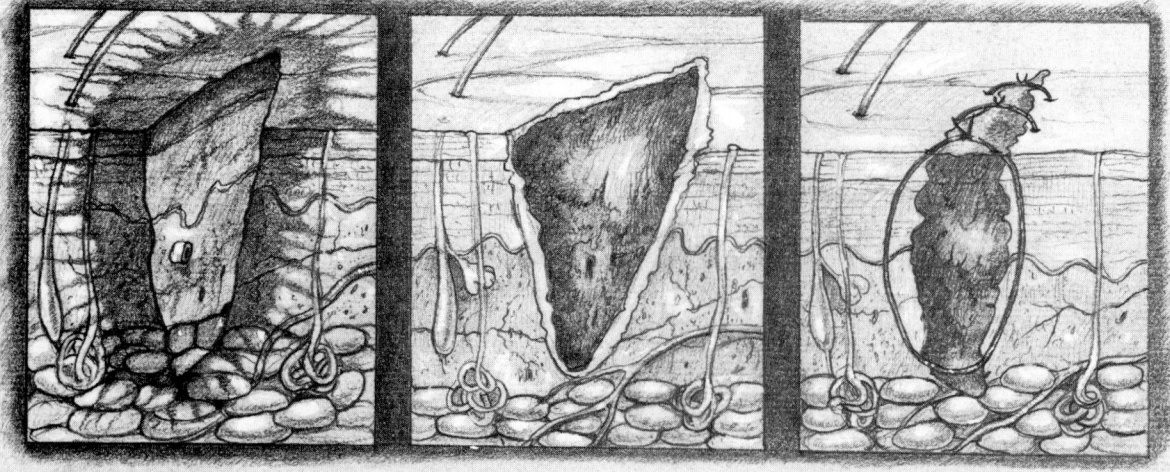

Infected wound   Granulation   Closure with wide scar

An infected wound may be left open until all evidence of infection has subsided. The wound is then closed surgically.

FIGURE 16–24. The three types of wound healing. (From Ignatavicius, D., Bayne, M. V. [1991]. *Medical-surgical nursing: A nursing process approach* [p. 479]. Philadelphia: W. B. Saunders.)

362

tissue (Atkinson and Kohn, 1986, p. 325). Third-intention healing is the slowest of all the healing processes.

Sutures

The surgeon and the RNFA have an extensive assortment of sutures at their disposal (Table 16–3). Sutures are either absorbable or nonabsorbable. However, both absorbable suture and nonabsorbable suture are foreign bodies. Another characteristic of suture is the filament. A monofilament suture consists of a single suture strand. Because of the single strand, it requires more knots to prevent slippage. Multifilament suture consists of strands of braided suture. It is easier to tie and the knotting is more secure. A disadvantage, however, is the possible harboring of bacteria in the braided structure of the suture strand (Nora, 1991, pp. 10–11).

The surgeon and RNFA choose suture materials based on the type of body tissues being sutured. To prevent suture breakage, the surgeon and RNFA consider the strength of the suture material. They must understand the nature of the suture material, the biological forces in the healing wound, and the interaction of the suture and the tissues. Table 16–4 should guide the surgeon and RNFA in suture selection (Ethicon, 1988, p. 37).

Needles

The surgeon and RNFA should carefully select suture needles. The use of inappropriate needles may prolong

TABLE 16–3. SUTURE MATERIALS

Suture	Filament	Absorption	Uses
Catgut 　Plain		5–70 d	Ligature 3–0 Ophthalmology
Chromic		20–90 d	Gastrointestinal anastomoses 3–0, 4–0 Fascia 0 Skin, oral mucosa, genitourinary tract Ophthalmology
Polyglactin 910 (Vicryl)	Braided	40–90 d	Ligature 3–0 Fascia 0 Subcutaneous tissue 3–0 Peritoneum 2–0 Urinary tract Microsurgery 8–0, 11–0 Ophthalmology
Polydioxanone	Monofilament	90–200 d	Abdominal and thoracic closure Subcuticular Colorectal Orthopedic
Silk	Braided	Nonabsorbable	Ligature 3–0 Gastrointestinal anastomoses 3–0 Skin 4–0 Blood vessel 5–0
Cotton	Twisted	Nonabsorbable	Fascia No. 30 Subcutaneous tissue No. 50 Skin No. 80
Wire	Monofilament	Nonabsorbable	Skin Nos. 34, 36 Fascia Nos. 30, 32 Retention No. 28 Tendons Neurosurgery Orthopedic
Nylon	Monofilament	Nonabsorbable	Skin 6–0, 5–0, 4–0 Fascia 0 Retention 0 Microsurgery 8–0, 11–0 Vascular
Polypropylene (Prolene)	Monofilament	Nonabsorbable	Skin 6–0, 5–0, 4–0 Fascia 0 Retention 0 Microsurgery 8–0, 11–0 Vascular 6–0 Tendons Ophthalmology
Polyester fiber 　Mersilene 　Ethibond	 Braided Braided	 Nonabsorbable Nonabsorbable	 Same as silk Same as silk

From Nora, P. F. (1991). *Operative surgery: Principles and techniques* (3rd ed.) (p. 11). Philadelphia: W. B. Saunders.

TABLE 16–4. PRINCIPLES OF SUTURE SELECTION

Principle	Rationale
When a wound has reached maximal strength, sutures are no longer needed.	Tissues that ordinarily heal slowly such as skin, fascia and tendons should usually be closed with nonabsorbable sutures. Tissues that heal rapidly such as stomach, colon and bladder may be closed with absorbable sutures.
Foreign bodies in potentially contaminated tissues may convert contamination to infection.	Avoid multifilament sutures which may convert a contaminated wound into an infected one. Use monofilament or absorbable sutures in potentially contaminated tissues.
Where cosmetic results are important, close and prolonged apposition of wounds and avoidance of irritants will produce the best result.	Use the smallest inert monofilament suture materials such as nylon or polypropylene. Avoid skin sutures and close subcuticularly whenever possible. Under certain circumstances, to secure close apposition of skin edges, skin closure tape may be used.
Foreign bodies in the presence of fluids containing high concentrations of crystalloids may act as nidus for precipitation and stone formation.	In the urinary and biliary tract, use *rapidly absorbed sutures.*
Selecting suture size.	Use the finest size, commensurate with the natural strength of the tissue. If the postoperative course of the patient may produce sudden strains on the suture line, reinforce it with retention sutures. Remove them as soon as the patient's condition is stabilized.

From *Ethicon wound closure manual* (1988). (pp. 37–38). Somerville, NJ: Ethicon, Inc.

the operation and damage the structural integrity of tissues and may lead to necrosis of the tissue, as well as the possibility of infection. In addition, approximation of the wound may fail if the wrong suture needle is used. Tables 16–5 and 16–6 show needle body shapes and points and their typical applications.

Closure Methods

Primary Closure

When doing a primary closure, the RNFA brings each layer of tissue into correct approximation. This means that like tissues are brought together: fascia to fascia, muscle to muscle, subcutaneous tissue to subcutaneous tissue, and skin edges to skin edges. Approximation of like tissues and elimination of all dead space allow each layer to heal properly. Figure 16–25 shows correct and incorrect appositions of tissues.

Pulling the tissues together with the correct amount of tension is crucial for a successful closure. If sutures

are too tight, the tissue blanches and then strangulates, causing it to die for lack of adequate blood supply. Likewise, if sutures slip or become loose, dead space may form and fluid may seep into the wound, thus causing poor wound healing (Fig. 16–26).

Common Techniques. A continuous suture, also called a running stitch, is used to close a tissue layer by passing one strand of suture back and forth between the two edges of the wound (Fig. 16–27). The surgeon ties the suture at the end of the suture line. A continuous suture line is strong because tension is evenly distributed along the full length of the wound. If, however, the suture breaks, the whole suture line is disrupted. In addition, a continuous suture uses less suture material, thus leaving less foreign body in the wound. For a continuous suture in the presence of infection, use a monofilament suture to avoid harboring microorganisms in the interstices of a multifilament suture (Ethicon Wound Closure Manual, 1988, p. 11).

An interrupted suture line is a series of singly placed stitches (Fig. 16–28). As each suture is placed, it is tied and cut. The technique is used more often, even though it takes more time, because the integrity of the suture line remains intact if a suture breaks. In addition, if infection is present, microorganisms are less likely to travel along the primary suture line of interrupted stitches (Ethicon, 1988, p. 11).

Figure 16–29 and Table 16–7 show the common suturing techniques and describe commonly used stitches.

Secondary Closure

The presence of an infection or gross contamination necessitates a secondary closure. This allows access to the contaminated tissue for cleaning and enables the tissue to recover from the infection before final closure. During the first stage of a secondary closure, the RNFA closes the deep tissue, such as the peritoneum and fascia, with a monofilament suture material. The next tissue layers remain open, which permits irrigation of the wound and instillation of antibiotics during dressing changes. Figure 16–30 shows secondary (delayed) closure of a traumatic wound. In this illustration, sutures of No. 30 wire are inserted to close the subcutaneous tissue and skin. Note that the sutures are not tied, rather they are held down with adhesive.

Some surgeons insert skin sutures during a secondary closure. This technique allows the incision edges to pull together, thus reducing the amount of tension placed on the incision. The amount of scar tissue that forms from this type of closure is also decreased. The RNFA places the skin sutures far apart to allow the proper healing process.

Retention Suture

In the presence of gross contamination, obesity, tissue loss, or excessive tissue damage, such as the type seen with massive trauma, the surgeon may use retention suture. Approximating the incision or damaged tissue

Text continued on page 369

TABLE 16–5. NEEDLE BODY SHAPES AND TYPICAL APPLICATIONS IN ANATOMIC SITES AND TISSUES

Shape	Typical Applications
Straight	Gastrointestinal tract, Nasal cavity, Nerve, Oral cavity, Pharynx, Skin, Tendon, Vessels
Half-curved	Skin, rarely used
1/4 circle	Eye, primary application, Microsurgical procedures
3/8 circle	Aponeurosis, Biliary tract, Dura, Eye, Fascia, Gastrointestinal tract, Muscle, Myocardium, Nerve, Perichondrium, Periosteum, Peritoneum, Pleura, Tendon, Urogenital tract, Vessels
1/2 circle	Biliary tract, Eye, Gastrointestinal tract, Muscle, Nasal cavity, Oral cavity, Pelvis, Peritoneum, Pharynx, Pleura, Respiratory tract, Skin, Subcutaneous fat, Urogenital tract
5/8 circle	Cardiovascular system, Nasal cavity, Oral cavity, Pelvis, Urogenital tract, primary application
Compound Curved	Eye, anterior segment

From *Ethicon wound closure manual* (1988). (p. 42). Somerville, NJ: Ethicon, Inc.

TABLE 16–6. NEEDLE POINTS AND BODY SHAPES WITH TYPICAL APPLICATIONS

Needle Point and Body Shape	Typical Application
Conventional Cutting	Ligament Nasal cavity Oral cavity Pharynx Skin Tendon
Reverse Cutting	Fascia Ligament Nasal cavity Oral mucosa Skin Tendon sheath
MICRO-POINT. Reverse Cutting Needle	Eye
Precision Point Cutting	Plastic or cosmetic procedures Skin
Side-cutting Spatulated	Eye, primary application Microsurgical procedures Reconstructive ophthalmic procedures
TAPERCUT. Surgical Needle	Bronchus Perichondrium Calcified tissue Periosteum Fascia Pharynx Ligament Tendon Nasal cavity Trachea Oral cavity Uterus Ovary Vessels, sclerotic
Taper	Aponeurosis Nerve Biliary tract Peritoneum Dura Pleura Fascia Subcutaneous fat Gastrointestinal tract Urogenital tract Muscle Vessels Myocardium
Blunt	Blunt dissection through friable tissue Kidney Liver Spleen Uterine cervix for ligating incompetent cervix

From *Ethicon wound closure manual* (1988). (p. 73). Somerville, NJ: Ethicon, Inc.

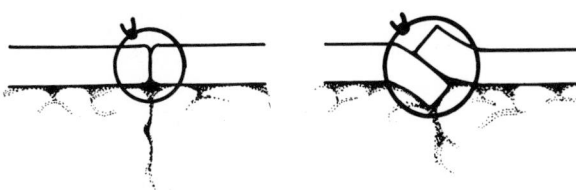

FIGURE 16–25. Correct (*left*) and incorrect (*right*) approximation of tissues. (Redrawn from Nealon, T. F. [1971]. *Fundamental skills in surgery*. Philadelphia: W. B. Saunders.)

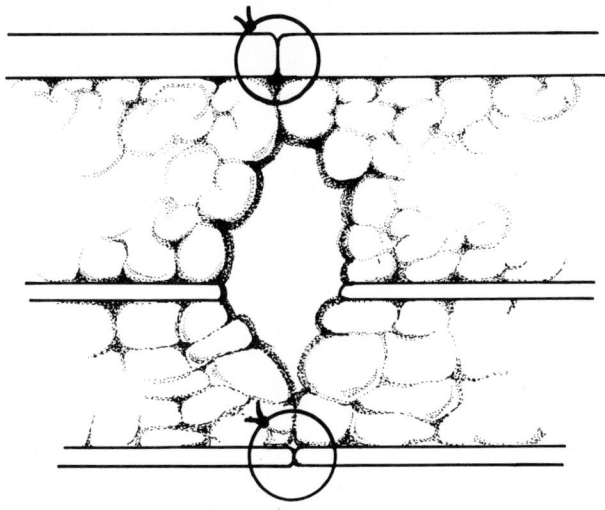

FIGURE 16–26. Dead space in a wound. (Redrawn from Nealon, T. F. [1971]. *Fundamental skills in surgery*. Philadelphia: W. B. Saunders.)

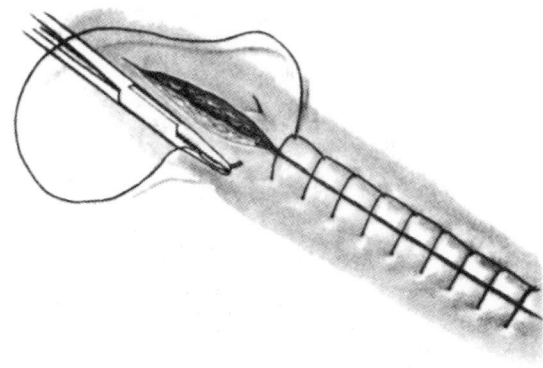

FIGURE 16–27. Continuous suture. (From *Ethicon wound closure manual* [1988]. Somerville, NJ: Ethicon, Inc.)

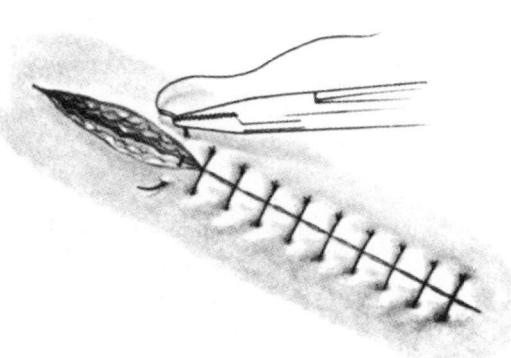

FIGURE 16–28. Interrupted sutures. (From *Ethicon wound closure manual*. [1988]. Somerville, NJ: Ethicon, Inc.)

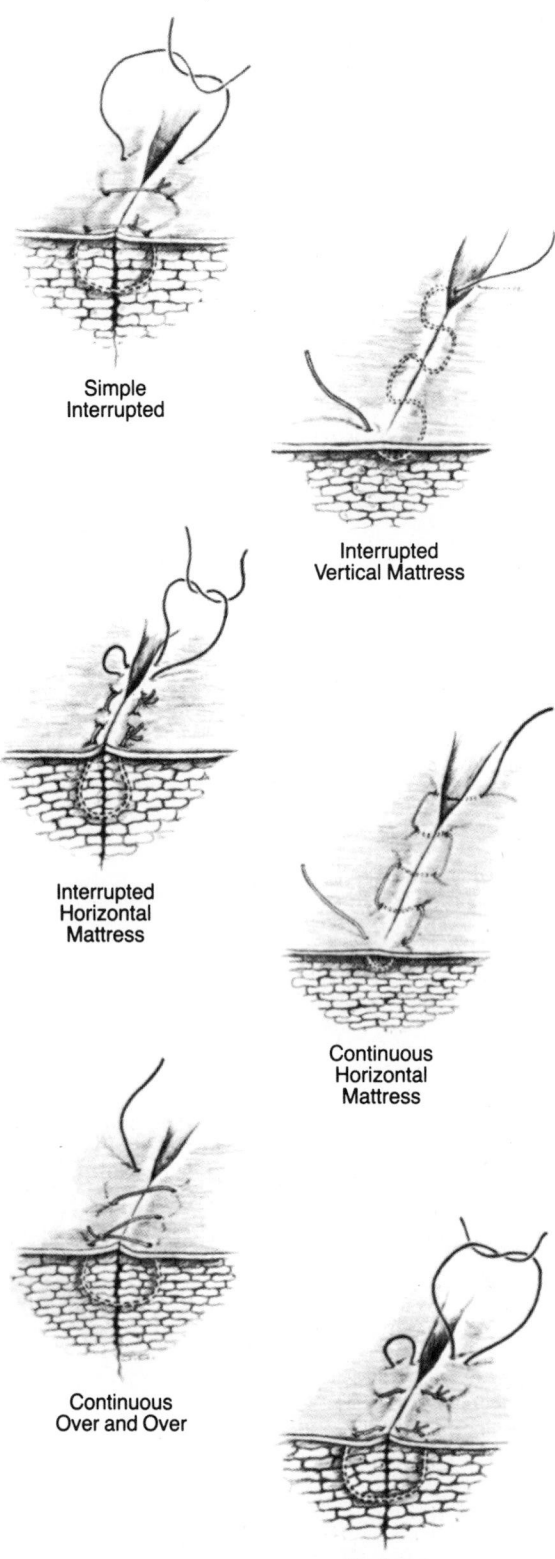

Simple
Interrupted

Interrupted
Vertical Mattress

Interrupted
Horizontal
Mattress

Continuous
Horizontal
Mattress

Continuous
Over and Over

Continuous
Subcuticular

FIGURE 16–29. Common suturing techniques. (From *Ethicon wound closure manual*. [1988]. Somerville, NJ: Ethicon, Inc.)

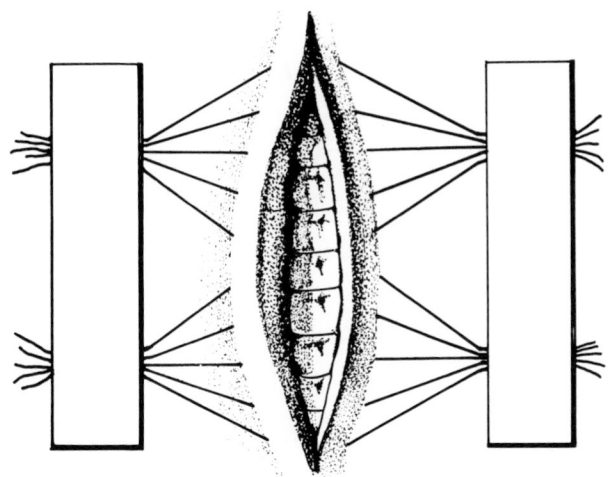

FIGURE 16–30. Delayed closure of a traumatic wound (see text). (From Nealon, T. F. [1991]. *Fundamental skills in surgery*. Philadelphia: W. B. Saunders.)

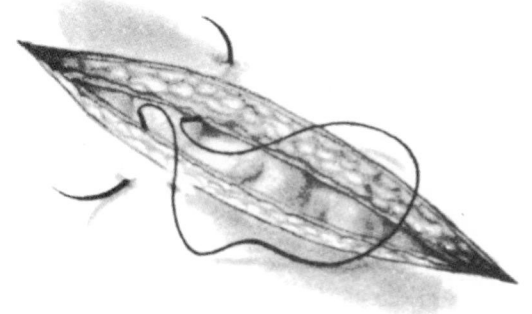

FIGURE 16–31. Through-and-through retention sutures. (From *Ethicon wound closure manual* [1988]. Somerville, NJ: Ethicon, Inc.)

with a large through-and-through nonabsorbable suture material reduces tension and holds incision edges together until healing is complete.

The surgeon places retention sutures about 2 inches away from each edge of the wound. When placing the retention suture, the surgeon selects one of the following closure techniques: through-and-through retention sutures or buried coaptation-retention sutures (Ethicon, 1988, p. 12).

Through-and-through retention sutures are inserted before the peritoneum is closed (Fig. 16–31). The surgeon places the suture from inside the peritoneal cavity. The suture is inserted through the peritoneum, all abdominal layers, and the skin using a simple interrupted or a figure-of-eight stitch. The surgeon then closes the wound in layers for a distance of about three fourths the length of the wound. Next, the surgeon draws the retention sutures together and ties them. While tying, the RNFA should place a finger in the abdominal cavity to prevent strangulation of the viscera during closure. Closure of the remainder of the wound continues in a similar manner (Ethicon, 1988, p. 12).

Buried coaptation-retention sutures are inserted after the peritoneum is closed (Fig. 16–32). The suture is placed through the fascia and then the skin. The surgeon places these retention sutures "approximately two centimeters apart in the posterior rectus sheath and peritoneum in the so-called 'far-and-near' or 'far-near-near-far' fashion." After inserting the retention sutures, the surgeon closes the wound in layers and then ties the retention sutures (Ethicon, 1988, p. 12).

Figure 16–33 shows a wound closed with retention suture and bolsters. Note how bolsters are used to prevent the heavy suture materials from cutting into the skin (Ethicon, 1988, p. 33).

Use of the Needle Holder

Learning correct use of a needle holder takes coordination and time to get the feel of the instrument. When passing a needle holder, the scrub nurse should place it with feeling in the palm of the assistant's hand (Fig. 16–34). Note how the RNFA receives the needle holder with the needle point toward the thumb. This prevents unnecessary wrist motion. To prevent dragging of the suture across the sterile field, the suture is held by the scrub nurse (Ethicon, 1988, p. 51). After receiving the needle holder, the RNFA grasps it firmly and inserts the thumb and fourth finger (ring finger) through the rings of the instrument. This technique enables the RNFA to use the index and middle fingers to control

TABLE 16–7. **COMMONLY USED STITCHES**	
Continuous Suture	**Interrupted Sutures**
To Appose Skin and Other Tissue	
Over and over	Over and over
Vertical mattress	Vertical mattress
Horizontal mattress	Horizontal mattress
Subcuticular	
To Invert Tissue	
Lembert	Lembert
Cushing	Halsted
Connell	Pursestring
To Evert Tissue	
Horizontal mattress	Horizontal mattress

From *Ethicon wound closure manual* (1988). (p. 13). Somerville, NJ: Ethicon, Inc.

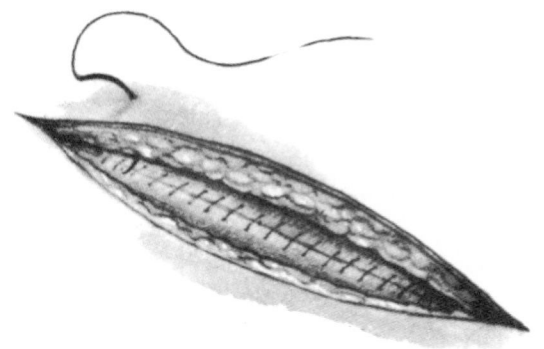

FIGURE 16–32. Buried coaptation-retention sutures. (From *Ethicon wound closure manual* [1988]. Somerville, NJ: Ethicon, Inc.)

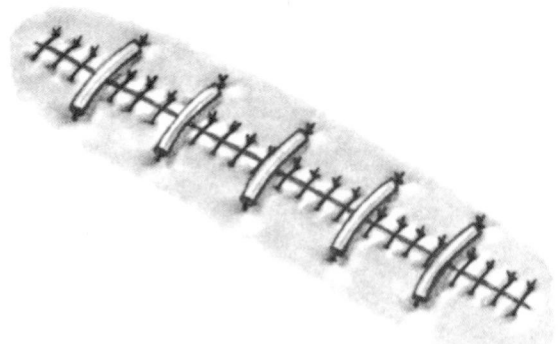

FIGURE 16–33. Retention suture with bolsters. (From *Ethicon wound closure manual* [1988]. Somerville, NJ: Ethicon, Inc.)

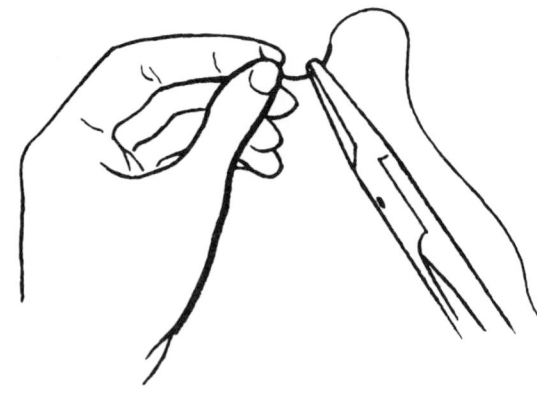

FIGURE 16–35. Loading the needle holder. (From *Ethicon wound closure manual* [1988]. Somerville, NJ: Ethicon, Inc.)

and push the needle through the tissue. When inserting the needle, the RNFA rotates the wrist, thus pushing the needle through the tissue with one smooth easy motion.

Palming is another way to handle a needle holder. With this technique, the RNFA places only the fourth finger through the ring of the instrument, which permits opening and closing of the needle holder without having to place the thumb into the ring. Many prefer this technique because it allows the assistant to handle the needle holder more quickly.

Loading of the Needle Holder

Correct placement of the needle in the needle holder prevents it from turning when entering the tissue during suturing (Fig. 16–35). Place the needle in the jaws just below the point where it flattens out (Fig. 16–36).

Placement of Sutures

When inserting the needle, place the point at a right angle to the tissue (Fig. 16–37). This technique allows the needle a clean and smooth entry through the tissue. After inserting the needle, release it, and grasp down from the point and pull it through. Unless there is no other way to pull the needle through the tissue, avoid grasping the point. Grasping the needle at the point

dulls and bends it out of shape. A dull or damaged needle point not only makes suturing more difficult but also causes unnecessary trauma to the tissue.

Getting the needle and suture through both sides of the incision usually requires two motions. After pulling the needle through one side, reposition it in the needle holder and place the point in the tissue so that it exits the tissue at a right angle. To bring the incision edges properly together, keep the suture at the same level in the tissue. Next, advance the suture through the tissue by using a smooth, uninterrupted, and gentle pulling motion. When suturing, bring like tissues together: peritoneum to peritoneum, muscle to muscle, fascia to fascia, subcutaneous tissue to subcutaneous tissue, and skin to skin. Many surgeons use the Smead-Jones stitch when closing the abdomen (Fig. 16–38). This stitch simultaneously approximates peritoneum, muscle, and fascia. When suturing, the free end of the suture is easily contaminated if not controlled. The RNFA can control the free end by placing the suture to the right of the needle holder when using the right hand and to the left when using the left hand.

When using a straight needle for closure, grasp the skin edges gently but firmly with a tissue forceps. Lifting the edge of the incision aids in placing the needle point in the tissue. After the needle is through one side, repeat the procedure with the opposite incision edge. Place the suture at an equal depth and distance from the skin edges.

If not actually performing the closure, the RNFA

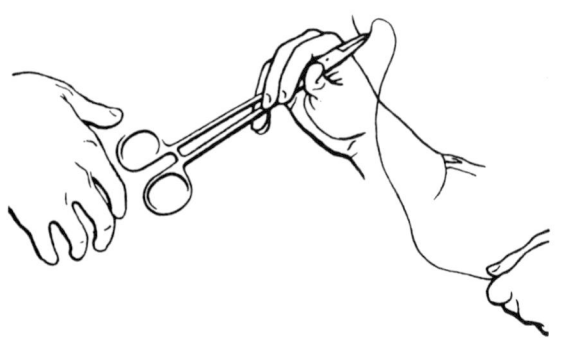

FIGURE 16–34. Passing a needle holder. (From *Ethicon wound closure manual* [1988]. Somerville, NJ: Ethicon, Inc.)

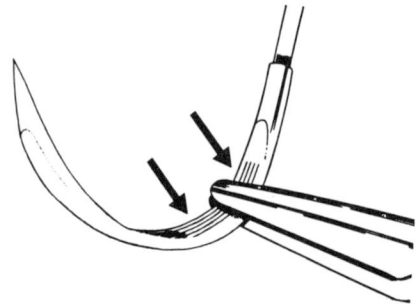

FIGURE 16–36. Correct placement of the needle in the needle holder. (From *Ethicon wound closure manual* [1988]. Somerville, NJ: Ethicon, Inc.)

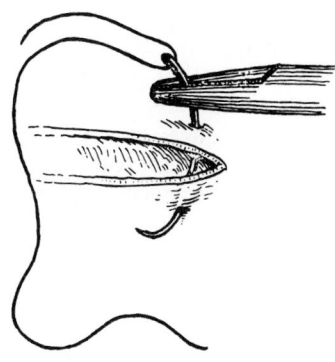

FIGURE 16–37. Inserting a suture needle. (From Nora, P. F. [1991]. *Operative surgery: Principles and techniques* [3rd ed.] [p. 19]. Philadelphia: W. B. Saunders.)

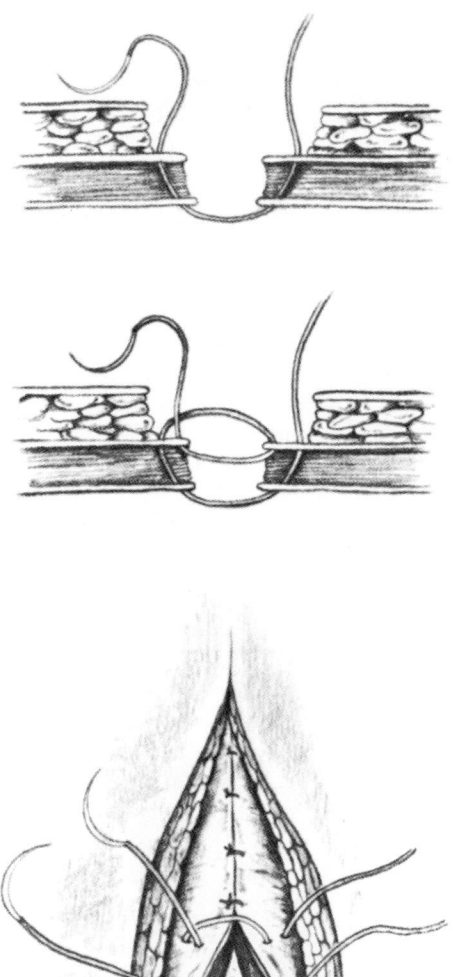

FIGURE 16–38. Smead-Jones far-and-near technique for abdominal wound closure. (From *Ethicon wound closure manual* [1988]. Somerville, NJ: Ethicon, Inc.)

handles the ends of the suture during closure. The RNFA prevents knots and redundant suture from getting in the way of the surgeon by keeping the suture taut and straight. Placing tension on the suture also aids in controlling the tissue during the closure by holding the tissue edges up or apart. This maneuver not only makes placement of the next suture easier but also provides the necessary exposure for the surgery to proceed smoothly.

Staples

Skin staples are frequently used for skin closure (Fig. 16–39). Unless used properly, however, complications in healing can interfere with the desired cosmetic results.

The two basic requirements for apposing skin [with skin staples] are that:

1) The edges of the cuticular and subcuticular layers are everted, that is, aligned with the edges slightly raised in an outward direction. As it heals, the tissue will tend to flatten out and form an even surface.

2) The skin edges must be aligned as close to their original configuration on the horizontal plane as possible. If one edge is allowed to slide or to be placed in a location other than its original one, the best cosmetic results will not be obtained and unnecessary scars can form (Ethicon, 1988, p. 57).

Before placing the skin staples, the RNFA forces the skin edges together with one tissue forceps until the edges evert or picks up each wound edge individually with two tissue forceps and approximates the edges. Next, tension is applied to either end of the incision until the tissue edges begin to approximate themselves (Ethicon, 1988, p. 57).

Surgical Knots

Knots keep vessels closed and hold tissues together (Table 16–8). When suturing, the RNFA uses the simple or overhand knot, square knot, granny knot, and surgeons' knot (Fig. 16–40). The simple knot is the first step of basic knot tying, whereas the square knot is a complete and true knot. Unless requested by the surgeon, avoid the granny knot. This slip knot does not provide the security necessary to ensure that tissue holds together and vessels remain closed. Maintain tension or traction on the tissue with the surgeons' knot. This knot does not slip after the first throw is in place.

Most assistants use the square knot because it provides a secure and competent knot in or around the tissue. Although it is possible to tie a square knot using the one-hand technique (Figs. 16–41 and 16–42), many surgeons and assistants prefer to tie using the two-hand technique (Figs. 16–43 and 16–44). This technique gives the assistant better control over knot placement and aids in maintaining proper knot tension.

Because it usually stays in place after the first throw is made, the surgeon's knot is used to maintain the proper position of the tissue, particularly when working in deep tissue. In addition, the surgeon's knot helps control the tissue. After making the double wrap, the RNFA ensures proper placement and tension of the knot on the tissue by following the knot down with the tip of the finger. The square knot is another knot of choice if the surgeon's knot is not required.

An area that requires a deep tie may also need a suture ligature. The surgeon places a suture ligature,

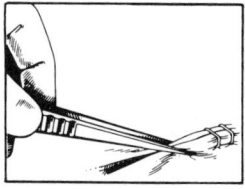
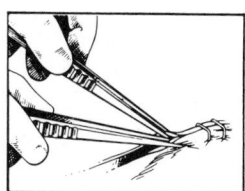

1. Evert and approximate skin edges as desired with one or two tissue forceps.

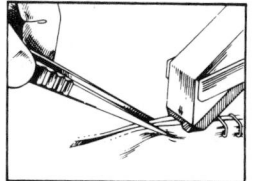
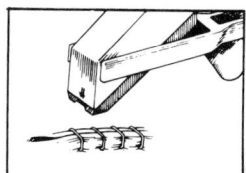

2. Position stapler very lightly over everted skin edges and squeeze trigger.

3. Back stapler off the staple.

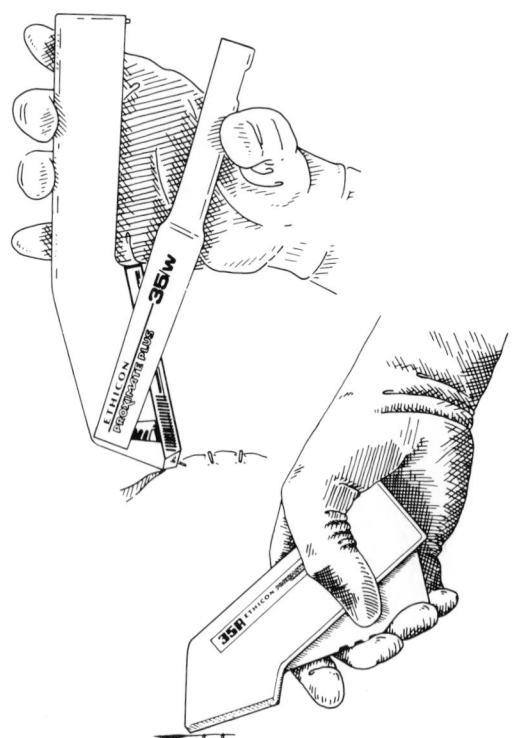

4. Both stapler configurations can be fired from any angle.

FIGURE 16–39. Stapling the skin with a disposable skin stapler. (From *Ethicon wound closure manual* [1988]. Somerville, NJ: Ethicon, Inc.)

TABLE 16–8. GENERAL PRINCIPLES OF KNOT TYING

1. Tie the knot firmly to minimize slippage.
2. Use a simple knot.
3. Tie a small knot and cut the ends as short as possible to minimize foreign body tissue reaction.
4. Avoid sawing one strand of suture down over another strand when tying the knot. This may weaken the suture and result in breakage when the second throw is made.
5. Avoid excessive tension when using finer-gauge suture materials. To tie the knot securely and avoid breakage, pull the two ends of the suture in opposite directions with uniform rate and tension.
6. Do not attach clamps or hemostats to suture that will remain in situ. Avoid the crushing or crimping application of surgical instruments, such as needle holders and forceps, to the strand, except when grasping the free end of the suture during an instrument tie.
7. Do not tie suture for tissue approximation too tightly, as this causes tissue strangulation.
8. To avoid loosening of the knot, after tying the first loop maintain traction on one end of the strand for control.
9. Avoid extra throws when tying the knot. They do not add to the strength of the knot; they only contribute to its bulk.

From *Ethicon wound closure manual* (1988). (p. 13). Somerville, NJ: Ethicon, Inc.

and then the RNFA ties the knot using the same process as described above. After insertion of the suture ligature, the suture is brought back to the opposite side of the hemostat and the knot is completed.

When making a deep tie, use a needle holder to complete the tie. Loop the suture around the end of the holder, grasp the other end of the suture, and pull it through the loop; this starts the knot. To complete the knot, wrap in the opposite direction to form a square knot.

Applying Knot Tension

Securing the knot prevents it from falling out of the tissue. Using the correct amount of tension when tying the knot prevents slipping when the final knot is in place. The knot tension holds the tissue together and keeps the vessel closed. This tension should approximate, not strangulate or tear, the tissue.

The RNFA can maintain firm and steady tension during knot tying by holding one end of the suture still while tying the knot. Steady tension prevents the suture material from breaking during the tie. Jerking, sawing, or snapping the suture may cause it to break during the procedure. Because tissues swell when placing knots, use only the necessary number of throws to complete the knot. This reduces the bulk of the suture left in the patient. When tying deep knots, to ensure proper placement of the tie on the tissue, always carry the suture down to the tissue with the tip of the finger.

Keeping the vessel closed or the tissue in place necessitates properly placed, firmly set, and squared knots. Different types of tissue require different amounts of tension to provide the correct closure. If the tension is too loose, the incision gaps. If the tension is too tight, the tissue strangulates, thus creating the potential for necrosis.

Cutting of Sutures

When cutting sutures, run the tip of the scissors down the length of the suture strand to the knot. If surgical gut has been used, cut the strand 6 mm from the knot. Cut synthetic sutures 3 mm from the knot to minimize the amount of foreign material left in the wound. Before cutting the suture, ensure that the tips of the scissors are in sight to avoid cutting tissue. As sutures are cut, remove the ends from the operative site (Ethicon, 1988, p. 14).

Cutting Tissue

Scalpels

The modern scalpel consists of a handle that is designed to receive a variety of disposable blades. The

Text continued on page 378

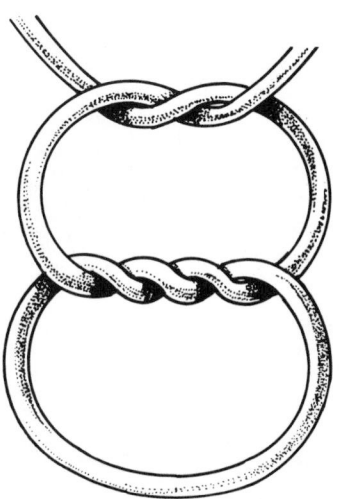

FIGURE 16–40. Surgeon's knot. (Redrawn from Nealon, T. F. [1991]. *Fundamental skills in surgery*. Philadelphia: W. B. Saunders.)

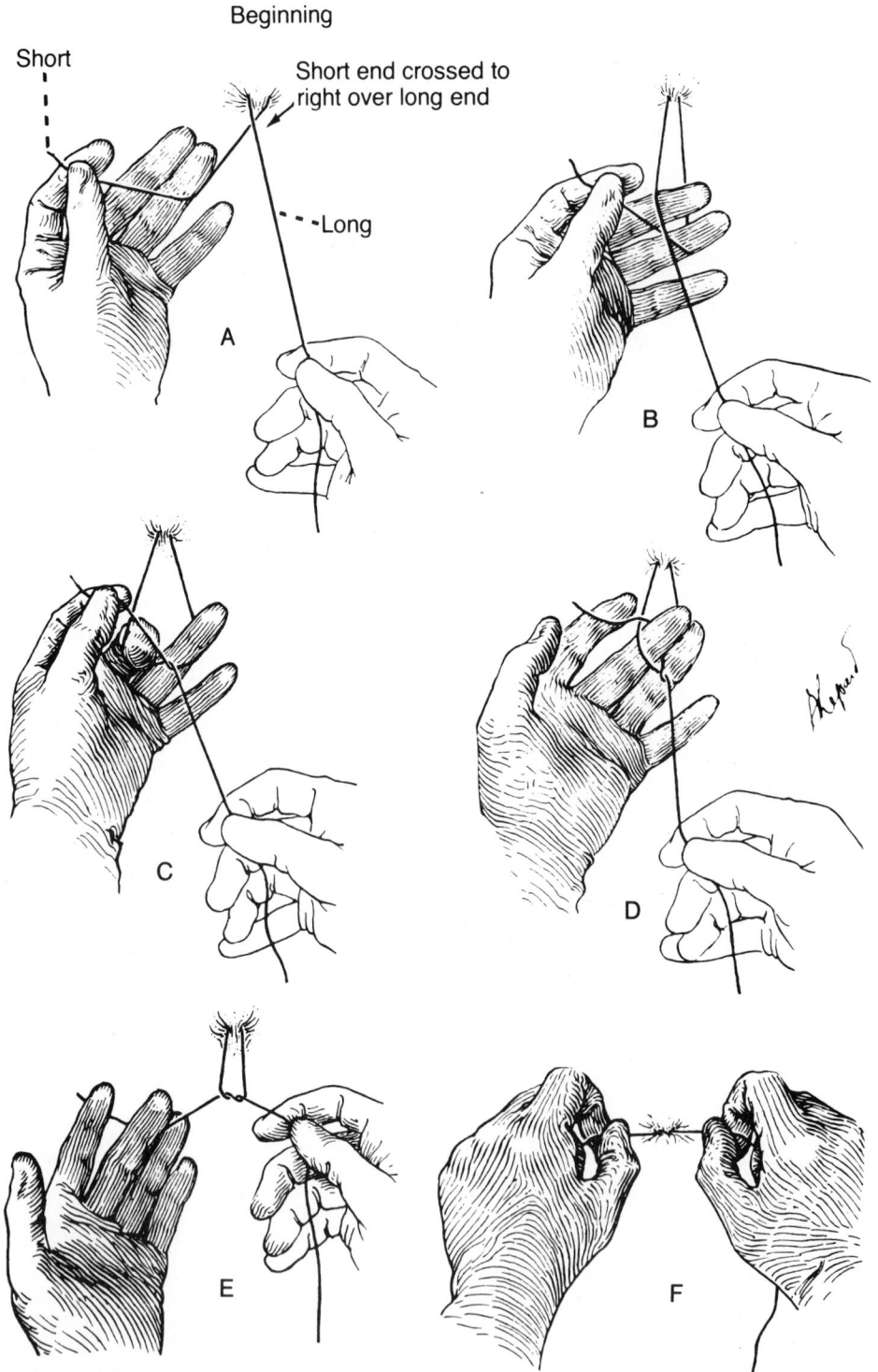

FIGURE 16–41. One-hand method of tying a square knot. First half-hitch. (From Nora, P. F. [1991]. *Operative surgery: Principles and techniques* [3rd ed.] [p. 17]. Philadelphia: W. B. Saunders.)

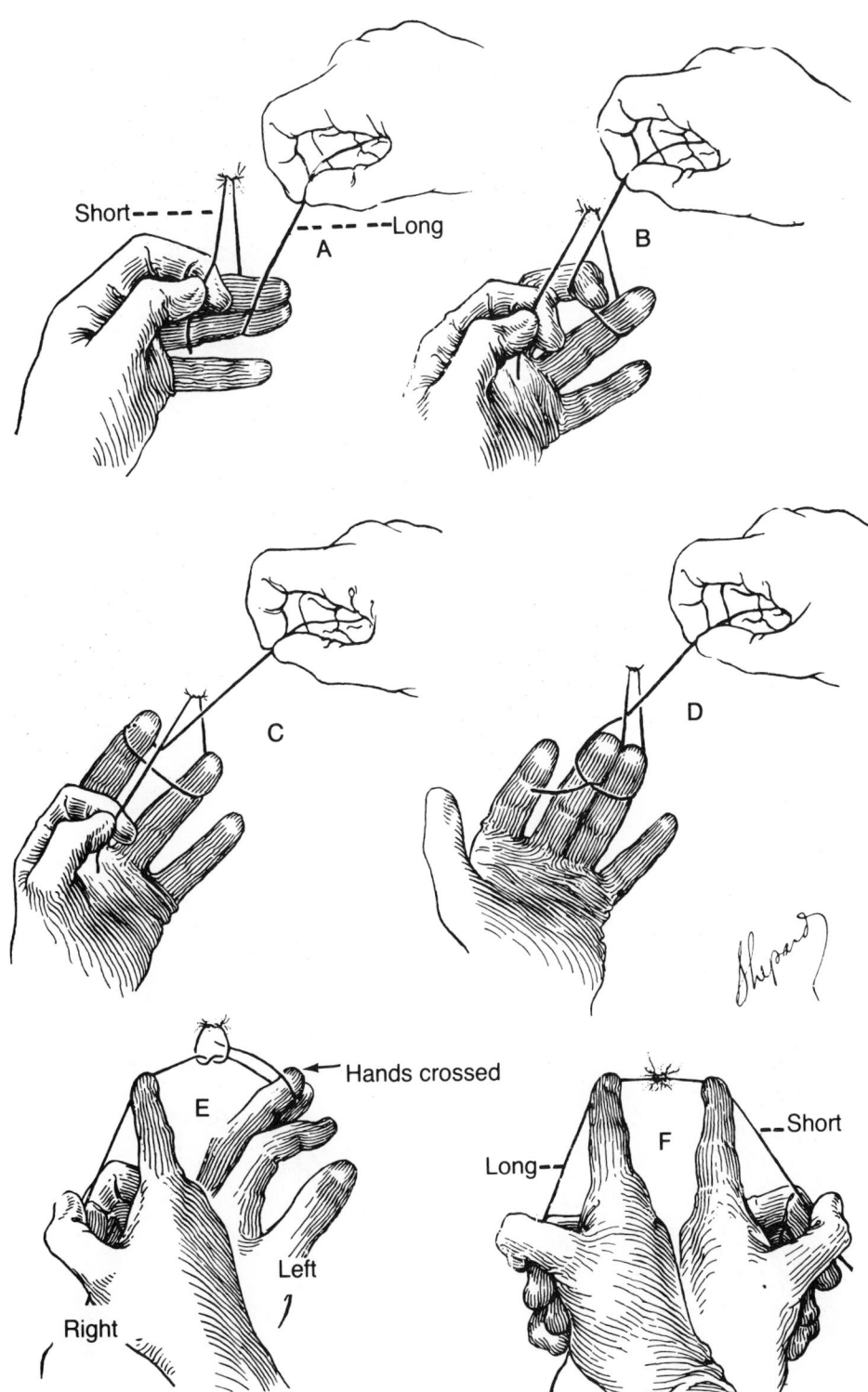

FIGURE 16–42. One-hand method of tying a square knot. Second half-hitch. (From Nora, P. F. [1991]. *Operative surgery: Principles and techniques* [3rd ed.] [p. 18]. Philadelphia: W. B. Saunders.)

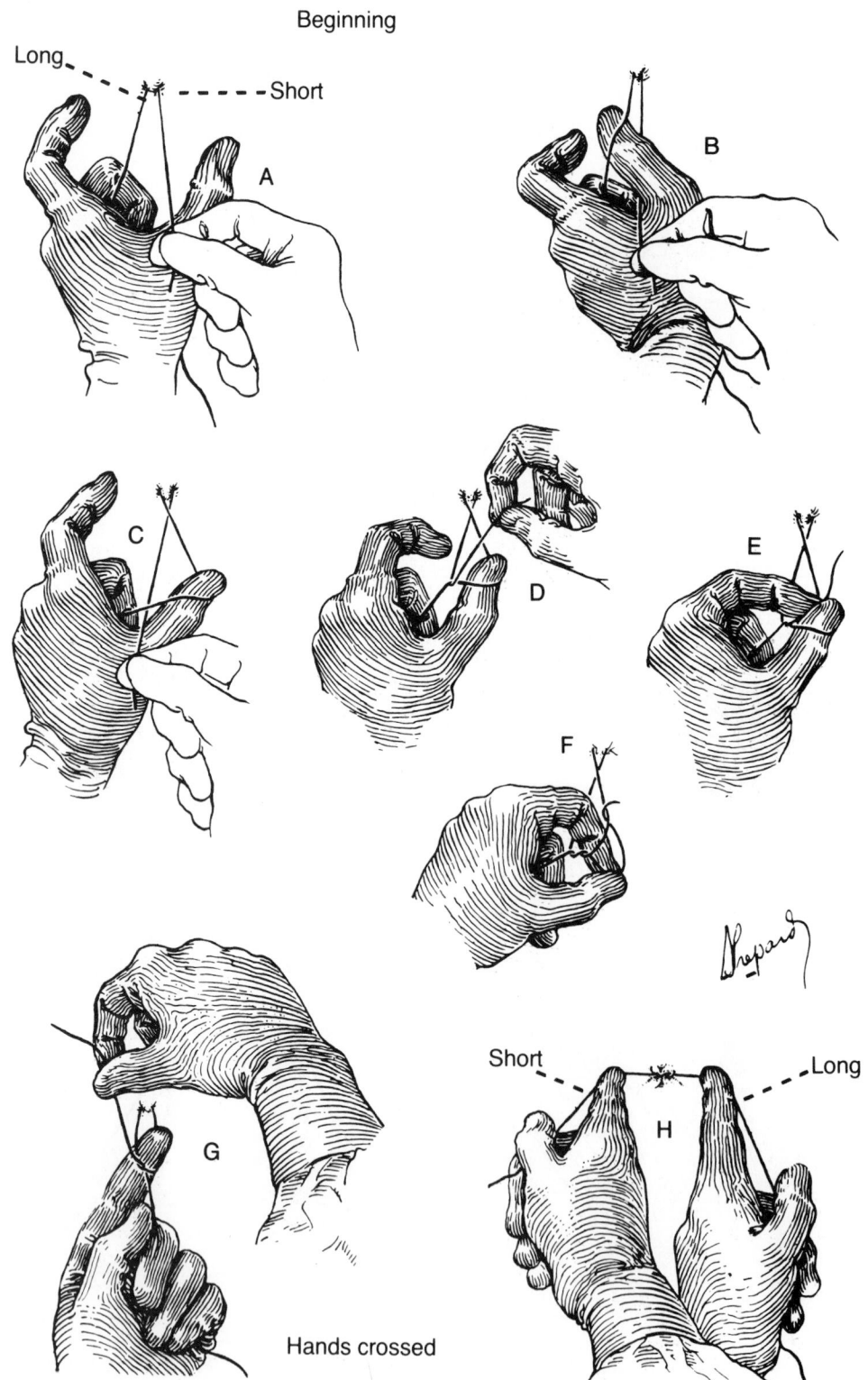

FIGURE 16–43. Two-hand method of tying a square knot. First half-hitch. (From Nora, P. F. [1991]. *Operative surgery: Principles and techniques* [3rd ed.] [p. 14]. Philadelphia: W. B. Saunders.)

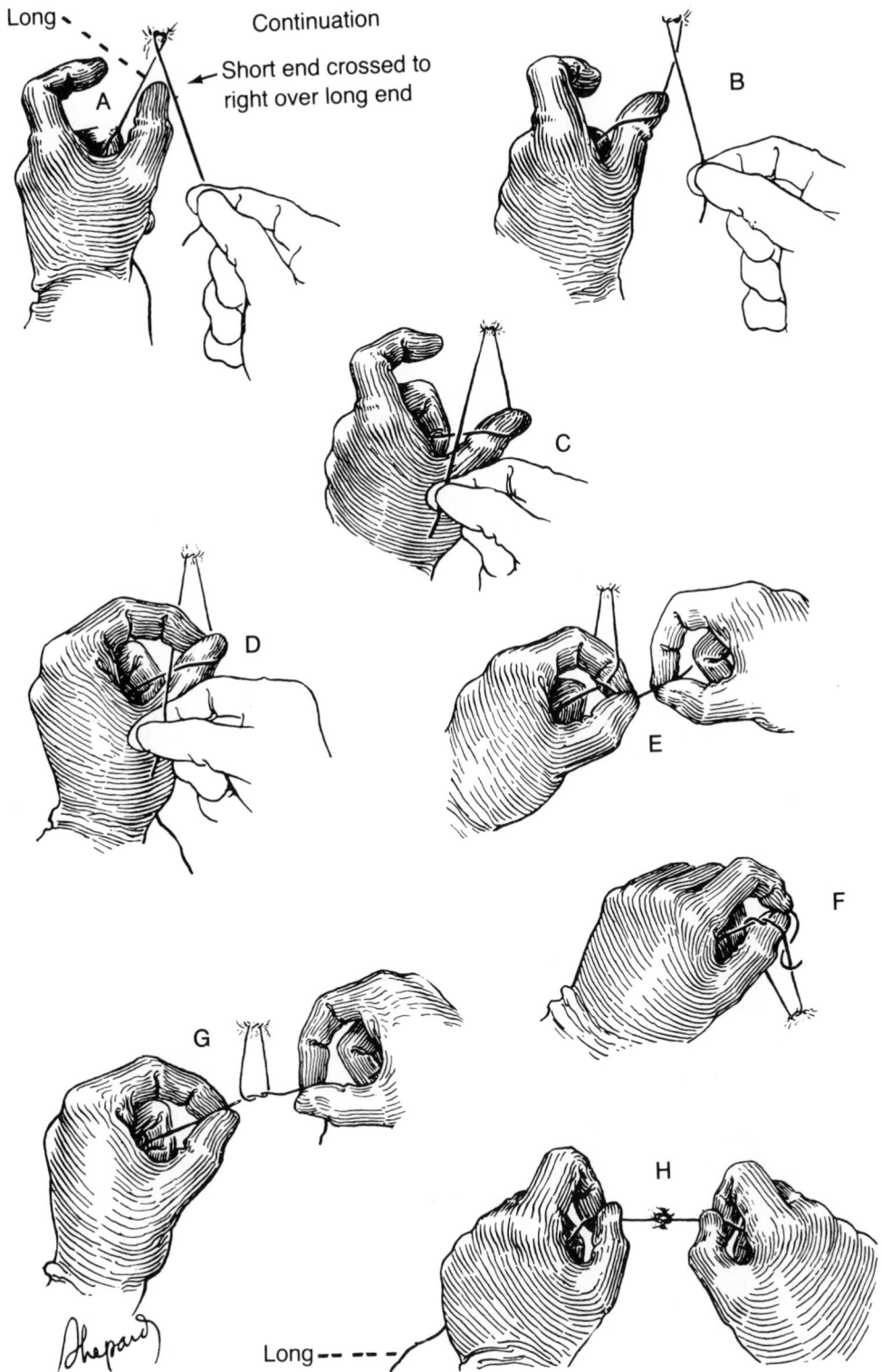

FIGURE 16–44. Two-hand method of tying a square knot. Second half-hitch. (From Nora, P. F. [1991]. *Operative surgery: Principles and techniques* [3rd ed.] [p. 15]. Philadelphia: W. B. Saunders.)

blade is changed as soon as it becomes dull, as the edge must be sharp and smooth. The type of operation and the patient's size determine not only the size and location of the initial incision but the type of blade as well. An incision must be just long enough to provide adequate space to perform the operation. For large incisions, the scalpel handle is held against the palm with the thumb and fingers gripping it from above. This is known as the power grip.

The blade should be vertical to the skin to prevent beveling and should cut dermis and epidermis quickly with a single stroke, applying even pressure. This technique promotes precision approximation of skin, which promotes wound healing. The depth of the incision is controlled by downward pressure of the index finger. A wide blade such as the No. 10 or 20 is commonly used. Figure 16–45 shows the proper scalpel angle. Note how the scalpel is at a 90-degree angle to the skin. This allows the sides of the wound to be of equal height and facilitates proper closure.

The No. 15 blade has a small curve and short cutting surface and is used for small incisions and dissecting fine tissue. It can also be used with a pencil-like grip. The No. 11 blade tapers to a fine point and requires a gentle, constant pressure. In the precision grip, the scalpel handle is held like a pencil and the hand is stabilized by providing light contact with the patient with the fingers. It can be used to make a small skin incision and is often used to puncture an abscess, cut a vessel wall, or make a sharp cut in small structures such as the fallopian tube. Many different sizes and shapes of blades are required for specific purposes. The right-angled scalpel blade may be used to cut tissues at the bottom of a deep hole. A crescent-shaped No. 12 blade with a pointed tip can be used in a hole when the surgeon may impale tissue with the tip as she or he cuts it.

Scissors

Scissors are used for dissecting tissue, severing clamped blood vessels, and cutting suture. Figure 16–46 shows a Metzenbaum scissors, which is used for dissecting during surgical procedures. When using a scissors, control is maintained by inserting the thumb and fourth (ring) finger through the handle rings. The index and third fingers are then used to stabilize the scissors as it cuts. In Figure 16–47, Metzenbaum scissors are used to divide nerve fibers below the submandibular ganglion during a radical neck dissection. Mayo scissors are used to open the peritoneum (Fig. 16–48).

Electrical Cutting Devices

Several instruments can be used to cut and coagulate tissue at the same time. The electrosurgical unit uses high-frequency electrical energy to produce heat to coagulate and a more intense heat to cut tissue. Held like a pencil, it is used for both dissection and hemostasis. Care must be used to touch only the tissue to be coagulated, as surrounding tissue can be damaged. This method is widely used to control bleeding. It is valuable to coagulate small vessels that are difficult to ligate owing to their size or location.

These units can be used on monopolar and bipolar

Text continued on page 383

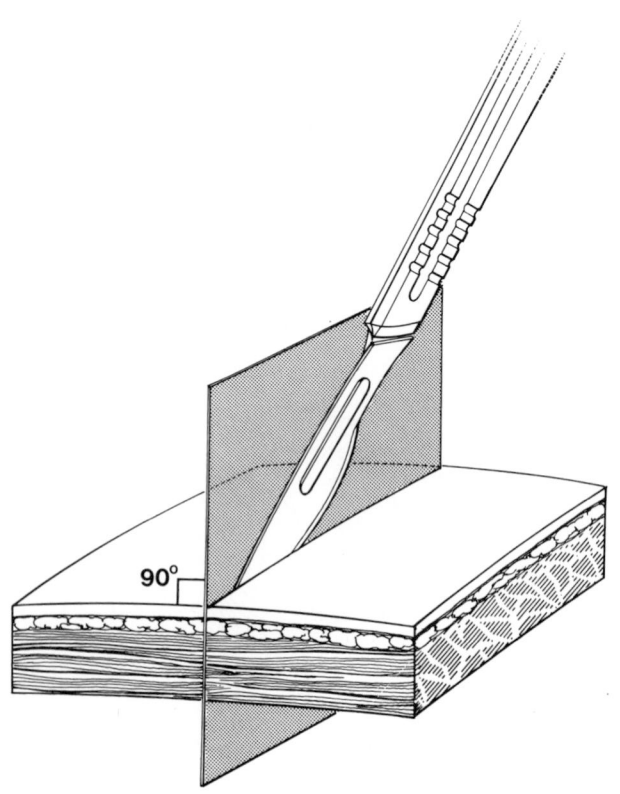

90°

FIGURE 16–45. Proper scalpel angle. (From Nora, P. F. [1991]. *Operative surgery: Principles and techniques* [3rd ed.] [p. 80]. Philadelphia: W. B. Saunders.)

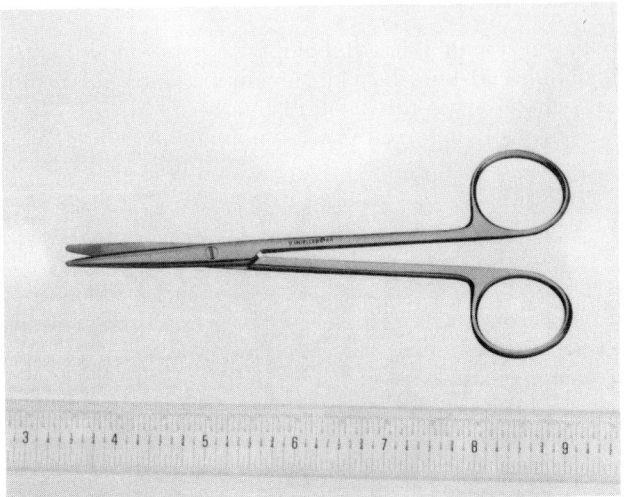

FIGURE 16–46. Metzenbaum dissection scissors. (Courtesy of Baxter Healthcare Corporation, McGaw Park, IL.)

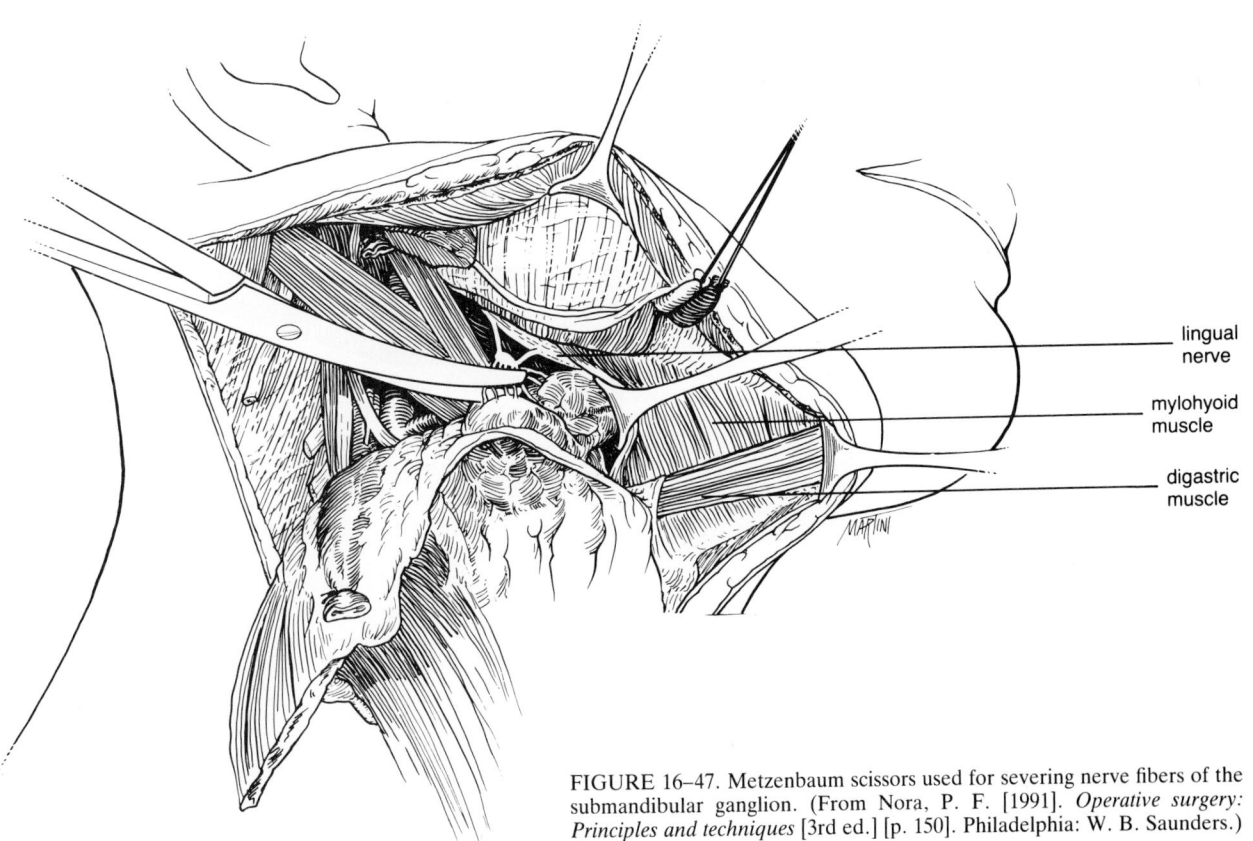

lingual nerve

mylohyoid muscle

digastric muscle

FIGURE 16–47. Metzenbaum scissors used for severing nerve fibers of the submandibular ganglion. (From Nora, P. F. [1991]. *Operative surgery: Principles and techniques* [3rd ed.] [p. 150]. Philadelphia: W. B. Saunders.)

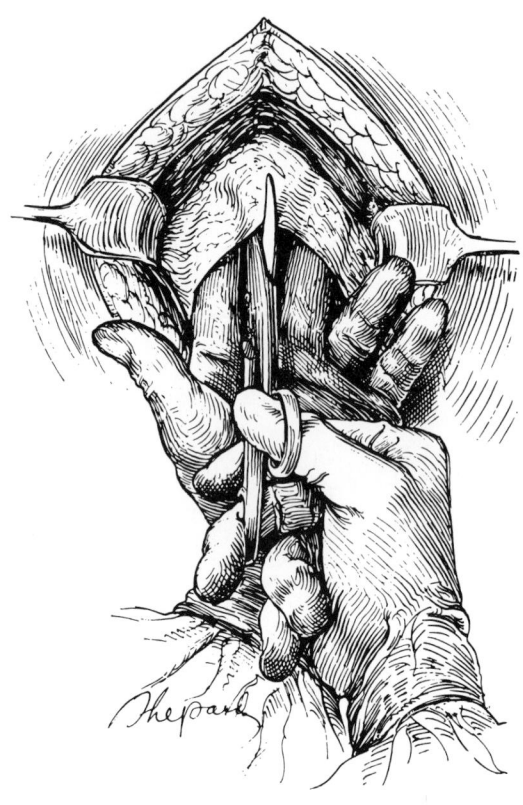

FIGURE 16–48. Opening the peritoneum with Mayo scissors. (From Nora, P. F. [1991]. *Operative surgery: Principles and techniques* [3rd ed.][p. 445]. Philadelphia: W. B. Saunders.)

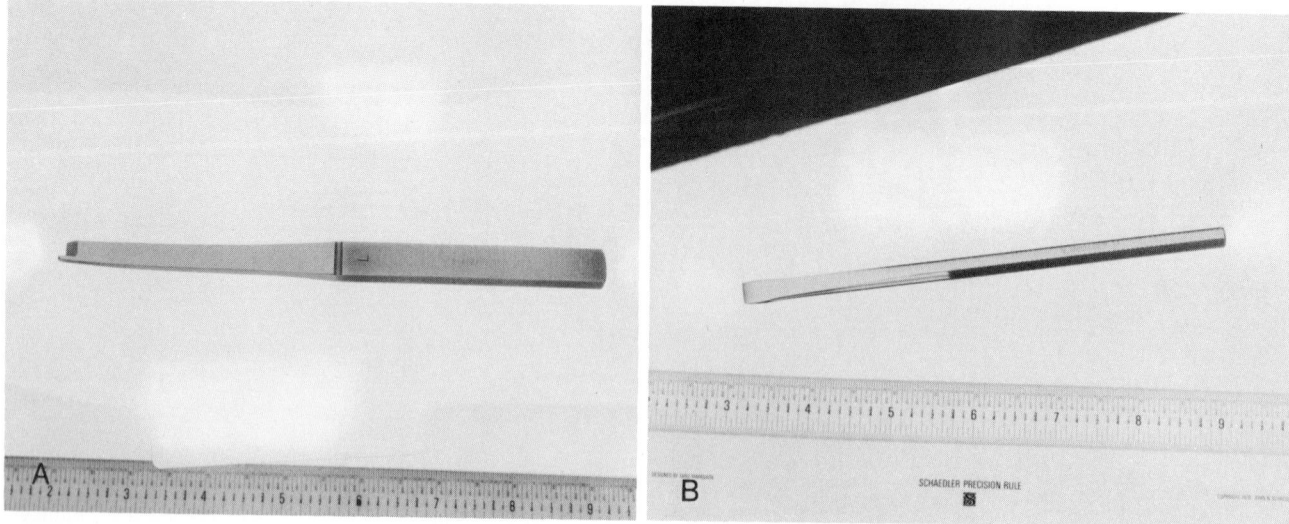

FIGURE 16–49. Standard bone chisels. *A*, Converse chisel. *B*, J.E. Sheehan chisel. (Courtesy of Baxter Healthcare Corporation, McGaw Park, IL.)

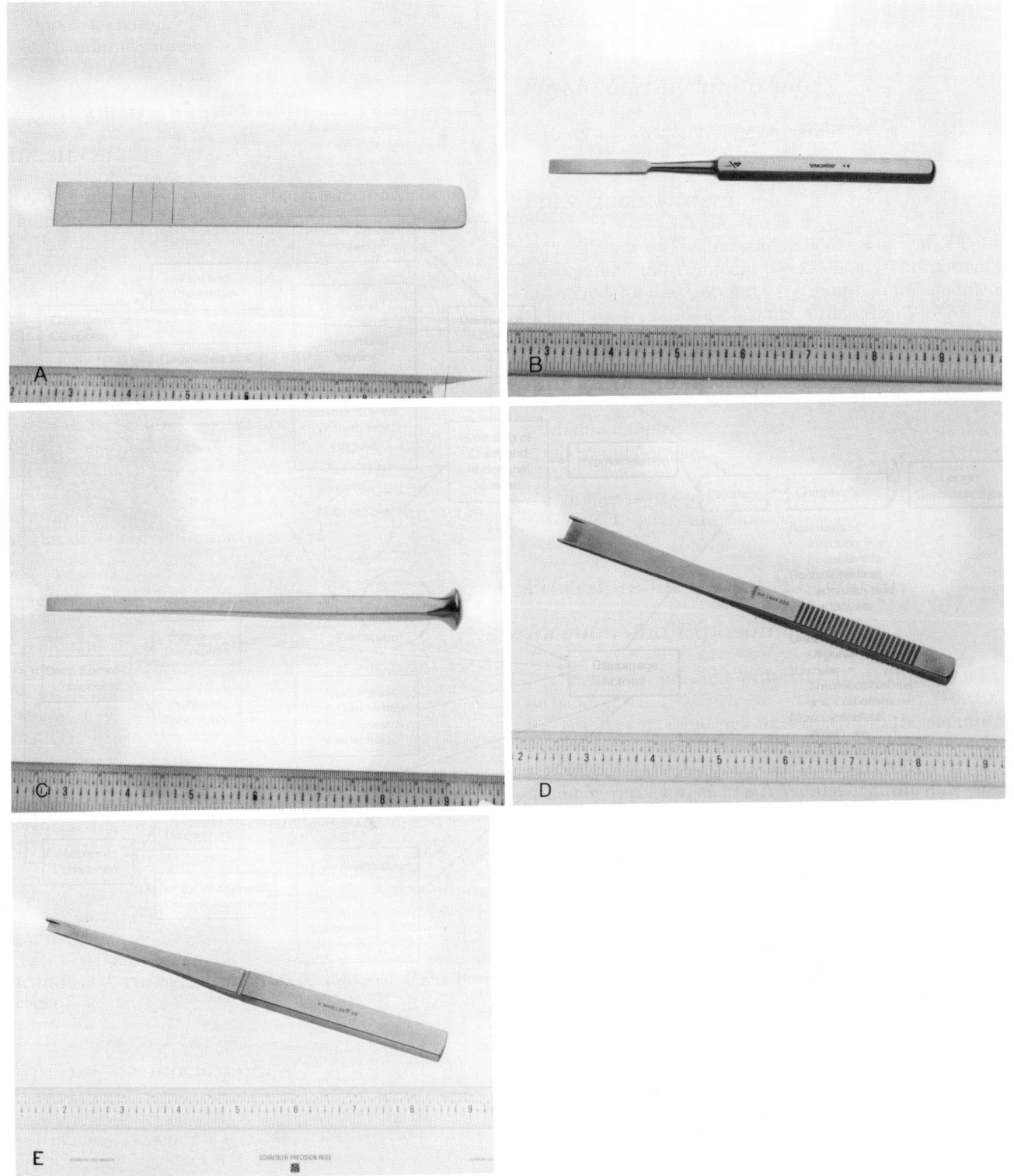

FIGURE 16–50. Stainless steel osteotomes. *A*, Straight osteotome. *B*, Hoke osteotome. *C*, U.S. Army osteotome. *D*, Cinelli osteotome. *E*, Converse osteotome. (Courtesy of Baxter Healthcare Corporation, McGaw Park, IL.)

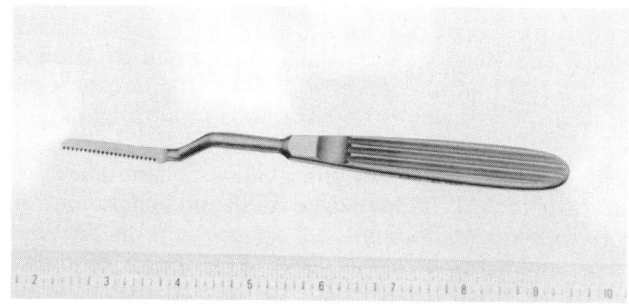

FIGURE 16–51. Nasal saw. (Courtesy of Baxter Healthcare Corporation, McGaw Park, IL.)

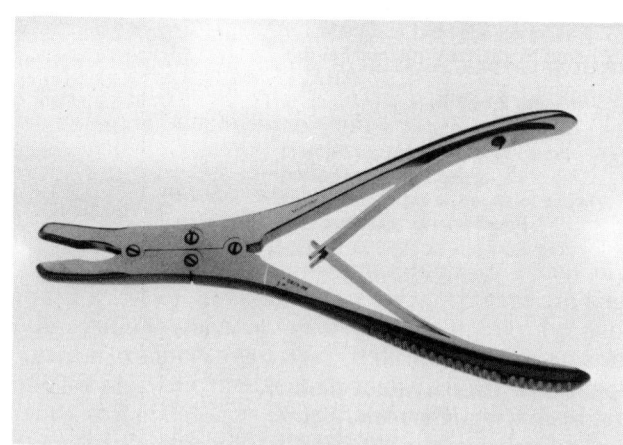

FIGURE 16–52. Double-action rongeur forceps. (Courtesy of Baxter Healthcare Corporation, McGaw Park, IL.)

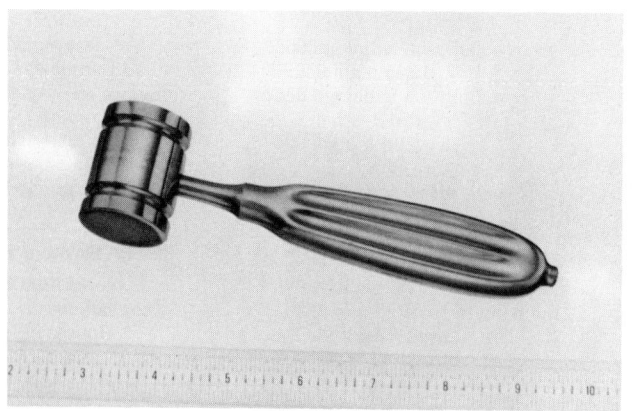

FIGURE 16–53. Surgical mallet. (Courtesy of Baxter Healthcare Corporation, McGaw Park, IL.)

settings. When the monopolar setting is used, the patient must be grounded and the pencil kept in its holder to avoid inadvertent burn to the patient. The Shaw scalpel is a heated blade that seals small blood vessels as it cuts. It is a slow process and is often used in delicate surgery such as infertility procedures in which bleeding must be well controlled.

Orthopedic and Other Cutting Devices

Orthopedics and specialities such as otolaryngology, plastics, and neurosurgery use instruments designed for cutting bone. Some of the more common instruments are chisels, curets, bone cutters, gauges, elevators, and osteotomes. Figure 16–49 shows examples of a Converse chisel and a J.E. Sheehan chisel. Osteotomes are shown in Figure 16–50: straight 22-mm, Hoke, U.S. Army type, Cinelli, and Converse. The Joseph nasal saw is shown in Figure 16–51. Figure 16–52 shows a Ruskin rongeur forceps, and a Crane mallet is shown in Figure 16–53. Saws and drills, reamers, and screwdrivers driven by compressed nitrogen or electricity are widely used. Powered tools generate high heat and should be used for only short periods of time. Because this heat damages adjacent tissue, cool saline is used to drip onto the blade or drill whenever it is in use. The nurse and the assistant must take care not to obstruct the surgeon's view when irrigating.

SUMMARY

As reimbursement patterns change, fewer physician first assistants will be available to provide exposure and clamp, grasp, and suture tissue during a surgical procedure. RNFAs will be called on to handle tissue with instruments during surgery.

Bibliography

Atkinson L. J., Kohn, M. L. (1986). *Berry and Kohn's introduction to operating room technique* (6th ed.). New York: McGraw-Hill.
Ethicon wound closure manual (1988). Somerville, NJ: Ethicon, Inc.
Fuller, J. R. (1993). *Surgical technology: Principles and practice* (3rd ed.). Philadelphia: W. B. Saunders.
Gordon, M. (1987). *Manual of nursing diagnosis: 1986–1987*. New York: McGraw-Hill.
Groah, L. K. (1983). *Operating room nursing: The perioperative role*. Reston, VA: Reston Publishing.
Nora, P. F. (1991). *Operative surgery: Principles and techniques* (3rd ed.). Philadelphia: W. B. Saunders.
Rothrock, J. C. (1987). *The RN first assistant: An expanded perioperative nursing role*. Philadelphia: J. B. Lippincott.

Providing Hemostasis

Vicki J. Fox

DEFINITION

The term *hemostasis* means prevention of blood loss (Guyton, 1991). Because hemostasis is essential to successful wound management, applying hemostatic techniques is one of the critical tasks done by the registered nurse first assistant (RNFA).

MEASURABLE CRITERIA

The RNFA demonstrates competency to provide hemostasis by

- recognizing alterations in clotting mechanisms that put the patient at risk for experiencing intraoperative and postoperative bleeding
- recognizing hypovolemic shock
- applying mechanical methods to control bleeding
- applying thermal methods to control bleeding
- applying chemical methods to control bleeding

ROLE OF THE REGISTERED NURSE FIRST ASSISTANT

Providing hemostasis is an ongoing process throughout the surgical procedure. Usually, the surgeon determines the appropriate hemostatic technique and the RNFA performs or assists in performing the technique. The accomplished RNFA, however, determines the appropriate technique for many situations, recommends treatment modalities, and acts accordingly. The RNFA should know all the hemostatic options available in an institution, anticipate the patient's needs and request that the circulating nurse have specific supplies and equipment available, and make recommendations to the surgeon. The circulating nurse is responsible for most of the nursing activities that ensure patient safety when using electrical equipment. Besides providing and preparing the necessary equipment and supplies for hemostasis, the scrub nurse is occasionally asked to assist in accomplishing hemostasis.

CONSIDERATIONS

This chapter presents potential nursing diagnoses related to alterations in the patient's clotting mechanism and the application of hemostatic techniques. Scrub nurses and circulating nurses, as well as perioperative nurses practicing as RNFAs, will find the outcome standard and potential nursing diagnoses useful as they assess the patient for risk factors, plan care, apply interventions to control bleeding, and evaluate the effectiveness of the interventions.

Mechanism of Clotting

Understanding the mechanism of blood coagulation aids the RNFA in assessing the patient's clotting abilities and applying mechanical, thermal, and chemical hemostatic techniques.

Depending on the type of trauma, a blood vessel either contracts or constricts when damaged (Fig. 17–1). If cut, the vessel wall contracts. Direct trauma to the muscle in the vessel wall, however, causes it to constrict for several centimeters, resulting in vascular spasm. The greater the trauma, the greater the degree of vasospasm. For example, sharply cut vessels usually result in greater blood loss than crushed vessels.

After damage is incurred, plugging of the disrupted vessel with platelets begins. Platelets are normally oval or round disks. When platelets contact the collagen fibers of a damaged vessel wall, they swell and assume irregular shapes with protuberances. They also become sticky and secrete enzymes that activate adjacent platelets. The cumulative effect is the formation of a loose platelet plug.

Next, the blood clot forms. This event occurs in three steps:

1. Prothrombin activators form in response to vessel trauma (extrinsic pathway) or damage to the blood cells (intrinsic pathway).
2. Aided by the activators, prothrombin is converted to thrombin (calcium ions are essential to this process).
3. Thrombin converts the fibrinogen to fibrin.

The fibrin threads then enmesh with the platelets in the platelet plug and remaining blood components to form a tight, unyielding plug. Later, the clot retracts, closing the vessel even more.

After clot formation, fibroblasts invade the clot and organize into connective tissue. During this process, the proteolytic enzyme called plasmin, or fibrinolysin, is activated to digest the fibrin threads. Eventually, the clot dissolves (Guyton, 1991).

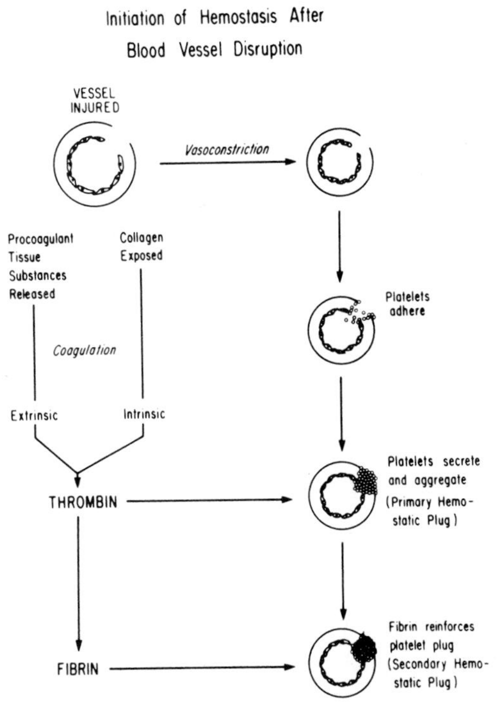

FIGURE 17–1. Formation of primary and secondary hemostatic plugs after blood vessel injury. (From Polk, H. S., Stone, H. H., Gardener, B. [Eds.]. [1987]. *Basic surgery* [3rd ed.] [p. 544]. East Norwalk, CT: Appleton-Century-Crofts.

RECOGNIZING HYPOVOLEMIC SHOCK

Hypovolemic shock, one of the complications of excessive blood loss, is an important concern for the RNFA. Depletion of the vascular volume caused by hemorrhage limits heart filling and decreases cardiac output. Hypovolemic shock can be mild to severe.

The patient experiencing mild, hypovolemic shock has lost 20% or less of blood volume. The patient's skin perfusion is poor especially the feet, which may be pale, cool, and clammy. The subcutaneous veins on the foot collapse. If the patient is in a supine position, the blood pressure and pulse remain normal. With sitting or standing rapidly, however, the blood pressure falls and the pulse rises. Urine output is normal. The patient may complain of being cold or thirsty.

In *moderate* shock, the patient has lost 20 to 40% of circulating volume. Look for pale skin and a low urine output. Many patients maintain a normal blood pressure and pulse in a supine position. A few, however, have a drop in pressure and a rise in pulse rate.

Hypotension, oliguria, and tachycardia indicate that the patient has lost 40% or more of blood volume and is experiencing *severe* shock. Skin perfusion is poor, and as the hypovolemia worsens or persists, the patient shows changes in the electrocardiogram (an indication of myocardial ischemia). As circulation decreases to the brain, the patient may become agitated, restless, or obtunded.

Skin pallor due to vasoconstriction is the first sign of hypovolemia. The RNFA should note that, although skin pallor is a sensitive physical sign, it is nonspecific. Fear, hypothermia, and hypoglycemia also produce poor skin perfusion. Impaired skin integrity from hypovolemia is unlikely except in severe shock; at that point, restoration of blood circulation to the heart and the brain is of greater priority (Polk et al., 1987). Table 17–1 presents the progression of hypovolemic shock.

OUTCOME STANDARD

Providing hemostasis does not compromise or cause injury to the patient.

Criteria

Depending on the patient's health status, the patient is free from evidence of

- postoperative infection related to the use of intraoperative thermal and chemical hemostatic techniques
- injury related to the use of intraoperative mechanical, chemical, and thermal hemostatic techniques
- intraoperative or postoperative fluid volume deficit

ASSESSING THE PATIENT'S CLOTTING MECHANISMS

Before surgery, the RNFA should assess the patient's clotting mechanisms. When a patient's history or physical examination suggests bleeding or clotting difficulties, the physician orders platelet and coagulation studies. If no studies have been obtained on these patients, the RNFA should recommend appropriate tests: platelet count, prothrombin time (PT), partial thromboplastin time (PTT), thrombin time, quantitative platelet counts, and bleeding time. PT measures the extrinsic clotting mechanism. PTT measures the activity of the intrinsic

TABLE 17–1. STAGES OF HYPOVOLEMIC SHOCK

Peripheral venous constriction	Trunk cooling
Poor capillary filling	Agitation
Pallor	Decreased pain sensation
Peripheral cooling	Loss of deep tendon reflexes
Oliguria	Acidotic breathing
Increased pulse rate	Deep pallor
Thirst	Loss of consciousness
Increased respiratory rate	Death
Hypotension	

From Polk, H. S., Stone, H. H., and Gardener, B. (Eds.). (1987). *Basic surgery* (3rd ed.) (p. 56). East Norwalk, CT: Appleton-Century-Crofts.

clotting mechanisms. Thrombin time detects abnormalities in converting fibrinogen to fibrin. Compare coagulation study results to the control study results. Quantitative platelet counts less than 60,000/mm³ indicate that the patient may have an occult thrombocytopenia, either acquired or congenital. A lack of platelets prolongs bleeding time (Polk et al., 1987).

Thrombocytopenia develops with decreased platelet production, as in bone marrow aplasia, infiltration, and suppression (e.g., by drugs and radiation) or vitamin B_{12} deficiency. Increased destruction of platelets by autoantibodies (e.g., in idiopathic thrombocytopenic purpura) or alloantibodies (e.g., from transfused blood), prosthetic devices, disseminated intravascular coagulation, cavernous hemangiomas, or thrombotic thrombocytopenic purpura also cause thrombocytopenia. Additional causes are hypersplenism, massive transfusions, and cardiopulmonary bypass (Polk et al., 1987).

The RNFA should suspect qualitative platelet defects if the patient takes antiplatelet drugs. For example, aspirin prolongs bleeding time, an effect that can last up to 3 to 5 days. Currently, there is no available agent to reverse this action. Dipyridamole (Persantine), sulfinpyrazone (Anturane), nonsteroidal anti-inflammatory drugs (sulindac [Clinoril], ibuprofen [Motrin], piroxicam [Feldene]), and antihistamines also have antiplatelet action, but to a lesser degree than does aspirin.

High doses of dextran also cause qualitative platelet abnormalities. Dextran coats the platelet surface and interferes with platelet aggregation. Patients with renal failure are at risk because qualitative platelet abnormalities increase proportionally with the degree of uremia. Other patients who may experience qualitative platelet abnormalities include those with myeloproliferative diseases and bone marrow replacement (Polk et al., 1987).

The RNFA may encounter patients with acquired bleeding disorders. Severe liver disease, such as cirrhosis and hepatitis, impair clotting factors, especially vitamin K–dependent factors. Additionally, the liver fails to remove the enzymes that activate fibrinolysis. Malnutrition, obstructive jaundice, antibiotic sterilization of the gastrointestinal tract, or malabsorption such as ulcerative colitis or Crohn's disease should also alert the RNFA to the possibility of vitamin K depletion. In such cases, the patient has a prolonged PT and PTT.

Because vitamin K plays an essential role in the activity of most clotting factors, depletion of this vitamin has serious consequences for the surgical patient. In the event of a vitamin K deficiency, the RNFA should alert the surgeon. Parenteral administration of vitamin K can improve clotting times in 8 to 12 hours. In the presence of liver disease, however, the degree to which it helps the patient depends on the extent of parenchymal cell damage (Guyton, 1991).

During the preoperative assessment, the RNFA should note if the patient takes anticoagulant drugs such as coumarin compounds (sodium warfarin [Coumadin]). These drugs, although having no anticoagulating effect in vitro, work by inhibiting the synthesis of vitamin K–dependent factors and prothrombin. The effects of coumarin compounds diminish in 5 to 10 days. Administration of parenteral vitamin K, however, restores the PT to safe levels in about 12 hours. A PT of less than two times the control value reduces the risk of intraoperative and postoperative hemorrhage. If the patient takes heparin, use the PTT to monitor the drug effects. Because heparin has a short plasma half-life, cessation of drug administration for about 2 hours returns the PTT to normal. If necessary, protamine sulfate can immediately reverse the effects of heparin (Polk et al., 1987).

Less common bleeding problems include mixed coagulation and platelet defects. During the preoperative assessment, the RNFA should identify patients at risk for disseminated intravascular coagulation. Risk factors include widespread metastatic disease, massive trauma or burns, gram-negative or gram-positive sepsis, and some viral and malarial infections. Exposure to incompatible blood products, retroplacental hemorrhage, and snake bites also place the patient at risk. This syndrome results from the diffuse consumption of clotting factors, platelet aggregation, fibrin formation, and secondary fibrinolysis. The surgeon usually treats the patient with heparin while pursuing the underlying cause of the syndrome (Polk et al., 1987).

Potential Alterations in Functional Health Patterns

Nutritional-Metabolic Pattern

Diagnosis

High risk for fluid volume deficit related to intraoperative or postoperative blood loss

Definition

Presence of risk factors for the patient to experience intraoperative or postoperative blood loss secondary to alterations in clotting mechanisms

Risk Factors

- Vitamin K deficiency
- Renal failure
- Myeloproliferative diseases
- Bone marrow replacement
- Severe liver disease, such as cirrhosis and hepatitis
- Malnutrition, obstructive jaundice, antibiotic sterilization of the gastrointestinal tract, or malabsorption
- Mixed coagulation and platelet defects
- Widespread metastatic disease, massive trauma or burns, gram-negative or gram-positive sepsis, and some viral and malarial infections
- Retroplacental hemorrhage
- Incompatible blood products
- Aspirin, dipyridamole, sulfinpyrazone, nonsteroidal anti-inflammatory drugs (sulindac, ibuprofen, piroxicam) and antihistamine use

- Anticoagulant drug use (coumarin [Coumadin] compounds [sodium warfarin] and heparin)
- High doses of dextran
- Snake bites

Expected Outcome

The patient is free from intraoperative or postoperative fluid deficit (bleeding) related to alterations in clotting mechanisms. There is no evidence of

- uncontrollable intraoperative bleeding
- postoperative bleeding, hematoma development, and excessive wound drainage

CONTROLLING BLEEDING BY MECHANICAL METHODS

The RNFA applies pressure, hemostatic clips, clamps, and sutures as mechanical methods to control bleeding.

Regardless of the rate of blood flow, and whether it is from a denuded surface or a pulsatile artery, mechanical methods usually work. This discussion describes how to use pressure and apply hemostatic clips to control bleeding. Chapter 16 describes the application of clamps and suture.

Potential Alterations in Functional Health Patterns

Health Perception—Health Management Pattern

Diagnosis

High risk for injury related to the use of mechanical methods to achieve hemostasis

Definition

Presence of risk factors for the patient to experience injury related to the use of pressure and the application of hemostatic clips to achieve intraoperative hemostasis

Risk Factors

- Adhesions
- Obesity (excessive tissue mass impedes exposure of the operative field, which may interfere with the use of pressure or the application of hemostatic clips)
- Poor operative exposure
- Use of packs to stop bleeding
- Application of inappropriate-sized clip
- Defective clip appliers
- Improper identification of anatomical structures before clipping

Expected Outcome

The patient is free from injury related to the use of mechanical methods to achieve hemostasis. There is no evidence of

- intraoperative fluid deficit: hemorrhage due to the improper use of pressure or application of hemostatic clips
- postoperative infection or pain related to retained packing sponges
- postoperative pain or neurological deficit related to inadvertent clipping of nerves surrounding the bleeding site
- impaired tissue integrity; damaged or destroyed integumentary and subcutaneous tissue related to inadvertent use of excessive pressure or clipping of tissue surrounding the bleeding site

Pressure

Pressure is the direct or indirect exertion of force on a surface to stop bleeding. The RNFA applies direct pressure with one or more fingers to the site of bleeding. When applying indirect pressure, however, the RNFA uses the fingers or palm to compress the area adjacent to the site of active bleeding. The RNFA also uses laparotomy sponges or other materials, such as a pack, to apply pressure. Achieving hemostasis with packs, however, is not as reliable as ligating the bleeding vessels. The supplies needed for applying pressure are dry laparotomy sponges or other suitable packing materials.

Perioperative Nursing Interventions

- Before using pressure, assess the need for hemostasis and determine the appropriateness of using pressure on the anatomical structure requiring hemostasis.
- After the skin is incised, apply moderate pressure all along the incised surface.
- Control subcutaneous bleeding with a dry laparotomy sponge. Place the sponge on the bleeding surface and press with the fingertips; this provides hemostasis and countertraction. The surgeon often does the same on the opposite surface. If necessary, the RNFA may use two dry laparotomy sponges, one for each side of the wound, and pull on both sides on the incised surface in opposite directions.
- Use a dry laparotomy sponge to apply direct digital pressure to the area of active bleeding. If the site of bleeding is hidden from view or direct pressure is unsuccessful or is impractical, apply indirect pressure or pressure to adjacent structures. For example, pressure on the scalp slows the bleeding from the dermis after an incision. Pressure on the femoral artery slows blood flow from a severed popliteal artery.
- For sudden and profuse bleeding, apply direct dig-

ital pressure. Exert only enough pressure to stop or slow the blood flow. Use pressure as a temporary measure until bleeding is controlled by other means, such as ligatures and clips.
- Inform the scrub nurse and the circulating nurse of the location and number of laparotomy sponges used as packs. Report when the sponges are removed. Use only radiopaque packing materials.
- Before closing the wound, recheck areas that were packed for hemostasis.

Hemostatic Clips

The RNFA uses hemostatic clips to ligate blood vessels. Quick and easy to apply, clips are efficient and effective for achieving hemostasis. Nonabsorbable clips made of stainless steel or titanium are easily seen on x-ray films. Stainless steel clips, however, can severely interfere with a computed tomographic image. Titanium clips also interfere with computed tomographic images, but to a lesser degree than stainless steel clips. Metal clips are available in various sizes. Absorbable clips are made of polyglycolic acid, which hydrolyzes in about 8 weeks. The equipment and supplies needed for clip application are tissue forceps, clip appliers, and clips.

Perioperative Nursing Interventions

- Before using clips, assess the need for hemostasis and determine the appropriateness of using the clips on the anatomical structure requiring hemostasis.

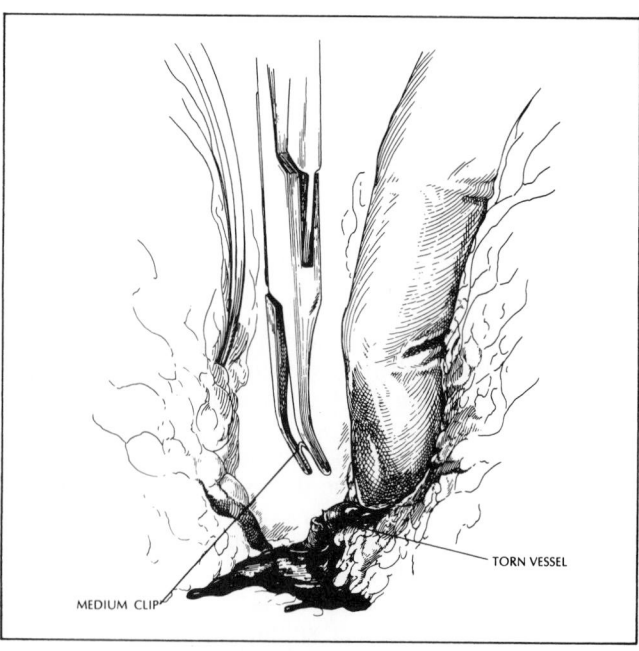

FIGURE 17–2. Application of clips to a traumatized vessel. (From *Weck Hemoclip surgical occluding clip.* [1985, August]. Research Triangle Park, NC: Edward Weck & Company.)

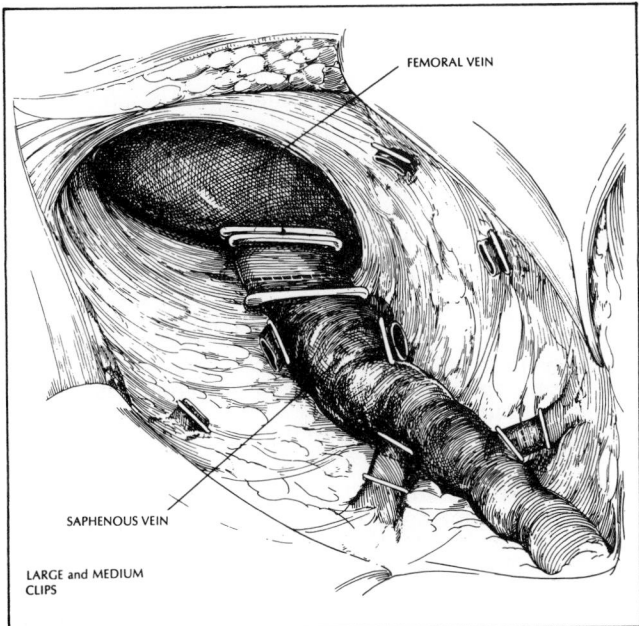

FIGURE 17–3. Clip the saphenous vein distally and proximally, then divide between the clips. (From *Weck Hemoclip surgical occluding clip*. [1985, August]. Research Triangle Park, NC: Edward Weck & Company.)

- Check clip appliers to ensure proper functioning. Look for symmetrical jaws that securely hold the clip and close without overlapping.
- In the event of bleeding, isolate the severed vessel and apply direct digital pressure with a dry laparotomy sponge to control bleeding. Next, slowly roll the sponge off the incised vessel and grasp it with a nontraumatic tissue forceps. Apply the clip to a skeletonized vessel (Fig. 17–2). Avoid clipping the tissue surrounding the vessel.
- After skeletonizing a vessel, apply two clips and then cut the vessel between the clips. Avoid clipping the tissue surrounding the vessel. For example, the RNFA clips the saphenous vein distally and proximally and then cuts the vein (Fig. 17–3).

Documentation and Communication Procedures

Except in extraordinary circumstances, the RNFA usually does not document or report the use of pressure to control bleeding. The use of clips, however, is documented in the intraoperative nurse's notes.

CONTROLLING BLEEDING BY THERMAL METHODS

The RNFA uses heat from an electrical current or a laser as thermal methods to control bleeding. Thermal methods of hemostasis effectively control bleeding from small blood vessels and denuded surfaces. These methods, however, are not reliable for controlling large venous or large pulsating arterial bleeding. This discussion describes the use of electrocautery, a plasma scalpel, and a laser to control bleeding.

Before using a thermal hemostatic method, the RNFA should assess the need for hemostasis and determine the appropriateness of using the particular method on the anatomical structure requiring hemostasis. Indiscriminate use of thermal hemostatic methods can result in permanent damage to vital structures, such as nerves. The implementation of appropriate safety precautions for the patient and the surgical team is essential when using thermal methods to provide hemostasis (Association of Operating Room Nurses [AORN], 1992).

Potential Alterations in Functional Health Patterns

Health Perception–Health Management Pattern

Diagnosis

High risk for injury related to the use of electrocautery to achieve hemostasis

Definition

Presence of risk factors for the patient to experience skin damage, hemorrhage, hematoma formation, postoperative pain, and neurological deficit related to the use of electrocautery to achieve intraoperative hemostasis

Risk Factors (AORN, 1992, *III*:5–2—5–3)

- Excessive body hair, scar tissue, or damaged tissue at dispersive electrode sites
- Presence of internal prosthetic devices at the dispersive electrode site
- Obesity (excessive subcutaneous tissue does not conduct electricity as well as muscle tissue)
- Poor tissue mass, especially over bony prominences
- Perspiration at dispersive electrode site
- Use of inflammable agents to prepare the operative site
- Use of electrocardiographic leads and rectal temperature probes
- Improper identification of anatomical structure before cauterizing
- Inappropriate use of electrocautery to stop bleeding
- Exposed metal touching the patient's skin
- Defective electrosurgical dispersive pad
- Inappropriate placement of electrosurgical dispersive pad
- Tension of the active and dispersive electrode cords
- Poor exposure of the operative field

Expected Outcome

The patient is free from injury related to the application of electrocautery to achieve intraoperative hemostasis. There is no evidence of

- impaired skin integrity at dispersive electrode and electrocardiographic lead sites
- intraoperative fluid deficit hemorrhage due to ineffective cauterization of blood vessels
- postoperative impaired tissue integrity hematoma formation due to ineffective cauterization of blood vessels and deep tissue burns
- postoperative pain or neurological deficit related to inadvertent cauterization of nerves surrounding the bleeding site

Diagnosis

High risk for injury related to the use of a laser to achieve hemostasis

Definition

Presence of risk factors for the patient to experience skin damage around the operative site and corneal burns related to the use of a laser to achieve intraoperative hemostasis

Risk Factors (AORN, 1992, III:10–1—10–3)

- Movement during laser operation
- Use of inflammable agents to prepare the operative site
- Use of inflammable draping material
- Poor exposure of the operative field
- Use of reflective instruments
- Use of dry sponges during a laser operation
- Inadequate eye protection for the patient
- Use of non–laser safe endotracheal tube during respiratory or digestive tract surgery
- Exposed tissue around the operative field

Expected Outcome

The patient is free from injury related to the use of laser equipment to achieve intraoperative hemostasis. There is no evidence of

- impaired tissue integrity surrounding the operative site
- corneal burns

Diagnosis

High risk for infection related to the use of electrocautery

Definition

Presence of risk factors for the patient to experience infection related to the use of electrocautery to achieve intraoperative hemostasis

Risk Factors

- Existing infection
- Immunosuppression secondary to blood transfusions
- Contaminated wound
- Retained blood products in the subcutaneous layer (provides a growth medium for bacteria)
- Excessive use of electrocautery resulting in large areas of tissue injury and necrosis, especially in the subcutaneous layer
- Charring of tissue during the cauterization of blood vessels
- Hematoma formation due to inadequate cauterization of blood vessels

Expected Outcome

The patient is free from infection related to the use of electrocautery to achieve intraoperative hemostasis. There is no evidence of

- chills and fever
- redness, warmth, and swelling around the incision or open wounds
- unusual wound drainage
- abnormal white blood cell count and positive cultures from wound drainage

Electrocautery

The hemostatic mechanism of electrocautery is heat. Electrical current flows into the tissue and produces heat that desiccates tissue and coagulates blood. Electrosurgical units (ESUs) consist of a generator, a foot switch and active electrode (a hand-controlled active electrode combines the two), and the electrical plug, cord, and connections. Many units have two modes of functioning: monopolar (also called unipolar) and bipolar. In the monopolar mode, current flows from the generator, through the patient, and back to the generator via the dispersive electrode pad. With the bipolar mode, however, current flows from the generator between two tips of a forceps and back to the generator. The current does not flow through the patient; therefore, a dispersive electrode pad is unnecessary (AORN, 1992). The equipment and supplies needed are dry laparotomy sponges, appropriate tissue forceps, the ESU, and an active electrode. Monopolar units require a dispersive electrode.

The RNFA uses the ESUs for coagulation, cutting, and fulguration. Frequently used, the coagulation mode achieves hemostasis by sealing a blood vessel with heat. The cutting mode uses a higher-frequency current that produces continuous hot sparks. Cells in contact with the hot active electrode explode and tissue is separated. Some ESUs have a blend mode for the cutting and coagulation functions. With this mode, the RNFA can simultaneously cut tissue and stop bleeding. Fulguration destroys tissue by continuous electrical sparks. Deep tissue necrosis, however, is likely to occur with fulguration (Kneedler and Dodge, 1987; Rothrock, 1987).

Hemostasis with electrocautery is not as reliable as ties or suture ligatures; therefore, the RNFA should use it only on small vessels. Hemostasis of large vessels must be accomplished with ties, clips, or suture ligatures. Tissue density and the amount of fluid in or surrounding the tissue also affects the amount of current and the time necessary to produce hemostasis.

A defective ESU can cause burns or electrical shocks of the patient and the surgical team and increases the risk of fire and explosion hazards. The RNFA should not use the ESU in the presence of inflammable agents such as alcohol. The depth of tissue injured by the heat produced through electrocautery is difficult to predict and to control. When one is using electrocautery, injury to adjacent nerves or other anatomical structures can easily occur. Electrical burns can occur at the site of the dispersive electrode, under electrocardiographic leads, at temperature probe entry sites, at positional pressure points, and at sites where the patient's skin comes in contact with grounded metal, such as the OR bed (AORN, 1992). Burns of the skin edges may occur if a noninsulated portion the active electrode inadvertently contacts the skin while the electrocautery is applied to a deeper structure.

Perioperative Nursing Interventions

- Follow institutional protocols regarding ESU safety and apply the AORN recommendations for electrocautery (AORN, 1992).
- After positioning the patient so that the skin has no contact with metal, apply the dispersive electrode to clean, dry skin over a large muscle mass. Place the electrode as close to the operative site as feasible. Avoid bony prominences, hairy surfaces, scarred areas, implanted metal devices, or prostheses. Ensure that the pad has even contact with the skin. Check all connections to ensure that they are intact. Repeat the inspection whenever the patient's position is changed. Set the ESU to the operator's specifications. Confirm settings verbally with the operator. Keep settings at the lowest levels possible.
- Use isolated electrocardiographic leads and do not place the leads between the operative site and the dispersive electrode.
- Before using the ESU, assess the need for hemostasis and determine the appropriateness of using the instrument on the anatomical structure requiring hemostasis by evaluating vessel size. If the vessel is large, use a ligature or clips to control the bleeding.
- Check the active electrode (pencil) before use. Look for frayed cords and ensure that the tip of the active electrode is securely seated. Activate the electrode by depressing and then releasing the appropriate switches. The unit should immediately activate when the switch is depressed and deactivate when the switch is released.
- Do not indiscriminately activate the electrode. Identify the cautery site and adjacent structures. Do not cauterize adjacent nerves or tissue unless their destruction is intended.
- In the event of bleeding, isolate the severed vessel and apply direct digital pressure with a dry laparotomy sponge to control bleeding. Next, slowly roll the sponge off the severed vessel and touch the vessel with the activated electrode for as long as it takes to blanch the tissue. Charring the tissue is usually not necessary. When using tissue forceps, grasp the end of the vessel with the forceps and touch the activated electrode to the tissue forceps for as long as it takes to blanch the tissue. Avoid grasping the surrounding tissue with the forceps. If the scrub nurse operates the active electrode, verbally indicate when to begin the electrical current. Stop the flow of current by releasing the tissue from the grasp of the forceps.

Laser

Laser is an acronym for light amplification by stimulated emissions of radiation. Carbon dioxide, argon, and yttrium-aluminum-garnet are used to create the laser beam. Each substance produces a different light with its own specific wavelength. The water in cells evaporates so quickly that the cell explodes and vaporizes. This thermal effect cuts, cauterizes, and sterilizes tissue. The equipment and supplies needed for laser surgery are damp laparotomy sponges, dull nonreflective instruments, and appropriate eye protection devices that stop beam transmission. The temperatures generated by the laser beam are high.

Perioperative Nursing Interventions
(AORN, 1992, *III*:10–1—10–3)

- Cooperate with the circulator in applying the AORN recommendations for laser use in the operating room (AORN, 1992) when preparing the room, the surgical team, and the patient for laser surgery.
- Place warning signs at all entrances to the room.
- Wear eye protection appropriate to the laser being used.
- Tape saline-moistened pads to the closed eyelids of the anesthetized patient or provide eye protection if the patient is awake.
- Apply damp laparotomy sponges to the tissue surrounding the operative site.
- Use flame-resistant or moistened drapes.
- Use dulled, ebonized, or nonreflective anodized finished instruments near the site of laser use.

- Use wet tongue blades or quartz or titanium rods as a backstop for the beam. This prevents the beam from inadvertently hitting underlying tissue.
- Inform the circulator when the laser is not in use so she or he may set the laser on standby.
- Evacuate the noxious fumes and laser plume with appropriate scavenging devices.

Plasma Scalpel

The heated cutting blade of the plasma scalpel achieves hemostasis by heat sealing the blood vessels as they are cut. The system consists of three components: the power unit, which provides control and calibrating functions; the reusable scalpel handle, which is connected to the power unit by a cable; and the disposable blade, which comes in sizes similar to those of the No. 10 and No. 15 blades. The equipment and supplies needed when using the plasma scalpel are the three components of the system and dry laparotomy sponges.

Tissue damage is minimal with the plasma scalpel because only a thin layer of tissue is heated by the cutting blade. Studies have shown that infection resistance of wounds made with the plasma scalpel is the same as that of those made with a cold blade and slightly better than that of those made with electrocautery. The plasma scalpel blade is heated by electrical microcircuitry. Because the current does not pass into the patient, a grounding pad is not needed. A plasma scalpel cannot conduct electrocautery current to clamps or tissue forceps. Serious damage to the power unit can result if the blade comes in contact with an activated electrocautery tip. The surgeon selects the temperature of the cutting blade on the basis of tissue requirements. Some systems provide a hand-controlled switch that, when depressed, causes the blade to become hotter. During use, heat dissipates in pooled blood or other body fluids. Most handles require ethylene oxide sterilization.

Perioperative Nursing Interventions

- Before using the plasma scalpel, assess the need for hemostasis and determine the appropriateness of using the instrument on the anatomical structure requiring hemostasis.
- Request the appropriate temperature settings (110°C for skin incisions). For other tissues, the temperature setting is usually between 180 and 240°C).
- Maintain a dry operative field by blotting blood and other body fluids with dry laparotomy sponges.
- When using the blade, make long slow strokes to prevent the onset of bleeding. Blood vessels 2 mm and smaller should seal as they are cut. For larger vessels, exert light pressure on the bleeder with the flat of the blade.
- During the procedure, occasionally clean the blade

with a dry laparotomy sponge to prevent thermal isolation.
- Do not allow an activated electrocautery tip to come in contact with the blade.
- Do not use the heated blade to make skin incisions through plastic adhesive drapes.
- Do not rest the blade on the drapes or on the patient when activated.
- Do not immerse the handle in liquid.

Documentation and Communication Procedures

When using *electrocautery*, document the generator number, power settings, and electrocardiographic electrode and dispersive plate placement in the intraoperative nurse's notes. In addition, document the condition of the skin at the site of the dispersive plate and electrocardiographic electrodes before and after the procedure and note any skin lesions postoperatively that were not apparent preoperatively.

When using a *laser*, document the unit number, power setting, and safety precautions used in the intraoperative nursing notes. Include a description of the preoperative and postoperative condition of the skin surrounding the operative site.

Document *plasma scalpel* use by including the number of the power unit in the intraoperative nurse's notes. If they occur, note the presence of thermal burns.

CONTROLLING BLEEDING BY CHEMICAL METHODS

Direct topical application of chemical agents such as microfibrillar collagen, hemostat gelatin sponge, collagen sponge, and oxidized cellulose to areas of active bleeding are chemical methods to control bleeding.

The RNFA uses chemical agents as an adjunct to hemostasis when controlling bleeding by ligatures or when other conventional methods are ineffective or impractical. Successful use of chemical agents entails a slow rate of blood flow, as in denuded, oozing surfaces of the gallbladder bed or liver abrasions. The use of chemical agents on pulsating arterial bleeding is contraindicated (PDR, 1992). The RNFA should determine the appropriateness of using a chemical agent on the anatomical structure requiring hemostasis. In addition, the RNFA should consider wound classification before using a chemical agent because the use of most agents is ill advised or contraindicated in contaminated wounds. To use chemical agents when blood or other fluids submerge the bleeding site, the bleeding must be visible. Chemical agents are not designed to act as a tampon or a plug in a bleeding site (PDR, 1992). The patient should have no known allergies to the agent being used or to the substance from which the agent was derived.

Potential Alterations in Functional Health Patterns

Health Perception–Health Management Pattern

Diagnosis

High risk for infection related to the use of microfibrillar collagen hemostat, gelatin sponge, and oxidized cellulose

Definition

Presence of risk factors for the patient to experience postoperative infection related to the use of microfibrillar collagen hemostat, gelatin sponge, and oxidized cellulose to achieve hemostasis

Risk Factors

Microfibrillar Collagen Hemostat
- Suppressed immune system secondary to blood transfusions
- Retained blood products in the subcutaneous tissue (retained blood products provide an excellent growth medium for bacteria)

Gelatin Sponge
- Allergy to gelatin products
- Inflammation of the operative site, wound contamination, or infection
- Application to wound edges

Oxidized Cellulose
- Contaminated wound
- Suppressed immune system secondary to blood transfusions
- Retained blood products in the subcutaneous tissue (retained blood products provide an excellent growth medium for bacteria)

Expected Outcome

The patient is free from postoperative infection related to the use of microfibrillar collagen hemostat, gelatin sponge, and oxidized cellulose to achieve intraoperative hemostasis. There is no evidence of

- chills and fever; redness, warmth, and swelling around the incision or open wounds; and unusual wound drainage
- abnormal white blood cell count and positive cultures from wound drainage

Diagnosis

High risk for injury related to the use of microfibrillar collagen hemostat

Definition

The presence of risk factors for the patient to experience abscess and hematoma formation, bone and tissue injury due to insecure orthopedic prosthesis, nonhealing of wound skin edges, bowel adhesion, compromised urinary output, aspiration, blood contamination, and allergic response related to the use of microfibrillar collagen hemostat to achieve intraoperative hemostasis

Risk Factors

- Use of a microfibrillar collagen hemostat (significantly reduces the bonding strength of methylmethacrylate)
- Application to wound edges
- Failure to remove excess amounts of agent
- Use of blood scavaging systems
- Allergy to bovine products

Expected Outcome

The patient is free from injury related to the use of microfibrillar collagen hemostat to achieve intraoperative hemostasis. There is no evidence of

- abscess and hematoma formation
- failure of orthopedic prosthesis due to a reduction of bonding strength of methylmethacrylate
- nonhealing of wound skin edges
- bowel adhesion
- compromised urinary output due to mechanical pressure against the ureter
- aspiration of microfibrillar collagen hemostats
- blood contamination with microfibrillar collagen hemostat particles
- allergic response to microfibrillar collagen hemostat

Diagnosis

High risk for injury related to the use of collagen sponge

Definition

Presence of risk factors for the patient to experience hematoma formation, pain, and neurological deficit related to the use of collagen sponge to achieve intraoperative hemostasis

Risk Factors

- Allergy to materials of bovine origin
- Use in urological, ophthalmological, and neurological replacement procedures
- Use in the presence of methylmethacrylate
- Application to wound edges

Expected Outcome

The patient is free from injury related to the use of collagen sponge to achieve intraoperative hemostasis. There is no evidence of

- hematoma formation due to vascular oozing from improper application or use of gelatin sponge
- formation of adhesions
- allergic reactions
- postoperative pain or neurological deficit

Diagnosis

High risk for injury related to the use of oxidized cellulose for hemostasis

Definition

Presence of risk factors for the patient to experience interference with callus formation in bone defects, stenosis of vascular structures, headaches, sneezing, and burning and stinging sensations to localized application areas related to the use of collagen sponge to achieve intraoperative hemostasis

Risk Factors

- Orthopedic surgery
- Spinal cord and optic nerve surgery
- Vascular surgery
- Nasal surgery (polypectomy) when used for packing
- Hemorrhoidectomy, skin graft donor sites, and dermabrasion

Expected Outcome

The patient is free from injury related to the use of oxidized cellulose for hemostasis. There is no evidence of

- impaired bone healing
- vascular stenosis
- headaches
- sneezing, burning and stinging sensations to localized application areas

Nutritional-Metabolic Pattern

Diagnosis

High risk for impaired tissue integrity related to the use of gelatin sponge

Definition

Presence of risk factors for the patient to experience nervous, integumentary, and subcutaneous tissue damage related to the use of gelatin sponge to achieve intraoperative hemostasis

Risk Factors

- Inappropriate application of gelatin sponge, resulting in bleeding after closure
- Use during neurosurgery and tendon repairs
- Application to wound edges
- Presence of tissue inflammation

Expected Outcome

The patient is free from damage to nervous, integumentary, or subcutaneous tissue related to the use of gelatin sponge to achieve intraoperative hemostasis. There is no evidence of

- hematoma formation due to vascular oozing from improper application or use of gelatin sponge
- postoperative pain or neurological deficit related to inappropriate use of gelatin sponge

Microfibrillar Collagen Hemostat

Microfibrillar collagen hemostat (Avitene) is a purified bovine corium (dermal) collagen. It is a fibrous, water-insoluble partial hydrochloric salt. Microfibrillar collagen hemostat is prepared in a loose fibrous form and in a compacted nonwoven web form. When microfibrillar collagen hemostat comes in contact with a bleeding surface, platelets are attracted to it and adhere to the fibrils. The platelets then aggregate, beginning the clotting phenomenon (PDR, 1992).

Because it is a foreign substance, microfibrillar collagen hemostat may potentiate wound infections and formation of abscesses. Microfibrillar collagen hemostat may significantly reduce the bonding strength of methylmethacrylate. When applied to wound edges during the closure of incisions, it interferes with the healing of the skin edges. Failure to remove excess microfibrillar collagen hemostat may result in bowel adhesion or mechanical pressure significant to compromise the ureter. Failure to remove excess microfibrillar collagen hemostat in otolaryngological procedures may result in aspiration of particles. Fragments of microfibrillar collagen hemostat may pass through filters of blood scavenging systems. Microfibrillar collagen hemostat is contraindicated in patients sensitive to materials of bovine origin.

Equipment and supplies needed when using microfibrillar collagen hemostat are dry tissue forceps free of blood, dry lap sponges, and suction.

Microfibrillar collagen hemostat is inactivated by autoclaving. Sterilization by ethylene oxide is contraindicated. Ethylene oxide reacts with the bound hydrochloric acid in microfibrillar collagen hemostat to form ethylene chlorohydrin. Microfibrillar collagen hemostat adheres to wet gloves, instruments, and tissue surfaces. Furthermore, moistening microfibrillar collagen hemostat with saline or thrombin impairs its ability to act as a hemostatic agent. Microfibrillar collagen hemostat cannot control bleeding due to systemic disorders. The effect of microfibrillar collagen hemostat on platelet adhesion and aggregation, however, is not inhibited by heparin.

Perioperative Nursing Interventions

- Assess the need for the use of microfibrillar collagen hemostat to provide hemostasis
- Ascertain if the patient has any known allergies to bovine derivatives.
- Determine the adequacy of primary efforts at hemostasis (clamping, electrocautery, tying, and suturing) before using microfibrillar collagen hemo-

stat. Evaluate the rate of blood flow. Ascertain if the bleeding site can be made visible and accessible.

- Determine the appropriateness of microfibrillar collagen hemostat to the anatomical structure on which it would be used.
- Keep microfibrillar collagen hemostat away from skin edges when closing the incision.
- Do not use microfibrillar collagen hemostat on bone surfaces to which prosthetic devices are to be attached with methylmethacrylate.
- Determine the appropriateness of microfibrillar collagen hemostat in light of the wound classification. Using microfibrillar collagen hemostat is ill-advised in the presence of contaminated or infected wounds.
- When applying or assisting in the application of microfibrillar collagen hemostat, suction or sponge the area dry. Provide additional exposure as needed. With clean dry tissue forceps, such as Mayo forceps, apply microfibrillar collagen hemostat to the bleeding site. Using moderate pressure, hold a dry lap sponge on the bleeding site. Hemostasis usually occurs in about 1 minute. The time will vary depending on the force and severity of the bleeding. Three to 5 minutes may be required for brisk bleeding such as splenic lacerations or arterial suture lines. Additional microfibrillar collagen hemostat may be used as needed. Apply the nonwoven web form of microfibrillar collagen hemostat in small squares to the bleeding site. Cover the site with a dry cottonoid for small areas or lap sponge for larger areas. A suction tip may be used to hold pressure on the cottonoid. Pack microfibrillar collagen hemostat firmly into the spongy bone surface to control oozing from cancellous bone. Avoid spilling microfibrillar collagen hemostat on nonbleeding surfaces, particularly in the abdominal or thoracic viscera.
- Remove excess microfibrillar collagen hemostat from all surfaces by gently teasing with blunt forceps and irrigation before closing the wound.
- Avoid the reintroduction of blood from operative sites treated with microfibrillar collagen hemostat. Notify the circulating nurse to discontinue the use of blood scavenging equipment once microfibrillar collagen hemostat is used.
- Discard unused microfibrillar collagen hemostat.
- Do not resterilize microfibrillar collagen hemostat.

Absorbable Gelatin Sponge

Gelatin sponge (Gelfoam) is a pliable sponge of purified gelatin, which can hold several times its weight. The sponge liquefies in 2 to 5 days after application to the bleeding mucosa of the rectum, the vagina, or the nasal passages and is absorbed in 4 to 6 weeks without excessive scar formation. Heating gelatin sponge, however, affects absorption time (PDR, 1992).

Because gelatin sponge absorbs fluid, it expands and exerts pressure on adjacent structures. Implantation in the brain or around the spinal cord may result in compression of these structures owing to the accumulation of sterile fluid around the sponge. Gelatin sponge interferes with the healing of the skin edges when used in the closure of incisions and has caused excessive fibrosis when used during tendon repairs. Adverse effects have occurred when gelatin sponge is used in areas of intense inflammation (PDR, 1992). In addition, when gelatin sponge is used in the presence of gross contamination or infection, bacteria can become enmeshed in the gelatin sponge and thus cause the formation of an abscess.

The equipment and supplies needed are straight Mayo scissors, dry tissue forceps free from blood, dry laparotomy sponges, suction, and the gelatin sponge.

Perioperative Nursing Interventions

- Determine the appropriateness of using gelatin sponge on the anatomical structure requiring hemostasis. Evaluate the appropriateness of the gelatin sponge on the basis of the wound classification. Do not use during neurosurgery, for tendon repairs, and in the presence of inflammation. Recommend the use of another agent.
- Before using gelatin sponge, evaluate the effectiveness of hemostasis by mechanical and thermal methods. Look at the rate of blood flow and, if possible, make the site accessible by clearing away blood with suction or a dry sponge.
- Provide additional exposure as needed.
- Cut pieces of gelatin sponges into the desired size.
- For dry application, compress each piece between the fingers and then use a clean tissue forceps to apply it to the bleeding site. Using moderate pressure, hold it with a dry laparotomy sponge on the bleeding site for 10 to 15 seconds.
- The RNFA may apply a wet or damp piece. For wet application, the scrub nurse should have the sponges prepared for use by immersing the cut pieces in saline, squeezing out the air bubbles, and then placing the pieces back in the saline until used. For damp application, blot the piece of gelatin sponge on a dry laparotomy sponge. Using moderate pressure, hold the gelatin sponge in place with a dry laparotomy sponge for at least 10 to 15 seconds. Capillary action draws the blood into the gelatin. Wet the laparotomy sponge with saline to avoid pulling the gelatin off the site when removing the sponge.
- An alternative method of using wet or dry gelatin sponge is to apply suction to the laparotomy sponge while holding the gelatin in place. This technique draws blood into the gelatin and seems to hasten clotting.
- Pack gelatin loosely in closed spaces or cavities because it swells as it absorbs fluid. Apply light pressure in cavities or closed spaces.
- To prevent recurrent bleeding, leave the gelatin

sponge in place. If desired, the RNFA may close the wound with the gelatin sponge left in place.
- Keep gelatin away from skin edges when closing the incision; gelatin interferes with wound healing.
- Discard unused gelatin sponges; do not resterilize.

Absorbable Collagen Sponge

The collagen sponge (Instat, Hemopad) is a purified and lyophilized (freeze-dried) bovine dermal collagen. It is prepared as a lightly cross-linked spongelike pad. The collagen protein has a helical structure, which is preserved in the manufacturing process. Collagen's inherent hemostatic action is dependent on this helical structure. When blood comes in contact with collagen, platelets aggregate and release clotting factors. Collagen sponge is absorbed in 8 to 10 weeks (PDR, 1992).

Because collagen sponge absorbs fluid and may expand, exerting pressure on adjacent structures, it is not recommended for use in neurological, urological, and ophthalmological procedures. Collagen sponge reduces the bonding strength of methyl methacrylate and interferes with the healing of the skin edges. Formation of adhesions, foreign body reactions, and allergic reactions are among the most serious adverse effects of collagen sponges. Heating inactivates the collagen sponge.

The equipment and supplies needed are straight Mayo scissors, dry tissue forceps free from blood, dry laparotomy sponges, suction, and the collagen sponge.

Perioperative Nursing Interventions

- Before surgery, determine if the patient has allergies to collagen sponges or bovine derivatives.
- Determine the appropriateness of using collagen sponge on the anatomical structure requiring hemostasis. In addition, evaluate the appropriateness of the collagen sponge on the basis of the wound classification. Avoid the use of collagen sponges in neurological, urological, and ophthalmological procedures and in the presence of methyl methacrylate.
- Before using collagen sponge, evaluate the effectiveness of hemostasis by mechanical and thermal methods. Look at the rate of blood flow, and, if possible, make the site accessible by clearing away blood with suction or a dry sponge.
- Provide additional exposure as needed.
- Pack collagen loosely in closed spaces or cavities because it swells as it absorbs fluid. Compression of adjacent structures can occur as the collagen swells. Do not use collagen sponges on bone surfaces to which prosthetic devices are to be attached with methyl methacrylate.
- Cut pieces of collagen sponges into the desired sizes. It is most effective when used dry. With clean tissue forceps, apply it to the bleeding site. Hold it with a dry lap sponge on the bleeding site using

moderate pressure. Hemostasis usually occurs in 2 to 5 minutes. Remove excessive collagen before closing the wound.
- Keep collagen away from skin edges when closing the incision.
- Discard unused gelatin sponges and do not resterilize.

Oxidized Regenerated Cellulose

Oxidized cellulose (Surgicel, Surgicel Nu-Knit) is an absorbable, white, knitted fabric, which has a faint caramel odor. It can be sutured or cut without fraying. Oxidized cellulose is stored at room temperature. Performance is not affected by the cellulose's age, but discoloration may occur. When saturated with blood, it swells into a dark gelatinous mass, which aids in the formation of clot. The mechanism of how oxidized cellulose works is not clearly understood. It appears to have a local physical effect, rather than altering normal clotting mechanisms (PDR, 1992).

Autoclaving causes physical breakdown of oxidized cellulose. The hemostatic effect of oxidized cellulose is unaffected by the addition of thrombin. The activity of thrombin, however, is destroyed by the low pH of oxidized cellulose. The hemostatic effect of oxidized cellulose is diminished when it is moistened with water, saline, other hemostatic agents, or anti-infective agents.

Oxidized cellulose is bactericidal to a wide range of gram-positive and gram-negative aerobes and anaerobes. In contrast to other chemical hemostatic agents, it has not been shown to potentiate infections in experimental studies. Even so, it is not recommended as a replacement for prophylactic or therapeutic antibiotics. Because it is a foreign body, its use in contaminated wounds can potentiate infection.

Oxidized cellulose may interfere with callus formation when used in bone defects, such as fractures. Additionally, it absorbs fluid and may expand, exerting pressure on adjacent structures. This is especially true when it is used around the spinal cord in laminectomies and around the optic nerve. The rate at which it is absorbed is dependent on the amount used, the extent of blood saturation, and the tissue bed. Encapsulation and foreign body reactions can occur if oxidized cellulose is left in the wound. Stenosis of vascular structures may occur if oxidized cellulose is used to wrap a vessel tightly. The low pH of oxidized cellulose may cause burning or stinging sensations, headaches, and sneezing when it is used as a pack for epistaxis. It may also account for burning or stinging when cellulose is used after the removal of a nasal polyp, hemorrhoidectomy, and application to wound surfaces such as donor sites, venous stasis ulcerations, and dermabrasions.

Use oxidized cellulose only in the presence of whole blood. Oozing of other body fluids, such as serum, does not react with oxidized cellulose to produce satisfactory hemostasis. In addition, do not use oxidized cellulose as a wound-packing material.

The equipment and supplies needed are straight Mayo scissors, dry tissue forceps free from blood, dry laparotomy sponges, suction, and the oxidized cellulose.

Perioperative Nursing Interventions

- Determine the appropriateness of using oxidized cellulose on the anatomical structure requiring hemostasis. In addition, evaluate the appropriateness of the oxidized cellulose on the basis of the wound classification.
- Before using oxidized cellulose, evaluate the effectiveness of hemostasis by mechanical and thermal methods. Look at the rate of blood flow and, if possible, make the site accessible by clearing away blood with suction or a dry sponge.
- Provide additional exposure as needed.
- Avoid its use in fractured bones, as it may interfere with callus formation.
- Avoid wrapping structures such as blood vessels and ureters.
- Cut pieces of oxidized cellulose into the desired size.
- Use only the amount necessary to achieve hemostasis.
- Apply it, dry, with clean tissue forceps to the bleeding site. Hold it with a dry laparotomy sponge on the bleeding site, using moderate pressure until

- If possible, remove oxidized cellulose before closing the wound. It may, however, be left in place with no adverse effects if it is properly applied and is present in small amounts.
- Do not use it as a packing material for bleeding wounds.
- Discard unused oxidized cellulose and do not resterilize.
- Evaluate the patient postoperatively for signs of stinging and burning, sneezing, or headaches when oxidized cellulose was used for epistaxis. Look for postoperative burning or stinging when used after the removal of a nasal polyp, hemorrhoidectomy, and application to wound surfaces such as donor sites, venous stasis ulcerations, and dermabrasions. If it is causing the patient difficulty, recommend removal.

Documentation and Communication Procedures

Document the use of microfibrillar collagen hemostat, gelatin sponge, collagen sponge, and oxidized cellulose in the intraoperative nurse's notes. Inform postoperative nurses if oxidized cellulose is used for packing or is applied to wound surfaces.

SUMMARY

The RNFA plays an important role in providing hemostasis during a surgical procedure. Knowledge of the mechanisms of clotting and how to assess the patient's clotting mechanisms will enable the RNFA to implement methods to control bleeding by mechanical, thermal, and chemical methods.

ACKNOWLEDGEMENT
The author wishes to thank Sherroll Neill, M.D., Tyler, TX, general and vascular surgeon, friend, mentor, and critic for his technical review of the text.

Bibliography

Association of Operating Room Nurses. (1992). *Standards and recommended practices for perioperative nursing*. Denver.

Fay, M. F. (1987). Drainage systems: Their role in wound healing. *AORN Journal, 46*, 442–455.

Guyton, A. C. (1991). *Textbook of medical physiology* (8th ed.). Philadelphia: W. B. Saunders.

Kneedler, J. A., Dodge, G. H. (Eds.) (1987). *Perioperative nursing care: The nursing perspective* (2nd ed.). Boston: Blackwell Scientific.

1992 Physicians' desk reference (46th ed). Montvale, NJ: Medical Economics Company.

Polk, H. S., Stone, H. H., Gardener, B. (Eds.). (1987). *Basic surgery* (3rd ed.). East Norwalk, CT: Appleton-Century-Crofts.

Regis, M. L., Hill, S. B., Schmidt, C. V. (1986). Wolff-Parkinson-White syndrome: Cryosurgical ablation of accessory pathways. *AORN Journal, 44*, 742–756.

Rothrock, J. C. (Ed.). (1990). *Perioperative nursing care planning*. St. Louis: C.V. Mosby.

Rothrock, J. C. (Ed.). (1987). *The RN first assistant: An expanded perioperative nursing role*. Philadelphia: J. B. Lippincott.

Salvatiarra, O. (1986). Donor-specific transfusions in living-related transplantation. *World Journal of Surgery, 10*, 361–368.

CHAPTER 18

Facilitating Postoperative Care

Vicki J. Fox

DEFINITION

Facilitating postoperative care refers to the activities performed by the registered nurse first assistant (RNFA) during the postoperative period to make the patient physically and psychologically ready to begin convalescence and rehabilitation.

MEASURABLE CRITERIA

The RNFA demonstrates competency to facilitate postoperative care by

- recognizing postoperative wound complications.
- recognizing fever, tachycardia, pulmonary complications, thrombophlebitis, urinary tract infections, and adynamic ileus
- assessing postoperative comfort level
- assessing nausea and vomiting

- ensuring the proper functioning of devices employed to assist recovery

ROLE OF THE REGISTERED NURSE FIRST ASSISTANT

Because practice settings vary, the involvement of the RNFA in postoperative care varies. The postoperative phase of care begins with admission of the patient to the postanesthesia care unit (PACU) and ends with the resolution of postoperative sequelae (*A job analysis for the RN first assistant*, 1992). The RNFA's activities during the postoperative phase should complement the nursing care the patient receives in the PACU, the nursing unit, the clinic, and the home.

CONSIDERATIONS

To facilitate postoperative care, the RNFA must understand the critical variables that affect convales-

TABLE 18–5. TYPICAL APPEARANCE TIMES OF COMPLICATIONS AFTER MAJOR ABDOMINAL SURGERY

Type of Complication	Postoperative Day									
	1	2	3	4	5	6	7	8	9	10
Pulmonary	X	X								
Ear, nose, and throat	X	X	X							
Urinary tract			X	X	X					
Thromboembolic					X	X	X	X	X	X
Wound infection, deep abscess				X	X	X	X	X	X	X
Anastomotic leaks and abscess						X	X	X		

Adapted from Polk, H. S., Stone, H. H., Gardener, B. (Eds.). (1987). *Basic surgery* (3rd ed.) (p. 706). East Norwalk, CT: Appleton-Century-Crofts.

- Absence of frequency or burning on urination
- Return of bowel sounds and function in an appropriate amount of time
- Normal breath sounds and respiratory rate
- Heart rate within normal limits
- Absence of pain and swelling in the extremities

Standard IV

The patient experiences physiological and psychological comfort after surgery.

Criteria

The following demonstrate an acceptable comfort level:

- Absence of nausea, vomiting, and hiccups
- Verbalization of adequate pain relief
- Relaxed facial expression
- Gradual increase in activity level

RECOGNIZING POSTOPERATIVE WOUND COMPLICATIONS

The experienced RNFA should be able to recognize the signs of wound complications, identify the underlying cause, and recommend and initiate appropriate treatment. The most common wound complications are infection, abscess, seroma, gas gangrene, wound dehiscence, and nonhealing wounds.

Infection

Infections manifest themselves in a variety of ways. However, these signs of infection are always present:

- Pain and tenderness due to irritation of local nerve endings
- Increased temperature of the area involved
- Redness in response to the vascularization process
- Swelling due to edema and inflammatory exudate

Wound complications frequently have systemic manifestations, such as elevated temperature and tachycardia. A clue to the type of pathogen involved is the postoperative day on which the infection becomes apparent (Table 18–6).

Streptococcus and *Staphylococcus aureus* usually cause cellulitis. This diffuse inflammatory response, without tissue necrosis or purulent exudate, exhibits all the signs of an infection and may involve a large area of skin surface. Sometimes, the skin has the texture of an orange peel. The patient may also be febrile. When the inflammation has small focal areas of tissue necrosis and multiple tiny pockets of pus, the infection is called *phlegmon*. The inoculum is a combination of *Streptococcus* and *S. aureus*, or an aerobic gram-negative rod. If the infection has spread to the lymph system, the condition is known as *lymphangitis*. The treatment of both is the administration of a parenteral antibiotic effective against gram-positive cocci. The physician may order an antibiotic according to what typically causes this type of infection. Cultures may also be ordered. If the correct antibiotics are administered, the condition of the wound improves rapidly, usually within 24 hours.

The use of heat to promote wound vasodilation is unnecessary; local vessels are already maximally dilated (Polk et al., 1987). Heat, however, seems to increase patient comfort. If these measures do not improve the condition of the wound soon, the RNFA should suspect an underlying abscess, which would necessitate drainage.

Potential Alterations in Functional Health Patterns

Health Perception–Health Management Pattern

Diagnosis

High risk for postoperative wound infection

Definition

The presence of risk factors for the patient's wound to be invaded by pathogenic organisms

Risk Factors (see Table 18–3)

Expected Outcome

The patient is free from a postoperative wound infection. There is no evidence of

- chills and fever
- redness, warmth, and swelling around the incision or open wounds
- unusual wound drainage
- abnormal white blood cell count and positive cultures of wound drainage

Perioperative Nursing Interventions

- Assess the wound for cellulitis, phlegmon, or lymphangitis.

TABLE 18–6. POSTOPERATIVE WOUND INFECTIONS			
Onset (Postoperative Day)	Usual Pathogen	Wound Appearance	Other Signs
1–3	*Clostridium perfringens* and related species	Brawny, hemorrhagic, cool, occasional gaseous crepitation, putrid dishwater exudate, intense local pain	High sustained fever (39–40°C), irrational, leukocytosis >15,000/mm³, occasional jaundice
2–3	*Streptococcus*	Erythematous, warm, tender, occasionally hemorrhagic with blebs, serous exudate	High spiking fever (up to 39–40°C), irrational at times, leukocytosis >15,000/mm³, rare jaundice
3–5	*Staphylococcus*	Erythematous, warm, tender, purulent exudate	High spiking fever (up to 38–39°C), irrational at times, leukocytosis 12,000–20,000/mm³, rare jaundice
>5	Gram-negative rod	Erythematous, warm, tender, purulent exudate	Sustained low-grade to moderate fever (38–39°C), rational, leukocytosis 10,000–16,000/mm³
>5	Symbiotic	Erythematous, warm, tender, focal necrosis, purulent, putrid exudate	Moderate to high fever (38–40°C), mentation variable, leukocytosis >15,000/mm³, occasional jaundice

From Polk, H. S., Stone, H. H., Gardener, B. (Eds.). (1987). *Basic surgery* (3rd ed.) (p. 151). East Norwalk, CT: Appleton-Century-Crofts.

- Look for systemic infection.
- Determine the patient's comfort level and assess the skin condition.
- Assess the wound for gas formation (most common sites are the extremities after traumatic injury).
- Monitor the white blood cell count.
- Culture the wound if necessary.
- Refer for medical treatment if indicated.
- In the event of infection, implement measures to reduce pain such as elevating the affected area to decrease edema and applying moist heat for patient comfort.
- Administer antibiotics as ordered.
- If antibiotics have not been ordered, recommend an appropriate antibiotic to the physician.
- Implement patient education measures regarding the status of infection and its treatment.
- Reevaluate the affected area after 24 hours of antibiotic therapy.
- Document findings and activities according to institutional policy.

Abscess

An abscess forms when the inflammatory process becomes suppurative, is confined within a single anatomical space, and is surrounded by granulation tissue. The abscess consists of purulent materials, necrotic host tissue, and bacteria. *S. aureus*, gram-negative rods, and a variety of anaerobic strains working synergistically with gram-negative rods are the bacteria usually found in an abscess.

The abscessed area is usually tender to the touch. If touched in this area, the patient most likely indicates pain. The patient may be febrile. Taut skin and tissue necrosis further confirm the presence of an abscess.

The treatment of an abscess is drainage. Afterward, the surgeon may loosely pack the wound or insert a drain to keep it open and drained. If a drain is used, after the cavity is completely collapsed, the RNFA may gradually withdraw it during several days (Polk et al.,

1987). When packing the wound, the RNFA should moisten the material with normal saline. Studies have shown that hydrogen peroxide, 1% povidone-iodine, 0.25% acetic acid, and 0.5% sodium hypochlorite are toxic to human fibroblasts (Lineweaver et al., 1985; Viljanto, 1980). These agents also severely reduce a wound's ability to resist infections (Rodeheaver et al., 1982). The RNFA should change the packs frequently, especially with heavy drainage. If there is a large amount of purulent drainage, the RNFA should attach a wound drainage appliance. This protects the skin surrounding the drainage site. The enterostomal therapy nurse is an extremely valuable resource in caring for problem wounds. The RNFA can and should rely heavily on the enterostomal therapy nurse's expertise. The surgeon may order antibiotics; their role, however, is secondary to drainage and meticulous wound care.

Potential Alterations in Functional Health Patterns

Nutritional–Metabolic Pattern

Diagnosis

High risk for impaired tissue integrity related to abscess formation

Definition

Presence of risk factors for the patient to experience damage to the integumentary or subcutaneous tissue owing to the formation of an abscess

Risk Factors

- Presence of pus in the wound
- Inadequate wound drainage
- Use of agents such as hydrogen perioxide, 1% povidone-iodine, 0.25% acetic acid, and 0.5% sodium hypochlorite to clean the wound
- Poor wound care

Expected Outcome

The patient is free from impaired tissue integrity related to abscess formation. There is no evidence of damage to integumentary or subcutaneous tissue.

Perioperative Nursing Interventions

- Assess the patient for signs of abscess.
- Look for systemic signs of infection.
- Determine the patient's comfort level.
- Assess the skin condition.
- Monitor the white blood cell count.
- Culture the wound if necessary.
- Refer for medical treatment if indicated.
- Implement measures to reduce pain as described for infection.
- Administer antibiotics as ordered.

Interventions for Abscess

- Implement wound care measures after the abscess has been drained.
- When repacking the wound, loosely pack it with material moistened in normal saline.
- Initiate measures to protect the skin from irritating drainage, tape, or chemicals.
- Daily assess the skin around the drainage site for signs of irritation or breakdown.
- Counsel the patient about her or his abscess, the planned treatment, and the probable clinical course.
- Show the patient how to care for his or her wound.
- Document findings and activities according to institutional policy.

Seroma

Seromas are common in obese patients and in wounds with areas of undermined skin flaps. They consist of blood and protein-rich fluid. Usually, seromas are sterile in the beginning but are susceptible to infections. The local swelling associated with a seroma may make the patient uncomfortable. The skin over and surrounding a seroma is usually not inflamed or compromised (Polk et al., 1987).

Seromas may require drainage. The surgeon or RNFA can do this at the bedside by needle aspiration. A persistent seroma, however, may necessitate the insertion of an indwelling closed drainage system, which uses suction to keep the fluid evacuated and the cavity collapsed. The RNFA should have these treatments prescribed by a physician or should recommend to the physician that they be done.

Potential Alterations in Functional Health Patterns

Health Perception-Health Management Pattern

Diagnosis

High risk for infection related to seroma formation in the postoperative wound

Definition

Presence of risk factors for the patient to experience a postoperative wound infection after the formation of a seroma

Risk Factors

- Obesity
- Surgical wound with areas of undermined skin flaps

Expected Outcome

The patient is free from postoperative wound infection related to seroma formation. (See discussion of potential for infection related to postoperative wound.)

Perioperative Nursing Interventions

- Assess the wound for signs of a seroma.
- Determine the patient's comfort level.
- Assess the skin condition.
- Monitor the white blood cell count.
- Culture the wound if necessary.
- Refer for medical treatment if indicated.

Interventions for Seroma

- Implement measures to reduce pain.
- Administer pain medication as ordered.
- Aspirate the seroma.
  1. Collect the supplies necessary to aspirate the seroma: 20- to 35-ml syringe, 16- or 18-gauge needle, skin preparation solution, adhesive bandage (Band-Aid), 0.5 ml local anesthetic (optional), 3-ml syringe, and 25-gauge needle.
  2. Prepare the skin with alcohol or an antiseptic of preference.
  3. After anesthetizing the skin with 0.5 ml of local anesthetic, insert the large-gauge needle attached to the large syringe and evacuate fluid until the cavity has collapsed.
  4. After withdrawing the needle, cover the site with an adhesive bandage to keep fluid from leaking from the needle wound.
- Assist in inserting a suction wound drainage device.
  1. Collect the supplies necessary to insert the suction wound drainage device: skin preparation solution, wound drainage device of choice, four drape towels, No. 15 or 11 blade and No. 3 knife handle, hemostat, needle holder, suture scissors, 10-ml syringe, 18- and 25-gauge needles, and 10 to 20 ml of local anesthetic agent, dressing sponges, tape, and sterile gloves.
  2. Prepare the skin with alcohol or an antiseptic of preference.
  3. Don sterile gloves and prepare supplies.
  4. Draw up local anesthetic agent with an 18-gauge needle.
  5. Cut the drain to the proper length and attach it to the reservoir.
  6. Square off the area with sterile drapes.
  7. Numb the skin and track site to the seroma with the 25-gauge needle and local anesthetic agent.

8. Make an incision approximately 2 cm in size well below the seroma site. With a hemostat, make a track through the subcutaneous layer to the seroma. Fluid may leak out at this point.

9. Insert the drain through the track into the seroma cavity with a hemostat.

10. Close the incision and secure the tubing with suture. Dress the wound. Reassess the wound daily and check the amount of drainage.

● Counsel the patient about the seroma, the treatment, and the probable clinical course.

● Teach the patient how to care for the wound.

● Document findings and activities according to institutional policy.

Gas Gangrene

Gas gangrene is often caused by a combination of two processes. One is the action of microbial enzymes in contact with healthy tissue. The other is the action of microbial enzymes indirectly by causing thrombosis of blood vessels supplying the tissue with nutrients. Destruction of tissue can be extensive, often producing visible tissue necrosis. The extent of tissue destruction and the rate at which the process spreads are functions of the resistance of the host and the species of bacteria involved.

Three types of gas gangrene exist: aerobic, anaerobic, and synergistic. Extremely virulent strains of hemolytic streptococci usually cause aerobic gangrene. The gas bacillus Clostridium perfringens and related species cause anaerobic gangrene. For both types, the onset is sudden, marked by high fever, intense local pain, and an incredibly foul odor. The tissue is crepitant, dark, and cool. Hemorrhagic areas may appear at the margin of the infection. The patient may also exhibit signs of jaundice, confusion, moribundity, tachycardia, and dyspnea. If untreated, gas gangrene leads to septic shock.

Several bacterial species, usually one aerobic and one anaerobic, cause synergistic gangrene. With the combination of bacteria, the results are more destructive than with either species alone. Meleney ulcer is one such infection.

The surgeon treats gas gangrene with wide débridement of all necrotic tissue, administration of parenteral antibiotics, and delayed wound closure. The RNFA can assist with surgical débridement. The hyperbaric oxygen chamber has been a promising adjunctive treatment (Polk et al., 1987).

Potential Alterations in Functional Health Patterns

Nutritional-Metabolic Pattern

Diagnosis

High risk for impaired tissue integrity related to the formation of gas gangrene

Definition

Presence of risk factors for the patient to experience damage to the integumentary or subcutaneous tissue owing to the formation of gas gangrene

Risk Factor

● Wound contamination with hemolytic streptococci or C. perfringens

Expected Outcome

The patient is free from impaired tissue integrity related to the formation of gas gangrene.

Perioperative Nursing Interventions

● Assess the wound for signs of gas gangrene.
● Check for signs of systemic infection.
● Assess the patient's comfort level.
● Assess the patient's skin.
● Check the wound for crepitus.
● Assess the mental status.
● Check the white blood cell count.
● Culture the wound if necessary.
● Refer for medical treatment as indicated.

Interventions for Gas Gangrene

● Implement measures to reduce pain.
● Implement safety measures if the patient is confused.
● Administer antibiotics as ordered.
● If antibiotics have not been ordered, recommend an appropriate antibiotic to the physician.
● Counsel the patient about the infection, the treatment plan, and the probable clinical course.
● Show the patient how to care for the wound.
● Follow institutional policies regarding the isolation of patients with gas gangrene.
● Assist with the surgical débridement of the wound.
● Document findings and activities according to institutional policy.

Wound Dehiscence and Evisceration

If it happens, wound dehiscence usually occurs about the fifth postoperative day. Infection is the precipitating factor in 50% of cases. Wound edge ischemia and wound closure under extreme tension are other usual causes of wound dehiscence. Before dehiscence occurs, the patient has serosanguineous drainage. After the wound begins to separate, evisceration may occur. The patient often reports that "something gave way." The treatment of wound dehiscence or evisceration is surgical closure.

Potential Alterations in Functional Health Patterns

Health Perception–Health Management Pattern

Diagnosis

High risk for potential for infection related to wound dehiscence or evisceration

Definition

Presence of risk factors for the patient to experience wound infection and peritonitis related to wound dehiscence and evisceration after surgery

Risk Factors

- Inadequate wound closure
- Wounds closed under undue tension
- Compromised wound healing

Expected Outcome

The patient is free from wound infection and peritonitis.

Perioperative Nursing Interventions

- During the first 5 to 6 days of convalescence, check the wound for signs of impending separation.
- Look for serosanguineous drainage.
- Assess the patient's level of comfort.
- Refer for medical treatment immediately in case of dehiscence or evisceration.
- If evisceration occurs, implement measures to ensure patient safety.
  1. Place the patient in a supine position.
  2. Cover the wound with sterile towels moistened with saline.
  3. Implement measures to prevent hypovolemic shock.
  4. Prepare the patient for surgical closure.
- Counsel the patient about the wound, the treatment plan, and the probable clinical course.
- Assist with the surgical closure of the wound.
- Document findings and activities according to institutional policy.

Nonhealing Wounds

Infection, hematomas, seromas, retained foreign substances, underlying disease or conditions, and alteration in tissue perfusion due to excessive wound tension, adjacent scarring, or trauma may cause the patient to have a nonhealing wound (Kneedler and Dodge, 1987; Rothrock, 1987) (Table 18–7). The treatment is specific to the cause.

Potential Alterations in Functional Health Patterns

Nutritional-Metabolic Pattern

Diagnosis

High risk for impaired skin integrity: nonhealing wound

Definition

Presence of risk factors for the patient to experience impaired wound healing after surgery.

Risk Factors

- Infection
- Hematomas

TABLE 18–7. CAUSES OF NONHEALING WOUNDS

Cancer
    Basal cell carcinoma
    Leukemia
    Melanoma
    Squamous cell carcinoma
Chronic trauma
    Factitious ulcer
    Hyperactivity
    Peripheral neuropathy
    Poor hygiene
    Proximal nerve injury
    Pruritus
Drug therapy
Infections
Inadequate nutrition
    Starvation (protein depletion)
    Inflammatory bowel disease (malabsorption syndromes)
Radiation
    Locally irradiated tissues
    Radiation enteritis
Vascular disorders
    Arterial ischemia and atherosclerosis
    Diabetes
    Decubital ulcers
    Arteritis

Adapted from Rothrock, J. C. (Ed.). (1987). *The RN first assistant: An expanded perioperative nursing role* (p. 194). Philadelphia: J. B. Lippincott.

- Seromas
- Retained foreign substances
- Underlying diseases or conditions
- Alteration in tissue perfusion due to excessive wound tension
- Adjacent tissue scarring or trauma
- Altered circulation to the affected area due to swelling
- Exudates irritating to the skin
- Use of cytotoxic substances to clean the wound
- Chemical irritation of substances used to clean an open wound
- Altered nutritional state
- Obesity
- Use of tape
- Pressure from drain tubes

Expected Outcome

The patient experiences optimal wound healing.

Perioperative Nursing Interventions

- Assess the wound for signs of nonhealing.
- Review preoperatively and postoperatively the patient's history for risk factors.
- Assess the white blood cell count.
- Culture the wound if necessary.
- Refer for medical treatment if indicated.
- Implement measures to reduce discomfort, if present.
- Implement measures to eliminate infection, hematomas, seromas, and retained foreign substances.
- Do not use cytotoxic substances and chemicals to clean the wound. Use normal saline.

- Counsel the patient about the wound, the treatment plan, and the probable clinical course.
- Show the patient how to care for the wound.
- Document findings and activities according to institutional policy.

RECOGNIZING FEVER, TACHYCARDIA, PULMONARY COMPLICATIONS, THROMBOPHLEBITIS, URINARY TRACT INFECTIONS, AND ADYNAMIC ILEUS

The experienced RNFA recognizes postoperative complications other than wound complications, identifies underlying causes, and recommends treatment. When appropriate, the RNFA also initiates treatment. Fever, tachycardia, thrombophlebitis, urinary tract infection, prolonged ileus, and pulmonary problems such as atelectasis, infiltration, and effusions are the most common postoperative complications.

Fever

Elevated temperature can occur at any time postoperatively. Transient low-grade postoperative fever, however, is considered normal. Some patients experience fever from pyrogens in blood if given blood intraoperatively. If inflamed tissue was removed during surgery, the RNFA should expect a constantly elevated temperature 3 to 5 days postoperatively. Gradually, the temperature returns to normal. A spiking temperature, one that is intermittently high, may mean a more serious problem, such as bacterial seeding into the blood stream. Determining the source is crucial. Spiking temperatures during the first 2 days postoperatively are usually pulmonary in origin. The primary treatment is increased ambulation. From the fourth to the seventh day, suspect wound complications. Fevers on the sixth to the ninth days are commonly attributable to intraabdominal abscesses or anastomotic leaks. Thrombophlebitis can cause a fever from the sixth to the 10th day. After the cause is determined, the appropriate treatment may be recommended.

Potential Alterations in Functional Health Patterns

Nutritional-Metabolic Pattern

Diagnosis

High risk for postoperative hyperthermia (fever)

Definition

Presence of risk factors for the patient to experience an elevated temperature after surgery

Risk Factors

- Intraoperative blood administration
- Removal of inflamed tissue during surgery

- Decreased ambulation
- Wound complications
- Intraabdominal abscesses or anastomotic leaks
- Thrombophlebitis

Expected Outcome

The patient is free from postoperative fever.

Perioperative Nursing Interventions

- Implement interventions to eliminate, attenuate, or modify the risk factors associated with fever
- If a patient experiences a fever, perform the following:
  1. Evaluate its pattern and assess for the underlying cause.
  2. Refer for medical treatment when indicated.
  3. Implement measures to educate the patient regarding the elevated temperature, the treatment, and the probable clinical course.
  4. Document findings and activities according to institutional policy.

Tachycardia

Postoperative tachycardia, like postoperative fever, should be assessed on the basis of its underlying cause. The most frequent causes are fever; lack of a medication routinely taken by the patient, such as digitalis; relative hypotension (for example, if the patient is ordinarily hypertensive); inadequate pain relief; and apprehension. The treatment depends on the underlying cause.

Potential Alterations in Functional Health Patterns

Activity-Exercise Pattern

Diagnosis

High risk for alteration in postoperative cardiac rate (tachycardia)

Definition

Presence of risk factors for the patient to experience an increased cardiac rate after surgery

Risk Factors

- Fever
- Lack of a medication routinely taken by the patient, such as digitalis
- Relative hypotension
- Inadequate pain relief
- Apprehension

Expected Outcome

The patient exhibits a cardiac rate within normal limits.

Perioperative Nursing Interventions

- Implement interventions to eliminate, attenuate, or modify the risk factors associated with tachycardia.

- After it is established that the patient is tachycardiac, perform the following:
  1. Assess the patient for the underlying cause.
  2. Refer for medical treatment if indicated.
  3. Implement measures to educate the patient regarding tachycardia, the treatment, and the probable clinical course.
  4. Document findings and activities according to institutional policy.

Pulmonary Complications

Pulmonary complications usually appear during the first 2 days postoperatively. These can involve atelectasis, infiltrate, or effusions. They are usually accompanied by an elevated temperature, tachycardia, restlessness, elevated white blood cell count, lowered partial pressure of oxygen, increased partial pressure of carbon dioxide, dyspnea, increased respiratory rate, pallor, and shortness of breath. In severe cases, hypoxia can cause deterioration of mental status and level of consciousness and cyanosis.

Portions of the bronchial tree can become plugged with mucus if the patient cannot cough effectively. Pain and splinting is a major cause of ineffective cough. Adequate pain relief can assist the patient to move the secretions; however, narcotics can depress respiratory effort. Nonnarcotic methods of pain relief are encouraged and may be successful in some cases. For example, intrapleural catheters may be inserted intraoperatively during a thoracotomy. Postoperatively, the catheter is injected with a local anesthetic agent. The patient who smokes is at especially high risk for all postoperative pulmonary complications.

Segmental atelectasis can occur with bed rest or inadequate intraoperative ventilation. Bronchial obstruction, which frequently accompanies atelectasis, prevents transmission of breath and voice sounds during auscultation. The areas of atelectasis are dull when percussed.

The treatment is to increase activity, such as ambulation. In some cases, the use of the incentive spirometer, postural drainage, percussion, inspiration of humidified air, intermittent positive-pressure breathing treatments with mucolytic agents, and tracheal suction may also be employed. The patient should have adequate fluid intake.

If these conditions persist, the patient may experience pneumonia. The infiltrate can be seen on x-ray films. Breath sounds may be diminished, especially in the lower lobes. Crackles may also be heard. Pneumonia can develop as a result of massive or subtle aspiration. Sputum cultures may be positive. Antibiotics should be included in treatment measures discussed above. In severe or persistent cases, a therapeutic bronchoscopy may be required.

Postoperative pleural effusions can be caused by pneumonia, pulmonary embolus, congestive heart failure, or subdiaphragmatic abscess. The most common cause of pleural effusion is pneumonia (see above). Plural effu-

sions are often visible on chest x-ray films. The diaphragmatic markings are blunted on upright films. The fluid may layer on decubital views. Pleural fluids tend to muffle all sounds when auscultated. Percussion notes are dull; breath sounds are decreased or absent, especially in the lower lobes.

Pulmonary embolus presents with sudden chest or shoulder pain, dyspnea, tachycardia, hypotension, pallor, cyanosis, restlessness, and hypoxia. The pulse oximeter readings fall significantly and suddenly. The oxygen pressure is significantly lower, even reaching dangerous levels. Sudden death can occur. Immediate resuscitative intervention may be required. Mortality is high if not treated within 24 hours. Peripheral venograms, pulmonary arteriograms, and lung scans may be ordered to confirm an embolic event. Anticoagulants may be ordered as a continuous heparin infusion or intermittent heparin injections. Long-term oral anticoagulant therapy may be desirable. Measures to prevent pulmonary embolus are directed at preventing thrombophlebitis. Pulmonary embolectomy may be necessary in cases of massive embolus, if the patient survives the initial event. Radical treatment in documented cases of recurrent pulmonary embolus entails vena caval interruption by ligating, filtering, or performing umbrella lysis of the vena cava.

Postoperative fluid overload can lead to congestive heart failure. It is characterized by vascular congestion and the inability of the heart to pump enough blood to meet the body's metabolic needs. Careful monitoring of the patient's intake and output and daily weights is essential, especially in patients with preexisting congestive heart failure. It may be difficult to differentiate between overhydration and third spacing of fluids. Central venous pressure monitoring is inadequate for this complication. Monitoring pulmonary wedge pressures with a Swan-Ganz catheter is more appropriate. Diuretics and inotropic drugs may be used in the treatment of overhydration.

Subdiaphragmatic abscesses irritate the diaphragm, creating a pleural effusion. The patient experiences pain on light palpation of the subcostal margin of the affected side. Abscesses produce a dull sound when percussed. Arterial blood gas measurements and pulse oximeter readings gradually deteriorate. Abscesses are readily seen with sonography or computed tomography. The treatment is surgical or percutaneous drainage of the abscess. The effusion may be aspirated. If the effusion is severe enough, the surgeon may choose to insert a chest tube to drain the effusion.

Potential Alterations in Functional Health Patterns

Activity-Exercise Pattern

Diagnosis

High risk for ineffective airway clearance during the postoperative period

Definition

Presence of risk factors for the patient to experience ineffective removal of secretions from the airway owing to poor cough after surgery

Risk Factors

- Bed rest
- Poor cough associated with narcotics, anesthesia, pain, fatigue, tenacious secretions, tracheal edema due to endotracheal intubation, surgical procedures around the trachea such as thyroidectomy and carotid end arterectomy, and abdominal distention
- Presence of a nasogastric tube intraoperatively or postoperatively

Expected Outcome

The patient's airway is maintained.

Diagnosis

High risk for ineffective breathing pattern during the postoperative period

Definition

Presence of risk factors for the patient to experience respirations inadequate to maintain sufficient oxygen supply for cellular requirements during the postoperative period

Risk Factors

- Ineffective airway clearance
- Stasis of pulmonary secretions
- Aspiration
- Smoking
- Hypoventilation during anesthesia (e.g., deflated lung during pulmonary resection)
- Intraoperative handling of pulmonary tissue, leading to edema or alveolar damage

Expected Outcome

The patient is free from alterations in breathing patterns after surgery as evidenced by

- normal breath sounds
- resonant percussion over the lung field
- pulse and respiratory rates within normal limits
- maintenance of afebrile status
- respiratory rate within normal limits (16–20 breaths/minute)
- cough productive of clear mucus only
- absence of pleuritic pain
- white blood cell count remaining within normal limits
- arterial blood gas values or pulse oximeter readings within normal limits
- retention of usual mental status
- maintenance of usual skin color

Perioperative Nursing Interventions

- Implement interventions to eliminate, attenuate, or modify the risk factors associated with pulmonary complications.
- Assess pulmonary complications.

- Assess the patient's activity level and ability to ambulate.
- Monitor arterial blood gas values and pulse oximeter readings.
- Evaluate the effectiveness of cough.
- Evaluate the use of respiration-depressing drugs.
- Monitor intake and output.
- Monitor pulmonary wedge pressures.
- Refer for medical treatment, if indicated, or immediately in the event of a pulmonary embolus.
- In the event of pulmonary complications, recommend appropriate diagnostic and/or treatment modalities.
- Assess the effectiveness of measures to prevent pulmonary infiltrates and pneumonia.
- Assess the effectiveness of measures to prevent pulmonary embolus.
- Implement measures to educate the patient regarding her or his role in preventing pulmonary complications.
- If complications occur, educate the patient regarding the treatment and the probable clinical course.
- Document findings and activities according to institutional policy.

Thrombophlebitis

Thrombophlebitis results from inactivity with venous stasis in the lower extremities or as a complication of intravenous catheters. Prolonged venous cannulation or chemical reaction from intravenous medications can cause a peripheral vein to thrombose.

By far the most serious form of thrombophlebitis occurs in the deep veins of the legs. This can be precipitated by pelvic edema resulting from surgical procedures (e.g., hysterectomy and hip procedures), intraoperative positioning that restricts venous return, or postoperative bed rest. The patient may experience pain, local tenderness, swelling in the calf and foot, and transient fever. If a clot embolizes to the pulmonary circulation, sudden death can occur.

Deep thrombophlebitis can be palpated. With the leg flexed at the knee and relaxed, press the calf muscles against the tibia with the fingertips. Feel for increased firmness or muscle tension. Thrombophlebitis is prevented by maintaining high venous flow. This is accomplished by the application of elastic stockings, elevation of the legs, and muscular exercise. The patient should avoid having the legs in a dependent position unless he or she is ambulating. The physician may prescribe continuous heparin infusions or intermittent heparin injections.

Potential Alterations in Functional Health Patterns

Activity-Exercise Pattern

Diagnosis

High risk for acute pulmonary embolus

Definition

The presence of risk factors for the patient to experience a deficit in blood supply to the pulmonary circulation related to pulmonary embolus secondary to thrombophlebitis after surgery

Risk Factors

- Venous stasis from immobility
- Positioning during surgery and in the PACU
- Abdominal distention
- Intraoperative trauma to the pelvic veins

Expected Outcome

The patient is free from deep vein thrombosis. There is an absence of

- tenderness and pain in the calf
- edema in the lower extremities
- fever

Perioperative Nursing Interventions

- Implement interventions to eliminate, attenuate, or modify the risk factors associated with thrombophlebitis.
- Assess for venous thrombosis.
- Implement measures for patient comfort.
- Encourage early ambulation.
- Implement measures to educate the patient regarding his or her role in preventing thrombophlebitis.
- If complications occur, perform the following:
  1. Refer for medical treatment.
  2. Educate the patient regarding the treatment and the probable clinical course.
  3. Assess the effectiveness of measures to treat thrombophlebitis.
- Document findings and activities according to institutional policy.

Urinary Tract Infections

Urinary tract infections can be diagnosed by the patient's description of the problem. Patients may express an urgent and frequent need to evacuate small amounts of urine. They may also verbalize bladder fullness, burning on urination, and suprapubic distention. Urine may be foul smelling or cloudy. The patient may have chills and fever. Urinalysis shows many white blood cells in the urine. A culture produces bacteria. Infections can be treated with the administration of sulfas or antibiotics if necessary. Absence of urination with suprapubic distention means urinary retention. Measures to prevent urinary retention are activities that facilitate voiding, such as running water, assisting male patients in standing to void, and offering a bedpan or assistance to the bathroom every 2 to 3 hours. If these measures prove inadequate, a catheter should be inserted intermittently or be indwelling.

Potential Alterations in Functional Health Patterns

Health Perception–Health Management Pattern

Diagnosis

High risk for postoperative urinary tract infection

Definition

Presence of risk factors for the patient to experience a urinary tract infection after surgery

Risk Factors

- Dehydration
- Urinary retention
- Indwelling urinary catheter

Expected Outcome

The patient remains free from a urinary tract infection as evidenced by

- clear urine
- no unusual odor to urine
- absence of frequency, urgency, or burning on urination
- absence of chills or fever
- inconsequential number of white blood cells or bacteria in urine
- negative urine culture

Perioperative Interventions

- Implement interventions to eliminate, attenuate, or modify the risk factors associated with urinary tract infection.
- Assess for signs of urinary tract infection.
- In the event of urinary tract infection, perform the following:
  1. Refer for medical treatment.
  2. Implement measures for patient comfort.
  3. Educate the patient regarding the treatment and the probable clinical course.
  4. Assess the effectiveness of measures to treat urinary tract infection.
- Document findings and activities according to institutional policy.

Adynamic Ileus

By far the most common occurrence of adynamic ileus is after abdominal surgery. The bowel remains flaccid for several days. Intestinal motility is ineffective in moving contents along the tract or it stops entirely. Adynamic ileus is frequently associated with thoracic, retroperitoneal, and abdominal trauma, as well as spinal cord injuries. Less frequent causes are metabolic and vascular. Low serum potassium levels paralyze the smooth muscle of the bowel. An example of an ileus caused by vascular insufficiency is venous or arterial occlusion of mesenteric vessels producing ileus followed by bowel death. Surgical intervention with resection of the ischemic bowel and restoration of the blood supply is urgent. Adynamic ileus, unaccompanied by mesenteric vascular insufficiency or peritonitis, exhibits diminished to absent bowel sounds, abdominal distention, nontender abdomen, nausea, vomiting, and signs of extracellular fluid loss. Generally, the patient is not concerned about the abdomen because it is not tender. The patient may express "feeling full."

Postoperative ileus in the absence of metabolic or vascular insufficiencies is a self-limiting condition. The treatment of adynamic ileus is to withhold oral intake until bowel function returns. The patient may be relieved by the insertion of a nasogastric tube to evacuate the stomach contents. The first sign of returning bowel function is active sounds or the passage of flatus. If adynamic ileus is persistent, the RNFA may suspect peritonitis, potassium depletion, or wound dehiscence.

Potential Alterations in Functional Health Patterns

Elimination Pattern

Diagnosis

High risk for altered postoperative bowel function

Definition

Presence of risk factors for the patient to experience prolonged ileus after surgery

Risk Factors

- Manipulation of intestines intraoperatively
- Decreased activity
- Administration of medications (i.e., narcotics for pain relief)
- Peritonitis
- Septicemia
- Hypovolemia
- Hypokalemia

Expected Outcome

The patient does not experience prolonged adynamic ileus as evidenced by

- soft, nondistended abdomen
- absence of nausea and vomiting
- return of bowel sounds in an appropriate amount of time, depending on the surgical procedure
- passage of flatus or stool

Perioperative Nursing Interventions

- Implement interventions to eliminate, attenuate, or modify the risk factors associated with adynamic ileus.
- Assess the patient for signs of prolonged ileus.
- Assess the comfort level.
- In the event of prolonged adynamic ileus, perform the following:
  1. Refer for medical treatment.
  2. Implement measures for patient comfort.
  3. Implement measures to educate the patient regarding the reasons for ileus and when bowel function is expected to return.
- Document findings and activities according to institutional policy.

ASSESSING POSTOPERATIVE COMFORT LEVEL

The RNFA should be able to assess the patient's postoperative comfort level, identify causes of alterations in comfort, and then recommend and initiate appropriate treatment. Postoperative pain, nausea, and vomiting are the most common causes of alteration in comfort.

Postoperative pain is caused by injured nerve fibers in incised or traumatized tissue. The assessment of pain is an ongoing process that often begins as the patient returns to consciousness in the PACU. Figure 18–1 presents a flow chart for the management of postoperative pain. Pain is believed to be an interaction between physiological and psychological systems. It is a highly subjective experience and, therefore, difficult to evaluate. The RNFA cannot know how intense pain may be for the patient. The use of a pain intensity scale to assess the patient's pain is very helpful (Fig. 18–2). Many factors influence the patient's perception and reaction to painful stimuli. Fear and the expectation of pain seem to intensify one's response to pain. Cultural systems develop different expressions of pain, methods of coping with pain, and fears and beliefs regarding pain (Martinelli, 1987). Patients who cope with chronic pain tend to have a higher tolerance for pain (Kneedler and Dodge, 1987).

Severity of pain is related to the type of surgical procedure. For example, knee and rectal procedures seem to create intense pain. Severity of pain is also associated with the type of anesthetic agent used. Patients who have had regional anesthesia may not experience pain in the PACU but may do so later. Whether an anesthetic-reversing agent was used affects immediate postoperative pain (Kneedler and Dodge, 1987). Figure 18–3 illustrates the potential detrimental effects of pain on the patient. The RNFA must become adept at recognizing the signs and symptoms of pain. Kim and Moritz (1982) characterized pain by describing the following behaviors:

- guarding or protective behavior
- self-focusing
- altered time perception
- withdrawal from social contact
- impaired thought processes
- distraction behavior
- crying
- moaning
- restlessness
- facial mask of pain
- eyes dull
- fixed or scattered movement
- grimace
- alteration in muscle tone (may be listless to rigid)
- autonomic responses not seen in stable chronic pain
- diaphoresis
- blood pressure and pulse rate change
- pupillary dilation
- increased or decreased respiratory rate

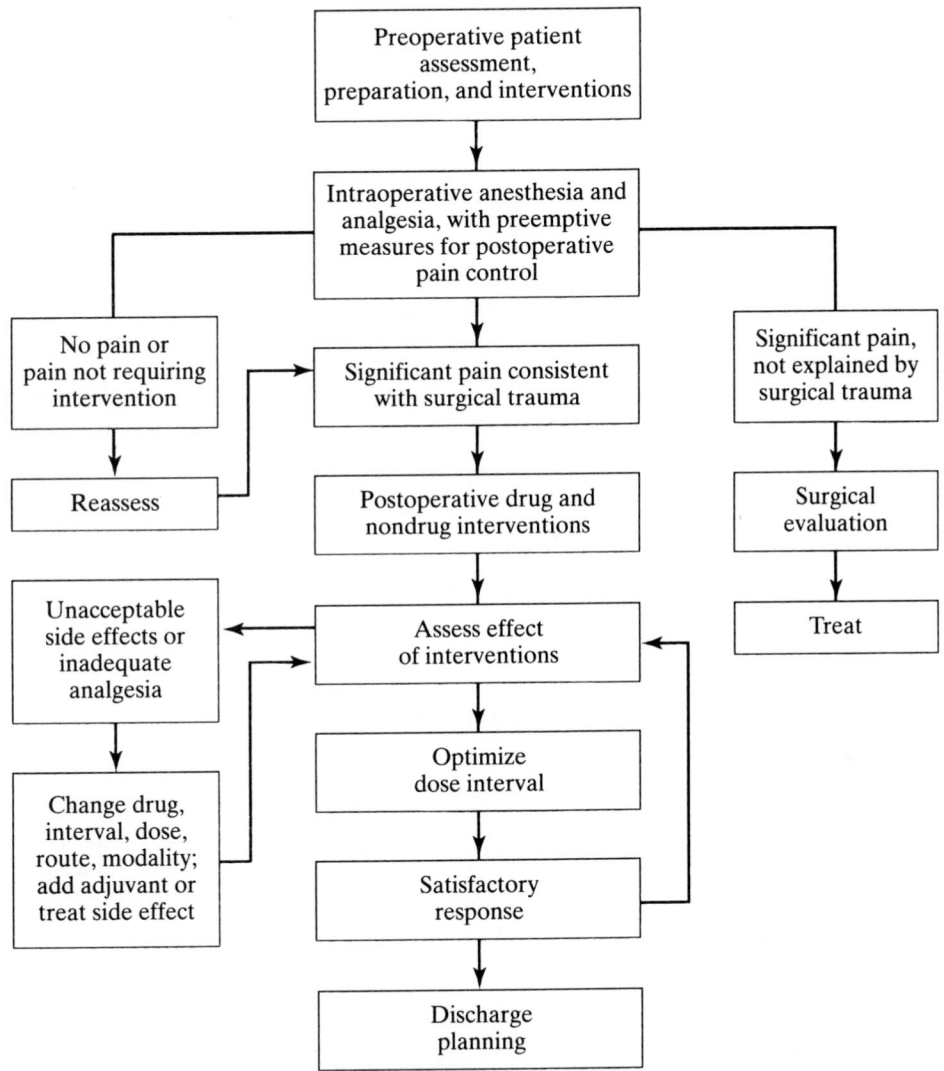

FIGURE 18–1. Flow chart depicting postoperative pain management. (Adapted from *Acute pain management in adults: Operative procedures. Quick reference guide for clinicians.* AHCPR Pub No. 92-0019. (1992). (p. 4). Rockville, MD: Agency for Health Care Policy and Research, Public Health Service, U.S. Department of Health and Human Services.)

Simple Descriptive Pain Intensity Scale[1]

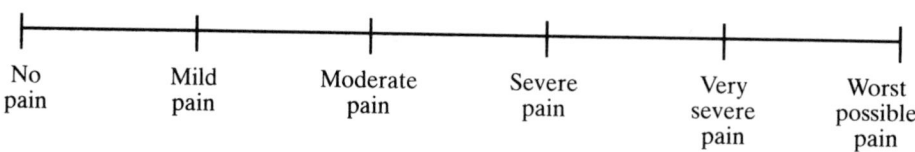

0–10 Numeric Pain Intensity Scale[1]

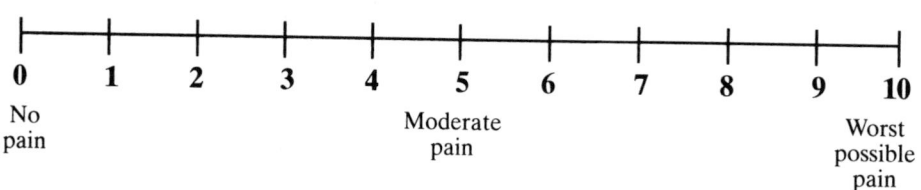

Visual Analog Scale (VAS)[2]

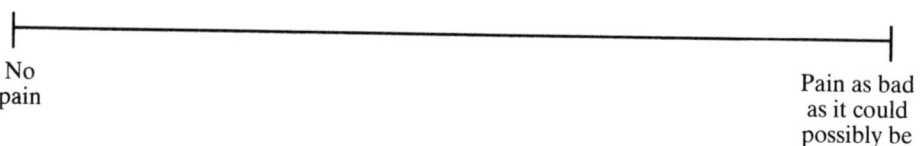

[1]If used as a graphic rating scale, a 10 cm baseline is recommended.

[2]A 10 cm baseline is recommended for VAS scales.

FIGURE 18–2. Examples of pain intensity scales. (Adapted from *Acute pain management in adults: Operative procedures. Quick reference guide for clinicians*. AHCPR Pub No. 92-0019. (1992). (p. 14). Rockville, MD: Agency for Health Care Policy and Research, Public Health Service, U.S. Department of Health and Human Services.)

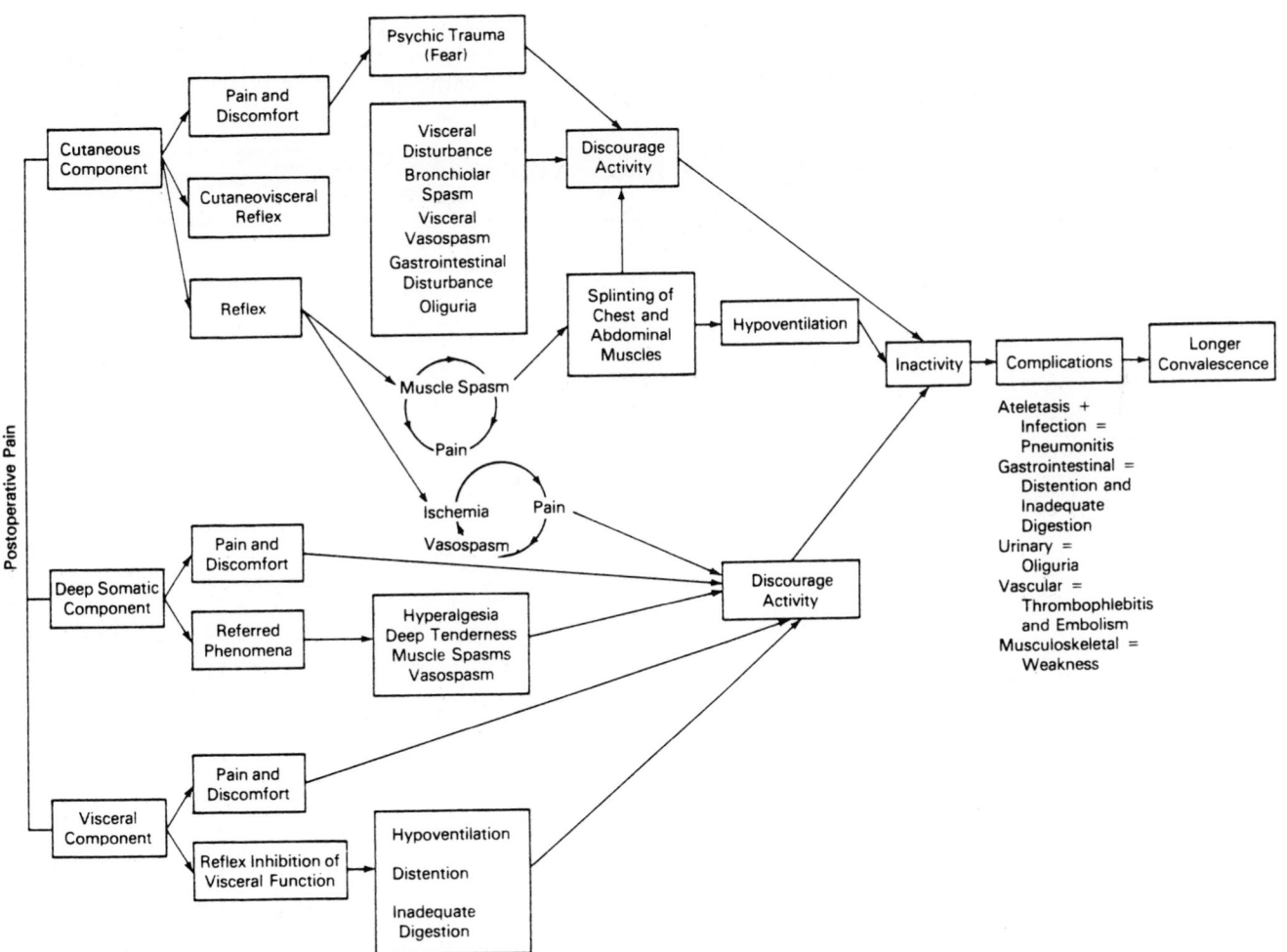

FIGURE 18–3. Possible effects of postoperative pain. (From Bonica, J. J. [1953]. *The management of pain* [p. 1241]. Philadelphia: Lea & Febiger.)

The RNFA should also know the recommended dose and effects of medication given to control or relieve pain (Tables 18–8 and 18–9). A common side effect of narcotics is respiratory depression. An occasional patient exhibits a previously unknown allergy to the drug being used. These are easily recognized by patient reports of itching and a generalized rash. The patient may also report tightness in the throat. Nausea and vomiting are also common side effects of narcotics (see below).

Traditionally, acute pain has been managed with intramuscular injections of narcotics. Today, there are several alternatives to the traditional approach. For example, injecting the surgical wound with a long-acting local anesthetic such as 0.5% bupivacaine (Marcaine) during closure can keep the patient virtually pain free for 4 to 6 hours. Table 18–10 presents scientific evidence for interventions to manage pain in adults. Epidural catheters are used to instill tiny doses of long-acting morphine (Starten and Cullen, 1986). Small doses are required to achieve pain relief with virtually no respiratory depression. A dose of 2 to 3 mg can last from 8 to 12 hours. However, there are inherent dangers with the use of epidural catheters. These include epidural hemorrhage and infections. The result can be paraplegia. If the medication injected drifts to higher levels on the spinal cord, respiratory arrest can result. These patients must be closely monitored for these complications while the catheter is in place.

It is common practice to keep the patient in the surgical intensive care unit until the catheter is removed. Intrapleural catheters may be inserted intraoperatively

TABLE 18–8. DOSING DATA FOR NONSTEROIDAL ANTI-INFLAMMATORY DRUGS (NSAIDs)

Drug	Usual Adult Dose	Usual Pediatric Dose[1]	Comments
Oral NSAIDs			
Acetaminophen	650–975 mg q 4 hr	10–15 mg/kg q 4 h	Acetaminophen lacks the peripheral anti-inflammatory activity of other NSAIDs
Aspirin	650–975 mg q 4 h	10–15 mg/kg q 4 h[2]	The standard against which other NSAIDs are compared. Inhibits platelet aggregation; may cause postoperative bleeding
Choline magnesium trisalicylate (Trilisate)	1000–1500 mg bid	25 mg/kg bid	May have minimal antiplatelet activity; also available as oral liquid
Diflunisal (Dolobid)	1000 mg initial dose followed by 500 mg q 12 h		
Etodolac (Lodine)	200–400 mg q 6–8 h		
Fenoprofen calcium (Nalfon)	200 mg q 4–6 h		
Ibuprofen (Motrin, others)	400 mg q 4–6 h	10 mg/kg q 6–8 h	Available as several brand names and as generic; also available as oral suspension
Ketoprofen (Orudis)	25–75 mg q 6–8 h		
Magnesium salicylate	650 mg q 4 h		Many brands and generic forms available
Meclofenamate sodium (Meclomen)	50 mg q 4–6 h		
Mefenamic acid (Ponstel)	250 mg q 6 h		
Naproxen (Naprosyn)	500 mg initial dose followed by 250 mg q 6–8 h	5 mg/kg q 12 h	Also available as oral liquid
Naproxen sodium (Anaprox)	550 mg initial dose followed by 275 q 6–8 h		
Salsalate (Disalcid, others)	500 mg q 4 h		May have minimal antiplatelet activity
Sodium salicylate	325–650 mg q 3–4 h		Available in generic form from several distributors
Parenteral NSAID			
Ketorolac tromethamine (Toradol)	30 or 60 mg IM initial dose followed by 15 or 30 mg q 6 h Oral dose following IM dosage: 10 mg q 6–8 h		Intramuscular dose not to exceed 5 days

Note: Only the above NSAIDs have FDA approval for use as simple analgesics, but clinical experience has been gained with other drugs as well.
[1]Drug recommendations are limited to NSAIDs where pediatric dosing experience is available.
[2]Contraindicated in presence of fever or other evidence of viral illness.
Adapted from *Acute pain management in adults: Operative procedures. Quick reference guide for clinicians.* AHCPR Pub No. 92–0019. (1992). (pp 18–19). Rockville, MD: Agency for Health Care Policy and Research, Public Health Service, U.S. Department of Health and Human Services.

during a thoracotomy. A 20-gauge epidural catheter is placed percutaneously through the intrapleural space immediately below the incision. Postoperatively, the catheter is injected with a local anesthetic agent. A 20- to 30-ml dose of 0.5% bupivacaine (Marcaine) with 1:200,000 epinephrine can be injected every 4 to 6 hours with no respiratory depression. A continuous drip has also been shown to be effective and safe (McIlvaine et al., 1988). After injection of the bupivacaine hydrochloride, the patient should be assessed not only for level of comfort, but also for signs of blood pressure, respiratory, or heart rate depression. The RNFA can discuss the insertion of such pain control methods with the anesthetist and the surgeon intraoperatively.

Intravenous narcotics via patient-controlled pumps have gained widespread acceptance (Kresl, 1988). Studies have shown that patients use less medication overall with this method than patients who are given intramuscular injections. There are several reasons for this. Narcotics given intravenously require a relatively small dose to work (3 to 5 mg of morphine). Small doses given at relatively frequent intervals maintain a more constant level of relief. Patients tend to use the medicine at increasingly longer intervals (taper off) after the first 24 hours.

The RNFA should also be aware of nonnarcotic methods to relieve pain (see Table 18–10). These may be used in conjunction with narcotics or alone if the patient finds the level of pain control acceptable. Deep breathing relaxation has been shown to be effective (Miller, 1987), with the added advantage of improving respiratory effort. Transcutaneous electrical nerve stimulation has been helpful in some patients. Another method is teaching the patient how to splint the wound with a pillow when moving or coughing. Position changes can relieve discomfort. Diversional techniques such as back rubs, quiet conversation, and distractions can assist the patient in becoming more comfortable. The patient should have a restful environment.

Potential Alterations in Functional Health Patterns

Cognitive-Perceptual Pattern

Diagnosis

High-risk for alteration in comfort (postoperative pain)

Definition

Presence of risk factors for the patient to experience acute pain after surgery

Risk Factors

- Surgical incision
- Pressure on nerve endings from edema or purulent substances
- Tissue necrosis from infection
- Chemical irritation from substances used to clean the wound
- Reflex muscle spasm
- Excessive tissue trauma
- Aggressive tissue retraction and manipulation

Expected Outcome

The patient experiences minimal postoperative wound pain as evidenced by

- verbalization of the presence of adequate pain control
- relaxed facial expression and body positioning
- gradual increase in activity level
- decreasing use of pain medications

Perioperative Nursing Interventions

- Implement interventions to eliminate, attenuate, or modify the risk factors associated with postoperative pain.
- Assess the patient for level of pain relief (see Fig. 18–2).
- Assess how the patient responds to pain.
- In the event of inadequately controlled postoperative pain, perform the following:
  1. Refer for medical treatment if indicated.
  2. Implement measures to educate the patient regarding his or her role in pain control.
  3. Implement nonpharmacological measures for pain relief.
- Document findings and activities according to institutional policy.

ASSESSING NAUSEA AND VOMITING

The RNFA should be able to assess the patient's comfort level relative to nausea and vomiting. The RNFA should be able to differentiate between nausea and vomiting that are narcotic induced and nausea and vomiting caused by postoperative adynamic ileus and postoperative complications. Narcotic-induced nausea and vomiting usually occur shortly after the medication has been administered. The patient may state that she or he thinks the pain medicine is making her or him sick. The treatment is to administer an antiemetic and change the type of or eliminate the narcotic. A nasogastric tube is rarely necessary for narcotic-induced nausea and vomiting.

Potential Alterations in Functional Health Patterns

Cognitive-Perceptual Pattern

Diagnosis

High risk for alteration in comfort related to nausea and vomiting

TABLE 18–9. DOSING DATA FOR OPIOID ANALGESICS		

Drug	Approximate Equianalgesic Oral Dose	Approximate Equianalgesic Parenteral Dose
Opioid Agonist		
Morphine[1]	30 mg q 3–4 h (around-the-clock dosing) 60 mg q 3–4 h (single dose or intermittent dosing)	10 mg q 3–4 h
Codeine[2]	130 mg q 3–4 h	75 mg q 3–4 h
Hydromorphone[1] (Dilaudid)	7.5 mg q 3–4 h	1.5 mg q 3–4 h
Hydrocodone (in Lorcet, Lortab, Vicodin, others)	30 mg q 3–4 h	Not available
Levorphanol (Levo-Dromoran)	4 mg q 6–8 h	2 mg q 6–8 h
Meperidine (Demerol)	300 mg q 2–3 h	100 mg q 3 h
Methadone (Dolophine, others)	20 mg q 6–8 h	10 mg q 6–8 h
Oxycodone (Roxicodone, also in Percocet, Percodan, Tylox, others)	30 mg q 3–4 h	Not available
Oxymorphone[1] (Numorphan)	Not available	1 mg q 3–4 h
Opioid Agonist-Antagonist and Partial Agonist		
Buprenorphine (Buprenex)	Not available	0.3–0.4 mg q 6–8 h
Butorphanol (Stadol)	Not available	2 mg q 3–4 h
Nalbuphine (Nubain)	Not available	10 mg q 3–4 h
Pentazocine (Talwin, others)	150 mg q 3–4 h	60 mg q 3–4 h

Note: Published tables vary in the suggested doses that are equianalgesic to morphine. Clinical response is the criterion that must be applied for each patient; titration to clinical response is necessary. Because there is not complete cross tolerance among these drugs, it is usually necessary to use a lower than equianalgesic dose when changing drugs and to retitrate to response.

Caution: Recommended doses do not apply to patients with renal or hepatic insufficiency or other conditions affecting drug metabolism and kinetics.

[1]For morphine, hydromorphone, and oxymorphone, rectal administration is an alternate route for patients unable to take oral medications, but equianalgesic doses may differ from oral and parenteral doses because of pharmacokinetic differences.

[2]Caution: Codeine doses above 65 mg often are not appropriate due to diminishing incremental analgesia with increasing doses but continually increasing constipation and other side effects.

Definition

Presence of risk factors for the patient to experience discomfort during the postoperative period due to nausea and vomiting

Risk Factors

- Visceral irritation
- Postoperative adynamic ileus
- Narcotics
- Anesthetic agents

Expected Outcome (Ulrich et al., 1986)

The patient does not experience postoperative discomfort due to nausea or vomiting as evidenced by

- absence of vomiting
- absence or stated relief of nausea

Perioperative Nursing Interventions

- Implement interventions to eliminate, attenuate, or modify the risk factors associated with postoperative nausea and vomiting.
- Assess the patient for the causes of nausea and vomiting.
- Refer for medical treatment if indicated.
- Document findings and activities according to institutional policy.

ENSURING THE PROPER FUNCTIONING OF DEVICES TO ASSIST RECOVERY

Several devices are commonly used to assist the patient in recovering from surgical intervention. These include nasogastric tubes, dressings, chest tubes, closed drainage systems, and open drains. The RNFA should be aware of how these devices function, their purpose, how to check if they are functioning properly, and how to remove them after they have served their purpose.

The purpose of a nasogastric tube is to keep the stomach evacuated. It is used to treat nausea and vomiting with distention from ileus. The patient with a nasogastric tube may be restricted to nothing by mouth; therefore, the output should be made up almost entirely of gastric secretions. Normally, the stomach secretes up to 500 to 1000 ml/day. After the nasogastric tube output has dropped below this level, it is no longer therapeutic and should be removed. Severe ear pain can mean acute otitis media if the nasogastric tube occludes the eustachian tube. The nasogastric tube should be removed immediately. It may be repositioned to the other nostril if necessary.

The purpose of dressings is to provide a clean environment for the incision, thus preventing the introduction of pathogens into the wound before the wound edges can seal. Wound edges seal to bacteria within 4 hours. Dressings also wick drainage up and away from

TABLE 18–9. DOSING DATA FOR OPIOID ANALGESICS *Continued*

Recommended Starting Dose (adults more than 50 kg body weight)		Recommended starting dose (children and adults less than 50 kg body weight)[3]	
Oral	*Parenteral*	*Oral*	*Parenteral*
30 mg q 3–4 h	10 mg q 3–4 h	0.3 mg/kg q 3–4 h	0.1 mg/kg q 3–4 h
60 mg q 3–4 h	60 mg q 2 h (intramuscular/subcutaneous)	1 mg/kg 3–4 h[4]	Not recommended
6 mg q 3–4 h	1.5 mg q 3–4 h	0.06 mg/kg q 3–4 h	0.015 mg/kg q 3–4 h
10 mg q 3–4 h	Not available	0.2 mg/kg q 3–4 h[4]	Not available
4 mg q 6–8 h	2 mg q 6–8 h	0.04 mg/kg q 6–8 h	0.02 mg/kg q 6–8 h
Not recommended	100 mg q 3 h	Not recommended	0.75 mg/kg q 2–3 h
20 mg q 6–8 h	10 mg q 6–8 h	0.2 mg/kg q 6–8 h	0.1 mg/kg q 6–8 h
10 mg q 3–4 h	Not available	0.2 mg/kg q 3–4 h[4]	Not available
Not available	1 mg q 3–4 h	Not recommended	Not recommended
Not available	0.4 mg q 6–8 h	Not available	0.004 mg/kg q 6–8 h
Not available	2 mg q 3–4 h	Not available	Not recommended
Not available	10 mg q 3–4 h	Not available	0.1 mg/kg q 3–4 h
50 mg q 4–6 h	Not recommended	Not available	Not recommended

[3]Caution: Doses listed for patients with body weight less than 50 kg cannot be used as initial starting doses in babies less than 6 months of age.
[4]Caution: Doses of aspirin and acetaminophen in combination opioid/NSAID preparations must also be adjusted to the patient's body weight.
Adapted from *Acute pain management in adults: Operative procedures. Quick reference guide for clinicians.* AHCPR Pub No. 92-0019. (1992). (pp. 20–21). Rockville, MD: Agency for Health Care Policy and Research, Public Health Service, U.S. Department of Health and Human Services.

the skin. Other functions are to provide pressure, hemostasis, support to the wound, or débridement of the wound (Fay, 1987). Although pressure dressings may offer some benefit in reducing edema, the risk of tape burns of the skin is high. Dressings for hemostasis are inappropriate. The control of bleeding is best achieved intraoperatively. Pressure dressings should be limited to immobilizing and supporting the wound. One appropriate use of the pressure dressing is on skin grafts. Pressure ensures that the donor skin stays in contact with the blood supply at the graft site. Wounds may be débrided by the frequent changing of dressing materials loosely packed into an open wound.

The purpose of chest tubes is to evacuate air, fluid, or pus from the pleural space so that the lung can completely inflate. Chest tubes are inserted intraoperatively after thoracic procedures. Chest tubes may be used in case of spontaneous pneumothorax, which can occur while the patient is being mechanically ventilated. Iatrogenic pneumothorax (penetration of the pleural space with a needle while inserting a subclavian catheter) is also treated with chest tubes. Pleural effusions (causes discussed above) are drained via chest tubes. A variety of chest drainage systems are on the market. The RNFA should be well acquainted with those most often used in an institution.

If the skin at the insertion site is not well closed, air may be pulled into the chest around it. A reliable method to prevent this is to place three sutures intraoperatively. The first two close the incision around the tube and secure the tube in place. The third suture is placed to be tied to close the skin when the chest tube is removed. A frequently used, but less reliable, method to make the seal around the tube airtight is to apply petroleum jelly (Vaseline)–impregnated gauze at the insertion site. Pursestring sutures in the skin around the tube provide an airtight seal; however, they are likely to cause necrosis of the skin.

The decision to remove the chest tube depends on its function. If its purpose is to drain fluid and superlative exudate, it may be removed when less than 200 ml/day is draining from the chest. If the purpose is to evacuate air, it may be removed when there is no evidence of an air leak. An air leak is present if, when the patient coughs, air bubbles appear in the water seal of the system.

Philosophies differ widely regarding the use of drains. Some physicians believe that drains are more likely to cause infections than to prevent them. These physicians usually remove drains much earlier than those who believe drains to be highly beneficial. The RNFA should have a working knowledge of the types of systems available to make recommendations to the surgeon. The RNFA should also know how to properly assemble, insert, and activate each system, as well as how to remove them when no longer needed.

Closed drainage systems are placed to evacuate fluid that may accumulate or that has already accumulated in a wound. Closed drains are used more often in nonsuppurative wounds than in suppurative wounds. Closed systems are composed of a collection unit, extension tubing, and drainage tubing. Drainage tubing is available

TABLE 18–10. SCIENTIFIC EVIDENCE FOR INTERVENTIONS TO MANAGE PAIN IN ADULTS

Intervention[1]	Type of Evidence	Comments
Pharmacologic Interventions		
NSAIDs		
Oral (alone)	Ib, IV	Effective for mild to moderate pain. Begin preoperatively. Relatively contraindicated in patients with renal disease and risk of or actual coagulopathy. May mask fever.
Oral (adjunct to opioid)	Ia, IV	Potentiating effect resulting in opioid sparing. Begin preop. Cautions as above.
Parenteral (ketorolac)	Ib, IV	Effective for moderate to severe pain. Expensive. Useful where opioids contraindicated, especially to avoid respiratory depression and sedation. Advance to opioid.
Opioids		
Oral	IV	As effective as parenteral in appropriate doses. Use as soon as oral medication tolerated. Route of choice.
Intramuscular	Ib, IV	Has been the standard parenteral route, but injections painful and absorption unreliable. Hence, avoid this route when possible.
Subcutaneous	Ib, IV	Preferable to intramuscular for low-volume continuous infusion. Injections painful and absorption unreliable. Avoid this route for long-term repetitive dosing.
Intravenous	Ib, IV	Parenteral route of choice after major surgery. Suitable for titrated bolus or continuous administration (including PCA), but requires monitoring. Significant risk of respiratory depression with inappropriate dosing.
PCA (systemic)	Ia, IV	Intravenous or subcutaneous routes recommended. Good, steady level of analgesia. Popular with patients but requires special infusion pumps and staff education. See cautions about opioids above.
Epidural and intrathecal	Ia, IV	When suitable, provides good analgesia. Significant risk of respiratory depression, sometimes delayed in onset. Requires careful monitoring. Use of infusion pumps requires additional equipment and staff education.
Local Anesthetics		
Epidural and intrathecal	Ia, IV	Limited indications. Expensive if infusion pumps employed. Effective regional analgesia. Opioid sparing. Addition of opioid to local anesthetic may improve analgesia. Risks of hypotension, weakness, numbness. Use of infusion pump requires additional equipment and staff education.
Peripheral nerve block	Ia, IV	Limited indications and duration of action. Effective regional analgesia. Opioid sparing.
Nonpharmacologic Interventions		
Simple Relaxation (begin preoperatively)		
Jaw relaxation Progressive muscle relaxation Simple imagery	Ia, IIa, IIb, IV	Effective in reducing mild to moderate pain and as an adjunct to analgesic drugs for severe pain. Use when patients express an interest in relaxation. Requires 3–5 min of staff time for instruction.
Music	Ib, IIa, IV	Both patient-preferred and "easy listening" music are effective in reducing mild to moderate pain.
Complex Relaxation (begin preoperatively)		
Biofeedback	Ib, IIa, IV	Effective in reducing mild to moderate pain and operative site muscle tension. Requires skilled personnel and special equipment.
Imagery	Ib, IIa, IIb, IV	Effective for reduction of mild to moderate pain. Requires skilled personnel.
Education/Instruction (begin preoperatively)	Ia, IIa, IIb, IV	Effective for reduction of pain. Should include sensory and procedural information and instruction aimed at reducing activity related pain. Requires 5–15 min of staff time.
TENS	Ia, IIa, III, IV	Effective in reducing pain and improving physical function. Requires skilled personnel and special equipment. May be useful as an adjunct to drug therapy.

[1]Insufficient scientific evidence is available to provide specific recommendations regarding the use of hypnosis, acupuncture, and other physical modalities for relief of postoperative pain.

Type of Evidence—Key
Ia Evidence obtained from meta-analysis of randomized controlled trials.
Ib Evidence obtained from at least one randomized controlled trial.
IIa Evidence obtained from at least one well-designed controlled study without randomization.
IIb Evidence obtained from at least one other type of well-designed quasi-experimental study.
III Evidence obtained from well-designed nonexperimental descriptive studies, such as comparative studies, correlational studies, and case studies.
IV Evidence obtained from expert committee reports or opinions and/or clinical experiences of respected authorities.

Note: References are available in the *Guideline report. Acute pain management: Operative or medical procedures and trauma.* AHCPR Pub. No. 92–0001. Rockville, MD: Agency for Health Care Policy and Research, Public Health Service, U.S. Department of Health and Human Services. 1992.
Adapted from *Acute pain management in adults: Operative procedures. Quick reference guide for clinicians.* AHCPR Pub No. 92–0019. (1992). (pp. 16–17). Rockville, MD: Agency for Health Care Policy and Research, Public Health Service, U.S. Department of Health and Human Services.

in a variety of sizes and styles. Most rely on some form of vacuum to facilitate the evacuation of fluid. These may be pumping devices that are stationary (wall suction with regulator), a line-powered pump (Gomco), or a manually activated device. Vacuum pressure is fixed for manually controlled systems, whereas it can be regulated with stationary or line-powered devices. The most common reasons for failure of closed drainage systems are inadequate diameter of the tube, improper placement or displacement of tube, loss of vacuum pressure, occlusion of the drain fenestration with clot or tissue, and retrograde contamination of the wound during emptying (Fay, 1987).

Open drains are used for the same reasons as closed systems. They are used more often in suppurative than in nonsuppurative wounds. Open drains ensure that the wound stays open for the drainage of thick suppurative and necrotic materials. Open drains can be soft latex or rigid plastic or Silastic tubing in a variety of styles, sizes, and lengths. These drains are secured with a safety pin or sutured to the skin. This prevents the drain from becoming dislodged and being pulled either into or out of the wound. A common practice with an open drain is to remove it gradually over several days. This allows the abscess cavity to drain and collapse as the drain is removed.

The drainage can be irritating to the skin. Frequent dressing changes with continuous assessment of the surrounding skin are necessary with open wounds. Wound drainage bags protect the skin when there is a large amount of drainage. The enterostomal therapy nurse is an extremely valuable resource in dealing with problem wounds.

Potential Alterations in Functional Health Patterns

Nutritional-Metabolic Pattern

Diagnosis

High risk for injury related to devices used to assist patient recovery

Definition

Presence of risk factors for the patient to experience bodily injury (i.e., impaired skin integrity, damage to internal organs) from devices used to assist during recovery

Risk Factors

Malfunctioning or improperly applied:
- nasogastric tube
- taped pressure dressings
- chest tubes
- closed wound drainage devices
- open wound drainage devices

Expected Outcome

The patient remains injury free, as evidenced by the maintenance of skin integrity and absence of damage to internal organs.

Perioperative Nursing Interventions

Nasogastric Tube

- Check proper functioning of the nasogastric tube.
- Check for proper positioning.
- Inject 10 to 20 cc of air and auscultate the stomach for the sound of air bubbles.
- Reposition if necessary.
- Note output.
- Check for patency.
- Irrigate with about 30 ml of saline.
- Check the suction unit.
- Place suction tubing in water.
- Assess the skin condition where the tube is secured.
- Assess the patient's comfort level.
- Implement measures to relieve dryness of mucous membranes.
- Remove when no longer therapeutic.

Dressings

- Remove soiled dressings.
- Redress the wound only when drainage is present or if the purpose of the dressing is to débride the wound.
- Assess the skin condition under dressings and tape.
- Inspect wounds and the skin condition under splints and redress to continue support of the wound.
- Check that casts are intact.

Chest Tubes

- Check the proper functioning of the system.
- Note whether the suction regulator is properly set.
- Note the amount and nature of the drainage.
- Ask the patient to cough.
- Note air bubbles in the water seal, which indicate there is an air leak into the pleural space.
- Note if air is being pulled into the chest at the insertion site.
- Assess the skin condition around the insertion site.
- Remove when no longer therapeutic.

Removal of Chest Tubes

Equipment and Supplies

Suture scissors
Sterile gloves
Sponges
2–0 or 3–0 silk suture on a cutting needle if a suture to tie has not been placed intraoperatively

Optional Supplies

3-ml syringe
2 to 3 ml of 1% lidocaine (Xylocaine)
25-gauge needle

Procedure

Open supplies.
Don the gloves.
Remove the dressing.
Cut the sutures securing the tube to the skin.
Ask the patient to inhale deeply and hold the breath.
With a sponge and the fingertips, apply slight pressure to the skin above the insertion site as the tube is removed to prevent air from being pulled into the chest.
Remove the tube in one steady motion.
Apply firm pressure above the insertion site until the incision is closed.
Tie the remaining suture to close the incision.
Tell the patient that she or he may breathe normally.
Inject local anesthetic, if indicated.
Close with 2–0 or 3–0 silk on a cutting needle if no suture has been placed intraoperatively.
Dress the wound.

Closed Drainage Systems

- Check the proper functioning of the system.
- Check if the vacuum is engaged.
- Note the amount of drainage collected in the past 24 hours.
- Compare daily amounts of drainage.
- Note the color, consistency, and odor of drainage.
- Check the patency of tubing.
- Ensure that the tubing is properly connected and free from kinks and that the system is airtight.
- Note the amount of drainage around the insertion site.
- Assess the skin condition at the insertion site.
- Remove when closed drainage is no longer therapeutic.

Removal of Closed Drainage Systems

Equipment and Supplies

Suture scissors
Gloves
Sponges
Tape

Procedure

Open supplies.
Don the gloves.
Remove the dressing.
Cut the suture securing the drain to the skin.
Remove the drain in one steady motion.
Dress the wound.

Open Drainage Systems

- Note if the drain is secured so that it does not come out or is not pulled into the wound.
- Check and compare the amount of drainage with that on previous days.
- Assess the color, consistency, and odor of drainage.
- Assess the skin condition around the insertion site.
- Gradually remove the drain.

Removal of Open Drainage Systems

Equipment and Supplies

Suture scissors
Gloves
Sponges

Optional Equipment and Supplies

Wound drainage bag or tape
Safety pin or 4–0 nylon suture
3-ml syringe
2 to 3 ml of 1% lidocaine
25-gauge needle

Procedure

Open supplies.
Don the gloves.
Cut the suture, if any.
Remove the drain about 5 cm.
Reapply the safety pin, if applicable.
Instill local anesthetic, if indicated.
Suture the drain to the skin with nylon.
Clean the skin around the wound.
Apply the dressing or wound drainage bag.
Remove drain when no longer therapeutic.

SUMMARY

The RNFA plays an important role in the recovery of the patient. Recognizing postoperative wound complications, the signs of fever, tachycardia, pulmonary complications, thrombophlebitis, urinary tract infections, and adynamic ileus; assessing the patient's postoperative comfort level; and ensuring the proper functioning of devices employed to assist recovery are skills that facilitate the recovery of the patient.

ACKNOWLEDGEMENT

The author wishes to acknowledge Sherroll Neill, M.D., general and vascular surgeon, friend, and mentor, for his technical review of this chapter.

Bibliography

Association of Operating Room Nurses. (1992). *Standards and recommended practices for perioperative nursing.* Denver.
Fay, M. F. (1987). Drainage systems: Their role in wound healing. *AORN Journal 46,* 442–455.
A Job Analysis for the RN First Assistant. Denver, CO: The National Certification Board: Perioperative Nursing, Inc.
Kim, M., Moritz, D. (Eds.). (1982). *Classification of nursing diagnosis* (p. 258). New York: McGraw-Hill.
Kneedler, J. A., Dodge, G. H. (Eds.). (1987). *Perioperative patient care: The nursing perspective* (2nd ed.). Boston: Blackwell Scientific.
Kresl, J. S. (1988). Patient-controlled analgesia: A new system for pain management. *AORN Journal 48,* 481–487.
Lineweaver, W., Howard, R., Soucy, D., et al. (1985). Topical antimicrobial toxicity. *Archives of Surgery,* 120, 267–270.

Martinelli, A. M. (1987). Pain and ethnicity: How people of different cultures experience pain. *AORN Journal 46*, 273–281.

McIlvaine, W. B., Knox, R. F., Fennessey, P. V., Goldstein, M. (1988). Continuous infusion of bupivacaine via intrapleural catheter for analgesia after thoracotomy in children. *Anesthesiology, 69*, 261–264.

Miller, K. M. (1987). Deep breathing relaxation: A pain management technique. *AORN Journal 45*, 484–488.

Polk, H. S., Stone, H. H., Gardener, B. (Eds.). (1987). *Basic surgery* (3rd ed.). East Norwalk, CT: Appleton-Century-Crofts.

Rodeheaver, G., Bellamy, W., Kody, M., et al. Bactericidal activity and toxicity of iodine-containing solutions in wounds. *Archives of Surgery, 117*, 181–185.

Rothrock, J. C. (Ed.). (1987). *The RN first assistant: An expanded perioperative nursing role.* Philadelphia: J. B. Lippincott.

Starten, E. D., Cullen, M. L. (1986). Collective review: Epidural catheter analgesia for the management of postoperative pain. *Surgery, Gynecology and Obstetrics 162*, 389–404.

Ulrich, S. P., Canale, S. W., Wendell, S. A. *Nursing care planning guides: A nursing diagnosis approach.* Philadelphia: W. B. Saunders.

Viljanto, J. (1980). *Disinfection of surgical wounds without inhibition of normal wound healing. Archives of Surgery, 115*, 253–256.

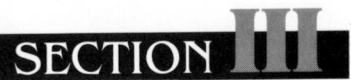

CLINICAL APPLICATIONS

CHAPTER 19

Assisting the Anesthetist

Rebecca P. Fairly and Ruth P. Shumaker

DEFINITION

Anesthesia care may be given by an anesthesiologist or a certified registered nurse anesthetist working under the direction and supervision of an anesthesiologist or a physician (Gruendemann and Meeker, 1987). In this chapter, the term anesthetist refers to an anesthesia provider.

HISTORY

Ancient humans sought relief from pain with the use of plant and herb extracts. Intoxicants such as wine and whiskey were also used to produce insensibility (Gruendemann and Meeker, 1987). Lotions, ointments, and occasionally even brute force were used. The effects of these potions and drugs were not fully understood, and many people were overdosed and died as a result of the potency and action of these agents.

One of the first medical breakthroughs in anesthesia occurred in 1772: Joseph Priestley, an English naturalist, prepared nitrous oxide. Dr. Humphrey Davy described its properties and suggested that it was capable of destroying physical pain and could be used in surgical operations. Early uses of ether were documented by Drs. Crawford W. Long and William J. Morton. The delivery of ether was difficult and many problems were encountered. Sir William Macewan devised the idea of passing a tube into the trachea. The anesthesia could then be directed into the respiratory tract without obstruction from the tongue. Anesthesia techniques and agents have improved from those early years and go far beyond the relief of pain. The well-being of the entire patient is now considered.

ROLE OF THE PERIOPERATIVE NURSE

The team approach is an important concept when a patient is receiving anesthesia. Each individual must recognize his or her responsibility yet remain aware of the role of the other team members.

Staffing of individual hospitals determines the extent of participation of the perioperative nurse with anesthesia. The perioperative nurse should be familiar with medications and techniques used to assist anesthesia personnel effectively.

The perioperative nurse should reassure and comfort the patient. Providing support to patients alleviates their anxiety. The nurse should convey a genuine concern for the patient's safety and well-being. A quiet environment must be maintained. The perioperative nurse should keep movement and noise in the operating room to a minimum after the patient is brought to the room.

PREOPERATIVE ASSESSMENT

A preoperative assessment by the anesthetist and a member of the perioperative team is ideal. Establishing good rapport with the patient and the family is important.

A preoperative visit is done by anesthesia personnel to evaluate the patient's health and conduct a medical history. The preoperative medication and the type anesthetic best suited to each patient can thus be determined. Discussing and explaining special monitoring or procedures should be done with the patient and the family. This allows the patient and family members to voice concerns and ask questions. Many fears can be alleviated during the preoperative visit.

One tool developed to determine the patient's risk for side effects while undergoing anesthesia is the American Society of Anesthesiology's physical status classification:

Class 1: A patient with no organic, physiological, biochemical, or psychiatric disturbances.
Class 2: Mild to moderate systemic disturbances caused by a condition to be treated surgically or by a pathophysiological process. Example: hypertension or diabetes.
Class 3: Severe systemic diseases with more than one system involved. Example: hypertension and cardiac disease or cardiac disease and pulmonary problems.
Class 4: Severe systemic disease or disturbances that are life threatening. Examples: heart disease with cardiac insufficiency, persistent angina; advanced degrees of pulmonary, hepatic, renal, or endocrine insufficiency.
Class 5: A patient who has little chance of survival. Surgery may be a resuscitative measure with little anesthesia. Examples: a ruptured abdominal aneurysm or major cerebral trauma with rapidly increasing intracranial pressure.
Emergency surgery: Any patient in one of the classes listed who undergoes surgery in an emergency situation.

TYPES OF ANESTHESIA

Anesthesia is the loss of sensation with or without the loss of consciousness. There are two main categories of anesthesia. General anesthesia produces an unconscious state in the patient, and regional anesthesia produces a loss of feeling in some area of the body (Groah, 1990). The goal of anesthesia is a total elimination of pain and awareness at a level safe for each patient.

General Anesthesia

General anesthesia may be induced by inhalation or intravenous injection. In each technique, the patient passes through various stages. These stages were first developed by Guedel in 1920 (Dripps, 1988) and define the depth of anesthesia:

● Stage I: This stage begins with the administration of the anesthetic agent and continues until loss of consciousness.
● Stage II: State of delirium, or "excitement phase," begins when the patient loses consciousness and continues until stage III. During this stage, respiration is irregular and breath holding is common.
● Stage III: State of surgical anesthesia extends from the onset of regular respiration until respiration ceases. This stage is divided into four planes:
    1. Respiration is regular and the patient is no longer excited.
    2. The eyes become fixed; all muscles of respiration are still functioning.
    3. Intercostal muscles are paralyzed and breathing is purely diaphragmatic.
    4. Depressed respiration occurs; paralysis of the diaphragm is present.
● Stage IV: State of respiratory paralysis begins with the weakened respiration from plane 4 and ends with circulatory collapse and death (Miner, 1990).

During each stage of anesthesia, the perioperative nurse must assume responsibility for keeping the noise in the operating room to a minimum and providing reassurance to the patient.

Vomiting and regurgitation can occur and the perioperative nurse must be available to assist anesthesia personnel with suctioning and calm the patient if necessary. The perioperative nurse should offer assistance during the intubation. Handing the endotracheal tube to the anesthesia personnel is helpful. If the intubation is difficult, the perioperative nurse may need to help the anesthetist visualize anatomical landmarks. Firm direct compression of the trachea downward can assist in visualizing the trachea. If the patient's trachea deviates from the midline, the perioperative nurse may manipulate the trachea toward the midline. This deviation is common in patients who have tumors or injuries to the neck that involve swelling.

Good suction should always be available and checked before anesthesia induction. Repeated attempts at visualization of the trachea can cause an increase in secretions.

Inhalation Anesthesia

During inhalation anesthesia, a mask is placed over the patient's nose and mouth. The patient inhales the vapors of anesthetic gas mixed with oxygen. These gases pass into the respiratory tract, reach the blood stream, and saturate the brain.

Inhalation inductions are slower than intravenous inductions and the excitement phase is longer. The perioperative nurse should stay at the patient's side and keep the environment as professional and quiet as possible. The last sense to leave is hearing, and some patients may still be aware even though they appear to have a deep level of anesthesia.

A common occurrence during inhalation anesthesia is loss of the airway. The perioperative nurse may need to help with repositioning the patient's head or lifting the lower jaw, as directed by the anesthesia personnel.

There are two types of inhalation anesthesic agents: anesthetic gas and the volatile anesthetics, or those that are liquid at room temperature. Nitrous oxide is one of the most commonly used inhalation anesthetics. Nitrous oxide gas has myocardial depressant effects and can cause significant decreases in blood pressure. It is administered in combination with oxygen, narcotics, and muscle relaxants to provide balanced anesthesia.

The most common volatile anesthetics are isoflurane (Forane), halothane (Fluothane), enflurane (Ethrane), and desflurane (Suprane). All the volatile anesthetics are associated with potent respiratory depression and should never be administered unless anesthesia personnel are present.

Isoflurane depresses respiration. It provides good muscle relaxation, which is desirable in many surgical procedures. Isoflurane is associated with a low incidence of renal or hepatic damage and offers good cardiovascular stability. The use of isoflurane results in a greater incidence of coughing, breath holding, and laryngospasm than that of the other volatile agents. This is because of its pungent odor (Miller, 1990).

Halothane is a potent respiratory depressant; therefore, ventilation must be supported. Halothane rarely irritates the larynx and does not increase respiratory secretions. Halothane has more prominent cardiovascular depressant effects than other agents that decrease heart rate and arterial blood pressure. Cases of hepatitis have been reported after administration of halothane. Halothane should not be administered to patients with abnormal liver functions. Halothane sensitizes the heart to catecholamines. Epinephrine administration with halothane anesthesia should be monitored closely (Joyce, 1990). Anesthesia personnel should be notified when epinephrine is being used in the surgical field.

Enflurane has marked central nervous system action. Seizure activity has been associated with its use. Enflurane should not be given to patients with a history of seizures.

Desflurane is an agent with a strong odor. It allows for a much faster inhalation anesthesia induction and emergence. Desflurane offers good cardiovascular stability.

The most critical times during anesthesia are the induction and the emergence. The perioperative nurse must be alert for possible problems during those times and be available to assist the anesthesia personnel. The environment should be kept as quiet as possible. No procedures should be performed during induction until the anesthetist gives permission.

The perioperative nurse and anesthesia personnel should be in constant communication. The perioperative nurse should be aware of routine anesthesia procedures. The alert perioperative nurse is able to anticipate and assist with those procedures.

Intravenous Anesthesia

Intravenous anesthesia allows for a more rapid and pleasant induction. Metabolism, redistribution, and excretion rid the patient's system of its effects. Often, patients request this technique. Patients enjoy the short euphoric period during induction. Frequently, intravenous anesthetics are mixed with inhalation anesthetics.

Dissociative Anesthesia

Dissociative anesthesia produces a loss of consciousness and profound analgesia. It is frequently associated with vivid and unpleasant dreams. Hallucinations are common postoperatively (Gilman et al., 1990). Ketamine hydrochloride (Ketalar) is used in dissociative anesthesia. The perioperative nurse must be aware of the potential problems and keep the environment as quiet as possible. The patient must be protected from injury.

Regional Anesthesia

Regional anesthesia is the loss of sensation without the loss of consciousness. Subarachnoid (or spinal) blocks, epidural blocks, and regional field blocks are done.

Subarachnoid blocks involve the injection of a local anesthetic into the subarachnoid space. Absorption of the drug takes place rapidly in the nerve fibers. There is loss of neural sensation and controlled movement. For administration of a block, the patient may be placed in a sitting position or lying on one side. The perioperative nurse should reassure the patient and help with positioning. The perioperative nurse should stand in front of the patient to help stabilize her or him during administration of the block. Monitoring equipment should be placed on the patient before administration of the block. The perioperative nurse can help monitor changes in blood pressure or heart rate during the administration of the block. The perioperative nurse may need to shave or prepare the area where the block will be done.

A lumbar dural puncture is done with a small-bore needle, spinal fluid is returned, and accurate placement is determined. The local anesthetic is then injected. Subarachnoid blocks may last 30 minutes to 3 hours. Epinephrine can be added to prolong the effect by decreasing the absorption rate of the medication.

Hypotension is the most common complication of spinal anesthesia. The subarachnoid block causes a peripheral vasodilation. This dilation causes hypovolemia and a fall in blood pressure. This hypotension usually responds quickly to treatment with intravenous fluid replacement (Miller, 1990). Headaches can result from the dural puncture and loss of spinal fluid. Treatment usually consists of increased intake of fluids and bed rest.

Epidural anesthesia is done by injecting local anesthetic agents into the space between the ligamenta flava and the dura. A single dose of medication can be administered and a catheter may be placed for repetitive dosing (Miner, 1990). Epidural anesthesia does not block the motor function and there is little incidence of headache. There is less hypotension associated with epidural anesthesia.

Epidural blocks are used in labor and delivery. The catheter may be placed before general anesthesia and used for postoperative management of pain. Epidural narcotics can be given and patients must be monitored for respiratory depression.

Peripheral, or field, blocks can be done on almost any area of the body. The local anesthetics block conduction through the nerve fibers and have little systemic effect on the patient. The perioperative nurse should reassure and support the patient during regional anesthesia.

The most common peripheral block is a Bier block, or intravenous regional block. The perioperative nurse and the anesthetist must have a good working knowledge of the double tourniquet. The tourniquet must be applied correctly to avoid damage to the patient. Improper use of the tourniquet can affect the block, and a potentially dangerous overdose of medication may occur. The perioperative nurse should check with the surgeon or the anesthetist for the desired tourniquet pressure. The tourniquet is usually set 100 mm Hg above systolic blood pressure to avoid leakage. Documentation should include tourniquet application, pressure setting, and inflation and deflation times. The surgeon should be notified of the tourniquet time approximately every 30 minutes.

When the surgery is over, the tourniquet is deflated and the local anesthetic is circulated into the blood stream. A seizure may occur if the medication has not been metabolized and a toxic blood level is reached. Intermittent deflation of the tourniquet is frequently done to avoid this complication. The perioperative nurse should assist the anesthetist in administering oxygen and sedatives, such as diazepam (Valium), if a seizure occurs. The perioperative nurse should check with the anesthesia personnel before deflating the tourniquet in intravenous regional anesthesia.

The perioperative nurse must monitor the environment in the operating room during regional anesthesia. Patients are awake and aware of the environment. Intravenous sedation can be given to relieve anxiety. Reassurance and a concerned attitude are important to convey to the patient.

MEDICATIONS

Preoperative medications are ordered for various reasons and should be individualized for each patient. Preoperative medications may be given to relieve anxiety and pain, reduce reflexes, decrease secretions, and eliminate the possibility of awareness.

The physical and mental status of the patient determine the amount of premedication necessary. The more critically ill, elderly, and inactive the patient, the smaller the requirement for premedication.

Sedatives, Tranquilizers, and Hypnotics

Sedatives, tranquilizers, and hypnotics encompass a large variety of medications. They have general depressant effects on the central nervous system, which can allay anxiety, provide sedation, and induce amnesia. These groups have little association with nausea and vomiting. Respiratory depression can occur.

Barbiturates are used for intravenous induction of anesthesia. They are relatively short acting and depress the central nervous system (Gilman et al., 1990). Barbiturates have some cardiovascular depressant effect. Doses must be individualized and titrated to achieve the desired effect in individual patients. The most common barbiturates used in anesthesia are thiopental (Pentothal), sodium thiamylal (Surital), and methohexital sodium (Brevital).

Propofol (Diprivan) is an intravenous hypnotic agent used for induction and maintenance of general anesthesia. It can also be used for intravenous sedation during monitored anesthesia (see below). Propofol is a white oil-in-water emulsion. This medium supports bacterial growth and strict aseptic technique should be used. Propofol can cause pain on injection and may necessitate pretreatment with lidocaine.

Narcotics

Narcotics are used preoperatively and intraoperatively. All narcotics depress respiration, and the perioperative nurse should be aware of the patient's sedation level when receiving the patient in the operating room.

Common narcotic premedications are meperedine hydrochloride (Demerol), morphine sulfate, and hydromorphone hydrochloride (Dilaudid).

Narcotics used during induction and maintenance of anesthesia are shorter acting and more potent than narcotics given for premedication. Respiratory depression is pronounced with these narcotics and respiratory support should be available. Common intraoperative narcotics are alfentanil (Alfenta), sufentanil citrate (Sufenta), and fentanyl citrate (Sublimaze).

Individual hospital requirements for the procurement of controlled drugs vary. The perioperative nurse who obtains narcotics and sedatives must document usage and wasting of these drugs with the anesthesia personnel.

Neuromuscular Blockers

Neuromuscular blockers or muscle relaxants are necessary in many operations. Neuromuscular blockers temporarily paralyze the patient. They prevent coughing, breathing, and moving. Muscle relaxation is necessary in most abdominal surgery. The patient's ventilation must be supported.

Muscle relaxation is used for intubation of most patients. Intubation is usually done with short-acting muscle relaxants: succinylcholine (Anectine or Quelicin).

If muscle relaxation is desired after the induction longer-acting muscle relaxant can be used. The most frequently used neuromuscular blockers are atracurium (Tracrium), vecuronium bromide (Norcuron), pancuronium bromide (Pavulon), and doxacurium chloride (Neuromax). These medications are usually metabolized by the end of the operation. Occasionally, their effects may still be present and reversal of their effect is necessary. The perioperative nurse should be familiar with the location of these medications.

MONITORING OF PATIENTS RECEIVING LOCAL ANESTHESIA

Monitored anesthesia care is a term used to describe local anesthetic operations that require anesthesia personnel in attendance. Local anesthetics are usually administered by the surgeon. Anesthesia personnel monitor the patient's blood pressure, heart rate, and breathing and can give intravenous sedations, if necessary.

Perioperative nurses need the necessary monitoring skills when assigned to local anesthesia cases. Patients receiving local anesthesia may have serious health problems. When preparing for these cases, the perioperative nurse needs to assess the patient's history and physical examination findings, laboratory results, and electrocardiograms. Immediately before surgery may be the first opportunity the nurse has to assess the patient's needs.

Before the surgical procedure, necessary equipment and medications should be obtained. Equipment consists of an electrocardiographic monitor, a pulse oximeter, and a blood pressure cuff. The perioperative nurse should be prepared to provide oxygen therapy, intravenous therapy, and pharmacological measures and/or emergency measures, as directed, if an adverse reaction occurs. The nurse should ensure the availability of resuscitative equipment. Optimal practice entails a nurse, other than the circulating nurse, to monitor patients receiving local anesthesia; however, this practice may not be possible in all settings. The Association of Operating Room Nurses (AORN, 1992, *III*:11–3) provides recommendations for monitoring the patient receiving local anesthesia. These are intended as achievable recommendations representing what is believed to be an optimal level of practice. Policies and procedures set by each institution determine to what degree the recommended practice can be fulfilled.

The perioperative nurse must have a working knowledge of monitoring equipment and must be able to interpret the data. Abnormalities should be reported to the surgeon. Continuous documentation provides a clear picture of the patient's response to local anesthesia and the surgical intervention. Documentation should include continuous monitoring of medications and their dose, route and time of administration, and effects. When administering drugs, the nurse should be familiar with the dosage, duration, and action (Table 19–1). The patient should be monitored for allergic and abnormal reactions to medications. The patient's level of awareness should be monitored and recorded. For intravenous therapy, the site and rate of administration and the

TABLE 19–1. **LOCAL ANESTHETICS**		
Generic (Trade) Name	**Anesthetic Use**	**Maximal Dose**
Benzocaine (Americaine)	Topical (ointment or aerosol)	
Cocaine	Topical	200 mg
Dibucaine (Nupercaine)	Spinal	100 mg
Lidocaine (Xylocaine)	Infiltration	500 mg
	Peripheral nerve block	
	Epidural	
	Spinal	
	Topical	
Procaine hydrochloride (Novocain)	Infiltration	1000 mg
	Spinal	
Bupivacaine hydrochloride (Marcaine)	Infiltration	200 mg
	Peripheral nerve block	
	Epidural	
Chloroprocaine hydrochloride (Nesacaine)	Infiltration	1000 mg
	Peripheral nerve block	
	Epidural	
Etidocaine hydrochloride (Duranest)	Infiltration	300 mg
	Peripheral nerve block	
	Epidural	
Mepivacaine hydrochloride (Carbocaine)	Infiltration	500 mg
	Peripheral nerve block	
	Epidural	
Prilocaine hydrochloride (Citanest)	Infiltration	900 mg
	Peripheral nerve block	
	Epidural	
Tetracaine (Pontocaine)	Spinal	200 mg

effect are documented. If oxygen is administered, the rate and effect should be recorded.

Signs may be posted that local anesthesia is in progress and that the patient is awake. A quiet environment helps to alleviate the patient's anxiety and fear.

POSITIONING

Positioning the patient for surgery is a shared responsibility. The perioperative nurse and the anesthetist should communicate to determine special positioning needs. After the induction of anesthesia, the perioperative nurse should ask the anesthetist when the patient can be positioned safely.

Preoperatively, the perioperative nurse should obtain attachments or special equipment needed and be familiar with their use to minimize delays.

The position of the patient should offer the surgeon optimal exposure without damage to the patient. Adequate ventilation and circulation should be checked and documented when the final position is achieved.

When the patient is in the supine position, arm boards are frequently used and should be self-locking to prevent movement during surgery (Gruendemann and Meeker, 1987). The patient's arms should be at less than a 90-degree angle with the palms up and padding under the elbows and wrists. If the patient's extremity does not lie flat, padding should be added to keep the extremity within the patient's anatomical range of motion. The position of the arms and the padding should be rechecked during longer procedures to ensure that no displacement has occurred. The patient's fingers should be kept in sight when the position of the operating room bed is changed to prevent pinching them in the breaks of the bed (Gruendemann and Meeker, 1987).

Before placing the patient in or removing the patient from the lithotomy position, the perioperative nurse must consult the anesthetist. Lowering the legs too rapidly may cause a significant decrease in blood pressure as flow returns to the legs.

Before placing the patient in the lateral position, the perioperative nurse needs to make an axillary roll of the correct size to place at the level of the axilla. Padding of the bony prominences should be done. The arms should be carefully positioned and secured away from the operative field. Circulatory checks of all four extremities should be carried out and documented.

The prone position calls for more attention to achieve the safest position for the patient. Chest supports should not prevent venous return from the neck. The head should be supported and the patient's eyes and ears protected from pressure. Periodic changes in the head position during longer procedures are necessary to prevent necrosis. Hyperextension of the ankles should be avoided and pressure should be kept off the toes (Gruendemann and Meeker, 1987).

Placing a patient in the sitting position can be a lengthy process. The patient must be secured and padding placed at every possible pressure area. The patient must be secured to prevent sliding on the operating room bed during surgery. The perioperative nurse should be able to operate the operating room bed to achieve the proper position. The perioperative nurse should be aware of complications that can arise with the patient in the sitting position. Surgery done with the patient in the sitting position usually requires invasive monitoring. The perioperative nurse can help with the placement of these monitors under the direction of the anesthetist. (See Chapter 12 for further discussion of positioning the patient for surgery.)

EMERGENCY SURGERY

Emergency operations present with little or no notice. The perioperative nurse and the anesthesia personnel must work together quickly and effectively. Preoperative assessment may not be possible, except when moving the patient to the operating room bed. Many unforeseen complications can arise.

Induction of anesthesia for emergency surgery must be done quickly and safely. If access to the airway is difficult and trauma of the neck is involved, this presents a difficult intubation (see below).

Rapid-sequence inductions are usually done in emergency surgery. Any patient who is considered to have increased gastric contents, or a full stomach, should have a rapid-sequence induction. Patients with trauma, intestinal obstruction, active gastrointestinal bleeding, hiatial hernia, pregnancy, or active nausea and vomiting should be treated as having a full stomach. Any patient who has consumed fluid or solid food 6 hours before surgery should also be considered to have a full stomach. The rationale for this is that the stomach empties its contents into the duodenum 2 to 6 hours after eating or drinking, and gastric emptying ceases when a person sustains significant trauma. These conditions affect the rate of digestion, gastric secretions, intraabdominal pressure, and risk of aspiration (Fezer, 1987).

A rapid-sequence induction is usually done with the administration of rapid-acting intravenous agents and muscle relaxants and the application of cricoid pressure. The perioperative nurse must be able to assist with this induction.

Cricoid pressure is routinely administered by the perioperative nurse and can enhance a safe, rapid intubation. When cricoid pressure is applied, the esophagus is compressed between the cervical vertebrae and the trachea. This occludes the esophagus and is the most effective measure to prevent the risk of aspirating gastric contents (Fezer, 1987). Aspiration pneumonitis carries a significant morbity and mortality rate. Morbidity depends on the volume and acidity of the aspirated material. Aspiration pneumonitis can cause acute respiratory compromise, cyanosis, acidosis, hypotension, and cardiac arrest. Prevention of aspiration should be a primary goal (Fezer, 1987).

Communication between the anesthetist and the perioperative nurse is essential during anesthesia induction and intubation. The nurse stands at the patient's side (usually the right side). The patient is usually placed in reverse Trendelenburg position and 100% oxygen is administered for 3 to 5 minutes, if possible. During this time, the nurse identifies the anatomical features of the neck and landmarks for applying cricoid pressure (Fezer, 1987). The thyroid cartilage is made of two fused plates that form the larynx and give it a triangular shape. The cricoid cartilage is the first tracheal cartilage and is located one fingerbreadth below the thyroid cartilage prominence (Adam's apple) (Fezer, 1987). After locating the cricoid cartilage, the perioperative nurse places his or her thumb and second finger on either side of the cricoid cartilage and the index finger over the cricoid cartilage—one fingerbreadth below the thyroid cartilage prominence. This finger placement prevents lateral movement of the trachea, which may distort the anatomical features and make intubation more difficult. Cricoid pressure is performed by applying *downward* pressure with the thumb, index finger, and second (long) finger. Some nurses prefer to place one hand behind the patient's neck as they apply pressure (Fezer, 1987).

The nurse should reassure the patient while standing at his or her side. Apply cricoid pressure as soon as the patient loses consciousness and maintain that pressure until intubation is accomplished, the endotracheal tube cuff is inflated, and placement of the endotracheal tube is verified. Premature release can be followed by regurgitation before the airway is secured (Fezer, 1987).

If intubation is not accomplished on the first attempt, the nurse should maintain pressure during additional attempts and follow instructions from the anesthetist to aid in securing the airway. Suction apparatus should be available and the perioperative nurse should not leave the patient's side until the airway is secured. If the patient vomits, the nurse must release cricoid pressure and help position the patient on his or her side or with the head down so the mouth can be suctioned. Cricoid pressure during active vomiting can lead to esophageal rupture (Fezer, 1987).

The perioperative nurse performs a vital function through the proper administration of cricoid pressure. It is necessary to perform this procedure effectively to prevent aspiration (Fezer, 1987). Anesthesia personnel should demonstrate this procedure to perioperative nurses who are unsure of the proper application before emergency surgery and rapid-sequence induction are necessary.

Positioning a patient with multiple trauma should be done carefully to prevent further injury. Documentation of all noted injuries should be maintained for future reference.

The temperature of the patient during emergency surgery poses a major problem. All attempts should be made by the perioperative nurse, the anesthesia personnel, and the surgeon to maintain the patient's temperature. Intravenous warmers, blanket warming, and the warming of intraabdominal irrigation fluids may help. The perioperative nurse should increase the room temperature, if possible.

BLOOD COMPONENT THERAPY

During the past few decades, blood and blood components have been increasingly recognized as medications rather than innocuous fluids to replace modest blood loss. Hemotherapy focuses on the benefit and risk in the administration of blood and blood components (Dripps, 1988).

The sympathetic nervous system functions to prevent blood loss and maintain vital functions. It causes vascular smooth muscles to contract and reduces the vascular bed, by vasoconstriction, to maintain intravascular volume when necessary. However, when blood loss exceeds what a patient can tolerate, cardiovascular instability can occur (Dripps, 1988).

Intravenous fluid therapy and the administration of volume expanders such as dextran can be used to maintain intravascular volume. These may help the patient to avoid receiving blood or blood products.

When blood therapy is indicated, there are two types of red blood cell replacement. Packed red blood cells are used to increase the red blood cell mass in anemic patients and those requiring blood replacement during and after surgery. Packed red blood cells can increase the hematocrit 2 to 4% or the hemoglobin concentration by 1 g/dl of blood. The infusion should be slow but may be given as rapidly as necessary to maintain intravascular volume during rapid blood loss. Packed red blood cells are preferred to whole blood because they provide the same oxygen-carrying capacity but a lower immunological response. Washed or frozen red blood cells are used to minimize the risk of febrile and allergic reactions in previously sensitized patients (Dripps, 1988).

Whole blood is used to increase both the red blood cell mass and plasma volume, simultaneously restoring blood volume and oxygen-carrying capacity. The usual indication for whole blood is massive blood loss. Rapid infusion of whole blood can trigger congestive heart failure (Dripps, 1988).

Autologous donation of blood occurs when patients predeposit blood for their own use at a later time. This is done for elective surgery, in which the risk of blood loss is frequently high and replacement usually necessary. Autologous donation should occur about 32 days before surgery. The risks involved are anemia, hypovolemia, and untoward reactions during the donation procedure. Autologous donations may result in fewer objections to transfusion by various religious groups; for example, some Jehovah's Witnesses permit autologous donation (Dripps, 1988).

Machines called cell savers are available for intraoperative cell salvage. Cell savers retrieve the blood, process the blood and remove debris, and return the blood for infusion to the patient. Intraoperative salvage is especially indicated in patients with rare blood types, autoimmunized patients with multiple antibodies, and patients with a history of severe transfusion reaction (Dripps, 1988).

A designated donor option has arisen out of fear regarding transfusion. Patients may feel more secure in receiving blood from people they know. There is no evidence that designated donor blood is safer than blood collected from a volunteer donor by licensed, accredited blood banks (Dripps, 1988).

The perioperative nurse must give conscientious attention to verification of the patient's identification, proper labeling of blood products, and documentation of blood products being checked before administration.

Signs and symptoms of transfusion reactions are listed in Table 19–2. The perioperative nurse and the anesthetist should communicate and work together if a transfusion reaction occurs and the following steps should be taken:

1. Discontinue administration of the blood product.
2. Maintain the intravenous catheter site with normal saline.
3. Notify the blood bank and the surgeon.
4. Initiate therapy as necessary: support blood pressure, maintain hydration, maintain renal function, and treat febrile episodes.
5. Send newly collected, labeled, and clotted specimens to the blood bank.
6. Send urine specimens to the laboratory for hemoglobin analysis.

COMPLICATIONS

Hypotension

Hypotension is frequently seen and is usually a minor event. Hypotension can be caused by many factors. Excessive premedication, spinal or epidural anesthesia, vascular absorption of local anesthetics, hemorrhage or plasma loss, increased airway pressure, surgical maneuvers, and changes in position can cause hypotension. These hypotensive episodes usually respond well to increasing the intravenous fluids and placing the patient in Trendelenburg position.

If hypotension does not respond to these measures, vasoconstrictors, such as ephedrine, can be given. If the patient is hypovolemic blood or plasma expanders may be necessary to replace intravascular volume (Dripps, 1988).

The perioperative nurse must stay atuned to the patient's condition. If assistance is needed to treat prolonged hypotension, anesthesia personnel and the perioperative nurse must work together quickly to obtain medications, intravenous fluids, or blood. Hypotension can lead to myocardial infarctions, especially in the elderly patient and patients with cardiac disease. Rapid restoration of blood pressure is essential (Dripps, 1988).

Hypertension

Hypertension is a common preexisting medical problem. Hypertensive patients should continue taking antihypertensive medications up to the time of surgery. Blood pressures can vary greatly under anesthesia. Preoperatively, the patient may be anxious and worried. Anesthesia may treat hypertension to some degree.

Many patients arrive in surgery with undiagnosed hypertension. Intraoperative hypertension can occur in any patient whose response to pain is not obtunded. A crisis can occur if hypertension continues. A cerebrovascular accident, heart failure, pulmonary edema, myocardial infarction, and hemorrhage can occur. Therapy must be prompt (Dripps, 1988). Perioperative nurses must be available for assistance. They should be able to locate necessary medications and supplies quickly.

Coughing and Laryngospasm

Coughing is a protective mechanism to foreign substances in the respiratory tract. Coughing is a relatively frequent occurrence and is usually treated without adverse outcomes. Coughing can lead to laryngospasm. Coughing and laryngospasm may be caused by pharyngeal secretions, early stimulation of the airway, or peripheral stimulation such as touching or examining the patient. Suctioning the patient too deeply during light planes of anesthesia can cause vomiting and laryngospasm (Dripps, 1988).

Laryngospasm can be a serious event. During laryngospasm, little air is able to enter the lungs. One may hear a high-pitched stridor, or there may be complete closure of the glottis, in which no exchange of oxygen occurs. Positive airway pressure usually breaks laryngospasm. If the laryngospasm persists, an additional dose of succinylcholine may be necessary to provide relaxation and ventilation of the patient. Laryngospasm can lead to anoxia, cyanosis, and cardiac arrest if untreated. Occasionally, intubation of the patient must be done to provide adequate ventilation (Dripps, 1988).

TABLE 19–2. TRANSFUSION REACTIONS

Type of Reaction	Awake Patient	Anesthetized Patient
Acute hemolytic	Pain at infusion site, anxiety, chest pain, dyspnea, chills, headache, flank pain	Fever, hemoglobinemia, hemoglobinuria, shock, disseminated intravascular coagulation
Febrile	Chills, faintness	Fever, shock (rare)
Hypervolemic	Dyspnea, headache, palpitations	Pulmonary edema, hypertension, arrhythmias
Allergic	Pruritus, hoarseness, faintness, urticaria	Urticaria, stridor, hypotension
Delayed hemolytic	Fever, malaise, falling hematocrit, increased indirect bilirubin level, increased urine urobilinogen level	Not applicable

The perioperative nurse must assist the anesthetist when laryngospasm occurs and intubation is necessary. Good suction should be available. The perioperative nurse may need to gather medications and laryngoscopes for possible intubation of the patient.

Difficult Intubations

Airway assessment is a routine part of the anesthesia assessment. Preparing for the intubation ahead of time is critical.

Patients may have head or neck trauma. This trauma may lead to swelling or bleeding around the airway that makes intubation difficult. Many patients with cervical injuries cannot have their neck position changed without the risk of further damage or paralysis. If it is determined that the patient's condition or airway may be compromised by attempts at intubation, a tracheostomy should be performed (Dripps, 1988).

Awake intubations are frequently performed for patients with compromised airways. This type of intubation allows the patient to continue spontaneous breathing during the intubation. Intravenous sedation may be used in small amounts. Awake intubations may be achieved orally or nasally. Topical anesthetics should be applied to produce vasoconstriction of mucous membranes and decrease coughing and gagging reflexes.

The perioperative nurse may need to help accumulate equipment and medications necessary to assist with these intubations. The nurse should stand at the patient's side to reassure the patient and assist the anesthesia personnel. Awake intubation necessitates patient cooperation. Fiberoptic flexible laryngoscopes are utilized and can make awake intubations less traumatic to the patient. Visualization of the airway during intubation can prevent improper placement of the endotracheal tube. Flexible fiberoptic laryngoscopes allow visualization without manipulation of the neck (Miller, 1990).

The perioperative nurse, positioned at the patient's side, may hold the endotracheal tube in place as the flexible fiberoptic laryngoscope is advanced. Suction should be available to attach to the flexible fiberoptic laryngoscope, and lubrication should be applied before insertion. After the anesthesia personnel have identified the trachea, the fiberoptic laryngoscope is advanced into the trachea and used as a guide for the endotracheal tube to slide over. The endotracheal tube placement is verified, and the anesthetic induction proceeds as rapidly as possible.

Cardiac Arrest

Cardiac arrest in the operating room may occur at any time. The patient's preoperative evaluation may alert the anesthesia personnel of potential problems. The patient may need invasive monitoring before sur-gery. Arterial blood pressure and Swan-Ganz catheters may be placed for monitoring during surgery. The perioperative nurse may assist anesthesia personnel in preparing the patient for these procedures when necessary.

For local anesthesia when intravenous sedation is given, the airway must be monitored closely for obstruction. Airway obstruction usually occurs if the patient is oversedated. The tongue is frequently the cause of obstruction, and the airway can be reestablished by the head tilt and neck lift maneuver or the jaw thrust maneuver. Oxygen may be administered if the patient becomes obtunded. If the airway cannot be effectively reestablished, hypoxia occurs and can lead to cardiac arrest.

With general anesthesia, the airway is usually secured and the patient is well oxygenated. If cardiac arrest occurs, the perioperative nurse must have the defibrillator and the emergency drug cart brought to the operating room. A cardiac board should be placed under the patient. All available personnel should report to the operating room for instructions.

The surgeon usually begins cardiac compression, and drug therapy may also be started. All perioperative nurses should have basic cardiac life support certification. The perioperative nurse may be asked to assist with cardiac compression if the surgeon tires.

Proper positioning of the hands on the patient's chest is important for successful external cardiac massage. The hands of the provider must be positioned so the maximal impulse of the compression is over the patient's cardiac ventricles, but not on the xiphoid process or the rib cage. The provider's elbows should be straight and the weight of the upper body used for compression. It takes approximately 100 pounds of force to depress the sternum of an adult 1.5 to 2 inches, which is the amount necessary for adequate cardiac compression (Miller, 1990).

Drug therapy is aimed at the specific cause of the arrest. Correction of hypoxia, correction of respiratory and metabolic acidosis, increase of perfusion pressure, suppression of ventricular ectopy, stimulation of a more forceful myocardial contraction, and acceleration of cardiac rate are desirable. Defibrillation may be necessary. The perioperative nurse must be familiar with the function of the defibrillator. Conductive pads or jelly is applied to protect the patient from electrical burns. The surgeon usually holds the paddles and the perioperative nurse charges the defibrillator.

Documentation is difficult during a cardiac arrest. One nurse is usually responsible for charting and other nurses help mix and administer the medications.

When the patient's condition stabilizes, the patient should be monitored in the intensive care unit. The intensive care unit should be notified of the patient's expected arrival, cardiovascular condition, and any special needs such as ventilators and medication pumps.

The perioperative nurse should communicate with the surgeon and the anesthesia personnel any specific postoperative needs to avoid delays in care.

Malignant Hyperthermia

Malignant hyperthermia is a potentially fatal hypermetabolic syndrome that can be induced by all of the currently used inhalation anesthetics or by the injection of succinylcholine. Malignant hyperthermia is characterized by muscle rigidity, increasing carbon dioxide concentration, tachycardia, and a rapid rise in temperature. Malignant hyperthermia occurs about once in every 40,000 cases of adult anesthesia and once in every 15,000 pediatric surgical cases (Dripps, 1988). Predisposition to malignant hyperthermia is an autosomal dominant hereditary trait. It is more frequent in male patients. It almost always occurs under general anesthesia but can be brought on by stress, trauma, and strenuous exercise.

Early symptoms include an unexplained elevation in the patient's expired carbon dioxide concentration, tachycardia, unstable blood pressure, tachypnea, muscle rigidity, and cyanosis (Wlody, 1989). Elevation in temperature is usually a late sign and results from a hypermetabolic state of the skeletal muscle and results in an oxygen consumption of two to three times the normal amount. If malignant hyperthermia is not treated, the temperature may rise 1°C every 5 minutes (Wlody, 1989). Tachycardia is one of the first signs of malignant hyperthermia. There can be rapid ventricular arrhythmias such as frequent premature ventricular contractions or ventricular tachycardia. Rigidity of the muscles may or may not occur. Muscle rigidity is usually seen in the jaw first and may occur in the chest or the extremities. The perioperative nurse should report any rigidity noted during positioning or preparing the patient for surgery.

Fever is a late clinical sign and may not occur if the patient is treated promptly with dantrolene sodium. Mortality is related to the maximal temperature reached. Temperatures of 42.8° to 44°C (109°–111°F) have been reported (Wlody, 1989). The temperature elevation may be manifested by hot flushed skin and excessive heat in the tissues around the wound. The perioperative nurse may notice excessive warmth during preparation of the patient for surgery.

Malignant hyperthermia usually occurs within 30 minutes after induction of anesthesia. It can occur or reoccur 2 to 3 hours postoperatively (Wlody, 1989).

Patients develop a rosy flushed appearance owing to the increased energy use, which produces body heat. This heat causes vasodilation and the skin may become mottled or cyanotic. The surgeon is notified and surgery and anesthesia are discontinued. The patient is hyperventilated with 100% oxygen to help meet the increased oxygen consumption.

All rubber goods on the anesthesia machines should be changed as quickly as possible. The perioperative nurse may need to gather a clean breathing circuit and soda lime and assist with these changes.

The treatment of malignant hyperthermia is straightforward. The entire surgical team must work together for the safety of the patient. Dantrolene sodium is the treatment for malignant hyperthermia. Large amounts of diluent are necessary to mix dantrolene. Dantrolene is not readily dissolved and mixing takes time. The pharmacy should be notified so that mixing may take place more quickly.

The perioperative nurse should bring the emergency cart and defibrillator to the operating room. Ventricular arrhythmias are treated as necessary. Sodium bicarbonate administration and hyperventilation can treat acidosis.

Monitoring of arterial blood gas values may be necessary and the perioperative nurse may assist the anesthesia personnel in positioning of the wrist and gathering equipment for monitoring the arterial catheter.

Administration of intravenous fluids must be maintained. Increased systolic blood pressure causes flushing of the kidneys and promotes diuresis. Insulin and glucose may be given to reduce the serum potassium ion concentration. The perioperative nurse should know the location of medications such as dantrolene, insulin, and potassium chloride. When cooling the patient becomes necessary, iced saline intravenous fluids, cooling blankets, and iced nasogastric lavages are used. Ice packs may be placed against the groin, in the axillae, and on the patient's head (Gruendemann and Meeker, 1987). The perioperative nurse should have designated personnel report to the operating room for instructions.

Assessment and early treatment are key factors in the patient's survival. The perioperative nurse and the anesthetist should communicate any malignant hyperthermia concerns and be prepared for treatment.

SUMMARY

When a patient is receiving anesthesia, the perioperative nurse has the opportunity to demonstrate and practice critical care skills. The perioperative nurse should assume the responsibility for the review and practice of skills in areas of identified deficiency. A self-assessment of these skills and proficiency should be evaluated. Policies and procedures for the patient receiving anesthesia should be included in the orientation and ongoing education of all nurses in the practice setting (AORN, 1992). The ability to plan, organize, and communicate with anesthesia personnel and other health care providers should result in a positive outcome for the surgical patient.

Bibliography

American Society of Anesthesiologists. (1992). *Relative value guide. Physical status classification.* Chicago.

Association of Operating Room Nurses. (1992). *Standards and recommended practices for perioperative nursing.* Denver.

Dripps, R., Eckenhoff, J., Vandam, L. (1988). *Introduction to anesthesia: The principles of safe practice.* Philadelphia: W. B. Saunders Co.

Fezer, S. J., III. (1987). Cricoid pressure: How, when and why. *AORN Journal, 45*(6), 1374.

Gilman, A. G., Rall, T. W., Taylor, P., Neis, A. S. (1990). *The pharmacological basis for therapeutics* (8th ed.). New York: Pergamon Press.

Groah, L. K. (1990). *Operating room nursing: Perioperative practice* (2nd ed.). East Norwalk, CT: Appleton & Lange.

Gruendemann, B. J., Meeker, M. (1987) *Alexander's care of the patient in surgery* (8th ed.). St. Louis: C. V. Mosby.

Joyce, J. L. (1990). Inhalation anesthetic: Comparing nitrous oxide, isoflurane, halothane, and enflurane. *AORN Journal, 52,* 77–83 .

Miller, R. D. (1990). *Anesthesia* (3rd ed.). New York: Churchill Livingstone.

Miner, D. G. (1990, August). Anesthesia: The perioperative nurse's role. *Todays O.R. Nurse, 12*(8), 24–25.

Wlody, G. (1989). Malignant hyperthermia: Potential crisis in patient care. *AORN Journal, 50,* 286–297.

CHAPTER 20

General Surgery

Joyce M. Stengel

DEFINITION

The primary focus of general surgery is the gastrointestinal tract and the breast. *General* refers to a variety of surgeries. The discussion in this chapter includes the stomach, the liver, the small and large intestine, and the breast, as well as laparoscopic surgeries.

ANATOMY

The stomach is a curved muscular organ that receives food from the esophagus (Fig. 20–1). The stomach is divided into four areas: the cardia, the fundus, the body, and the pylorus. Each of these portions secretes fluids that aid in the digestion of food. The stomach both mixes and initiates peristalsis of food and secretions so that they are driven into the small intestine.

The small intestine joins the stomach at the pylorus, which is the lower opening. In the small intestine, digestion of all ingested foods is completed. The small intestine is about 500 cm long and consists of the duodenum, the jejunum, and the ileum. The duodenum houses the pancreatic and common bile ducts, which provide the digestive fluids. The jejunum is supplied with blood from the mesentery, which contains fat, blood vessels, lymph vessels, lymph nodes, and nerves. The mesentery also supplies blood to the ileum, or last portion of the small bowel.

The large intestine or colon extends from the end of the ileum to the rectum. The large intestine is about 5 feet long and is divided into the right and left sides of the colon. The right side of the colon consists of the cecum, the ascending colon, the hepatic flexure, and the proximal transverse colon. The left side of the colon consists of the distal transverse colon, the splenic flexure, the descending colon, the sigmoid, and the recto-

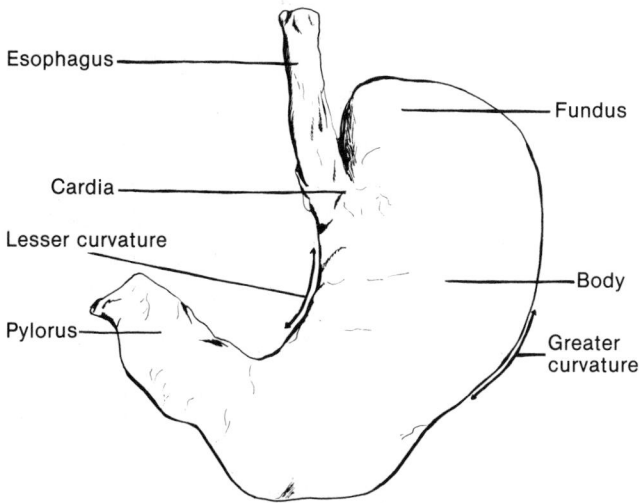

FIGURE 20–1. Stomach anatomy.

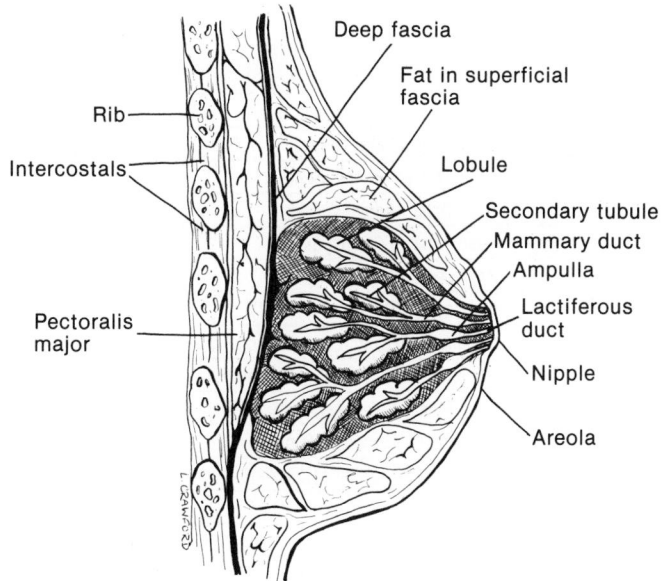

FIGURE 20–3. Breast anatomy.

sigmoid colon. The large intestine is responsible for maintaining the patency of the gastrointestinal tract by eliminating and removing all indigestible materials.

The liver is one of the largest organs in the body, representing 2% of the total body weight. It is located in the upper right portion of the abdomen just beneath the diaphragm. The liver consists of two principal lobes. These two lobes, the left and the right, are separated by the falciform ligament (Fig. 20–2). The liver has many functions, including storage and filtration of blood, secretion of bile, conversion of sugars into glycogen, and many other metabolic activities.

The gallbladder is a pear-shaped organ measuring 3 to 4 inches long. It is located below the liver and actually divides the liver into the right and left lobes. The gallbladder's main function is the storage of bile; it can hold about 50 ml of bile when fully distended. The

gallbladder is divided into four portions: the fundus, the body (which serves as the storage area), the infundibulum, and the neck, which connects with the cystic duct. The cystic duct continues and is joined with the common duct.

The anatomical structure of the gastrointestinal tract is complex. The above discussion describes briefly the anatomical features of the organs involved in the surgical procedures considered below. The breast is also described in this chapter because it is a major focus of general surgery.

The mammary glands lie in the front of the chest over the pectoral muscles (Fig. 20–3). Each mammary gland consists of multiple lobes, which are separated by adipose tissue. Adipose tissue contributes to the size of the breasts. At the tip of each breast is an area called the areola. At the center of the areola is the nipple. Breasts have multiple ducts, which empty into the nipple. The breast produces milk after childbirth as well as functioning as a secondary sex organ.

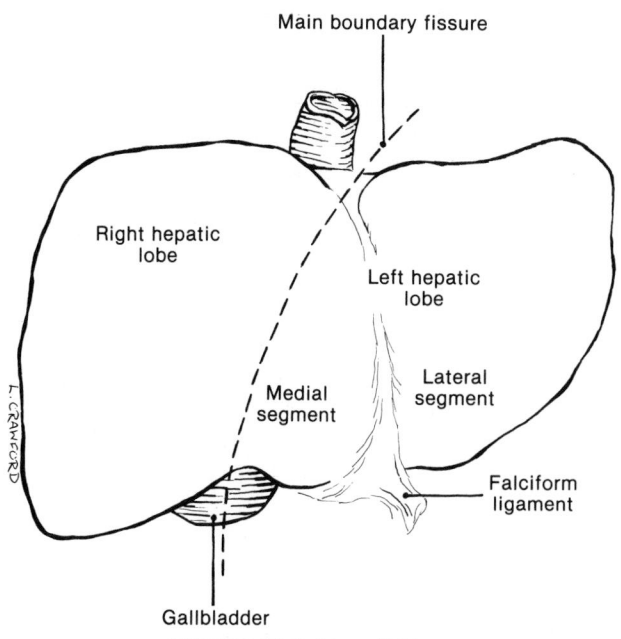

FIGURE 20–2. Liver divisions.

SPECIAL INSTRUMENTS, SUPPLIES, AND EQUIPMENT

General surgery is usually an operating room nurse's first experience in perioperative care. General surgery utilizes basic instruments and supplies. A major instrument set (laparotomy set) is the instrument set used for general surgical procedures within the abdominal cavity. The instruments incorporated in a major instrument set include various scissors, forceps, and clamps, both crushing and noncrushing. Noncrushing clamps are used when less damage to tissue is warranted, whereas crushing clamps execute the opposite. Dozens of clamps are available for general surgery and many are surgeon specific. Tables 20–1 through 20–5 show examples of instrument sets for general surgery.

TABLE 20–1. MAJOR INSTRUMENT SETS

8ea	Backhaus Towel Forceps, 5¼in
4ea	Halsted Mosquito Forceps, 5in, Curved
10ea	Crile Artery Forceps, 6¼in
6ea	Pean Artery Forceps, 6¼in
2ea	Pean Artery Forceps, 8in
2ea	Kantrowitz Thoracic Clamp, 7½in
2ea	Kantrowitz Thoracic Clamp, 9½in
4ea	Ochsner Artery Forceps, Straight, 6¼in
2ea	Ochsner Artery Forceps, Straight, 8in, 1 x 2
4ea	Allis Tissue Forceps, 6in, 5 x 6 Teeth
2ea	Allis Tissue Forceps, 7½in
4ea	Babcock Tissue Forceps, 6¼in
2ea	Babcock Tissue Forceps, 8in
2ea	Foerster Sponge Forceps, 9½in
1ea	Vital® Mayo-Hegar Needle Holder, 6in
2ea	Vital® Mayo-Hegar Needle Holder, 7in
2ea	Vital® Mayo-Hegar Needle Holder, 9in
1ea	Vital® Mayo 6¾in, Curved, Dissecting
1ea	Vital® Metzenbaum Tonsil Scissors, 7in, Curved
1ea	Vital® Metzenbaum Dissecting 9in Scissors, Curved
1ea	Vital® Mayo 6¾in, Straight, Dissecting
6ea	Halsted Mosquito Forceps, Straight, 5in
2ea	Vital® Crile-Wood Needle Holder, 6in
1ea	Russian Tissue Forceps, 10in
1ea	Russian Tissue Forceps, 6in
1ea	DeBakey Tissue Forceps, 7¾in, Delicate
2ea	DeBakey Tissue Forceps, 9½in, Delicate
1ea	Tissue Forceps, 5in, 1 x 2 Teeth
2ea	Adson Forceps, 4¾in, 1 x 2 Teeth
2ea	Surgical Handle #3
1ea	Surgical Handle #7
1ea	Mueller-Balfour Abdominal Retractor, 12in
2ea	Goelet Retractor, Double ended, 1¼in
1st	USA Retractor, Double ended, 2/set 8in
1ea	Richardson Retractor, 1½in, x
1ea	Kelly Retractor, 2in x 2½in
1ea	Kelly Retractor, 2½in x 3in
2ea	Walter-Deaver Retractor #4, 1in x 13in
1ea	Walter-Deaver Retractor #5, 2in x 12in
1ea	Harrington Retractor, Large, 12½in, Splanchnic
1ea	Harrington Retractor, Small, 12½in, Splanchnic
2ea	Gelpi Perineal Retractor, 7in
1ea	Flexsteel Ribbon Retractor, 1in x 13in
1ea	Flexsteel Ribbon Retractor, 1¼in x 13in
1ea	Flexsteel Ribbon Retractor, 2in x 13in
1ea	Yankauer Suction Tube, Half-Curved
1ea	Pool Abdominal Suction Tube, Straight, 30Fr.

From *The surgical armamentarium* (1988). McGaw Park, IL: Baxter-V. Mueller (p. L 1).

TABLE 20–2. MINOR INSTRUMENT SETS

8ea	Backhaus Towel Forceps, 5¼in
4ea	Halsted Mosquito Forceps, 5in, Curved
10ea	Crile Artery Forceps, Curved, 6¼in
2ea	Carmalt Artery Forceps, Curved, 6¼in
2ea	Pean Artery Forceps, 6¼in, Curved
2ea	Ochsner Artery Forceps, Straight, 6¼in
4ea	Allis Tissue Forceps, 6in, 5 x 6 Teeth
2ea	Babcock Tissue Forceps, 6¼in
2ea	Kantrowitz Thoracic Clamp, 7½in
1ea	Foerster Sponge Forceps, 9½in
1ea	Vital® Mayo-Hegar Needle Holder, 6in
2ea	Vital® Mayo-Hegar Needle Holder, 7in
1ea	Vital® Mayo 6¾in, Straight, Dissecting Scissors
1ea	Vital® Metzenbaum Tonsil Scissors, 7in, Curved
1ea	Vital® Mayo 6¾in, Curved, Dissecting Scissors
1ea	Tissue Forceps, 5in, 1 x 2 Teeth
1ea	Russian Tissue Forceps, 6in
1ea	DeBakey Tissue Forceps, 7¾in, Delicate
2ea	Adson Forceps, 4¾in, 1 x 2 Teeth
2ea	Surgical Handle #3
1ea	Surgical Handle #7
2ea	Senn Retractor, 6¼in
2ea	Volkmann Retractor. Sharp, 4 prongs
2ea	Goelet Retractor, Double ended, 1¼in
1st	USA Retractor, Double ended, 2/set 8in
1ea	Richardson Retractor, 1½in
1ea	Kelly Retractor, 2in x 2½in
2ea	Gelpi Perineal Retractor, 7in
1ea	Flexsteel Ribbon Retractor, 1 x 13in
1ea	Flexsteel Ribbon Retractor, 1¼in x 13in
1ea	Yankauer Suction Tube, Half-Curved
1ea	Adson Suction Tube. Curved, 11Fr.

From *The surgical armamentarium* (1988). McGaw Park, IL: Baxter-V. Mueller (p. L 1).

TABLE 20–3. PEDIATRIC LAPAROTOMY INSTRUMENT SETS

8ea	Backhaus Towel Forceps
1ea	Pool Suction Tube
2ea	Micro Line Scissors
1ea	Mayo Scissors
1ea	Mayo Scissors
2ea	Adson Tissue Forceps
2ea	Adson Dressing Forceps
2ea	Semken Dressing Forceps
2ea	Semken Tissue Forceps, 1 x 2 Teeth
2ea	Babcock Intestinal Forceps
1ea	Crile-Wood Needle Holder
4ea	Hartmann Mosquito Forceps
4ea	Allis Pediatric Forceps
2ea	Richardson Retractor
2ea	Deaver Retractor
1ea	Mayo-Collins Retractor
1ea	Balfour Retractor
1ea	Ribbon Retractor
1ea	Surgical Handle #3
1ea	Surgical Handle #3L
1ea	Tissue Forceps, 5½in
1ea	Dressing Forceps, 6in
1ea	Vital® Metzenbaum Dissecting Scissors, Curved, 5¾in
1ea	Vital® Metzenbaum Dissecting Scissors, Curved, 7in
12ea	Halsted Mosquito Forceps, Curved, 5in
6ea	Crile Micro-Line® Artery Forceps, 5½in, Curved
4ea	Crile Micro-Line Artery Forceps, 5½in, Straight
4ea	Pean Micro-Line Artery Forceps, 5½in
4ea	Kocher Artery Forceps, 1 x 2 Teeth, 5½in
4ea	Ballenger Sponge Holding Forceps, 7in
1st	USA Retractor, Double ended, 8in
1ea	Senn Retractor, Delicate, 6¼in
2ea	Vital® Mayo-Hegar Needle Holder, 6in
1ea	Frazier Suction Tube, 10Fr.

From *The surgical armamentarium* (1988). McGaw Park, IL: Baxter-V. Mueller (p. L 2).

TABLE 20–4. GALLBLADDER INSTRUMENT SETS

2ea	Jorgenson Scissors, Curved, 9in
1ea	Metzenbaum Scissors, Curved, 11in
1ea	Metzenbaum Scissors, Curved, 9in
4ea	Ochsner Artery Forceps, Curved, 8in
2ea	Lahey Gall Duet Forceps, 7½in
2ea	Elliott Gall Bladder Forceps, 8in
2ea	Rochester Gall Stone Forceps, 8½in
2ea	Judd-DeMartel Gall Bladder Forceps, 6¼in
2ea	Allis Tissue Forceps, 7½in
2ea	Babcock Intestinal Forceps, 8in
1ea	Mayo Common Duct Probe, 15Fr.
1ea	Mayo Common Duct Probe, 18Fr.
1ea	Mayo Common Duct Probe, 20Fr.
1ea	Bakes Common Bile Duct Dilators, 9/set
1ea	Fenger Gall Duct Probe
1ea	Mayo Common Duct Scoop #1, Small
1ea	Mayo Common Duct Scoop #2, Medium
1ea	Mayo Common Duct Scoop #3, Large
2ea	Mayo Cystic Duct Scoop
1ea	Ochsner Trocar 14Fr.
1ea	Ochsner Trocar 20Fr.
1ea	Boettcher Artery Forceps, 7¼in
1ea	Kantrowitz Clamp, 10½in

From *The surgical armamentarium* (1988). McGaw Park, IL: Baxter-V. Mueller (p. L 3).

TABLE 20–5. INTESTINAL INSTRUMENT SETS

2ea	Kocher Intestinal Forceps, 9¾in
2ea	Kocher Intestinal Forceps, 9½in
1ea	Carter Resectional Clamp, 10in, Straight
1ea	Glassman Anterior Resectional Clamp, 3in
2ea	Boettcher Tonsil Artery Forceps, 7¼in
2ea	Allen Intestinal Clamp, 8in, 1 x 2 Teeth
6ea	Judd-Allis Intestinal Forceps, 7½in
6ea	Carmalt Artery Forceps, 8in, Curved
1ea	Glassman Non-crushing Gastrointestinal Clamp, 9¼in
1ea	Glassman Non-crushing Gastrointestinal Clamp, 9in
1ea	Furniss Anastomosis Clamp
1ea	Dennis Anastomosis Clamp
1ea	Foss Resection Clamp, 11½in
1ea	Payr Resection Clamp, 13¾in
1ea	Payr Resection Clamp, 11in
1ea	Payr Resection Clamp, 8in

From *The surgical armamentarium* (1988). McGaw Park, IL: Baxter-V. Mueller (p. L 3).

Exposure is an important aspect of general surgery and is provided with the use of retractors. There are multiple hand-held retractors such as Deaver and malleable retractors. Self-retaining table-mounted retractors may also be employed. The self-retaining table-mounted retractors allow optimal exposure for the surgical procedure.

A perioperative nurse's experience in general surgery would not be complete without the use of surgical staples. Intestinal staplers have a wide range of applications, especially in general surgery, facilitating resection, anastomosis, and fascia and skin closure. Equipment for general surgery is specific for each procedure planned. Hepatic resections sometimes employ the use of a Cavitron ultrasonic aspirator, which aspirates diseased liver tissue through an ultrasonic handpiece. Other equipment includes an argon beam coagulator, which allows enhanced electrocoagulation using argon beam gas, and an ultrasonic neoprobe, which enables the surgeon to detect metastatic tissue intraoperatively.

The most recent advance in general surgery is the introduction of endoscopic procedures. Equipment for laparoscopic surgery includes video monitors, a printer, a videocassette recorder camera, a light source, a carbon dioxide insufflator, suction irrigation apparatus, laparoscopes, and instruments to enter the abdomen endoscopically and those for dissecting, grasping, and cutting.

GASTRECTOMY

Definition

Gastrectomy refers to the removal of the stomach (total gastrectomy) or a part of it (subtotal gastrectomy).

Indications

A gastrectomy is performed for the treatment of malignant disease or for chronic ulcers that do not respond to a medical regimen. If a partial gastrectomy is performed, 70 to 80% of the stomach is removed and an anastomosis is made from the remaining stomach to a loop of intestine, usually the jejunum. A total gastrectomy involves an anastomosis of the end of the esophagus to the jejunum. The goal of both types of surgeries is to maintain the patency and continuity of the gastrointestinal tract.

Perioperative Nursing Implications

Anesthesia

The choice for abdominal surgery is usually a general anesthetic. General anesthesia enables the surgeon to have complete relaxation of the organs and muscles involved. An epidural anesthetic (regional block) may also be used. The epidural catheter is placed before surgery, and anesthetics can be infused at intervals or at the end of the operation. The block aids in decreasing postoperative pain. Unlike narcotics, regional anesthesic agents do not depress the cough reflex, and comparative studies have shown that respiratory dynamics are better when pain is treated with an epidural block (Way, 1983). The patient is usually given a preoperative antibiotic for control of infection and promotion of wound healing. Other drugs such as sedatives and smooth muscle relaxants may be given preoperatively.

From the time of anesthesia induction, the anesthetist must constantly monitor the following functions: setting of the flowmeters and vaporizers of the anesthesia machine; movements of the reservoir bag or ventilator; the sounds of air movement in the respiratory passages; the quality of the pulse; heart sounds; blood pressure; tissue color and perfusion; overt movements; pupil size and reactivity; and tear flow (Way, 1983). The anesthetist also monitors the patient hemodynamically. Many patients undergoing abdominal surgery require adjuvant blood therapy.

Position

The patient is placed in a supine position. An eggcrate or soft mattress is placed under the patient before surgery for comfort and prevention of pressure ulcers. These mattresses are used when surgery is estimated to be lengthy. The arms are placed at the patient's sides or extended on arm boards. The decision of arm position is determined by the surgeon and/or the anesthetist.

Pneumatic compression stockings are applied to both legs for the prevention of emboli and venous thrombosis. Thermal drapes can be used for warmth and temperature control.

Creation and Maintenance of the Sterile Field

All members of the surgical team are responsible for maintaining the integrity of the sterile field during the operative procedure. The patient is prepared from the clavicle to the groin. The surgical area is cleansed with povidone-iodine (Betadine) or soap solution. This is done immediately before surgery. The patient is covered with sterile drapes. The only area left undraped should be the operative site. The scrub nurse creates the sterile field by making sure all instruments are sterile. The nurse positions the instrument tables close to the surgical field to minimize contamination. The team should constantly be alerted to breaks in technique that create an unsterile environment.

Equipment and Supplies

A major instrument set is used for a gastrectomy, along with retractors (Deaver, Army-Navy, Bookwalter), gastric and bowel staplers, and surgeon-specific instruments. These may include gastric clamps and long instruments, such as Judd-Allis forceps, Babcock tissue forceps, and Mixter forceps. Suture is preferred but chromic, polyglactin 910 (Vicryl), and silk are normally used. The nurse also needs culture tubes, drains, a Foley catheter, suction equipment, electrocautery equipment, sponges, and blades.

All instruments and supplies should be functional. The nurse should be alerted to any problems with the equipment during the procedure.

Drugs and Solutions

Normal saline
Antibiotics for irrigation

Physiological Monitoring

A Foley catheter is placed for constant bladder drainage to establish urine output. A nasogastric tube, usually a Levin 12 to 18 Fr., is placed for decompression of the gastrointestinal tract. A nasopharyngeal tube is placed to monitor the temperature of the patient. Hemodynamic monitoring may be used if there is a chance of marked blood loss. Arterial catheterization, usually of the radial artery, is done for monitoring blood pressure and obtaining blood gas measurements during and after the operation.

Physician's Orders, Laboratory and Diagnostic Studies

Preoperative studies for the patient undergoing a gastrectomy sometimes include a gastric analysis, gastrointestinal radiographic series such as a barium test, and gastrointestinal x-ray films. Physician's orders also include a chest x-ray film, complete blood count study, electrocardiogram, and skin and bowel preparation. The patient is instructed to take nothing by mouth after midnight. Prophylactic antibiotics may be ordered, and the administration of all other medications that the patient is taking should be continued, unless otherwise indicated.

Procedure

Incision and Exposure

An upper midline incision is made with a No. 10 blade. Electrocautery is used for dissection and control of any bleeding sites. The peritoneum is grasped by the surgeon and the assistant to facilitate entering the abdomen. After the abdomen is fully opened, a general exploration is initiated. Exposure is attained by the use of retractors.

Details

The stomach is mobilized by ligating and dividing the omental vessels. Scissors, suture ties, and hemoclips aid in mobilization. Hemoclips are titanium or stainless steel clips that are used for ligating vessels. Two hemoclips ligate the vessel, and a scissors or a knife blade divides the vessel between the clips. Suture ties enhance ligation. An intestinal stapling instrument is used to close the duodenum. Before removing the instrument, the surgeon places a gastric clamp (Payr, Glassman) on the specimen side to prevent oozing when the duodenum is transected. Another intestinal stapling instrument is used to close the gastric pouch. The surgeon places the stapling instrument around the stomach at the level of the transection. Again, a gastric clamp is used on the specimen side before firing the stapling instrument. The remaining gastric pouch is anastomosed to the proximal jejunum.

The gastrojejunostomy is created by using another stapling instrument. The GIA instrument has two cartridge forks containing staples (Fig. 20–4). Two double rows of staples join the tissue, and a knife blade cuts between the two, creating a stoma. The surgeon inspects all areas of anastomosis for hemostasis.

The surgery described is also called Bilroth II gastric resection. In a Bilroth I resection, the remaining gastric pouch is anastomosed to the duodenum; a total gastrectomy entails anastomosis of the esophagus and the jejunum.

Closure

When hemostasis is controlled, all retractors and sponges are removed. A final inspection of the abdomen is made, ensuring that no abnormalities have been overlooked. The abdomen is irrigated with a warm normal saline solution and drains are placed. The peritoneum, fascia, subcutaneous fat, and skin are then reapproximated and closed using chromic, Vicryl, or

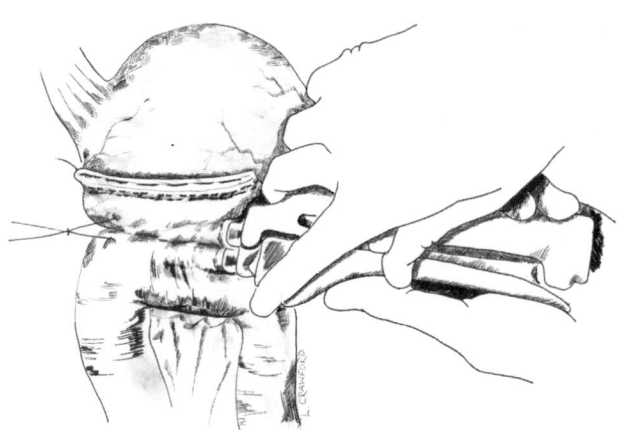

FIGURE 20–4. Gastrojejunostomy using GIA instrument for anastomosis.

polyproplyene (Prolene) suture. A sterile dressing is applied.

Postoperative Care

Patients are observed in the postanesthesia care unit (PACU) until they are conscious and vital signs are stable. Routine postoperative orders include urine output measurements, administration of fluids and electrolytes, dressing changes, inspection and suctioning of drainage tubes, respiratory care, and administration of medications such as antibiotics, sedatives, and narcotics for pain relief.

Potential Surgical Complications

Dumping syndrome (rapid emptying of the gastric contents into the small intestine)
Hemorrhage
Infection
Gastric retention due to edema of the stoma or organic obstruction

HEPATIC RESECTION

Definition

Hepatic resections are done to remove a portion of the liver. The resection is based on the surgical anatomy (e.g., right hepatic lobectomy, left hepatic lobectomy, wedge resection, trisegmentectomy, and left lateral and left medial segmentectomy). Liver transplant surgery is the removal of the entire liver. The following discussion concerns hepatic resections.

Indications

Hepatic resections are done to remove primary or secondary malignant tumors, benign tumors, traumatic ruptures, cysts, and abscesses. The perioperative functional status of the liver is important. Cirrhosis is a relative contraindication for hepatectomy because the limited reserve of the residual cirrhotic liver is usually insufficient to meet essential metabolic demands and the cirrhotic liver has little capacity for regeneration (Way, 1983).

Perioperative Nursing Implications

Anesthesia

In addition to anesthesia implications already mentioned, the nurse may need to use cell-saving equipment (autologous transfusion) and a rapid-injection blood infusion pump. This is accomplished by placement of a 14- or 16-gauge intravenous catheter for rapid administration of blood, fluids, or medications. A central venous pressure monitor may be required for assessment of the circulation, and a Swan-Ganz catheter may be inserted for assessment of cardiac function and output. Blood warming units should also be available.

Position

For most elective major hepatic resections, the nurse should raise the patient's right shoulder approximately 30 degrees from the horizontal; this allows thoracic extension of the primary abdominal incision. The patient's hips remain flat to facilitate laparotomy. The patient is positioned to allow elevation of the kidney rest. This will facilitate exposure of the liver hilum (Nora, 1990).

See the discussion for gastrectomy above.

Creation and Maintenance of the Sterile Field

The patient is prepared from the nipples to the groin. An impervious split drape is used to cover the surgical site. The nurse anticipates an intraoperative blood loss and has available multiple drapes and bath blankets, which may be placed under the operating room bed.

Equipment and Supplies

Hypothermia can be a problem and the nurse places a thermal blanket on the operating room bed. Additional suctioning equipment should be available. In addition to a laparotomy set, the nurse has a vascular set on the instrument table. Vascular control is necessary in any hepatic resection to provide a bloodless field and decrease the risk of hemorrhage (Steuer, 1990). The nurse should be aware of specific clamps that are preferred by the surgeon. A large hepatic clamp should be available to occlude the segment of the liver that is being transected. The surgeon may perform a cholecystectomy at the time of resection, and gallbladder instruments should be on the surgical field. Chest instruments should also be available if the incision needs to be extended. The argon beam coagulator and Cavitron ultrasonic aspirator should be available (see above). In addition to suture used for a gastrectomy, a chromic suture on a large needle is used for bleeding hepatic vessels.

Drugs and Solutions

Normal saline
Gelatin sponge (Gelfoam)
Oxidized regenerated cellulose (Surgicel)
Topical thrombin
Antibiotics

Physiological Monitoring

Refer to the discussion of gastrectomy and see under anesthesia above.

Physician's Orders

In addition to typical admission orders for patients having abdominal surgery, serum albumin levels should be monitored as well as serum glutamic-oxaloacetic transaminase and serum glutamic-pyruvic transaminase. These levels are normally elevated in patients with hepatic disease.

Laboratory and Diagnostic Studies

Laboratory and diagnostic studies include liver biopsy, arteriography, liver function studies, hepatic angiography, and computed tomography.

Procedure

Incision and Exposure

Most hepatic lobectomies are performed through an abdominal incision, but some surgeons prefer a thoracoabdominal approach for right lobectomies.

After the abdomen is entered, a retractor (Bookwalter) is placed for optimal exposure. The surgeon may use an extension of the Bookwalter retractor for retraction of the rib cage. Exposure is maintained for the procedure. Abdominal packs may also be placed for retraction of other organs.

Details

Dissection begins on the vessels and ducts surrounding the liver and the gallbladder. These hilar vessels are divided and ligated. Scissors, hemoclips, and suture ties (chromic or silk) are used for the dissection. An automatic, reloadable hemoclip applier is also used for ligation. It enables the surgeon to have better visualization and control hemostasis. The scrub nurse prepares the Cavitron ultrasonic aspirator and has it ready for the transection. A hepatic clamp is placed on the lobe to be resected. The clamp occludes the blood flow and marks the line of resection. The aspirator or electrocautery is used to transect the lobe. During the resection, hemostasis is achieved with hemoclips and suture ligatures of hepatic vessels. After the specimen has been removed, it is sent to the pathology department for diagnosis and study.

Hemostasis is controlled by electrocautery, thrombin, gelatin sponge, or oxidized regenerated cellulose. Many times, all of these agents are employed. Massive hemorrhage can be a complication after resection of the liver. The surgeon can also temporarily pack the abdomen with laparotomy sponges to provide compression.

Closure

When hemostasis is attained, the abdomen is irrigated with warm saline, drains are placed, and the abdomen is closed with Vicryl and Prolene suture. Dressings are applied and the patient is transferred to the surgical intensive care unit.

Postoperative Care

The patient requires close monitoring and metabolic support postoperatively. Blood glucose levels are checked frequently. Vitamin K and fresh-frozen plasma are administered to supply clotting factors. If hypoalbuminemia occurs, albumin is given and the serum bilirubin level is assessed daily.

Potential Surgical Complications

Wound and pulmonary infections
Fever of unknown origin
Abscess formation
Residual liver failure
Stress ulcers
Ascites
Coma
Varices
Hepatic encephalopathy

RIGHT-SIDED COLECTOMY

Definition

A *right-sided colectomy*, or hemicolectomy, refers to a removal of a segment or whole portion of the right side of the colon.

Indications

A right-sided colon resection is performed for patients with an obstruction, cancer, polyps, diverticular disease, volvulus, ulcerative colitis, and Crohn's disease.

Perioperative Nursing Implications

Anesthesia

Refer to the discussion of gastrectomy.

Position

Refer to the discussion of gastrectomy.

Creation and Maintenance of the Sterile Field

Refer to the discussion of gastrectomy.

Equipment and Supplies

See discussion of equipment and supplies for gastrectomy, above.

Drugs and Solutions

Normal saline
Antiobiotic solution for irrigation

Physiological Monitoring

Refer to the discussion of gastrectomy.

Physician's Orders

In addition to orders for all patients having abdominal surgery, a patient having a colectomy is ordered to have a bowel preparation. It is advisable to eliminate the fecal mass and reduce the number of bacteria as much as possible before the operation (Way, 1983). The patients receive clear liquids usually 48 hours before surgery. Cathartics and enemas can be also ordered.

Laboratory and Diagnostic Studies

Laboratory and diagnostic studies include abdominal x-ray films, fiberoptic colonoscopy and sigmoidoscopy, barium enema examination, and determination of baseline carcinoembryonic antigen levels. Carcinoembryonic antigen is a protein found in cell membranes of many tissues, including colorectal cancer. A blood hemoglobin determination is done for anemia, and a stool examination can be useful.

Procedure

Incision and Exposure

The patient is prepared from the nipples to the pubis, and drapes are placed, leaving only the surgical area exposed. The abdomen is opened using a midline incision. Wound hemostasis is established using hemostats or cautery. Suture ties and ligatures (chromic) are used to ligate any bleeding vessels. The peritoneum is grasped with two hemostats to facilitate entering the abdomen, and retractors are placed.

Details

The abdomen is explored by the surgeon for metastatic lesions, abnormalities, and other disease. Biopsy is performed for any suspicious areas. The surgeon inspects and palpates the small bowel along its length. The right half of the omentum is separated from the left and is included in the resected specimen. Sometimes, an umbilical tape is tied on the transverse colon proximal to the area of resection to lessen the spread of malignant cells.

The major branches of the superior mesenteric artery are ligated and divided using hemoclips, scissors, and suture ties. The large and small bowel (ileum) are grasped on the specimen side with crushing clamps (such as Allen intestinal clamps or Kocher intestinal forceps) and with noncrushing clamps (Glassman gastrointestinal clamps) on the anastomotic side. The large and small bowel are divided and the specimen is removed. The right-sided colon specimen is sent to the pathology department for diagnosis and study.

Towels or laparotomy sponges are placed to isolate the areas to be anastomosed, restricting contamination by bowel contents. The gastric-intestinal stapling instrument is used to perform the ileocolostomy. A fork of the instrument is inserted into each bowel lumen. The instrument is closed and fired. The knife in the instrument is used to create the stoma between both lumina. A stapling instrument is then used to close the opening of the two ends of lumina. A row of silk sutures is placed for reinforcement of anastomosis.

Closure

The abdomen is irrigated with warm saline and closed as described above.

Postoperative Care

In addition to routine postoperative care, the patient receives parenteral therapy until gastric motility is resumed. Adjuvant therapy may be started (e.g., radiation and/or chemotherapy).

Potential Surgical Complications

Obstruction
Perforation
Bleeding
Infection

MASTECTOMY (PARTIAL OR MODIFIED RADICAL)

Definition

A *partial mastectomy* is an excision of a segment of the breast that is malignant or suspicious for tumor. A *modified radical mastectomy* is a total removal of the breast plus axillary dissection.

Indications

Presence of a dominant mass
Abnormal mammogram with suspicious lesion
Nipple discharge
Red, indurated breast

Perioperative Nursing Implications

Anesthesia

A patient who is having a partial mastectomy is usually admitted the day of surgery. An anesthetist interviews the patient by telephone the night before or the day of surgery. The patient is given a local anesthetic such as lidocaine 1%. Epinephrine can be added to prolong the anesthetic effect and reduce bleeding. Supplemental sedation can also be given. Monitoring includes vital signs, heart rhythm, and oxygenation status.

General anesthesia is preferred for patients having a modified radical mastectomy because of the length and extent of the surgery. The nurse assists the anesthetist with placing an intravenous catheter on the unaffected side to maintain fluid volume and administer necessary medications (Stein and Zera, 1991). All laboratory values should be within normal limits. Preoperative medications and antibiotics may be given.

Position

The patient is positioned supine on the operating room bed. The arm on the affected side is extended laterally; one should be careful not to adduct it more than 90 degrees (to avoid branchial plexus injury). The unaffected arm can be placed along the side of the patient or extended laterally.

Creation and Maintenance of the Sterile Field

The affected breast and axilla are cleansed with povidone-iodine solution or soap. The arm should be prepared to the elbow, and a sterile stockinet is used to isolate the hand and the forearm. Sterile drapes are used to cover the patient, leaving only the breast and axilla exposed.

Equipment and Supplies

A dissecting set is used for a partial mastectomy. Instruments include hemostats; Allis tissue forceps, Kocher forceps, and Kelly forceps; scissors; and tissue (thumb) forceps. A minor instrument set is also suitable for a partial mastectomy. A major instrument set is used for modified radical mastectomy. Suture for breast surgery includes chromic, Vicryl, and Prolene. Elastic (Ace) wraps or a therapeutic breast support are used for dressing the surgical site.

Drugs and Solutions

Local anesthetic
Normal saline
Antibiotics for irrigation

Physiological Monitoring

Refer to discussion of gastrectomy.

Physician's Orders

Physician's orders include a chest x-ray film, electrocardiogram, and complete blood count. The patient is instructed to have nothing by mouth after midnight. Perioperative antibiotics can be ordered.

Laboratory and Diagnostic Studies

Mammography
Chest radiography
Bone scan
Cytological examination of nipple discharge if evident
Complete physical examination

Procedure for Partial Mastectomy

Incision and Exposure

The area is injected with a local anesthetic and an incision is made with a No. 10 or 15 blade. The skin incision descends through the fat layer to the superficial plane of the breast (Fowble et al., 1991). The fat is retracted by the use of Allis tissue forceps or a self-retaining retractor such as a Weitlaner retractor.

Details

The tissue surrounding the abnormality is freed by using scissors, knife, or cautery. The suspicious tissue is then excised widely. If the lesion is suspicious for carcinoma, more breast tissue is removed. The tissue is immediately placed on ice and sent to the pathology department for diagnosis. Specimens are sent on ice when an assessment of hormone receptors is needed. Sixty percent of patients with metastatic breast cancer respond to hormonal manipulation if these tumors contain estrogen receptors (Way, 1983).

Closure

After hemostasis is attained, the subcutaneous fat layer is closed with a Vicryl suture. The skin incision is closed with a subcuticular suture material such as nylon and Prolene.

Procedure for Modified Radical Mastectomy

Incision and Exposure

An elliptical (oval) incision is made, including the areola and the nipple. Skin flaps are retracted with Allis tissue forceps or towel clips, and the breast tissue is dissected with Metzenbaum scissors or cautery.

Details

The dissection continues to the smaller pectoral minor muscle, which is ligated and excised. Removal of the pectoral muscle allows axillary exposure. The axillary vein is dissected free from vessels and nerves, except for the thoracodorsal, long thoracic, and intercostobrachial nerves (Fowble et al., 1991). Further dissection is along the serratus muscle, and the axillary contents are then excised along with the breast (Fig. 20–5).

Closure

The chest is irrigated with warm saline, and suction drains are placed in the axilla and over the pectoral muscle. Closure is attained by approximating the skin flaps with Vicryl suture. The skin is closed with a subcuticular stitch.

Postoperative Care

Postoperative care includes mobilization of the arm to prevent limitation of motion and the avoidance of intravenous fluid and medication administration and treatment on the affected side. Follow-up care should be done for life to detect local and distant recurrences.

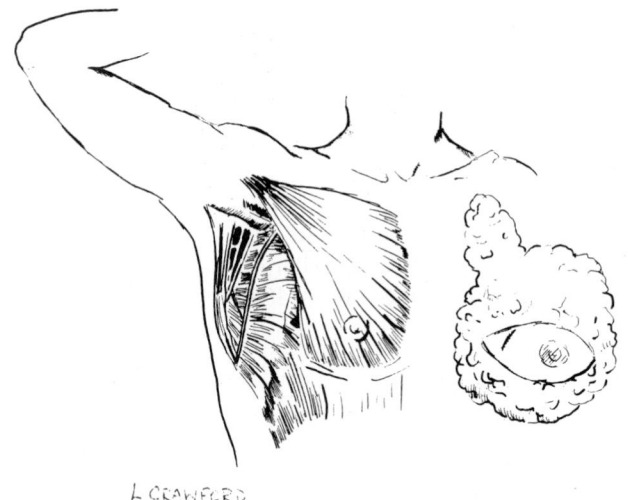

L CRAWFORD

FIGURE 20–5. Modified radical mastectomy.

Potential Surgical Complications

Hematoma
Infection
Brachial plexus injury from overabduction of the arm
Lymphedema

SURGICAL ENDOSCOPIC PROCEDURES

The introduction of high-resolution video cameras to the established techniques of laparoscopy has ushered in an era of minimally invasive surgery (Dent et al., 1991). This chapter discusses three endoscopic surgeries: cholecystectomy, herniorrhaphy, and appendectomy.

Definition

Laparoscopic *cholecystectomy* is the removal of the gallbladder endoscopically instead of through a laparotomy. A laparoscopic *appendectomy* is the removal of the appendix via the same technique, and a *herniorrhaphy* is performed endoscopically instead of via an abdominal incision at the inguinal site.

Indications

Indications for laparoscopic procedures are essentially the same as those for open procedures. Patients are told before surgery that an open procedure may be performed if complications arise. Indications for a laparoscopic cholecystectomy include cholelithiasis and cholecystitis. An endoscopic appendectomy is performed for patients with appendicitis, and laparoscopic herniorrhaphies are performed for patients with a hernia.

Perioperative Nursing Implications

Anesthesia

A general anesthetic is used. The abdominal wall muscles must be relaxed to allow distention during insufflation.

Position

The patient is placed in a supine position. Both arms are extended on arm boards for the cholecystectomy. This position enables the surgical team members to stand on both sides of the arm boards for manipulation of the camera and instruments. It also enables surgical team members to view the video monitors, which are located at each side of the patient's head.

The position of choice for laparoscopic herniorrhaphies and appendectomies is supine also, but the patient's arms are positioned at the patient's sides because the surgical team is located toward the upper end of the operating room bed.

Creation and Maintenance of the Sterile Field

The abdomen is prepared from the nipples to the symphysis pubis. If the patient is having a hernia repair, the groin and top portion of the thighs are prepared. If the patient has a lot of abdominal hair, a shave may be required. Surgical drapes are applied, keeping the abdomen exposed. Endoscopic procedures involve a lot of equipment around the operative field. It is important that the surgical team maintain a sterile environment. Traffic in the operating room should be kept to a minimum during the setup and the procedure.

Equipment and Supplies

In addition to a laparotomy set, a laparoscopic cholecystectomy set is used. This set contains a laparoscope, a camera, a light cord, carbon dioxide tubing, and laparoscopic instruments. These instruments must be available and functional. Scissors, graspers, and dissectors are crucial to the operation and can be either disposable or reusable.

An insufflation needle, used to establish pneumoperitoneum, surgical trocars (used for laparoscopic guidance), and an endoscopic clip applier are placed on the field.

During an endoscopic appendectomy, an endoscopic GIA surgical stapler with refills must be available. An instrument called a patch spreader lays the mesh inside the hernia sac. Refer to the discussion of special instruments, supplies, and equipment above for additional video equipment.

Drugs and Solutions

Normal saline solution
Bupivacaine hydrochloride (Marcaine) 0.5%
Iothalamate meglumine (Conray)

Physiological Monitoring

Refer to the discussion of gastrectomy.

Physician's Orders, Laboratory and Diagnostic Studies

The physician's orders and laboratory and diagnostic studies differ little from the preoperative work-up of patients undergoing an open procedure. The preoperative work-up for patients having a laparoscopic cholecystectomy includes an abdominal ultrasound study to confirm the presence of gallstones, and if common bile duct stones are suspected, endoscopic retrograde cholangiopancreatography is done. If stones are present at endoscopic retrograde cholangiopancreatography, a stone extraction is done.

A bowel preparation is ordered for patients with appendicitis. Other physician's orders are as discussed for gastrectomy.

Procedure for Laparoscopic Cholecystectomy

Incision and Exposure

Initial entry is made using an insufflation needle at the umbilicus. The needle is inserted through a small skin incision. Pneumoperitoneum is established using carbon dioxide gas through a high-flow electronic insufflator (Fig. 20-6A). The abdomen is filled with 3 to 4 L of carbon dioxide gas until the intraabdominal pressure is 12 to 14 mm Hg. The insufflation needle is then removed and a 10- or 11-mm trocar is inserted in the umbilical incision. A laparoscope is then inserted in the umbilical incision and a video camera and light source are hooked up to the laparoscope (Fig. 20-6B). The general surgeon operates directly from the monitor. Two monitors are used during the procedure and are placed on both sides of the patient. An observation of the peritoneal cavity is then performed.

Two 5-mm incisions are made on the right side of the body below the dome of the liver. Surgical trocars are inserted through these incisions. Laparoscopic graspers, dissectors, and scissors are then inserted to manipulate and dissect the gallbladder. Another incision is made on the midline and this is used as the main operative site.

Details

Grasping forceps are inserted, grasping the gallbladder. The gallbladder is then retracted superiorly. The peritoneum is dissected from the gallbladder, exposing the cystic artery, the cystic duct, and the common bile duct. It is important to recognize that the cephalad traction of the gallbladder often distorts the normal anatomy of the common bile duct, sometimes causing it to become "tented up" at its junction with the cystic duct. Such distortion may result in inadvertent injury to the common bile duct if the operator is not aware of this potential abnormal appearance (Zucker and Bailey, 1990). An endoscopic clip applier is then introduced through the 11-mm trocar to ligate both the cystic duct and the artery. Two clips are applied to each structure, and scissors or a laser are then used to transect the cystic duct and artery.

If there is evidence of gallstones, an operative cholangiogram may be done. Microscissors create the hole in the cystic duct, and a cholangiographic instrument is used to insert the catheter and hold it in place.

The gallbladder is dissected from the liver bed via laser or electrocautery. The area is irrigated and checked for hemostasis. The laparoscope is removed from the

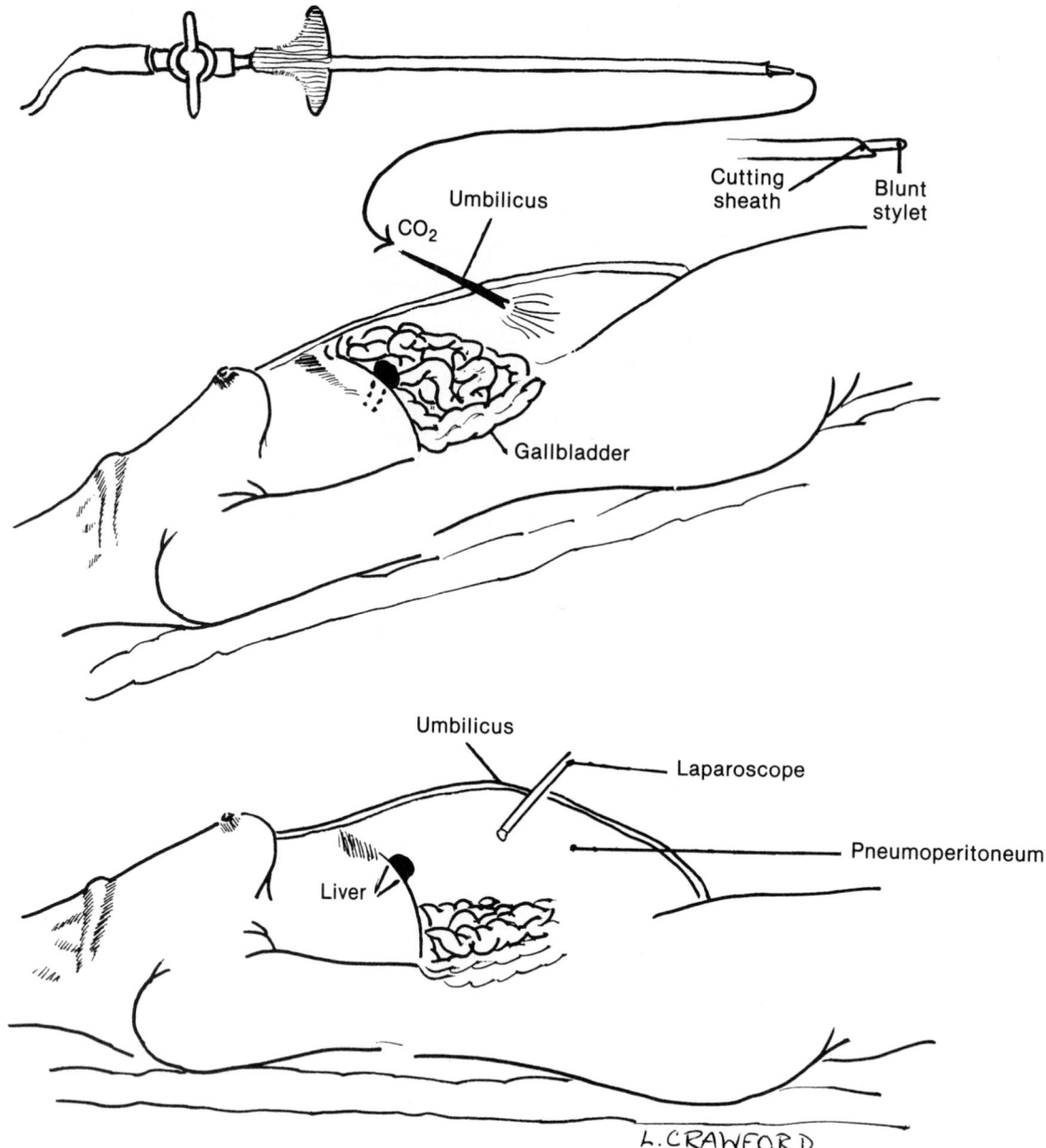

FIGURE 20–6. *A*, Surgical trocar insufflating carbon dioxide through the umbilicus for pneumoperitoneum. *B*, Laparoscope insertion after insufflation is completed.

umbilical site and placed in the midline incision. The gallbladder is then removed from the umbililical site using an 11-mm claw forceps. The gallbladder is removed intact. If the gallbladder cannot fit through the incision, bile can be drained or the incision can be made larger.

Closure

After removing the trocar sheaths, the umbilical incision is closed with a Vicryl fascia stitch followed by a subcuticular suture. All other puncture wounds are secured by either suture or adhesive strips. Dressings are then applied, completing the procedure.

Postoperative Care

The Foley catheter and nasogastric tube are usually removed in the PACU, barring any problems with urinary retention and nausea. Pain medications are given as needed, although postoperative pain is usually minimal, with pain normally described at the trocar site.

Potential Surgical Complications

Common bile duct injury
Hepatic artery injury
Abscess

Bile leak
Retained common bile duct stones
Shoulder pain from air under the diaphragm
Hernia from the port site
Wound infection

Procedure for Laparoscopic Herniorrhaphy

Incision and Exposure

In addition to use of the same exposure as in a cholecystectomy, a 12-mm trocar and sheath are inserted so the endoscopic hernia stapler, endoscopic patch spreader, and mesh can be introduced.

Details

After pneumoperitoneum is attained, the hernia orifice is located and identified. Mesh is applied to close the defect of the hernia. The mesh, the nature of which varies according to the surgeon's choice, may be placed inside the sac in the form of a "cigarette" roll or as a loose pack (Ger, 1991). The mesh is introduced into the abdomen via the 12-mm sheath and is spread over the defect by the endoscopic patch spreader. It is secured down by the endoscopic hernia stapler.

Closure

Refer to the discussion of laparoscopic cholecystectomy.

Postoperative Care

Refer to the discussion of laparoscopic cholecystectomy.

Potential Surgical Complications

Recurrence of hernia
Incomplete closure of the stapler
Meralgia paresthetica (traumatization of the lateral femoral cutaneous nerve, which passes through the inguinal ligament)

Procedure for Laparoscopic Appendectomy

Incision and Exposure

Three surgical trocars are used for an appendectomy: one for the umbilical site; one as an accessory port used for dissection, irrigation, and suctioning; and a main operative trocar that the endoscopic intestinal stapling device is used through.

Details

The appendix is dissected from the colon using cautery, scissors, and dissecting instruments. The mesoappendix is dissected along its base and the appendiceal artery is ligated with an endoscopic clip. Intentional separation of the mesoappendix from the appendix is performed to minimize the appendiceal mass of tissue, which must be removed through the 10-mm laparoscopic port (Geis et al., 1992).

The base of the appendix is closed and transected using an endoscopic GIA stapling device.

Closure

Refer to the discussion of laparoscopic cholecystectomy.

Postoperative Care

Refer to the discussion of laparoscopic cholecystectomy.

Potential Surgical Complications

Bowel obstruction
Wound infection
Incomplete closure of staples

ACKNOWLEDGEMENT
The author wishes to acknowledge gratefully Laura Crawford, the graphic artist who provided the drawings.

Bibliography

Aufses, A. H., Block, G. E. (1986). *Surgical management of granulomatous inflammatory bowel disease.* New York: LTI Medica.

Dent, T. L., Ponsky, J. L., Berci, G. (1991). Minimal access general surgery: The dawn of a new era. *American Journal of Surgery, 161,* 323.

Fowble, B., Goodman, R. L., Glick, J. H., Rosato, E. F. (1991). *Breast cancer treatment.* St. Louis: Mosby Year Book.

Geis, W. P., Miller, C. E., Kokoszka, J. S. (1992). Laparoscopic appendectomy for acute appendicitis: Rationale and technical aspects. *Contemporary Surgery, 40*(1), 13–19.

Ger, R. (1991). The laparoscopic management of groin hernias. *Contemporary Surgery, 39*(4), 15–19.

Jackson, D. C., Martin, T., Evans, M. M., Rubio, P. A. (1990). Endoscopic laser cholecystectomy. A new approach to gallbladder removal. *AORN Journal, 51,* 1546–1552.

Jarrell, B. E., Carabasi, R. A., III. (1986). *Surgery.* Media, PA: Harwal Publishing.

Jeejeeboy, K. (1980). *Gastrointestinal diseases.* Garden City, NY: Medical Examination Publishing.

Nora, P. F (1990). *Operative surgery: Principles and Techniques* (3rd ed). Philadelphia: WB Saunders Co, p. 787.

Polk, H. C., Harbrecht, P. J., Martin, L. F. (1983). Right colon resection. *Surgical Profiles, 2,* 83, 1–21.

Reddick, E. J., Olson, D. O. (1990). *Reddick laparoscopic cholecystectomy.* KTP/532 Clinical Update, 31.

Stapling techniques general surgery (3rd ed.). (1988). Norwalk, CT: United States Surgical Corporation.

Stein, P., Zera, R. T. (1991). Breast cancer. *AORN Journal, 53,* 938–963.

Steuer, K. (1990). Hepatic resection: Indications, procedures, patient care. *AORN Journal, 52,* 230–250.

Tortora, G. J., Anagnostakos, N. P. (1984). *Principles of anatomy and physiology.* New York: Harper & Row.

Way, L. (1983). *Surgical diagnosis and treatment.* Los Altos, CA: Lange Medical Publications.

Wells, M. (1987). *Decision making in perioperative nursing.* Philadelphia: B. C. Decker.

Zucker, K. A., Bailey, R. W. (1990). *Atlas of endo cholecystectomy.* Norwalk, CT: United States Surgical Corporation.

CHAPTER 21

Vascular Surgery

Donna S. Watson and Beverly W. Ejsing

DEFINITION

The early beginnings of vascular surgery included efforts to stop hemorrhage from large vessels. The first tools consisted of only a knife and cautery. It was not until Ambroise Paré, who perfected the use of ligature for controlling bleeding, that the techniques and technology of the 20th century began to evolve.

Vascular surgery is surgery on one or more blood vessels in the body, or surgery to treat disease of any of the blood vessels of the body. Patients often have more than the usual amount of preoperative anxiety. Their quality of life depends on the success of the surgical procedure. Many patients face eventual loss of one or both limbs, the possibility of a stroke, or death resulting from uncontrolled bleeding. The surgical team is the most important component of a successful surgical outcome. Each member is responsible for being knowledgeable of the procedure and able to anticipate the

451

expected course of action. The following discussion of procedures outlines key information for the assistant in vascular surgery.

ANATOMY

Arterial disease affects the arterial system of the human body by impairing the flow of blood. Impairment of the blood flow may be related to (1) the total or partial obstruction of the vessel lumen related to plaque, (2) the actual structure of the vessel lumen (e.g., narrow vessel lumen), or (3) trauma to the vessel. This chapter discusses primarily surgical interventions for effects of obstruction of the vessel lumen.

Obstruction of the vessel lumen is related to *athero-sclerosis*, which is the process of plaque development. This silent disorder progresses for years before clinical manifestations become noticeable. The clinical manifestations result from "(1) chronic ischemia due to plaque enlargement great enough to reduce blood flow, (2) acute ischemia due to arterial embolism of plaque-associated platelet thrombi or atheromatous debris, and (3) acute ischemia produced by thrombosis of arteries at sites of advanced plaques" (Zwolak and Cronenwett, 1990, p. 8). The most common sites of atherosclerotic plaque development occur in the "coronary arteries, the carotid bifurcation, the infrarenal abdominal aorta, the iliac arteries, and the superficial femoral artery" (Zwolak and Cronenwett, 1990, p. 11). Figure 21–1 illustrates the effect of atherosclerosis on some major vessels and the possible complications. This chapter discusses surgical interventions for some of the complications—carotid endarterectomy, resection of an abdominal aneurysm, femoropopliteal bypass graft, and amputation.

The major artery of the body, the aorta, originates at the aortic valve of the heart, arches away from the heart, and flows downward through the body. In the pelvis, it bifurcates into the iliac arteries, which develop branches through which blood flows to the legs (see Fig. 21–1). The venous system is much the same as the arterial, with the major vessel in the body being the vena cava.

SPECIAL INSTRUMENTS, SUPPLIES, AND EQUIPMENT

Vascular instruments are designed to minimize trauma to the vessel. Because the instruments are delicate, many are wrapped individually to avoid damage. Vascular surgery can be complicated in only a few minutes by the absence of pedal pulses or the inability of the patient to move an extremity. For this reason, instruments should never be allowed to become contaminated until the patient leaves the operating room.

Special supplies include peanut dissectors, Fogarty inserts, vessel loops, suture boots, and an assortment of

vascular suture. Hemostatic agents (e.g., topical thrombin) to control oozing from the anastomosis site should be readily available. Anticoagulation during the procedure can be accomplished with the administration of heparin sulfate and reversal with protamine sulfate.

The diseased vessel may be replaced with a manufactured fabric graft, a vessel harvested from the patient, or a bovine graft. Grafts come in different sizes and shapes and should be immediately available, with one back-up, before the beginning of the procedure. The types of grafts include woven, which do not leak blood through the walls and do not need to be preclotted; and knitted, which necessitate preclotting with the patient's blood before heparin is administered to prevent the graft from leaking. If a bovine graft is inserted, care must be taken to rinse the preserving solution thoroughly from the graft. This is accomplished by rinsing the graft three times in normal saline, discarding the saline after each rinsing.

CAROTID ENDARTERECTOMY

Definition

Carotid endarterectomy is the removal of atherosclerotic plaque or emboli from the carotid artery. The lesion is most frequently located at the carotid bifurcation and may restrict blood flow and/or be embolic (Sandmann, 1992). The main goal is prevention of the major potential complication of this surgical intervention—stroke. The expertise, skills, and knowledge of the surgical team are essential for this delicate procedure.

Indications

Indications for a carotid endarterectomy are listed in Table 21–1. Because of the potential complication of stroke during the procedure, the risk of surgical intervention versus conservative treatment must be considered. The symptomatic patient may have a *transient ischemic attack*, which "is a transient or temporary episode of neurologic dysfunction commonly manifested

TABLE 21–1. **INDICATIONS FOR CAROTID ENDARTERECTOMY**

Carotid territory transient ischemic attack
Amaurosis fugax
Completed stroke with minimal to moderate neurological deficit
Central retinal artery occlusion
Asymptomatic high-grade stenosis
Vertebrobasilar transient ischemic attack
Acute stroke (in hospital)
Stroke in evolution

From Eldrup-Jorgensen, J., O'Donnel, T. F. (1990). Extracranial cerebral vascular disease. In P. F. Nora (Ed.), *Operative surgery: Principles and techniques* (3rd ed.) (p. 959). Philadelphia: W. B. Saunders.

Affected site

Cerebral vessels

Carotid arteries

Aorta

Coronary arteries

Renal arteries

Iliac arteries

Femoral arteries

Tibial arteries

Complication

Stroke
Transient ischemic attacks
Chronic ischemic brain disease

Stroke
Ischemic attacks

Aneurysm

Heart attack
Angina

Hypertension

Peripheral vascular disease

Peripheral vascular disease

Peripheral vascular disease

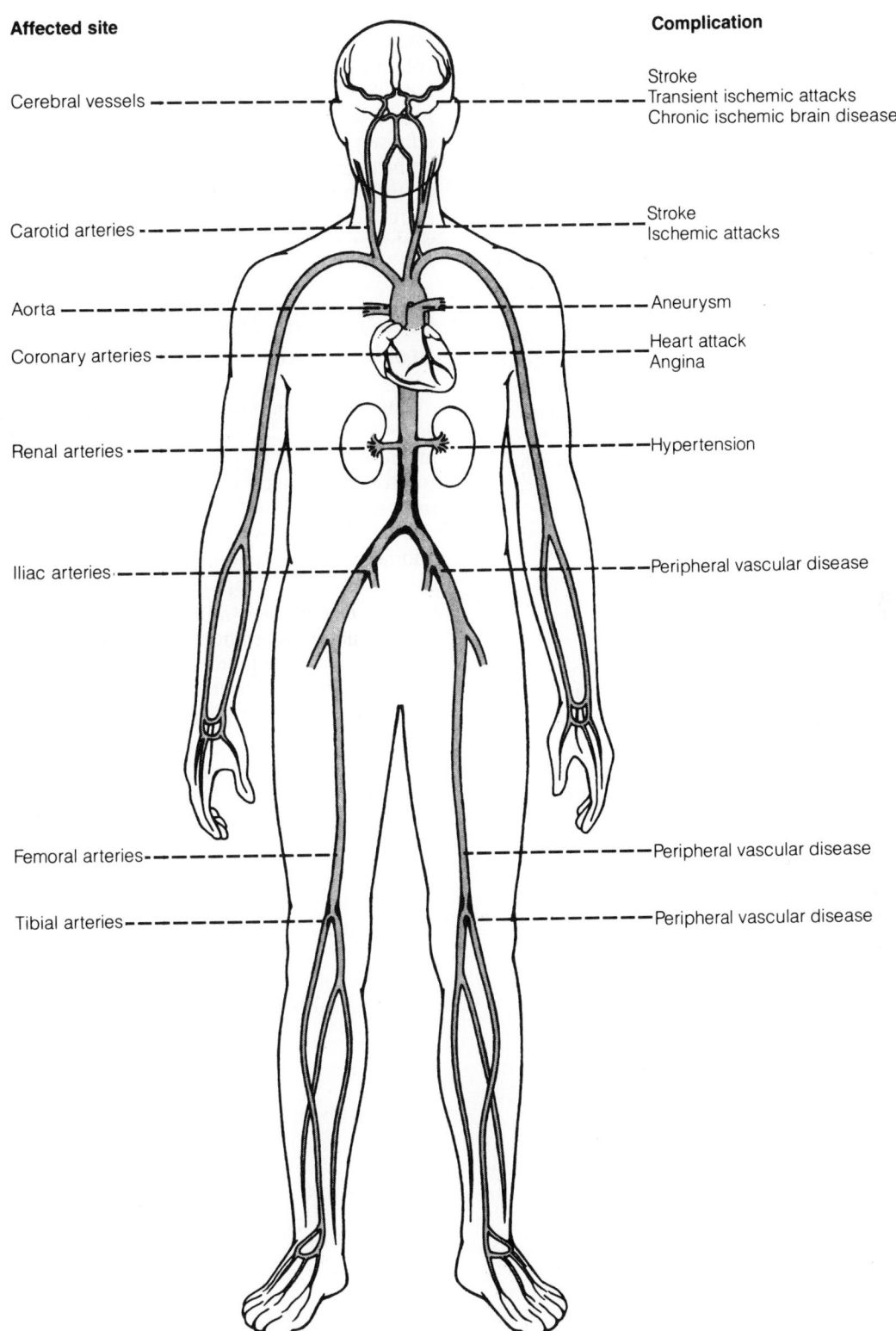

FIGURE 21–1. Major arterial blood vessels affected by atherosclerosis. (From *Report of the 1977 Working Group to Review the Report by the National Heart and Lung Institute Task Force on Arteriosclerosis: Arteriosclerosis* [DHEW Publication No. NIH 78–1526]. 1977, Washington, DC: U.S. Government Printing Office.)

by a sudden loss of motor, sensory, or visual function, lasting a few seconds or minutes but no longer than 24 hours" (Brunner and Suddarth, 1984, p. 1306). Other symptoms may include dysphasia, aphasia, hemiplegia, sensory or motor deficit, ataxia, dizziness, diplopia, dysarthria, weakness, and amaurosis fugax. *Amaurosis fugax* is monocular blindness related to an ophthalmic artery embolus; generally, this condition is temporary.

If the patient has a stroke that includes permanent neurological loss, the decision for surgical intervention must weigh key factors. These include assessing the patient's remaining neurological function and determining that the benefits of surgical intervention are greater than the potential risks. The goal is to preserve any remaining neurological function.

In the United States, a large number of carotid endarterectomies are performed on asymptomatic patients (Handelsman, 1991). However, there is controversy about surgical intervention for these patients. Research is needed to study the outcomes of surgical intervention versus conservative treatment for asymptomatic patients.

Related Surgical Procedures

Coronary artery bypass grafting

Perioperative Nursing Implications

Anesthesia

Anesthesia for the carotid endarterectomy patient is critical, because myocardial infarction during the perioperative phase is most frequently a contributing cause of death (Kennedy and Wasnick, 1990). A thorough preoperative assessment includes a cardiac, pulmonary, and neurological history. Cardiac and neurological risks are explained to the patient by the anesthesiologist.

The procedure can be performed under regional or general anesthesia. Although there is much controversy about the advantages of the regional technique, the main advantage is the ability to monitor the patient's neurological status during the surgery. A deep cervical plexus block is most frequently used. The technique varies from a single-injection interscalene approach to multiple injections of the transverse processes of C2, C3, and C4. The amount of local anesthetic agent administered depends on the type, which is based on the anesthetist's preference and the patient's size.

There is no clear evidence that the use of one anesthetic agent for general anesthesia is recommended instead of another for carotid endarterectomy patients. Instead, the choice of anesthetic agent is based on the patient's preexisting medical conditions. Youngberg and Gold (1991) identified that "the choice of a specific general anesthetic technique may be of less importance than ensuring that adequate cerebral and coronary blood flow is maintained" (p. 347).

Position

The patient is placed in supine position with the arms tucked to the side. The surgical site is exposed by rotating the patient's head toward the unaffected side approximately 60 degrees (Fig. 21–2). The head is supported with a foam or a plastic head holder. Wide adhesive tape may be applied from one side of the bed, be brought across the patient's forehead, and be secured on the opposite bed side to ensure the patient's position. A rolled blanket or foam padding is placed under the shoulders to hyperextend the neck.

Creation and Maintenance of the Sterile Field

The skin preparation usually involves iodophor scrub and solution, or gel. Bone wax or a cotton ball is placed in the ear canal to prevent pooling of the preparation solution. The neck is prepared starting at the incision site, working down to the clavicle level to the chest midline, continuing from the incision site up to the middle of the ear, and including all areas of the posterior neck. Drapes are applied and may be secured with staples. The right or the left lower leg is prepared in case a saphenous vein patch is necessary.

Equipment and Supplies

Instruments contained in a minor vascular set are listed in Table 21–2. These instruments should be updated periodically to reflect the needs of the surgical team.

Drugs and Solutions

Intravenous heparin sulfate
Normal saline

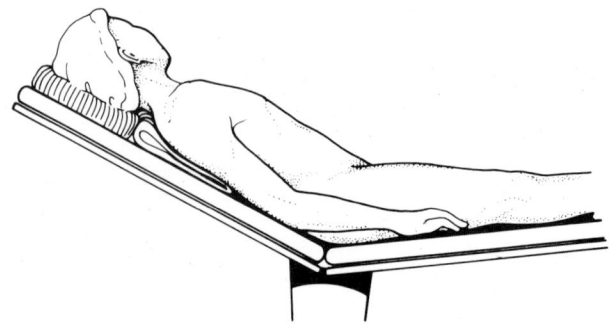

FIGURE 21–2. Position of the patient for carotid endarterectomy. (From Sandmann, W. [1992]. Carotid endarterectomy. In P. R. F. Bell, C. W. Jamieson, C. Vaughan Ruckley [Eds.]. *Surgical management of vascular disease* [p. 674]. Philadelphia: W. B. Saunders.)

TABLE 21–2. MINOR VASCULAR INSTRUMENTATION

Retractors

2 shallow Deaver	2 thyroid rakes
2 Army-Navy	2 Weitlaner
3 right-angled	1 Oschner
3 bands	1 Henley
2 Cushing vein	2 Henley blades
1 Richardson	

Suction and Other Items

1 short No. 12 Frazier	1 nerve hook
1 short No. 4 Frazier	1 ruler

Hemoclip Applier

2 small
2 medium
1 Freer elevator

Knife Handles

2 No. 3
1 No. 7

Scissors

1 regular Metzenbaum	1 nurses
1 long Metzenbaum	1 suture
1 Church	1 large suture
1 No. 7 Potts	

Forceps

2 short smooth	4 Allis
2 Adson toothed	12 towel clips
2 Atragrips, 7 inch	2 Crile
2 titanium Rhoton, 7 inch	2 Mixter
2 short toothed	1 sponge stick
4 Jackson	1 Beck clamp
8 curved mosquito	1 Cooley clamp
8 straight mosquito	1 long Kelly
12 curved hemostats	4 curved Fogarty
6 straight hemostats	4 straight Fogarty
4 short Kelly	1 super Crafoord
4 Kocher	1 Rumel

Carotid Clamps

1 large
1 small
2 Berkowitz special

Fine Vascular Instruments (Wrapped)

2 small Potts scissors	2 coronary bulldogs
2 small iris scissors	2 cannulas
4 fine vascular forceps, 5 inch	5 small vascular clamps
2 Castroviejo needle holders	5 coronary dilators

Mueller Bulldogs (Wrapped)

2 straight
1 curved

Needle Holders (Wrapped)

2 Mayo-Hegar, 9 inch	2 Ravdin
2 Sarot	2 Mayo-Hegar, 6 inch

Physiological Monitoring

Basic monitoring methods for all endarterectomy patients include electrocardiogram (ECG), intraarterial catheters, monitors of cerebral perfusion, and pulse oximetry. Continuous monitoring of blood pressure is essential, because sudden changes in the blood pressure may occur during the procedure. Central venous pressure catheters and a pulmonary arterial catheter are generally not indicated unless warranted by the patient's condition.

Specimens and Cultures

Specimens are collected and saved until after the operative procedure. The specimen is labeled and placed into formalin and sent to the pathology laboratory for examination. Cultures are not routinely taken during this procedure.

Physician's Orders

Typical admission orders include a medical examination with emphasis on cardiovascular and neurological assessment, arteriography, and techniques to evaluate the extent of carotid artery disease (e.g., computed tomography and magnetic resonance imaging). The patient has nothing by mouth (NPO) after midnight. A shave preparation is ordered on the correct side to the level of the earlobe. Male patients are usually permitted to shave themselves. A blood sample is ordered for type and cross-match for 2 U of whole blood. If the patient is receiving a continuous infusion of heparin sulfate preoperatively, an activated partial prothrombin time, a hematocrit and hemoglobin count, and a platelet count are most likely ordered. The night before surgery, aspirin, 325 mg orally, is administered.

Laboratory and Diagnostic Studies

Recommended laboratory tests include ECG, chest x-ray film, electrolyte determinations, coagulation studies, and angiography.

Procedure

Incision and Exposure

A vertical incision is made along the anterior border of the sternocleidomastoid muscle (Fig. 21–3). The arteriogram is used to determine the incision site, and the length of the incision is based on its location and the size of the plaque. Electrocautery is used to provide hemostasis and divide the platysma muscle. Blunt-edged self-retaining retractors may be applied by the surgeon or the assistant to provide better exposure. The facial vein, which lies across the carotid bifurcation, is divided and ligated with suture. Identification and exposure are provided for the vagus nerve, the internal jugular vein, the common carotid artery, the internal carotid artery, the external carotid artery, the hypoglossal nerve, and the superficial thyroid arteries. The internal and external

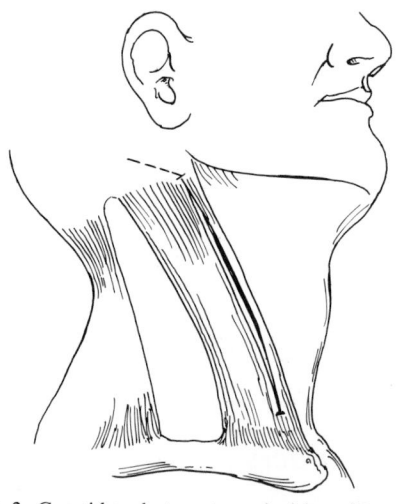

FIGURE 21–3. Carotid endarterectomy incision. (From Eldrup-Jorgensen, J., O'Donnel, T. F. [1990]. Extracranial cerebral vascular disease. In P. F. Nora [Ed.]. *Operative surgery: Principles and techniques* [3rd ed.] [p. 960]. Philadelphia: W. B. Saunders.)

carotid arteries are carefully dissected with minimal manipulation to prevent dislodging the plaque.

Details

The common carotid artery is dissected, exposing the artery and its branches. The assistant should be prepared to assist with the application of vessel loops and carotid clamps. After the artery is dissected and before the artery is clamped, anticoagulation therapy is initiated with the administration of heparin sulfate, 75 U/kg. Instruments that should be readily available include carotid clamps, a knife with a No. 11 or a No. 15 blade, vascular scissors, vascular forceps, an angled vascular clamp, an elevator, and possibly a carotid shunt.

Controversy exists about the use of a carotid shunt. Opponents of shunting cite "increased operative time, decreased ease of endarterectomy, increased trauma to the distal carotid artery, and increased risk of intraoperative embolism" (Walsh and McDaniel, 1990, p. 51). Advantages include cerebral perfusion and a less hurried procedure for the surgeon. In an investigation by Sandmann (1992) of 503 carotid endarterectomy patients assigned to random treatment groups with and without shunting, severe perfusion ischemia occurred in only 4% of those undergoing shunting during 40 minutes of shunting. Neurological monitoring (electroencephalography and somatosensory evoked potential monitoring) was applied to each patient. Sandmann advocated electroencephalographic and somatosensory evoked potential monitoring during clamping and the use of carotid shunt for high-risk patients (e.g., those with an unstable cardiorespiratory status) and intraoperative changes in neurological monitoring variables.

The carotid artery is clamped, and an arteriotomy is made with a No. 11 or a No. 15 blade and extended with Potts scissors. The extent of the plaque may be identified by the color of the atherosclerotic artery. If plaque is present, it appears yellowish compared with a bluish color where no plaque exists. Plaque may be removed with a Penfield endarterectomy blade (Fig. 21–4). The plaque is removed first at the proximal end of the common carotid artery and then the most distal. Special care is taken to irrigate with heparinized saline to remove any loose remnants of plaque and identify any that remains (Fig. 21–5). If any plaque remains that cannot be removed, it is carefully tacked down with a 7–0 nonabsorbable suture.

Closure

The arteriotomy is closed with nonabsorbable suture such as a 6–0 polypropylene (Prolene) suture. Closure is done with a continuous running stitch. If a patch is needed for closure, a synthetic graft or the saphenous vein may be used. Before complete closure, the carotid shunt, if inserted, is removed. Unclamping proceeds with the distal clamp first, allowing back bleeding and flushing, followed by removal of the proximal clamp. The suture lines are examined for leaks. To aid in controlling bleeding, leaks may be repaired with suture patches and/or oxidized regenerated cellulose (Surgicel).

The sternocleidomastoid fascia and the platysma muscle are closed with either a continuous or an interrupted suture. To facilitate drainage, a temporary drain may

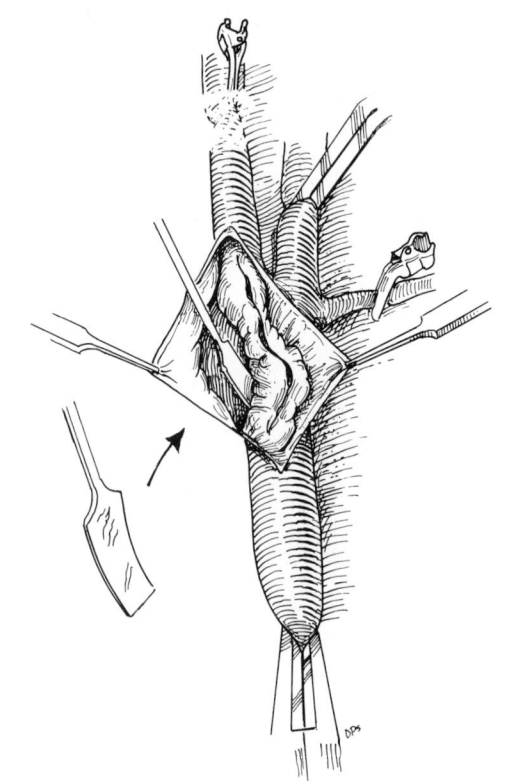

FIGURE 21–4. Removal of plaque with a Penfield dissector. (From Eldrup-Jorgensen, J., O'Donnel, T. F. [1990]. Extracranial cerebral vascular disease. In P. F. Nora [Ed.]. *Operative surgery: Principles and techniques* [3rd ed.] [p. 962]. Philadelphia: W. B. Saunders.)

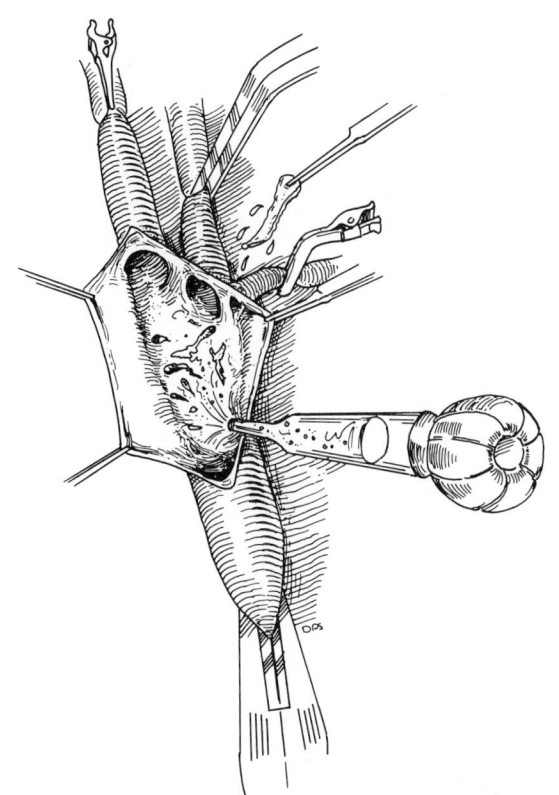

FIGURE 21–5. Irrigation and inspection of the operative field. (From Eldrup-Jorgensen, J., O'Donnel, T. F. [1990]. Extracranial cerebral vascular disease. In P. F. Nora [Ed.]. *Operative surgery: Principles and techniques* [3rd ed.] [p. 965]. Philadelphia: W. B. Saunders.)

be inserted. Skin is closed with a continuous absorbable suture or staples. Gauze is applied over the incision and secured with tape. A bulky dressing is avoided because of the possibility of concealing a hematoma postoperatively.

Postoperative Care

The patient is transferred to the postanesthesia recovery area for routine monitoring. Depending on the patient's cardiopulmonary status, he or she may be transferred to the nursing floor or the intensive care unit. To decrease the incidence of complications of kinking of the artery, bleeding, and thrombosis, flexion and turning of the patient's neck are avoided. The head is elevated 20 degrees and maintained in straight alignment and secured with towel rolls or sandbags to prevent flexion and turning for 12 hours postoperatively. The patient's blood pressure is frequently monitored and should not exceed 160 mm Hg owing to the possibility of intracerebral hemorrhage. The surgeon should be notified of a systolic blood pressure greater than 160 mm Hg or less than 120 mm Hg. Neurological status should be assessed every hour, including that of the vagus and hypoglossal nerves. Monitor closely for signs of neck hematoma. The patient is discharged in 3 to 5 postoperative days.

Potential Surgical Complications

Infection
Stroke
Emboli
Cranial nerve injuries
Myocardial infarction
Neck hematoma

RESECTION OF ABDOMINAL AORTIC ANEURYSM, AORTIC BIFURCATION GRAFT

Definition

Resection of an abdominal aortic aneurysm involves the removal of atherosclerotic plaque from the aorta that has been weakened and may even be bulging from the accumulation of plaque. A vascular graft is inserted to strengthen or replace the diseased aorta. The disease process may include the renal arteries and the mesenteric artery.

Indications

Clinical manifestations of an abdominal aneurysm depend on the size, location, and rate of growth. At present, 80% of all aneurysms are diagnosed in the asymptomatic stage compared with 50% in the 1960s (Millis et al., 1992). A familial predisposition is noted; it occurs in a 9:1 ratio of male to female, and usually after the age of 60 years. The patient may have a pulsating abdominal mass, abdominal pain, or low back pain. Other manifestations include claudication after walking one or two blocks and, in severe cases, even less distance.

There is controversy about when to operate electively on a patient with an abdominal aneurysm. The debate concerns the likelihood of rupture of an aneurysm 6 cm or larger. Some surgeons choose to operate only if the aneurysm is greater than 5 cm.

Related Surgical Procedures

Carotid endarterectomy
Coronary artery bypass grafting

Perioperative Nursing Implications

Anesthesia

The most acceptable technique is general anesthesia, although the use of epidural and regional techniques have been reported. Anesthesia may be induced with thiopental or other drugs of choice. If the patient has cardiovascular compromise, the drug most often administered is etomidate owing to its mild effects on the cardiovascular system. A state of general anesthesia is maintained by inhalation or intravenous technique, depending on the status of the patient and the individual choice of the anesthesiologist.

Because of the type of surgery, the patient is at risk for potential blood loss and significant swings in blood pressure. Minimal monitoring methods include arterial and central venous pressure catheters and the insertion of a urinary catheter. Although blood is ordered, the patient should be protected from multiple blood transfusions if at all possible. The cell saver is a device that collects all blood suctioned during the procedure, washes the cells in a heparinized saline solution, separates the plasma, and collects the cells to be readministered intravenously as autologous packed cells. This device should be readily available.

Position

The patient is placed in the supine position. To allow more room at the operative site, each arm is secured on a padded arm board and positioned at a less than 90-degree angle.

Creation and Maintenance of the Sterile Field

The patient is shaved and prepared with iodophor scrub and solution, or gel, from the nipple line to the midthigh. If the disease process extends to the renal or mesenteric arteries, a portion of the ankle over the saphenous vein may also be prepared in case a vein graft is needed. The patient is draped to expose the abdomen and midthigh areas. The genitalia are isolated with adhesive drapes to prevent contamination of the field if the incision is extended into the femoral areas.

Equipment and Supplies

Instruments should include those in the major vascular set listed in Table 21–3. In addition, the following items should be immediately available: a selection of aortic vascular grafts in multiple sizes, aortic bifurcated vascular grafts in multiple sizes, vessel loops, vascular clamps, vascular suture, a cell saver, the surgeon's choice of abdominal retractor, a large Foley catheter with a 75-ml bag, nasogastric tubes of various sizes and suction, and a beanbag to aid in positioning the patient if necessary.

Ensuring that all types and sizes of grafts are available is critical. If the disease extends past the bifurcation of the aorta, a bifurcated vascular graft is used. If not, a tubular vascular graft is used. The types of grafts include woven, which do not leak blood through the walls and do not need to be preclotted; and knitted, which neces-

---

TABLE 21–3. MAJOR VASCULAR INSTRUMENTATION

Deaver Retractors

2 shallow
2 deep
3 broad

Retractors

1 malleable	2 Army-Navy
2 bands	1 large Richardson
2 Cushing vein	2 Weitlaner

Suction and Other Items

2 short No. 9 Frazier	1 probe
2 short No. 10 Frazier	1 grooved director
2 long No. 11 Frazier	1 ruler
1 nerve hook	

Hemoclip Appliers

1 small
2 medium
2 large

Knife Handles

3 No. 3
1 No. 7
3 long No. 3

Scissors

1 regular Metzenbaum	1 suture
2 long Metzenbaum	1 Church
1 extralong Metzenbaum	1 Potts, 7 inch
1 long suture	1 Lincoln
1 nurses	

Forceps

2 vascular, 7 inch	6 Crile
3 Atragrip, 11 inch	4 long Kelly
3 long smooth	6 Mixter
2 short smooth	2 sponge stick
2 Adson toothed	8 towel clips
2 Russian	2 Shod Craford
2 titanium Rhoton, 7 inch	1 super Craford
2 short toothed	1 long straight Fogarty
2 Jackson	1 long angled Fogarty
6 curved mosquito	4 Harken aortic clamps
6 straight mosquito	1 super flat-back
12 curved hemostats	Satinsky
6 straight hemostats	2 Beck clamps
4 Kelly	1 Cooley clamp
6 Kocher	4 short straight Fogarty
6 Allis	4 short curved Fogarty
	3 Berkowitz

Needle Holders

2 black-handled, 10 inch	2 Ravdin
1 Mayo-Hegar, 6 inch	2 Sarot
2 French-eye	4 Mayo-Hegar, 9 inch
2 long French-eye	

Fine Vascular Instruments (Wrapped)

2 small Potts scissors	5 vascular bulldog
2 small iris scissors	clamps
4 fine vascular forceps, 5 inch	2 cannulas
2 Castroviejo needle holders	3 coronary bulldogs

Mueller Bulldogs (Wrapped)

2 straight
1 curved

sitate preclotting with the patient's blood before heparin is administered to prevent the graft from leaking.

A urinary catheter with a 75-ml bag is used in case the aortic aneurysm ruptures during the procedure. This is considered an emergency, and every effort must be made to get the bleeding under control as quickly as possible. The catheter is inserted into the intact portion of the aorta and the bag inflated with normal saline to prevent the escape of blood. With the bleeding controlled, the procedure can proceed as usual.

Drugs and Solutions

Heparin sulfate solution
Protamine sulfate

Physiological Monitoring

Because the patient is at risk for unexpected blood loss, swings in blood pressure, and possible pulmonary dysfunction, monitoring is critical to the successful outcome of this procedure. Routine monitoring includes the insertion of a pulmonary arterial catheter to monitor left ventricular pressure, cardiac output, and systemic vascular resistance. An arterial catheter is inserted to monitor arterial blood pressure readings and allow direct access to arterial blood for continuous monitoring of arterial blood gases.

Specimens and Cultures

Specimens are collected and saved until after the operative procedure. The specimen is labeled and placed into formalin and sent to the pathology laboratory for examination. Cultures are not routinely taken.

Physician's Orders

Typical admission orders include a complete blood count (CBC) with electrolyte determinations, platelet count, prothrombin time (PT), partial thromboplastin time (PTT), creatinine level, pulse status, urinalysis, resting ECG, and posteroanterior and lateral chest films. If the patient has been receiving diuretics, the potassium level is checked. A blood sample is drawn for cross-matching, and 6 U of packed cells is ordered. If the patient is scheduled for an angiogram, creatinine and serum potassium determinations are ordered the following morning.

The night before surgery, the patient is ordered a depilatory from the nipples to the knees. The patient is requested to shower with chlorhexidine gluconate (Hibiclens). The patient may be given magnesium citrate, one bottle orally at 8 PM, or polyethylene glycol–electrolyte solution (GoLYTELY), 4 L to start at 6 PM the night before surgery. A Fleet enema is ordered the night before surgery. The patient is NPO after midnight.

Laboratory and Diagnostic Studies

The results of laboratory and diagnostic studies ordered (see above) should be reviewed. All results should be available and present on the chart before surgery. Any abnormal values or reports that would affect the outcome of surgery should be reported to the surgeon.

Procedure

Incision and Exposure

An abdominal midline incision is made from the xiphoid to the pubis. Electrocautery may be used to dissect to the fascia. The fascia and the peritoneum are opened with scissors. The abdomen is carefully checked for any other disease process that might cause the procedure to be aborted. A bowel nodule, diverticulitis, and accidental entry into the bowel are causes of possible contamination of a graft and reasons to abort the surgery. The small bowel is lifted from the abdominal cavity and placed into a plastic intestinal bag. The surface of the aneurysm is carefully exposed.

Details

After exposure of the aorta, vessel loops may be used to identify and mobilize the renal and mesenteric arteries, if necessary. Exposure of the iliac or femoral arteries is accomplished in much the same manner. Vessel loops are used to control and mobilize these vessels.

Heparin sulfate, 4000 to 5000 U, is administered before clamping of the aorta. After heparinization, the aorta is clamped with a vascular clamp of the surgeon's choice (e.g., DeBakey aortic clamp). To prevent back bleeding, the femoral or iliac arteries are also clamped with vascular clamps (e.g., Fogarty vascular clamps). The aneurysm is incised longitudinally with either a No. 10 or a No. 11 knife blade (Fig. 21–6). The incision is extended with Mayo scissors (Fig. 21–7). The thrombus and the plaque are carefully removed from the aneurysm lumen (Fig. 21–8).

The graft chosen by the surgeon is sewn into place at the proximal end with either 3–0 or 4–0 nonabsorbable suture. A clamp is placed on the graft itself to test the suture line for leaks. Leaks are repaired with the same suture used for the anastomosis. Tension is then placed on the graft, and the graft is cut and sutured to the aortic bifurcation (Fig. 21–9).

If the aneurysm extends below the bifurcation and involves the common iliac arteries, punctures are made in the artery with a No. 11 knife blade and extended with small vascular scissors. In rare cases, an endarterectomy is necessary to clear the vessel completely. A bifurcation graft is used and the graft is trimmed to ensure appropriate fit. The anastomosis is completed with either 4–0 or 5–0 nonabsorbable vascular suture.

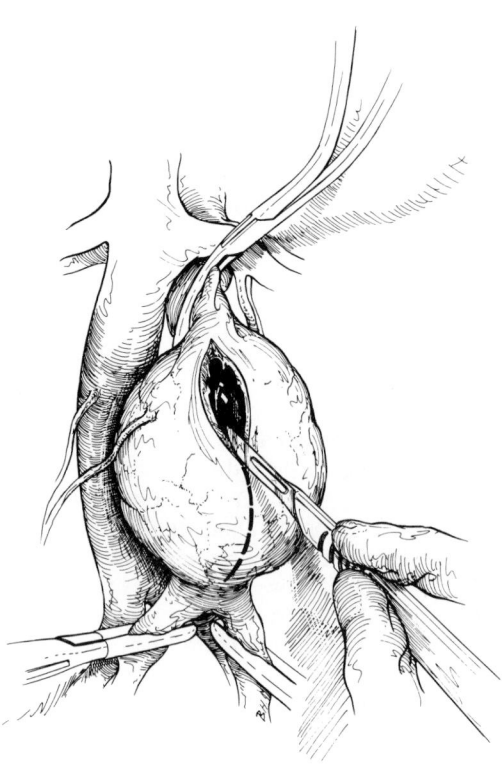

FIGURE 21–6. Clamping and dissecting of the aneurysm. (From Hollier, L. H. [1989]. Technical modifications in the repair of thoracoabdominal aortic aneurysms. In R. M. Greenhalgh [Ed.]. *Vascular surgical techniques: An atlas* [2nd ed.] [p. 154]. Philadelphia: W. B. Saunders.)

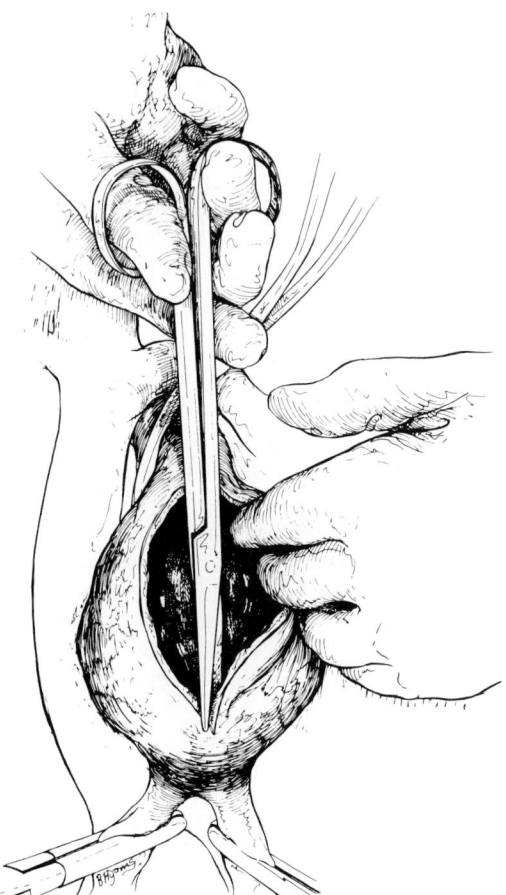

FIGURE 21–7. Extending the incision of the aneurysm with Mayo scissors. (From Hollier, L. H. [1989]. Technical modifications in the repair of thoracoabdominal aortic aneurysms. In R. M. Greenhalgh [Ed.]. *Vascular surgical techniques: An atlas* [2nd ed.] [p. 154]. Philadelphia: W. B. Saunders.)

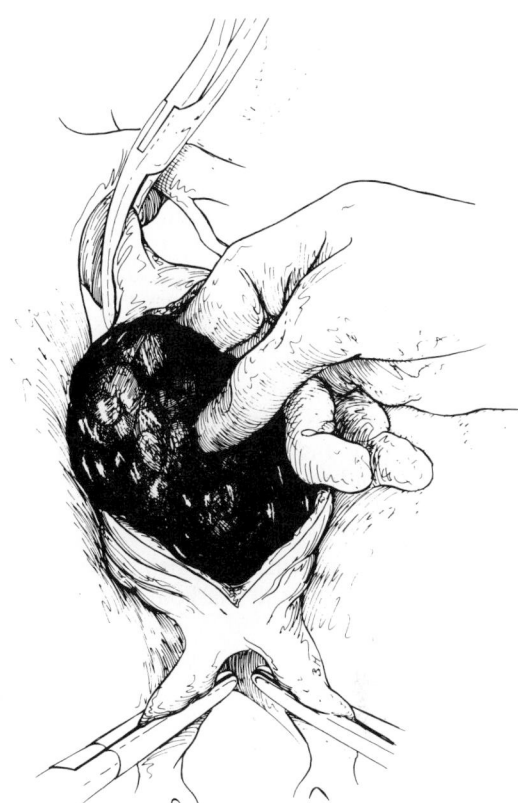

FIGURE 21–8. Removal of a thrombus and loose arteriosclerotic debris. (From Hollier, L. H. [1989]. Technical modifications in the repair of thoracoabdominal aortic aneurysms. In R. M. Greenhalgh [Ed.]. *Vascular surgical techniques: An atlas* [2nd ed.] [p. 155]. Philadelphia: W. B. Saunders.)

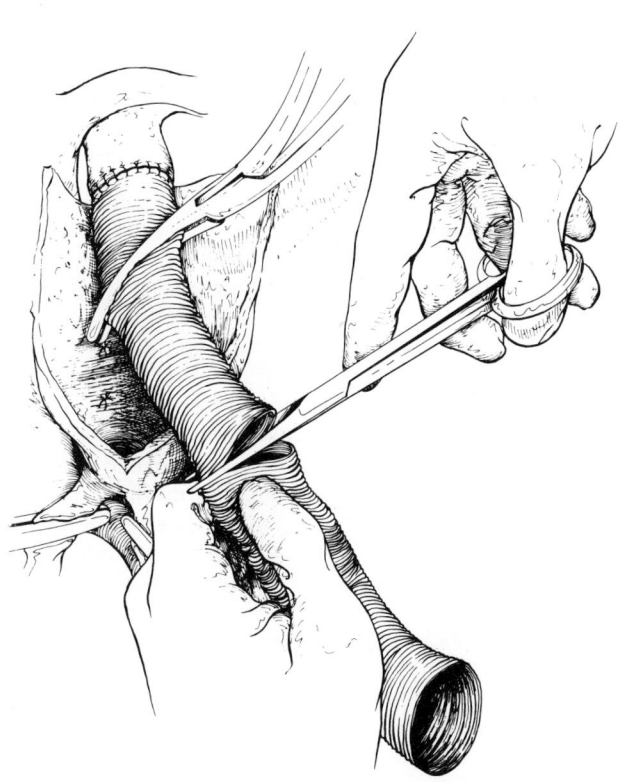

FIGURE 21–9. Final anastomosis to aortic bifurcation. (From Hollier, L. H. [1989]. Technical modifications in the repair of thoracoabdominal aortic aneurysms. In R. M. Greenhalgh [Ed.]. *Vascular surgical techniques: An atlas* [2nd ed.] [p. 157]. Philadelphia: W. B. Saunders.)

The vascular clamp is removed, and leaks are handled in the same manner as at the proximal end. The procedure for the other leg is completed in the same manner. If either or both renal or mesenteric arteries are involved with disease, a vein graft can be taken from the prepared lower leg. This is sewn into place with either 5–0 or 6–0 nonabsorbable vascular suture. After the release of all vascular clamps, the action of heparin sulfate is reversed with the administration of protamine sulfate and all suture anastomoses are checked closely for bleeding.

Closure

The abdomen is closed with No. 2 or other nonabsorbable suture and without a drain to prevent contamination and subsequent infection. A visceral retainer may be used temporarily during the closure. The skin may be stapled or sutured. The genitalia incisions are handled in the same manner, also without a drain. Pedal pulses are assessed and marked with a skin marker. If no pulses are present and no improvement in the color or warmth of the legs is noted, the incision is reopened.

Postoperative Care

The patient is admitted to the surgical intensive care unit for 1 or 2 days after surgery. Routine vital signs are assessed. Urinary output is monitored and if it is less than 30 ml/hour, the surgeon is notified. Peripheral pulses are assessed every 4 hours. Antibiotics and pain medication are ordered by the surgeon. Extensive laboratory data are collected during the patient's stay in the surgical intensive care unit. Ambulation is allowed on the first postoperative day. If there are no complications, the patient is transferred to the nursing unit on the first or second postoperative day. The patient is discharged 7 to 10 days postoperatively.

Potential Surgical Complications

Infection
Suture failure
Weakness of the arterial wall
Excessive tension of the graft
Faulty surgical technique

FEMOROPOPLITEAL BYPASS GRAFT

Definition

Femoropopliteal bypass graft involves bypassing atherosclerotic arterial occlusion of the femoral artery with a graft. The procedure planned may not necessarily be the procedure performed, because of the unpredictable condition of the patient's donor veins. Because the patency rate is higher with the autologous saphenous vein, it is generally the surgeon's first choice. The saphenous vein in either the same leg or the opposite leg may be unavailable because it is occluded, too small, or varicosed. This may necessitate the use of other graft materials, which include other autologous veins (e.g., arm veins), human umbilical cord vein, Dacron, or expanded polytetrafluoroethylene (Gore-Tex).

Indications

The patient faces the potential loss of a limb with atherosclerotic occlusion of the femoral artery. The patient may have claudication, calf tenderness, mottling, discoloration, and even gangrene of the foot of the affected leg. Flinn and Yao (1990) identified the following therapeutic alternatives: "(1) noninvasive, nonsurgical (medical treatment); (2) invasive, nonsurgical (percutaneous transluminal angioplasty, laser-assisted angioplasty); and (3) invasive, surgical" (p. 945). The decision on treatment is based on the severity of symptoms and extent of arterial occlusion. The degrees of ischemia and severity include "(1) ischemic rest pain, (2) ischemic ulceration, and (3) cutaneous gangrene" (Flinn and Yao, 1990, p. 943). The greater the severity, the greater is the extent of involvement of other arterial segments of the leg.

Related Surgical Procedures

Aortic bifurcation graft

Perioperative Nursing Implications

Anesthesia

The choices of anesthesia for patients undergoing peripheral vascular surgery include general anesthesia, regional nerve blocks, and epidural or spinal anesthesia. There has been little research conducted that supports one technique instead of another. The choice of anesthesia technique depends on the cardiopulmonary status of the patient, and the technique that would least compromise this status is usually chosen.

General anesthesia is the most frequent choice, particularly if the patient has any type of cardiac compromise. In such an instance, monitoring methods usually include the use of pulmonary and arterial catheters to monitor closely hemodynamic status. To minimize the effects on the cardiovascular system, narcotics and nitrous oxide are administered.

A regional block may be applied to the sciatic, femoral, or obturator nerves. The use of this technique depends on the expected length of surgery and the patient's condition. If the procedure is expected to be lengthy and complex, general anesthesia is usually chosen instead of a regional block.

Spinal and epidural techniques are chosen if the

patient's condition permits. Advantages include an awake patient and greater pain control and patient management in the postoperative recovery period.

Position

The patient is placed in the supine position. Each arm is secured on a padded arm board and positioned at a less than 90-degree angle or tucked to the patient's side.

Creation and Maintenance of the Sterile Field

The patient is shaved and prepared with iodophor scrub and solution, or gel, from the lower rib cage to the toes on the operative side, from the patient's midline to the bed line on the abdomen, and circumferentially around the leg. Any other site that may be used as a potential vein donor site (e.g., arms, unaffected leg) should also be included. The genitalia are isolated with adhesive drapes to prevent contamination of the field.

The patient is draped to expose the lower abdominal quadrant of the operative side and the entire leg. If there is gangrene present on the foot, the foot should be wrapped in a sterile towel or placed in a sterile plastic bag at the time of draping to prevent contamination of the operative site.

Equipment and Supplies

The instruments needed are included in the minor vascular set listed in Table 21–2. In addition, grafts of all sizes and types, hemoclip applicators, Silastic vessel loops, vascular suture, and hernia tape should be available.

Drugs and Solutions

Heparin sulfate solution

Physiological Monitoring

Because peripheral vascular surgery generally does not include risks related to significant blood pressure swings, large blood loss, and fluid shifts, monitoring depends on the patient's condition, the anesthesia technique, and the surgeon's preference. Routine monitoring variables include ECG, blood pressure, respiratory rate and pattern, pulse oximetry, and temperature. A urinary catheter may be inserted to monitor output throughout the procedure.

Specimens and Cultures

Cultures and specimens are not routinely taken during this procedure.

Physician's Orders

Blood is typed and cross-matched for 2 U of whole blood. The patient is requested to shower with chlorhexidine gluconate, and a depilatory is applied from the umbilicus to the toes. The patient is given aspirin, 325 mg orally, the night before surgery. Aspirin is administered long term for the anticoagulation effects and is found to maintain a better patency rate for polytetrafluoroethylene grafts. The patient is NPO after midnight. If an ischemic ulcer is present, an orthopedic bed frame with trapeze and sheepskin is ordered. To prevent decubital ulcers of the heel, protective padding is ordered.

Laboratory and Diagnostic Studies

Routine laboratory tests include urinalysis, CBC, panel 7, PT, PTT, platelet count, resting ECG, posteroanterior and lateral chest films, and blood bank sample. Pulses are assessed and recorded; an ultrasonic flow detector (e.g., Doppler) may be used to assess patency of vessel and ankle pressures. An arteriogram is ordered. The results of all laboratory and diagnostic studies ordered should be reviewed. All results should be available and present on the chart before surgery. Any abnormal values that would affect the outcome of surgery should be reported to the surgeon.

Procedure

Incision and Exposure

Incisions are made over the skin of the femoral and popliteal arteries, proximally and distally to the obstruction. The incisions may be medial, lateral, or posterior approaches. Tissue is dissected down to the vessels, which are held with hernia tape or vessel loops for identification and mobilization.

Details

The patient is heparinized to prevent clotting of clamped vessels. The femoral artery is clamped and punctured with a No. 11 knife blade and the puncture is extended with vascular scissors. The distal end of the vein graft is anastomosed to the femoral artery using 5–0 or 6–0 nonabsorbable suture. The clamp is removed for a few seconds, with a clamp placed distal to the anastomosis, to test for leaks. Leaks are repaired with the same type of suture used for the anastomosis.

A tunnel is made to feed the graft down to the popliteal artery. It is important not to twist or kink the graft. In addition, the graft should be positioned so that normal leg motion does not twist or kink the graft. Careful measuring ensures that the graft is not left too long or too short.

The popliteal artery is clamped distal to the expected graft site, and a puncture is made with a No. 11 knife blade. The puncture wound is extended with small vascular scissors. The anastomosis is made with 5–0, 6–0, or 7–0 nonabsorbable vascular suture. When the entire graft is opened to blood from the femoral artery, it is inspected for leaks at both anastomoses. The patency of the graft can be documented with an intraoperative arteriogram. Contrast material is injected into the artery and the x-ray film documents its travel to the foot. A Doppler monitor with a sterile probe tip is placed directly on the vessel to assess its patency. The sound of the flowing blood is confirmed. Pedal pulses should also be assessed.

Closure

Subcutaneous tissue is closed with absorbable suture and the skin is either sutured or stapled. Dressings are applied and taped lengthwise.

Postoperative Care

Depending on the cardiopulmonary status of the patient, the patient is transferred to the surgical intensive care unit or to the nursing unit. The legs are maintained in straight alignment for 24 hours. The patient is usually maintained NPO for several hours after surgery to ensure that the graft is patent and reexploration is not indicated. Routine vital signs are assessed. Femoral and popliteal pulses are palpated every hour. A foot cradle and heel protectors are usually applied. The patient ambulates on the second postoperative day. Low-dose heparin administration is discontinued when the patient is ambulatory and aspirin, 325 mg, is continued daily. If there are no complications, the patient is discharged 7 to 10 days postoperatively.

Potential Surgical Complications

Hemorrhage
Thrombosis
Infection
Graft stenosis
Graft occlusion

FEMOROFEMORAL BYPASS

Definition

Femorofemoral bypass is done to bypass an occlusion below the bifurcation of the aorta, but above the femoral artery. The graft shunts blood from one femoral artery to the other, allowing complete blood flow to both legs.

Indications

The primary indications for this procedure are limb ischemia and claudication. The following factors should be considered when choosing surgical intervention: (1) the extent of the arterial run-off, (2) the adequacy of the arterial run-off, (3) the type of graft material to use, and (4) the patient's general medical condition.

Perioperative Nursing Implications

Anesthesia

See the discussion of femoropopliteal bypass graft.

Position

The patient is placed in the supine position. Each arm is secured on a padded arm board and positioned at a less than 90-degree angle or tucked to the patient's side.

Creation and Maintenance of the Sterile Field

The patient is shaved and prepared with iodophor scrub and solution, or gel, from the umbilicus to the groin and extended to the knees. The genitalia may be isolated with adhesive drapes to prevent contamination of the field.

Equipment and Supplies

The instruments needed are included in the minor vascular set listed in Table 21–2. In addition, grafts of all sizes and types, hemoclip applicators, Silastic vessel loops, vascular suture, and hernia tape should be available.

Drugs and Solutions

Heparin sulfate solution

Physiological Monitoring

Because peripheral vascular surgery generally does not include risks related to significant blood pressure swings, large blood loss, and fluid shifts, monitoring depends on the patient's condition, the anesthesia technique, and the surgeon's preference. Routine monitoring variables include ECG, blood pressure, respiratory rate and pattern, pulse oximetry, and temperature. A urinary catheter may be inserted to monitor output throughout the procedure.

Specimens and Cultures

Cultures and specimens are not routinely taken during this procedure.

Physician's Orders

Blood is typed and cross-matched for 2 U of whole blood. The patient is requested to shower with chlorhexidine gluconate, and a depilatory is applied from the umbilicus to the toes. The patient is given aspirin, 325 mg orally, the night before surgery and is NPO after midnight. If an ischemic ulcer is present, an orthopedic bed frame with a trapeze and sheepskin is ordered. To prevent decubital ulcers of the heel, protective padding is ordered.

Laboratory and Diagnostic Studies

Routine laboratory tests include urinalysis, CBC, panel 7, PT, PTT, platelet count, resting ECG, posteroanterior and lateral chest films, and blood bank sample. Pulses are assessed and recorded; an ultrasonic flow detector (e.g., Doppler) may be used to assess patency of vessel and ankle pressures. An arteriogram is ordered. The results of all laboratory and diagnostic studies ordered should be reviewed. All results should be available and present on the chart before surgery. Any abnormal values that would affect the outcome of surgery should be reported to the surgeon.

Procedure

Incision and Exposure

Inguinal incisions are made over the deep and superficial femoral arteries. Vessel loops may be used to identify and mobilize the femoral arteries on either side (Fig. 21–10). After the donor femoral artery is located,

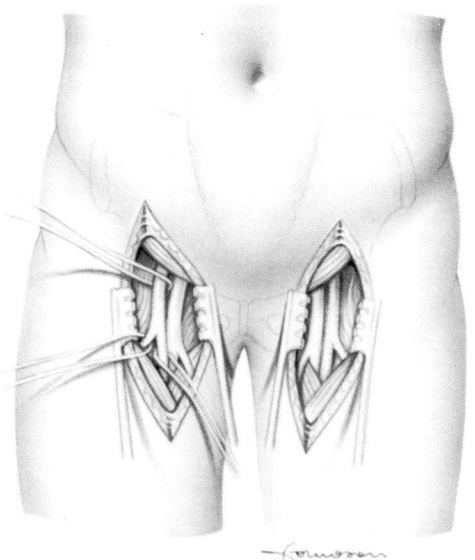

FIGURE 21–10. Inguinal incisions. (From Fiorani, P., Faraglia, V., Taurine, M., et al. [1989]. Femorofemoral bypass. In R. M. Greenhalgh [Ed.]. *Vascular surgical techniques: An atlas* [2nd ed.] [p. 180]. Philadelphia: W. B. Saunders.)

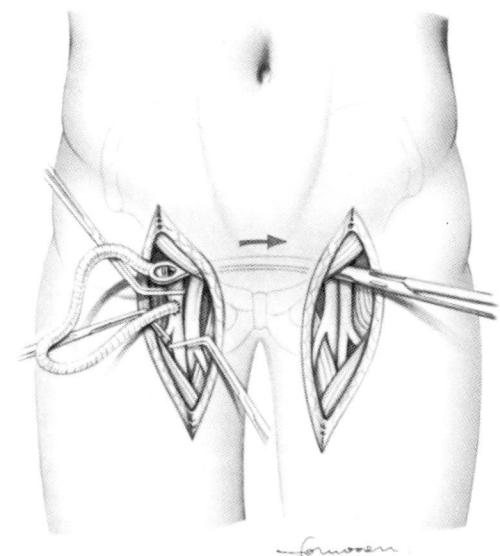

FIGURE 21–11. Tunneling of the graft. (From Fiorani, P., Faraglia, V., Taurine, M., et al. [1989]. Femorofemoral bypass. In R. M. Greenhalgh [Ed.]. *Vascular surgical techniques: An atlas* [2nd ed.] [p. 182]. Philadelphia: W. B. Saunders.)

heparin sulfate is administered to prevent clotting while the vessels are clamped.

Details

A vascular clamp is placed on the unaffected femoral artery proximal to the proposed anastomosis site, the vessel is punctured with a No. 11 knife blade, and the puncture is extended with small vascular scissors. The graft is sutured to the femoral artery using 5–0 or 6–0 nonabsorbable vascular suture. The graft can be clamped and the femoral clamp removed to test for leaks. These can be repaired using the same suture used for the anastomosis.

A tunnel should be made across the pubis through which the graft should be fed, using care not to twist or kink it (Fig. 21–11). It should be cut at exactly the length needed to ensure proper placement. A vascular clamp is placed on the femoral artery on the affected side if necessary to prevent back bleeding. The vessel is punctured with a No. 11 knife blade and extended with small vascular scissors. The anastomosis is accomplished in the same manner as for the other side using the same type of suture. When all clamps are removed, leaks can be identified and patched (Fig. 21–12). A Doppler monitor may be used to document blood flow through the graft.

Closure

The subcutaneous tissue is closed with 3–0 absorbable suture. Skin is closed with staples or suture. Popliteal and pedal pulses are noted and marked with a skin marker on the affected leg. Dressings and tape are applied.

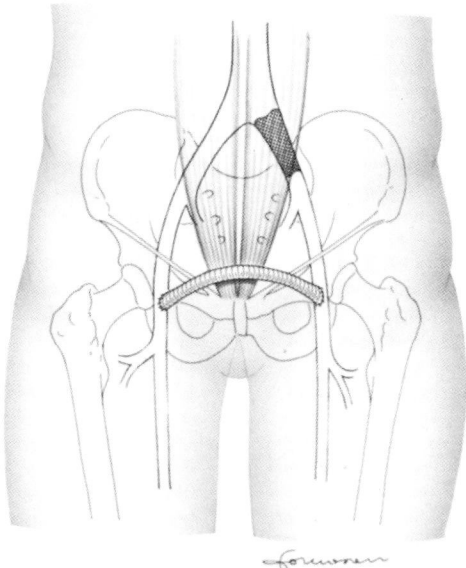

FIGURE 21–12. Completed anastomosis. (From Fiorani, P., Faraglia, V., Taurine, M., et al. [1989]. Femorofemoral bypass. In R. M. Greenhalgh [Ed.]. *Vascular surgical techniques: An atlas* [2nd ed.] [p. 182]. Philadelphia: W. B. Saunders.)

Postoperative Care

Depending on the cardiopulmonary status of the patient, the patient is transferred to the surgical intensive care unit or to the nursing unit. The legs are maintained in straight alignment for 24 hours. The patient is usually maintained NPO several hours after surgery to ensure that the graft is patent and reexploration is not indicated. Routine vital signs are assessed. Femoral and popliteal pulses are palpated every hour. A foot cradle and heel protectors are usually applied. The patient ambulates on the second postoperative day. The administration of low-dose heparin is discontinued when the patient is ambulatory and aspirin, 325 mg, is continued daily.

Potential Surgical Complications

Hemorrhage
Thrombosis
Infection
Graft stenosis
Graft occlusion

ABOVE-KNEE AMPUTATION

Definition

Amputation is removal of a limb that cannot be salvaged. In the past, amputations were primarily performed by orthopedic surgeons. However, today nearly two thirds of all lower limb amputations are performed by general and vascular surgeons owing to the compli-

cations of peripheral vascular disease and/or diabetes mellitus (Burgess and Malone, 1990). An above-knee amputation is less likely for patients with peripheral vascular disease and generally is indicated only when skin and muscle tissue necrosis occurs beyond the lower third of the leg (Burgess and Malone, 1990).

Indications

Amputation is a last resort for the patient with continuous pain at rest, previous bypass surgery, existent gangrene, complications related to diabetes mellitus, or infection unresponsive to conservative therapy (e.g., administration of antibiotics, débridement). Other indications for amputation of the lower extremity include trauma, burns, and frostbite.

Related Surgical Procedures

Below-knee amputation

Perioperative Nursing Implications

Anesthesia

The choices of anesthesia for the patient undergoing amputation include general, regional block, epidural, and spinal methods. General anesthesia is preferred; however, if the patient's existing medical condition does not permit general anesthesia, other methods may be applied.

Position

The patient is placed in the supine position. Each arm is secured on a padded arm board and positioned at a less than 90-degree angle or tucked to the patient's side.

Creation and Maintenance of the Sterile Field

The patient is shaved and prepared with iodophor scrub and solution, or gel, from the umbilicus to the groin on the affected side to the toes. The genitalia may be isolated with adhesive drapes to prevent contamination of the field. If the foot is infected or gangrenous, it is wrapped in a sterile towel or a plastic bag as described for femoropopliteal bypass grafting.

Equipment and Supplies

In addition to the instruments needed as listed in the minor vascular set (see Table 21–2), a bone cutter, elevators, rongeurs, and a bone file are needed. The surgeon's preference of saws should be immediately available (e.g., hand saw, Gigli saw, powered saw).

Drugs and Solutions

Normal saline
Antibiotic irrigation solution

Physiological Monitoring

Because amputation generally does not include risks related to significant blood pressure swings, large blood loss, and fluid shifts, monitoring depends on the patient's condition, the anesthesia technique, and the surgeon's preference. Routine monitoring variables include ECG, blood pressure, respiratory rate and pattern, pulse oximetry, and temperature.

Specimens and Cultures

After the amputation is completed, the assistant hands off the limb to the circulator. The limb is wrapped in plastic wrapping, labeled, and taken to the pathology department for analysis. If infection is present, cultures should have been previously taken and generally are not taken during the procedure.

Physician's Orders

Routine laboratory tests include urinalysis, CBC, panel 7, PT, PTT, platelet count, resting ECG, postero-anterior and lateral chest films, and blood bank sample. An arteriogram is ordered. The results of all laboratory and diagnostic studies ordered should be reviewed. All results should be available and present on the chart before surgery. Any abnormal values that affect the outcome of surgery should be reported to the surgeon.

Laboratory and Diagnostic Studies

To assist in determining the level of amputation, the following diagnostic studies are conducted: angiogram, ankle and popliteal systolic pressures assessed with a Doppler monitor, and transcutaneous oximetry studies.

Procedure

Incision and Exposure

The level of the amputation is 4 to 6 inches above the knee joint. This type of stump allows later rehabilitation with the application of a prosthesis. The incision is made circumferentially around the leg, leaving a longer posterior portion of skin and fatty tissue to be used as a flap, bringing the postoperative suture line to the ante-

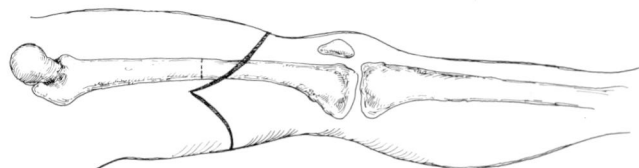

FIGURE 21–13. Above-knee outline of skin flaps and the level of bone division. (From Burgess, E. M., Malone, J. M. [1990]. Major amputations. In P. F. Nora [Ed.], *Operative surgery: Principles and techniques* [3rd ed.] [p. 1255]. Philadelphia: W. B. Saunders. Redrawn from Slocum, O. [1949]. *An atlas of amputation.* St. Louis, C.V. Mosby.)

rior surface of the leg or the thigh and providing a cushion for the bone stump if a prosthesis is used (Fig. 21–13). Tissue and the fascia femoris are dissected, followed by dissection of the muscles down to the bone using electrocautery.

Details

The nerves and vessels are ligated and allowed to retract upward between the muscles. The bone is severed with a hand saw or a powered saw. The exposed bone is rounded with a fine bone rasp. Flap tissue is brought forward and secured with absorbable suture.

Closure

The fascia is closed with interrupted sutures owing to the possibility of healing complications. A suction drain and/or a Penrose drain is inserted deep into the wound. The subcutaneous layer and skin are closed with interrupted sutures with minimal tension. The stump is dressed with a fluffed gauze dressing and wrapped with an elastic bandage or bias stockinet.

Postoperative Care

After recovery in the postanesthesia care area, the patient is usually transferred to the nursing unit. The patient is transferred to the postanesthesia care unit on an orthopedic bed frame with a trapeze. The patient is frequently assessed for pain and drainage from the dressing. Subcutaneous heparin, 5000 U, is ordered every 12 hours until the patient is out of bed. If drains are inserted, they are removed on the second or third postoperative day. Physical therapy personnel are consulted and the patient is generally discharged on the 11th postoperative day.

Potential Surgical Complications

Failure to heal
Residual limb infection
Pain
Flexion contractures

Pulmonary complications
Thromboembolic complications
Stump revision

BELOW-KNEE AMPUTATION

Definition

Below-knee amputation has major advantages over above-knee amputation in the rehabilitation process. It is the most useful and preferable for lower extremity amputation.

Indications

See the discussion of above-knee amputation.

Related Surgical Procedures

Above-knee amputation

Perioperative Nursing Implications

Anesthesia

The choices of anesthesia for the patient undergoing amputation include general, regional block, epidural, and spinal methods. General anesthesia is preferred; however, if the patient's existing medical condition does not allow general anesthesia, other methods may be applied.

Position

The patient is placed in the supine position. Each arm is secured on a padded arm board and positioned at a less than 90-degree angle or tucked to the patient's side.

Creation and Maintenance of the Sterile Field

See the discussion of above-knee amputation.

Equipment and Supplies

In addition to the instruments listed in the minor vascular set (see Table 21–2), a bone cutter, elevators, rongeurs, and a bone file are needed. The surgeon's preference of saws should be immediately available (e.g., hand saw, Gigli saw, powered saw).

Drugs and Solutions

Normal saline
Antibiotic irrigation solution

Physiological Monitoring

Because amputation generally does not include risks related to significant blood pressure swings, large blood loss, and fluid shifts, monitoring depends on the patient's condition, the anesthesia technique, and the surgeon's preference. Routine monitoring variables include ECG, blood pressure, respiratory rate and pattern, pulse oximetry, and temperature.

Specimens and Cultures

After the amputation is completed, the assistant hands off the limb to the circulator. The limb is wrapped in plastic wrapping, labeled, and taken to the pathology department for analysis. If infection is present, cultures should have been previously taken and generally are not taken during the procedure.

Physician's Orders

See the discussion of above-knee amputation.

Laboratory and Diagnostic Studies

To assist in determining the level of amputation, the following diagnostic studies are conducted: angiogram, ankle and popliteal systolic pressures assessed with a Doppler monitor, and transcutaneous oximetry studies.

Procedure

Incision and Exposure

Utilizing the long posterior flap technique, the level of the anterior incision is approximately 8 to 12 cm below the tibial tubercle and extends circumferentially for two thirds of the leg; this area is the base for the posterior flap (Fig. 21–14). The lateral incision is extended distally 5 inches posterior to the line of the fibula and directed distally; this area is the flap. The anterior incision is incised to the tibia. Vessels are ligated with suture. The nerves and vessels are ligated and allowed to retract upward between the muscles. The tibial and fibular periosteum each is cut gently and retracted and the tibia and fibula are transected. Each bone is smoothed with a bone rasp. The posterior muscle mass

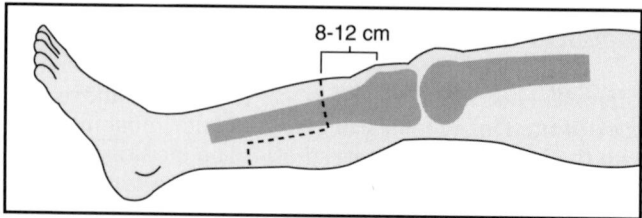

FIGURE 21–14. Below-knee outline of the skin incision and the level of bone section.

is cut along the incision lines, completing the amputation. Care is taken to ligate all nerves and vessels. If posterior muscle mass is muscular, the gastrocnemius-soleus group of muscles may be trimmed to reduce excessive muscle bulk. The posterior muscle mass is sutured to the anterior tibial fascia and tibial and fibular periosteum.

Details

The nerves and vessels are ligated and allowed to retract upward between the muscles. The bone is severed with a hand saw or a powered saw. The exposed bone is rounded with a fine bone rasp. Flap tissue is brought forward and secured with absorbable stuture.

Closure

The fascia and skin are closed with interrupted non-absorbable monofilament sutures owing to the possibility of healing complications. A suction drain and/or a Penrose drain is inserted deep into the wound. The stump is dressed with a rigid plaster dressing or a fluffed gauze dressing and wrapped with an elastic bandage or bias stockinet. On occasion, after dressings are applied, the prosthetist is brought into the operating room and a postsurgical prosthesis is applied to the stump, preventing deformities of knee flexion and providing comfort on movement.

Postoperative Care

After recovery in postanesthesia recovery area, the patient is usually transferred to the nursing unit. The patient is transferred to the postanesthesia care unit on an orthopedic bed frame with a trapeze. The patient is frequently assessed for pain and drainage from the dressing. If the patient has a plaster dressing and verbalizes significant pain or if fever is present, the cast is removed and the wound assessed. Subcutaneous heparin, 5000 U, is ordered every 12 hours until the patient is out of bed. If drains are inserted, they are removed on the second or third postoperative day. Physical therapy personnel are consulted and the patient is generally discharged on the 11th postoperative day.

Potential Surgical Complications

Failure to heal
Residual limb infection
Pain
Flexion contractures
Pulmonary complications
Thromboembolic complications
Stump revision

LIGATION AND STRIPPING OF VARICOSE VEINS

Definition

Ligation and stripping of varicose veins entails surgical removal of varicose veins of the leg.

Indications

The patient with varicose veins often has cosmetic concerns. Deformities of the vein valves and weakness within the vessel walls have caused them to bulge, discolor, or even rupture beneath the skin. Swelling and night cramps may be caused by varicose veins, and the patient may experience pain, fatigue, or aching of the legs, which is worse with prolonged periods of standing.

Related Surgical Procedures

None

Perioperative Nursing Implications

Anesthesia

The choices of anesthesia for the patient undergoing ligation and stripping of varicose veins include general, regional block, epidural, and spinal methods. If the patient is scheduled for same-day surgery, spinal anesthesia is not administered, because of the long recovery period.

Position

The patient is placed in the supine position. Each arm is secured on a padded arm board and positioned at a less than 90-degree angle or tucked to the patient's side.

Creation and Maintenance of the Sterile Field

The patient is shaved and prepared with iodophor scrub and solution, or gel, from the umbilicus to the groin on the affected side to the toes. The genitalia may be isolated with adhesive drapes to prevent contamination of the field.

Equipment and Supplies

The instruments needed include the minor vascular set listed in Table 21–2 and internal and external vein strippers. Depending on the surgeon's preference and the location and type of veins, a tourniquet may be applied.

Drugs and Solutions

Normal saline

Physiological Monitoring

See Below-Knee Amputation.

Specimens and Cultures

Specimens are collected and saved until after the operative procedure. The specimens are labeled and placed into formalin and sent to the pathology department for examination. Cultures are not routinely taken.

Physician's Orders

Routine laboratory tests include urinalysis, CBC, panel 7, resting ECG, and posteroanterior and lateral chest films. The results of all laboratory and diagnostic studies ordered should be reviewed. All results should be available and present on the chart before surgery. Any abnormal values that would affect the outcome of surgery should be reported to the surgeon.

Laboratory and Diagnostic Studies

In addition to the laboratory studies ordered by the physician, the patient is assessed with Doppler ultrasound examination and often phlebography.

Procedure

Incision and Exposure

Preoperatively, the varices are marked with a skin marker, with the patient in a standing position (Fig. 21–15). Bergan (1990) identified the following basic principles to increase the success of the procedure: "(1) Incision at the ankle and groin are transverse, and incision on the leg and thigh are vertical. (2) Careful subcutaneous closure of wounds, close attention to detail in approximation of skin edges, and search for and obliteration of all varicosities are essential. (3) Cutaneous nerves must be avoided at anteromedial and posterolateral ankle incisions."

With these principles in mind, several incisions are made along the path of the affected vein. The fascia is dissected and a self-retaining retractor is applied. Blunt dissection using nontoothed dissecting forceps and a peanut forceps is used to dissect tissue around the affected vein.

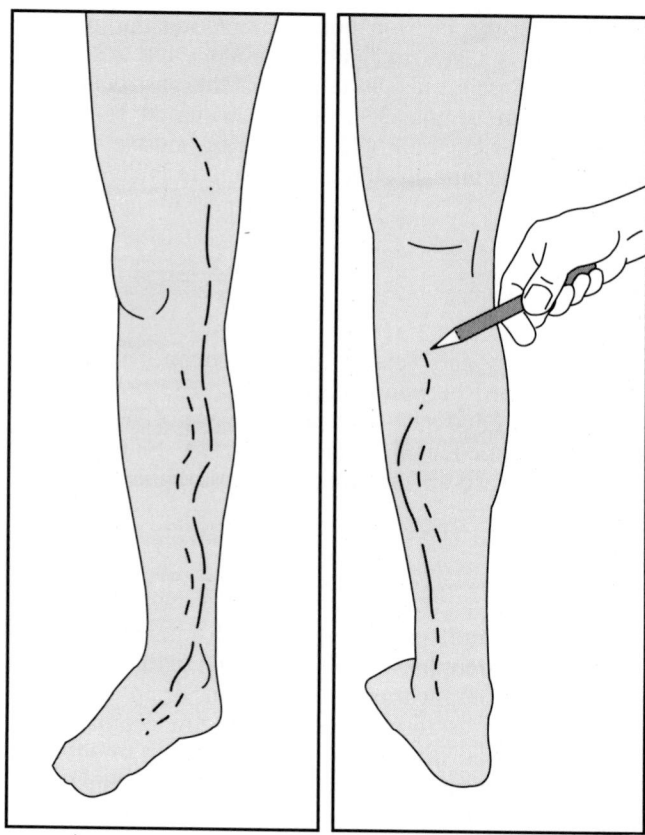

FIGURE 21–15. Preoperative marking of varices performed with the patient in a standing position. (Redrawn from Royle, J. P. [1992]. Treatment of primary varicose veins. In P. R. F. Bell, C. W. Jamieson, C. Vaughn Ruckley [Eds.], *Surgical management of vascular disease* [p. 1245]. Philadelphia: W. B. Saunders.)

Details

The steps in a saphenous vein stripping are diagrammed in Figure 21–16. The stripping and ligation of any vein include mobilization of the vein. The proximal end of the vein is ligated and divided. A stripper is introduced and fed through the vein as far as possible. An incision is made over the distal portion of the stripper, exposing the vein, which is ligated, cut, and tied to the end of the stripper. When gentle traction is applied to the stripper, the vein should dislodge and come out with the stripper. If it cannot be passed the entire length of the affected vessel, the stripper should be cleaned off by removing the tie at the distal end and peeling the vein from it. It is reinserted after further mobilization of the vessel until the entire length of the affected vein has been removed. This may be necessary on the tributaries of the vein that also are distended from pooled blood.

Closure

The multiple incisions are closed with 3–0 absorbable suture and skin with paper tape incisional closure. Soft dressings are applied and the leg is wrapped in an elastic bandage.

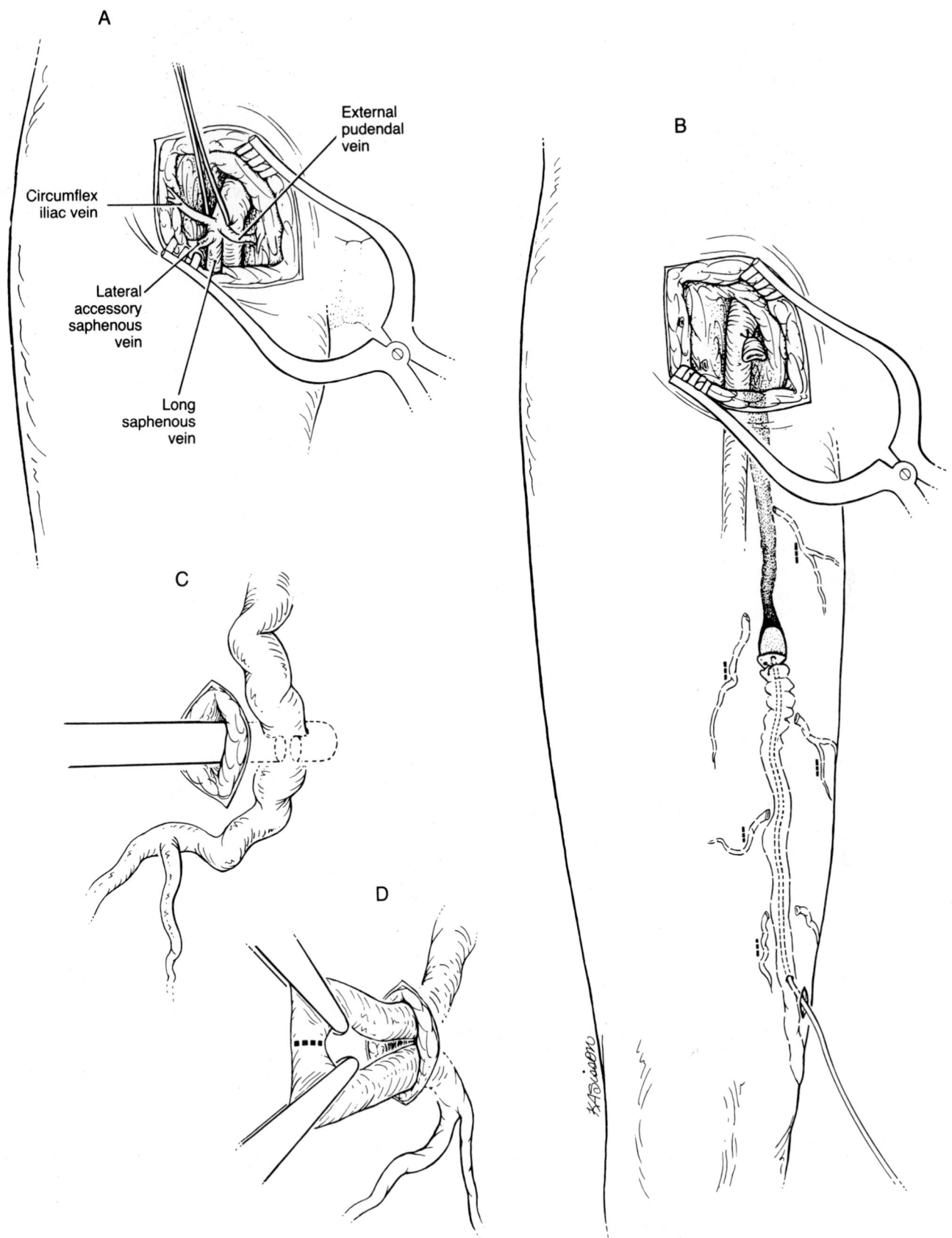

FIGURE 21–16. Steps in saphenous vein stripping. (From Bergan, J. J. [1990]. Surgery of the veins of the lower extremity. In P. F. Nora [Ed.]. *Operative surgery: Principles and techniques* [3rd ed.] [p. 995]. Philadelphia: W. B. Saunders.)

Postoperative Care

Unless the patient's condition indicates otherwise, the procedure is done on an outpatient basis. After recovery in the postanesthesia care area, the patient is discharged with written instructions specific to wound care, monitoring of infection, administration of pain medication, and ambulation and activity.

Potential Surgical Complications

Saphenous nerve damage
Sural nerve damage
Patches of numbness
Lateral popliteal nerve palsy
Damage to the femoral vein
Arterial stripping
Hemorrhage
Superficial thrombosis
Deep venous thrombosis
Unsightly scar
Lymphatic leak
Infection

Bibliography

Bergan, J. J. (1990). Surgery of the veins of the lower extremity. In P. F. Nora (Ed.). *Operative surgery: Principles and techniques* (3rd ed.). Philadelphia: W. B. Saunders.

Brunner, L. S., Suddarth, D. S. (1984). *Textbook of medical-surgical nursing* (5th ed.). Philadelphia: J. B. Lippincott.

Burgess, E. M., Malone, J. M. (1990). Major amputations. In P. F. Nora (Ed.). *Operative surgery: Principles and techniques* (3rd ed.). Philadelphia: W. B. Saunders.

Eldrup-Jorgensen, J., O'Donnel, T. F. (1990). Extracranial cerebral vascular disease. In P. F. Nora (Ed.). *Operative surgery: Principles and techniques* (3rd ed.). Philadelphia: W. B. Saunders.

Flinn, W. R., Yao, J. S. T. (1990). Occlusive arterial disease—Femoral, popliteal, and tibial. In P. F. Nora (Ed.), *Operative surgery: Principles and techniques* (3rd ed.). Philadelphia: W. B. Saunders.

Handelsman, H. (1991). *Carotid endarterectomy (revised)* (DHHS Publication No. AHCPR 91–0029). Rockville, MD: Agency for Health Care Policy and Research.

Kennedy, S. K., Wasnick, J. D. (1990). Cerebrovascular surgery. In M. P. Yeager, D. D. Glass (Eds.). *Anesthesiology and vascular surgery*. Norwalk, CT: Appleton & Lange.

Millis, J. M., Brown, S. L., Busuttil, R. W. (1992). Thoracic and abdominal aneurysms. In P. R. F. Bell, C. W. Jamieson, C. Vaughan Ruckley (Eds.). *Surgical management of vascular disease*. Philadelphia: W. B. Saunders.

Sandmann, W. (1992). Carotid endarterectomy. In P. R. F. Bell, C. W. Jamieson, C. Vaughan Ruckley (Eds.). *Surgical management of vascular disease*. Philadelphia: W. B. Saunders.

Walsh, D. B., McDaniel, M. D. (1990). Surgical technique and judgement: The vascular surgeon at work. In M. P. Yeager, D. D. Glass (Eds.). *Anesthesiology and vascular surgery*. Norwalk, CT: Appleton & Lange.

Youngberg, J. A., Gold, M. D. (1991). Carotid artery surgery: Perioperative anesthetic considerations. In J. A. Kaplan (Ed.). *Vascular anesthesia*. New York: Churchill Livingstone.

Zwolak, R. M., Cronenwett, J. L. (1990). Pathophysiology of vascular disease. In M. P. Yeager, D. D. Glass (Eds.). *Anesthesiology and vascular surgery*. Norwalk, CT: Appleton & Lange.

Cardiac Surgery

Susan K. Fisher

DEFINITION

Cardiac surgery refers to all surgical procedures involving the heart and proximal great vessels. The goal of cardiac surgery "is to restore or preserve adequate cardiac output and circulation of blood to the brain and tissues throughout the body" (Atkinson and Kohn, 1986).

ANATOMY

Heart

The heart is located approximately in the middle of the chest between the lungs. The muscle that forms the walls of the heart is called the *myocardium* and is distinct from smooth and skeletal muscle. The heart is divided into right and left halves. Each half is made up of two cavities. The atrial cavity empties into the ventricle on each side. The two sides of the heart are separated by a septum. The entire heart is encased in pericardium, which is a fibrous sac containing a small amount of fluid called *pericardial fluid*.

Between each atrium and ventricle is a valve that permits one-way blood flow from the atrium to the ventricle (Fig. 22–1). On the right side of the heart is the tricuspid valve. The mitral valve is on the left. Valves also control blood flow from the ventricles. The pulmonary valve controls the flow of blood from the right ventricle to the pulmonary artery. The aortic valve controls blood flow from the left ventricle to the aorta.

Great Vessels

Blood from the systemic circulation returns to the heart via the inferior and superior venae cavae, which empty into the right atrium. The blood enters the right ventricle through the tricuspid valve, exits via the pulmonary valve, flows into the pulmonary artery, and then enters the lungs. The oxygenated blood returns via the pulmonary veins to the left atrium. Flow continues through the mitral valve into the left ventricle and then through the aortic valve into the aorta and into the systemic circulation.

The right and left coronary arteries emerge from the aorta, distal to the aortic valve. These vessels initiate the arterial system, which provides nutrients to the myocardium (Fig. 22–2). The left main coronary artery, which supplies the left ventricle, quickly divides to form the left anterior descending and circumflex branches. The right coronary artery serves the right ventricle and terminates in the posterior descending artery.

The heart's conduction system coordinates pumping action. Cardiac muscle cells depolarize independently.

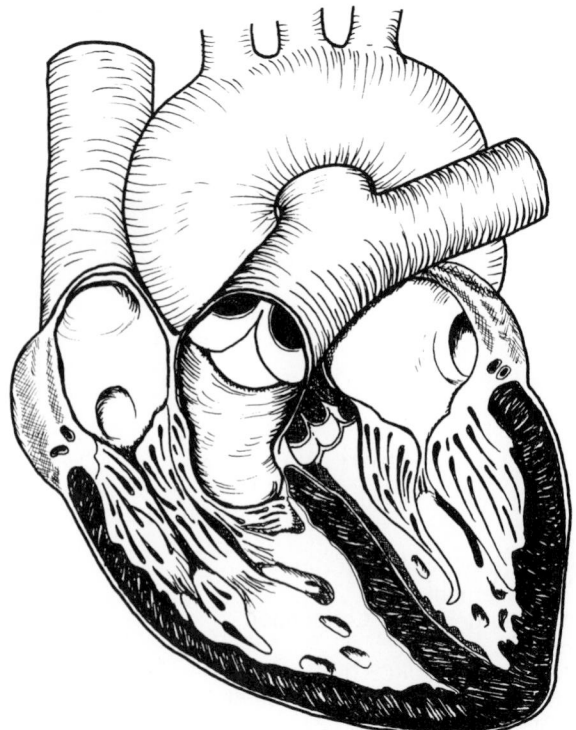

FIGURE 22–1. Heart, showing the valves and the great vessels. (Courtesy of Linda Eggers, Philadelphia, PA.)

Consequently, cells with the fastest rate control the depolarization rate of the remaining cardiac cells. These pacemaking cells are called the sinoatrial node and are located in the right atrial wall. From the sinoatrial node, the wave of excitation passes from cell to cell until it

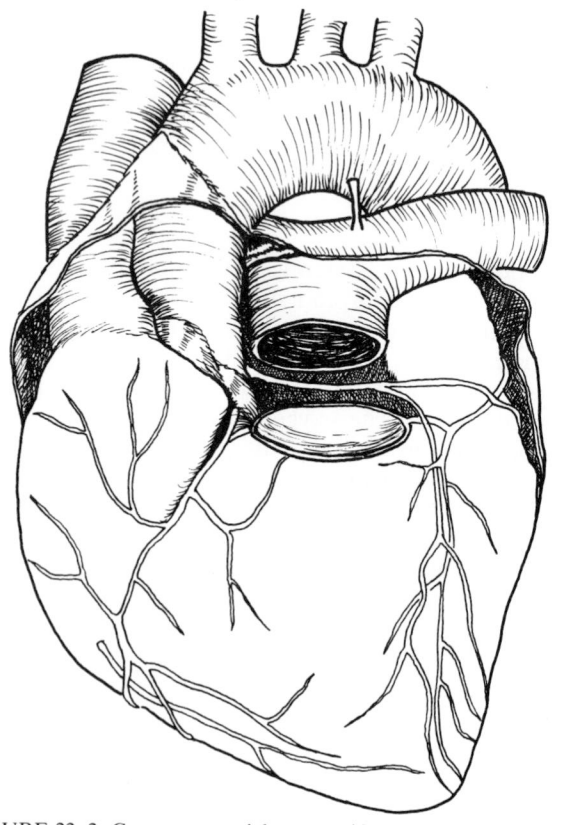

FIGURE 22–2. Coronary arterial system. (Courtesy of Linda Eggers, Philadelphia, PA.)

474

encounters a second mass of specialized cells called the atrioventricular node. The atrioventricular node delays the action potential for 0.1 second, which allows the atria to contract and empty blood into the ventricles before ventricular contraction occurs. From the atrioventricular node, the action potential travels though fibers called the bundle of His, which divides into right and left bundle branches and terminates in the Purkinje fibers, thereby completing the conduction cycle and ensuring a coordinated ventricular contraction (Luciano et al., 1978).

INDICATIONS

Indications for cardiac surgery are related to the symptoms of the patient. Symptomatic indications include angina that is not controllable with medication, chronic dyspnea and orthopnea, and arrhythmias. Many diagnostic studies are performed to determine the problem and evaluate the appropriateness of surgery. Diagnostic studies include cardiac catheterization, echocardiography, electrocardiography (ECG), and transesophageal echocardiography to diagnose valvular disease. Treatment decisions are usually made jointly between the cardiologist and the cardiac surgeon.

Cardiac Catheterization

Cardiac catheterization is a diagnostic procedure usually performed on the potential cardiac surgery patient to determine appropriate therapeutic intervention. The procedure is done percutaneously by inserting a catheter through a large vein, usually the femoral, and guiding it into the heart. The catheter is used to detect cardiac and pulmonary pressures, cardiac output, and cardiac ejection fraction and to inject radiopaque dye into the coronary arteries. When dye is injected, fluoroscopy is used to establish coronary anatomy and determine the presence of coronary lesions. Cardiac catheterization data provide evidence of conditions such as valvular, pulmonary artery, and coronary artery disease (Mark et al., 1986).

In angioplasty, angioplasty balloons are used to dilate narrowed coronary arteries. Another innovative treatment modality is the use of laser beams to clear arteries of plaque.

Patients undergoing cardiac catheterization are sedated and given local anesthesia during the procedure. The femoral puncture site must have pressure applied and be monitored after the procedure for bleeding.

SPECIAL INSTRUMENTS, SUPPLIES, AND EQUIPMENT

A dedicated heart set is the instrument set most frequently used for cardiac surgery. A vascular set with special cardiac clamps can also be used; however, a dedicated heart set is preferable because it is easier to monitor the location of the set in the event of an emergency.

Basic laparotomy instruments and vascular clamps are used for cardiac surgery. The essential vascular clamps include a cross-clamp for the aorta; a partial occlusion clamp, which is also used for the aorta; a DeBakey, or C-clamp, which is occasionally used for cannulation and for exposure of the vena cava; and small Fogarty clamps for femoral cannulation. Other types of vascular clamps should also be available. The cardiac set should also include vascular and fine coronary forceps, fine needle holders such as coronary and Castroviejo, and sternal wire needle holders. Pacing cables are needed for use with the pacing wires placed in the heart at the conclusion of the surgery. Scissors include fine vascular scissors, such as Potts, iris, Church, and Metzenbaum scissors. Wire cutters for sternal wires, Rumel tourniquets for cannulation suture, a Beaver knife, and chest retractors complete the heart set. Table 22–1 lists the instruments in a basic open heart set.

Sterile supplies include the sternal saw, 1-L cups for topical cooling, and the cannulas specific to the operation. Chest drainage and chest tubes are needed at the conclusion of the procedure. Internal defibrillator paddles should also be available on the surgical field.

Equipment for cardiac surgery includes a saw motor, a defibrillator, and an electrosurgical unit. It is helpful to have two electrosurgical units for coronary artery bypass procedures, one for the chest and one for vein harvest from the legs. For surgery entailing cardiopulmonary bypass, a pump and autotransfusion unit is needed. Anesthesia equipment includes the anesthesia machine, a monitor for central venous pressure, a cardiac output monitor, and an activated clotting time calculator. An atrial-ventricular pacemaker should also be available in the room.

SURGICAL PROCEDURES NECESSITATING EXTRACORPOREAL CIRCULATION

Cardiopulmonary Bypass

Definition

The most significant advance in the field of cardiac surgery was *extracorporeal circulation* (McGoon, 1985). This procedure refers to the diversion of systemic blood away from the heart and lungs (cardiopulmonary bypass) to a mechanical pump or oxygenator. The pump returns the blood to the body via a cannula in the aorta.

Because many cardiac procedures are similar in technique to the point of establishing cardiopulmonary bypass, the procedure for entering the chest cavity and establishing cardiopulmonary bypass is described below.

Indications

Cardiopulmonary bypass is indicated for surgery on the heart or great vessels in which a bloodless field is

needed, the activity of the heart must be temporarily stopped, or movement of or pressure on the heart would cause difficulty in heart function. The goal of cardiopulmonary bypass is to provide a motionless and bloodless operative field without creating myocardial necrosis (Lazar and Roberts, 1985). Cardiopulmonary bypass can be partial or complete. With partial cardiopulmonary bypass, there is a small amount of blood circulating through the heart and lungs. Complete cardiopulmonary bypass diverts most of the venous blood to the pump before entering the heart (Kirklin and Barratt-Boyes, 1986). Hypothermia is usually combined with cardiopulmonary bypass. There is no set core temperature. Temperature varies from patient to patient, depending on the condition of the heart and the anticipated length of the procedure. Cooling reduces the metabolic demands of the heart during the period when there is no blood flowing through the heart.

The heart is stopped during cardiopulmonary bypass by the use of cooling or cardioplegia solution. Potassium is the common component of cardioplegia solution. The solution causes cardiac arrest. Other components of cardioplegia solution are magnesium, procaine, glucose, oxygen, bicarbonate, phosphate, and calcium. Mixed together, these elements safely stop the heart, meet the energy demands of the heart in the absence of coronary blood flow, provide membrane stability, and act as a buffer to metabolic acidosis. Depending on the surgeon's preference, cardioplegia solution may be prepared as an asanguineous solution or as a blood mixture.

Figure 22–3 illustrates the mechanism by which blood bypasses the heart and lungs. The large venous cannula, which is inserted into the right atrium, diverts the blood returning from the systemic circulation via the superior and inferior venae cavae to the heart-lung machine. Roller pumps draw the blood through filters and an oxygenator. The blood then flows back to the patient through the cannula that has been placed in the aorta. This cannula is inserted distal to the aortic occlusion

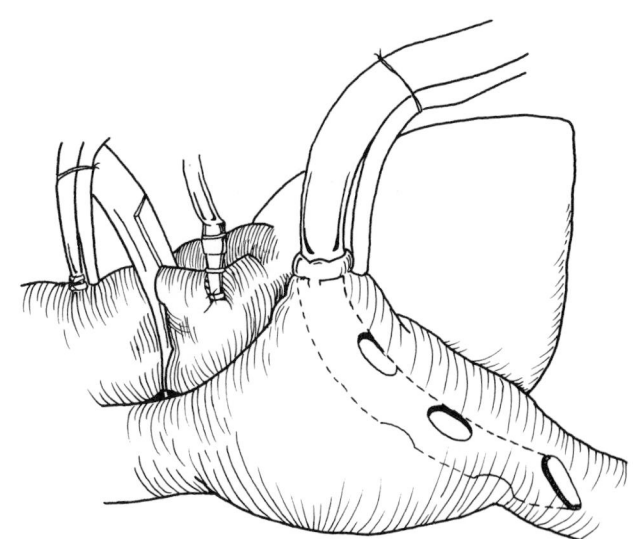

FIGURE 22–3. Cannulated heart. (Courtesy of Linda Eggers, Philadelphia, PA.)

TABLE 22–1. BASIC OPEN HEART SET

24ea	Mosquito Forceps, Curved
24ea	Crile Forceps, 5½in, Curved
8ea	Crile Forceps, 6¼in, Curved
6ea	Pean Forceps, 8in, Curved
10ea	Sarot Forceps
6ea	Cardiovascular Forceps, 7½in, Curved
2ea	Ochsner Forceps, 8in, Curved
10ea	Ochsner Forceps, 8in, Straight
20ea	Towel Clips, Large
20ea	Towel Clips, Small
2ea	Mosquito Forceps, Straight
6ea	Allis Clamps (6)
2ea	Babcock Forceps, Small Jaws, 7½in
1ea	Vital® Baumgarten Wire Twister
2ea	Potts-Smith Scissors, Angled 45°
1ea	Cooley Scissors
1ea	Metzenbaum Scissors, 9in
1ea	Metzenbaum Scissors, 11in
1ea	Mayo-Harrington Scissors, 11¾in
1ea	Wire Cutter, Angular Blades
1ea	No. 4 Knife Handle
1ea	No. 3 Knife Handle
1ea	No. 7 Knife Handle
1ea	No. 3 Knife Handle
2ea	Kantrowitz Clamp, 7½in
1ea	Kantrowitz Clamp, 9½in
4ea	Sponge Sticks, Straight
1ea	Sponge Sticks, Curved
1ea	Bandage Scissors, Large
1ea	Cooley Graft Suction
2ea	Large Multi-Holed Suctions
1ea	Cooley Intracardiac Suction Tube
1ea	Yankauer Suction Tube
2ea	Anthony Tip Suctions
2ea	U.S. Army Retractors
2ea	Gelpi Retractors
1ea	Sharp Rake Retractor
1ea	Blunt Rake Retractor
2ea	Senn Retractors
2ea	Kelly Retractors, Small
1ea	Kelly Retractor, Medium
1ea	Kelly Retractor, Large
2ea	Baby Deaver Retractors
2ea	Narrow Deaver Retractors
3ea	Large Deaver Retractors
2ea	Baby Ribbon Retractors
2ea	Narrow Ribbon Retractors
2ea	Medium Ribbon Retractors
1ea	Large Ribbon Retractor
2ea	Rumel Stylets
1ea	Bailey Approximator

2ea	Vein Retractors
1ea	Cooley Clamp
2ea	Cooley Clamps
2ea	Glover, Small (Baby) Clamps
4ea	Cooley "Alligator" Clamps
1ea	Cooley Anastomosis Clamp
1ea	Internal Carotid Clamp
1ea	Cooley Clamp
1ea	Cooley Aortic Clamp, Large
1ea	1 Set Rubber Tourniquets
1ea	Semb Ligature Carrier
2ea	Cooley Iliac Clamps, Short
2ea	Cooley Iliac Clamps, Long
1ea	Cooley Renal Clamp
2ea	Cooley Curved Glovers
2ea	Cooley Straight Glovers
4ea	Medium Dressing Forceps
2ea	Long Dressing Forceps
2ea	Cooley Vascular Tissue Forceps, 8in
2ea	Cooley Vascular Tissue Forceps, 9½in
2ea	Cooley Vascular Tissue Forceps, 6in
2ea	Small Tissue Forceps, Toothed
2ea	Adson Tissue Forceps, Toothed
2ea	Cushing Tissue Forceps, No Teeth
2ea	Cooley Patent Ductus Clamps, Straight
1ea	Cooley Patent Ductus Clamp, Angled 15°
1ea	Cooley Patent Ductus Clamp, Angled 30°
1ea	Cooley Carotid Clamp
1ea	Cooley Anastomosis Clamp
3ea	Vital® Crile-Wood Needle Holder, 8in
3ea	Vital® Crile-Wood Needle Holder, 7in
1ea	Vital® Cooley Intracardiac Needle Holder, 9in
2ea	Gemini Mixter Clamp
1ea	Cooley Sternotomy Retractor, Adult
1ea	Cooley Atrial Retractor, Right
1ea	Cooley Atrial Retractor

From *The Surgical Armamentarium* (1988). McGaw Park, IL: Baxter Health Care Corp.

clamp. The left ventricular vent cannula is placed through the superior pulmonary vein and left atrium and then into the left ventricle. Blood flowing through the left ventricular vent cannula is removed by the pump, filtered, oxygenated, and combined in a reservoir with blood from the venous cannula. The cardioplegia needle is inserted proximal to the aortic cross-clamp. Cardioplegia solution is cooled by the heart-lung machine and delivered to the coronary arteries through a 14-gauge angiocath that has been inserted into the aorta proximal to the aortic cross-clamp.

Perioperative Nursing Implications

Anesthesia

During cardiopulmonary bypass, cardiac output (actually pump output), systemic venous pressure, pulmonary venous pressure, arterial blood oxygen and carbon dioxide content, and temperature are controlled externally and monitored by the perfusionist, who works under the direction of the cardiac surgeon.

General endotracheal anesthesia is used for cardiac surgery necessitating cardiopulmonary bypass. The patient is routinely premedicated with morphine and scopolamine to allow for an easier anesthesia induction. Usually, an arterial catheter is placed in the radial artery before induction. If radial artery placement is impossible, the catheter is placed in the femoral artery. Swan-Ganz and central venous pressure catheters are also placed before induction.

Anesthesia is induced using a combination of drugs. Fentanyl and pancuronium are commonly used. If inhalation agents are used for intubation, they include nitrous oxide, halothane, and enflurane. Muscle relaxants are given to prevent shivering during core cooling.

Blood products may be needed during the surgery, especially if the patient has a low blood volume or hematocrit preoperatively. Arterial blood gas samples are frequently sent for analysis during cardiopulmonary bypass. The anesthetist also monitors the patient's activated clotting time.

Position

The patient is placed in a supine position by the circulating nurse. The arms may be tucked straight at the patient's sides. If the arms are tucked, toboggans may be used for arm positioning. These positioning aids help prevent injury to the brachial plexus and allow the surgical team to operate. A rolled sheet may be placed under the shoulders to elevate the chest for good exposure. Because the patient for cardiac surgery is commonly prepared from the chin to the toes, the grounding pads should be placed on the buttocks. The head is held in a cloth-covered foam support.

Creation and Maintenance of the Sterile Field

The skin preparation usually involves iodophor scrub and solution, or gel. The chest is prepared from the chin to the groin. Both sides of the groin are prepared for possible femoral cannulation. The groin should be free from hair. Both legs may also be prepared. A disposable cardiovascular drape is used to provide a visible operative field. The circulating nurse should be available during the draping procedure to dispose properly of the paper backing of the plastic drape and to position the instrument tables and equipment. The Mayo stand is positioned over the patient's feet, with the larger instrument table at the scrub nurse's right. The electrosurgical unit is placed at the foot of the operating room (OR) bed. Light sources for surgical headlights should be placed behind each surgeon. The sternal saw motor is placed behind the surgeon, with the foot pedal in easy reach. After the instrument tables and equipment are positioned, the perfusion team moves the heart-lung and suction machines into place to the left of the patient and near the operative team.

Equipment and Supplies

Suture varies according to the surgeon's preference. Silk or braided polyester are commonly used. Cannulation suture and pericardial stay suture are the only suture needed to enter the chest and begin cardiopulmonary bypass. Myocardial pacing wires are needed during the warming phase of cardiopulmonary bypass. A No. 10 skin blade is used to open the chest and a No. 11 blade is used for aortic cannulation. A No. 11 blade, or a No. 12 hook blade, may be used for venous cannulation. Large laparotomy sponges and 4 × 8 inch gauze sponges are used. Two or three chest tubes and chest drainage devices are used after surgery.

Attention to detail is critical during the establishment of cardiopulmonary bypass. The scrub nurse should ensure that all instruments and equipment are operational before starting the procedure. Cannulas should be checked for patency before starting surgery. Instruments and suture for cannulation should be on the Mayo stand. These include hemostats, Crile artery forceps, Mixter forceps, ties, cross-clamp, Rumel tourniquets, tissue forceps, Metzenbaum scissors, and knife blades.

Drugs and Solutions

Cardioplegia solution
Lactated Ringer's solution
Normal saline

Physiological Monitoring

Before preparing the skin, a Foley catheter is inserted to monitor urine output. A rectal or bladder probe is used to monitor temperature. A nasopharyngeal temperature probe is often used to monitor temperature and is placed by the anesthetist.

Specimens and Cultures

Specimens are usually not taken when establishing cardiopulmonary bypass.

Physician's Orders

Typical admission orders include a complete blood count with electrolyte, blood urea nitrogen, creatinine, and clotting studies. A blood sample is taken for the cross-matching. Occasionally, pulmonary function tests and arterial blood gas measurements are ordered. The administration of previously ordered medications is continued. The patient is instructed to take a shower the evening before surgery with an antimicrobial soap. If not contraindicated because of allergies or skin sensitivities, a depilatory is also used on the operative area. The patient maintains nothing by mouth (NPO) status after midnight.

Laboratory and Diagnostic Studies

A chest x-ray film is routinely taken on admission. This should demonstrate lungs free from disease as well as the position and size of the heart. For a second operation, the x-ray film also shows the position of sternal wires that are removed after the skin is incised.

The results of previously ordered laboratory studies should be reviewed. All blood values should be within normal limits. Correction of abnormal values should take place before surgery.

Procedure

Incision and Exposure

A midline skin incision is made from one fingerbreadth below the suprasternal notch to 3 cm below the xiphoid process. The midline of the sternum, along with any bleeding sites from the incision, is cauterized. The assistant should apply retraction to the upper angle of the skin incision to provide exposure. The suprasternal ligament is cut with heavy scissors or cautery and a right-angled clamp is passed over and behind the sternum and spread to create space for the sternal saw. The reciprocating saw is placed in this space and the sternum is cut down the midline. While cutting, the surgeon hugs the toe of the saw up against the sternum. The assistant should be ready with suction. After the sternum is split, a thin layer of bone wax may be placed over the edges of the periosteum, which may be cauterized. The chest retractor is inserted and opened gradually with the dissection of fascia. The thymus is separated to the level of the innominate vein. While the surgeon and assistant each pull upward on the pericardium with forceps, the surgeon cuts longitudinally into the pericardium. The pericardium is dissected from the heart and aorta and held up to fashion a basket using pericardial stay sutures.

Details

After the pericardial reflection is dissected from the aorta, heparin is given by the anesthetist, and the aortic cannulation suture is introduced. Two concentric pursestring sutures are placed in the adventitia and a Rumel tourniquet of 22 Fr. red rubber is slung on the suture.

Another pursestring suture is placed in the right atrial appendage, and a pursestring suture is placed for the cardioplegia apparatus in the aorta, if used. To cannulate the aorta, an incision is made with the No. 11 blade. The aorta may be dilated before the insertion of the aortic cannula. The pursestring sutures are tightened around the cannula using the tourniquet and a hemostat, and the cannula is attached to the latex or Silastic pump tubing supplied by the perfusionist. A tie or stitch of heavy silk is usually used to secure the aortic cannula.

Because the atrium has an appendage, it may be opened in a number of ways. Commonly a C-clamp, or DeBakey clamp, is placed on the appendage; the appendage is then opened with scissors or blade and tissue forceps, or a Crile artery forceps is placed on the opposing edges. The venous cannula is advanced as the clamp is removed, and the pursestring suture is tightened as described above. The cannula is then attached to the venous pump line. At this point, tubing clamps may be removed from the lines and the bypass initiated. The vent pursestring suture is placed in the superior pulmonary vein and the left ventricle is vented using a No. 11 blade. A Crile artery forceps is used to open the hole, and the vent cannula is connected to the pump vent tubing. The vent cannula is inserted while the patient is undergoing bypass. It would be unsafe to insert the cannula without cardiopulmonary bypass because the heart must be pushed to one side to expose the cannulation site. In addition, the patient's heart may not tolerate low pressure and a beating heart may suck in air.

After the predetermined flow rate is reached, cooling begins by decreasing the temperature in the pump heat exchanger to 4°C. At the point of ventricular fibrillation, the aortic cross-clamp is placed along with the cardioplegia apparatus, and cardioplegia solution is instilled into the coronary arteries. Iced lactated Ringer solution is also poured on the heart for topical cooling. This is continued until the patient reaches the desired temperature, approximately 25°C, and there is no electrical activity in the heart. After the field is motionless and bloodless, the repair may begin.

Closure

The surgeon instructs the perfusionist to rewarm the blood approximately 10 minutes before he or she is ready to remove the aortic cross-clamp. The perfusionist turns the heat exchanger to 38 to 40°C and warm blood begins to flow to the patient. When the cross-clamp is removed, the scrub nurse should use warm saline to assist in warming the patient. When the nasopharyngeal temperature reaches 37°C, bypass may be stopped. Usually, as the patient is warmed, electrical activity returns to the heart. This may be in the form of ventricular fibrillation, which may need to be corrected by electrical defibrillation. Atrial and ventricular pacing wires, if needed, are usually placed at this point and are brought out through the skin and secured with a skin suture. If the patient's rhythm and pressures remain stable after termination of bypass, the vent and venous cannulas are removed, the cardioplegia needle having been removed previously. Protamine is given to reverse the anticoagulant properties of heparin. The activated clotting time is checked after the protamine has acted. Because protamine causes hypotension in some patients and life-threatening allergic reaction in others, the aortic cannula is left in place until well after the protamine is given. If the patient remains stable, the aortic cannula is removed, and the pursestring suture is tied down to close the cannulation site.

The main goal after terminating bypass is to maintain hemostasis. All cannulation and suture lines should be inspected. Polypropylene (Prolene) suture with or without polytetrafluoroethylene (Teflon) felt pledgets is used for bleeding sites. The pericardium may be left open to avoid tamponade after chest tubes are inserted, and the chest is closed. Stainless steel wires are placed through the sternum, tightened to approximate the bone, and twisted down. Absorbable suture is used to close the muscle, fascia, and subcuticular skin layers.

Postoperative Care

The patient is immediately transported to the intensive care unit. Typical postoperative orders include intake and output measurement, cardiac output measurement, central venous pressure catheter care, and ventilator care. The ventilator may be removed from the patient as soon as the first postoperative night. To avoid infection, chest tubes are removed as soon as drainage is minimal. Pacing wires are removed before the patient is discharged from the hospital. If there are no complications, the patient is transferred to the stepdown unit on the first or second postoperative day.

Potential Surgical Complications

Infection
Coagulopathy due to the platelet destruction by the pump
Kidney failure from poor perfusion during bypass
Changes in red blood cells and plasma proteins
Emboli from particulate matter

Coronary Artery Bypass Grafting

Definition

Coronary artery bypass grafting (CABG) is done to establish a conduit to bypass a narrowed or obstructed portion of a coronary artery and thus provide blood flow to a potentially ischemic portion of myocardium.

Indications

CABG is performed on patients with arteriosclerotic coronary artery disease. This disease process is similar to arteriosclerotic disease in other vessels of the body. It refers to a focal intimal accumulation of lipids, complex carbohydrates, blood products, fibrous tissue, and calcium deposits that results in narrowing of the coronary artery and eventually limits blood flow to the myocardium (Kirklin and Barratt-Boyes, 1986).

Indications for CABG include chronic stable and acute unstable angina with demonstrated coronary artery lesions by cardiac catheterization. Usually patients with continued angina and abnormal electrocardiograms (ECGs) or stress test results after 3 months of medication are candidates for CABG (Lytle and Loop, 1985). The objective of surgery is to establish a bypass graft distal to the obstruction in the coronary artery. Usually, the reversed saphenous vein is the conduit of choice, and increasingly, the internal mammary artery is used to provide blood flow to a diseased left anterior descending artery. Lesions greater than 50% are usually chosen to be bypassed.

Related Surgical Procedures

Coronary endarterectomy

Perioperative Nursing Implications

Anesthesia

Refer to the discussion of cardiopulmonary bypass.

Position

In addition to positioning the patient for cardiopulmonary bypass place the patients legs, after preparing and draping, on a rounded pillow or cushion and in frog leg position. Care must be taken to avoid pressure on the popliteal vessels.

Creation and Maintenance of the Sterile Field

In addition to the chest and the groin, both legs are prepared circumferentially from the groin to and including the ankle areas. These areas should also be without hair, from either preoperative depilatory or shave. The cardiovascular drape is used to expose the entire body, except feet, genitalia, and pubic areas.

After the completion of draping, the scrub nurse should organize and pass off the field the electrosurgical unit active electrode and suction lines. If the mammary retractor is used, the scrub nurse assists the surgeon in setting it up. In the absence of internal mammary grafting, the perfusion cannulas are passed up to the field and organized before the skin incision is made.

Because of vein harvesting from the patient's legs, the Mayo stand is placed to the extreme right of its usual position. After the vein is harvested and the incision closed, the Mayo stand is moved back over the patient's legs.

Equipment and Supplies

In addition to pericardial pursestrings suture and suture for cannulation, 5-0, 6-0, and 7-0 (and occasionally 8-0) double-armed Prolene sutures are needed to perform the anastomosis. Larger 3-0 and 4-0 Prolene sutures, with and without Teflon pledgets, are needed to repair any bleeding sites after decannulation. For closure, the surgeon uses No. 5 or 6 sternal wires, absorbable suture, and skin clips or suture.

A 4- or 4.8-mm aortic punch is used to establish proximal access for the grafts. Cardiotomy suction cannulas are attached to the cardiotomy tubing, which is passed from the pump. Cannulas for cannulation as described above should be available at the beginning of the procedure, as should sterile internal defibrillator paddles.

A small rounded scalpel is used for dissection. This blade, along with an umbilical tape, peanut dissectors, and vessel loops are passed to the scrub nurse during the setup for the procedure.

At the conclusion of the operation, a sterile chest drainage device is passed to the scrub nurse along with two or three chest tubes. After the scrub nurse hands the connected chest drainage device off the field, the circulating nurse should connect it to suction. The wound is dressed with gauze sponges and tape. Often, the leg is wrapped with an elastic bandage for compression.

In addition to those instruments needed for cardiopulmonary bypass, the scrub nurse should have within reach fine coronary instruments, including forceps, scissors, dilators, and needle holders as described under special instruments, supplies, and equipment above. Table 22-2 lists the instruments in a coronary artery bypass set. In addition, a partial occlusion clamp is used for the proximal anastomosis upon removal of the aortic cross-clamp. Peanut dissectors on clamps should be available for blotting the coronary artery when opened, as should saline syringes with Webster cannulas. Small and medium ligation clips are used for the vein harvest as well as the dissection of the internal mammary artery. Small 5-0 and 3-0 ties are also used for the vein harvest. After the scrub nurse provides the surgeon harvesting the vein with the necessary instruments (knife, scissors, mosquito hemostats, ties, clips, and vessel loops and forceps), his or her primary attention should be directed toward the surgical team members operating at the chest.

Drugs and Solutions

Heparinized saline
Papaverine hydrochloride
Cefoxitin or other antibiotics
Oxidized regenerated cellulose (Surgicel) or absorbable gelatin sponge (Gelfoam)
Methylene blue
Warm and cool normal saline
Iced lactated Ringer solution

Specimens and Cultures

In addition to a possible culture, if the surgeon performs a coronary endarterectomy, the plaque recovered should be sent to the pathology department.

Physician's Orders

In addition to typical admission orders for patients having cardiac surgery while undergoing bypass, the administration of digoxin should be discontinued 36 hours before surgery unless atrial fibrillation occurs. The administration of propranolol or calcium channel blockers should be continued to avoid the possibility of a myocardial infarction.

Laboratory and Diagnostic Studies

The cardiac catheterization findings should be reviewed before surgery. For additional information, refer to the discussion of cardiac catheterization.

Procedure

Incision and Exposure

When harvesting the greater saphenous vein, the skin incision is routinely made lateral to the medial malleolus, and blunt dissection is achieved to the level of the vein. The vein should be freed in one segment. The assistant ligates and divides branches as it is cleared. The skin incision should continue proximally up the leg without creating flaps. When the desired length of vein is freed, it should be ligated at the distal end after being clamped. The free end of the vein should be clearly

	TABLE 22-2. CORONARY ARTERY BYPASS SET
1ea	Delicate Potts Scissors
1ea	Delicate Potts Reverse Cutting Scissors
2ea	Vital® Cooley Intracardiac Needle Holder
2ea	Vital® Cushing Tissue Forceps, 7in
1ea	Cooley Reverse Cutting Scissors
1ea	Cooley Coronary Dilators
1ea	Garrett Vascular Dilators
1ea	Mills Mammary Forceps
1ea	Mills Saphenous Forceps
1ea	Parsonnet Retractor
1ea	Micro Bulldog Clamp, Curved
1ea	Micro Bulldog Clamp, Straight
1ea	Micro Bulldog Clamp, Curved
1ea	Micro Bulldog Clamp, Straight
1ea	Vital® Cooley Micro Needle Holder, 6in
1ea	Vital® Cooley Micro Needle Holder, 6¾in
1ea	Vital® Cooley Micro Needle Holder, 8in

From *The Surgical Armamentarium* (1988). McGaw Park, IL: Baxter Health Care Corp.

marked with a suture or vein cannula and the clamped end suture ligated. The vein should then be distended with heparinized saline to check for any leaks, which are repaired with ties, clips, or 6–0 Prolene suture. Adventitial bands on the vein should be removed. Often, the length of vein is marked with methylene blue to avoid twisting during the anastomosis. After the vein is prepared, the proximal end is clamped and cut, and the clamped portion is suture ligated. The leg is then closed with several layers of continuously run absorbable suture and sometimes skin clips.

After the chest is opened and before cannulation, the internal mammary artery may be mobilized. This dissection is done with forceps, cautery, and Metzenbaum scissors. A special retractor is placed, which allows elevation of only one side of the chest. The OR bed is rotated to expose the left underside of the sternum. Starting at the sixth rib, a pedicle of internal mammary artery, fat, and muscle is dissected away from the chest to the level of the first rib. The distal portion is divided obliquely and a papaverine solution of 60 mg in 500 ml of saline is injected onto and into the artery to prevent vasospasm. Bleeding should be brisk from the transected end. Clips are used for ligation. The internal mammary artery is prepared by dissecting the pedicle from the distal 1 cm of the artery. It is grafted in the usual distal anastomosis fashion, having been passed over or through the pericardium. The pedicle is secured with a few interrupted sutures.

Details

After the beginning of cardiopulmonary bypass, the heart is positioned using cold, wet sponges or other equipment of the surgeon's preference. Distal anastomoses may be performed first, with those to the back of the heart done at the outset. While the assistant provides traction, the surgeon incises the epicardium with the rounded scalpel, brushing the anterior surface of the artery to clear it. The vessel is entered obliquely with the blade to avoid cutting into the back wall of the artery. The arteriotomy is enlarged using fine-angled scissors to 4 to 6 mm in length. The vessel is then probed to determine size and patency. The vein graft end is cut and beveled to cover the circumference of the artery with fine scissors and coronary forceps. The end-to-side anastomosis is completed with 6–0 or 7–0 double-armed Prolene suture. Before the suture line is tied, the vein is infused with cardioplegia solution or saline to check for any leakage at the anastomosis.

After all distal anastomoses are completed, and the patient is warming, the cross-clamp is removed. It is replaced with a partial occlusion clamp, which allows some blood to eject into the aorta but prevents blood flow to the area of surgery. The area proximal and lateral to the ascending aorta is the region of the proximal anastomosis. The vein graft is distended with cold cardioplegia solution to determine appropriate length, then cut and beveled. A stab is made with a No. 11 blade, into which an aortic punch is introduced to cut a rounded opening for anastomosis. This is performed with a 5–0 or 6–0 double-armed Prolene suture.

While the suture is tied, the opening may be marked with a small metal ring or clip that delineates the area of grafting if there is a later cardiac catheterization.

After all anastomoses are completed and observed for bleeding, cardiopulmonary bypass may be stopped and decannulation started.

Closure

Closure of the chest is accomplished as described above. A third chest tube is inserted into the left pleura if it was entered during dissection of the internal mammary artery.

Postoperative Care

In addition to receiving the postoperative care for the bypass, the patient undergoing CABG should be referred to both the surgeon and the cardiologist for follow-up care.

Potential Surgical Complications

Electrolyte imbalances
Arrhythmias
Cardiac tamponade
Hypothermia
Impaired gas exchange
Neuropsychological disturbances
Pain
Sleep disturbances

Valve Replacement

Definition

Valve replacement refers to removing the patient's natural valve and substituting a mechanical or prosthetic tissue valve.

Indications

Valve replacement is performed for the patient whose natural valve is damaged or dysfunctional. The most common valves involved are the mitral and aortic valves. Diseased valves become stenotic or regurgitant. Stenotic valves are stiff and unable to close securely. Regurgitant valves are unable to prevent backflow while shut. Causes of valve disease include rheumatic fever, bacterial endocarditis, atherosclerosis, and calcification. The decision for surgery is based on symptoms presented as well as data obtained from echocardiograms and cardiac catheterization studies.

More than 50 different designs for prosthetic valves are available. Boncheck (1985) described the ideal characteristics of a prosthetic valve:

1. is able to transmit physiological blood flows without pressure gradient or leaks

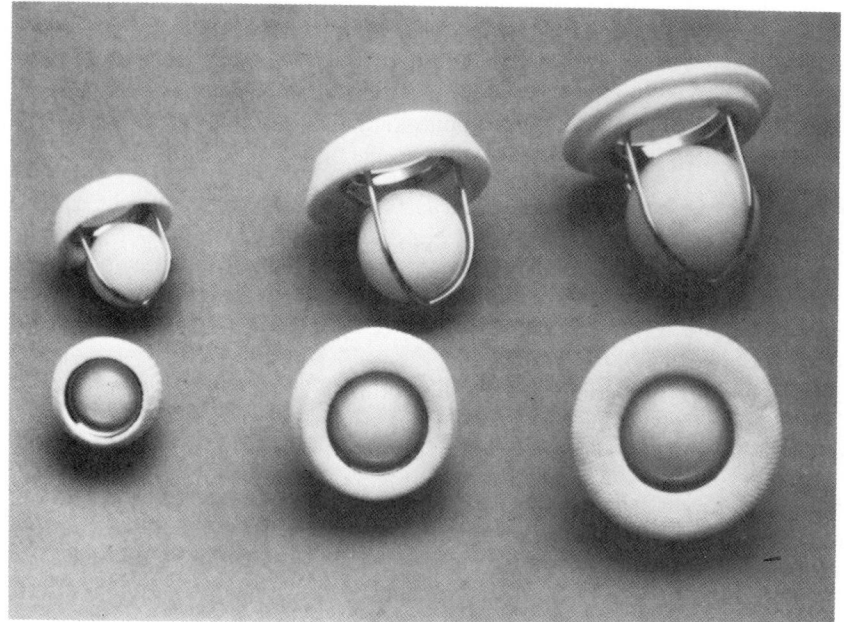

FIGURE 22–4. Starr-Edwards valves. (From Morgan, R. J., Davis, J. T., Fraker, T. D. [1985]. Current status of valve prosthesis. *Surgical Clinics of North America, 65*, 706.)

2. is durable
3. is thrombosis resistant
4. has host compatibility
5. is relatively easy to insert
6. functions quietly

Of the mechanical valve designs, the most popular are the ball-and-cage model (Fig. 22–4) and the hinged carbon polymer tilting disk model (Fig. 22–5). The most commonly used biological valve is the porcine xenograft (Fig. 22–6).

Related Surgical Procedures

Valve repair, such as commissurotomy
Placement of an annuloplasty ring in any of the four heart valves

Perioperative Nursing Implications

Anesthesia

In addition to routine procedures for cardiac anesthesia described above, the head of the OR bed may need to be raised during preparation if there is concurrent pulmonary hypertension. Supplemental oxygen should be given. Before cardiopulmonary bypass, the patient's heart rate should be kept within a narrow range that provides an adequate cardiac index while not exceeding a rate that prevents blood flow across stenotic valves.

Position

Refer to the discussion of cardiopulmonary bypass.

Creation and Maintenance of the Sterile Field

The creation and maintenance of the sterile field is done as described for cardiopulmonary bypass.

Equipment and Supplies

In addition to supplies needed for cardiopulmonary bypass, suture for valve replacement is needed. This is often double-armed, polyester suture, sometimes with Teflon felt pledgets. Additional Prolene suture with and without felt pledgets and a 4 × 4 inch piece of Teflon felt are cut and used to close the aortotomy and atriotomy.

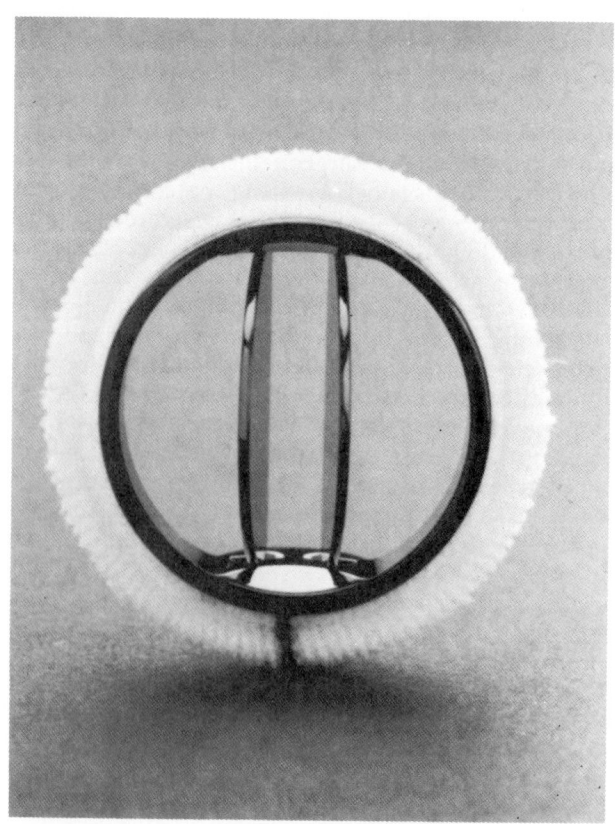

FIGURE 22–5. St. Jude valve. (From Morgan, R. J., Davis, J. T., Fraker, T. D. [1985]. Current status of valve prosthesis. *Surgical Clinics of North America, 65*, 708.)

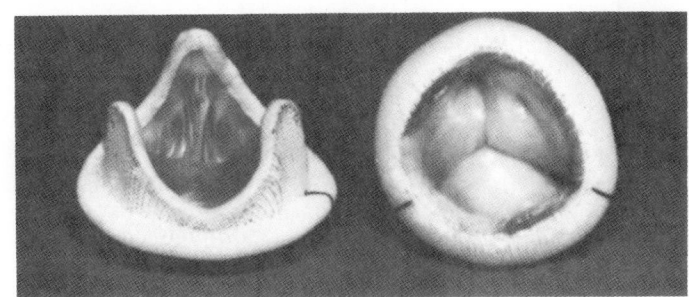

FIGURE 22–6. Carpentier-Edwards valve. (From Morgan, R. J., Davis, J. T., Fraker, T. D. [1985]. Current status of valve prosthesis. *Surgical Clinics of North America, 65*, 709.)

It is the circulating nurse's responsibility to pass the desired valve to the sterile field and record the data. The patient's chart should contain the information of the valve manufacturer, size, and serial number.

In terms of cannulation, there are two alternatives for valve surgery. If an aortotomy is performed, specialized cardioplegia perfusors are used to perfuse directly into the coronary ostia. If a mitral valve replacement is done, there are two venous cannulas, one in the inferior and one in the superior vena cava. In this instance, an umbilical tape is often passed around the cannula and kept in place with a tourniquet.

In addition to instruments for cardiopulmonary bypass, specialized valve instruments are needed. These include special retractors such as an aortic leaflet retractor and vein retractor used for aortotomy exposure and small Kelly-Richardson and Cooley retractors for mitral exposure. Chordae retractors are also used for exposure. Long instruments, including scissors, forceps, and knife handles, are useful for work deep in the chest, such as in mitral valve replacement. If the valve is calcified, a pituitary rongeur is used to débride the area. Three small basins for saline are needed if a porcine valve is used. These valves are soaked for 2 minutes in each basin to rinse the glutaraldehyde, which is used for preservation. Finally, valve sizers appropriate to the type of valve to be used are needed.

Drugs and Solutions

Normal saline
Iced lactated Ringer solution
Antibiotic solution

Specimens and Cultures

A swab from the patient's natural valve and/or a piece of the valve may be sent for culture. The removed natural valve should be sent to the pathology department for analysis.

Physician's Orders

In addition to orders for all patients undergoing bypass, recommended procedures preoperatively include a complete dental examination, with any diseased teeth removed. An infection in the teeth could have serious effects on the valve prosthesis.

Laboratory and Diagnostic Studies

Cardiac catheterization and echocardiographic results should be reviewed in addition to results of studies performed for cardiopulmonary bypass.

Procedure

Incision and Exposure

After initiating bypass, the aorta is opened for aortic valve replacement and the left atrium opened vertically for mitral valve replacement. For an aortic valve replacement, the first assistant retracts the fat pad at the atrioventricular groove and the opened aorta with a vein retractor. If the left atrium is opened, a small Kelly-Richardson or other atrial retractor is used. Before the aortic valve is excised, a small gauze sponge is packed in the aorta to prevent calcium emboli formation. The valves are excised with scissors, forceps, blades, and rongeurs. Sutures are placed to mark the commissures. The sutures are tagged with clamps. Next, the valve is sized with the appropriate type of sizers.

Details

After the prosthetic valve is prepared, it is sewn with interrupted 2–0 (for aortic) or 1–0 (for mitral) polyester (Dacron) suture with or without felt pledgets. After all the valve sutures are sewn through the prosthetic valve cuff and the annulus, the suture is wetted and the valve passed down and seated into place. The sutures are then tied down and seated into place. During a mitral valve replacement, a 14 Fr. Foley catheter is passed through the valve and the balloon inflated to act as a frustrator during atrial closure.

Closure

Both the aortic and atrial closures are completed with 3–0 double-armed Prolene suture. Felt strips may be used. The incision is closed with two sutures. One oversews the aorta or atrium in one direction; the second oversews in the opposite direction. Before the repair is tied closed, the patient is placed in Trendelenburg position with positive pressure applied to the lungs, and a large-gauge needle is placed in the apex of the left ventricle to remove air from the heart. The closure is completed and bypass terminated and the chest is closed as described above.

Postoperative Care

In addition to receiving routine postoperative care, the patient with a mechanical valve is started on a regimen of anticoagulation therapy on the second postoperative day. Sodium warfarin (Coumadin) or aspirin is used and continued throughout the lifetime of the patient with a mechanical valve. The patient with a biological prosthesis is temporarily anticoagulated for approximately 1 month.

Potential Surgical Complications

Infection
Bleeding disorders
Thrombus or embolus formation
Valve failure

Resection Surgeries for Conduction Disorders

Definition

Resections for conduction disorders are surgical procedures done using cardiopulmonary bypass to excise or ablate selected portions of endocardium or subendocardium.

Indications

Resection surgeries for conduction disorders are performed for patients with tachyrhythmias to interrupt or remove conduction bypass or reentry tracts. Reentrant arrhythmias occur when a closed electrical circuit allows repetitive self-sustaining activation to occur. An example of this is Wolff-Parkinson-White syndrome. With this syndrome, there are accessory atrioventricular pathways that make possible the continuous electrical excitement of the heart, resulting in supraventricular tachycardia (Smith et al., 1985). This results in inadequate ventricular filling time. Supraventricular tachycardia can lead to sudden death. These disorders are diagnosed with ECG and electrophysiological studies in which electrode catheters are used to map the atrioventricular area in an effort to locate the accessory pathways. Figure 22–7 provides visual explanation of the reentry pathway present in Wolff-Parkinson-White syndrome.

Related Surgical Procedures

Wolff-Parkinson-White syndrome ablation
Subendocardial resection
Ventricular tachycardia mapping and ablation

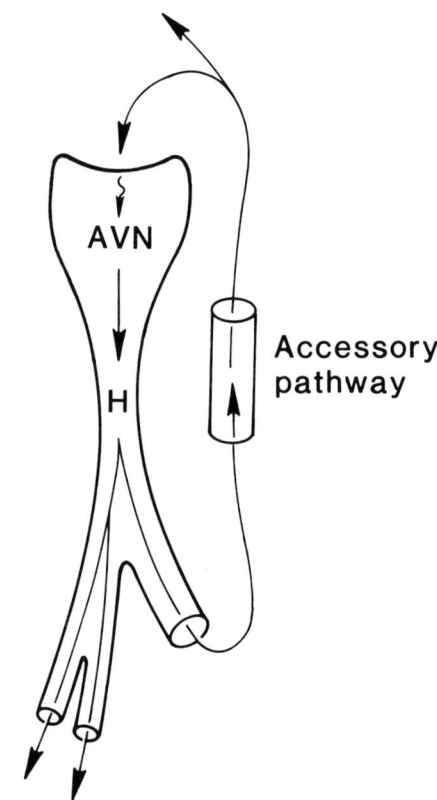

FIGURE 22–7. Accessory pathway in Wolff-Parkinson-White syndrome. AVN, atrioventricular node; H, His bundle. Arrows indicate the directions of activation, including continuous activation through the accessory pathway. (From Smith, P. K., Holman, W. L., Cox, J. L. [1985]. Surgical treatment of supraventricular tachyarrhythmias. *Surgical Clinics of North America, 65*, 554.)

Perioperative Nursing Implications

Anesthesia

Refer to the discussion of cardiopulmonary bypass.

Position

Refer to the discussion of cardiopulmonary bypass.

Creation and Maintenance of the Sterile Field

Preparing and draping are done as described for cardiopulmonary bypass. In addition to the OR furniture listed for cardiopulmonary bypass, electrophysiological monitoring equipment must also be in the room. Because this equipment is large, a dedicated OR is usually identified for these procedures. If cryoablation is to be done, this machine must also be placed close to the sterile field.

After draping is performed, the scrub nurse should pass the connection for the internal defibrillator paddles to the circulating nurse immediately, as they will be needed during the mapping process when arrhythmias may be induced.

Equipment and Supplies

In addition to instruments and supplies for cardiopulmonary bypass, sterile epicardial electrodes and additional pacing wires are needed, as well as the hand-held probe used to "read" electrical activity.

There are many leads and probes passed to the sterile table. The scrub nurse should be careful to keep these untangled and organized so that they may be passed to the surgeon when needed.

Drugs and Solutions

Warm and cool normal saline
Iced lactated Ringer solution
Antibiotic solution

Physiological Monitoring

Refer to the discussion of cardiopulmonary bypass.

Specimens and Cultures

If endocardial resection is performed, the excised endocardium is sent for examination.

Physician's Orders

In addition to undergoing procedures in preparation for cardiopulmonary bypass, on admission the patient should be scheduled for cardiac catheterization to determine any coronary artery or valve disease that may be corrected during surgery. The administration of antiarrhythmic drugs, such as amiodarone, should be discontinued, as it may interfere with defibrillation of induced ventricular tachycardia or cause fibrillation intraoperatively.

Laboratory and Diagnostic Studies

The cardiac catheterization results should be reviewed as well as the electrophysiological studies done by the cardiologist, which may indicate the area of accessory pathways.

Procedure

Incision and Exposure

Refer to the discussion of cardiopulmonary bypass.

Details

After bypass is established, the heart is kept warm and electrodes are sutured onto the heart at various locales. The recordings of the readings of these electrodes provide a picture of the timing of electrical events in the heart. A hand-held probe is used to locate pathways and identify the earliest ventricular activity. Electrical stimulation is used to induce arrythmia to assist in identifying the origin. Atrial mapping may also be done to demonstrate any retrograde conduction.

In Wolff-Parkinson-White syndrome ablation, the pathway is destroyed by isolating the atrium from the ventricle at the determined areas of the bypass tract. This is done by dissection and may also be done with cryoablation at −60°C. In other endocardial resections, the area of identified preexcitation is dissected and/or cryoablated, and the area of incision is closed with Prolene suture.

Closure

Before bypass is terminated, the mapping procedure is repeated. If no bypass tract is identified, closure is continued in the routine manner.

Postoperative Care

Postoperative care is similar to that for other patients after cardiopulmonary bypass. Strict attention, however, must be paid to ECG abnormalities and to bleeding immediately postoperatively, as the nature of the resection potentiates the possibility of bleeding problems.

The patient is usually transferred to the cardiology service before discharge from the hospital for predischarge electrophysiological studies. Some hospitals doing this procedure have a team of electrophysiologists (cardiologists) who specialize in this clinical area.

Potential Surgical Complications

Intraoperative and postoperative hemorrhage
Myocardial infarction
Stroke
Infection
Pulmonary complications
Return of arrhythmias

SURGICAL PROCEDURES NOT NECESSITATING EXTRACORPOREAL CIRCULATION

Pacemaker Insertion

Definition

Pacemaker insertion involves the implantation of cardiac pacing leads and a generator for the purpose of providing the heart with external electrical stimulation.

Indications

Pacemakers are indicated for the treatment of patients with heart block and conduction disorders (Kowey et al., 1985). This includes patients with sick sinus syndrome, in which there is sinoatrial node dysfunction, and patients who experience second-degree atrioventricular block or complete heart block after myocardial infarction.

A person with a heart rate less than 40 beats/minute usually becomes symptomatic and is at risk for sudden death (Moses et al., 1987). Therefore, chronic or episodic inadequate cardiac output secondary to bradycardia is also an indication for pacemaker insertion. Diagnosis is confirmed with ECG or ambulatory 24-hour ECG monitoring.

Related Surgical Procedures

Pacemaker surgery is often scheduled according to the type of pacemaker to be used. Pacemakers are classified into universally accepted categories. In this three-letter system, the first letter refers to the chamber paced, the second to the chamber sensed, and the third to the method of activation. The following letter codes are used:

A—atrium
V—ventricle
D—dual
O—synchronous
T—triggered
I—inhibited

Two of the most common types of pacemakers used are the VVI and DDD. As demonstrated by the letter codes, the VVI pacemaker senses and paces the ventricle and operates in an inhibition manner. In other words, if the pacemaker senses the ventricle firing, it inhibits its own stimulation. The DDD pacemaker senses and paces both the atrium and the ventricle and can operate in both modes, inhibition and triggered.

Perioperative Nursing Implications

Anesthesia

Local anesthesia with some intravenous sedation (usually fentanyl) is the choice for pacemaker insertion. The usual anesthetic is lidocaine 1%. If present, the anesthetist may operate the pacemaker analyzer. In the absence of a qualified anesthesia provider, the cardiologist operates the pacemaker analyzer. Venous access and ECG monitoring are established on the patient's entry to the OR. Supplemental oxygen is provided.

Position

The patient is in the supine position with the right arm extended for better exposure of the subclavian vein area. Any areas of pressure should be padded and the patient's head may be elevated and oxygen administered if necessary.

Creation and Maintenance of the Sterile Field

The right lower neck and chest are prepared to the midline down to the nipple and laterally to the shoulder with iodophor solution and draped. The electrocautery unit is placed close to the field and the suction tubing is attached to the suction canister. The electrosurgical

dispersive pad should be placed on the patient's right buttock or thigh.

After draping is performed, pacing cables are passed to the anesthetist or cardiologist and the electrocautery cord and suction apparatus are passed off the field in a manner so as not to cross the field and impede the use of fluoroscopy. A small table is placed to the patient's right (no Mayo stand is needed) so that the fluoroscopy C-arm can enter the field from the left.

Equipment and Supplies

Suture needed for pacemaker insertion is minimal. Silk or polyester ties (1–0 and 3–0), 3–0 silk or polyester (Dacron) suture on a taper needle for tacking down the leads, and absorbable suture for a two-layer closure are the only suture needed. A skin (No. 10) blade for the skin incision and a No. 11 blade for incising the vein are used. Small gauze sponges and dressings are needed. A minor dissection instrument set is used with the addition of vascular scissors and forceps and pacing cables for connection to the pacemaker analyzer. Finally, the pacing leads and generator chosen by the surgeon should be available in the OR (Fig. 22–8). Additionally, a fluoroscopy C-arm is used with the appropriate OR bed.

The scrub nurse and other members of the surgical team should don lead aprons before scrubbing and gowning. Local syringes and needles are needed for the anesthetic. The scrub nurse also covers the C-arm with a clear sterile cover before its use.

Drug and Solutions

Lidocaine 1%
Warm normal saline
Antibiotic irrigation

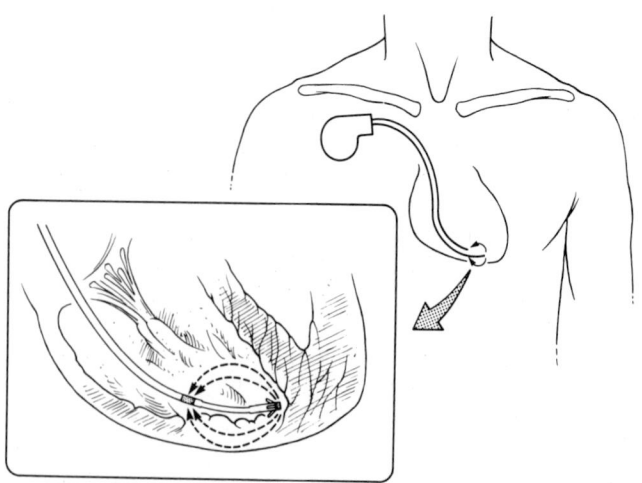

FIGURE 22–8. Placement of pacemaker generator and lead. Inset shows the flow of electrons during the pacemaker spike from distal to the electrode, through the endocardium, to the proximal electrode. (From Moses, H. W., Taylor, G. J., Schneider, J. A., Dove, J. T. [1987]. *A practical guide to cardiac pacing* (2nd ed.). Boston: Little, Brown.)

Physiological Monitoring

Cardiac monitoring is crucial during pacemaker insertion. In the absence of an anesthesia provider, the perioperative nurse must have the skill necessary to interpret normal and abnormal ECG readings during the procedure. Blood pressure monitoring as well as pulse oximetry is essential.

Specimens and Culture

Specimens and cultures are rare.

Physician's Orders

Typical preoperative orders include complete blood count with determination of electrolyte values and bleeding times, chest x-ray film, preoperative shower with an antimicrobial soap and depilatory, ECG, and NPO status after midnight.

Laboratory and Diagnostic Studies

Any electrolyte disturbances should be corrected before surgery. The chest x-ray film should demonstrate a clear chest.

Procedure

Incision and Exposure

An incision is made obliquely into the deltopectoral groove. With the registered nurse first assistant providing traction with small retractors, the surgeon dissects until the cephalic vein is exposed. The cephalic vein is ligated distally and a 1–0 tie is passed around the vein for control. The vein is opened and probed for patency. An opening of 3 mm is necessary for the lead to pass.

Details

The pacing lead, with stylet, is passed into the cephalic vein and advanced under fluoroscopy to the right atrium, through the tricuspid valve, and into the right ventricle. Some leads are made with a coil spring, which is embedded into the myocardium. Others are lined with soft barbs at the electrode end.

The implanted lead is then connected to the pacing cable to be analyzed for its thresholds for sensing electrical activity and for pacing. The pacing threshold is the smallest amount of delivered voltage that causes depolarization. For the ventricular lead, the optimal pacing threshold is 0.3 v (Moses et al., 1987).

If used, the atrial lead is placed next. It is placed through the subclavian vein as described above and tested in the same manner.

Both leads are either secured with the provided small plastic sleeves to the vein and fascia or anchored simply with nonabsorbable suture. After the leads are secured, the patient is asked to breathe deeply and cough while the lead positions are examined under fluoroscopy for possible dislodgment.

The generator pocket is then made by separating the pectoral muscle fascia from the overlying subcutaneous tissue. Because blood is conductive, the leads are cleaned of blood with a moist sponge and connected to the selected generator. The generator most commonly used has a lithium battery. This battery has a life expectancy of 5 to 10 years, depending on the frequency of discharge. The generator is placed into the pocket and the area is irrigated with antibiotic solution.

Closure

After the ECG is verified, the fascia and skin layers are closed with absorbable suture.

Postoperative Care

Patients receiving intravenous sedation are transported to the postanesthesia care unit for monitoring. A postoperative chest x-ray film is taken to confirm the position of the pacemaker. The patient is given prophylactic antibiotics for 24 hours and pain medication as needed. Ambulation and a full diet may be resumed when the patient is fully recovered from intravenous sedation. The patient may be discharged the day after surgery if there are no complications. Follow-up care should be confirmed with the cardiologist.

Potential Surgical Complications

Bleeding
Infection
Arrythmia
Lead migration
Cardiac tamponade
Lead-generator disconnection or malfunction
Electrode fracture
Generator failure

Automatic Implantable Cardioverter/Defibrillator Insertion

Definition

The automatic implantable cardioverter/defibrillator (AICD) consists of leads placed on or near the heart and a generator power source (Fig. 22–9). This device provides constant protection for the tachyrhythmic patient as a result of its ability to detect and correct arrhythmias (Flores and Hilderbrant, 1984) by delivering a 28-J defibrillating electrical shock to the heart.

Indications

The AICD is indicated for survivors of sudden cardiac death not associated with a myocardial infarction and patients whose inducible arrhythmias are not controlla-

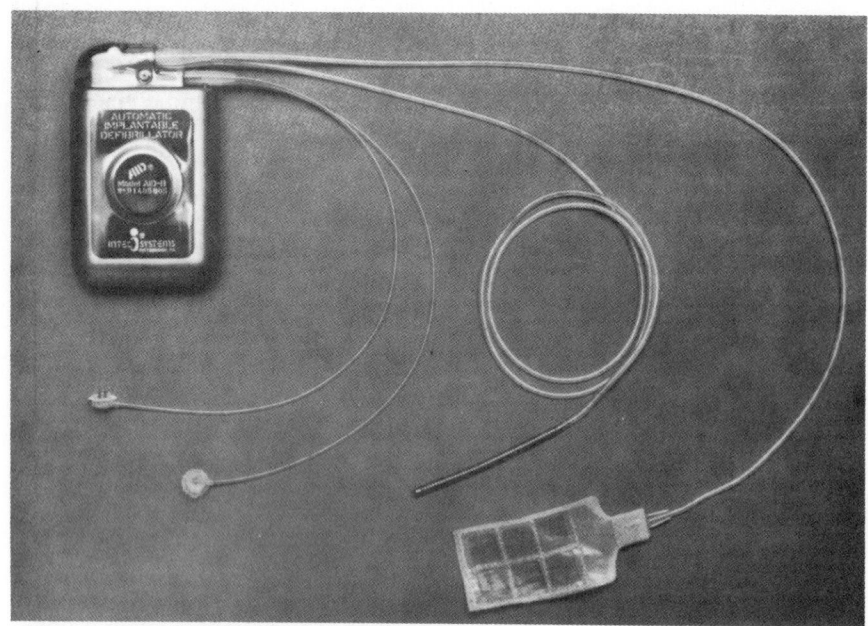

FIGURE 22–9. AICD generator and leads. (From Echt, D. S., Winkle, R. A. [1985]. Management of patient with the automatic implantable cardioverter/defibrillator. *Clinical Progress, 3,* 6.)

ble by drugs (Cannom and Winkle, 1986). It is recommended in place of ablation or resection surgery in patients with ejection fractions less than 40% or patients with infrequent ventricular tachycardia.

The system includes a titanium-encased generator, consisting of a sensing device, batteries, and energy storage capacitors weighing 292 g, and several types of leads. The optional spring lead is placed in the superior vena cava. One or two patch leads are used, which are sutured to the epicardium and consist of a titanium mesh surface, which measures a maximum of 20 cm². Two unipolar epicardial screw-in leads provide a bipolar signal for rate counting by the device. The generator provides up to 4 shocks during an episode of arrythmia and is capable of 100 to 150 shocks in its lifetime. The specific generator is chosen according to the patient's maximal heart rate and required energy level (Winkle et al., 1984).

Perioperative Nursing Implications

Anesthesia

General anesthesia is chosen for all cases of AICD insertion. Monitoring is determined by the patient's condition and may include a central venous pressure catheter and Swan-Ganz catheter. An arterial catheter is always inserted. ECG leads are placed outside the operative field. If arrhythmias occur during induction, they are not treated with drugs, which would cause difficulty in inducing arrhythmias during surgery.

Position

Because this procedure can be done from a number of approaches, there are different positioning possibilities. If a midline incision and sternotomy are to be performed, the patient is supine with a rolled sheet beneath the shoulders and with the arms tucked at the sides with toboggans. Only plastic toboggans should be used if a spring lead will be inserted, as fluoroscopy will be used. If a thoracotomy approach is used, the patient will be positioned laterally, and sandbags, pillows, and a double arm board will be used as positional aids. If an anterior thoracotomy or subcostal approach is used, the patient is slightly lateral with a rolled sheet placed longitudinally behind the patient's left side.

Creation and Maintenance of the Sterile Field

With the patient in the supine position, the chest and groin areas are prepared and draped, excluding the genitalia and pubic area. For thoracotomy, the lateral chest is prepared to the midline in front and back. Iodophor solution is used in both instances. The operative area should be hairless.

After draping is performed, tables are moved to the field and the scrub nurse is positioned at the patient's right. The Mayo stand is placed over the patient's legs. Defibrillator cables should be passed off the field and connected to the defibrillator to be ready. If external paddles are to be used, the scrub nurse should keep moist gauze sponges over the area of contact. If a fluoroscopy C-arm is used, the scrub nurse drapes it in a sterile fashion with a plastic sheet.

Equipment and Supplies

Silk and Prolene suture of varying sizes and several needle types are used, as well as sternal wires for sternotomy and heavy polyester suture for thoracotomy. Absorbable suture is used for the three-layer closure. Routine No. 10 and 11 blades and large and small sponges are needed. Chest tubes are routinely inserted.

Also needed are sterile internal and/or external paddles, the multiple cables to connect the recorder and the generator, and monitoring leads with adaptor pins. The AICD check probe and subclavian puncture set are needed. The defibrillator is placed near the field. The cardiologist uses a multichannel physiological recorder as well as a pacing analyzer to study arrhythmias and their response.

If a sternotomy is performed, a major vascular instrument set is needed with the additional chest retractor. If a thoracotomy or subcostal incision is made, an instrument set appropriate for lung resection is needed.

Drugs and Solutions

Warm normal saline
Antibiotic irrigation

Specimens and Cultures

Specimens and cultures are rare.

Physician's Orders

If preadmission electrophysiological studies have been performed, the patient may be admitted 1 day before surgery. Pulmonary function testing should be done on the day of admission to confirm lung status. Blood testing ordered should include a complete blood count with electrolyte and bleeding time determinations. A chest x-ray film should be ordered, along with a 12-lead ECG. The patient should be ordered NPO after midnight and a preoperative shower with antimicrobial soap should be taken.

Laboratory and Diagnostic Studies

Results of all ordered tests should be reviewed before surgery. A treadmill stress test is routinely done before admission and the result should be reviewed, as this is an assessment of maximal heart rate, which is used to make generator choice.

Procedure

Incision and Exposure

If a spring lead is to be used, a small skin incision is made under the left clavicle and the subclavian vein is entered with a standard needle. A guide wire is positioned in the right atrium under fluoroscopy and a sheath is placed over the wire. The lead is then passed through the sheath and secured with the supplied lead and anchor.

If a thoracotomy is to be done, the patient is then repositioned and a standard thoracotomy is performed through the fifth or sixth intercostal space. Blunt dissection is used to free the cardiac apex.

If a sternotomy is performed, it is done as described for cardiopulmonary bypass, up to the point of place-

ment of pericardial stay sutures (Cannom and Winkle, 1986).

Details

The large patch lead is sewn over the left ventricle with six or eight sutures of silk or Prolene. A second large or small patch may be placed posteriorly. Epicardial leads are placed within 2 cm of each other also on the left ventricle. A pocket is then formed from a horizontal skin incision in the left abdominal wall below the level of the umbilicus. The leads are tunneled down to this area using a straight chest tube. The leads are connected to sterile cables passed to the recording machine, which analyzes the quality of the sensed ECG. Defibrillation thresholds are then determined after inducing ventricular fibrillation and tachycardia. This threshold should be at least 10 J less than the maximal energy of the selected generator (Cannom and Winkle, 1986).

Before the generator is passed to the field, it is checked and deactivated by the cardiologist. When passed to the field, it is reactivated using the magnet, then again inactivated by placing the magnet over it for 30 seconds. The generator then emits a continuous tone. The magnet is held over the generator while the arrhythmia is induced. When the magnet is removed, the generator activates and senses the arrhythmia. By keeping the AICD check probe on the generator during this time, the cardiologist can determine the time for the generator to charge after sensing the arrhythmia. The generator is inactivated before closure.

Closure

The generator pocket is irrigated with antibiotic solution and closed with absorbable suture in two layers. The chest is closed after the insertion of chest tubes appropriate to the manner of surgery. A sternotomy is closed with No. 6 sternal wire and absorbable suture of the muscle, fascia, and skin layers. A thoracotomy incision is closed with heavy paracostal stitches of polyester, then in three layers with absorbable suture.

Postoperative Care

The patient should be transferred to an intensive care unit bed directly from the OR and then to a telemetry unit. The AICD is kept inactive in the early postoperative period and antiarrhythmic drugs withheld, except during acute arrhythmias. When the patient's hemodynamic status is stable and he or she is ambulatory, the administration of antiarrhythmic drugs is begun by the cardiologist and the AICD is activated. A Holter monitor is recommended during the first 24 hours of AICD activation to determine any missed arrhythmias. Before AICD activation, the patient may undergo external cardioversion without damaging the device. Prophylactic antibiotics and pulmonary care are ordered. Chest tubes are removed as soon as drainage is minimal, at about the second postoperative day, and surgical dressings are changed. Before the patient is discharged on the fifth to seventh day, final electrophysiological testing is done.

Potential Surgical Complications

Lead migration
False positive shocks
Lead fracture
Infection
Generator failure

Bibliography

Atkinson, L. J., Kohn, M. L. (1986). *Berry & Kohn's introduction to operating room technique* (p. 570). New York: McGraw-Hill.

Boncheck, L. I. (1985). The basis for selecting a valve prosthesis. In K. M. McCauley, A. N. Brest, D. C. McGoon (Eds.), *McGoon's cardiac surgery: An interprofessional approach to patient care* (pp. 103–116). Philadelphia: F. A. Davis.

Cannom, D. S., Winkle, R. A. (1986). Implantation of the automatic implantable cardioverter defibrillator: Practical aspects. *PACE, 9,* 793–809.

Flores, B. T., Hildebrandt, M. (1984). The automatic implantable defibrillator. *Heart and Lung, 13,* 608–613.

Gordon, M. (1987). *Manual of nursing diagnosis: 1986–1987.* New York: McGraw-Hill.

Kirklin, J. W., Barratt-Boyes, B. G. (1986). *Cardiac surgery: Morphology, diagnostic criteria, natural history, techniques, results, and indications.* New York: John Wiley.

Kowey, P. R., Mullan, D. F., Wetstin, L. (1985). Pacemaker therapy. *Surgical Clinics of North America, 65.* 592–612.

Lazar, H. L., Roberts, A. J. (1985). Recent advances in cardiopulmonary bypass and the clinical application of myocardial protection. *Surgical Clinics of North America, 65,* 455–476.

Luciano, D., Vander, A., Sherman, J. (1978). *Human function and structure.* New York: McGraw-Hill.

Lytle, B. W., Loop, F. D. (1985). Elective coronary surgery. In K. M. McCauley, A. N. Brest, D. C. McGoon (Eds.), *McGoon's cardiac surgery: An interprofessional approach to patient care* (pp. 31–48). Philadelphia: F. A. Davis.

McGoon, D. C. (1985). From whence? In K. M. McCauley, A. N. Brest, D. C. McGoon (Eds.), *McGoon's cardiac surgery: An interprofessional approach to patient care* (pp. 1–8). Philadelphia: F. A. Davis.

Mark, D. B., Califf, R. M., Stack, R. S., Phillips, H. R. (1991). Cardiac catheterization. In D. C. Sabiston (Ed.), *Textbook of surgery: The biological basis of modern surgical practice* (14th ed.) (pp. 2135–2164). Philadelphia: W. B. Saunders.

Moses, H. W., Taylor, G. J., Schneider, J. A., Dove, J. T. (1987). *A practical guide to cardiac pacing* (2nd ed.). Boston: Little, Brown.

Smith, P. K., Holman, W. L., Cox, J. L. (1985). Surgical treatment of supraventricular tachyarrythmias. *Surgical Clinics of North America, 65,* 553–570.

Wetstein, L., Landymore, R. W., Herre, J. M. (1985). Current status of surgery for ventricular tachyarrythmias. *Surgical Clinics of North America, 65,* 571–594.

Winkle, R. A., Stinson, E. B., Echct, D. S., et al. (1984). Practical aspects of automatic cardioverter/defibrillator implantation. *American Heart Journal, 108,* 1335–1346.

CHAPTER 23

Transplantation Surgery

Susan A. Garruto

DEFINITION

Transplantation surgery is the art of explanting an organ or tissue from the body and implanting it into the body of the same or a different individual.

HISTORY

Transplant surgery is recorded in the literature as early as Homer's *Iliad*. In this work, he describes the monstrous Chimaera, which was a remarkable creature created by the gods consisting of the body of a goat, the head of a lion, a serpent at the rear, and a goat's head rising from its back. The word *chimera* is used to describe individuals who have hybrid characteristics such as the circulating cells of both donor and recipient after bone marrow transplantation.

The earliest evidence of grafting was found in the trephine holes of a Bronze Age skull. A large defect was evidently filled by reimplanting the removed fragment.

491

Ancient Hindu surgeons developed techniques of grafting to repair defects of the nose and ears. In the *Sushruta Samhita*, a document written about 700 BC, a technique for nasal reconstruction is recorded.

John Hunter, a Scottish surgeon, is rightfully known as the father of experimental surgery. He pioneered several procedures involving transplantation. One of his most famous autografts was performed by transplanting a cock's claw into its comb. The claw survived the autografting and continued to grow. In a xenograft experiment, Hunter transplanted a tooth into the comb of a cock. These techniques left him unable to distinguish allografting from autografting on the basis of graft survival.

TYPES OF TISSUE AND ORGAN TRANSPLANTATION

Although the terminology for organ transplantation was first communicated by Alexis Carrel in 1905, the preferred nomenclature has changed a bit. An *autograft* is an organ or tissue that is transplanted from one part of the body to another part of the body in the same individual. Vein grafts are among the most commonly employed autografts. *Isograft,* also known as isogeneic graft, is a tissue or organ graft between individuals of the same species who are genetically identical. An *allograft,* formerly called a homograft, denotes a transplant between nonidentical members of the same species. A *xenograft* (in the past called a heterograft) is a transplant done between members of different species. These are usually tissue grafts such as pigskin. Depending on the site of implantation, grafts are termed orthotopic or heterotopic. *Orthotopic* grafts are surrounded by the same tissues and located in the same part of the body after transplantation (e.g., liver transplant). *Heterotopic* grafts are sometimes implanted into privileged sites (e.g., kidney transplant).

Frequent failures with allografts and xenografts raised questions as to the incompatibilities of species and individuals. The entire focus of transplantation of body parts or whole organs began to shift from technical to biological investigation in the latter part of the 19th century.

PROBLEMS WITH REJECTION

It was not until the 20th century that rejection was acknowledged as a major biological phenomenon and accepted as the rule rather than the exception. Today, rejection remains by far the major cause of transplant failure, regardless of the tissue or organ grafted. Human leukocyte antigen (HLA) matching, antilymphocytic serum use, and thoracic duct drainage have all proved to be positive steps in an attempt to resolve the rejection problem. The use of cyclosporine has given great optimism to those in the field of transplantation but its

benefits have been limited owing to its undesirable side effects.

The nature of the host immune responsiveness to foreign antigens is complex. Optimal donor-recipient matching for the HLA haplotype has a great impact on reducing graft rejection. This is especially apparent in living related donors for kidney, pancreas, and bone marrow transplantation. Because of the large volume of cadaver transplants performed, the range of the matches resulting from extensive donor organ sharing has caused controversy regarding the benefit of HLA matching in cadaver transplants.

Many other clinical, host, and donor variables can affect the reaction to allografts. Studies have shown that patients with better matched grafts have retained a higher percentage of transplants with less immunosuppression (Terasaki, 1989). It was believed that cyclosporine immunotherapy could overcome poor matching; however, it is now established that the beneficial effects of good matching are pronounced regardless of cyclosporine therapy (Terasaki, 1989). The use of cyclosporine has altered kidney transplantation. Poorly matched local donors can undergo transplantation and be maintained on a regimen of cyclosporine, bypassing the need to share organs with another institution and possibly a better matched patient.

The importance of HLA matching for other organ transplants is unclear. Owing to the urgent nature of these transplants (heart, liver, lung) in the absence of an alternative means of therapy (such as dialysis), HLA matching seems less practical. Stronger immunosuppression is usually used, thereby making the influence of HLA matching hard to assess. For cadaver donor transplantation, the time and expense involved in testing donor-recipient compatibility are technically impractical because these organs have relatively short preservation periods. Standard practice includes the use of ABO-compatible and cross-match–negative donors for all solid organ transplants (vascularized). In some cases of heart and liver, the cross-match is considered optional.

After a patient undergoes transplantation, he or she becomes sensitized from the cadaver organ. If the graft is rejected, this broad sensitization can increase the risk of rejection of future transplants. The exact mechanism (whether cellular and/or humoral alloantigens) is not clear.

The paramount indicator of all types of graft rejection is inflammation. The intensity, pattern, and type of inflammation mark the clinical and pathological changes as well as the proper classification of rejection. The time after transplantation and the speed of development are often useful indicators of the type of rejection process involved. Rejection is commonly classified in three ways: hyperacute, acute, and chronic. The terminology can be misleading because the terms chronic and/or acute not only may suggest the speed of onset or the time after transplantation but also can imply the nature of the inflammatory reaction.

Hyperacute rejection usually occurs within hours or days of transplantation. The presumptive mechanism is humoral presensitization, because there is a high correlation with the presence of preformed cytotoxic antibodies to the blood group or HLA antigens of the donors. It is an irreversible process that rapidly leads to organ death.

Acute rejection usually occurs within days or months after transplantation and is of rapid onset. Early signs and symptoms include fever, graft tenderness, and swelling. There are subtypes of acute rejection to separate cellular from humoral immune mechanisms or to differentiate interstitial from vascular damage. The common histological pattern seen is thought to be a combination of antibody and cellular reactions leading to the destruction of epithelial structures of the organ.

Chronic rejection is usually seen several months or years after transplantation. Its pattern is similar to that of cellular rejection; however, it is a vascular form of antibody-mediated rejection resulting in subintimal foam cell deposition in the arteries. Eventually, scarring and ischemic changes are present. The late onset of chronic rejection could be due to adequate immunosuppression, because the reaction is against weaker histocompatibility disparities.

Rejection is usually diagnosed via a biopsy so that the therapy can be prescribed accordingly. For patients receiving cyclosporine, the biopsy can help differentiate between toxicity and rejection, which is important in determining whether the dose of drug should be decreased or increased. There are many other reasons for performing biopsies of the allografts, all intricately related to defining the antibodies and characterizing the rejection as to extent and type.

Immunotherapy is used to reduce donor-specific alloreactivity, while still preserving the remaining functions of the immune system, which protect the host from infection. Although immunosuppressive therapy often provides long-term graft survival, owing to the global effect of the drugs, the patients are still exposed to a high risk of infection. These infections are often life threatening, as are the complications and side effects of the drugs used. Cyclosporine is known to be nephrotoxic. Two histopathological changes attributed to cyclosporine are perimyocyte fibrosis (referred to as the cyclosporine effect) and interstitial mononuclear infiltrates, which are diffuse in specimens not otherwise diagnostic of rejection. Much work is being done toward being able to predict accurately impending rejection. Because the expression of rejection can vary (cellular versus humoral) and not all rejection is manifested systemically, many challenges still exist for researchers.

GRAFT PRESERVATION AND STORAGE AND ARTIFICIAL LIFE SUPPORT SYSTEMS

Simple Cooling

Simple cooling through induction of hypothermia retains tissue viability in the absence of circulation 10 times longer than at normal body temperature. Simple cooling, also referred to as cold storage, has demon-

strated that kidneys can safely be preserved for 30 hours. Collins solution or the modified Euro-Collins solution is the primary flush-out solution used for renal allograft cold storage. The solution's composition "1. minimizes hypothermic induced cell swelling, 2. prevents intracellular acidosis, 3. prevents the expansion of the interstitial space during the flush-out period, 4. prevents injury from oxygen free radicals (especially during reperfusion), and 5. provides substrates for regenerating high-energy phosphate compounds during reperfusion." (Belzer and Southard, 1988). Collins solution contains a high concentration of glucose (130 mmol/L), which is impermeable to the cell; this reduces the tendency for the cell to swell. Intracellular acidosis is also an important consideration in cold storage. The ischemia, even though cold, stimulates glycolysis and glycogenolysis and increases the production of lactic acid and hydrogen ions. Adding a buffer causes an alkaline pH and improves the storage, especially for livers and pancreas.

To be effective, the flush-out solution should contain substances that create colloidal osmotic pressure, which allows free exchange of the constituents in the solution but does not expand the interstitial space.

Oxygen consumption should be preserved, especially in lung and intestine transplants. Oxygen-free radicals caused by the high endogenous activity of superoxide dismutase can cause injury.

The last property that needs consideration is energy metabolism. Organ reperfusion necessitates the rapid regeneration of the sodium pump. Adenosine triphosphate degrades into adenosine, inosine, and hypoxanthine to which the plasma is freely permeable. These precursors are important for successful organ preservation.

Simple cooling is achieved by flushing the allograft with cold isosmolar or hyperosmolar (buffered) solution and then storing at 0 to 4°C. This simple method has been particularly useful in preserving skin, cornea, kidney, liver, pancreas, heart, and lung. All these organs have different metabolisms; these differences influence how well they are preserved and for how long they can be preserved.

The liver has a greater capability to metabolize glucose than does the kidney; therefore, glucose is not an effective agent to prevent cell swelling, and glucose could stimulate acidosis in the liver.

On the basis of this consideration, Belzer and Southard have designed a cold-storage solution that provides consistent 76-hour preservation for the pancreas, 72-hour storage for the kidney, and 30-hour or longer preservation of the liver (Belzer and Southard, 1988). Conceptually, there are important differences between this solution and the one developed by Collins. Glucose was replaced by an impermeant anion (lactobionate), with a molecular mass of 358 daltons, to prevent cell swelling. Raffinose, a trisaccharide of 594 daltons, was added to further suppress cell swelling. Hydroxyethyl starch, which is a stable nontoxic colloid, was added to prevent the expansion of extracellular space. Many other components can be added or deleted from the solution, depending on the organs to be preserved. However, this universal cold storage solution appears to be equally effective for initial cooling during in situ flushing of donor organs and for their subsequent cold storage.

Freezing

The technique of freezing is most widely used for bone, cartilage, heart valves, and saphenous vein. Freezing produces anaerobic hypothermic ischemia. Ultralow-temperature freezing is theoretically the only means of obtaining truly long-term preservation (i.e., from months to years). The problem that is inherent to freezing is the thawing process. Currently, no available technique prevents the formation of ice cystals and retains the viability of the organ.

Bone is harvested under sterile conditions, wrapped in plastic and cloth, and frozen to $-80°C$. At present, there is not a definite expiration date placed on frozen bone. Freeze-drying bone takes the frozen bone and sublimates it in a vacuum until residual moisture is reduced to 5% or less. This bone can then be stored indefinitely in a vacuum at room temperature.

Heart valves are harvested using sterile technique and placed in an antibiotic treatment medium. After the antibiotic treatment stage, the tissue is packaged, and the low-temperature preservation protocol is started and finally is completed after the tissue reaches $-196°C$ in liquid nitrogen. The tissue valves are frozen in liquid nitrogen and flown to their destination. The thawing procedure takes 14 minutes in a bath of $42°C$; maximal tissue viability is maintained at this precise time.

Chemical Inhibition of Metabolism

Chemical inhibition of metabolism in cardioplegia solution is used for cardiac transplantation and many other open heart procedures. A motionless and bloodless field is necessary to perform open heart surgery. Several processes are incorporated in maintaining myocardial hypothermia at $10°C$: myocardial precooling, systemic hypothermia, rapid administration of cold potassium cardioplegia solution, and careful attention to topical hypothermia.

Systemic hypothermia is induced via the perfusate solution, which is passed through the aortic and venous bypass circulation. Hypothermia is initiated by taking $24°C$ perfusate and reducing the pump inflow temperature to a minimum of $16°C$ until the measured myocardial temperature falls below $20°C$. At this point, the aorta is cross-clamped and $4°C$ cardioplegia solution is infused into the aortic root. The aim of cardioplegia solution is to produce rapid cardiac arrest and reduce the energy demands on the heart to a low level, while preserving the myocardium. The instillation of the $4°C$ cardioplegia solution produces a quick chemical arrest and an immediate reduction in myocardial temperature to $8°C$. Prolonged chemical arrest is maintained by the combination of potassium and magnesium in the cardioplegia solution, combined with hypothermia. Pericardial

lavage is begun before cardiac arrest by dumping cold slush of Ringer irrigation or saline around the heart.

Maximal reduction in myocardial metabolism is maintained throughout the ischemic period, through the use of topical cold and periodic reinfusion of cardioplegia solution.

Tissue Culture

Tissue cultures of autologous components of skin can now be grown. Donor skin cells are taken and those without antigenetic determinants can be isolated and grown into sheets in vitro. Scientists have also been able to mix in melanocytes for dark-skinned patients. These sheets can then be transferred and grown on second- and third-degree burns. The long-term results of these grafts are not satisfying, however, because the graft is thinner and lacks a normal dermis. Traumatic fissures and scar tissue are the most common complications.

Pancreatic islet transplantation is a growing field. It is believed that prompt reversal of hyperglycemia could be observed after islet transplantation in patients with diabetes. The major limitations to clinical human pancreatic islet transplantation are the lack of availability of adequate quantities of donor islets and the difficulty in preventing islet graft rejection.

Islet culture experiments of Anderson, Hellerstrom, and Lazaraw have documented the survival of cultured islets and the separation of islets from exocrine cells (Reemtsma and Weber, 1981). Expansion of donor islet cell population has been done in vitro in tissue culture. Cultures are also useful in assessing the islet function before transplantation.

Cryopreservation of islets was developed by Kemp and Rajotte, and it allows survival of long-term frozen-thawed islets (Reemtsma and Weber, 1981). Ideally, a method combining cryopreservation storage and islet culture will be perfected in the future.

Organ Perfusion

There has been a resurgence of interest in perfusion preservation of kidneys. Continuous perfusion supplies the organ with oxygen and nutrients and removes the end products of metabolism. The method utilizes a machine that delivers a perfusate (e.g., Belzer solution) at low flow and low pressure while maintaining hypothermic conditions of the perfusate and organ temperature of 6 to $10°C$. The kidney has been satisfactorily preserved for up to 72 hours.

The advantages of continuous perfusion are extending preservation time, allowing the surgeon to perform the transplant on an elective rather than an emergency basis, providing a way to perfuse and preserve an organ that has been exposed to warm ischemia, supporting metabolism by regulating various processes and products and by adding potentially beneficial agents to the organ, and eliminating vasospasm, to name a few. Overall, the extended preservation time is not useful in obtaining a better match for the organ.

Some disadvantages of pulsatile perfusion include the expense of preservation equipment and the personnel necessary to run it, the possibility of technical failure of the pump, the possible removal of necessary cell constituents, and the possible physical disruption of the vascular architecture of the kidney.

At present, Miami, Minnesota, Ohio, and Wisconsin Universities are using pulsatile perfusion. The overall belief is that it reduces the acute tubular necrosis rate.

Artificial Vital Organs

The artificial kidney, commonly referred to as dialysis, was developed by William Kolff about the time of World War II. George Thorn and Carl Walter working from 1947 to 1950 (and with Benjamin Miller and John Merrill later) made dialysis (peritoneal) part of standard therapy for renal failure in the United States. The longer patient survival provided by dialysis allowed physicians time to prepare patients for renal transplantation.

Dialysis plays a central role in preparing patients with end-stage renal disease for renal transplantation. The goals of dialysis are to alleviate the metabolic and hemodynamic consequences of uremia. At present, two methods of dialysis exist. Peritoneal dialysis uses the peritoneal membrane to exchange fluid and electrolytes. Hemodialysis separates the blood and fluid using a cellophane-like membrane that allows ultrafiltration and clearance. Dialysis regimens can be made specific to each patient. Knowledge of the risks and benefits as well as the patient's experience are necessary for determining whether to use hemodialysis or peritoneal dialysis.

The End-Stage Renal Disease program, supported by funding of the United States government since 1973, has allowed any medically suitable patient to be considered for hemodialysis or peritoneal dialysis (Garovoy and Guttmann, 1986). Equipment and medical personnel in dialysis centers as well as home treatment are now widely available throughout the United States.

The only diseases that preclude a patient from being accepted for long-term dialysis are advanced metastatic carcinoma, severe cerebrovascular disease, and hepatorenal syndrome. It is best to evaluate and prepare patients before their actual need for dialysis or transplantation. Experience shows that treatment should begin with the first signs of renal insufficiency, and transplantation and/or dialysis should be initiated at the earliest sign of uremia.

Because the organ donor is such a rare resource, between 20 and 40% of the patients listed for a heart transplant die each year before a suitable donor can be found. As the safety and effectiveness of cardiac transplantation has been demonstrated, more and more centers are claiming an interest in performing this operation. This has led to the identification of a larger recipient population in a severely limited donor field. Even if a potential donor is identified, organs often cannot be used for a number of reasons. Thus, there is a need for interim treatment for the cardiac transplant candidate waiting for the proper donor.

Currently, there are multiple centers throughout the world where new engineering and design ideas for artificial hearts and assist devices are being implemented for circulatory support. In use are the intraaortic counterpulsation balloon pump, ventricular assist devices, and the partial or total artificial heart.

The intraaortic counterpulsation balloon pump has limited application. It is best used to support a failing left ventricle after cardiopulmonary bypass. Some other indications include cardiogenic shock and unstable angina. This device is not useful in stabilizing patients with other types of cardiac disease.

Ventricular assist devices are designed to take the oxygenated blood from the left atrium or ventricle and return it under pressure to the aorta. However, the minimally pulsatile or nonpulsatile characteristics fail to duplicate the physiology of the normal circulation. There are many disadvantages and factors limiting the use of ventricular assist devices; an alternative for inflow is a left ventricular apex cannula. Patients awaiting transplant usually have dilated myopathy, and apex cannulation is suitable. Thrombus and infection present the greatest continuous risk during the implantation period. The exact length of time an assist device can remain implanted has yet to be defined.

Total artificial hearts are attached to the atrial and vascular cuffs after excision of the native ventricles. The action is complete replacement of ventricular function. The pumps are implanted and connected to their power source by transthoracic pneumatic drive lines. Improvements and refinements have been made in the pneumatic pumps. The total artificial heart takes over the entire circulation. It has no limitation to the ability to eject blood during systole, and through improvements in design and drive adjustments, the inefficiency of diastolic filling will be overcome. Initiating circulatory support should follow strict criteria as does listing patients for transplantation. Most of the patients undergoing interim mechanical support have idiopathic or ischemic cardiomyopathy manifested through severe end-stage left ventricular failure often associated with high ventricular failure. Many patients do well with the total artificial heart and actually recover from the end-stage damage from heart failure, are weaned from the ventilator, and even begin ambulation and oral nutrition before heart transplantation.

There are many disadvantages of the total artificial heart. It is large and often does not fit in the mediastinum; obstruction of return (systemic or pulmonary venous) can occur if there is insufficient room. The risk of embolism, particularly stroke, has been the greatest complication. The use of anticoagulants has led to worsened bleeding complications. Other major disadvantages include infection and total dependence on the artificial heart.

SPECIAL INSTRUMENTS, SUPPLIES, AND EQUIPMENT

In most cases in which other organs are harvested from cadavers, the kidneys are also recovered. Procedures, equipment, and supplies vary according to recovery teams. The instruments needed include

Major laparotomy pack
    2 self-retaining Balfour retractors
    2 Harrington retractors
    2 Deaver retractors (long blades, standard width)
    2 suction tips
Vascular instruments
    Aortic clamps (Satinsky and DeBakey—2 each)
    Vein retractors
    Electrocautery—2 each
    Hemoclips (small, medium, and large)
Suture
    1–0, 2–0, and 3–0 silk ties and suture
    4–0 and 5–0 polypropylene (Prolene) suture
    1–0 silk on a large cutting needle for closing
Sterile containers to send bilateral ureteral cultures for routine culture and sensitivity testing, 6 to 8 L of chilled lactated Ringer solution for irrigation, 4 to 6 sterile containers for tissue typing specimens, 5 red- and 5 green-topped blood tubes for blood specimens
4 to 6 intestinal bags
Vessel loops
Ice (unsterile)
4 bottle jets (sterile pour spouts)

A separate back table for preparing kidneys for preservation should have the following:

Intravenous (IV) pole
Spotlight or satellite light
Laboratory basin
4 mosquito hemostats (2 straight, 2 curved)
2 pair of vascular forceps
2–0 silk ties
4–0 and 5–0 braided nonabsorbable suture ligature
1 small Metzenbaum scissors
1 angled Potts scissors
2 50-ml syringes
Irrigating tips for syringes
14-gauge polyethylene intravenous cannula

If a heart or liver recovery is being done, a hyperthermia blanket is needed. Additional supplies for heart recovery include a rib spreader, bone wax, a sternal saw and motor or Lebshe knife and mallet, additional large vascular clamps (DeBakey or Satinsky), straight and angled Potts clamps, an extra IV pole, a pressure bag for infusion of cardioplegia solution, an additional back table, and laboratory basins.

Needs and procedures vary with individual recovery teams. If special equipment or supplies are needed, they are generally brought by the recovery teams (e.g., renal perfusion fluid, cardioplegia solution, and Collins solution). Otherwise, the operating room (OR) staff at the donor hospital supplies the OR with the necessary instruments, supplies, and equipment.

KIDNEY TRANSPLANTATION FROM A LIVING RELATED DONOR

Definition

Kidney transplantation from a living related donor is currently the treatment of choice for a patient with end-stage renal disease. The results have been superior in both patient and graft survival after living related donor transplantation. Because the supply of cardaveric organs cannot meet the demands of those people with end-stage renal disease needing a transplant, every effort should be made to increase the living related transplantation rate, because transplantation costs are less than the maintenance costs of continued long-term dialysis.

Indications

The most common diseases leading to an eventual need for transplantation are glomerulonephritis and pyelonephritis. The quality of life is far superior after successful transplantation; however, the short-term risks of transplantation (as with any surgery) are greater than the risk of long-term dialysis. Long-term cumulative risks of dialysis are at least as great as those of transplantation.

The justifications for using living related donors for kidney transplantation are that (1) a normally functioning, anatomically normal, and readily obtainable organ is available without an indefinite waiting period for a cadaveric kidney and (2) the long-term allograft and recipient survival is better with the use of such kidneys than with cadaveric organs (Barker et al., 1986).

The administration of cyclosporine in particular has improved the survival of grafts and patients in cadaveric kidney transplantation but has not diminished the difference in graft survival statistics between living related donors and cadaveric donors. Furthermore, donor-specific transfusions have improved haplotype-mismatched donor recipient combinations to achieve results that are equivalent to those with HLA identical siblings. Although donor-specific transfusions were popular several years ago, they are not used much at present.

Related Surgical Procedures

The donor operation can be approached from a thoracotomy (flank) incision or transperitoneally through a midline abdominal incision. This operation is similar to a nephrectomy or an adrenalectomy. The recipient operation approach is through a retroperitoneal incision, and then the kidney is placed in the right or left lower quadrant just above the inguinal ligament.

Perioperative Nursing Implications

Before preparing the patient receiving the kidney, the circulator takes 1 ml of neomycin and polymyxin B (Neosporin GU irrigant) in 500 ml of normal saline and instills it via the Foley catheter (which is then clamped) to distend the bladder and facilitate its identification and dissection.

The circulator is the key person in communicating between ORs during a living related transplant. The circulator can greet both patients and let them have time to say good-bye before the donor is taken into the OR. She or he then relays messages back and forth from the ORs as to the progress of the procedures and the estimated time when the kidney will be available versus when the recipient will be ready.

Anesthesia

Recipient

If the recipient has been undergoing dialysis before surgery, dialysis is performed 12 to 36 hours before transplantation to control volume, blood pressure, potassium level, and acidosis (Flye, 1989). The choice of anesthetic technique is influenced by the adequacy and timing of dialysis. Fortunately, many patients for living related transplant are still making minimal amounts of urine and have not yet been dialyzed. Because living related kidney transplant grafts usually function immediately, these patients are given crystalloid as if they were going to have normal renal function at the end of the case.

Many transplant recipients who have been undergoing dialysis have a fistula in their arm; the other arm should be used for a peripheral IV catheter and blood pressure cuff. Use of the arm with a fistula poses the risk of failure to obtain a true pressure reading as well as thrombosis of the fistula.

Epidural anesthesia in conjuction with general anesthesia has been considered. This allows the delivery of epidural narcotics and diminishes the need for neuromuscular blockers, which are metabolized unpredictably in uremic patients. General anesthesia is maintained with nitrous oxide and isoflurane or halothane. Methoxyflurane and Ethrane are contraindicated in patients with renal dysfunction and in recipients of fresh kidney allografts because of their potential nephrotoxicity (Garovoy and Guttmann, 1986). The sole use of a regional anesthetic is contraindicated because of the potential for emesis resulting from the high doses of azathioprine (Imuran) and methylprednisolone (Solu-Medrol) given intraoperatively. The choice of nondepolarizing muscle relaxant is based in part on the site of metabolism and elimination. Atracurium or vecuronium is preferred to drugs such as pancuronium or curare. Finally, all anesthetic agents can produce hypotension; thus, optimal intraoperative fluid management with the maintenance of normal blood pressure often requires addition of colloidal solutions such as albumin to maintain renal perfusion (Garovoy and Guttmann, 1986).

Intraoperative immunosuppressive, antibiotic, and diuretic doses are dictated by the surgeon. Large doses of furosemide are given, and often, the patients have mild acute tubular necrosis postoperatively. However, any urine output is acceptable, even with a specific gravity of 10.

Donor

The kidney transplant donor is a unique patient in that he or she has consented to major surgery with no expectation that some specific pathological condition will be corrected. These patients are in an optimal state of health. Any invasive monitoring not necessary for patient monitoring or management is not used. All modalities for the treatment of postoperative pain are offered. Epidural narcotics or intercostal blocks have been the most effective treatments. The single invasive procedure deemed necessary for the surgery is bladder catheterization; the urine output is monitored by anesthesia personnel. To maximize the quality of the renal graft, its donor gets large doses of furosemide before the vessels are clamped; therefore, the administration of diuretics necessitates the use of a Foley catheter.

Position

Donor

The patient is placed in lateral decubitus position, with extreme kidney posture for greater exposure. A sandbag is placed behind the back and a pillow is placed between the legs. The safety strap is placed across the thighs, and some surgeons also use 2-inch tape across the patient's iliac crest and attach the tape to the OR bed, to ensure stability. A pillow is also placed between the arms or a double arm board can be used.

Recipient

The recipient is placed in a supine position with a safety strap across the thighs; the arms can be tucked at the patient's sides or left extended on arm boards.

Creation and Maintenance of the Sterile Field

The donor is prepared anteriorly from the midline, posteriorly from the vertebral column, superiorly from the scapula, and inferiorly from the iliac crest. This entire area is shaved preoperatively.

The recipient is shaved preoperatively on the operative side. The preparation is done over the entire abdomen from the xiphoid to the symphysis pubis.

Donor

The donor is draped to provide good exposure. The folded towels are placed and then a large sterile incise drape. Because the patient is in a lateral position, it is hard to keep things from falling on the floor. Therefore, the Mayo stand should be brought in as close to the field as possible, to give the surgeons a place to put the instruments. All other furniture is simply placed where it is most convenient for the scrub nurse.

Recipient

The recipient is draped, exposing only the operative side, although both sides are prepared. The nonoperative side is covered by sterile towels. Occasionally, a bump is placed under the back on the operative side to aid exposure. The Mayo stand is positioned over the patient's legs. The perfusion table is usually set up in the OR for the recipient procedure. It is positioned behind the back table so the surgeons have room to sit or stand and work on the donor kidney.

Equipment and Supplies

Donor

Patient drapes; gowns; a back table cover; a Mayo stand cover; a basin set; Fogarty inserts (small); vessel loops; 50-ml and 10-ml syringes; suture booties (small); a needle counter; light handles; electrocautery and extension tip; a magnetic pad; suction tubing; large and small laparotomy sponges; 4 × 8 sponges; Nos. 10, 11, and 15 blades; pushers; a Foley catheter; and a urinary drainage system are needed.

Suture. 3–0 and 5–0 braided nonabsorbable suture ties, 2–0 chromic ties, 2–0 silk ties, 3–0 braided nonabsorable suture on a taper needle, 2–0 chromic suture on a taper needle, 6–0 and 5–0 polypropylene, 1–0 polydioxanone absorbable monofilament suture (PDS) on a taper needle, 1–0 polyglactin 910 on a taper needle, 3–0 polyglactin 910, and skin staples of 4–0 polyglactin 910 are needed.

Recipient

A patient drape; gowns; a Mayo stand cover; a back table cover; a basin set; suction tubing; electrocautery; peanut dissectors; large and small laparotomy sponges; 4 × 8 sponges; 50-ml syringe; suture booties (small); small Fogarty inserts; vessel loops; Nos. 10, 11, and 15 blades; a needle counter; light handles; No. 24 Fr. Foley catheter with three-way connection; an irrigation set-up; a urinary drainage bag; a disposable aortic punch (4.0); and bone wax are used.

Suture. 3–0 plain ties, 3–0 and 5–0 braided nonabsorbable suture ties, 3–0 braided nonabsorbable suture on a taper needle, 2–0 chromic ties, 2–0 chromic suture on a taper needle, 5–0 and 6–0 double-armed polypropylene, 6–0 double-armed polyglactin 910 or PDS, 4–0 polyglactin 910 or PDS on a taper needle, 1 PDS pop-off, No. 1 polypropylene, 3–0 polyglactin 910, and skin staples are used.

The instruments necessary for the donor and recipient operations are the same, with the exception of an adult chest retractor, which is needed for the donor operation:

a major vascular set containing vascular forceps, scissors, needle holders, and clamps, as well as basic instruments and retractors. For the recipient operation, either a Bookwalter or a Balfour retractor is used to get adequate exposure. Extradeep and elephant Deaver retractors should also be available.

Drugs and Solutions

The solutions needed are 1 ml of neomycin and polymyxin B (Neosporin GU irrigant) in 500 ml of normal saline for instillation into the bladder of the recipient and cold Ringer irrigation for preserving the donor kidney and cold renal perfusion fluid with 5000 U of heparin for flushing the kidney after it is removed.

Physiological Monitoring

A nasal temperature probe is used by anesthesia personnel to monitor the patient's temperature. Anesthesia personnel also monitor the urine output. The circulating nurse monitors blood loss by weighing sponges and measuring the products in the suction container.

Specimens and Cultures

Occasionally, a urine culture is collected from the recipient after insertion of the Foley catheter. A time zero biopsy may be taken of the donor kidney before implantation. This is put in fixative and sent for evaluation in less than 24 hours.

Physician's Orders

Donor

Preliminary evaluation is done to qualify the donor. This includes routine work-up for renal or medical diseases precluding donation, tissue typing, mixed leukocyte culture, urinalysis, urine culture and sensitivity testing, creatinine clearance, IV pyelogram, and arteriogram. All females of childbearing age must have a pregnancy test.

Admission and preoperative orders for the living related donor include (1) admission 2 days before surgery; (2) laboratory studies: complete blood count (CBC), SMA-7 (serum electrolytes, blood urea nitrogen, creatinine), calcium phosphate, prothrombin time (PT), partial thromboplastin time, type and cross-match for 4 U of packed red blood cells, and final cross-match and tissue typing; (3) electrocardiography (ECG); (4) chest x-ray film; (5) the evening before surgery: (a) Fleet enema, (b) nothing by mouth (NPO) after midnight, and (c) signed operative consent; and (6) available in the OR, cefazolin 1 g IV (unless the patient is allergic).

Recipient

The patient is admitted 2 days before surgery; if he or she is undergoing continuous ambulatory peritoneal dialysis (CAPD) or intermittent peritoneal dialysis (IPD), this continues after admission. If hemodialysis is needed, it is scheduled for the first nursing shift of the day, the day before surgery.

Preoperative laboratory studies (for hemodialysis, can be done while patient is undergoing dialysis): (1) CBC; (2) SMA-7; (3) calcium phosphate; (4) liver function tests; (5) hepatitis B surface antigen; (6) PT and PTT; (7) type and cross-match of 4 U of packed red blood cells; (8) final cross-match; (9) ECG; (10) corrected sedimentation rate; (11) administration of medications: (a) azathioprine (Imuran), 10 mg/kg orally the evening before transplant surgery, (b) cyclosporine, 14 mg/kg orally the evening before transplant (for HLA-identical transplants: 15 mg/kg intravenously intraoperatively), (c) methylprednisolone, 15 mg/kg, (d) cefazolin, 1 g IV (unless the recipient is allergic); (12) notation on the patient's chart of the recipient's daily urine output at present, hepatitis B surface antigen status, and any bladder abnormalities; (13) notification of the surgeon of the final cross-match result (in the event of a positive cross-match, the transplant would be cancelled); and (14) donor arteriogram ordered and brought to the OR with the donor.

Laboratory and Diagnostic Studies

Donor

The results of the studies must show that the donor has two normal kidneys. A study has been conducted to estimate the long-term status of the remaining kidney after a unilateral nephrectomy; no indication of diminished renal function has been found (Flye, 1989).

The related donor is selected on the basis of the histocompatibility factor. Inheritance of the major histocompatibility complex means two siblings have a 25% chance of being HLA identical (i.e., having inherited the same chromosome 6 haplotype from each parent), a 50% chance of sharing one haplotype, and a 25% chance of sharing neither haplotype. Parent-to-child donation always involves a one-haplotype identity. The outcome of a related donor transplant is correlated with the degree of histocompatibility. Donor-specific transfusions are deliberate transfusions of blood from the prospective living related donor. They are used for one haplotype–matched recipients to achieve results equivalent with those with HLA-identical siblings. However, these transfusions are associated with a 30% risk of inciting positive cytotoxic antibodies, thus precluding transplant from the selected renal donor.

Procedure

Incision and Exposure

Donor

The patient is lying on his or her side, the OR bed is fully flexed, and the kidney bar is raised. The left kidney is chosen, if possible, because the renal vein is longer, facilitating the recipient operation. A flank incision is made between the 11th and 12th ribs. Some surgeons remove the 12th rib, but the procedure can be done almost as readily and with less risk of entering the pleura through a subcostal incision, without removing the rib. The chest retractor, with scapula blades attached, is used for exposure (a Bookwalter retractor can also be used). With the use of electrocautery, Metzenbaum scissors, and vascular forceps, Gerota fascia is incised. The greater curvature of the kidney and upper pole are dissected free and the hilar structures are exposed with care.

Recipient

Good relaxation is needed for the recipient operation owing to the tediousness of the anastomosis. An oblique incision is made just above the inguinal ligament. Electrocautery, along with hemostats, is used to maintain hemostasis as the external and internal oblique muscles are divided. The transverse abdominal muscle and transverse fascia are also divided. The Balfour retractor with one deep and one shallow blade or the Bookwalter retractor is positioned.

Details

Donor

On the left side, the adrenal and gonadal veins are ligated so the entire length of the renal vein can be utilized. Care must be taken not to manipulate the renal artery, causing spasm and decreased renal perfusion (Fig. 23–1). If there are accessory donor renal arteries present, they should be preserved, because occlusion of these end arteries causes renal infarcts. Great care should also be taken not to skeletonize the ureter. It should be freed up along with its blood supply and fat. The ureter is divided close the bladder after ligating the distal end. Mannitol is administered to ensure adequate urine output; if the donor is well hydrated, urine should be seen coming from the proximal end of the divided ureter.

At this point, coordination of timing with the recipient operation (which is performed simultaneously by a separate team) is confirmed. When the recipient iliac vessels and bladder have been prepared, the donor renal artery and vein are clamped and divided in that order. Beck clamps are used most often. The kidney is taken to the OR for the recipient procedure and immediately per-

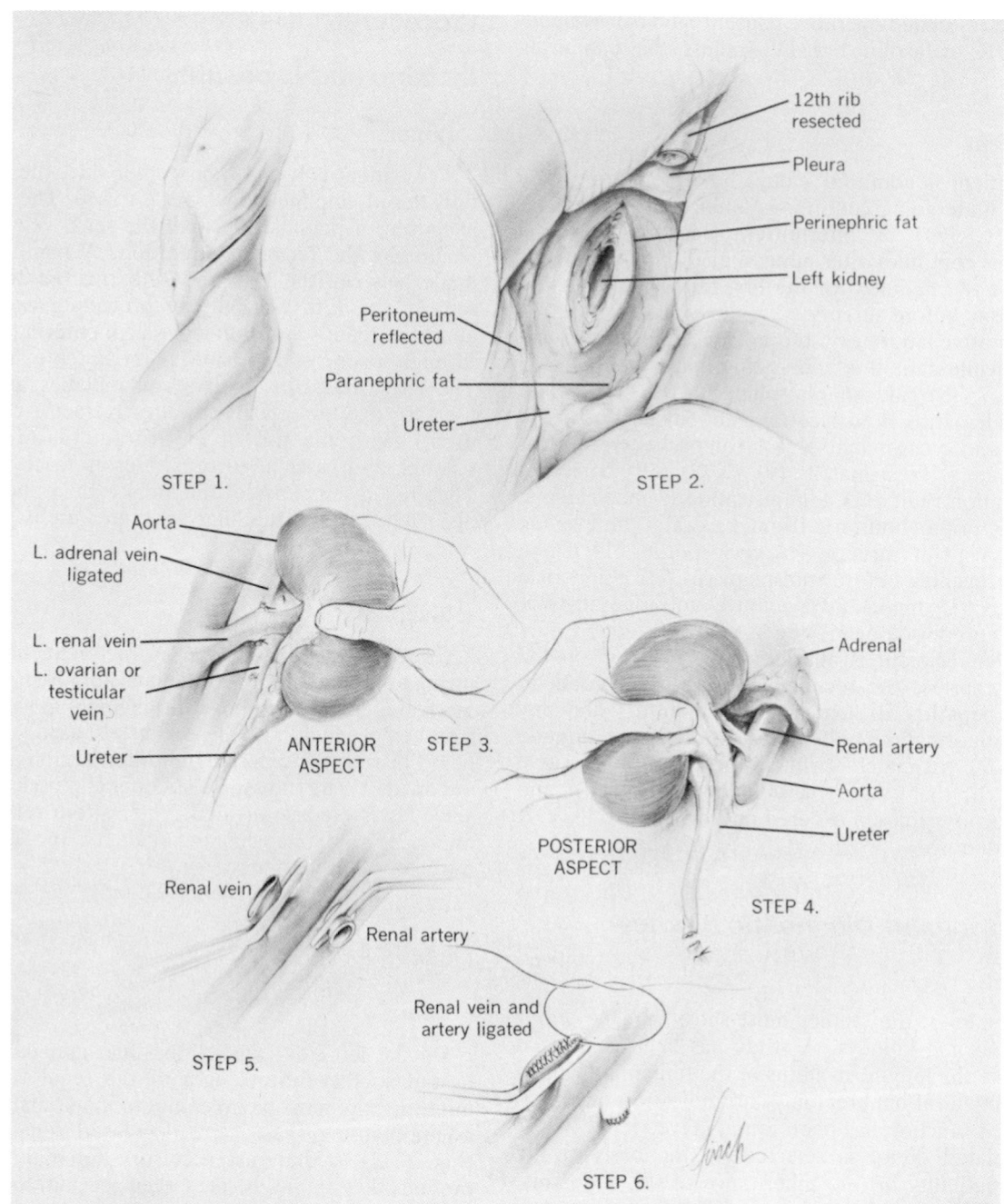

FIGURE 23–1. Nephrectomy from a living related donor takes place via an extraperitoneal flank incision. A portion of the 12th rib may be resected for additional exposure (*step 2*). The renal vein and artery stumps are oversewn after removal of the kidney. (From Simmons, R. L., Kjellstrand, C. M., Najarian, J. S. [1972]. Section II. Technique complications and results. In J. S. Najarian, R. L. Simmons [Eds.]. *Transplantation* [p. 450]. Philadelphia: Lea & Febiger.)

fused with several hundred milliliters of cold intracellular solution (renal perfusion fluid with heparin) to remove the formed blood elements and to reduce its core temperature. It is immersed in a basin of Ringer irrigation cooled to 4°C. The donor vessels are oversewn with 6–0 and 5–0 Prolene sutures for the artery and the vein, respectively. The cavity is irrigated with warm saline irrigation, and the incision is closed without drainage.

Recipient

The iliac vessels are exposed retroperitoneally through an oblique incision just above the inguinal ligament (Fig. 23–2). The lymphatics are divided using 3–0 braided nonabsorbable suture on a taper needle and 3–0 braided nonabsorbable suture ties. This division is necessary to expose the iliac vessels, and great care is

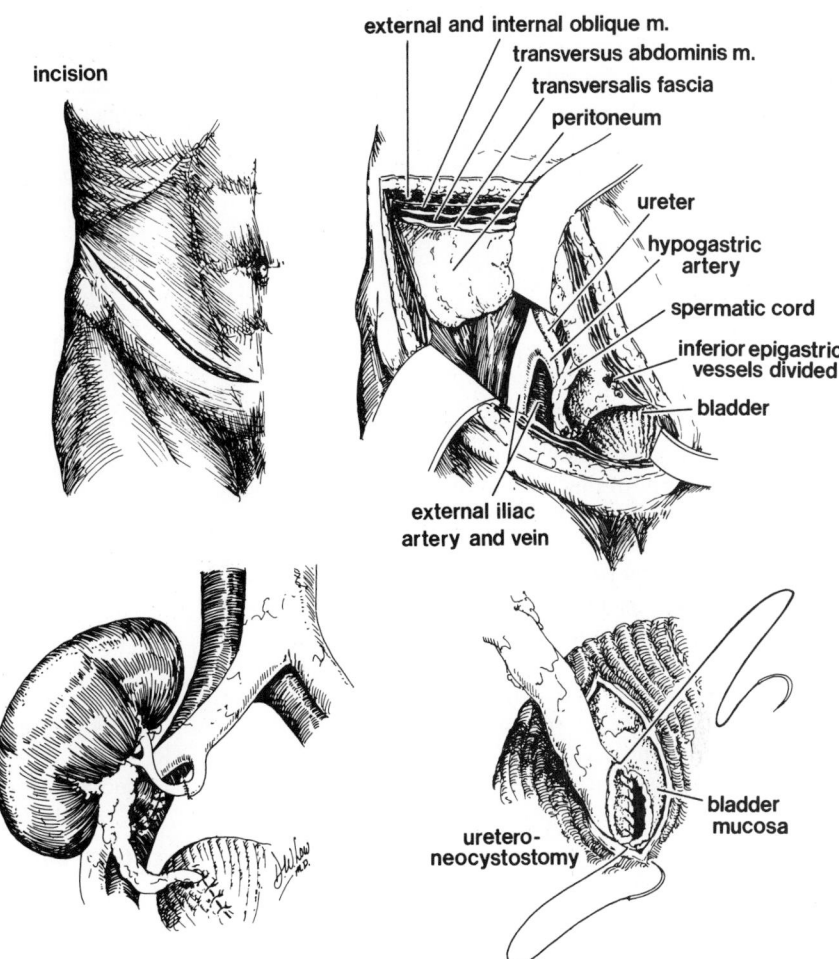

incision

external and internal oblique m.
transversus abdominis m.
transversalis fascia
peritoneum
ureter
hypogastric artery
spermatic cord
inferior epigastric vessels divided
bladder

external iliac artery and vein

ureteroneocystostomy
bladder mucosa

FIGURE 23–2. In the renal recipient operation, the vessels for revascularization are exposed through an extraperitoneal incision, and urinary continuity is reestablished with a ureteroneocystotomy. (From Barker, C. F., Naji, A., Perloff, L. J. [1986]. Renal transplantation. In D. C. Sabiston Jr. [Ed.]. *Textbook of surgery* [p. 413]. Philadelphia: W. B. Saunders.)

taken to prevent lymph leak or lymphocele, which might obstruct the collecting system. Exposure of the bladder is facilitated by dividing the inferior epigastric vessels and, in women, the round ligament. Because the bladder has been distended preoperatively, it is easy to identify.

If there are multiple renal arteries present while the kidney is still sitting in the cold solution, the end of the smaller renal artery is anastomosed to the side of the largest renal artery. Revascularization in the recipient can then be accomplished by a single anastomosis.

Anastomosis of the end of the transplant renal artery to the proximal end of the recipient's divided internal iliac artery is completed using a continuous 6–0 polypropylene suture. An end-to-side anastomosis of the renal artery to the external iliac artery should be used if there is significant disease of the internal iliac artery or if this method is preferred. The venous anastomosis is completed by attaching the end of the transplant vein to the side of the recipient's external iliac vein; a continuous 5–0 polypropylene suture is used. After both anastomoses are completed, the clamps are removed and the kidney is observed for perfusion.

The ureterovesical anastomosis is next performed, usually by ureteroneocystostomy. In males, the ureter should pass beneath the spermatic cord to avoid obstruction. A small incision is made in the dome of the bladder

through the mucosa with a No. 11 blade. A short length of spatulated transplant ureter is anastomosed end to side to the mucosa using a continuous 6–0 polyglactin 910 or PDS suture. Several interrupted 4–0 polyglactin 910 or PDS sutures are used to cover this anastomosis with bladder muscle.

Because of the coagulopathy and susceptibility to infection of uremic immunosuppressed patients, meticulous surgical technique and hemostasis are particularly important.

Closure

Donor

The incision is approximated simply by unflexing the OR bed and lowering the kidney bar. The fascia is closed with interrupted 1–0 PDS suture. If there is subcutaneous tissue, it is closed with 3–0 polyglactin 910. Skin staples are used to close the skin or a 4–0 polyglactin 910 subcuticular running stitch is used.

Recipient

The abdominal musculature is closed with interrupted 1–0 PDS; the external and internal oblique muscles are closed with interrupted 1–0 PDS. The subcutaneous tissue is closed with interrupted 3–0 polyglactin 910, and the skin is closed with either subcutaneous 4–0 continuous polyglactin 910 or skin staples.

Often, the Foley catheter is irrigated with antibiotic irrigation solution to deter any obstruction in the flow of urine attributable to clot formation.

Postoperative Care

Donor

The donors are kept NPO for approximately 24 hours and then advanced to clear fluids and a regular diet. An IV catheter is kept in place for 24 hours until the patient is tolerating oral intake of fluids; it is then converted to a heparin lock. The Foley catheter is removed the morning after surgery. A chest x-ray film is obtained while the patient is in the recovery room to rule out conditions such as pneumothorax, and coughing, deep breathing, and incentive spirometry are begun the first postoperative day. Often, these patients have a great deal of postoperative pain and are medicated for such. Living related donors can be discharged on an average of 5 to 7 days postoperatively.

Recipient

Postoperatively, the patient is taken to the recovery room until she or he is adequately stable and oriented; then the patient is admitted to the transplant floor. Vital signs are taken every 15 minutes until the patient's condition is stable, then every 30 minutes for 4 hours, every hour for 2 hours, and then every 4 hours. A staff physician is notified if

temperature is greater than 100.5°F orally
urine output is less than 30 ml/hour
systolic blood pressure is greater than 180 or less than 100 mm Hg
pulse rate is greater than 120 beats/minute

The patient is kept NPO, then advanced to clear liquids and then to a regular diet (with fluid sodium and potassium restrictions, depending on renal function).

The nurse performs the following:

Weighs the patient daily.
Obtains input and output measurements.
Assists the patient to cough, turn, and deep breathe every hour while awake.
Performs spirometer care per respiratory care recommendations.
Connects the Foley catheter to straight drainage, measures the hourly urine output, and discontinues the use of Foley catheter after 48 hours, unless specified for longer use (e.g., during difficult ureteroneocystostomy). Gently irrigates the Foley catheter with 20 ml of sterile saline as needed for lack of urine flow.

Obtains urine culture and sensitivity testing weekly and as needed.
Institutes fistula and shunt precautions.
Restricts the patient to bed rest for 12 hours then allows out of bed.
Administers IV fluids: replaces the prior hour's urine output volume milliliter for milliliter with normal saline (0.45% sodium chloride) and 1 ampule of sodium bicarbonate; after 6 hours, if the urine output is 100 to 200 ml/hour, reduces to half replacement.
Administers medications:
  Morphine sulfate given intramuscularly (IM) or through epidural catheter (if present)
  Codeine sulfate IM
  Alutabs, 2 tablets orally four times daily
  Multivitamins, 1 tablet orally daily
  Nystatin (Mycostatin) mouthwash, 5 ml in 10 ml of water three times daily, swish and swallow.
  Docusate sodium (Colace), 100 mg orally twice daily
  Cefazolin, 1 g IV every 8 hours for 48 hours (unless the patient is allergic)
  Laxative, per physician or ward regimen
  Sedative
Checks the immunosuppression orders daily.
Resumes the administration of necessary preoperative medication (phenytoin [Dilantin]).

Study Orders

1. Daily CBC and platelet count
2. Daily measurement of electrolytes, potassium, creatinine, blood urea nitrogen, glucose, calcium, and phosporus levels for 3 days after transplantation, then weekly
3. Renal nuclear medicine scan on the first postoperative day
4. Weekly liver function tests
5. Hepatitis B surface antigen measurement every 1st and 15th of the month
6. Cytomegalovirus antibody titer weekly
7. Histocompatibility testing weekly
8. Cyclosporine level
9. Flow cystometric analysis three times a week and as necessary

Immunosuppression Protocol

1. Cyclosporine—Begin 14 mg/kg/day orally on first postoperative day. If oliguria is present, start a lower dose of cyclosporine (10 mg/kg/day). Subsequent doses are determined by cyclosporine levels.
2. Prednisone regimen—Begin on first postoperative day 1.5 mg/kg/day (rounded off to nearest 10). Taper as per protocol.
3. Azathioprine—In recipients with diuresing kidney transplant (receiving cyclosporine), the dose is 1 mg/kg/day after tapering daily from the loading dose. Aziothioprine is ordered on a daily basis depending on the CBC. Dose may be given orally or IV.

Patients are watched closely for any signs or symptoms of postoperative complications. If the postoperative course goes well, living related recipients could be discharged in 10 days.

Potential Surgical Complications

Donor

In addition to pain and the usual morbidity factors associated with an operation of this magnitude, there is an operative mortality of 0.05%. Some complications that have been experienced by this group are urinary tract infection, pneumothorax, blood transfusion reactions, wound infection, atelectasis, and incisional hernia. Overall, these patients do extremely well and are happy with their decision to donate.

Recipient

Complications in the first few hours or days after transplantation are commonly related to technical problems in establishing vascular and urinary continuity or to damage that occurs during donor nephrectomy or graft preservation.

Arterial obstruction must be considered promptly if the transplant inexplicably fails to function initially or if established diuresis suddenly ceases in the first few hours, especially in living related transplants, in which prompt graft function should be the rule. Immediate reoperation without waiting for diagnostic studies allows the best chance for salvaging a graft with strongly suspected ischemia, because only a few minutes of total vascular occlusion can be tolerated without irreversible damage.

Hemmorhage due to imperfect hemostasis in the setting of uremic coagulopathy or anticoagulation for preoperative hemodialysis is the usual cause of early postoperative bleeding. Usually, the arterial anastomosis needs to be examined and sometimes redone.

Renal transplant artery stenosis is usually confirmed by arteriogram to distinguish stenosis from rejection. The cause is usually technical (e.g., improper anastomosis, injury of the intima of the renal artery during perfusion, and kinking at the anastomotic site from redundancy or twisting of the arteries). At present, percutaneous transluminal angioplasty is advocated for most instances of renal transplant artery stenosis.

Venous thrombosis, although rare, can occur owing to technical errors such as kinking, an injury from the clamping of the vein, or compression of the transplant. Usually, standard anticoagulant treatment is effective.

Urinary tract complications can occur. The most common cause of sudden cessation of urine output immediately postoperatively is a clot in the bladder or urethral catheter, which should be corrected by irrigation. Other causes of urinary obstruction are more serious, including vascular occlusion, acute tubular necrosis, and rejection. A ureteroneocystostomy may become occluded by a hematoma at the junction of the ureter and the bladder or by a technically unsatisfactory anastomosis. Treatment must be planned and individualized.

Acute tubular necrosis is a technical difficulty that occasionally leads to an ischemic insult to a kidney from a related donor. Oliguria in the early transplant period should be treated with aliquots of fluid and colloid to exclude hypovolemia. Mannitol and furosemide are given IV to increase output but are probably not going to alter the course of true acute tubular necrosis. Because there is no specific treatment, one must await the return of function within the usual 1 to 4 weeks, meanwhile trying to maintain adequate but safe immunosuppression and good general condition, if necessary by dialysis.

PANCREAS TRANSPLANTATION

Definition

A pancreas transplant aids in the normalization of carbohydrate metabolism, which it is hoped will stabilize if not reverse some of the ravaging complications such as neuropathy, retinopathy, vasculopathy, and enteropathy. It is best to perform a pancreas transplant early, to prevent secondary complications.

Indications

Most pancreas transplant patients have advanced secondary complications of diabetes before transplantation. Because immunosuppression is necessary, patients whose secondary complications of diabetes are or will be more serious than the potential side effects of immunosuppressive therapy are the best candidates. However, pancreas transplantation in the early stages of the disease is advocated.

Pancreas transplantation may be recommended for nonuremic nonkidney transplant patients, those with preproliferative retinopathy who are thus at great risk for loss of vision, or those with albuminuria who thus have early but progressive diabetic nephropathy.

Joint stiffness or measurement of insulinlike growth factors might identify diabetic patients who are at high risk for the development of secondary complications.

Diabetic patients who have impaired counterregulatory mechanisms and who are at high risk for hypoglycemic reactions while receiving intensive insulin therapy benefit from pancreas transplant.

Controversy exists as to the benefits of a simultaneous pancreas and kidney transplant versus those of the two-stage procedure.

Candidates must be carefully selected because of the limited success and potential morbidity and mortality. Diabetic individuals for whom the potential benefits of transplantation outweigh the risks of transplantation or continued standard treatment are also pancreas transplant candidates. Some standard criteria identified during a history and physical examination include the presence of insulin-dependent diabetes mellitus (usually juvenile onset), a serum C-peptide level less than 0.2 mg/ml, and insulin dependence for longer than 10 years. It is important for the physician doing the history and physical examination to document the stage of the diabetes. Most of these patients have multiple complications related to the diabetes. Neuropathy persists and they lose sensation in their hands and feet.

Complications of peripheral vascular disease, including carotid artery disease and claudication, are present. In addition, these patients get retinopathy and have poor vision.

- *Established diabetic nephropathy:* Proteinuria: 150 mg/24 hours, but less than 3 g/24 hours with adequate creatinine clearance at least 60 ml/minute.
- *Autonomic neuropathy:*
  1. Abnormal radionuclide gastric emptying study and symptoms consistent with gastroparesis
  2. Multiple blood pressure determinations supporting severely symptomatic orthostatic hypotension
  3. Abnormal cardiovascular autonomic reflexes
- *Labile diabetes or failure of insulin therapy:*
  1. More than 90 days of hospitalization for difficulty with glucose control during the previous year.
  2. During the previous year, six or more hypoglycemic episodes in 1 month necessitating emergency medical attention despite an appropriate insulin regimen
  3. During the preceding year, four or more unexplained episodes of diabetic ketoacidosis (DaFoe, 1988)

Candidates should be between 18 and 50 years of age. Patients with an existing renal allograft must have demonstrated stable renal function for at least 6 months defined as serum creatinine level less than 3 mg/dl with no significant increase during the past several weeks.

Patients with end-stage diabetic nephropathy are not good candidates because end-stage diabetic nephropathy is accompanied by major morbid events (blindness, amputation, stroke, myocardial infarction, severe heart failure). Coronary artery disease is also common in the diabetic patient with end-stage diabetic nephropathy and accounts for one third of deaths in these patients. Patient survival rates are significantly higher in patients without end-stage diabetic nephropathy.

Patients should be selected to maximize the potential benefits of pancreas transplant, without the risks that exceed those of standard treatment. It is well established that total endocrine therapy for insulin-dependent diabetes mellitus can be accomplished by a functioning vascularized pancreas allograft.

The rationale for pancreas transplant is that the microangiopathic and other lesions associated with diabetes mellitus are likely to be secondary to disordered carbohydrate metabolism and that perfect control of blood glucose levels may prevent the development or halt the progression of lesions affecting the eye, the kidney, and the nervous systems. The imperfect control that can be achieved with conventional insulin therapy allows the progression of complications in a large portion of patients.

Potential benefits include possible elimination of the metabolic problems of insulin-dependent diabetes mellitus, possible elimination of the need for insulin injections, and possible prevention of additional damage to the blood vessels (microangiopathy) and other organs from the complications of diabetes.

An advantage of performing pancreas transplantation in diabetic patients who have or will require a kidney transplant is that the risks associated with immunosuppressive therapy are obligatory. There is still controversy about the sequence of the procedures. In most recipients of a kidney and pancreas allograft, both organs have been grafted simultaneously. However, synchronous transplants have been associated with relatively high complication rates. Those groups that still favor simultaneous kidney and pancreas transplantation suggest that, because the organs come from the same donor, close monitoring of renal allograft function may facilitate early diagnosis of pancreas graft rejection (Garovoy and Guttmann, 1986). At present, dyssynchronous procedures are more commonly performed for patients with end-stage diabetic nephropathy. (All of the patients are already receiving routine immunosuppressive medications.) This discussion addresses dyssynchronous transplantation using the whole pancreas. Centers performing pancreas transplants usually have thoroughly instructed the potential recipients of the magnitude of the operation and its complications, including the need for lifetime follow-up. The patients need to be highly motivated individuals with strong support systems for reassurance.

Related Surgical Procedures

The procedure for the pancreas transplant is similar to that for the kidney transplant, in that the donor organ artery is attached to the recipient external (or internal) iliac artery and the donor organ vein attaches to the recipient internal iliac vein. Both organs are attached to the bladder, although the pancreas can be drained in a number of other ways.

Perioperative Nursing Implications

The major focus of the circulating nurse is patient care preoperatively. These patients are nervous and need hand-holding support and reassurance. Of course, they are ecstatic to be called in for the transplant but they need a vote of confidence. The circulator is responsible for having the three-way Foley catheter and antibiotic solution ready to insert into the bladder. In addition, the slush machine should be turned on and priming of the cold solution is performed before the patient enters the room.

Anesthesia

The circulator assists the anesthetist with placement of all intravascular lines and monitoring devices preoperatively. Usually, these patients are sick. They have vascular disease as a result of long-standing diabetes. The patient's electrolyte values, especially the potassium level, are usually abnormal. Depending on the patient, the anesthetist could be dealing with several ongoing problems. For a cadaver transplant, the patient could have a full stomach. For a combined procedure (kidney and pancreas transplant), the relationship to dialysis is important to anesthesia personnel. If the patient has not undergone dialysis, he or she may have an increased potassium level, therefore limiting the use of succinylcholine, which is thought to increase the serum potassium concentration. If patients have been dialyzed or have a functioning kidney, they have a contracted or normal blood volume. The condition of diabetics may be poor (e.g., hypertension with no time preoperatively for correction). The anesthetist tries to maintain the blood glucose level at 150 to 200 mg/dl for the duration of the procedure, either doing individual sticks or inserting an arterial catheter to obtain blood samples for the serum glucose determination.

If the patient has a shunt or fistula, the other arm is used for blood pressure monitoring and peripheral IV catheter placement. If they have shunts in both arms and one is nonfunctioning, it is often not possible to get a pressure reading. No invasive monitoring is used for pancreas transplants.

Epidural anesthesia in combination with general anesthesia has been advocated. The epidural catheter is used to deliver epidural narcotics. This diminishes the need for neuromuscular blockers, which are metabolized rather unpredictably in the uremic patient (i.e., patients with poor renal function). Further, they do not seem to work as well in the uremic patient; the temptation is to give more than normal doses, which cannot be reversed, and thus the patient cannot breathe adequately postoperatively. This causes the patient to be held in the OR until the anesthetist is satisfied with the respirations.

The patient is maintained with epidural and a light general anesthetic combining oxygen with nitrous oxide and enflurane or halothane. Generally, anesthetists are not comfortable with using enflurane (Ethrane) because metabolism of the drug yields the 50 ppm concentration of free fluoride ions during a 4-hour procedure. This concentration can cause renal failure in the normal kidney, therefore it is better not to stress the kidney at risk.

Premedication is individualized, and usually, the surgeon determines immunosuppressive therapy and antibiotics. Intraoperatively, the surgeon again instructs the anesthesia personnel when to give more immunosuppressive and antibiotic drugs.

Anesthesia personnel monitor urine output through the Foley bag and the patient's temperature through a nasal temperature probe. It is important to keep in mind that neuromuscular blockers and reversal of their action are to some extent related to the temperature of the patient. Examples of drugs used in epidural anesthesia are lidocaine, bupivacaine, and morphine (4 to 8 mg). This epidural anesthesia reduces the number of narcotics needed postoperatively for the first 24 hours.

The only special equipment needed by anesthesia personnel is an IVAC pump for cyclosporine drips.

Position

The patient is positioned supine on the OR bed with both arms extended on armboards. The legs are covered, and a safety strap is placed across the thighs.

Creation and Maintenance of the Sterile Field

The patient is prepared from the nipples to the symphysis pubis. This area is shaved or a depilatory is used preoperatively.

The scrub nurse should be prepared in advance so that he or she can begin to make the slush solution and have the perfusion table ready for the arrival of the donor organ.

A duct is placed across the patient's thighs; side towels are used to square off the field. A large sterile incise drape is applied, covering all exposed skin. Roll and side sheets are used. The Mayo stand is pulled across the patient's lower legs. The large back table sits perpendicular to the OR bed and the slush machine is to the side of it. The perfusion table is perpendicular to the back table; it is draped with four layers.

Equipment and Supplies

Equipment and supplies needed for the procedure include drape packs and gowns; a basin set; a major vascular set; extralong instruments; a Mayo stand cover; an impervious drape sheet; elephant and extradeep Deaver retractors; a Balfour or Bookwalter retractor; a large sterile incise drape; suction tubing; electrocautery; a Babcock sponge; large and small laparotomy sponges; 4 × 8 sponges; a 50-ml syringe; small Fogarty inserts; suture booties (small); Nos. 10, 11, and 15 blades; vessel loops; a needle counter; a skin marker; pushers; bone wax; light handles; a drain; skin clips; sterile slush (Ringer irrigation); warm saline irrigation; a drape for the slush machine; and a scoop for the slush machine. Suture required for the procedure includes 1–0 silk ties; 3–0 plain ties; 2–0 chromic ties; 3–0 and 5–0 braided nonabsorbable suture ties; 2–0, 3–0, and 4–0 chromic on a taper needle; 3–0 braided nonabsorbable suture on a taper needle; 5–0 double-armed polypropylene; 5–0 single-armed polypropylene; 5–0 double- or single-armed polyglactin 910; 6–0 and 7–0 double-armed polypropylene; 0 polyglactin 910; No. 1 polypropylene; 3–0 polyglactin 910; 3–0 braided nonabsorbable suture on a Keith needle; and 3–0 double-armed polypropylene. For the perfusion table, 2–0, 3–0, and 5–0 silk ties; 5–0 braided nonabsorbable suture on a taper needle; and 4–0 silk pop-offs are needed.

Equipment needed for the perfusion table includes mosquito clamps, fine vascular forceps, scissors, 50-ml syringes (two), and a metal cannula needle.

A major vascular set, including vascular forceps, scissors, needle holders, and clamps, as well as general surgery instruments, is needed. Special additional instruments include a Balfour or Bookwalter retractor, elephant and extradeep Deaver retractors, long instrument pack, and long Castroviejo needle holders.

Drugs and Solutions

The drugs and solutions the circulator must prepare and pour include the following: For table irrigation, amphotericin, 50 mg (reconstituted with 10 ml of sterile water), is added to 1 L of normal saline for the Foley catheter. To distend the bladder, 1 ampule (1 ml) of neomycin and polymyxin B (Neosporin GU irrigant) is added to 500 ml of saline, and the bladder is filled before the bladder anastomosis is completed. Additional drugs needed by anesthesia personnel usually include cyclosporine, azathioprine, and hydrocortisone.

Physiological Monitoring

Both bloody sponges and bottled blood loss are measured by the circulating nurse. Urine output is monitored by anesthesia personnel.

Specimens and Cultures

A culture of the duodenum may be taken intraoperatively.

Physician's Orders

A complete physical examination and laboratory evaluation are performed as follows: Typical admission treatment and study orders for transplant evaluation include ECG; chest x-ray films (posteroanterior and lateral); urinalysis; urine culture and sensitivity testing; and 24-hour urine glucose, creatinine, and protein determinations. Blood studies include CBC, differential leukocyte count, platelet count, erythrocyte sedimentation rate, and SMA; determination of glucose (fasting and 2 hours postprandial), calcium, alkaline phosphatase, serum glutamic-oxalocetic transaminase (aspartate aminotransferase), serum glutamic-pyruvic transaminase (alanine aminotransferase), serum protein electrophoresis, uric acid, bilirubin, amylase, lipase, cholesterol, and triglycerides; PT and PTT; hepatitis profile, cytomegalovirus and HIV antibodies; blood group; Rh factor; and Coombs test (direct and indirect). Special studies include hemoglobin A_{1C}, C-peptide, insulin antibodies, and one red-topped tube for plasma renin activity and anti-HLA antibodies. Consultations include neurological evaluation and nerve conduction studies, routine ophthalmological evaluation and flourescein angiography, routine pretransplant psychiatric studies, and evaluation by nephrology, diabetology, nutritional support, and cardiology departments.

The patient's vital signs are taken during every shift and he or she is maintained on a constant test diet with greater than 150 g of carbohydrate. Routine administration of medications is continued.

Typical admission preoperative treatment orders for a pancreas transplant patient being admitted for surgery include determination of height, weight, previous renal transplant, HLA-identical or HLA-nonidentical status; evaluation for coronary artery disease; examination of double-voided urine for glucose and ketones; administration of Fleet enema; and administration of medications on admission:

mycostatin, 1 million Units
neomycin, 1 g orally
erythromycin, 1 g orally
IV 5% glucose in half-normal saline
on call to the OR, cefazolin sodium (Ancef), 1 g IV, and hydrocortisone, 100 mg IV
cyclosporine, 5 mg/kg/24 hours IV (start immediately) via continuous infusion
regular insulin dosage IV, on call to the OR

An operative consent for the cadaver pancreas transplant is verified in the chart.

Laboratory and Diagnostic Studies

Typical studies ordered preoperatively include baseline blood work, CBC, platelet count, SMA, coagulation profile, fibrinogen level, calcium phosphorus, C-peptide, final leukocyte cross-match to tissue typing, ECG if not done within 2 weeks, throat culture (routine *Candida*, viral), urine culture (routine *Candida*, viral), stool culture (*Clostridium difficile* and *C. difficile* toxin), and chest film (posteroanterior and lateral) (if not done within 2 weeks).

Procedure

Incision and Exposure

There are several approaches to implanting a pancreas graft. Some surgeons make a curved incision in the left iliac fossa; others use a straight midline incision. The author is familiar with the midline approach. After the incision is made and vessels cauterized, the Bookwalter retractor is positioned. Vascular forceps, Metzenbaum scissors, and Mixter and Crile clamps are used to dissect out the external iliac vessels. The lymphatics around the iliac vessels are ligated with 3–0 braided nonabsorbable suture ligatures. After the iliac vessels are exposed and isolated with vessel loops, the bladder is exposed.

Details

The donor pancreas should be in the room by this point. It is floated in the cold slush while being examined at the perfusion table. If a liver was harvested, the splenic artery and superior mesenteric artery are divided. A Carrel patch that combines the superior mesenteric and the celiac axis arteries is ideal. Also dependent on the harvesting technique is a decision as to how much duodenum to take. The preferred technique is to take en bloc a composite pancreaticoduodenal splenic graft. This allows a 4- to 6-inch segment of duodenum; it also maximizes islet mass in the pancreas graft by harvesting the whole organ (Fig. 23–3).

The pancreas graft vessels are anastomosed on the opposite side of the renal graft in patients who had previous kidney transplants. The portal vein (composed of the splenic, inferior mesenteric, and superior mesenteric veins) is anastomosed to the external iliac vein (which is clamped with Fogarty clamps) with a contin-

uous 5–0 Prolene suture. Fogarty clamps are applied to the external iliac artery in preparation for the donor artery anastomosis. If a Carrel patch is present, it is anastomosed to the external iliac artery using continuous 6–0 Prolene suture. If the aortic patch is not present, the splenic artery is attached to the internal iliac artery and the superior mesenteric artery is attached to the external iliac artery, which join at the common iliac artery. The clamps are then released on both the vein and the artery and the pancreas is revascularized.

Controversy exists about the best method for dealing with the pancreatic duct. To date, eight different methods have been used: cutaneous duodenostomy, pancreaticocutaneous fistula, duct ligation, open duct–intraperitoneal placement, pancreaticojejunostomy, pancreatic duct injection, pancreatic ductoureterostomy, and pancreaticocystostomy (Sutherland et al, 1984). All methods of duct management except ligation have served long-term graft function. The highest survival rates have been with duct injection and bladder drainage.

This discussion describes the pancreatic cystostomy. The duodenum is used and a peritoneal window is opened medially, and a side-to-side anastomosis is ac-

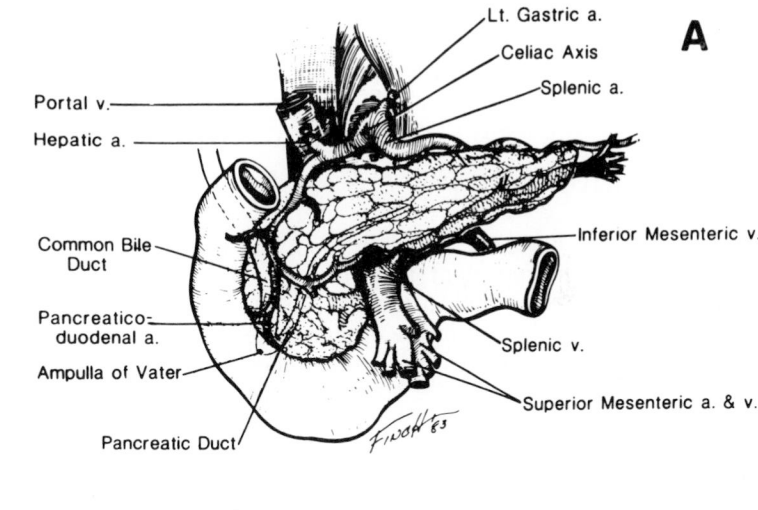

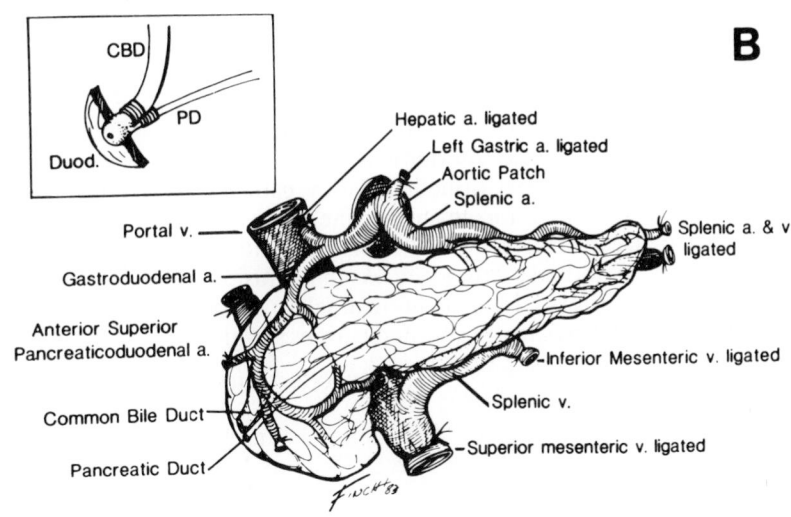

FIGURE 23–3. Technique for whole-pancreas transplantation. *A,* Pancreas anatomy in donor before excision. The duodenum can be excised en bloc with the pancreas graft for transplantation to the recipient. *B,* The pancreas can be separated entirely from the duodenum, or only the portion of the duodenum accompanying the ampulla of Vater can be retained (*inset*). CBD, common bile duct; PD, pancreatic duct. (From Sutherland, D. E. R., Chinn, P. L., Elick, B. A., et al. [1984]. Maximization of islet mass in pancreas grafts by near total or total whole organ excision without duodenum from cadaver donors. *Transplantation Proceedings, 16,* 115.)

complished in two layers, joining the duodenum to the bladder. Just before the bladder anastomosis, the bladder is distended with 1 ml of neomycin and polymyxin B (Neosporin GU irrigant) in 500 ml of normal saline, approximately 300 ml of irrigation. Because this is done under direct vision, the surgeon can tell the circulating nurse when the bladder is full. The bladder site is cleaned off, and an incision is made into the bladder with a No. 11 blade and extended with the Potts scissors. The anastomosis is done mucosa to mucosa and duodenal seromuscular layer to bladder detrusor muscle. Absorbable continuous 3–0 PDS suture is used for the inner layer, and 4–0 interrupted polypropylene suture is used for the outer layer. All of the anastomoses are checked for leaks and kinks.

The pancreatic transplant sits on the iliac fossa, and the surgeon checks its position. After the position is satisfactory, the surgeon checks the spleen to see if the blood flow is good, then a donor splenectomy is done. A splenectomy is indicated to prevent the possibility of graft-versus-host disease. Some surgeons insert a closed wound drain around the pancreatic graft and bring it through a separate incision. Others believe that this step is not necessary.

Closure

The fascia is closed with a running No. 1 polypropylene suture. The subcutaneous fat is closed with 3–0 braided absorbable suture; the skin is closed with clips.

Postoperative Care

These patients go to the recovery room and then are discharged to the transplant floor if they are stable. They have been extubated in the OR and usually are pain free owing to the use of the epidural anesthesia.

Typical postoperative treatment orders include measurement of vital signs every ½ hour until the patient is stable, then every hour for 6 hours, then every 2 hours for 24 hours, and then routinely. An oxygen mask is set depending on how the patient is oxygenating. Rectal temperature is taken immediately, then every 3 hours (the physician is notified of temperatures greater than 101°F). The patient should perform cough and deep breathing every 2 hours for 12 hours, ambulate on the first postoperative day, and remain NPO. A nasogastric tube is connected to low intermittent suction, guaiac testing of all stools is performed, a Foley catheter is connected to straight drainage, and urine glucose and ketone levels are measured every 4 hours. IV fluids (5% dextrose in half-normal saline) and insulin infusion (1 U of regular insulin to 1 ml of normal saline set at a rate to suit the patient) are given. Medications are given:

Morphine sulfate, 8 mg IM or IV, every 6 hours for pain.
Hydrocortisone, 100 mg IV and then 8 hours later; on postoperative day 1, 5 mg every 8 hours IV; on day 2, 25 mg every 8 hours IV; then discontinue.

Trimethoprim-sulfa, 1 tablet orally twice daily
Antacid, 30 ml every 2 hours
Docusate sodium (Colace), 200 mg orally twice daily
Dextran 40 (Rheomacrodex), 25 ml/hour (0.25 mg/kg/hour) for 14 days
Cefazolin sodium, 1 g IV every 8 hours for 5 days
For immunosuppression, cyclosporine, 4 mg/kg/24 hours IV; cyclosporine, 14 mg orally; prednisone, 15 mg/kg orally; azathioprine, 1 mg/kg orally; and antithymocyte globulin.

Study Orders

Typical postoperative study orders include the following:

Immediate. CBC and determination of platelets, electrolytes, creatinine, and blood urea nitrogen postoperatively, and every 4 hours for 24 hours; PT, PTT, and arterial blood gases immediately postoperatively and every 6 hours for 24 hours; fingerstick glucose measurement every hour for 24 hours, then every 2 hours for 24 hours. When the patient is taking oral medications at 8 AM, 4 PM, and 10 PM, fingersticks are obtained.

Daily. CBC and levels of platelets, electrolytes, coagulation factors, amylase, lipase, C-peptide, and cyclosporine are determined.

Weekly. Liver function tests (LFTs); determination of calcium, phosporus, and magnesium; examination of stool for *C. difficile* toxin; and urine and blood viral titers are done.

On the first postoperative day, a technetium renal and pancreas scan is obtained.

The hospital stay for a pancreas transplant averages about 50 days. The sutures (staples) are not removed for 3 weeks to allow healing of the incision. Because the objective of the treatment is to remove exogenous insulin therapy, the recipient uses home glucose monitoring on a daily basis while in the hospital.

Postdischarge Follow-up

Patients need to visit the transplant clinic daily initially, then twice weekly, and later at increasing intervals.

Monthly tests include sustacal challenge, IV glucose tolerance test, 24-hour serum and urine glucose determination (every 3 hours), and determination of hemoglobin A_{1C}. Repeat the evaluation at 3, 6, and 12 weeks, and then every 6 months thereafter. Subjectively, most patients have noted an improvement in neuropathy after transplantation, usually within 6 to 8 months, which is distinctly different from the case for patients with diabetes who have received renal transplants (Corry et al., 1986).

Potential Surgical Complications

Some potential technical failures in pancreas transplantation are thrombosis, infection, inadequate preservation, hemorrhage, and ascites. It is easy for a vascular thrombosis to occur because the pancreas is an organ with a relatively low blood flow rate. To avoid thrombosis, some surgeons heparinize intraoperatively with 5000 U of heparin. Postoperatively, all patients receive an IV infusion of low-molecular-weight dextrose (Rheomacrodex); the dosage is 25 ml/hour for 5 days. Nasogastric suction is used only for abdominal or gastric distention.

The best results occur when the grafts are flushed with cold (4°C) lactated Ringer solution (with heparin, 1000 U/L) and stored for up to 6 hours. Some institutions choose to store in a hyperosmolar silicon gel–filtered plasma solution, and these grafts last up to 24 hours.

Duct injection can contribute to technical failure because often fibrosis and islet loss are induced by the duct injection, causing rejection (Sutherland et al., 1984). Great care must be taken during the retrieval of the pancreas to avoid handling or traumatizing the pancreas, which might lead to subsequent pancreatitis in the recipient, resulting in graft thrombosis.

Some surgeons and physicians believe that graft survivals are dependent on matching HLA and using triple therapy (i.e., cyclosporine, azathioprine, and prednisone versus cyclosporine and prednisone).

LIVER TRANSPLANTATION

Definition

Liver transplantation is surgery performed for patients whose life is threatened by liver disease or whose life style is seriously affected by the disease. An orthotopic liver transplant is the last resort, considering all medical and surgical therapy. Patients with advanced liver disease should be considered as early as possible for a transplant to improve their chances of survival.

Indications

Candidates for transplant usually have cirrhosis from any one of multiple causes, including hepatitis B, non-A, non-B hepatitis causing postnecrotic cirrhosis, cryptogenic cirrhosis, and primary biliary sclerosis. Sclerosing cholangitis and inborn errors of metabolism are also indications for transplantation. On an experimental basis, transplant surgery is performed for tumor that is untreatable by any other method. In children 18 years or younger, biliary atresia is the most frequent medical diagnosis for transplant.

Related Surgical Procedures

The harvesting of the donor liver is a similar procedure because the entire liver is freed. In addition, a liver lobectomy or resection involves the same anatomical features.

Perioperative Nursing Implications

The circulator needs to know when the patient is due to arrive in the OR and the time the surgical incision is to be made. The availability of all the supplies necessary for the procedure should be ascertained. The perfusionists should be informed of the procedure and when they should arrive. Transport personnel should be notified of the need for a runner to carry blood specimens to the laboratory during the procedure.

Anesthesia

Because these procedures are labor intensive, many institutions have formed a liver transplant team in their anesthesia department. This has, in most cases, led to better managed patient care.

After being informed of a liver transplant, anesthesia personnel immediately begin to set up the room. The room temperature is raised to 80°F, the OR bed is checked and padded with eggcrate and sacral padding, and the hypothermia blanket (set at 32°C) is applied. All the intravenous lines are primed prior to the patient's arrival. The patient arrives approximately 1 to 1½ hours before the incision. The patient first gets one radial arterial and one peripheral IV catheter. Anesthesia is then induced, and the patient is intubated. Patients are considered to have a full stomach (owing to ascites and so on), so narcotic relaxants (fentanyl and sufentanil) and pancuronium bromide are used. Cricoid pressure is applied for intubation.

After the patient is anesthetized, the other radial arterial catheter is placed. Two 8½ Fr. venous ports (convert peripheral IV to 8½ Fr.) are placed for rapid infusion equipment, one in the right antecubital fossa, the other in the left internal jugular vein. The right internal jugular vein is used for the Swan-Ganz catheter for monitoring, including the central venous pressure, pulmonary arterial pressure, and cardiac output. The left arm is kept intact for venovenous bypass.

An esophageal temperature probe and a rectal temperature probe are inserted and monitored by anesthesia personnel. The anesthetist makes final checks by calling the blood bank to be sure that the whole blood, packed red blood cells, platelets, and cryoprecipitate have been ordered. He or she also checks to be sure that a runner is available to take blood gas specimens to the laboratory.

The procedure begins, and the patient is maintained on oxygen and a potent anesthetic agent, such as enflurane and isoflurane (Forane), narcotics, and a relaxant. A nasogastric tube is passed and kept on intermittent suction. Physiological monitoring is achieved through the arterial catheter; central venous pressure and pulmonary arterial pressure, through cardiac output monitoring; and temperature, through probes. The blood loss is controlled through the use of the organ beam coagulator. The cell saver is used to monitor and replace blood. The rapid infuser is used to replace large volumes of lost blood. Coagulation is monitored in several ways: the thromboelastogram enables assessment of the reaction time, the formation and lysis of thrombus, PT, and PTT; platelet and fibrinogen levels are also monitored. Anesthesia personnel then adjust their treatment according to these results and ascertain whether to give a blood product.

Before the anhepatic phase of the hepatectomy, venovenous bypass is used, if indicated. Indications include patients with marginal kidney function, reoperation for liver transplant, anticipated difficult anastomosis, and patients who cannot tolerate clamping of the vena cava. This system extracts blood from the lower part of the body and eliminates a large part of the venous circulation. With the axillary vein returning the arterial blood, the head is still perfused; however, the major venous drainage (vena cava and portal vein) is obstructed and it is easier to compress these vessels. The rapid infuser is used to support the circulation by giving large volumes of blood. Before the clamps are removed, the anesthetist anticipates a fall in cardiac output and peripheral resistance. The rapid infuser can deliver up to 1 L/minute or the pressure can be supported with inotropes (e.g., epinephrine). If citrate toxicity occurs in the blood, causing acidosis, high doses of calcium chloride and bicarbonate may need to be given.

At the end of the procedure, the patient is escorted to the intensive care unit and is intubated and ventilated for at least 24 hours.

Position

Proper positioning is paramount owing to the duration of the surgery. The OR bed is padded with an eggcrate mattress cut to fit the width of the bed. A warming blanket in a protective cover is placed on top of the eggcrate mattress. The control outlets are passed off at the upper right side of the OR bed. The heating blanket and eggcrate mattress are then covered with a bath blanket, which is tucked in under the mattress. A square piece of eggcrate padding is put in a pillowcase covered with a draw sheet and placed under the sacrum. A disposable safety strap is used across the thighs. The arm boards are also cushioned with eggcrate padding. Both arms are kept on arm boards for the entire procedure. ECG leads should be put on the patient's back. A Foley catheter and rectal probe are inserted and taped together to the inside of the thigh. An electrocautery pad and an argon beam grounding pad are placed on the thigh. Heel booties are applied to the feet. The legs are placed together with Webril bandages at the ankles so that the knees are slightly relaxed. A pillow is placed under the knees.

Creation and Maintenance of the Sterile Field

The patient is shaved and prepared from the neck to the thighs, including both axillae. A plastic drape is attached to the base of the OR bed by the circulating nurse to protect it from dripping blood. Bath blankets are taped to the floor around the OR bed to prevent blood pooling.

The OR furniture is strategically placed and the perfusionists set up on the left side of the OR bed. The Mayo stand goes over the patient's lower legs. The large back table is perpendicular to the OR bed. The large platform stool is in front of the back table. The small square drape table sits next to the back table. The medium-sized rectangular perfusion table runs parrallel to the OR bed. The ice machine (to make slush) is at the back of the scrub nurse's stools. The hypothermia or hyperthermia blanket is at the top right, along with the AG Bovie electrosurgical unit. The second AG Bovie electrosurgical unit is at the top left.

The scrub nurse's most important priority is to be scrubbed and set up early. It is an enormous task to set up and prepare the room for a liver transplant. Keeping up the pace is especially difficult for the circulator; therefore, if the scrub nurse sets up early, the circulator is free to help anesthesia personnel and the surgeons. Another important factor is thoroughly double checking that supplies and equipment needed are available either in the OR or on the liver cart just outside the room, again to ease the job of the circulator.

The patient is draped with double towels across the sternal notch, leaving the axillae exposed, down the nipple line, and to the midthigh. All towels are then clipped with towel clips. All subsequent drapes should be double sewn on with 2–0 silk cutting sutures (may substitute skin clips for sutures). Sterile incise drape strips are attached to the side of the patient to keep the drapes dry (this is optional). The scrub nurse should have extra drapes and gowns available throughout the procedure.

Equipment and Supplies

Impervious back table covers (two), a Mayo stand cover, towel packs (two), patient drape packs (two), laparotomy sponges, 4 × 8 sponges, dental rolls, an electrocautery pencil and extension tip, hand-held argon beam pencil, suction tubing, bulb syringes, a 10-ml control-top syringe, a 20-ml syringe, suture boots, vessel loops, Fogarty inserts, a sterile paper bag, a needle counter, a marking pen, labels, IV tubing (sterile), an ice machine drape and scoop, French-eye needles, a cholangiocatheter, T-tubes of various sizes, and French feeding tubes of various sizes are needed. A bile bag and (optional) closed suction reservoir drain are needed. A Foley catheter and urine drain set; Nos. 10, 11, and 15 blades; and No. 25 gauge, 5/8 inch needle are assembled. Skin clips and 4 × 4 inch dressings are needed.

Suture needs can vary, dependent on the presence of an incision from previous surgery. It is best to have a specialized cart with all the suture possibly needed for a liver transplant on it. To start the procedure one should have

1–0 and 2–0 silk ties

2–0 and 4–0 silk taper needle (pop-offs)

2–0 silk taper needle on cutting or staples—for drapes

2–0 polypropylene taper needle

3–0, 4–0, and 5–0 polypropylene taper needle, double-armed

6–0 and 7–0 polypropylene, double-armed on a cardiovascular needle

5–0, 6–0, and 7–0 single-armed sutures available for patches

Hernia tape, 36 inches

3–0 polyglactin 910 on a tapered needle

4–0 polyglactin 910 on a cutting needle

5–0 PDS

6–0 absorbable monofilament

Suture for closing the incision could be obtained at the end of surgery and should include

No. 2 polypropylene

0 braided nylon pop-off

1–0 PDS

3–0 polyglactin 910

Before the procedure begins, the circulator or scrub nurse attaches the self-retaining retractor clamps, upper hand, or iron interne retractors, on the patient's upper right and left side above the arm boards.

The required instruments include the self-retaining retractor clamps, upper hand, or Iron interne retractors, a liver set, elephant and extradeep Deaver retractors, extralong instrument pack, a sterile metal ice cube tray, a basin set, and a gallbladder pack under the table. In the liver set are several vascular clamps: they are Julian Potts, straight Potts coarctation, bronchus, Beck aortic, curved Potts, and large curved Potts clamps.

The perfusion table should be set up with four layers of drapes, and on it should be one large basin, one solution basin, two angled Potts clamps, one tenotomy scissors, one regular Metzenbaum scissors, two Sarot needle holders, two vascular forceps (7 inch), six rubber shodded mosquito forceps, six straight mosquito forceps, a Pomeroy adaptor with a 20-ml syringe, 4–0 silk ties (two packages), 4–0 silk pop-offs (eight each), 2–0 silk ties (two packages), 2–0 silk pop-offs (eight each), one Asepto syringe, and one needle counter.

The Mayo stand should be set up with staples or 2–0 silk taper needle (cutting) to sew drapes on, hernia tapes (10 each, 36 inches), 1–0 silk ties (two packages), 4–0 silk ties (two packages), right-angled clamp (two), Crile clamps (four), Potts dissecting scissors, and Rumel stylet with four rubber shods (4 inches each).

Drugs and Solutions

Ringer irrigation, 4 L for ice machine and 4 L on ice as back-up

1 bag of 1 L of lactated Ringer solution, alcohol, and sterile water to prime the ice machine

4 L of sterile or tap water to fill the reservoir in the hypothermia or hyperthermia blanket

Heparin (1 L) to mix in various concentrations

Normal saline solution for irrigation (have several liters warm, with bacitracin, 5000 U, and kanamycin, 0.5 g, each in a liter for irrigation)

Physiological Monitoring

Blood loss may be massive and is difficult to measure. Many sponges are wet and this must be taken into consideration. Often, on entering the peritoneum, the surgeon encounters ascites; usually, this fluid is measured separately from the actual blood loss. Blood loss can be extensive and suction liners need to be saved and tagged with the amount. To save time from constantly changing suction liners, use quadsuctions, which allow four canisters to fill before they need to be changed. The Foley catheter drainage is tracked by anesthesia personnel.

Specimens and Cultures

All nonscrubbed personnel in a liver transplant procedure should wear a protective gown and nonsterile gloves at all times. All specimens leaving the room should be double bagged and labeled as "blood and body fluid precautions" or "hepatitis precautions."

The donor liver is biopsied at the back (perfusion) table usually with a TruCut needle. This specimen is labeled time zero biopsy and placed in Bouin fixative and placed in the pathology laboratory refrigerator for evaluation in less than 24 hours. The vessels (vein and artery) that come with the donor liver are placed in the OR refrigerator with the recipient's name and date on the vial. These vessels are saved for 1 week in case a patch is needed for the artery or vein anastomosis. Lymph nodes from the donor have to be sent for tissue typing. Individual institutional policy determines how the tissue typing department is notified to receive the specimen. The native liver is double bagged in small plastic trash bags. It is kept fresh and placed in the pathology laboratory refrigerator for routine analysis. Any other blood samples to be transported or "mailed" via a pneumatic tube system should be bagged and labeled as "blood and body fluid precautions" or "hepatitis precautions." If a TruCut biopsy specimen is taken from the donor liver after it is sewn in, this is also fixed and put in the refrigerator for evaluation in less than 24 hours.

Physician's Orders

If the patient has never been evaluated for a liver transplant, she or he must be admitted as a liver transplant candidate. This involves a magnitude of tests, including CBC with differential leukocyte count, platelet count, sedimentation rate, reticulocyte count, iron level, total iron-binding capacity, PT, PTT, and levels of ferritin, carcinoembryonic antigen, calcium phosphorus, electrolytes, blood urea nitrogen, creatinine, glucose, magnesium, uric acid, amylase, ammonia, bilirubin (total and direct), serum glutamic-pyruvic transaminase, serum glutamic-oxaloacetic transaminase, lactate dehydrogenase, gamma-glutamyl transpeptidase (GGT), alkaline phosphatase, triglycerides, cholesterol, total protein, albumin, antinuclear antibodies, anti–smooth muscle antibody, alpha-fetoprotein, ceruloplasmin, alpha$_1$-antitrypsin, anti–hepatitis A virus, immunoglobulin G, immunoglobulin M, hepatitis B surface antigen and antibody, hepatitis B core antibody, and hepatitis C antibody. Testing for ABO type and screen, human immunodeficiency virus, coagulation profile, HLA typing, 24-hour urine for nitrogen, urinary sodium and potassium, and serum titers for cytomegalovirus, Epstein-Barr virus, and herpes virus is performed. Consultations with cardiology, pulmonology, psychiatry, gastrointestinal, nutritional support, anesthesia, and gynecology (Papanicolaou smear) departments are ordered. A chest x-ray film; ECG; computed tomographic scan of the abdomen to evaluate pancreas, portal vein, spleen size, focal liver disease, and calculate liver volume; ultrasound of the abdomen to evaluate portal vein potency, liver and spleen size, status of common bile duct, intrahepatic ducts and gallbladder, evidence of ascites or pancreatic disease; and a Doppler ultrasound of the portal system with a fatty meal per hospital protocol are obtained.

If the patient has already been evaluated and listed as a candidate by the transplant team, the following preoperative orders are instituted on admission:

1. Maintain the patient's NPO status.
2. Consult with the anesthesia department.
3. Obtain the patient's consent to the orthotopic liver transplant.
4. Type and cross-match for 20 U of packed red blood cells, 20 U of fresh-frozen plasma, and 20 U of platelets.
5. Send to the OR with the patient: ampicillin, 1 g IV; ceftriaxone, 1 g IV; and cyclosporine, 2 mg/kg IV.

Laboratory and Diagnostic Studies

Immediate preoperative studies include determination of CBC, electrolytes, blood urea nitrogen, creatinine, glucose, PT, PTT, platelets, total and direct bilirubin, serum glutamic-pyruvic transaminase, serum glutamic-oxaloacetic transaminase, gamma-glutamyl transpeptidase, lactate dehydrogenase, alkaline phosphatase, albumin, total protein, calcium, magnesium, and phosporus. An ECG and chest x-ray film (posteroanterior and lateral) are obtained. Blood is drawn for tissue typing (three green-topped and 1 red-topped tubes). Flow cytometry is performed. Viral cultures of blood, urine, and throat and serum titers for cytomegalovirus, herpes virus, Epstein-Barr virus, and human immunodeficiency virus are performed.

Procedure

Incision and Exposure

For cannulation, there are probably two teams of surgeons, one at the axilla and the other at the groin. They need 4 × 8 sponges, a No. 10 knife, electrocautery (two), and Weitlaner retractors (two) for exposing the axillary and groin incision. Potts dissecting scissors and vascular forceps (7 inch) along with Jackson clamps to expose the axillary and saphenous vein are used. Hernia tapes with Rumel tourniquets are applied to the vein and artery and hemostats are used to tag the hernia tapes.

A large bilateral subcostal incision with a midline extension is made on the abdomen. Because these patients have portal hypertension and active fibrinolysis, care must be taken to maintain hemostasis. Electrocautery and 2–0 and 4–0 silk suture ligatures are used. Potts dissecting scissors and vascular forceps, along with hemostats and Mixter clamps, are used for the dissection.

The side rails and traction bar of the self-retaining retractor are attached and adjusted vertically and horizontally. Two traction devices and crossbar are positioned with the largest retractor blades. The blades are positioned subcostally on the right and left sides of the chest. The dissection continues until the anterior and posterior aspects of the liver are freed up. An occasional 2–0 Prolene suture is used to patch holes made in the diaphragm. Long dental rolls on a long Kelly clamp may be used to free up the suprahepatic vena cava. Do not take down the hepatic artery until the donor liver is in the room. Do not take down the right triangular ligament until the patient is undergoing bypass.

The perfusionists should be in the room if bypass is to be used.

Details

Preparation of the Donor Liver

During the dissection, the donor liver is inspected and prepared at the back table by the harvesting surgeons. It is floated in a basin of Ringer irrigation slush. The temperature should remain constant at 4°C (room temperature or cold Ringer irrigation may need to be added to achieve the proper temperature). All vessels are checked for leaks. The inferior vena cava is clamped with an angled Potts clamp and flushed with Ringer solution in a bulb syringe. The same procedure is used for the suprahepatic vena cava. Leaks are patched with 2–0 and 4–0 silk ties and taper needles.

Cannulation

For venovenous bypass, the next phase includes cannulation. The Gott aneurysm shunt tubing is heparin bonded and comes in two sizes: 7 mm (two) and 9 mm (one). These cannulas are trimmed and primed using saline, then clamped with a tubing clamp to prevent

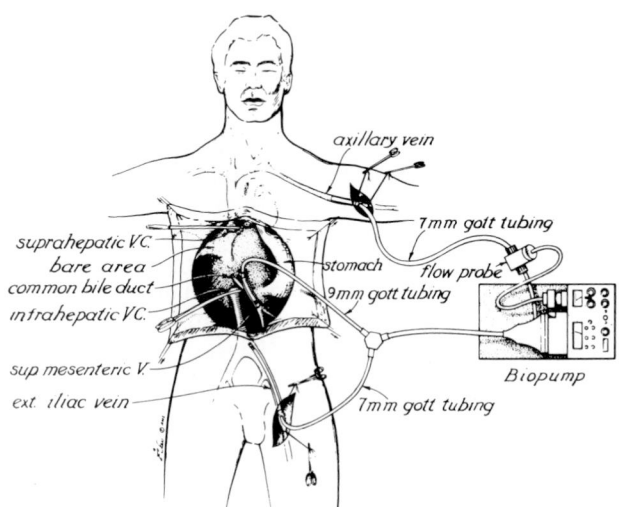

FIGURE 23–4. Anhepatic phase of orthotopic liver transplantation showing the use of venous bypass. Tubing circuits that are completely heparin bonded are now commercially available, obviating the use of Gott shunts. (From Flye, M. W. [1989]. *Principles of organ transplantation* [p. 359]. Philadelphia: W. B. Saunders.)

back bleeding after they are inserted. A 7-mm cannula is used to drain the blood from the inferior vena cava. The saphenous vein is tied off distally with a 2–0 silk tie; the No. 11 blade and angled Potts scissors are used for venotomy. The cannula is inserted up through the saphenofemoral venous junction to the common iliac vein junction. The second 7-mm cannula, which carries the return venous circulation, is inserted into the axillary vein using the same technique. A mini-Cooley clamp is used to clamp the axillary vein distally. The 9-mm cannula is used to pull the visceral blood via the portal vein. The technique for insertion is intense. A large Kelly clamp is placed on the proximal end of the portal vein, and the vein is ligated. The surgeon occludes the portal vein with her or his hand, removes the clamp, and then applies three Crile clamps to the cut end of the portal vein to triangulate it. The surgeon, still holding the vein, slides the clamped 9-mm cannula into the portal vein and then passes a hernia tape around the vein to secure the cannula. The cannulas are then filled with saline and connected with a plastic ⅜-inch Y-connector to the tubing coming from the centrifugal blood pump. All tubing clamps are removed, and the perfusionist is in charge of the flow. The cannulas are secured to the drapes with umbilical tapes and Kocher clamps. (This technique does not require systemic anticoagulation.)

Hepatectomy

After bypass, little dissection should be left. The triangular ligament is taken down using the electrocautery, 2–0 silk ties and taper needles, and 2–0 polypropylene taper needles (three) to ligate the deep vessels. The hepatectomy ensues: the suprahepatic vena cava is cross-clamped with a Potts gastrointestinal clamp, the infrahepatic vena cava is cross-clamped (with a large

angled Potts clamp), and the native liver is removed (Fig. 23–4). All major vessels are prepared for anastomosis using Potts scissors and vascular forceps to make the cuff.

Anastomosis

In preparation for the suprahepatic vena cava anastomosis, three 3–0 double-armed polypropylene sutures are placed in the recipient side of the vena cava first (Fig. 23–5). The donor liver is then brought up from the back table and held steady by several surgeons, while one surgeon completes the anastomosis. The infrahepatic vena cava is anastomosed with two 4–0 double-armed polypropylene sutures. When the anastomosis is half completed, the circulator places 1 liter of cold albumin (5%), which is connected to the field via sterile IV tubing that is passed off by the scrub nurse. The sterile end is hooked up to the plastic cannula that is in the donor liver. This albumin (approximately 500 to 800 ml) is used to flush out from the donor liver the potassium used in its preservation.

The surgeon then takes a tubing clamp and clamps the portal vein cannula to prevent air embolus through the venovenous bypass system. The portal cannula is then removed. A small angled Potts Cooley clamp is used to reclamp the actual portal vein. The vein is then flushed with saline and the anastomosis is completed using 6–0 double-armed polypropylene suture (four). (Systemic venovenous bypass continues via the saphenous and axillary cannulas.) After the portal vein anastomosis is completed, all vascular clamps are removed. The scrub nurse should have 4–0, 5–0, and 6–0 polypropylene suture ready. In conjunction with the anesthesiologist, the surgeon decides to terminate bypass. Have available three tubing clamps and many laparotomy sponges for packs.

The hepatic artery anastomosis is done next with two 7–0 or 6–0 double-armed polypropylene sutures. The surgeon may desire a Castroviejo needle holder. If the artery is in spasm, he or she may ask for papaverine

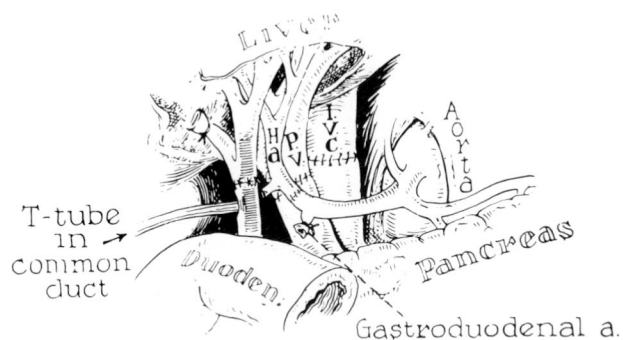

FIGURE 23–5. Most frequently used methods of vascular and biliary reconstruction in orthotopic liver transplantation. Most often, the arterial anastomosis is made in an end-to-end fashion between the donor celiac axis and the recipient common hepatic artery, proximal to the takeoff of the recipient gastroduodenal artery. (From Flye, M. W. [1989]. *Principles of organ transplantation* [p. 358]. Philadelphia: W. B. Saunders.)

injection (2 ml/10 ml of normal saline, or 30 mg/ml in a syringe with a 25-gauge needle). After this anastomosis is completed, the abdomen is packed and the incision is temporarily closed with simple large retention sutures. For the next ½ hour, the axillary vein is repaired with 6–0 and 7–0 polypropylene suture or ligated, and the saphenous vein is tied off. The groin and axillary incisions are closed in multiple layers of 3–0 polyglactin 910 and 4–0 polyglactin 910 interrupted subcuticular sutures. When the abdomen is reentered, the scrub nurse should have warm saline to irrigate.

Two methods of biliary reconstruction are used: a Roux-en-Y choledochojejunostomy and an end-to-end choledochocholedochostomy. The Roux-en-Y can be hand sewn or can use the gastrointestinal stapler. In either method, the jejunum is transected at a comfortable distance from the ligament of Treitz. The distal end is brought through a hole created in the transverse mesocolon ("retrocolic"). The proximal end is anastomosed end to side if hand sewn or side to side if stapled. The jejunum is clamped using Allen clamps, bowel clamps, or angled Potts clamps and is divided with electrocautery. Alternatively, the jejunum is transected with a gastrointestinal stapler. The anastomosis (usually end to side) is completed with a single layer of simple interrupted 5–0 or 6–0 absorbable suture (Wall et al., 1988). For a duct-to-duct repair, the donor and recipient common bile ducts are first approximated with full-thickness posterior stay sutures. An opening is made on the recipient's common bile duct for exit of the T-tube. Again, a simple but precise mucosa-to-mucosa anastomosis is performed with 5–0 absorbable suture. The scrub nurse should have a probe and French-eye needles available for this type of repair. A cholangiogram is taken via the T-tube, cholangiographic catheter, or French feeding tube to check the common bile duct anastomosis. Full-strength iothalamate meglumine (Conray) is used (no more than 5 ml). A cholecystectomy is performed on the donor liver.

Closure

All anastomoses are checked for leaks. If the surgeons are satisfied that there is no surgical bleeding, packs are removed and closure is begun. Warm antibiotic irrigation (bacitracin and kanamycin) is poured into the abdomen.

No. 2 polypropylene suture is used continuously to close the posterior rectus sheath and the peritoneum. Interrupted nylon suture is used to close the midline extension and the anterior rectus fascia. More antibiotic saline is instilled for irrigation. Braided absorbable 3–0 suture is used for subcutaneous fat and tissue. Clips are used on the skin.

The patient is thoroughly cleaned, and dressings are placed. The skin sutures holding the drapes need to be carefully removed, and the patient is again checked for cleanliness. Warm blankets are placed on top of the patient, and the patient is transferred to the surgical intensive care unit bed.

After the patient leaves the OR, all surfaces that came in contact with the patient's fluids are cleaned with 1:10 bleach (Clorox) solution instead of detergent. The instruments are either washed with glutaraldehyde (Cidex) solution or passed through the washer sterilizer. The OR floor is cleaned with bleach solution wherever one sees blood or fluid. The room is then cleaned thoroughly by the housekeeping department. The door to the room should remain labeled "hepatitis precautions." The eggcrate mattress and hypothermia blanket should be disposed of. (If the hypothermia blanket is reusable, it should be cleaned and double bagged and sent to the central supply department to be gas sterilized.) After the surgical case, the nurses can clean and restock the liver cart.

Postoperative Care

The postoperative care of these patients is extremely complicated. They have just undergone from 6 to 24 hours of surgery and are listed in critical condition. Their vital signs need to be taken every 15 minutes until their condition is stable, then hourly; hourly central venous pressure and intake and output measurements are obtained; they are kept NPO and on bed rest until they are extubated and then are allowed up as tolerated. They receive respiratory care according to the intensive care unit protocol; their Foley catheter is kept connected to closed gravity drainage. The T-tube is connected to closed drainage. The nasogastric tube is connected to low continuous suction and irrigated every 2 hours with 30 ml of normal saline solution. The patient is turned every 2 hours. Endotracheal suctioning is performed every 4 hours. Postural drainage and clamping are done every 4 hours. IV fluids (5% dextrose in half-normal saline) are given at 125 ml/hour. Medications include

Cyclosporine, 2 mg/kg IV per day as a continuous infusion
Methylprednisolone, 50 mg IV every 6 hours for four doses, 40 mg IV every 6 hours for four doses, 30 mg IV every 6 hours for four doses, 20 mg IV every 6 hours for four doses, 20 mg IV every 12 hours for two doses, and then 20 mg IV once per day
Azathioprine, 1.5 mg/kg day IV
Ampicillin, 1 g IV every 6 hours for 5 days
Ceftriaxone, 1 g IV every 12 hours for 5 days
Nystatin, 5 ml swish and swallow or via nasogastric tube four times daily
Magaldrate (Riopan), 30 ml via nasogastric tube every 2 hours

Keep 4 U of packed red blood cells on hold.

The postoperative study orders are similar to preoperative orders. Immediate laboratory testing is performed every 6 hours for 48 hours; more extensive laboratory testing is done daily. Chest x-ray films are obtained immediately postoperatively and then daily. A Doppler sonogram is ordered to check the patency of the hepatic artery. Daily cyclosporine levels are checked by high performance liquid chromatography (HPLC) ½ hour before the morning dose. A cytomegalovirus titer and post-transplant antibody determination are obtained weekly.

Potential Surgical Complications

Immediate postoperative complications include hemorrhage (first 24 hours), technical complications affecting the function of the liver, rejection, and infection. Hemorrhage is often cause for reoperation. Since liver transplants began, there have been scientific advances in decreasing mortality. The venovenous bypass technique has resulted in a marked decrease in intraoperative blood loss, and the rapid infusion pump has improved cardiodynamic stability during the anhepatic phase.

HEART TRANSPLANTATION

Definition

A heart transplant is the surgical removal of the native heart; usually it is performed for a person who is younger than 65 years old and has end-stage heart failure. There is agreement that all other medical and surgical modalities should have been exhausted. The ailing heart is then replaced with a healthy donated heart.

Indications

New York Heart Association class IV congestive heart failure that is refractory to maximal medical therapy and/or conventional surgery and expected survival of 6 months without a transplant are indications. A complete cardiac evaluation is required before a patient is listed for possible transplant. The results of the evaluation should show ejection fraction less than 20%, pulmonary vascular resistance less than 6 Wood units, and maximal oxygen consumption less than 12 ml/kg/minute. The majority of these patients have either end-stage coronary artery disease or cardiomyopathy.

Related Surgical Procedures

In heterotopic heart transplantation, the native heart is left in place and the new heart is "piggy-backed" onto the old heart, augmenting its function.

Perioperative Nursing Implications

The circulator should be informed as to the accurate time schedule for the procedure. She or he should be sure that health care team members from other disciplines (e.g., perfusionists and anesthesia personnel) are aware of the case. Some history regarding the recipient should be known (e.g., previous cardiac surgery, any special precautions needed, and whether the family is present). Have preparation solutions, a Foley catheter, and a rectal probe ready.

Anesthesia

Because patients often have failure of other organ systems secondary to heart failure, the integrity of renal, hepatic, and hemostatic functions is of particular importance in addition to routine anesthetic considerations. Because patients will be immunosuppressed, strict aseptic technique is critical, and invasive monitors that have been in place for more than 48 hours are routinely changed before anesthesia induction. Anesthetic premedication is rarely given because of the recipient's cardiac status; however, some sedation may be necessary because of the patient's anxiety level.

Most transplant recipients receive oral immunosuppressive agents (cyclosporine and azathioprine) preoperatively; therefore, they must be considered to have a full stomach. These patients have general anesthesia, but it is 95% narcotic induced (fentanyl, sufentanil); pancuronium bromide (Pavulon) is given for muscle relaxation. A Swan-Ganz catheter is preferentially placed via the left internal jugular vein to preserve the right internal jugular vein for postoperative endomyocardial biopsies. An 80-cm sheath is used to permit intraoperative withdrawal and repositioning. A radial arterial catheter and two peripheral IV catheters are inserted. Preoperative antibiotics (cefazolin or vancomycin) are given in the OR after establishing IV access.

Anesthesia is not induced until the procurement team inspects the donor heart. The time of induction is chosen so that the arrival of the heart and the initiation of bypass coincide. After anesthesia induction, the patient is intubated, nasopharyngeal temperature probe and a nasogastric tube are placed, and the Swan-Ganz catheter is withdrawn to 15 cm so it is removed from the surgical field. Heparinization, cannulation, and cardiopulmonary bypass commence.

After the new heart is attached, it is weaned from bypass slowly. The denervated, recently transplanted heart from a donor of different size and with different pulmonary and systemic afterloads usually necessitates customized pharmacological intervention. In addition, the recipient may demonstrate an elevated pulmonary vascular resistance and right-sided heart failure owing to this increased load on the transplanted heart. Anesthetics are titrated according to the left ventricular function, assuming that the new heart has normal coronary arteries. Isoproterenol is the drug of choice. Communication with the surgeon is imperative to diagnose and treat cardiac dysfunction. The Swan-Ganz catheter is repositioned in the pulmonary artery and heparin action is reversed. If coagulation abnormalities exist, they should be treated, usually with fresh-frozen plasma and platelets.

Position

The patient is supine with a safety strap across the thighs. The arms are tucked at the side and toboggans are used to protect them.

Creation and Maintenance of the Sterile Field

The patient's chest is shaved or, if time permits, a depilatory is used before transfer to the OR; both sides of the groin are also shaved. The patient is prepared from the chin to the midthigh down the nipple line. (Side towels are used.) Sterile towels are used to square off the field and a large impervious sheet is used to drape the entire body, with sterile incise drape segments for the chest and groins.

The scrub nurse sets up in plenty of time. The patients are often in critical condition and many times have had previous cardiac surgery. If this information is known ahead of time the necessary equipment, such as oscillating saw, bone hooks, and Fogarty clamps and inserts, can be obtained. The back (perfusion) table should be set up before the arrival of the heart.

The patient is draped with his or her head at anesthesia machine and his or her legs by the scrub nurse. The Mayo stand goes over the patient's legs; the large back instrument table is at the foot of the OR bed perpendicular to the OR bed; a square back table is kept with gowns and gloves; and an additional rectangular back table (perfusion table) is needed for preparing the donor heart.

Equipment and Supplies

Equipment needed for the procedure includes a sternal saw motor and foot switch, an electrocautery unit, a defibrillator with external and sterile internal paddles, a cell saver, and a heart-lung machine, headlight sources, standing stools, and kick buckets.

Supplies needed for the procedure include an open heart set; a sternal saw and cord; sterile light handles; Nos. 10, 11, and 15 knife blades; laparotomy sponges; 4 × 8 sponges; dissectors; electrocautery pencil and electrocautery pad; suction tubing; a needle counter; 16 Fr. Foley catheter; urine drain set; two No. 22 red rubber catheters; a 50-ml syringe; felt; alligator cables (for pacing); chest tubes (two angled and one straight); a disposable water seal drainage system; and gowns and drapes.

Suture needed for the procedure includes 1–0 braided polyester fiber suture taper needle, hernia tape, 1–0 braided nonabsorbable suture ties, pledgets, four temporary pacing wires, 3–0 and 4–0 polypropylene, No. 6 stainless steel wire, and 1–0, 3–0, and 4–0 braided absorbable suture.

The heart set should include a chest retractor (child and adult), vascular forceps, needle holders, scissors and clamps, basic laparotomy instruments, Rumel stylets, and a nerve hook.

Drugs and Solutions

Ringer irrigation, cold
Saline irrigation, cold

Physiological Monitoring

Blood loss is calculated by anesthesia personnel and the perfusionists; sponges need not be weighed. Urine output is monitored by anesthesia personnel. An external pacemaker is given to anesthesia personnel in case the heart needs to be paced as bypass is discontinued.

Specimens and Cultures

The native heart is double bagged and sent fresh to the pathology department.

Physician's Orders

Because heart transplants are complicated, there are several routes by which patients can be admitted to the hospital: they can be transferred from another facility, they can be admitted from home, or they can be inpatients transferred to the heart transplant service. Depending on where the patient is in the system, he or she is either admitted for a pretransplant evaluation or simply admitted to be transplanted because he or she was already placed on the active transplant list. All of the communication needs to start in the admissions office. The heart transplant coordinator should also be notified, and he or she can then contact the business office.

Preoperative orders include maintaining NPO status, except for medications. Depilatory preparation (for men and women) extends from the chin to midthigh and from anterior axillary line to anterior axillary line. Depilatory preparation includes both groin triangles; hair preparation areas are painted with povidone-iodine (Betadine). The patient urinates prior to coming to the OR. Weigh the patient and note it on the front of the chart. Cyclosporine and azathioprine doses are given orally with 50 ml of milk or juice. The preoperative studies ordered include type and cross-match of red blood cells. Laboratory studies that are ordered immediately include CBC, platelet count, PT, PTT, serum electrolytes, blood urea nitrogen, creatinine, glucose, and total bilirubin level. A portable anteroposterior chest x-ray film is taken.

Laboratory and Diagnostic Studies

Numerous studies are done before a patient is listed on the active transplant list. The actual pretransplant evaluation is done on an outpatient basis, unless the candidate needs a left-sided heart catheterization. Some of the highlights include history and physical examination, routine laboratory studies, congestive heart failure evaluation, pulmonary function tests, HLA typing, % of reactive antibodies, dental evaluation, psychiatric screening, financial screening, social work evaluation, cardiac catheterization, and various other tests and cultures when clinically indicated. After the results of theses studies are available, the transplant committee reviews the data and makes a recommendation to list or further study the transplant candidate.

Procedure

Incision and Exposure

After the patient is prepared and draped, the pump lines are passed up and attached to the sterile field. A standard median sternotomy incision is made approximately 1 hour before the estimated time of arrival of the donor heart. If the patient has had previous heart surgery, more time is allowed. An oscillating saw is used, and adhesions are dissected free. The chest retractor is inserted and the pericardium is opened. A pericardial basket is made using 1–0 braided polyester fiber sutures (Belzer, 1985).

Details

After heparin administration, the ascending aorta is cannulated near the innominate artery takeoff and a left atrial vent catheter is inserted into the left atrium–right superior pulmonary vein junction to decompress the recipient heart and prevent acute pulmonary edema. The venae cavae are encircled with hernia tape, and pursestring sutures are placed. Both venae cavae are cannulated on the right lateral borders of the caval-atrial junctions to provide an adequate right atrial cuff (Fig. 23–6).

The donor heart is kept cool. At the back table, the pulmonary veins on the donor heart are opened to form a continuous left atrial circumference. Cardiopulmonary bypass is instituted, and systemic cooling to 28°C is begun. Caval slings are tightened, and the aortic cross-clamp is applied. The heart is excised, beginning with the aorta and the pulmonary artery just above the semilunar valves. Both ventricles, atrial appendages (only), and the coronary sinus are excised. There are four anastomoses, all are completed with a continuous 3–0 polypropylene suture.

The left atrial anastomosis is started at the recipient left superior pulmonary vein and the donor left atrial appendage. Continuous external cold saline is used to bathe the heart. A second dose of cardioplegia solution may be given. A topical cooling device is placed against the heart to keep it cool. The right atrial anastomosis is started near the right atrial superior caval junction. The right atrial opening is enlarged by incising the donor right atrium from the inferior vena cava to the base of the donor atrial appendage. This opening is sewn to the recipient right atrial cuff. To avoid injury to the SA

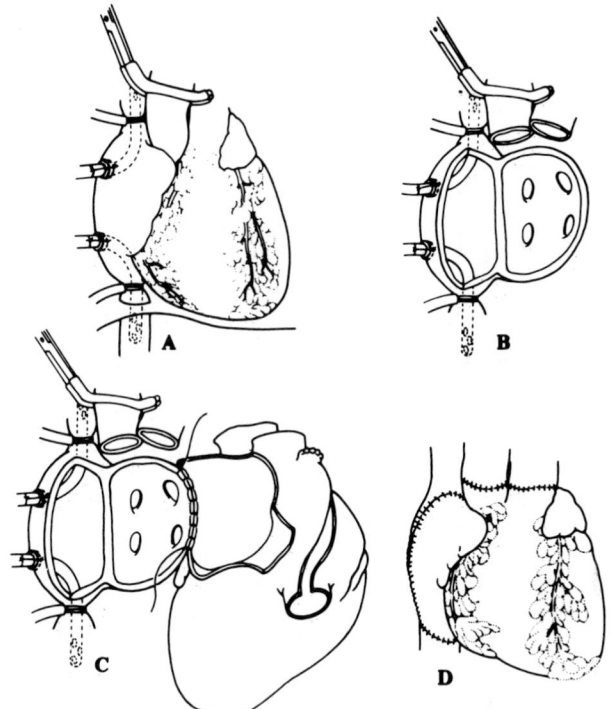

FIGURE 23–6. *A*, Cross-clamp applied and caval chokers tightened. *B*, Recipient atrial cuffs and great arteries. *C*, Left atrial anastomosis begun at the left superior pulmonary vein. *D*, Completed operation. (From Flye, M. W. [1989]. *Principles of organ transplantation* [p. 390]. Philadelphia: W. B. Saunders.)

node in the donor heart, the superior vena cava is ligated distal to the atrial-caval junction.

The pulmonary artery is anastomosed in an end-to-end fashion. Rewarming begins with the start of the aortic anastomosis. The aorta is anastomosed in an end-to-end-fashion. Caval slings are removed, and care is taken to remove air from the left side of the heart, the patient is positioned head down, and the aortic cross-clamp is removed. The heart is gradually resuscitated and the patient is weaned from cardiopulmonary bypass; two temporary pacing wires are placed on the donor right atrium and two on the ventricle. Internal paddles should be ready to perform cardioversion. An isoproterenol infusion (at 1 μg/minute) begins with the release of the aortic cross-clamp. When bypass stops, a dopamine infusion may be added. Nitroprusside is used as needed.

Closure

The aorta is decannulated and the site is oversewn with a 3–0 pledget of polypropylene suture. All anastomoses are checked for leaks, and 3–0 or 4–0 polypropylene suture is used for patching. The right pleural space is widely opened and drained with a No. 28 chest tube. The pericardial basket is released (and not closed). The edges of the pericardium and sternum are cauterized, and two mediastinal chest tubes are inserted. The Swan-Ganz catheter, placed before the operation, is repositioned in the pulmonary artery after that anastomosis is completed and before the chest is closed; it enables postoperative monitoring.

The sternum is closed with interrupted 6-gauge stainless steel wire. The fascia is closed so as to be watertight with a continuous 1–0 absorbable braided suture. The subcutaneous tissue is closed with a continuous 3–0 absorbable braided suture; the skin is closed with continuous 4–0 absorbable braided suture in a subcuticular fashion. Chest tubes are secured with 1–0 braided nonabsorbable suture. Chest tubes are connected to a closed water seal drainage system.

Postoperative Care

The heart transplant patient is admitted to a positive pressure room in the surgical intensive care unit. Personnel entering the room must wash their hands and wear masks. The patient wears a mask when he or she is out of the room. Gloves are worn when dealing with body fluids and wound care.

Vital signs are taken frequently; a nasogastric tube is connected to wall suction. Chest tubes are connected to a closed water seal drainage unit, which is set at −20 cm H_2O suction. A Foley catheter is connected to gravity drainage. Respiratory settings are determined by anesthesia personnel. Povidone-iodine is applied to the suture line daily. An attempt is made to limit total IV fluids, including vasoactive infusions.

Extubation should be accomplished as early as possible, usually on the first postoperative day. Early removal of chest tubes and catheters and early mobilization of the patient are desirable. Discharge depends on the postoperative course. Because multiple disciplines are involved in coordinating a transplant patient's care, discharge planning can be challenging. Medications and follow-up appointment, procedures, and tests are stressed. A close bond forms between the patients and the transplant coordinator; he or she is their resource person. Family support systems are imperative.

Potential Surgical Complications

Leaking anastomosis
Acute rejection

LUNG TRANSPLANTATION

Definition

Single-lung transplantation involves the removal of a diseased lung with subsequent replacement of an optimal functioning lung procured from an organ donor. It is a viable option for many patients suffering from various forms of end-stage lung disease and provides the recipient with adequate pulmonary function and normal pulmonary arterial pressures.

Indications

Single-lung transplantation is effective in the treatment of end-stage pulmonary fibrosis, chronic obstructive pulmonary disease, alpha-1 antitrypsin, and primary pulmonary hypertension, because it ensures that both ventilation and perfusion are preferentially diverted to the transplanted lung. Bilateral-lung transplantation is reserved for patients suffering from septic lung disease (i.e., cystic fibrosis). This discussion focuses on single-lung transplantation.

Related Surgical Procedures

Pneumonectomy is a major type of lung surgery that could be considered related to a lung transplant. Harvesting the lung from a cadaver is closely related to implantation in the recipient.

Perioperative Nursing Implications

The circulating nurses prepare the room by having the room temperature set at 65 to 68°F. They put the bean bag positioner on the OR bed and place 12 liters of saline irrigation in the freezer. The instrument sets, supplies, and equipment are placed in the room. Once the patient arrives, the nurse's priority is to see that he or she is comfortable and to offer reassurance. The nurses contact the perfusionists to prepare for the lung transplant procedure and the possibility of cardiopulmonary bypass.

Anesthesia

In preparation for transplantation, a Swan-Ganz catheter is positioned in the pulmonary artery on the opposite side from the transplant. The pulmonary arterial pressure, end-tidal carbon dioxide, and oxygen saturation are continuously monitored. An arterial catheter and large-bore peripheral venous catheters are inserted. Before anesthesia induction, the anesthetist prepares solutions of PGE_1 and dopamine, in addition to other routine resuscitation drugs. For a left lung transplant, a bronchus-blocking inflatable balloon is positioned and a standard endotracheal tube is used. For a right lung transplant, a left-sided Robert shaw double-lumen endotracheal tube is used. A double-lumen tube is used for either side. General anesthesia is achieved with high-dose fentanyl and pancuronium paralysis. The patient's temperature is monitored via a Foley temperature probe, and a nasogastric tube is placed.

Owing to the severe pulmonary disease that these patients have, often the ability to ventilate, oxygenate, and maintain cardiac output is compromised. Pulmonary fibrosis causes the lungs to be rigid and noncompliant, making it difficult to ventilate. Intraoperatively, when one lung needs to be collapsed in preparation for removal, the airway pressure increases and the function of the remaining lung may not be sufficient to maintain adequate ventilation. Owing to the reduction in the pulmonary vascular bed, pulmonary vascular resistance may increase to levels that might cause right ventricular failure and/or pulmonary edema.

Intraoperatively, anesthesia personnel deal with the problem of intrapulmonary shunt, which occurs when the transplanted lung's pulmonary vasculature is anastomosed. The lung is being perfused but not oxygenated. Consequently, the arterial saturation decreases; it can fall to an unacceptable level, depending on how diseased the native lung is. If the saturation level falls too low, the anesthesiologist can ask the surgeon to partially clamp the pulmonary artery to decrease the shunt or he or she can independently ventilate the transplanted lung using high-frequency jet ventilation.

Position

Depending on the way the surgeon plans to revascularize the bronchial anastomosis, the patient either is initially positioned supine then turned to full lateral decubitus position when an omental flap is taken, or is placed in full lateral decubitus position if a pedicled flap of intercostal muscle is used for structural reinforcement and early neovascularity. Proper care is taken to pad the legs and arms, and a safety strap is applied across the thighs.

Creation and Maintenance of the Sterile Field

The patient is turned onto his or her side for the thoracotomy incision and reprepared and redraped. The OR furniture is positioned to be most convenient for the surgical team.

The patient is draped in the thoracotomy position. A large sterile incise drape is applied to the chest. The groin is draped into the sterile field so that femoral cannulation can be performed if necessary. The magnetic pad is placed across the iliac crest to prevent instruments from falling. The Mayo stand is pulled across the patient's thighs.

The scrub nurse needs to know the sequence of the procedure. The scrub nurse should be prepared to assist with the initiation of cardiopulmonary bypass if it is needed.

Equipment and Supplies

A patient drape; a back table drape; gowns; a Mayo stand cover; basins; hernia tape; large sponges; Raytec sponges; a 50-ml syringe; electrocautery with extension tip; suture booties (small); a needle counter; a magnetic pad; suction tubing; Nos. 10, 11, and 15 blades; a Foley catheter and urine drain set; chest tubes; and a closed water seal drainage unit are assembled. Suture materials needed include 1–0 and 3–0 silk ties; 3–0 silk taper needle; 3–0, 4–0, and 5–0 double-armed polypropylene;

3–0 and 1–0 polyglactin 910 taper needle; 4–0 polyglactin 910; and skin staples.

A major chest set is needed, which should include chest retractors, vascular forceps, needle holders, and scissors. Also needed are bronchus clamps, lung clamps, vascular clamps (e.g., ductus arteriosus clamps, DeBakey clamps, and Crafoord clamps). Basic instruments are needed for exposure and hemostasis. Tubing clamps and Rumel stylets are needed if bypass is instituted. A set of extralong instruments should be kept sterile under the table. Because ischemic time is critical to the viability of the cadaver lung, the scrub nurse should set up well in advance, especially for a repeated chest incision (usually surgeons opt to use the opposite side; however, this also is dependent on which lung is being harvested and on the preoperative ventilation-perfusion lung scan in the recipient).

Drugs and Solutions

The only solution necessary is cold saline slush irrigation used to prevent warm ischemic injury in the donor lung.

Physiological Monitoring

Blood loss is calculated by the circulating nurse, who weighs the bloody sponges and totals the bottled blood loss. Anesthesia personnel monitor urine output, patient temperature, and hemodynamics.

Specimens and Cultures

Gram stains and cultures are taken from the donor lung before implantation. Antibiotic therapy is based on the results of these cultures. Until the results of these cultures are available, the recipient is treated prophylactically with a first-generation cephalosporin such as Ancef, 1 g every 8 hours.

Physician's Orders

Before a patient is listed for a transplant, there is an evaluation phase, which takes about 1 week and includes the collection of current pulmonary and cardiac function data as well as evaluation of renal and liver function. Because this surgery is severely donor limited, it is best to perform it when the likelihood of success is relatively high. The outcome of the evaluation usually predicts the probable success rate.

1. Respiratory Evaluation
   a. Complete pulmonary function tests with arterial blood gas
   b. Chest x-ray
   c. Sleep study if indicated
   d. Quantitative ventilation-perfusion lung scan
   e. Sputum culture

2. Cardiac Evaluation
   a. ECG
   b. Two-dimensional echocardiogram
   c. Gated nuclear angiogram
   d. Transesophageal echo (in patients with suspected interatrial communication)
   e. Cardiac catheterization
3. Evaluation of Exercise Tolerance
   a. 6-minute walk test
   b. Modified Bruce protocol
   c. Activities of daily living evaluation

Finally, after acceptance by a transplantation executive committee, the patient is placed on the active transplant list. These patients then begin a preoperative pulmonary rehabilitation on an outpatient basis. This program includes continuous monitoring while the patient is undergoing supervised treadmill walking, cycling, weight training, and performing light calisthenics. Patients are monitored continuously for oxygen saturation, pulse, respiratory rate, and perceived exertion. Continuous monitoring ensures that patients are exercising within safe limits and any deterioration is noted quickly. Preoperative exercise training optimizes the patient's functional ability, physical exercise tolerance, and emotional well-being during a difficult waiting period.

Once a suitable donor lung is identified the recipient is brought into the hospital. Before being taken to the operating room, the patient is given azathioprine 2 mg/kg IV and preoperative antibiotic. An ECG and chest x-ray are taken, and blood work and urinalysis are sent to the laboratory. Type and cross-match 6 to 8 U of blood.

Laboratory and Diagnostic Studies

Chemistry panel
CBC
Liver function test
Serologies
ABO
24-Hour urine for creatinine clearance

Procedure

Incision and Exposure

Once the patient is in the lateral decubitus position, a posterior lateral thoracotomy incision is made with subsequent excision of the fifth rib. The chest retractor is positioned. Single-lung ventilation is employed if tolerated by the patient.

Details

Extreme care is taken throughout the dissection to protect the phrenic nerve and the vagus nerve as well as its recurrent branch on the left side.

The pulmonary veins are isolated extrapericardially and the pulmonary artery as proximally as possible. On the right side, exposure is facilitated by division of the azygos vein and intrapericardial dissection of the right pulmonary artery posterior to the superior vena cava. On the left side, this is facilitated by the division of the ligamentum arteriosum. The main bronchus is encircled just proximal to its upper lobe division.

At this time, the pulmonary artery is test clamped to ensure that the patient can withstand a period on one lung. Anesthesia personnel have a PGE_1 infusion ready to aid the pulmonary vascular response. If the clamping creates significant instability, the clamp is removed and the femoral vessels are cannulated for partial venoarterial bypass. Patients with pulmonary hypertension are also placed on cardiopulmonary bypass. If hemodyamics remain stable during the test clamp and the donor lung is ready, the recipient's lung is removed.

The pulmonary veins are divided outside the pericardium. The first branch of the pulmonary artery and its descending branch are divided to leave as long a length on the pulmonary artery as possible. The bronchus is divided just proximal to the upper lobe takeoff; extreme caution is used to avoid dissecting tissue from around the recipient's main bronchus.

After removal of the lung, the pericardium is opened around the pulmonary veins and a clamp is placed on the left atrial cuff proximal to the veins. The ties previously placed on the venous stumps are removed, and an incision is made so that the superior and inferior pulmonary veins can be joined, thereby creating a generous cuff.

Lung Implantation

The donor atrial cuff and pulmonary artery are trimmed to match the recipient. The donor bronchus should be divided into two cartilaginous rings proximal to the upper lobe takeoff (Fig. 23–7).

The bronchial anastomosis is completed using interrupted 4–0 polypropylene suture for the cartilaginous portion and polyglactin 910 continuous sutures for the membranous portion. A pericardial patch is wrapped around the anastomosis and secured with two 4–0 silk sutures. Cold slush saline is placed on the lung throughout the procedure. The patient is maintained on one-lung ventilation unless cardiopulmonary bypass is required (rare for single-lung transplants unless the patient has pulmonary hypertension). After completion of the bronchial anastomosis, the lung is partially inflated and the bronchial closure is tested under water. The airway anastomosis is confirmed via fiberoptic bronchoscopy at the conclusion of the procedure.

The atrial anastomosis is done by sewing the back wall first from the inside out with a continuous 3–0 polypropylene suture. The front wall is then sewn with continuous polypropylene suture. The pulmonary artery is anastomosed at each end of the anastomosis using a series of individual sutures. Before completion of the pulmonary arterial anastomosis, the atrial clamp is grad-

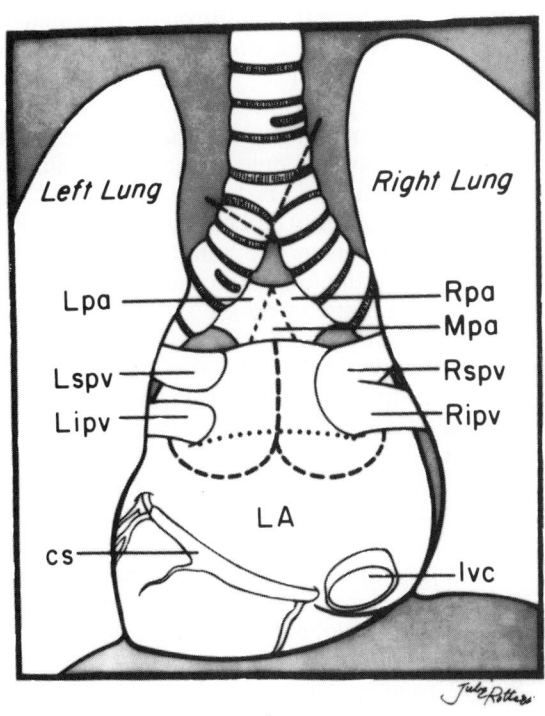
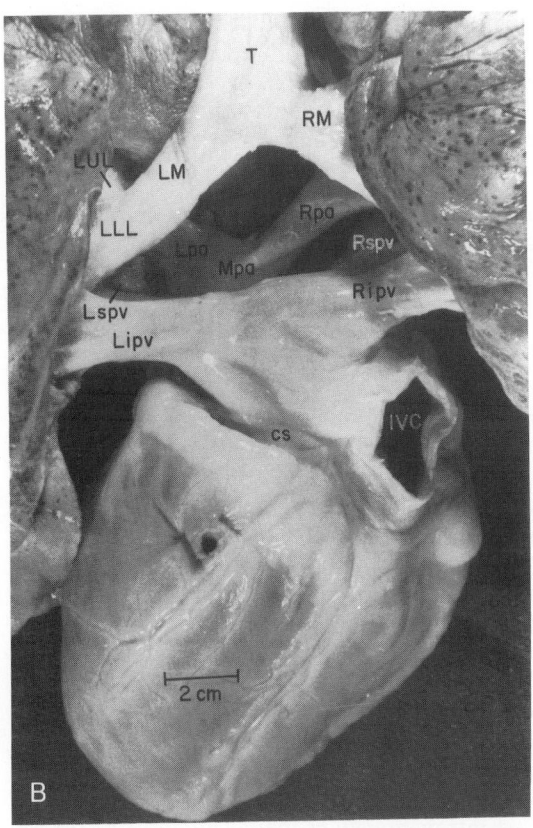

A

B

FIGURE 23–7. *A,* Posterior aspect of the left atrium, pulmonary arteries, and lower airway. Dashed lines (---) indicate sites of division of left and right mainstem bronchi, left and right pulmonary arteries, and atrial cuffs for left and right pulmonary veins when harvesting the heart and two lungs. All are suitable for separate organ. The dotted line (...) indicates the line of division made between the right and left inferior pulmonary veins when the heart alone is harvested by standard methods. This leaves insufficient tissue to facilitate single-lung transplantation. *B,* Posterior aspect of a human cadaver heart-lung bloc. Mediastinal tissues and pericardial reflections have been dissected from the specimen. Note closer proximity to the coronary sinus of the left inferior pulmonary vein than the right inferior pulmonary vein. T, trachea; LM, left mainstem bronchus; LUL and LLL, left upper and lower lobe bronchi; RM, right mainstem bronchus; Lpa and Rpa, left and right pulmonary arteries; Mpa, distal main pulmonary artery; Lspv and Rspv, left and right superior pulmonary veins; Lipv and Ripv, left and right inferior pulmonary veins; LA, left atrium; cs, coronary sinus; IVC, inferior vena cava. (From Flye, M. W. [1989]. *Principles of organ transplantation* [p. 424]. Philadelphia: W. B. Saunders.)

ually released. The pulmonary artery then back bleeds and the clamp on the pulmonary artery is opened momentarily to flush it. After the pulmonary arterial anastomosis is completed, both clamps are removed. The lung is perfused and both anastomoses are checked for leaks.

Closure

Sutures used for closure include

Pericostal area: No. 2 polyglactin 910
Muscle: 1–0 polyglactin 910
Subcutaneous tissue: 3–0 polyglactin 910
Skin: skin staples or 4–0 polyglactin 910

After the incision is closed, the single-lung transplant patient is kept in the lateral decubitus position. This facilitates optimal inflation, reduces edema, and prevents drainage into the new lung. It is during this initial hiatus between finalization of the operative procedure and the beginning of intensive care unit care when difficulties commonly occur.

Postoperative Care

After the patient is in the transplant care unit, protective isolation is enforced to provide the recipient with environmental protection during the time he or she is most susceptible to infection. A cautious use of diuretics and a low-dose inotrope ensures that hemodynamic stability is reached at the lowest possible left ventricular preload.

Respiratory Management

Under normal circumstances, a standard volume of cycled mechanical ventilatory support is supplied. The goals of respiratory management are to

1. Maintain the lowest possible peak airway pressure.
2. Maintain the lowest possible fraction of inspired oxygen.
3. Provide adequate pulmonary toilet.
4. Start chest physiotherapy early because a denervated airway results in a decreased cough reflex.

After the lung transplant patients are extubated and hemodynamically stable, they are transferred to the thoracic surgical floor in protective isolation. The goals of physiotherapy in the subacute stage of recovery are (1) to ensure maximal clearance of secretions, (2) to wean from supplemental oxygen, and (3) to increase exercise tolerance. During exercise sessions, an increase in the work of breathing and/or an unexpected decrease in oxygen saturation may indicate the beginning of a rejection episode. Diligent and careful monitoring of oxygen saturation during rest and exercise prevents unnecessary delays in the diagnosis and treatment of rejection. Weaning from supplemental oxygen and increasing exercise tolerance postoperatively takes about 2 to 5 weeks.

Immunosuppression

The recipient receives 1 to 2 mg/kg of body weight of azathioprine on returning from the OR. Cyclosporine is administered intravenously at 2 to 3 mg/hour based on the patient's weight. Adjustments are made until a level of 250 to 300 mg is achieved (if using an HPLC, whole blood method of measuring levels). The administration of steroids is avoided during the first week unless rejection occurs. Antithymocyte globulin is infused at 10 to 15 mg/kg of body weight after skin testing has been done. Subsequent dosage is adjusted on the basis of the absolute lymphocyte count, which is checked daily. If rejection occurs, the patient is treated with a 3-day course of high-dose bolus steroids, usually 1 g of Solu-Medrol on day 1, followed by 500 mg on day 2, and 250 mg on day 3.

Antimicrobial Treatment

Sputum Gram stains are repeated every 3 days while the patient is in the ICU. Readjustments in antibiotics are based on the recipient's postoperative course and subsequent sputum cultures.

Patients are placed on acyclovir if their HSV titer is positive. Also, they receive nystatin 500,000 U 3 times a day to prevent oral thrush. Once on the thoracic surgical floor, they start Bactrim 3 times a week to prevent pneumocystis pneumonia.

Potential Surgical Complications

The major complications that may occur include delayed bronchial healing, rejection, and infection. The bronchial anastomosis is threatened by ischemia and bronchial strictures. If an anastomotic stricture develops, it can be handled through repeated dilation or ultimately by using a short silicone stent placed endoscopically.

Signs and symptoms of rejection and infection are similar, making diagnosis difficult. In the absence of apparent sepsis, the development of a hilar infiltrate on the x-ray film and/or decline in arterial oxygenation suggests the onset of rejection. If rejection is suspected, the patient is given 1 g Solu-Medrol IV; expected improvement in the hilar infiltrate is within 12 hours. If no improvement is seen on the x-ray, a bronchoscopy may be performed to confirm the diagnosis of rejection and rule out infection.

The reimplantation response may develop and is evidenced by a perihilar and/or lower lobe air space beginning in the first 36 hours after transplantation. It varies in severity from a subtle perihilar haze to dense perihilar and basilar consolidation. This condition usually remains the same or worsens during the next 2 to 4 days and then begins to clear. Generally, the pattern of clearing involves a decrease in air space disease, with residual reticular interstitial disease, which finally clears completely. This reaction is possibly correlated with a prolonged ischemic time (longer than 4 hours) or more likely is related to decreased or absence of lymphatics in combination with the trauma of reimplantation.

BONE TRANSPLANTATION

Definition

Allograft implantation represents a biological solution to the problems raised by massive defects in the skeleton. "Despite the immune response, allograft material is generally well tolerated and non-toxic, it has the appropriate modulus and structure and is relatively easily shaped and implanted; it can be and frequently is incorporated by the host bone; the supply is theoretically unlimited: and if successful, it represents a permanent implant rather than a temporary spacer" (Mankin et al., 1987).

Indications

Bone for transplant can be obtained several ways. A bone autograft is transplanted from one part of a person's body to another. It is best used for small grafting as in a spinal fusion or nonunion repair.

A bone allograft is transplanted from a cadaver into the recipient. An important biological feature of an allograft is that healing does not necessitate a vascular anastomosis as do other organ transplants. For tumors that originate in the bone (giant cell osteosarcoma, chondrosarcoma, Ewing tumor, and some neoplasms) or for types of cancer that have spread to the bone from elsewhere in the body, large osteochondral allografts have been limb salvaging. Clinical use of bone allograft is not limited to skeletal reconstruction for tumor ablation, but includes maxillofacial reconstruction, spinal fusions, revision hip arthroplasties, repair of fracture nonunions, and replacement of benign cysts. Trauma is also an indicator for bone grafting, usually occurring in a young population.

Bone transplants offer a better solution than artificial prosthesis because bone graft can fuse directly to native bone. Custom prostheses take time to make and often need to be replaced. In the case of total joint procedures, the cement may loosen over the years. The major limitation to transplanting bone is that it does not grow if put into a child. Failure of a bone allograft is usually due to infection and/or fracture.

Related Surgical Procedures

Any orthopedic surgical procedure could be considered related to bone transplantation. In repairing a fracture or defect or replacing diseased bone, whether or not transplantation is required depends on the specific pathological condition.

Harvesting and preservation of bone allograft are similar to orthopedic procedures, except they are performed on cadaver donors. Keeping a hospital bone bank stocked can be a full-time job for many people. The harvests are performed using sterile technique, and generally the long bones of the arms and legs are taken. Accumulated research supports the idea that fresh-frozen and freeze-dried bone is decreasingly immunogenic, in that order. The antigen cells in the grafts are destroyed by freezing or freeze-drying (Czitrom et al., 1986).

Frozen allografts are first wrapped in layers of plastic, followed by cloth in a sterile fashion, and placed in a −80°C (Harris) freezer. Freeze-dried bone is lyophilized; this involves removing the moisture from the frozen bone to a residual of 3 to 5%. This bone can then be stored in glass or plastic evacuated containers at room temperature. This bone needs to be reconstituted in saline before use.

Perioperative Nursing Implications

The circulator must know in advance what the overall plan of the procedure involves: whether frozen, fresh, processed, or freeze-dried bone is to be used. She or he can then anticipate the equipment and supplies that are needed.

Anesthesia

The type of anesthetic used depends on the extent of the surgery to be performed. For larger allograft procedures, general anesthesia is preferred for several reasons. If the patient is awake, she or he could hear

discussion with pathology department personnel regarding the margins; if blood needs to be transfused rapidly, the vein distention can be painful to an awake patient. The patient is prepared as for any other major orthopedic surgery. Larger IV access (i.e., 7 Fr. and 1 standard) is needed. An arterial catheter is inserted and a Swan-Ganz catheter is placed if indicated (e.g., for older patients with heart disease). Tourniquet times are monitored by anesthesia personnel and the surgeon. For a patient with rheumatism, much care is taken to pad the OR bed and aid with positioning the patient comfortably.

Position

The patient can be positioned in a number of ways depending on where the allograft is to be placed. Normal precautions are taken to pad supports with Webril and secure the patient to the OR bed.

Creation and Maintenance of the Sterile Field

The patient is prepared using a typical orthopedic preparation consisting of povidone-iodine scrub (using brushes) followed by use of a povidone-iodine solution on sponges. The patient is shaved and prepared on the nursing unit the night before surgery and the affected limb is wrapped and kept sterile in an impervious stockinet.

After the patient is in the OR, special care is taken to apply several impervious split sheets around the base of the extremity to prevent strike through from the excessive irrigation and bleeding that occurs. The OR furniture is positioned however it is most comfortable for the scrub nurse, keeping in mind that a separate back table needs to be set up for preparation of the allograft.

It is important for the scrub nurse to set up early and be prepared with the allograft table for thawing or reconstituting the bone. The scrub nurse must also check the scheduled case (printed on the OR schedule) or verify the consented case with the surgeon and determine what type of power equipment the surgeon plans to use.

The draping requirements vary with the procedure. Usually, if a long bone of the legs or arms is being replaced, a stockinet is used to drape the extremity. The OR bed is draped in four layers. Often, after the removal of a tumor, the surgeons change gowns and gloves and redrape the sterile field, so as not to cross-contaminate the allograft. New instruments may also be opened.

Equipment and Supplies

Necessary equipment and medical-surgical supplies vary from case to case. Some standard items include a patient drape pack, a total joint drape pack, back table covers, a table drape pack, gowns, towel packs, Mayo stand covers, a cement gun, cement mixing bowl kit, cement, a funnel, a straight nozzle, laparotomy sponges, smaller sponges, impervious split sheets, impervious stockinet, Kling bandage, culture tubes, large closed drain suction reservoir, dressings, nonadhering dressing, disposable hemoclip appliers, lavage tubing, a long tip and shower head, a basin set, a long sterile basin (for soaking the allograft), suction tubing, a needle counter, light handles, electrocautery, Nos. 10 and 15 blades, skin staples, bulb syringes, a marking pen, and a grounding pad.

Suture needed for the procedure includes 1–0 and 2–0 silk ties, 2–0 silk pop-offs, No. 1 and 2–0 polyglactin 910, and 3–0 nylon.

The types of instruments needed are specific to each case. Generally, for bigger allograft transplants, a total hip set, osteotomes, gouges, reamers, vascular instruments, bone clamps (small and large), medium and small key elevators, an oscillating saw with a large blade, a reamer driver, Surgairetome with a pineapple burr, and two hoses are assembled. The types of prosthetic trialing device instruments depend on what part of the anatomy is being replaced.

Drugs and Solutions

Warm saline or Ringer irrigation is used to thaw the allograft. Polymyxin, 500,000 U, and bacitracin, 50,000 U, in 3000-ml bag of normal saline are used for irrigation. Tobramycin, 1.2-g vial mixed with cement, and thrombin spray, 20,000 U, are used for hemostasis.

Physiological Monitoring

Blood loss is calculated by weighing all sponges and keeping track of measured bottled blood loss. The Foley catheter drainage is measured by anesthesia personnel. If a tourniquet is used, the inflation and deflation times are monitored closely.

Specimens and Cultures

Numerous specimens are taken during the resection of a tumor. These segments are sent to the pathology department for frozen section examination, so that the surgeon knows when the margins are clear. Cultures and sensitivity testing of the allograft before its implantation are routinely performed.

Physician's Orders

Preoperatively, patients may undergo magnetic resonance imaging, computer tomography, and a series of radiographs (anteroposterior), depending on the indi-

cations. Magnetic resonance imaging is useful in defining the true intracompartmental extent of disease within a bone. Knowing the proximal and distal extent of a tumor preoperatively helps the physician decide on the appropriate type of surgical treatment.

Radiography is the most important tool for the surgeon planning allograft, because it allows him or her to size match the donor bone to within a few millimeters of the native bone. The radiographs are actually measured with a ruler to match up the inside and outside diameters and lengths.

Computed tomography and scintigraphy demonstrate the extent of the intramedullary disease and can also evaluate the possibility of lesions in other bones.

An arteriogram is ordered only when there is uncertainty about whether the vessels are involved in the limb salvage operation.

Laboratory and Diagnostic Studies

All patients are screened for infection through cultures and aspiration. Open biopsy of the diseased bone may be performed for tissue diagnosis.

Occasionally, these patients donate autologous blood preoperatively in case they need to be transfused.

Procedure

Incision and Exposure

The actual surgical technique depends on what part of the skeleton is being transplanted. First and foremost is selecting and preparing the bone to be used. This bone is unwrapped under sterile conditions, cultured, and rapidly thawed by soaking it in warm (45°C) antibiotic solution of lactated Ringer solution.

The actual surgery is done in two phases: phase one is the resection of the tumor, always being sure to include removal of the previous biopsy track; phase two is the implantation of the graft (Fig. 23–8).

Details

The first phase when dealing with bone tumors is the most important: to be sure that the margins are clear. Often, the surgeons regown and reglove, and so on, to avoid contamination from the tumor.

When implanting the allograft, attention to detail is important. Because these patients often are or will be receiving radiation therapy or chemotherapy, infection is a major threat to graft survival. The graft has already been sized, is cut to fit, and is inserted using compression plates and screws or intramedullary devices. The tendons, ligaments, and capsular structures are reattached to the graft, using nonabsorbable suture. Because the graft is actually dead bone, mistakes made in plating can lead to defects and early pathological fractures.

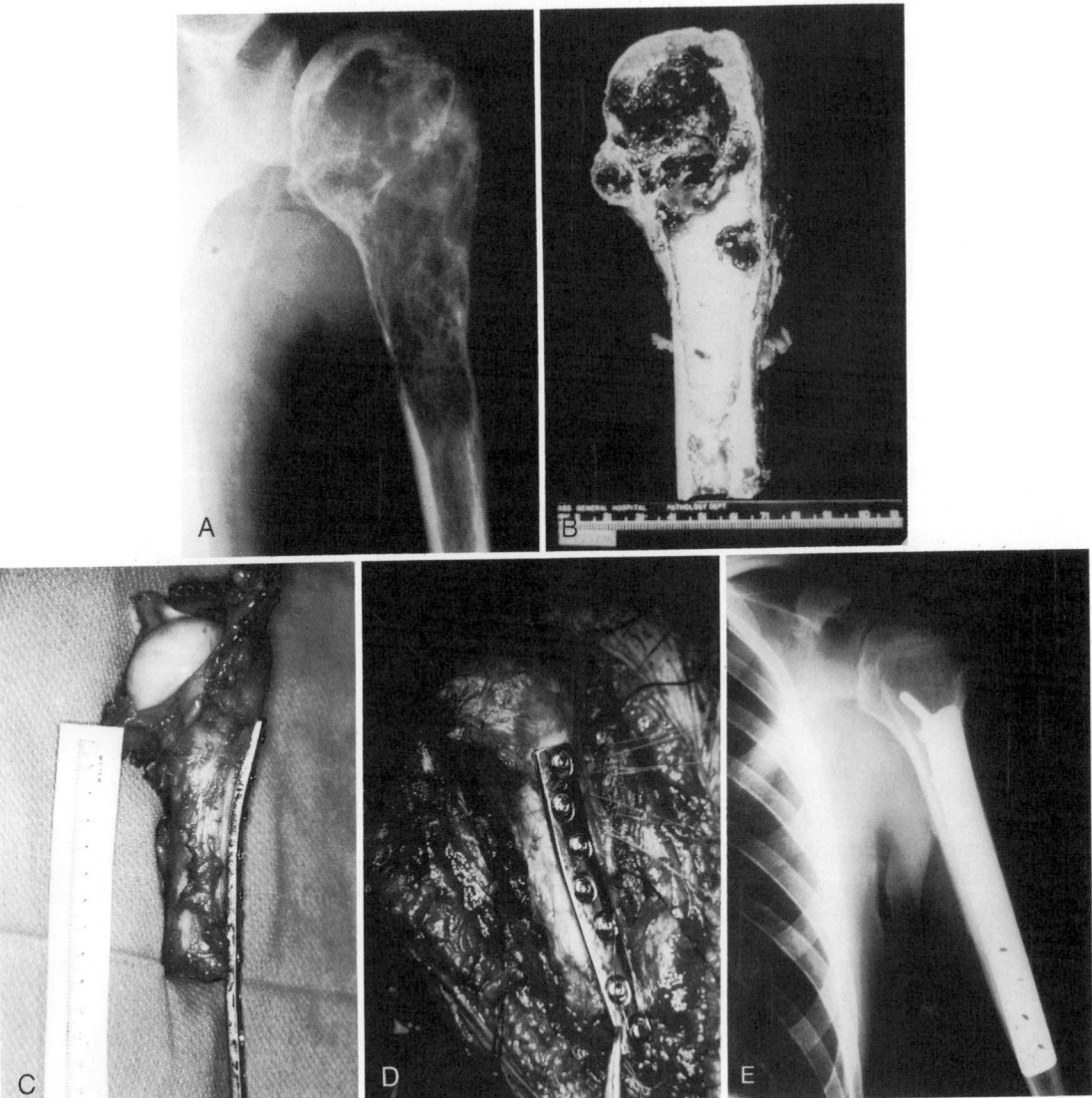

FIGURE 23–8. *A*, A 24-year-old man had a twice recurrent giant cell tumor of the proximal humerus. *B*, The lesion was resected. Note the extent of the lesion on the resected specimen. *C*, An allograft was sized and selected from the bank and prepared for insertion by application of a compression plate. Note that the capsular and rotator cuff insertions are retained on the graft. *D*, The graft is fixed in place with the plate and screws, and the rotator cuff is repaired with interrupted sutures. *E*, At almost 5 years after surgery, the host-donor junction site is well healed, and the graft-shoulder function is excellent except in the upper ranges. (From Flye, M. W. [1989]. *Principles of organ transplantation* [p. 444]. Philadelphia: W. B. Saunders.)

Closure

It is important that the allograft and hardware are well covered with subcutaneous tissue and skin. If necessary, a muscle flap should be used to avoid a skin slough. The wound is drained with closed drain suction reservoir for several days and the limb is kept immobilized to allow the reconstructed tendons and ligaments to heal.

The muscle and/or fascia is closed with interrupted No. 1 Vicryl, the subcutaneous tissue is closed with interrupted 2–0 Vicryl, and the skin is closed with interrupted 3–0 nylon suture.

Nonadhering dressings and gauze dressings are ap-

plied, and a plaster splint is used to immobilize the extremity.

Postoperative Care

Some physicians advocate maintaining the patient on a regimen of anticoagulants for several months. The administration of antibiotics is continued IV postoperatively for about 1 week and then orally for several months. After the swelling goes down, the limb is placed in a cast to allow the reconstructed ligaments and tendons to heal. A cast brace is then used until the host-graft junction site and the joint are stable, usually 6 months. While the patient is wearing the cast-type brace, supervised active and passive exercise programs are begun.

Radiographs are done routinely at 3-month intervals. Patients are followed closely for evidence of tumor recurrence, metastasis, infection, fracture, nonunion, or instability of the transplanted graft.

Potential Surgical Complications

The major complications are infection and rejection. Fortunately, these complications in the allograft can be treated by conventional means such as antibiotic therapy and rarely require a solution that seriously disables the patient. If the allograft has to be removed, the patient has not lost anything, he or she is just back where he or she started.

Rejection occurs in 3 to 15% of all cases. It is not treated with immunosuppressants. It is not wise to use a form of therapy with such potentially serious side effects for a problem that is not life threatening. Serious complications of rejection seem to correlate with the stage of the tumor, the extent of the resection, and the use of adjunctive chemotherapy and radiation. Many patients with tumors are already receiving chemotherapy; immunosuppressants would severely compromise their health. Rejection is also believed to mask itself in the form of fractures and nonunions.

Other potential surgical complications include pulmonary embolus, massive hemorrhage, and skin sloughing. Pulmonary embolus can be avoided through anticoagulation. Massive hemorrhage can be avoided if the anesthesiologist is prepared with the replacement blood volume and either the rapid infuser or the cell saver. Skin sloughing is seen more in late wound complications, and it can be disastrous.

The overall success of the procedure depends on the surgical technique. Attention must be paid to proper alignment, restoration of length, muscle balancing, cement technique, and bone preparation to achieve a good result.

Bibliography

Anderson, C. F., Velosa, J. A., Frohnert, P. P., et al. (1985). The risks of unilateral nephrectomy: Status of kidney donors 10 to 20 years post-operatively. *Mayo Clinic Proceedings, 60,* 367–374.

Bain, L. J. (1987, Fall). Bankers with inside investments. *Penn Medicine,* pp. 31–32.

Baldwin, J. C., Stinson, E. B., Oyer, P. E., et al. (1986). Technique of cardiac transplantation. In J. W. Hurst (Ed.), *The heart* (6th ed.) (pp. 2062–2075). New York: R. R. Donnelly.

Barker, C. F., Naji, A., Perloff, L. J. (1986). Renal transplantation. In D. C. Sabiston, Jr. (Ed.), *Textbook of surgery* (13th ed.) (pp. 407–429). Philadelphia: W. B. Saunders.

Belzer, F. O. (1985). Principles of organ preservation. *Transplantation Proceedings, 20*(Suppl. 1), 925–927.

Belzer, F. O., Southard, J. J. (1988). Principles of solid-organ preservation by cold storage. *Transplantation, 45,* 673–676.

Brown, K. L., Cruess, R. L. (1982). Bone and cartilage transplantation in orthopaedic surgery. *The Journal of Bone and Joint Surgery 64A*(2), 270–275.

Burchardt, H. (1987). Biology of bone transplantation. *Orthopedic Clinics of North America, 18,* 187–194.

Cerelli, J. G. (Ed.). (1987). *Organ transplantation and replacement.* Philadelphia: J. B. Lippincott.

Cooper, J. D., Pearson F. G., Patterson, G. A., et al. (1987). Technique of successful lung transplantation in humans. *Journal of Thoracic Cardiovascular Surgery, 93,* 173–181.

Corry, R. J., Nghiem, D., Schulak, J. A., et al. (1986). Surgical treatment of diabetic nephropathy with simultaneous pancreatic duodenal and renal transplantation. *Surgery, Gynecology and Obstetrics, 162,* 547–555.

Czitrom, A. A., Langer, F., McKee, N., Gross, A. (1986). Bone and cartilage allotransplantation. *Clinical Orthopaedics and Related Research, 208,* 141–145.

DaFoe, D. (1988). Pancreatic transplantation as treatment for IDDM. *Diabetes Care, 11,* 669–675.

DaFoe, D. C., Campbell, D. A., Marks, W. H., et al. (1985). Association of inclusion of the donor spleen in pancreaticoduodenal transplantation with rejection. *Transplantation, 40,* 579–584.

DeBoer, H. H. (1988). The history of bone grafts. *Clinical Orthopaedics, 226,* 292–298.

Dick, H. M., Malinin, T. I., Mnaymneh, W. A. (1985). Massive allograft implantation following radical resection of high-grade tumors requiring adjunct chemotherapy treatment. *Clinical Orthopaedics and Related Research, 197,* 88–95.

Diethelan, A. G., Sterline, W. A., Aldrete, J. S., et al. (1976). Retrospective analysis of 100 consecutive patients undergoing related living donor renal transplantation. *Annals of Surgery, 183,* 502–510.

Dunn, J. F., Nylander, W. A., Richie, R. E., et al. (1986). Living related kidney donors. *Annals of Surgery, 203,* 637–644.

Farrell, R. M., Stubenbard, W. T., Riggio, R. R., Muecke, E. C. (1973). Living renal donor nephrectomy: Evaluation of 135 cases. *The Journal of Urology, 110,* 639–642.

Flye, M. W. (1989). *Principles of organ transplantation.* Philadelphia: W. B. Saunders.

Friedlaender, G. E. (1985). Bone banking and clinical applications. *Transplantation Proceedings, 17*(Suppl. 4), 99–104.

Garovoy, M., Guttmann, R. D. (Eds.). (1986). *Renal transplantation.* New York: Churchill Livingstone.

Gebhardt, M. C., Lord, F. C., Rosenberg, A. E., Mankin, H. J. (1987). Treatment of adamantinoma of the tibia. *The Journal of Bone and Joint Surgery, 69A,* 1177–1188.

Goldman, M. H., Tilney, N. L., Vineyard, G. C., et al. (1975). A twenty year survey of arterial complications of renal transplantation. *Surgery, Gynecology and Obstetrics, 141,* 758–760.

Goldsmith, J., Kamholz, S. L., Montefusco, C. M., Veith, F. J. (1987). Clinical and experimental aspects of single lung transplantation of critical care. *Heart and Lung: The Journal of Critical Care, 16*(3), 231–236.

Griffith, B. P., Shaw, B. W., Hardesty, R. L., et al. (1985). Venovenous bypass without systemic anticoagulation for transplantation of the human liver. *Surgery, Gynecology and Obstetrics, 160,* 271–272.

Gross, A. E., Lavoe, M. V., McDermott, P., Marks, P. (1985). The use of allograft bone in revision of total hip arthroplasty. *Clinical Orthopaedics and Related Research, 197,* 115–122.

Harjula, A., Baldwin, J. C., Starnes, V. A., et al. (1987). Proper donor selection for heart-lung transplantation. *Journal of Thoracic and Cardiovascular Surgery, 94,* 874–80.

Hardesty, R. L., Griffith., B. P. (1987). Autoperfusion of the heart and lungs for preservation during distant procurement. *Journal of Thoracic Cardiovascular Surgery, 93,* 11–18.

Hart, M. M., Campbell, E. D., Karvin, M. G. (1986). Bone banking. *Clinical Orthopaedics and Related Research, 206,* 295–299.

Head, W. C., Berklacich, F. M., Malinin, T. I., Emerson, R. H. (1987). Proximal femoral allografts in revision–total hip arthroplasty. *Clinical Orthopaedics and Related Research, 225,* 22–36.

Head, W. C., Malinin, T. I., Berklacich, F. (1987). Freeze-dried proximal femur allografts in revision–total hip arthroplasty. *Clinical Orthopaedics and Related Research, 215,* 109–121.

Henry, M. L., Sommer, B. G., Ferguson, R. M. (1988). Improved immediate function of renal allografts with Belzer perfusate. *Transplantation, 45,* 73–75.

Higenbottom, T., Stewart, S., Penketh, A., Wallwork, J. (1988). Transbronchial lung biopsy for the diagnosis of rejection in heart–lung transplant patients. *Transplantation, 46,* 532–539.

Higenbottom, T., Stewart, S., Wallwork, J. (1988). Transbronchial lung biopsy to diagnose lung rejection and infection of heart–lung transplants. *Transplantation Proceedings, 20*(Suppl. 1), 767–769.

Harowitz, M. C., Friedlaender, G. E. (1987). Immunologic aspects of bone transplantation. *Orthopedic Clinics of North America, 18,* 227–233.

Lekander, B. J. (1988). Preventing complications for the heart-lung transplant recipient. *Dimensions of Critical Care Nursing, 7*(1), 18–26.

Lord, C. F., Gebhardt, M. C., Tomford, W. W., Mankin, H. J. (1988). Infection in bone. *The Journal of Bone and Joint Surgery, 70A,* 369–376.

McDermott, A. G. P., Langer, F., Pritzker, K. P. H., Gross, A. E. (1985). Fresh small-fragment osteochondral allografts. *Clinical Orthopaedics and Related Research, 197,* 96–102.

McDonald, J. C., Rohr, M. S., Tucker, W. Y. (1983). Recent experiences with autotransplantation of the kidney, jejunum and pancreas. *Annals of Surgery, 197,* 678–686.

Malinin, T. I., Martinez, O. V., Brown, M. D. (1985). Banking of massive osteoarticular and intercalary bone allografts—12 years experience. *Clinical Orthopaedics and Related Research, 197,* 44–57.

Malkowicz, S. B., Perloff, L. J. (1985). Urologic considerations in renal transplantation. *Surgery, Gynecology and Obstetrics, 160,* 579–588.

Mankin, H. J., Gebhardt, M. C., Tomford, W. W. (1987). The use of frozen cadaveric allografts in the management of patients with bone tumors of the extremities. *Orthopedic Clinics of North America, 18,* 275–289.

Merkel, F. K., Matalon, T. A. S. (1988). Intraperitoneal placement of renal transplants. *Transplantation Proceedings, 20*(Suppl. 1), 370–374.

Merrill, J. P., Murray, J. E., Harrison J., et al. (1984). Successful homotransplantation of the human kidney between identical twins. *JAMA, 251,* 2566–2573.

Meyers, M. H. (1985). Resurfacing of the femoral head with fresh osteochondral allografts. *Clinical Orthopaedics and Related Research, 197,* 111–114.

Nerstrom, B., Ladefoged J., Lund, F. (1973). Vascular complications in 155 consecutive kidney transplantations. *Scandinavian Journal of Urology and Nephrology, 6*(Suppl. 15), 65–74.

Patterson, G. A., Cooper, J. D., Dark, J. H., et al. (1988). Experimental and clinical double lung transplantation. *Journal of Thoracic and Cardiovascular Surgery, 95,* 70–74.

Reemtsma, K., Weber, C. J. (1981). Pancreas and pancreatic islet transplantation. In D. C. Sabiston Jr. (Ed.), *Textbook of surgery* (12th ed.) (pp. 537–542). Philadelphia: W. B. Saunders.

Salvatierra, O. (1985). Advantages of continued use of kidney transplantation from living donors. *Transplantation Proceedings, 17*(Suppl. 2), 18–22.

Sanfilippo, F., Vaughn, W. K., Spees, E. K., et al. (1984). Benefits of HLA-A and HLA-B matching on graft and patient outcome after cadaveric-donor renal transplantation. *New England Journal of Medicine, 311,* 358–364.

Sim, F. H., Beuirchamp, C. P., Choo E. Y. (1987). Reconstruction of musculoskeletal defects about the knee for tumor. *Clinical Orthopaedics and Related Research, 221,* 188–201.

Somerville, M. A. (1985). "Procurement" vs. "Donation"—Access to tissues and organs for transplantation: Should "contracting out" legislation be adopted? *Transplantation Proceedings, 17*(Suppl. 4), 53–68.

Steed, D. L., Brown, B., Reilly, J. J., et al. (1985). General surgical complications in heart and heart-lung transplantation. *Surgery, 98,* 739–744.

Sterioff, S. (1985). Unilateral nephrectomy in living related kidney donors is safe and beneficial [Editorial]. *Mayo Clinic Proceedings, 60,* 423–424.

Stewart, S., Higenbottom, T. W., Hutter, J. A., et al. (1988). Histopathology of transbronchial biopsies in heart-lung transplantation, *Transplantation Proceedings, 20*(Suppl. 2), 764–766.

Sundaram, M., McGuire, M. H., Herbold, D. R., et al. (1986). Magnetic resonance imaging in planning limb-salvage surgery for primary malignant tumors of bone. *Journal of Bone and Joint Surgery, 68,* 809–819.

Sutherland, D. E. R., Goetz, F. C., Najarian, J. S. (1979). Intraperitoneal transplantation of immediately vascularized segmental pancreatic grafts without duct ligation. *Transplantation, 28,* 485–491.

Sutherland, D. E. R., Goetz, F. C., Najarian, J. S. (1984). One hundred pancreas transplants at a single institution. *Annals of Surgery, 200,* 414–440.

Terasaki, P. I. (1989). Short and long term effects of HLA matching. In D. W. Gjertson (Ed.). *Clinical transplants* (pp. 353–360). Los Angeles: UCLA Tissue Typing Laboratory.

Toledo, P., Luis, H., Zammit, M., Valzie, K. (1978). Effect of glucagon and methlyprednisolone on pancreatectomized recipients of whole pancreas allografts. *Henry Ford Hospital Medical Journal, 26,* 41–45.

Toledo, P., Luis H. (1984). Pancreatic transplantation. *Surgery, Obstetrics and Gynecology, 157,* 49–56.

Tomford, W. W., Mankin, H. J., Friedlaender, G. E., et al. (1987). Methods of banking bone and cartilage for allograft transplantation. *Orthopedic Clinics of North America, 18,* 241–246.

Trumble, T. E., Friedlaender, G. E. (1987). Allogenic bone in the treatment of tumors, trauma, and congenital anomalies of the hand. *Orthopedic Clinics of North America, 18,* 301–310.

Vahey, T. N., Glazer, G. M., Francis, I. R., et al. (1988). Diagnosis of pancreatic transplant rejection. *AJR, 150,* 557–560.

Wall, W. J., Grant D. R., Duff, J. H. (1988). Biliary tract reconstruction using external cholecystostomy without stenting in liver transplantation. *Transplantation Proceedings, 20*(Suppl. 1), 541–543.

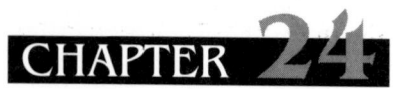

Plastic Surgery

Patricia S. Fritz

DEFINITION

The word *plastic* is derived from the Greek *plastikos,* which means to mold or give form. *Plastic surgery* therefore deals with the healing and anatomical restoration of patients with injury, disfigurement, or scarring that results from birth defects, trauma, or disease. Restoration of normal appearance and achievement of normal function are the goals of the plastic surgeon. These goals are obtained by surgeons with an active imagination, combined with fundamental surgical technical skills. A great deal of attention is given to the tiniest of details because the results of a large portion of plastic surgery are visible. Plastic surgery entails many anatomical systems.

ANATOMY

Integumentary System

The integument, or skin, forms a protective, pliable covering over the entire exterior of the body. At the

various openings on the body surface (the mouth, nares, anus, urethra, and vagina), the skin is continuous with mucous membrane linings. The integument is composed of a layer of closely packed cells (the epidermis), which rests on an inner fibrous layer (the dermis, or corium). The dermis is sometimes called the true skin.

There are also accessory skin structures: the hair, the nails, and integumentary glands.

The skin of an adult has a surface area of about 1.8 m² (3000 square inches) and a variable thickness. It is thickest on the palms, the soles, and the back, where it reaches about 6 mm. At the other extreme, on the tympanic membrane and over the eyelids, it is only 0.5 mm. The overall average is 1 to 2 mm.

The attachment of the skin varies from loose to tight. It is separated from the underlying structures in most parts of the body by a subcutaneous tissue called the *superficial fascia* (hypodermis). This tissue allows the muscles that underlie most of the skin to move freely. At some points where the superficial fascia is minimal and no muscles underlie the skin, as on the anterior surface of the tibia, the skin attaches to the periosteum of the bone. On the finger and toe pads and on the palms and plantar surfaces are seen alternating ridges and grooves that have a constant pattern—the fingerprints used for identicantion of individuals. They are called *friction ridges* because they prevent slippage when objects are grasped. The sweat glands open directly along the summits of these ridges but they are devoid of hair and sebaceous glands.

Skin color is caused in part by the pigment carotene (yellow), which is in the surface layer and in thin skin, and by the color of the circulating blood, which shows through to give the flesh appearance. The intensity of the flesh color depends on the state of contraction or dilation of the superficial vessels and on the extent of oxygenation of the blood. The difference in color among individuals and ethnic groups is due to the concentration of the pigment melanin.

Function

The functions of the skin are many. Basically, it stands as a protective barrier against the ever-changing and often adverse conditions of the external environment and adapts itself to them. Its receptors provide an awareness of this external environment. It adapts to wear by the thickening of the stratum corneum to form calluses if necessary. It prevents the body from drying.

Its oiled surface sheds water, and its pigment helps to protect the body from harmful ultraviolet radiation. It is an effective first line of defense against infectious organisms.

The integument is an important regulator of body temperature. This is accomplished through the coordinated activity of the nerve endings, the blood vessels, and sweat gland secretions; to a limited extent, excretion is a function of the skin. The skin has a limited capacity for absorption, especially when materials such as hormones, vitamins, and drugs are placed on the skin in a proper vehicle.

Structures

Epidermis

The *epidermis* is the outer and thinner layer of the skin. The epidermis is a stratified squamous epithelium, which comes about through the differentiation of the outer germ layer (the ectoderm). Where the skin is thick, four layers can be distinguished. They are, from outside inward, the stratum corneum, the stratum lucidum, the stratum granulosum, and the stratum spinosum. The cells of the *stratum spinosum* contain varying amounts of the brown pigment melanin. Only in albinos is the skin without melanin. The *stratum granulosum* consists of three to five layers of flattened cells whose cytoplasm contains many keratohyalin granules. The *stratum lucidum* is a clear homogeneous band outside of the stratum granulosum. It is composed of rows of flattened cells. The *stratum corneum*, the outermost layer, consists of flat, scalelike dead and cornified cells. They contain fibrous protein called *keratin*.

The surface cells are constantly being lost and are as constantly replaced from the moving up of cells from the underlying layers. They form a covering that is protective and that helps to prevent the excessive loss of moisture from the body surface.

Dermis, or Corium

The *dermis* is a layer of dense connective tissue derived from the mesoderm germ layer through the medium of mesenchyme. It consists of an outer papillary layer, which fits intimately into the underside of the epidermis, and an inner reticular layer. The dermis is thicker than the epidermis, ranging from 0.6 mm on the eyelids to as much as 3 mm on the soles and palms. The papillary layer is softer and contains more elastic and reticular fibers and fewer white fibers than the reticular layer. The connective tissue cells are also more common in this layer. Fat cells are scarce throughout the corium, although they are abundant in the hypodermis.

The reticular layer of the dermis has more bundles of collagenous fibers than the papillary layer, many running parallel to each other and more or less parallel to the skin surface.

The subcutaneous tissue, or hypodermis, while not a part of the skin, is closely associated with it. Where fat is abundant in it, it is called the *panniculus adiposus*. The layer varies in thickness from one part of the body to another. It is usually thicker than the dermis. It binds the skin loosely to underlying structures. Smooth muscles are also present in some areas of the subcutaneous tissue. Blood vessels and lymphatics travel through the subcutaneous tissue in going to and from the skin, and many sweat glands and hair follicles extend down into it.

Hair is more widely distributed over the body than many realize. Much of it is fine and soft and goes unnoticed. Only the palms, the soles, the dorsal sides of the terminal portions of the digits, the lips, the nipples of the breast, the umbilicus, and the skin portion of male and female genitalia are truly hairless. In cases of extensive burning or laceration of the skin, the epithelium of the hair follicles may play an important part in regeneration of the epidermis. Hair is a product of the epidermis and therefore of the ectoderm.

Glands

The integumentary glands are derived by invaginations of cords of the epithelium into the underlying mesenchyme. The important glands of the skin are the sebaceous, sudoriferous (sweat), and mammary glands.

The *sebaceous glands*, with few exceptions, develop from the epithelium in the necks of hair follicles. The secreting portions of the sebaceous glands are saclike masses of epithelial cells.

The *sudoriferous (sweat) glands* are in the form of simple coiled tubules extending down into the reticular layer of the dermis or in some cases into the subcutaneous tissue. They are found in most skin areas, being absent only on the margins of the lips, the concave surface of the external ear, the skin of the nipple, and skin portions of the genital organs. The secretion of the sweat glands is a thin, watery solution containing mainly sodium chloride and some sulfates, phosphates, and urea.

Mammary glands are paired glands of the integument that are rudimentary in the male and larger in the female. They are closely associated functionally with the reproductive system in the female.

Blood and Lymphatic Vessels

Arteries come into the skin through the subcutaneous tissue. They form a cutaneous plexus at the interface of the corium and the subcutaneous layers, from which branches go to the sweat and sebaceous glands, the deep part of the hair follicles, and the flat tissue.

The lymphatics begin as blind outgrowths or capillary networks in the dermal papillae. They join into a dense, flat meshwork of lymphatic capillaries in the papillary layer. From this point, the lymphatics form a deeper network at the boundaries of the corium and subcutaneous layers. The lymph leaves the skin area through lymphatics that travel alongside the arteries and veins.

Nerve and Nerve Endings

The integument is well supplied with nerves and nerve endings. Some of the nerves are afferent somatics for general sensations of pain, pressure, touch, heat, and cold. Others are efferent (motor and secretory) autonomic (sympathetic) fibers that go to the smooth muscle of blood vessels, to the myoepithelial cells of glands, and the arrector muscles of the hair follicles.

Afferent or sensory nerve endings (receptors) of the skin are varied and unequally distributed.

SPECIAL INSTRUMENTS, SUPPLIES, AND EQUIPMENT

All plastic surgery procedures can be done with some basic instrument trays. Modifications to the trays are made for each surgical procedure. All of the instruments used are common, except for maybe those that are used for craniofacial reconstruction.

Plastics tray
  No. 3 knife handles
  Suture scissors
  Sharp scissors
  Iris scissors
  Brown scissors
  Smooth Adson forceps
  Toothed Adson forceps
  Brown-Adson forceps
  Brown forceps
  Smooth forceps
  Plastic suction tip
  Frazier suction tip
  Ruler

  Skin hooks
  Brown needle holder
  Webster needle holder
  Straight and curved mosquito clamps
  Straight and curved hemostats
  Allis clamps
  Kocher clamps
  Small and large towel clips
  Small solution basin
  Small solution cup
Radical mastectomy pack
  Shallow Deaver retractors
  Band retractors
  Dull four-prong rakes
  Sharp four-prong rakes
  Small, medium, and large Richardson retractors
  Vein retractors
Forceps
  Toothed
  Smooth
  Dental
  Vascular
Scissors
  Metzenbaum
  Mayo
  Sharp
  Suture
  Wire cutter
  Small, medium, and large hemoclips
Suction tube
  Frazier
  Yankauer
  Abdominal

The rest of the mastectomy pack is made up of simple instruments.

Hose
Drills
  Reamer
  Oscillating
  Sagittal
  Reciprocating
Wrenches
Variety of burrs and blades
Rib pack
  Shallow Deaver
  Doyen costal elevators
  Weitlaner retractor
  Double-action rongeur
  Sharp four-prong rakes
  Large Tessier rib cutter
  Bone-holding forceps
  Double-ended periosteal elevator
Craniofacial set
  Mallet
  Monroe retractor
  Double-action rongeur
  Small bone-holding forceps
  Disimpaction forceps
  Bone scissors
  Bone bender
  Ramus retractor

Tessier retractor
    Down
    Reverse
Army-Navy retractors
Band retractors
Malleable retractors
Straight osteotome
Curved osteotome
Periosteal elevators (Tessier)
Curved periosteal elevators (Tessier)
Variety of suction tips
Mouth retractor
Straight and curved wire cutters
Variety of scissors
Kerrison rongeur
Pituitary rongeur
Lacrimal duct probes
Pick
Curved awl
Long awl
Medium awl
Small awl
Sponge stick
Wire twisters
Raney clip appliers

The rest of this set is a combination of two plastic trays.

REDUCTION OF MAXILLARY FRACTURE

Definition

Fracture detachments of the maxillas and/or associated bones are designated as fractures of the middle third of the facial skeleton and are commonly referred to as *midface fractures*.

Indications

Detachment of any midface bone or combinations of midface bones may produce a painful and annoying flail at the point of detachment, or the bones may become rigidly impacted and difficult to reduce. The separated midface fracture may vary from a horizontal detachment of the maxilla at the level of the floor of the nasal fossa to involvement of all combinations of facial segments above this arbitrary line.

Related Surgical Procedures

There can be unilateral or bilateral involvement with all combinations of segmental fracture patterns. The facial bony skeleton has to be restablished in a nearly symmetrical and normal attitude. After a relatively rigid mandible is established, the level of the midface fracture is determined, and the face is rebuilt from the mandible up to this level and fixed to the first stable bone

superiorly. The maxilla or multiple maxillary segments are brought forward, and the maxillary and mandibular teeth are fitted together in occlusion. Most cases of a horizontally detached maxilla at the level of the nasal fossa floor are handled satisfactorily by simply wiring the teeth in occlusion. This is a simple procedure.

The *zygomatic bones* are superficial bones of the face. The zygomatic bone is the cheek bone located at the upper and lateral part of the face. In addition to forming the prominence of the cheek, it enters into formation of part of the lateral wall and the floor of the orbital cavity. It articulates posteriorly with the zygomatic process of the temporal bone. This union forms the prominent zygomatic arch, which can be felt on the side of the face in front of the ear. *Maxilla* is the term used in reference to the upper jaw as a whole. However, there are actually two maxillas that fuse in the midline. Not only do the maxillas form part of the floor of the orbital cavities, but also the horizontal, or palatine, processes form the anterior three fourths of the roof of the mouth, or hard palate. Faulty union of these bones may result in a congenital deformity known as *cleft palate*.

Perioperative Nursing Implications

The circulating nurse must be able to anticipate by the fracture type what supplies (e.g., wire and arch bars) and equipment (e.g., air-powered drills, saws) are needed for the procedure.

Anesthesia

The type of anesthetic used depends on the extent of the injuries and the procedure to be performed. The anesthetic is given usually via nasotracheal tube or occasionally tracheostomy, depending and the type of fractures and the extent of injury.

Position

The patient is placed in routine supine position—the head is usually placed on a doughnut and netting is placed over the nasotracheal tube to keep it in place and out of the way.

Creation and Maintenance of the Sterile Field

The patient is prepared using povidone-iodine (Betadine) solution. The mouth is cleansed with peroxide solution.

It is important for the scrub nurse to be ready early, to have sterile suction available at all times, and to be conscientious about the sponge count and the insertion and removal of the throat pack.

The patient is draped with the usual four layers; the head and mouth area are draped with towels.

Equipment and Supplies

Necessary equipment and medical-surgical supplies vary from case to case. Some standard items include a patient drape pack, a table cover, gowns, a throat pack, 4 × 8 sponges, suction tubing, a disposable bulb syringe, No. 24 dental wire, rubber bands, and arch bars.

Osteotomy tray
Table pack
Patient drape
Gown pack
Hall drill
Burrs
Custom pack consisting of light handles, suture bag, needle counter, labels, marking pen
Suction tubings
Pushers
Paper Mayo stand cover
No. 24 wire
Arch bars with rubber bands
Lidocaine 2% (cartridges)
27-gauge needle
4 × 8 inch gauze
Bulb syringe
Nerve stimulator

Drugs and Solutions

Sterile normal saline solution is used for irrigation.

Physiological Monitoring

Blood loss is watched but it is usually minimal.

Specimens and Cultures

Usually, neither specimens nor cultures are obtained.

Physician's Orders, Laboratory and Diagnostic Studies

Preoperatively, a total battery of facial x-ray films is obtained.

Procedure

Details

If there is great comminution along the fracture lines and the maxilla is difficult to stabilize, all bony structures cephalad to this level are solid and can be used to attach fixation wires or appliances. After the teeth are wired in occlusion, the attached unit of maxilla can be moved vertically to the desired facial position. The fracture does not commonly produce great disturbance of the nasal airway. However, there are varying degrees of nasal mucosal edema and ecchymosis. Therefore, the airway should be monitored, as it is liable to become compromised by this edema or by possible hematoma formation.

Postoperative Care

Poor maxillary repositioning and dental occlusion are prevented by early reduction and fixation. Injury to the facial nerve causing loss of feeling can occur.

Preventing infection, ensuring an airway, and providing nourishment are the greatest postoperative nursing problems. Many patients experience an emotional reaction owing to distortion of the facial features.

Potential Surgical Complications

Immediate postoperative care for the patient includes measures to ensure the patient's comfort and safety. Because of the postoperative swelling that occurs around the orbits, the patient's vision might be impaired. Ice packs are used to reduce swelling and pain. Providing a means of communicating with the patient whose orbits are swollen and whose jaw is wired is another concern. The patient might become frustrated if unable to communicate.

Meticulous mouth care is extremely important. The drainage tends to crust in the mouth, and oral access is minimal owing to the wired jaw closure.

The patient's self-image is critical. The perioperative nurse assesses the patient for signs of body image disturbance; if signs are present, the nurse implements interventions, as described in Chapters 2 and 15.

BREAST RECONSTRUCTION WITH LATISSIMUS DORSI FLAP

Definition

The purpose of this procedure is to allow women as close to normal appearance as possible after a radical mastectomy for breast carcinoma.

Indications

No single reconstructive technique is suitable for every patient. The patient's desires and her general health, the availability of local tissue, and the surgeon's personal preference are considered. Many women grieve the loss of breast contour. Restoring the breast often improves the quality of the patient's life. Vastly improved cosmetic results have been obtained, and public awareness of and acceptance of available reconstructive techniques are increasing.

Related Surgical Procedures

The evolution of breast reconstruction began with the era of breast ablation. Before the 19th century, carcinoma of the breast was considered not amenable to surgical therapy. Other techniques related to this procedure are free adipose tissue graft, transfer of tissue from the buttock to the breast area, the use of a tubed abdominal flap, or the use of the opposite breast and the insertion of a silicone prosthesis.

Perioperative Nursing Implications

The circulator must know in advance the overall plan the case involves; she or he must be prepared with positioning aids and anticipate the equipment and supplies needed.

Anesthesia

General anesthesia is used for this procedure. The patient is intubated, and attention is given to proper positioning of the patient.

Position

The patient is placed in the midlateral position with the mastectomy site superior. A pillow is placed between the knees, and a roll is positioned below the dependent shoulder to prevent brachial plexus injury. A strip of wide adhesive tape secured to the operating room bed holds the hips in the correct position. The arm on the mastectomy side is extended in front of the patient and rests on a second Mayo stand, which has been well padded to avoid pressure on the ulnar nerve.

Creation and Maintenance of the Sterile Field

The skin of the upper arm and the anterior and posterior chest to beyond the midline is prepared with a povidone-iodine solution.

The draping varies with the preference of the surgeon. The area can be prepared and draped completely initially or reprepared and redraped after the first part of the procedure is completed. The arm is prepared and draped freely so it can be moved throughout the procedure.

Equipment and Supplies

Necessary equipment and medical-surgical supplies vary from case to case. Some standard items include a table cover, a patient drape, gowns, a basin set, towel packs, a Mayo stand cover, laparotomy sponges, tissue expanders, smaller laparotomy sponges, suction tubing, electrocautery, long electrocautery lips, rakes, a needle counter, light handles, Nos. 10 and 15 blades, bulb syringes, a grounding pad, a marking pen, Hemovac or other wound drain, and dressings.

Drugs and Solutions

Saline for irrigation is placed in a sterile basin.

Physiological Monitoring

Blood loss is calculated by weighing all sponges and keeping track of measured bottled blood loss.

Specimens and Cultures

There should be no specimens or cultures taken during this procedure.

Physician's Orders

Arrangements are made for the patient to have an oncology examination. This should include a mammogram of the contralateral breast, an alkaline phosphatase assay, a bone scan, and a liver scan when necessary. The patient is also advised to speak to others who have already undergone the operation. In some regions, the American Cancer Society is using reconstructed patients as volunteers.

Laboratory and Diagnostic Studies

Occasionally, these patients donate autologous blood preoperatively in case they need to be transfused.

Procedure

Incision and Exposure

Latissimus dorsi muscle is flat and triangular. It is situated below the scapula. The shape and position of this muscle is almost a mirror image of the anteriorly placed pectoralis major muscle. This anatomical similarity permits use of this flap in breast reconstruction after radical mastectomy. Immediately before surgery, the patient is placed in a sitting position and the proposed crease is marked. The anterior edge of the latissimus muscle can be felt by digital examination. The muscle is outlined on the skin with a marking pen, and this is used as the incisional line.

Details

The anterior edge of latissimus muscle is located. Sharp dissection may be necessary if scarring from a previous mastectomy makes the dissection difficult. Freeing up the flap, elevating the flap, and noting the thoracodorsal artery and vein and branches to the serratus anterior muscle are performed. A tunnel between the back wound and the anterior chest wound is formed. Tunneling of the flap is accomplished. The patient is then turned to a supine position with the flap pulled through the tunnel. The flap is then partly inset and a silicone implant is inserted below the contralateral inframammary crease. Sutures close off the cavity laterally.

Closure

The superior edge of the transferred latissimus muscle flap is sewn to the inferior edge of the pectoral muscle. Sutures usually are chromic swedge. The skin is closed with 3–0 nylon suture. The incisional lines are covered with a Xeroform, and a dressing gauze dressing is applied.

Postoperative Care

The patient is usually allowed out of bed the day after surgery. She will probably need some help. The dressings are checked. Pain associated with the reconstruction is usually mild to moderate. The patient resumes activities in about a week to 10 days.

Potential Surgical Complications

Infection of the breast cavity
Incorrect sizing and positioning of the implant

EXCISION OF GYNECOMASTIA

Definition

Gynecomastia, or enlargement of the male breast, occurs in a variety of diseases and clinical settings. The objective of treatment is to restore normal male contour and appearance, while leaving scars that are either concealed or inconspicuous.

Indications

The majority of cases that require surgical treatment occur in adolescent or young adult males and are without obvious cause. Embarrassment due to the female contour of the chest is the main concern, because except during the earliest stages, there is no pain, tenderness, nor any symptoms, except for the abnormal appearance.

Related Surgical Procedures

Incisions and approaches to the treatment of gynecomastia have been many and varied. The procedure for correcting gynecomastia can be compared with most of the breast procedures done for females.

Perioperative Nursing Implications

Anesthesia

The type of anesthetic used depends on the extent of the surgery to be performed. A small defect can be corrected with the use of a local anesthetic. For more extensive procedures, a general anesthetic is used.

Position

The patient is placed in the supine position, with the arms either at the sides or out straight, depending on the surgeon's preference.

Creation and Maintenance of the Sterile Field

The patient is prepared with a povidone-iodine solution; disposable towels are used. The draping is accomplished as for other breast surgery. If a Mayo stand is used, it is placed over the patient at about the knees. The operating room bed is draped with four layers of drapes.

Equipment and Supplies

Basic equipment is needed. Some standard items include a patient drape pack, a gown pack, table covers, extra towels, a dissecting set, some plastic surgery instruments, laparotomy sponges, suction tubing, electrocautery, light handles, a needle counter, a marking pen, a grounding pad, dressings, Nos. 10 and 15 blades, No. 25 short and No. 25 long 1½-inch needle with control-top syringe if local anesthetic is used.

Suture needed for the procedure includes 2–0 chromic ties and taper needles, 3–0 polyglactin 910 (Vicryl), and skin suture of surgeon's preference.

Drugs and Solutions

Saline solution is poured into a sterile basin on the sterile table to be used for irrigation. Lidocaine 1% with 1:100,000 epinephrine is used for local anesthesia in selected cases.

Physiological Monitoring

Depending on the extent of the procedure, blood loss may be monitored, as for mastectomy.

Specimens and Cultures

The only specimen is the breast tissue that is removed.

Physician's Orders, Laboratory and Diagnostic Studies

Preoperatively, the patient has routine electrocardiography, chest radiography, complete blood count, and urinalysis.

Procedure

Incision and Exposure

The actual surgical incision is entirely up to the surgeon. One possibility is the inconspicuous intraareolar incision.

Details

A semicircular (180-degree) incision just within the skin-areola junction is made down to the capsule of the breast. It is usually placed between the 3 and 9 o'clock positions, but its location may be varied to secure the best possible exposure. When the areola is small and the breast mass large, additional exposure may be needed. The skin below the incision is dissected from the face of the breast to a point beyond the periphery. The nipple and areola are undercut, leaving an attached button of breast tissue; the face of the breast above the nipple is released from the overlying skin and subcutaneous tissue. Hemostasis is secured by use of electrocautery. The gland, which is completely exposed on its outer face, may be removed from the underlying pectoral fascia by grasping its periphery and dissecting it free. The cavity, with its roof and floor, is trimmed free of any irregularities.

Closure

The cavity is irrigated copiously. A suction drain, Hemovac drain, or Jackson-Pratt drain is put in place and the wound is closed in layers. A light dressing permits inspection of the skin and nipple for circulation and enables detection of an expanding hematoma.

Postoperative Care

The patients are usually up and out of bed the night of surgery and home within a few days. If the procedure is limited, local anesthesia is used, and no drain is placed in the incision, the patient is able to go home the day of surgery.

Potential Surgical Complications

A complication could be acute bleeding into the large dead space despite suction drainage. If an extension in the areola approach had to be used, scar hypertrophy or keloid formation may occur.

ORBITAL-CRANIOFACIAL SURGERY

Definition

The purpose of orbital-craniofacial surgery is to provide the patient with binocular vision by moving the orbits closer together and provide the patient with a more acceptable appearance by moving the bones of the orbital-craniofacial skeleton into a more normal position.

An extracranial approach is possible, but an intracranial approach is used in most cases; therefore, a neurosurgeon as well as a plastic surgeon performs the operation through a bifrontal craniotomy approach.

Indications

A number of congenital anomalies involve the orbital-craniofacial skeleton. One of these is *Crouzon disease*, which includes premature closure of the cranial sutures resulting in an abnormally shaped skull, exophthalmos and hypertelorism, parrot's-beak nose, and maxillary hypoplasia.

Related Surgical Procedures

Preliminary assessment of a patient requiring surgical correction should be done by a craniofacial surgeon, a dentist, a neurosurgeon, an orthodontist, a speech pathologist, and a medical artist using drawings. All persons involved should first look at the degree of abnormal facial form but then they must consider the psychosocial impact on the patient. Difficulty with occlusion may be stated initially, but an interview may reveal that appearance is the chief concern. A variety of techniques must be considered to correct the malocclusion. Two basic premises underlie any technique chosen: (1) external incisions should never be used, and (2) all osteotomies required should be done in one operation. Some associated procedures are

Surgery for ocular hypertension
Correction of facial asymmetry
Medial and lateral canthal repair
Forehead advancement
Total vault reshaping

Perioperative Nursing Implications

The circulating nurse must know in advance what the overall plan of the case involves: whether neurosurgeons, plastic surgeons, and/or oral surgeons are to be involved. She or he can then anticipate what equipment and supplies will be needed.

When a deformity merits treatment, four factors affect the timing of the surgery: the age of the patient, the possible effect of further growth, the severity of the deformity, and the psychosocial effect on the patient and the family group. It is generally better to operate on a young patient, provided that it is technically feasible. Future growth does not improve a skeletal deformity and certain problems, such as exophthalmos and malocclusion, may become worse with growth. Some deformities are so severe that early surgery is necessary to have any hope for future rehabilitation. Early successful correction enables the patient to cope with the later recurrence of the deformity because she or he will know that it can be corrected again.

Guidelines for the timing of surgery can be given for some ages and conditions. Decisions concerning the timing of surgery and the specific procedures must not be made by one person, but by a health care team only after each member of the team presents and correlates findings with those of the other team members. The greatest benefit of the team conference concept lies in the achievement of successful long-term results.

Anesthesia

The anesthesiologist should be specialized in neuroanesthesia. She or he should be capable of producing hypotension and reducing brain size for hours. There must be close rapport between the anesthesiologist and the surgeon. Some principles are common to all procedures: The anesthetic is given either orally or via nasotracheal tube or sometimes via tracheostomy. The endotracheal tube should be polyvinyl chloride and have a high-volume, low-pressure cuff. An identical tube must be available because occasionally the tube can be cut by an osteotome. A stethoscope monitors the cardiac apex beat and the entry of air into the chest. Central venous and intraarterial pressures and heart rate function are recorded electronically with digital and waveform displays. Rectal temperature and airway pressure are monitored continuously. Urine output is monitored in operations of 4 hours or longer.

Position

The patient is supine. Positioning of the patient on the operating room bed so that all bony prominences are well padded. Pressure points on the occiput, scapulae, elbows, sacrum, and heels should be padded.

Creation and Maintenance of the Sterile Field

Head hair is best removed after the patient has arrived in the surgery department. The hair is first clipped with an electrical clipper, which is cleaned and disinfected after each use. The scalp is then shaved, using warm soapy water, with a disposable safety razor.

After shaving is performed, the skin is inspected carefully for any signs of inflammation or infection. An antiseptic skin preparation is applied after the patient is positioned and before draping. The agent or agents used are dictated by the hospital procedure. Three sites are used for the bone graft:

1. Cranial bone is used mainly in infants when open skull defects can be left to reossify spontaneously.
2. Rib grafts are used primarily because of the ease of removal; also, morbidity is lower than with iliac grafts.
3. Iliac grafts produce greater morbidity for the patient, but larger and more solid segments of bone are available.

The incisional line is marked with a marking solution or a scapel.

The operating room bed is positioned so that the anesthesiologist is to the side of the patient. This enables the surgical team to stand around the head of the bed table.

The draping requirements vary with the procedure and the donor graft site. The head is draped using a head drape. The scrub nurse is positioned at the head of the patient with the rest of the surgical team.

Equipment and Supplies

Necessary equipment and medical-surgical supplies vary from case to case. Some standard items include a table cover pack, a patient drape pack, back table covers, gowns, towel packs, Mayo stand covers, bulb syringes, 50-ml syringes, vials of injectable saline, vials of lidocaine 1%, epinephrine, sponges, 4 × 8 inch gauze, No. 19 hypodermic needle, a wire-passing burr, a contouring burr, air-powered drill and saw, electrocautery, a grounding pad, Nos. 10 and 15 blades, and a needle counter.

Rib pack
Craniofacial set
Craniotomy set

Plastic surgery instrument set
Air-powered drill set
Bulb syringe
Injectable saline 0.9%
Methylene blue
Cotton-tipped applicators
Raney clips
Lidocaine 1% with 1:100,000 epinephrine
22-gauge, 1½-inch needle
19-gauge needle
Gauze dressing
ABD bandage
Elastic (Ace) bandages, 6 inch
10-ml Luer-Lok syringes
Spray thrombin

Drugs and Solutions

Saline and povidone-iodine solution are used for irrigation of the wound.
Lidocaine 1% with 1:100,000 epinephrine is used to preinject the scalp area.

Physiological Monitoring

The patient has a Foley catheter inserted at the beginning of the procedure after being anesthetized. Controlled hypotension is needed for most of these procedures. Its use facilitates the surgery, decreases blood loss, and reduces the length of the operations considerably. Blood loss is difficult to measure accurately. Estimates can be made by measuring aspirates, weighing sponges, continually observing the surgery, and noting soiled drapes.

Specimens and Cultures

In most procedures, no specimens or cultures need to be taken.

Physician's Orders

Clinical examination must include an explanation to the patient of what will take place and to what extent the patient's cooperation will be required in the postoperative phase.

Laboratory and Diagnostic Studies

Laboratory investigations must include determination of hemoglobin level, red blood cell volume, blood urea nitrogen, blood glucose, and serum electrolytes and a coagulation screen to include platelet count, prothrombin time, partial thromboplastin time, and bleeding time. The patient is blood cross-matched for one and one half times the estimated blood volume loss. Laboratory facilities must be available during surgery to provide data on the levels of hemoglobin, serum electrolytes, blood gases, and specific blood components.

Procedure

Incision and Exposure

Skeletal exposure of the upper face and orbit is needed. A coronal incision is the most versatile approach and enables the entire facial skeleton down to the level of the maxillary alveolus to be exposed subperiosteally. This incision passes from one ear transversely to the other and can be extended down into the preauricular area. Hemostasis can be achieved either by inserting preincision blocking sutures—one polyglycolic acid (Dexon) swedge mattress suture is used as a hemostatic stitch—or by applying Raney clips immediately after the incision is made.

Details

The scalp is peeled forward to the level of the galea aponeurotica and the dissection continues down over the temporalis fascia to the level of the zygomatic arch. The periosteum is then divided and elevated using sharp elevators that dissect at the level of the cambium layer. The dissection continues forward to the superior orbital rim and laterally beneath the temporalis muscle. The separate pericranial flap can be used for soft tissue augmentation of cheeks. This is accomplished by dividing down the midline and transversely at the superior orbital rim. The subperiosteal dissection continues backward along the orbital roof, laterally down the lateral orbital rim, and over the root of the nose. Lateral dissection of the nasal bones should only pass to within 0.5 cm of the anterior lacrimal crest unless deliberate detachments of medial canthal ligaments is required. If extreme posterior visualization of the medial orbital wall is required, the anterior ethmoidal vessels can be cauterized with a bipolar cautery and then divided. Dissection of lateral nasal bones is extended laterally to enable visualization of the inferior orbital nerve and foramen. Dissection in the orbit continues from the orbital roof, down the lateral orbital, wall to the zygomatic arch. As the dissection continues medially across the orbital floor, it passes below the inferior orbital nerve. Dissections over the zygoma continue medially above and below the inferior orbital foramen and nerve and continues to the piriform margin. At the end of the procedure, the temporalis muscle must be reattached at the lateral orbital wall, the superior orbital rim, and the anterior part of the inferior temporal line.

If the lateral orbital wall was advanced or moved, the temporalis muscle is divided posteriorly and inferiorly.

It is rotated forward and reattached to drill holes in the lateral orbital wall and lateral superior orbital rim to prevent depression in this region. The frontal periosteum is replaced and the scalp is closed in one or two layers.

To obtain a rib graft, an oblique midaxillary incision is used. The incision should be no more than 4 to 6 cm long. Subcutaneous tissue and muscles are divided using cutting diathermy.

Rib periosteum is divided; the periosteum over the anterior rib surface is elevated, and in one area, the periosteum is stripped over the posterior surface. The posterior surface is then cleaned. The subperiosteal stripping is carried posteriorly as far as the angle of the rib; it is then divided with a curved rib cutter. The wound is filled with saline to demonstrate any pleural leaks.

The periosteum of each rib is sutured to promote uniform regeneration and then each muscle layer is sutured and the skin is closed with a subcuticular suture.

The region of the operative neurosurgical interest lies at the upper level of the supraorbital margins. Regardless of who turns down the desired scalp flap, the neurosurgeon removes cranial bones as required using standard craniotomy techniques. Onlay bone grafts are wired in place.

Closure

Craniofacial surgeons and neurosurgeons involved in the procedure must be familiar with one another's style. It is often advisable for the neurosurgeon to scrub and review the operative territory for bleeding and cerebrospinal fluid leakage just before final placement of bone grafts and scalp closure. After the skin is closed, the area is cleaned and compression dressing with gauze and Kling dressing are applied.

Postoperative Care

Postoperatively, all patients who undergo craniofacial surgery must be monitored in an intensive care unit. Neurological signs can be monitored as usual. Continual oozing of blood into the face and bone graft donor sites occurs for up to 24 hours postoperatively and may necessitate a blood transfusion. Good oral hygiene is mandatory.

Potential Surgical Complications

Blindness or visual impairment
Infection

Bibliography

Crooks, L. C. (1979). *Operating room techniques for the surgical team.* Boston: Little, Brown.

Crouch, J. E. (1972). *Function human anatomy* (2nd ed.). Philadelphia: Lea & Febiger.

Goldman, M. A. (1988). *Pocket guide to the operating room.* Philadelphia: F. A. Davis.

Groah, L. K. (1983). *Operating room nursing, The perioperative role.* Reston, VA: Reston Publishing.

Gruendemann, B. J., Meeker, M. H. (1983). *Alexander's care of the patient in surgery* (7th ed.). St. Louis: C. V. Mosby.

Jackson, I. T., Niunro, I. R., Salyer, K. E., Whitaker, L. A. (1982). *Atlas of craniomaxillofacial surgery.* St. Louis: C. V. Mosby.

Kneedler, J., Godge, G. (1983). *Perioperative patient care.* Boston: Blackwell Scientific.

McGibbon, B. M. (1984). *Atlas of breast reconstruction following mastectomy.* Baltimore: University Park Press.

Neurosurgery

Susan Puterbaugh

DEFINITION

Neurosurgery is defined as any surgery involving the nervous system. In practice, neurosurgery is primarily concerned with the central nervous system (brain, spinal cord, and supporting structures) and less frequently with the peripheral nervous system.

Neurosurgery is sometimes performed by general surgeons (vagotomy), orthopedic surgeons (laminectomy), or gynecologists (presacral neurectomy), or by neurosurgeons in cooperation with surgeons from other specialties such as head and neck or plastic surgeons (craniofacial surgery), orthopedic surgeons (laminectomy and spinal fusion), or general surgeons (ventriculoperitoneal shunt).

ANATOMY

The central nervous system is well protected by the bones of the skull and the vertebrae and by the cushioning effect of the cerebrospinal fluid (CSF). The periop-

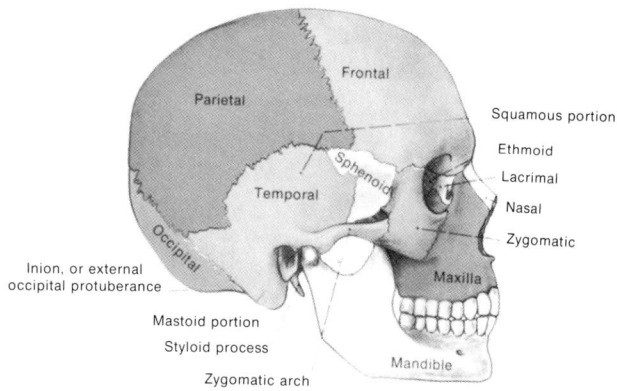

FIGURE 25–1. Bones of the right side of the skull. (From Jacob, S. W., Francone, C. A., Lossow, W. J. [1982]. *Structure and function in man* [5th ed.]. Philadelphia: W. B. Saunders.)

erative nurse should be familiar with basic neuroanatomy to anticipate the needs of the surgeon and to follow the progress of the surgical procedure.

Scalp

The brain is protected by several layers of tissue. The *scalp* consists of (1) a thick subcutaneous layer of fat, which is richly supplied with blood vessels, and (2) the galea aponeurotica, a thick fibrous tissue layer. The subaponeurotic space, under the galea, contains loose areolar tissue and blood vessels. The galea and subgaleal space provide the mobility of the scalp.

Skull

The *skull* is a rigid cavity with a volume of 1400 to 1500 ml. The bones forming the cranial cavity are frontal, parietal (two), occipital, temporal (two), eth-

moid, and sphenoid (Fig. 25–1). The irregular bony seams that join the bones are called *sutures*. The sutures most often used as landmarks in cranial surgery are the coronal, lambdoid, and squamous (Fig. 25–2).

The base of the skull consists of three cavities called *fossae*. The anterior fossa contains the frontal lobes. The middle fossa contains the temporal lobes, the upper brain stem, and the sella turcica, which holds the pituitary gland. The posterior fossa contains the brain stem (pons and medulla) and the cerebellar hemispheres. At the base of the skull is the foramen magnum, a large opening through which the brain stem joins the spinal cord. Other small openings, or foramina, in the skull permit the passage of the cranial nerves and blood vessels.

The skull itself is covered by a layer of periosteum called the *pericranium*. The bone consists of three layers. The outer table and inner table are solid hard bone. These layers are separated by soft, spongy cancellous bone that forms the diploetic space. This arrangement provides strength with a minimum of weight (Alspach and Williams, 1985).

Meninges

Under the skull lie the meninges, three layers of membrane that provide the covering for the brain.

The *dura mater* is a tough fibrous membrane lining the inner surface of the skull. The dura forms folds that divide the brain into four compartments. The falx cerebri is a midline fold that separates the hemispheres of the cerebrum. The falx cerebelli is a smaller vertical fold that separates the cerebellar hemispheres. The tentorium cerebelli is a transverse fold that forms a roof over the posterior fossa. This fold is the basis for describing areas of the brain as supratentorial or infratentorial. The brain stem and the cerebellum are infratentorial structures (Fig. 25–3).

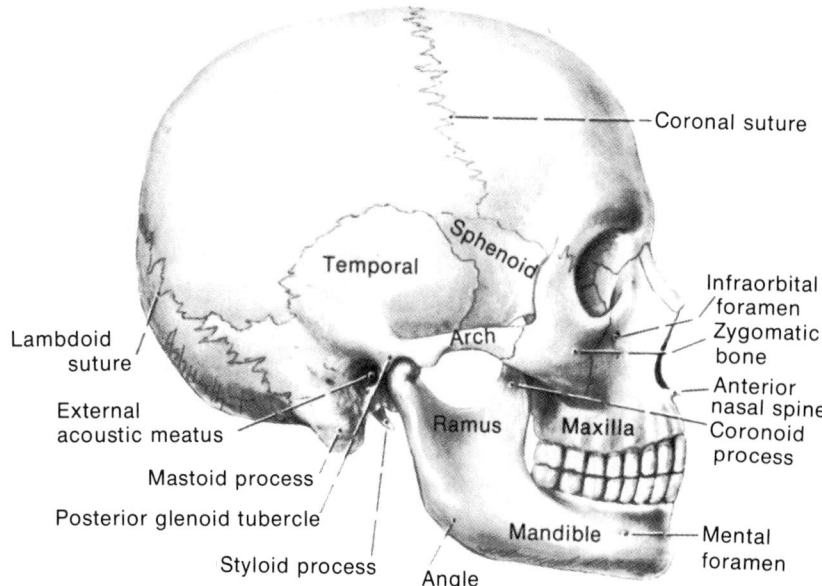

FIGURE 25–2. Sutures of the right side of the skull. (From Jacob, S. W., Francone, C. A., Lossow, W. J. [1982]. *Structure and function in man* [5th ed.]. Philadelphia: W. B. Saunders.)

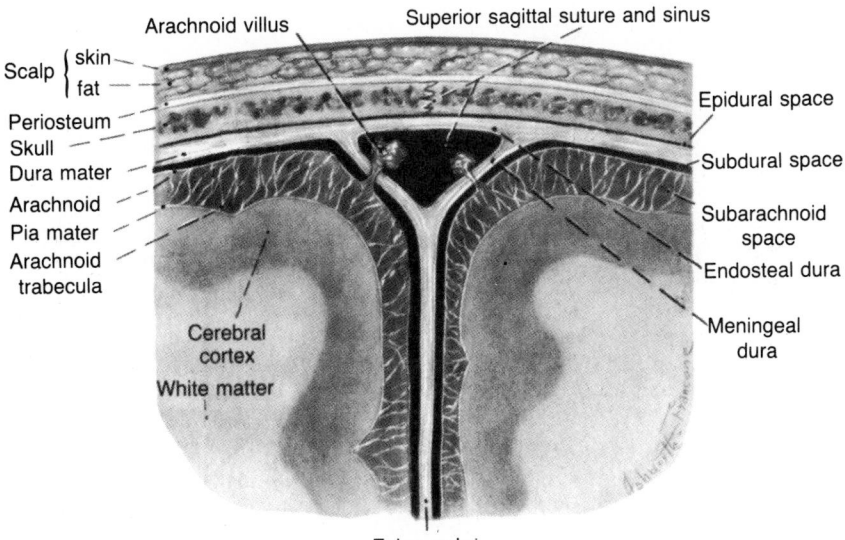

FIGURE 25–3. Coronal section of the skull, brain, meninges, and superior sagittal sinus. (From Jacob, S. W., Francone, C. A., Lossow, W. J. [1982]. *Structure and function in man* [5th ed.]. Philadelphia: W. B. Saunders.)

Layers of the dura separate at the folded areas to form venous sinuses. There are also several major arteries between the dural layers, the most important of which is the middle meningeal artery. Tearing of this artery due to trauma is often a cause of subdural hematoma.

Under the dura is a fine membrane known as the *arachnoid mater*. The inner surface of the arachnoid mater is separated from the layer below, the pia mater, by the subarachnoid space. This space is filled with CSF and large blood vessels. At the base of the brain, the spaces enlarge into cisterns. The arachnoid villi are projections of the arachnoid that absorb CSF into the venous system.

The meningeal layer closest to the brain is the *pia mater*. This delicate membrane follows the convolutions of the brain matter and contains numerous blood vessels. These blood vessels form part of the choroid plexus of the ventricles.

Brain

The *brain* is divided into several major segments: cerebrum, basal ganglia, thalamus, hypothalamus, midbrain, brain stem, and cerebellum.

The largest part of the brain is the *cerebrum*. It consists of two hemispheres divided longitudinally that are joined by the corpus callosum (Fig. 25–4). The lobes

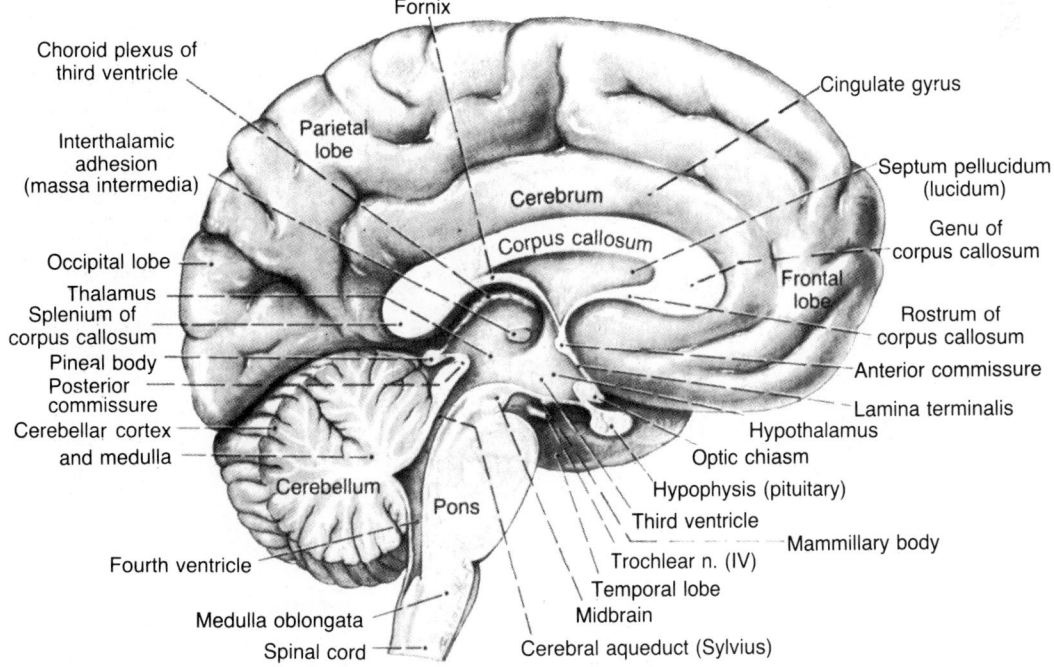

FIGURE 25–4. Sagittal view of the brain and spinal cord. (From Jacob, S. W., Francone, C. A., Lossow, W. J. [1982]. *Structure and function in man* [5th ed.]. Philadelphia: W. B. Saunders.)

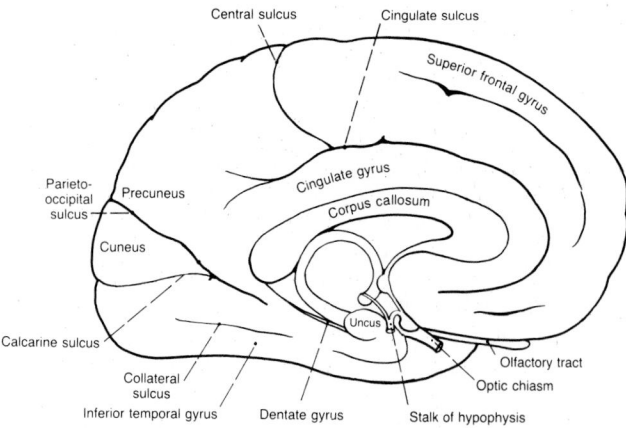

FIGURE 25–5. Major landmarks of the cerebral hemisphere. (From Jacob, S. W., Francone, C. A., Lossow, W. J. [1982]. *Structure and function in man* [5th ed.]. Philadelphia: W. B. Saunders.)

of the cerebrum are the frontal, parietal, temporal, and occipital, which correspond to the overlying bones of the skull. The surface of the cerebrum is marked by folds called *gyri* and small furrows called *sulci*. These markings are used as anatomical landmarks during cranial surgery (Fig. 25–5). The outer cerebral tissue is gray matter, or cerebral cortex, and the inner tissue is the white matter.

The *basal ganglia* are located near the corpus callosum

at the center of the cerebrum. They include the caudate nucleus, putamen, globus pallidus, claustrum, subthalamic nucleus, and substantia nigra.

The thalamus and hypothalamus are adjacent to the third ventricle. Together they are known as the *diencephalon*.

The *midbrain* lies between the cerebral hemispheres and the pons. It contains cerebral peduncles, nerve tracts, and nuclei.

The medulla oblongata and pons compose the *brain stem*, which lies below the midbrain.

The *cerebellum* is contained in the posterior fossa. It is divided in the midline to form two lobes that are marked transversely by small fissures. The tissue between the lobes is called the *vermis*.

The brain contains four chambers called *ventricles* (Fig. 25–6). There are two lateral ventricles, the third ventricle, and the fourth ventricle. They are lined with a membrane called the *ependyma*. Inside of each ventricle is the choroid plexus (Fig. 25–7), a vascular structure that produces the CSF by an osmotic filtration of fluid elements from the blood. This fluid circulates through the brain (Fig. 25–8) and around the spinal cord functioning as a liquid support and flotation device for the tissues. The CSF absorbs the shocks of external trauma.

The normal adult volume of CSF is 125 to 150 ml (Gruendemann and Meeker, 1987). The volume of fluid can fluctuate somewhat to maintain a consistent intracranial pressure, but space-occupying lesions and mechanical obstructions of flow can elevate intracranial

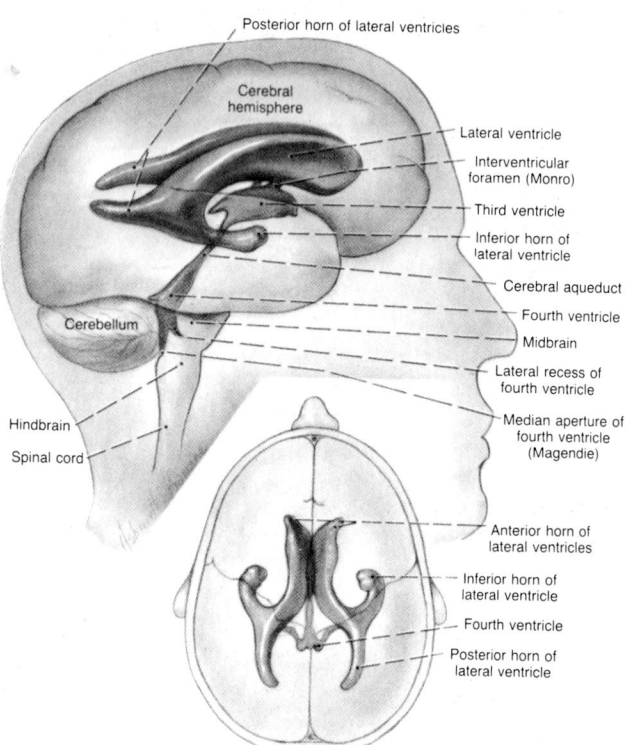

FIGURE 25–6. Ventricular system, lateral and superior views. (From Jacob, S. W., Francone, C. A., Lossow, W. J. [1982]. *Structure and function in man* [5th ed.]. Philadelphia: W. B. Saunders.)

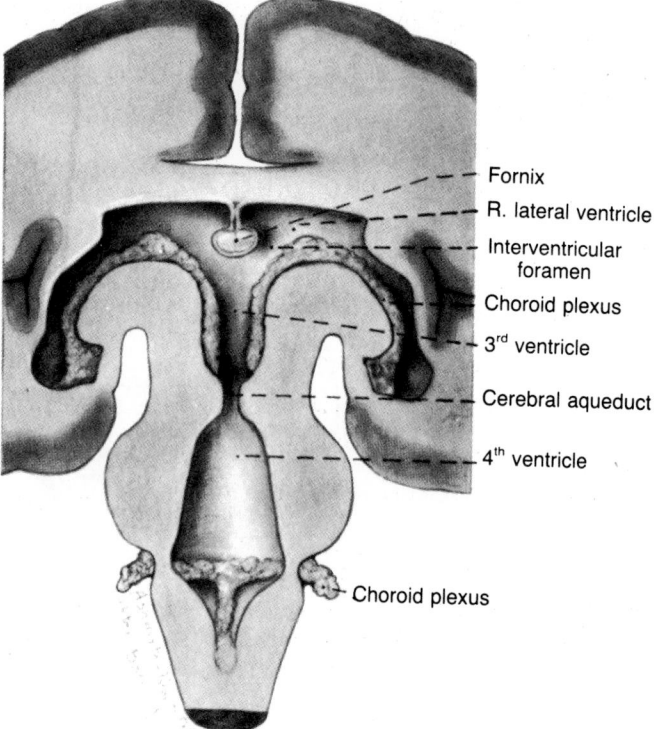

FIGURE 25–7. Ventricles of the brain with the choroid plexus. (From Basmajian, J. V. [1970]. *Primary Anatomy* [6th ed.]. Baltimore: Williams & Wilkins.)

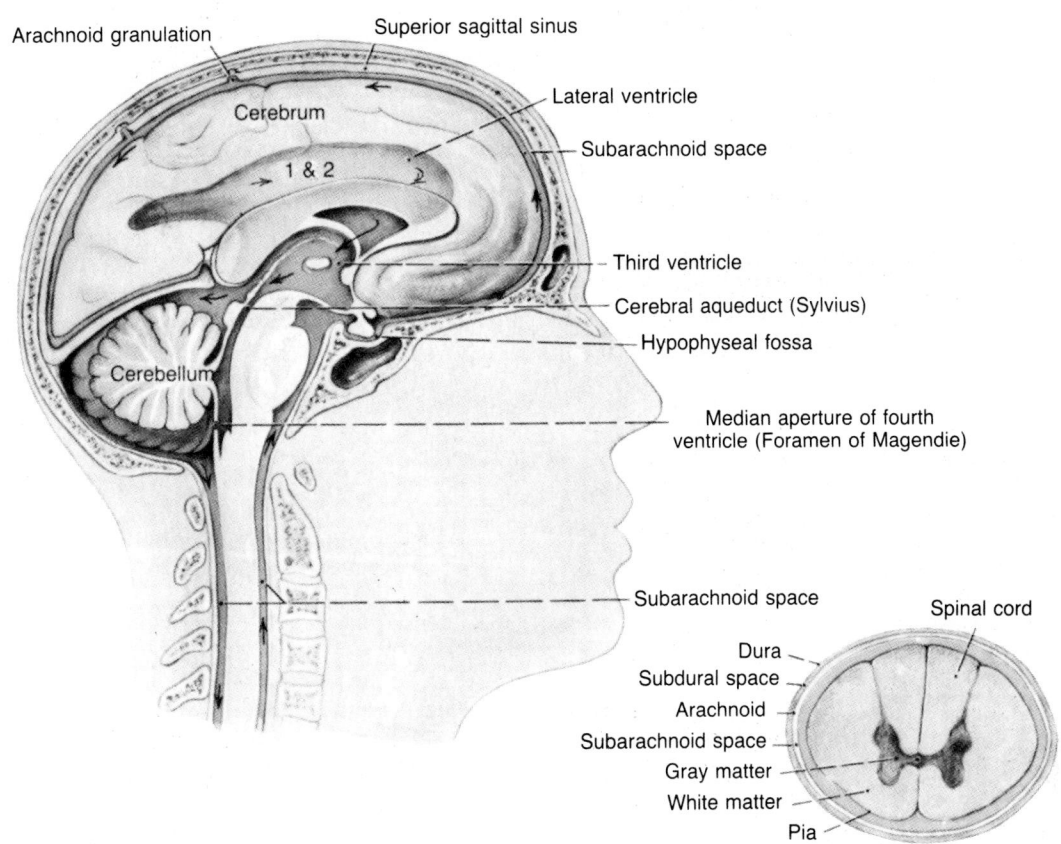

FIGURE 25–8. Circulation of the CSF in the brain and spinal cord. (From Jacob, S. W., Francone, C. A., Lossow, W. J. [1982]. *Structure and function in man* [5th ed.]. Philadelphia: W. B. Saunders.)

pressures. This elevation cannot always be compensated for.

Cerebral circulation is designed to support the oxygen requirements of the brain, even if there is an interruption in one of the supplying arteries. The arteries entering the brain are two internal carotid and two vertebral arteries. These arteries are connected by the basilar artery and the circle of Willis (Fig. 25–9). Branching from the circle of Willis are the anterior, middle, and posterior cerebral arteries. Venous drainage of the brain is effected via a network of veins that converge into the venous sinuses of the dura (Fig. 25–10). Blood is carried away from the brain via the jugular veins.

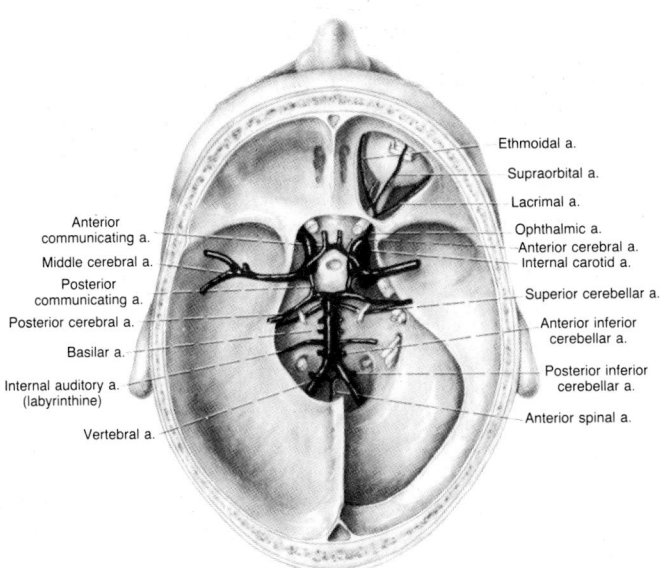

FIGURE 25–9. Arterial supply of the brain. (From Jacob, S. W., Francone, C. A., Lossow, W. J. [1982]. *Structure and function in man* [5th ed.]. Philadelphia: W. B. Saunders.)

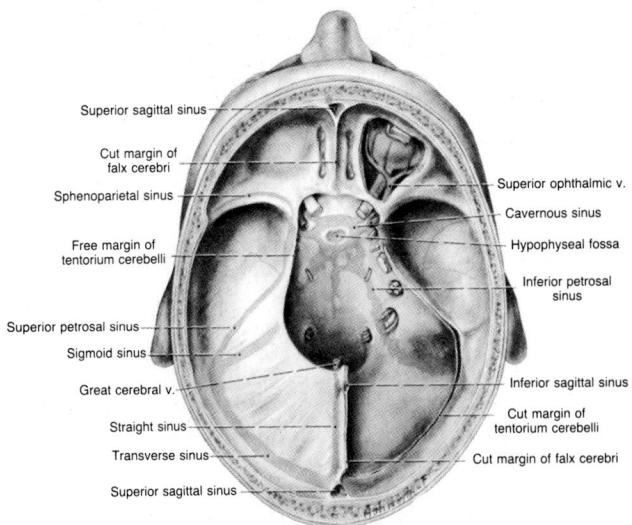

FIGURE 25–10. Venous drainage of the brain. (From Jacob, S. W., Francone, C. A., Lossow, W. J. [1982]. *Structure and function in man* [5th ed.]. Philadelphia: W. B. Saunders.)

Spine

The *vertebral column* is composed of 33 vertebrae, which are referred to by number and location: cervical vertebrae are numbered 1 to 7; thoracic, 1 to 12; and lumbar, 1 to 5. The sacrum is composed of five fused vertebrae, and the coccyx is made up of four small, fused vertebrae (Fig. 25–11). The structure of the vertebrae varies somewhat with their location, but the basic elements are common to all 33 (Fig. 25–12). Each vertebra has a body, which is a solid block of spongy bone lying anteriorly. The vertebral bodies are separated

from one another by an intervertebral disk of fibrocartilaginous material. The periphery of the disk is the tough annulus fibrosus, and the inner portion is a soft, gelatinous layer called the *nucleus pulposus* (Fig. 25–13). The vertebral arch consists of the most posterior segment, the spinous process, and the transverse processes, which are connected to the spinous process by the laminae. Articular surfaces, or facets, form the joints with the vertebrae above and below. The spinal column is held together by and forms support for muscles and ligaments.

The spinal cord is located in the spinal foramina,

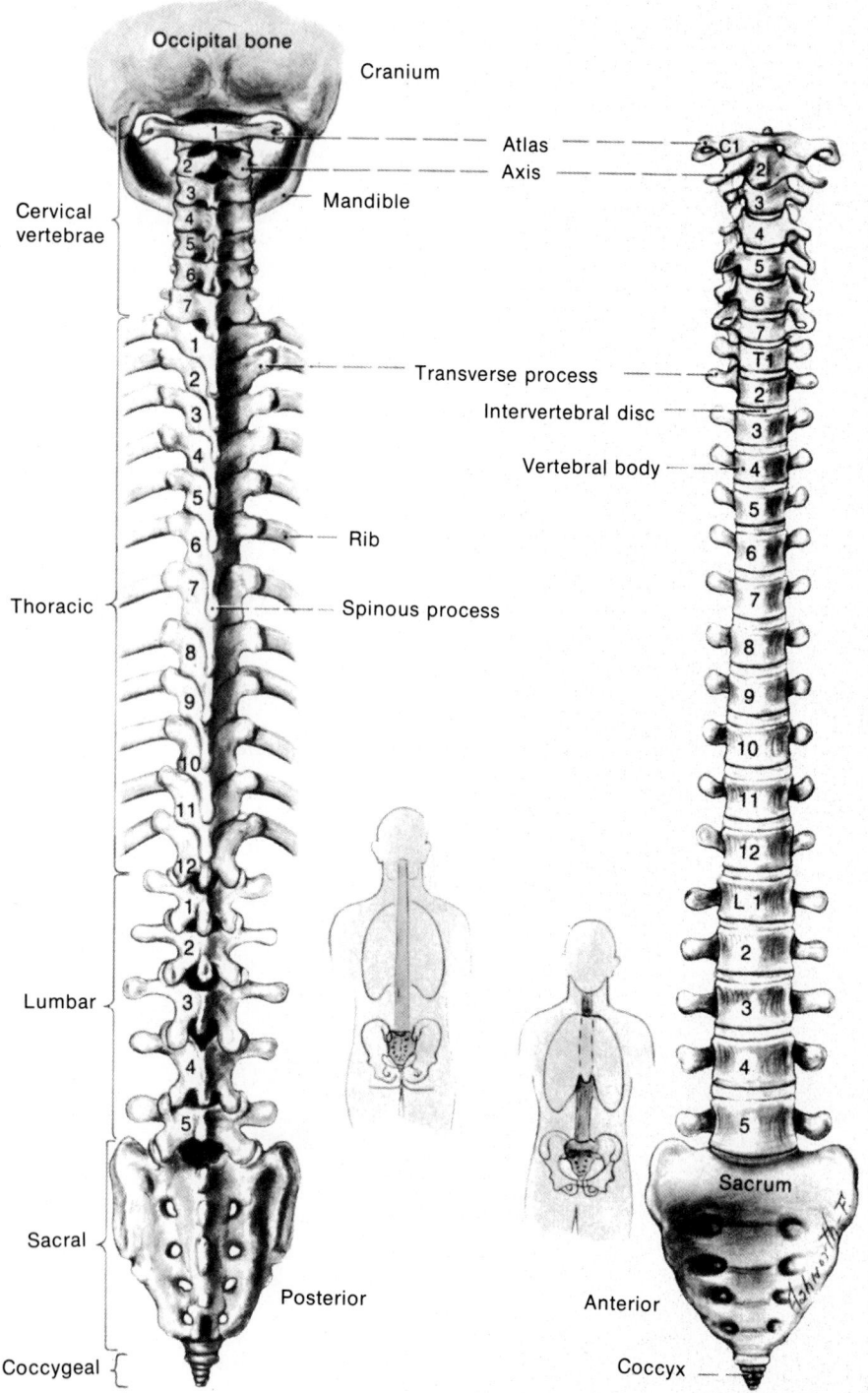

FIGURE 25–11. Posterior and anterior views of the vertebral column. (From Jacob, S. W., Francone, C. A., Lossow, W. J. [1982]. *Structure and function in man* [5th ed.]. Philadelphia: W. B. Saunders.)

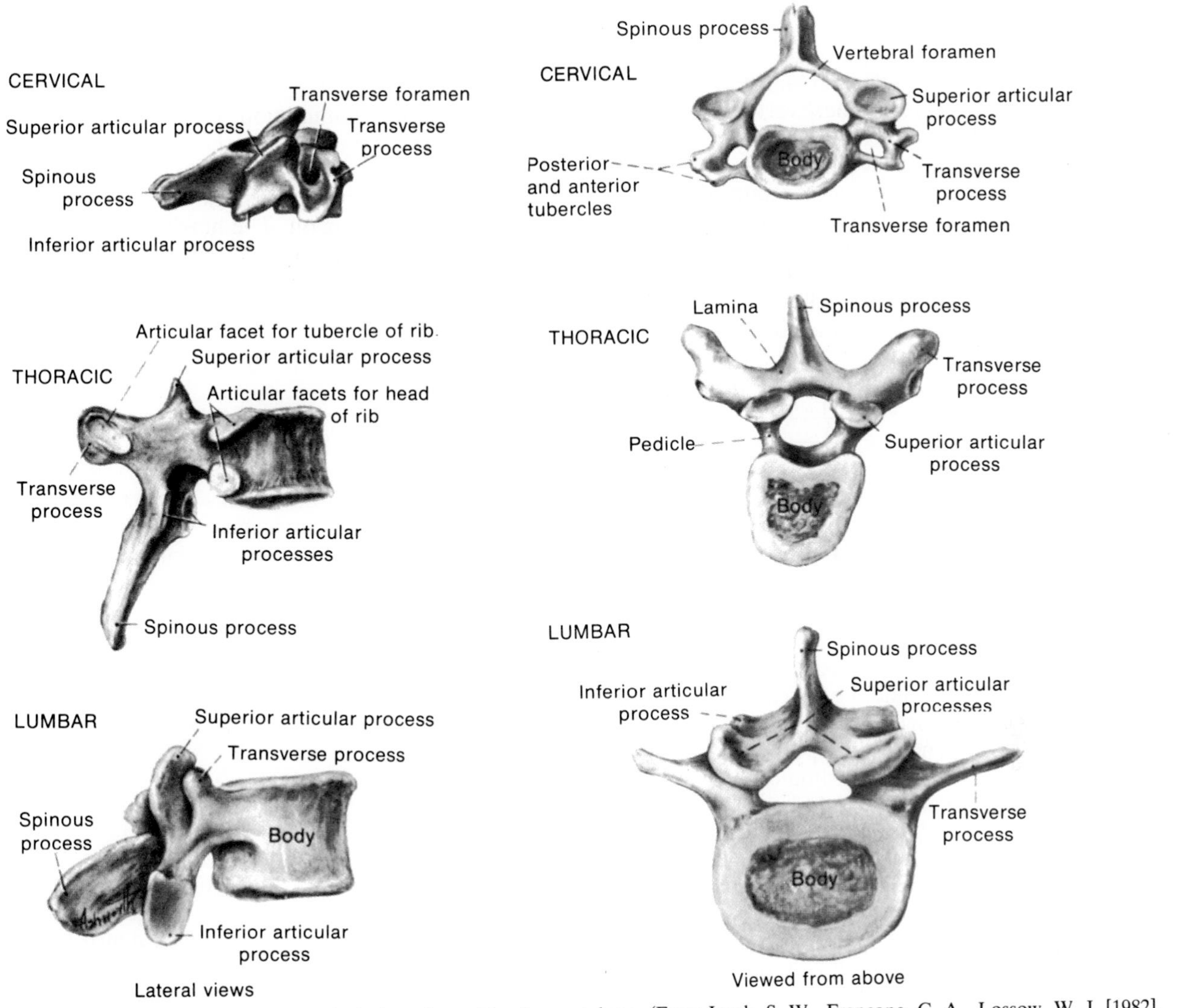

CERVICAL

Superior articular process

Spinous process

Inferior articular process

Transverse foramen

Transverse process

CERVICAL

Spinous process

Vertebral foramen

Superior articular process

Body

Posterior and anterior tubercles

Transverse process

Transverse foramen

THORACIC

Articular facet for tubercle of rib.

Superior articular process

Articular facets for head of rib

Transverse process

Inferior articular processes

Spinous process

THORACIC

Lamina

Spinous process

Transverse process

Pedicle

Superior articular process

Body

LUMBAR

Superior articular process

Transverse process

Spinous process

Body

Inferior articular process

Lateral views

LUMBAR

Spinous process

Inferior articular process

Superior articular processes

Transverse process

Body

Viewed from above

FIGURE 25–12. Lateral and top views of cervical, thoracic, and lumbar vertebrae. (From Jacob, S. W., Francone, C. A., Lossow, W. J. [1982]. *Structure and function in man* [5th ed.]. Philadelphia: W. B. Saunders.)

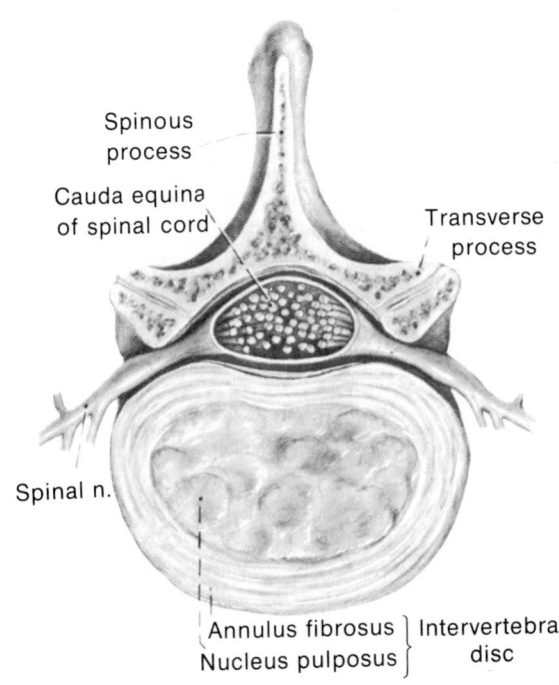

Spinous process

Cauda equina of spinal cord

Transverse process

Spinal n.

Annulus fibrosus — Intervertebral
Nucleus pulposus — disc

FIGURE 25–13. Normal relationship of the intervertebral disk to the spinal cord and nerve branches. (From Jacob, S. W., Francone, C. A., Lossow, W. J. [1982]. *Structure and function in man* [5th ed.]. Philadelphia: W. B. Saunders.)

545

collectively known as the *spinal canal*. The spinal cord is an extension of the brain stem and starts at the upper border of the atlas (first cervical vertebra) and ends at the upper border of the second lumbar vertebra as the conus medullaris. Spinal nerves exit the cord and pass out of the vertebral column via the intravertebral foramina at each vertebral level. In the lumbar area, a vertical bundle of spinal nerves forms the cauda equina. The spinal cord is covered by a dural sac that ends between the first and third sacral vertebrae. Under the dura is the arachnoid. The subarachnoid space contains the spinal fluid. Adhering to the cord is the delicate pia mater. The cord contains a central canal that is an extension of the fourth ventricle and is also filled with spinal fluid.

SPECIAL INSTRUMENTS, SUPPLIES, AND EQUIPMENT

Neurosurgery necessitates a large amount of specialized equipment and instruments. For this reason, a neurosurgical suite should be large and should have numerous electrical receptacles, at least three vacuum outlets, and a nitrogen line for operation of air-powered equipment. The surgical bed should be capable of accommodating neurosurgical headrest equipment and should move easily into a variety of positions.

Additional room furnishings should include a large back table, three preparation tables, one double-ring stand, two single-ring stands, two Mayo stands (or a large overbed instrument table), standing stools of various heights, sitting stools, and kick buckets.

Monitoring Equipment

The neurosurgical operating room (OR) should be equipped with all of the standard anesthesia equipment with the capability to monitor electrocardiographic patterns, arterial pressure, central venous pressure, and pulmonary arterial pressure. A pulse oximeter and the telethermometer are used routinely. At least two fluid or blood warmers are also necessary. A Doppler ultrasound should be available when cranial surgery is to be performed with the patient in the sitting position.

A cooling or heating mattress is usually necessary to maintain the patient's body temperature within normal limits. It may be placed under and/or on top of the patient.

Lighting

The overhead surgical illumination is best accomplished by a two-light system, either on two tracks or swiveling from a central point. This is especially helpful when the surgery involves two sites simultaneously. It is also advantageous when light coming from two angles provides superior visualization of a small, deep surgical wound, as in a craniotomy, or to a long wound, as in spinal surgery.

Additional illumination is provided by headlamps worn by the surgeons. The headlamp is connected by a fiberoptic cable to a light source. When properly adjusted, this lamp illuminates the exact spot that the surgeon is focusing on. The headlamp may be combined with magnifying loupes, or the loupes may be attached to frames worn independently of the headlamp.

Positioning Devices

The surgical bed should be padded with a foam flotation mattress, air mattress, or silicone gel mattress. Additional supportive and protective devices such as pillows, foam heel and elbow protectors, axillary rolls, chest rolls, doughnuts, bean bags, and arm boards should be available, as appropriate, for the anticipated surgical position. The perioperative nurse must meticulously position the neurosurgical patient because the length of the procedures places the patient at unusual risk for tissue injury and skin breakdown. Protective devices should be used to the fullest possible extent.

Positioning devices specific to neurosurgery provide support of the head and the spine during the surgical procedure.

The head section of the standard OR bed is replaced by a neurosurgical headrest when a craniotomy is to be performed. Neurosurgical headrests come in a variety of configurations, which are used according to the desired position and the surgeon's preference. One commonly used system is the Mayfield neurosurgical headrest. This consists of a basic unit that attaches to the OR bed and several different headrests. The general purpose headrest has rubber cups mounted in a half circle that support the head when the patient is supine. The horseshoe headrest is a horseshoe-shaped, sponge rubber–padded unit (Fig. 25–14) for use with the patient in the prone position. This headrest also has a pulley bar to be used when cervical traction is desired, for example, during a cervical fusion procedure.

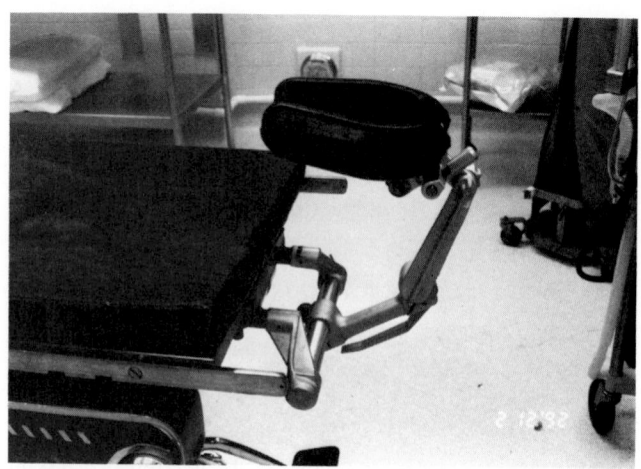

FIGURE 25–14. Mayfield Neurosurgical Headrest. (Courtesy of Codman and Shurtleff, Inc., Randolph, MA.)

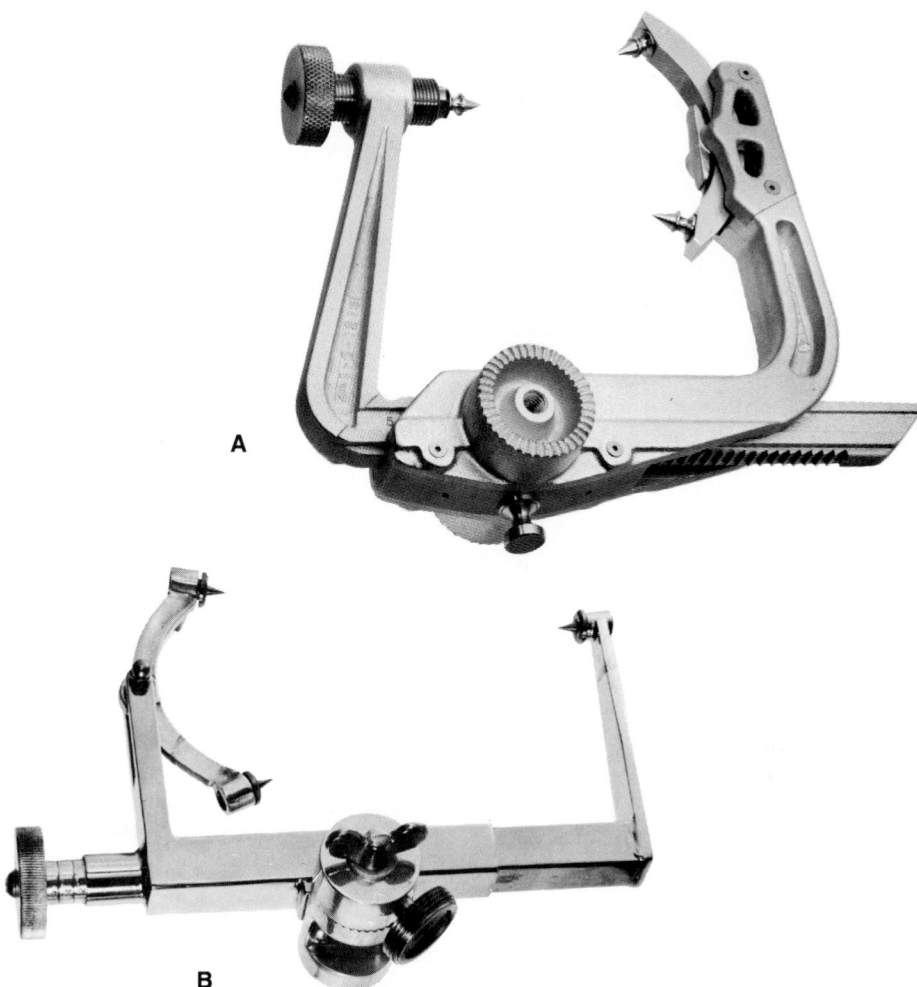

FIGURE 25–15. *A*, Mayfield skull clamp with detachable pins. *B*, Gardner skull clamp with detachable pins. (Courtesy of Codman and Shurtleff, Inc., Randolph, MA.)

The most commonly used head supportive device for craniotomy is the three-point rigid skeletal fixation clamp. The Mayfield and the Gardner are two common types (Fig. 25–15). Both of these types consist of a movable arc-shaped segment with places for pins on each end with a pin holder opposite. The cone-shaped pins are removable so that they can be sterilized. This device holds the head firmly (Fig. 25–16). It can be used with the patient in any position. The Mayfield cross-bar attachment arches across the surgical bed over the patient's legs. The cross-bar holds the head attachments when the patient is in a sitting position (Fig. 25–17).

For surgery on the spine, the Wilson frame or the Andrews frame may be used. An arm table is required for peripheral nerve surgery on the upper extremity. Further specifics of neurosurgical positioning are addressed relative to each procedure.

Other Equipment

Additional supplies and equipment necessary during the preparation phase of neurosurgery are hair clippers and razors to remove the patient's hair. Generally, the

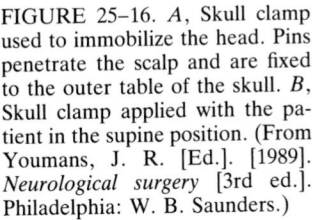

FIGURE 25–16. *A*, Skull clamp used to immobilize the head. Pins penetrate the scalp and are fixed to the outer table of the skull. *B*, Skull clamp applied with the patient in the supine position. (From Youmans, J. R. [Ed.]. [1989]. *Neurological surgery* [3rd ed.]. Philadelphia: W. B. Saunders.)

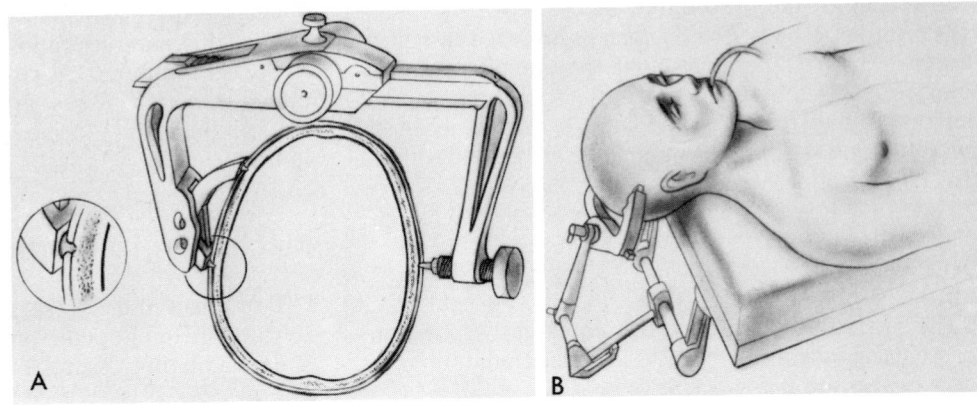

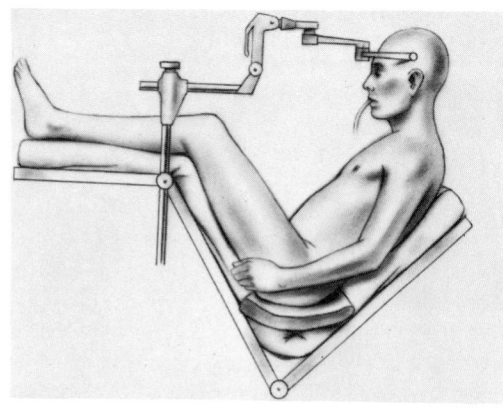

FIGURE 25–17. Head holder used with a crossbar attachment for a patient in the sitting position. (From Youmans, J. R. [Ed.]. [1989]. *Neurological surgery* [3rd ed.]. Philadelphia: W. B. Saunders.)

neurosurgeon prefers to perform this function personally. Sometimes hair removal is done in a preinduction area with the patient awake and other times inside the OR proper with the patient under anesthesia. The surgeon may want to complete the shave using a single-edge blade such as a Weck blade to achieve as much hair removal as possible.

Long immobility of the neurosurgical patient can create an environment for thrombus formation. Consequently, a variety of devices may be used intraoperatively to combat venous stasis. The legs may be wrapped with elastic bandages or antiembolism hose applied. Mechanical pneumatic compression devices can also be applied to the legs to promote venous circulation.

If a need to decrease the amount of CSF is anticipated, a spinal drain may be inserted. This procedure involves insertion of a catheter into the spinal canal. The catheter is connected to tubing with a stopcock that ends in a small drainage bag. When the surgeon so requests, the anesthetist or circulating nurse can open the stopcock to allow the spinal fluid to drain into the bag. This maneuver reduces the pressure in the brain.

Monitoring urine output is important during many neurosurgical procedures. When diuretics are administered, overdistention of the bladder is possible. When a large amount of blood loss is anticipated or when the patient has experienced trauma, urine output is an indicator of kidney function (Gruendemann and Meeker, 1987). Therefore, the perioperative nurse should anticipate the insertion of a Foley catheter in preparation for the procedure.

Several large pieces of equipment are used in neurosurgery. The perioperative nurse should be knowledgeable about this equipment so that the room arrangement can be planned to accommodate all of the necessary apparatus and so that the equipment can be used without difficulty intraoperatively.

Microscope

The operating microscope is used extensively in neurosurgical procedures. These include craniotomy for tumor removal and vascular surgery, lumbar and cervical diskectomy, and peripheral nerve repair. Use of the microscope can improve operative results by permitting better visualization of nerves and vascular structures, smaller incisions, less retraction of brain tissue, better hemostasis, and more accurate nerve and vascular repairs (Youmans, 1982). The microscope may be attached to a video system with a television monitor so that all team members can observe the procedure. A videocassette recorder may be used to document the procedure for further study and review.

Laser

A laser may be attached to the microscope or may be used under normal vision or with magnification provided by loupes. The carbon dioxide laser is used in brain surgery to ablate tumors. Brain tissue has a high water content. Because the carbon dioxide laser beam is absorbed by water, the laser radiation affects only a small area of brain tissue at a time (Walker, 1983). This provides a sharp zone of destruction and preserves normal brain tissue. As with any laser use, appropriate safety measures must be employed: warning signs on OR doors, eye protection for the patient and personnel, protection of the tissue surrounding the lesion with moist sponges, evacuation of the laser plume, and testing of the laser before use.

Ultrasound

Intraoperative ultrasound allows the surgeon to localize tumors with minimal dissection. The depth of the lesion can be measured precisely. This is especially useful during an open brain biopsy (Houston and Murphy-Irwin, 1986). The ultrasound waves are generated by a unit that has a screen for visualization of the image. A sterile probe is supplied to the scrub nurse, who hands off the end to the circulating nurse. The circulating nurse then connects the probe to the unit. The probe is applied directly to the brain tissue. This must be accompanied by continuous irrigation to eliminate air between the probe tip and the brain surface. Air interface degrades the quality of the image (Houston and Murphy-Irwin, 1986). The ultrasound unit may also have a videocassette recorder or an instant camera attached to document the results of the examination.

The ultrasonic irrigation-aspiration device is used to resect soft tumors. A vibrating handpiece breaks the tumor into tiny pieces. Irrigation and aspiration allow the specimen to be removed into a collection container in the device.

Electrosurgical Units

Two forms of electrosurgery are used in neurosurgery. A standard monopolar unit is needed for both cutting and coagulating tissue. A bipolar unit is used for coagulating fine vessels while minimizing the possibility of burns to adjacent tissues. The bipolar coagulator works by passing current through one side of a forceps electrode, across the tissue, and back through the opposite side of the forceps. No grounding of the patient is required with this unit. To work effectively, the forceps tips must be kept clean of charred tissue. Scraping the tips with a rough or sharp surface damages them; instead, they should be cleaned using a wet towel or sponge. There is also a unit available that provides continuous irrigation to the bipolar forceps tip. This prevents drying out of the tissue and therefore helps to keep the tissue from adhering to the forceps. Bipolar coagulators are available as an independent unit or incorporated in a monopolar unit. Various sizes of forceps are available, both straight and bayonet style, with tips of differing widths.

Nerve stimulators are used to identify nerve tissue and intraoperatively to evaluate nerve response. The device consists of a generator to which a sterile probe is connected. Sterile disposable self-contained nerve stimulators are also available.

Stereotaxic Equipment

Stereotaxic equipment entails specialized frames surrounding the head in three planes in conjunction with fluoroscopy or computed tomographic (CT) scans to locate specific areas within the brain. Stereotaxic technique can be used to pinpoint brain tumors so that biopsy can be performed through a burr hole under local anesthesia rather than a full craniotomy. It is also used to create lesions to achieve pain control, to relieve involuntary movements of parkinsonism, cerebral palsy, and Huntington chorea; and to control some types of seizures and to perform psychosurgery (Temple, 1984). Stereotaxic surgery has been used with guided endoscopy to localize tumors, which can then be vaporized by directing a laser beam through the endoscope. Stereotaxic endoscopy is also used for placement of radioactive isotopes (Koch and Poisson, 1989).

Power Equipment

A variety of air-powered equipment are used in neurosurgery. Powered equipment is useful because it decreases surgical time and reduces the fatigue of the surgeon. The most common is a craniotome. This device has several attachments. The cranial perforator creates burr holes in the skull. When used properly, the perforator stops automatically before the dura is penetrated. The saw blade with dural guard makes cuts in the skull between the burr holes. A wire pass attachment permits the drilling of small holes to reattach the bone flap.

Other types of bone drills and saws may be required when removing bone from the spine or when taking and shaping a bone graft. Several companies manufacture a pneumatic instrument system that is powerful and allows bone to be cut and sculpted rapidly. Manufacturer's

instructions for operation, maintenance, and sterilization of all power equipment should be carefully followed.

Materials to Provide Hemostasis

A number of items are used in neurosurgery to achieve hemostasis. The vascularity of the scalp necessitates special efforts to control bleeding when the incision is made. The surgeon may infiltrate the incision line with a local anesthetic agent to decrease bleeding. As the incision is made, scalp clips such as Raney, Leroy, and Michel clips may be applied over the edges of the incision on the scalp flap. The outer edge of the incision is secured by a series of hemostatic clamps such as Dandy and Crile clamps.

To minimize bleeding of the bone, cut edges are sealed with bone wax. This is a soft wax that is easily shaped and is rubbed on the bone edges in a thin layer. The scrub nurse should prepare the bone wax in small balls about 5 mm in diameter.

Besides the usual gauze sponges, neurosurgery requires special neurosurgical sponge material called Cottonoids. These are used on nerve tissue that might be injured by the coarse gauze sponge (Gruendemann and Meeker, 1987). Cottonoids are made from a compressed rayon material and are available in a variety of sizes and shapes. Strips are 6 inches long by ⅛, ¼, ½, ¾, or 1 inch wide. The strips have a radiopaque marker. Pattys or pledgets are small squares (¼ × ¼, ½ × ½, ¾ × ¾, or 1 × 1 inch) with a string and a radiopaque marker (Fig. 25–18). Cottonoids are always used moist. They should be displayed at the edge of the surgical field on a small metal tray or the bottom of a basin, arranged by size. The surgeon removes the Cottonoids from the tray using forceps. Because Cottonoids are

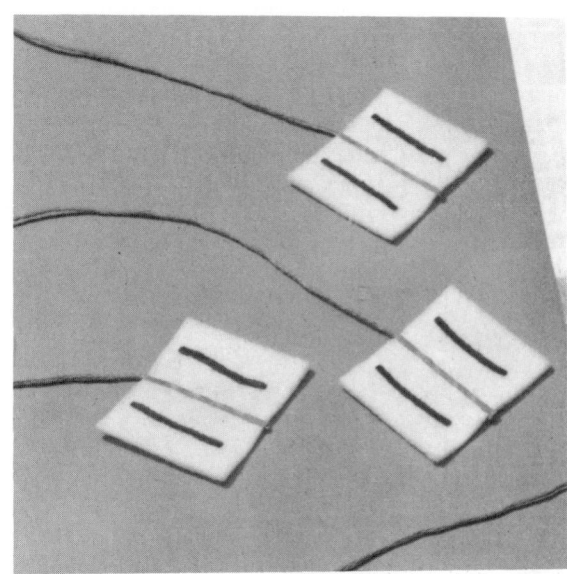

FIGURE 25–18. Cottonoid neurosurgical sponges. (Courtesy of Codman and Shurtleff, Inc., Randolph, MA.)

used to protect tissue and isolate areas and to provide hemostasis, numerous Cottonoids may be in the wound at any given time.

Cotton balls provide hemostasis in a deep area such as the bed of a tumor. Several wet cotton balls may be packed into the space to provide pressure. As the cotton balls are removed one by one, hemostasis is ensured. The scrub nurse is responsible for counting the cotton balls as they are placed into the wound and also for ensuring that they have all been removed.

Absorbable gelatin sponge (Gelfoam) is frequently used in neurosurgery. It is usually cut into sizes and shapes of the surgeon's preference and soaked in a solution of topical thrombin. The Gelfoam is then applied directly to the area of bleeding. It may be left in place but is usually removed before wound closure.

An absorbable knitted fabric of oxidized regenerated cellulose (Surgicel) is cut into the size desired by the surgeon and placed dry over bleeding areas. The Surgicel provides a substrate for clot formation. It should be removed after hemostasis has been achieved.

A microfibrillar collagen hemostat (Avitene) causes clotting when it is applied to a bleeding area. Because it adheres to a wet surface, it should be applied to the area using dry, smooth forceps. Excessive material should be removed after the bleeding has been stopped. Collagen sponges are also used as a hemostatic device.

Instruments

Specialized suction tips of many styles are used in neurosurgery. Suction tips are employed for retracting, dissecting, evacuating smoke, picking up Cottonoids, and removing blood and irrigation fluid. Suction tips that are also active electrodes are used for hemostasis. The scrub nurse should always be prepared to switch and clean suction tips. Frequently, they become clogged with bits of bone and tissue owing to their small diameter. Clearing the suction can be done using a stylet, but irrigation with a 10-ml syringe is often quicker and more effective in dislodging the blockage.

Microsurgical instruments consisting primarily of dissectors, forceps, needle holders, and scissors enable the performance of delicate procedures, but are useful only when in perfect working condition. These instruments must be maintained in exact alignment without nicks or burrs on the working areas. Proper care consists of washing by hand, sterilizing and storing in specialized

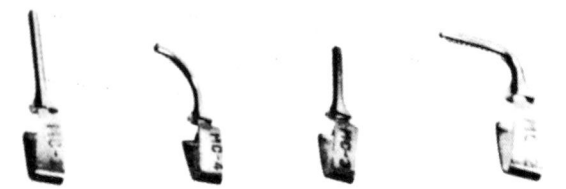

FIGURE 25–19. Aneurysm clips. (Courtesy of Codman and Shurtleff, Inc., Randolph, MA.)

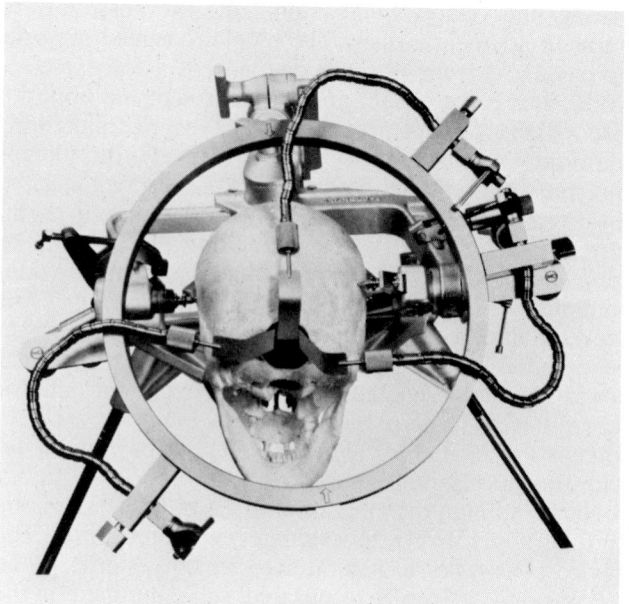

FIGURE 25–20. Budde-Halo Retractor. (Courtesy of Codman and Shurtleff, Inc., Randolph, MA.)

racks or cases and careful handling intraoperatively. The instruments should not be wiped with gauze intraoperatively because the fibers might snag and bend them. Instead, use special microsurgical cleaning pads.

Aneurysm clips come in many different sizes and configurations (Fig. 25–19). The type of clip used is according to the surgeon's preference. Each type of clip is used in a clip applier specifically designed for that clip. Aneurysm clips have delicate mechanisms designed to apply a specific amount of pressure when closed. Any experimental opening and closing of the clip can disrupt this mechanism; therefore, clips should be opened only by the clip applier. Temporary clips are applied to control bleeding without damage to the vessel and therefore exert less pressure than permanent clips. The scrub nurse needs to be aware of the difference between temporary and permanent clips and ensure that they are being used appropriately.

Several self-retaining retractors are especially designed for use during craniotomy. These are attached to the OR bed, the neurosurgical skull clamp, or the skull itself. The retractors hold brain spatulas on flexible arms and can be configured into a variety of positions. Common retractors of this type are the Leyla, Greenberg, and the Budde halo (Fig. 25–20). The Budde halo serves a dual purpose in that the supporting ring also acts as a handrest. This is especially useful in microsurgical procedures in which tremors caused by hand fatigue can be detrimental to the progress of the operation. Other self-retaining retractors such as the Weitlaner and the cerebellar retractor are also useful, especially for posterior fossa procedures.

Spinal procedures necessitate specialized retractors such as the Taylor and the Hibbs retractors. The Scoville retractor is a self-retaining retractor with a variety of detachable blades often used during laminectomy.

Following are several examples of instrument sets used for neurosurgery:

Craniotomy Instrument Set

Scissors
    1 Dandy trigeminal
    1 tenotomy
    1 Taylor
    1 Metzenbaum, 5½ inch
    1 Metzenbaum, 7 inch
    1 suture
    1 wire
Needle holders
    2 Sarot, 7½ inch
    2 Mayo-Hegar, 7 inch
    2 Crile-Wood
Clamps
    24 mosquitoes
    3 curved Crile
    3 straight Crile
    10 Allis
    2 Oschner
    2 Adson
    6 large towel clips
    6 small towel clips
    2 sponge sticks
    2 scalp clip appliers
Knife Handles
    2 No. 3
    2 No. 7
Forceps
    2 Adson with teeth
    2 Adson without teeth
    1 Cushing with teeth, 7¾ inches
    1 Cushing without teeth, 7¾ inches
    2 bayonet without teeth, 7¾ inches
    2 DeBakey vascular, 7¾ inches
Retractors
    2 Adson cerebellar curved
    2 Weitlaner cerebellar
    2 Gelpi
    2 brain retractors, 1 inch
    2 brain retractors, ¾ inch
    2 brain retractors, ⅝ inch
    2 brain retractors, ½ inch
    2 brain retractors, ⅜ inch
    2 brain retractors, ¼ inch
Suction tips
    1 each Adson Nos. 7, 9, and 11
    1 Adson straight
    1 each Frazier Nos. 7, 8, 10, and 12
1 sharp nerve hook
1 dull nerve hook
1 Langenbeck periosteal elevator
1 short dural separator
1 long dural separator
1 ruler
2 10-ml glass syringes
10 rubber bands

1 Hudson brace
1 D'Errico perforator
1 Cushing perforator
1 Hudson burr
1 Hudson twist drill
2 Gigli saw handle
2 cranial saw guides
2 Gigli saws
1 Cottonoid tray
1 each Penfield dissectors Nos. 1, 2, 3, 4, and 5
Rongeurs
    1 narrow-jawed Leksell double action
    1 wide-jawed Leksell double action
    1 Lempert
    1 Adson
    1 Love-Gruenwald
    2 3-mm Schlesinger (1 upbiting and 1 downbiting)
    2 5-mm Schlesinger (1 upbiting and 1 downbiting)
    1 3-mm angled Kerrison
    4 intervertebral disk rongeurs, assorted
Curets
    Angled Nos. 0 and 2
    Straight Nos. 0, 1, 2, and 3

Add to this set as needed:

    Rhoton suction tips
    Craniotome
    Monopolar and bipolar tips and cords
    Scalp clips
    Self-retaining brain retractor (Budde halo, Leyla, Greenberg)
    Microsurgical instruments
    Microvascular clips and appliers

Laminectomy Instrument Set

Clamps
    24 curved mosquitoes
    4 curved Crile
    4 straight Crile
    2 Adson
    4 Oschner
    2 sponge sticks
    12 towel clips
    6 Allis
Needle holders
    2 Mayo-Hegar, 7 inch
    2 Sarot, 7 inch
    2 Crile-Wood
Scissors
    1 Dandy
    1 Taylor
    2 Metzenbaum, 7 inch
    1 straight Mayo
    1 curved Mayo
Knife handles
    1 No. 4
    2 No. 3
    2 No. 7

Forceps
    1 Adson without teeth
    2 Adson with teeth
    2 Cushing bayonet, 7½ inch
    2 dressing, 6¼ inch
    1 Cushing with teeth, 7 inch
    1 Cushing with teeth, 8 inch
    1 DeBakey vascular, 7¾ inch
Suctions
    1 straight Adson
    1 each curved Adson Nos. 7, 9, and 11
    1 each Frazier Nos. 7, 8, 10, and 12
Retractors
    2 cerebellar curved Adson
    2 cerebellar Weitlaner
    2 Gelpi
    2 Hibbs
    2 Taylor
    2 6-prong rakes
    2 Cushing vein
    2 Army-Navy
    1 nerve root
Rongeurs
    1 5-mm double-action Leksell
    1 8-mm double-action Leksell
    1 4-mm gooseneck
    1 Adson
    1 Liston-Stille bone cutter
    3 Schlesinger, assorted
    1 angled Kerrison
    1 Love-Gruenwald
    5 disk rongeurs, assorted
2 medicine cups
1 each Penfield dissectors Nos. 1, 2, 3, 4, and 5
1 double-ended dissector
1 sharp nerve hook
1 dull nerve hook
1 Adson periosteal elevator
1 Langenbeck periosteal elevator
1 long dural elevator
1 short dural elevator
1 10-ml glass syringe
20 rubber bands
1 mallet
1 Cottonoid tray

Add to this set as needed:

Curved and straight curet sets
Curved and straight osteotomes
Gouges
Cobb elevators
Scoville retractor

Implantable Materials

Cranial surgery or trauma can cause defects or deformities that can be repaired for functional or cosmetic reasons using implantable materials. Defects of the dura can be covered with frozen or freeze-dried human cadaver dura or synthetic material. When a portion of the skull is missing, it can be repaired using a cranioplasty kit. This contains a slow-setting form of methyl methacrylate that can be molded into the correct shape and then trimmed to fit the defect exactly. The cranioplasty kit should be carefully differentiated from the aneuroplastic kit, which contains a fast-setting form of methyl methacrylate used for coating cerebral aneurysms. Burr hole covers made of silicone are sometimes used to fill the spaces left by burr holes.

CRANIOTOMY FOR ANEURYSMS OR ARTERIOVENOUS MALFORMATION

Definition

Cerebral aneurysms, which result from congenital, traumatic, arteriosclerotic, or infectious processes, are abnormal dilations of intracranial vessels (Gary, 1983). They may occur on the major intracranial vessels or the circle of Willis. Congenital aneurysms are the most common type and manifest themselves either by rupture, which results in subarachnoid hemorrhage, or by expansion, which causes pressure on surrounding structures (Gary, 1983). Most aneurysms are in the form of *berry* aneurysms and are so called because they have the form of a berry with a stem and a neck (Hickey, 1986). The other form is a dilation, or ballooning, of the vessel without a neck. This is called a *saccular* aneurysm. Most aneurysms occur at the bifurcation of arterial vessels. The majority of patients with aneurysms are asymptomatic until a rupture or bleed occurs. Survivors of an initial bleed have surgery for clipping or wrapping of the aneurysm.

An *arteriovenous malformation* is a nest of blood vessels that form an abnormal communication between the arterial and venous systems. Blood from the arteries is shunted directly into the venous system without passing through the usual capillary network. The result of this shunting is inadequate cerebral perfusion. This chronic ischemia results in cerebral atrophy, scarring, and focal infarction (Hickey, 1986). The scarring of the brain tissue that occurs is known as *gliosis*. The results of this process may be neurological deficit, seizures, hydrocephalus, or hemorrhage. Surgical excision of the lesion is the treatment of choice. Surgically inaccessible lesions can be treated by embolization, proton beam radiation, or stereotaxic laser therapy (Hickey, 1986).

Indications

The patient with a cerebral aneurysm is usually undiagnosed until a bleed occurs. The symptoms of a bleed are severe headache, meningeal irritation (rigid neck, mild fever, photophobia, blurred vision, irritability, and restlessness), and alteration in the level of consciousness. Baseline assessment includes classification of the patient by grading the symptoms according to the following criteria:

Grade I: alert, no neurological deficit, minimal signs of meningeal irritation
Grade II: alert, minimal neurological deficit, mild to severe headache, nuchal rigidity
Grade III: drowsy or confused, nuchal rigidity, possible mild deficit
Grade IV: stuporous, mild to severe deficit, nuchal rigidity
Grade V: deep coma, decerebrate rigidity, moribund appearance

Diagnosis of the aneurysm is made by detailed neurological examination, lumbar puncture, CT scan, and cerebral arteriography (Fig. 25–21).

Cerebral vasospasm is an important complication of ruptured cerebral aneurysm. Vasospasm alters the cerebral circulation and may cause neurological deficits and changes in the level of consciousness. Preventing vasospasm is a major consideration in the preoperative and postoperative care of these patients. Activities that cause an increase in blood pressure or intracranial pressure must also be avoided.

The surgical approach to both cerebral aneurysms and arteriovenous malformations varies according to the location of the lesion. The following discussion assumes a standard craniotomy with an approach involving a bone flap. Suboccipital or posterior fossa craniotomy is necessary for some aneurysm surgery. Special positioning requirements for this approach are discussed below. Much of the following discussion is applicable to perioperative nursing care for the craniotomy patient, regardless of the underlying pathological condition.

Perioperative Nursing Implications

Anesthesia

Craniotomy is performed under general anesthesia. The anesthetist utilizes invasive monitoring techniques

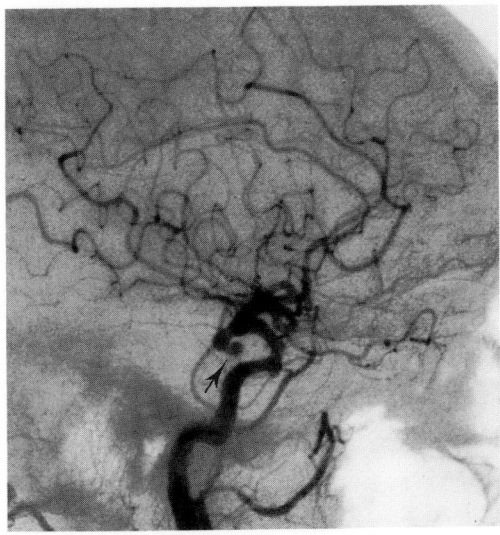

FIGURE 25–21. Lateral carotid angiogram illustrating aneurysm of the posterior communicating artery. (From Youmans, J. R. [Ed.]. [1989]. *Neurological surgery* [3rd ed.]. Philadelphia: W. B. Saunders.)

for this procedure, including the placement of arterial and central venous catheters. A pulmonary arterial catheter may also be required. Brain relaxation is achieved by placement of a lumbar drainage device, administration of medications (mannitol, furosemide, dexamethasone), and/or hyperventilation. Hyperventilation decreases the partial pressure of carbon dioxide, which causes vasoconstriction. Relaxation of the brain achieves a larger space for the operation and makes retraction easier (Gary, 1983).

Position

The circulating nurse should include a neurological assessment as part of the preoperative assessment routine. Documentation of any neurological deficits present preoperatively provides a basis for postoperative assessment. Knowledge of these deficits aids the nurse in planning the transfer to the OR bed and positioning intraoperatively.

Craniotomy is usually a lengthy procedure, so special care must be taken to position the patient to avoid trauma to the skin and the underlying tissue. The patient is usually placed in a supine position. The OR bed should have additional padding over the usual mattress. Foam heel protectors and elbow protectors should be used. The arm on the operative side is tucked in with the palm toward the patient's hip. The arm is secured with a lift sheet. The opposite arm is extended on a padded arm board. To prevent footdrop, support the soles of the feet with a pillow or a roll made of foam or a blanket. Warming blankets may be placed over and/or under the patient. If the blanket is on top of the patient, the nurse should ensure that it is not placing excessive weight on the toes.

The head is placed in a three-point head holder and turned as necessary. The nurse should supply sterile pins and ointment to go around the pin sites. The ointment provides a seal around the puncture wound to prevent the possibility of entrance of air into a venous sinus. Adequate personnel must be available when positioning the patient's head because this involves supporting the head while the head of the OR bed is removed and replaced with the neurosurgical head holder. Good body alignment must be ensured, with particular attention to the neck. If the head is turned far to one side, it may be necessary to place a support under the opposite shoulder to avoid excessive strain on the neck muscles.

The eyes should be protected with lubricant and eye patches taped in place. Covering the eye patches with transparent adhesive wound dressing material (Op-Site, Tegaderm) is a good method to ensure that the patches remain in place throughout the procedure. Eye goggles or shield devices that afford eye protection can also be used.

Creation and Maintenance of the Sterile Field

The entire head of the patient is shaved for this procedure. The skin preparation should include the area of the skull superior to the pins of the head holder. The ear on the operative side should be included if a temporal flap is planned. Care should be taken to exclude preparation solutions from the eyes and the ears.

After the patient is prepared, the scrub nurse supplies the surgeon with a sterile marking pen. The incision site is marked before draping because the flap is planned in relation to anatomical landmarks that are not visible after the drapes have been applied. If infiltration of the scalp for hemostasis is performed, it is done at this time. The head is draped with towels that are sutured or stapled in place. An adhesive incise drape is applied to the scalp. Alternatively, the adhesive drape is an integral part of a special disposable craniotomy drape. These drapes may also incorporate a pocket to collect fluids during the procedure. Drapes are positioned to cover completely the patient while forming a tent for the anesthetist so that the patient can be observed without encroaching on the sterile field. The tent is formed with a combination of Mayo stands and intravenous fluid poles to support the drapes. The scrub nurse then transfers the instrument-filled Mayo trays to the Mayo stands under the drapes. A suggested room arrangement is depicted in Figure 25–22. Suction and cautery cords are secured and handed off the field. The craniotome is connected to the power supply and tested for proper functioning.

Equipment and Supplies

Before the patient is draped, the operating microscope should be placed on the anesthesia side of the patient, and one or more undraped mayo stands are placed over the patient. Other special equipment includes craniotomy instruments, craniotome, microsurgical instruments, neurosurgical clips and appliers, marking pen, Cottonoids, suction, self-retaining retractor, monopolar and bipolar cautery, headlights, laser, and smoke evacuator.

All preoperative films should be in the room before the start of the procedure.

During the procedure, the scrub nurse should be cognizant of the following:

- Place instruments in the surgeon's hand in the position of function.
- Clean instruments after each use.
- Be prepared to accept instruments as the surgeon hands them back.
- Never bump the surgeon, the patient, the OR bed, or a retractor during the procedure (American Association of Neuroscience Nurses, 1980).

The scrub nurse must be aware that when the surgeon is working through the microscope, he or she cannot look away to accept or return an instrument. This requires attention from the scrub nurse at all times. Relief of the scrub nurse should be avoided during critical periods of the surgery.

Drugs and Solutions

The circulating nurse should obtain and dispense topical thrombin, hemostatic agents of the surgeon's choice, and warm saline for irrigation.

Physiological Monitoring

Blood loss should be monitored both on the sponges and in the suction. The nurse should establish the

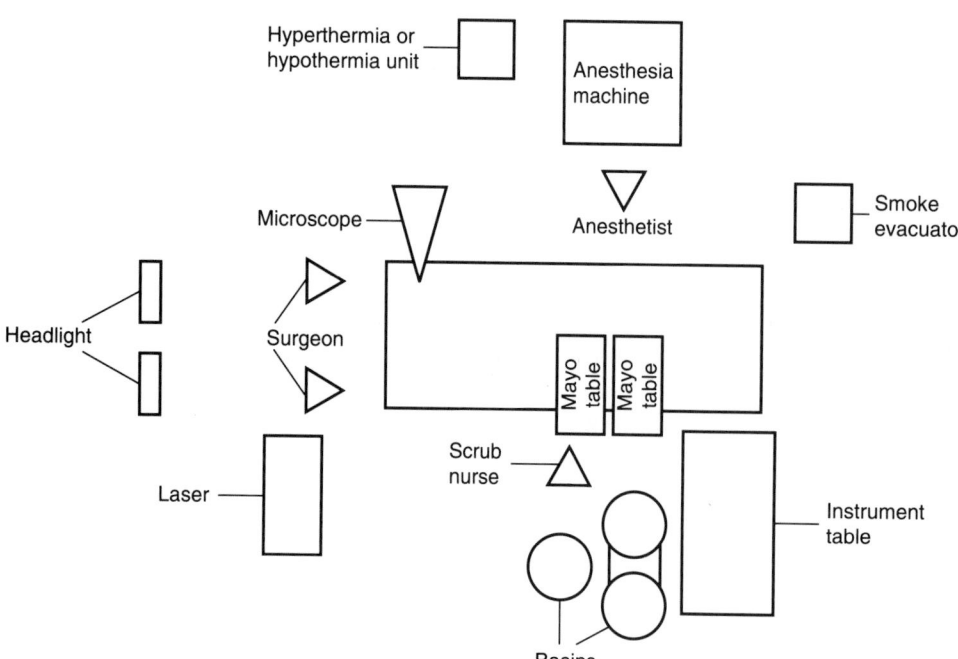

FIGURE 25–22. Room arrangement for craniotomy.

availability of blood before the start of surgery and be prepared to obtain blood and blood products at the request of the anesthetist. Urine output should be monitored via a Foley catheter.

During the procedure, the anesthetist usually requests periodic determination of arterial blood gas values, hemoglobin level, hematocrit values, and possibly clotting studies and electrolyte levels.

Specimens and Cultures

After excision of an arteriovenous malformation, the malformation itself is a specimen; aneurysm occlusion does not result in a specimen.

Physician's Orders

1. Ensure absolute bed rest with minimal stimulation.
2. Elevate the head of the bed 30 degrees.
3. Take blood pressure, pulse, respirations, and neurological vital signs every 30 minutes initially, increasing intervals as the patient's condition stabilizes.
4. Prevent activities that may cause increased intracranial pressure (e.g., Valsalva maneuver, coughing, sneezing, and vomiting).
5. Administer medications.

INDICATION OR TYPE	DRUG
Cerebral edema	Dexamethasone
Hypertension	Hydralazine hydrochloride
	Reserpine
Antipyretic or analgesic	Acetaminophen
Stool softener	Docusate sodium
Antifibrinolytic	Aminocaproic acid
Anticonvulsant	Phenytoin
Sedative	Phenobarbital
Vasospasm	Aminophylline
	Isoproterenol

The timing of aneurysm surgery is related to the possibility of rebleeding versus the danger of operating in the presence of vasospasm. At present, surgery is usually delayed 1 to 2 weeks to stabilize the patient's condition and reduce the possibility of vasospasm.

The patient with an arteriovenous malformation may also have symptoms of bleeding. Other initial symptoms are seizures, headache, bruit (rare), syncope, fainting, weakness, confusion, visual defects, and intellectual impairment resulting from chronic ischemia.

Preoperative care of the patient with arteriovenous malformation is the same as for the patient with cerebral aneurysm.

Laboratory and Diagnostic Studies

Diagnostic studies to document the arteriovenous malformation are CT scan and cerebral arteriogram.

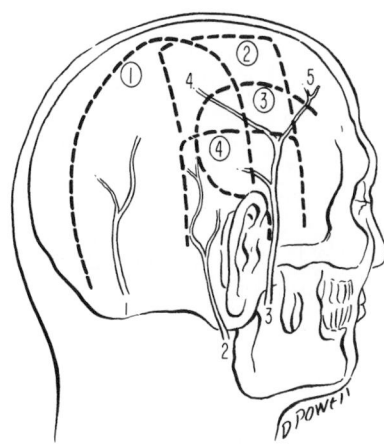

FIGURE 25–23. Basic craniotomy incisions: ①, occipital; ②, parietal; ③ and ④, temporal. Arteries: *1*, occipital; *2*, posterior auricular; *3*, superficial temporal; *4*, parietal branch; *5*, frontal branch. (From Wilkins, R. H., Odom, G. L. [1982]. Anesthesia and operative technique. In J. R. Youmans [Ed.]. *Neurological surgery* [2nd ed.]. Philadelphia: W. B. Saunders.)

Procedure

Incision and Exposure

The flap is planned according to the location of the lesion. The incision is placed within the hairline, using a broad-based pedicle with an adequate blood supply (Fig. 25–23). Finger pressure over gauze sponges is used to control bleeding as scalp clips or hemostats are applied along the skin edges (Fig. 25–24). Soft tissue is

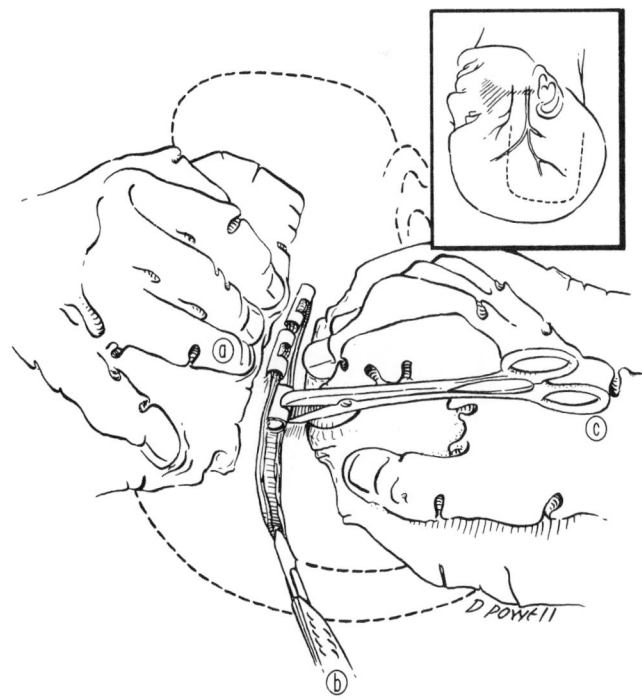

FIGURE 25–24. Craniotomy incision: digital compression *(a)*, scalp incision *(b)*, and application of scalp clips *(c)*. (From Wilkins, R. H., Odom, G. L. [1982]. Anesthesia and operative technique. In J. R. Youmans [Ed.]. *Neurological surgery* [2nd ed.]. Philadelphia: W. B. Saunders.)

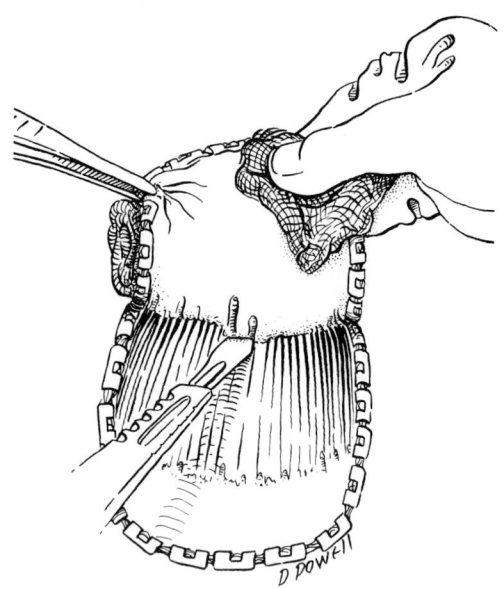

FIGURE 25–25. Reflection of a scalp flap. (From Wilkins, R. H., Odom, G. L. [1982]. Anesthesia and operative technique. In J. R. Youmans [Ed.]. *Neurological surgery* [2nd ed.]. Philadelphia: W. B. Saunders.)

separated from the underlying bone with a periosteal elevator. The scalp flap is reflected back over a sponge to minimize angulation that might compromise the blood supply (Fig. 25–25). Hemostasis is accomplished using electrocautery. The scalp flap is secured in position with Allis clamps or towel clips held by rubber bands that are then attached to the drapes.

Burr holes are accomplished with a cranial perforator. Four holes are placed at the corners of the incision (Fig. 25–26). Saline irrigation is used during the drilling process to reduce the heat generated by friction. Particles of bone produced are removed with an elevator and

small curet. This bone dust can be saved to fill in the burr hole defects at the time of closure. It can be scraped into a medicine cup and moistened with saline.

A dural separator is used in each burr hole to dissect the dura away from the bone. Cuts are then made between burr holes. This may be done by threading a Gigli saw between the holes using a dural guide and sawing manually or by using an air-powered craniotome incorporating the dural protector (Fig. 25–27). Again, the assistant should irrigate to avoid friction-generated heat and must also stabilize the head. The bone flap is elevated from the underlying dura using periosteal elevators and dissectors (Fig. 25–28). A small twist drill is used to make corresponding holes in the bone flap and the skull in preparation for closure (Fig. 25–29). A brain spatula is used under the skull edges to protect the brain during drilling. Closing sutures may be placed in the skull holes at this time. Central holes are drilled in the bone flap for suturing the dura up to the bone at closure. The bone flap is then wrapped in a moist sponge and placed in a basin to be stored on the back table until closure.

Some surgeons prefer to leave some muscle attached to the bone flap. In this situation, the bone is cut on only three sides and the side under the muscle is fractured and then smoothed using a rongeur (Fig. 25–30). The bone and muscle are wrapped in moist gauze and secured back in the same manner as the scalp flap.

After hemostasis is achieved with sponges, bone wax, and cautery, the dura is opened. The dura is elevated with a sharp hook and incised with a scalpel. The incision is continued around three sides within 1 cm of the circumference of the skull edges. Vessels are coagulated with bipolar cautery or ligated with clips (Fig. 25–31). Stitches of braided 4–0 nylon are placed to tack the

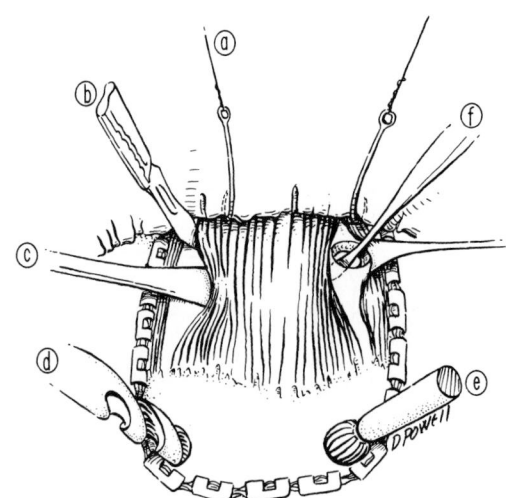

FIGURE 25–26. Retraction of a scalp flap *(a)*, incision of the muscle *(b)*, separation of muscle from bone with a periosteal elevator *(c)*, creation of burr holes *(d and e)*, and separation of the dura from the skull *(f)*. (From Wilkins, R. H., Odom, G. L. [1982]. Anesthesia and operative technique. In J. R. Youmans [Ed.]. *Neurological surgery* [2nd ed.]. Philadelphia: W. B. Saunders.)

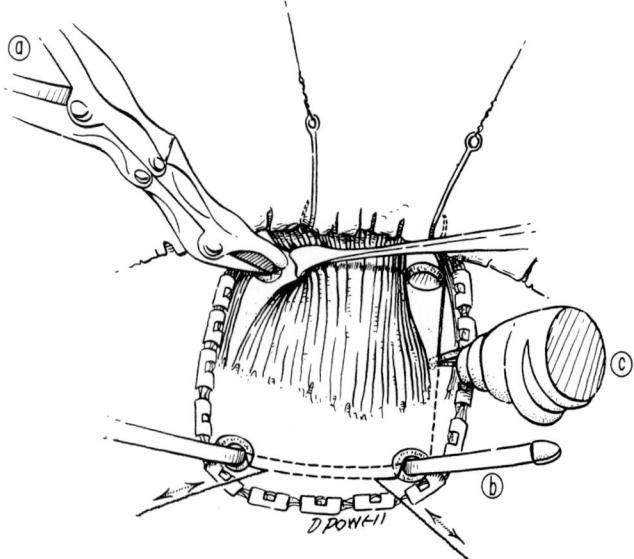

FIGURE 25–27. Craniectomy with a rongeur *(a)* and division of bone with a Gigli saw *(b)* or a craniotome *(c)*. (From Wilkins, R. H., Odom, G. L. [1982]. Anesthesia and operative technique. In J. R. Youmans [Ed.]. *Neurological surgery* [2nd ed.]. Philadelphia: W. B. Saunders.)

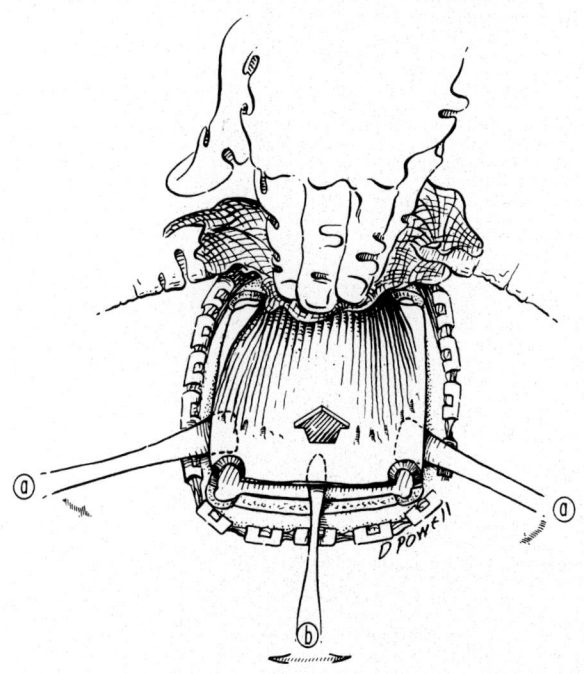

FIGURE 25–28. Elevation of the bone flap (a) and separation of the dura mater from the flap (b). (From Wilkins, R. H., Odom, G. L. [1982]. Anesthesia and operative technique. In J. R. Youmans [Ed.]. *Neurological surgery* [2nd ed.]. Philadelphia: W. B. Saunders.)

FIGURE 25–29. Waxing of the bone (a and b) and drilling of wire holes (c). (From Wilkins, R. H., Odom, G. L. [1982]. Anesthesia and operative technique. In J. R. Youmans [Ed.]. *Neurological surgery* [2nd ed.]. Philadelphia: W. B. Saunders.)

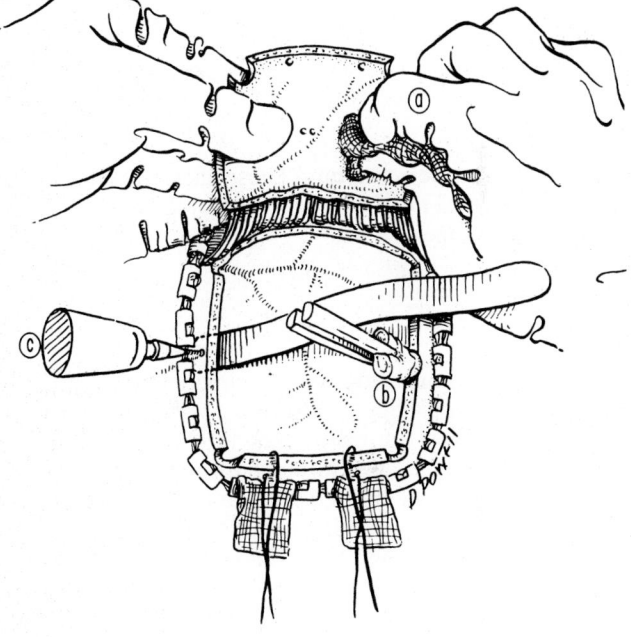

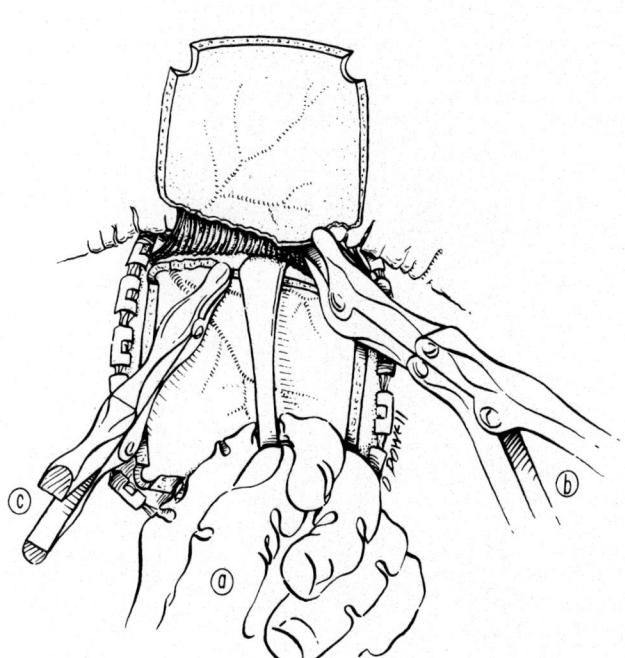

FIGURE 25–30. Separation of muscle from bone (a) and smoothing of the fractured bone edges (b and c). (From Wilkins, R. H., Odom, G. L. [1982]. Anesthesia and operative technique. In J. R. Youmans [Ed.]. *Neurological surgery* [2nd ed.]. Philadelphia: W. B. Saunders.)

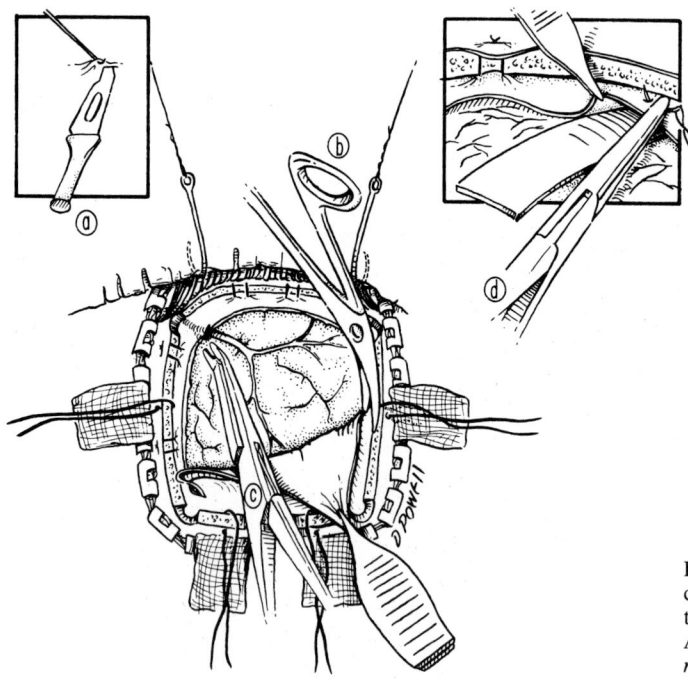

FIGURE 25–31. Incision and division of the dura mater (a and b), clip ligation of the dural vessels (c), and suturing of the dura mater to the pericranium (d). (From Wilkins, R. H., Odom, G. L. [1982]. *Anesthesia and operative technique.* In J. R. Youmans [Ed.]. *Neurological surgery* [2nd ed.]. Philadelphia: W. B. Saunders.)

dura up to the pericranium. These tack-up stitches aid in hemostasis. The dural flap is protected with moist Cottonoid sponges.

Details

When the lesion is located, the microsurgical portion of the procedure begins. Feeding vessels are isolated, care being taken to disrupt as little brain tissue as possible. Suction is always done through a Cottonoid, never directly on the brain tissue. Hypotension is usually induced at this time to minimize bleeding.

In the case of an aneurysm, the vessel is first dissected proximally so that, if a rupture occurs, the bleeding can be controlled. The neck of the aneurysm is visualized, and dissection necessary to allow clip placement is performed. The surgeon selects the appropriate clip and places it across the aneurysm neck. The body of the aneurysm is removed. The clip may be secured with a collar of muscle tissue or with acrylic cement. When clipping of the aneurysm is not possible, it may be wrapped or coated with an agent such as methyl methacrylate. This is done by placing the agent in a plastic syringe attached to a plastic angiocatheter cannula. The area around the aneurysm is isolated with moist Cottonoids before the substance is applied. After the aneurysm is occluded, hemostasis is ensured before closure.

Resection of arteriovenous malformation is similar to aneurysm occlusion in that involved vessels are identified and isolated. The vein draining the lesion is the last vessel to be ligated before the malformation is totally removed. Again, meticulous attention to hemostasis is given before closure.

Closure

The dura is closed (Fig. 25–32) using 4–0 braided nylon interrupted or running sutures. The dura is secured to the bone flap with a central tack-up stitch. If dural shrinkage has occurred, a dural graft may be necessary to achieve closure. The dural suture line should be watertight.

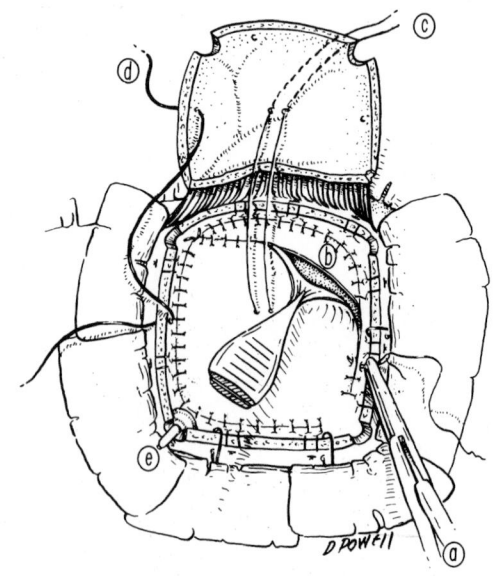

FIGURE 25–32. Suturing of the dura mater (a), dura graft (b), central tack-up suture (c), bone wires (d), and bottom of the silicone button (e). (From Wilkins, R. H., Odom, G. L. [1982]. *Anesthesia and operative technique.* In J. R. Youmans [Ed.]. *Neurological surgery* [2nd ed.]. Philadelphia: W. B. Saunders.)

The bone flap is replaced and secured with monofilament wire or nonabsorbable polypropylene suture. If wire is used, the ends are turned down into the drill holes. Bone dust may be packed into the burr holes at this time. The galea is closed with 2–0 polyglactin 910 sutures. The skin may be closed with suture or staples (Fig. 25–33). The incision is cleaned with hydrogen peroxide or saline and antibiotic ointment, and Telfa and 4 × 4 inch gauze are applied. The head is supported while the neurosurgical headrest is replaced by the head of the OR bed, and the drapes are removed. The dressing is secured with a head wrap of elastic gauze or a tubular elastic material. Ears contained within the dressing should be padded with cotton to avoid excessive pressure. The dressing may be anchored to the skin with tape.

Postoperative Care

After craniotomy, patients are admitted to an intensive care unit for close monitoring. The neurological condition can be assessed uniformly if a system of specific criteria such as the Glasgow coma scale is used. The head of the bed is kept elevated 30 degrees to decrease the intracranial pressure. The hemodynamic status is continuously assessed via electrocardiogram and arterial pressures. Arterial blood gas values indicate the adequacy of the respiratory effort, and central venous pressure and urine output indicate fluid balance.

As the patient's condition stabilizes, monitoring and supportive devices are removed. The patient is transferred to a postoperative unit. Normal diet is resumed and progressive activity is initiated. Rehabilitation for any residual neurological deficits is planned and implemented. Patients may be discharged from the hospital as early as 7 days after surgery or much later, depending on the patient's age, predisease condition, and residual problems.

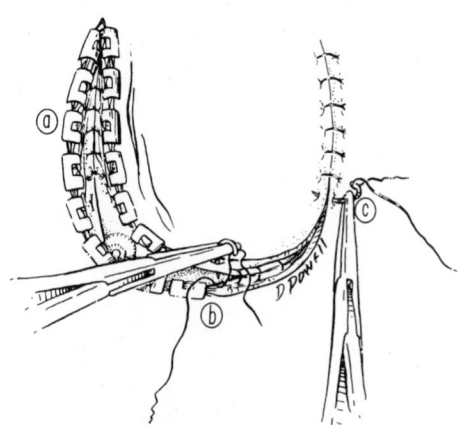

FIGURE 25–33. Sutures in fascia *(a)*, suturing the galea aponeurotica *(b)*, and suturing the skin *(c)*. (From Wilkins, R. H., Odom, G. L. [1982]. Anesthesia and operative technique. In J. R. Youmans [Ed.]. *Neurological surgery* [2nd ed.]. Philadelphia: W. B. Saunders.)

Potential Surgical Complications

The patient must be informed of the risks and hazards of craniotomy.

Additional loss of brain function, including memory
Recurrence or continuation of the condition that necessitated the operation
Stroke
Blindness, deafness, inability to smell, double vision, coordination loss, seizures, pain, numbness, and paralysis.

SUBOCCIPITAL CRANIOTOMY FOR NEOPLASTIC LESIONS OF THE POSTERIOR FOSSA

Definition

A neoplastic brain lesion is a tumor or mass that occurs within the brain.

Indications

Brain tumors may be benign or malignant, but any lesion that occurs within the cranium has the potential to create damage owing to compression, invasion, and infiltration of the surrounding structures. This can cause pathological changes, including edema, increased intracranial pressure, neurological deficits, seizures, alterations in pituitary function, and obstruction of flow of the CSF (Hickey, 1986). The incidence and severity of the pathophysiological condition is related to the size and location of the tumor. Lesions in the posterior fossa are approached via a suboccipital craniotomy. Tumors in the anterior and middle fossa are resected via a craniotomy that creates a bone flap for access. That procedure is the same as described above.

The signs and symptoms of a brain tumor are related to the size and location of the pathophysiological changes mentioned above. Typical symptoms are headache, vomiting, papilledema, personality changes, changes in the level of consciousness, seizures, ataxia, loss of coordination, visual changes, and pituitary dysfunction (Hickey, 1986).

Diagnosis of a brain tumor is established by a thorough neurological examination, skull films, electroencephalogram, carotid angiogram (Figs. 25–34 and 25–35), and CT scan (Figs. 25–36 and 25–37). Magnetic resonance imaging has enhanced the diagnosis of brain tumors by providing remarkably clear images of the tumor (Fig. 25–38). Additional preoperative orders are for routine chest radiograph, electrocardiogram, complete blood count, electrolyte determinations, chemistry, clotting studies, and urinalysis.

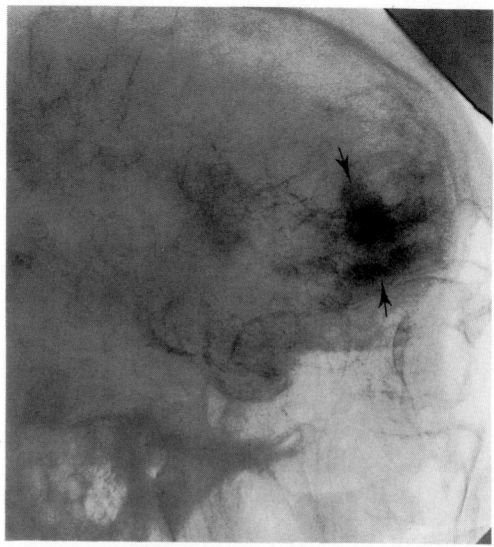

FIGURE 25–34. Carotid angiogram demonstrates tumor stain (TS). (From Youmans, J. R. [Ed.]. [1989]. *Neurological surgery* [3rd ed.]. Philadelphia: W. B. Saunders.)

Perioperative Nursing Implications

Anesthesia

Posterior fossa craniotomy is performed under general anesthesia. The usual monitoring devices are used, (e.g., electrocardiographic monitor, arterial pressure catheter, temperature probe, and pulse oximeter). If the procedure is performed with the patient in the sitting position, the possibility of air embolism must be anticipated. Air embolism occurs when there is a negative pressure

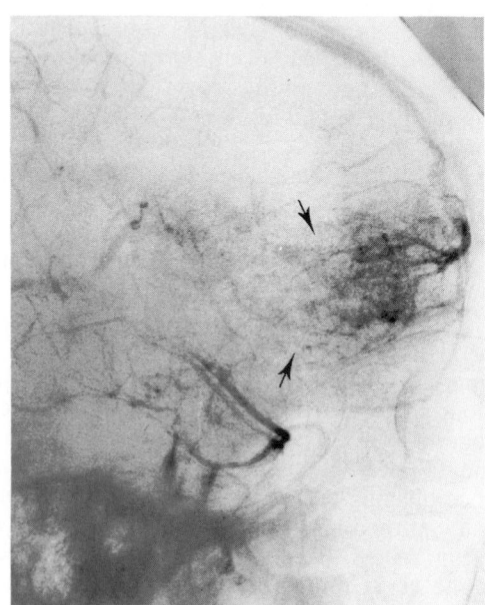

FIGURE 25–35. Carotid angiogram showing a halo of abnormal vessels surrounding a relatively avascular tumor mass. (From Youmans, J. R. [Ed.]. [1989]. *Neurological surgery* [3rd ed.]. Philadelphia: W. B. Saunders.)

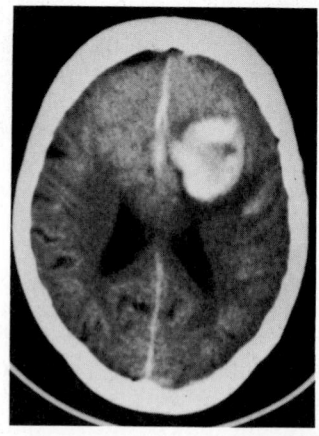

FIGURE 25–36. CT scan demonstrating a glioblastoma. (From Youmans, J. R. [Ed.]. [1989]. *Neurological surgery* [3rd ed.]. Philadelphia: W. B. Saunders.)

gradient between the right atrium and the venous sinuses or the diploetic veins. Entrainment of air can also occur from the soft tissue, bone edge, or dural edge (Temple and Katz, 1987). Usually, air embolisms are detected by an ultrasound Doppler placed over the heart. A turbulent sound indicates the presence of the embolism. A right atrial catheter must also be in place so that the embolism can be aspirated from the heart. Other methods for detecting air embolism are mass spectrometry, echocardiography, and capnography.

Position

This procedure may be done with the patient either prone or sitting, depending on the surgeon's preference. When the patient is sitting, the legs should be wrapped with elastic stockings or antiembolism hose. This reduces the pressure gradient between the head and the heart and also promotes venous return. Although the sitting position is ideal for respiration and visualization of the surgical site, it is not as good for circulation. As the patient is raised from supine to sitting, hypotension may occur.

The circulating nurse should collect all necessary equipment for positioning before the procedure starts.

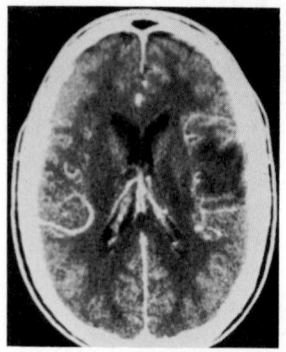

FIGURE 25–37. CT scan demonstrating an astrocytoma. Contrast-enhanced. (From Youmans, J. R. [Ed.]. [1989]. *Neurological surgery* [3rd ed.]. Philadelphia: W. B. Saunders.)

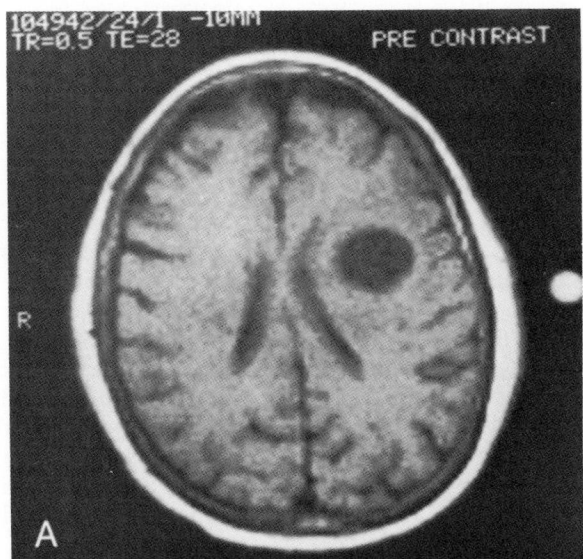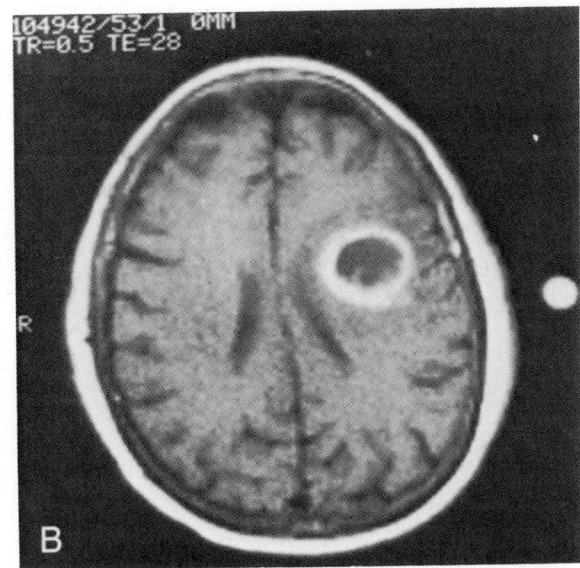

FIGURE 25–38. *A*, MRI scan of a glioblastoma. *B*, The same lesion with contrast. (From Kortman, K. E., Bradley, W. E., Jr. [1986]. Magnetic resonance imaging of central nervous system neoplasms. In F. A. Mettler, Jr., L. R. Muroff, M. V. Kulkarni [Eds.]. *Magnetic resonance imaging and spectroscopy*. New York: Churchill Livingston. By permission.)

This includes the pin head holder, the overtable attachment for the head holder, and the clamps to hold it to the sides of the table. Foam padding should be placed under the heels and under the elbows. Additional padding is also important under the buttocks, which supports most of the patient's weight. The feet should be supported by a footboard or roll. When the anesthetist is prepared, the head of the bed is slowly raised into the sitting position. The head is secured into the pin holder and the head section of the OR bed is removed. The neck should be in alignment and slightly flexed. Male genitalia should be checked to see that they are not compressed. A pillow is placed in the lap to support the arms, which are secured with adhesive tape.

If the surgery is to be done with the patient in the prone position, the patient is anesthetized and intubated while on the transport gurney. A Foley catheter is inserted. The OR bed is prepared with chest rolls appropriate to the size of the patient and foam padding under the knee area. The head of the bed is removed and replaced with the Mayfield headrest. Either the pin holder or the horseshoe head holder is used. The patient is turned onto the OR bed by at least four people. The anesthetist supports the head, usually assisted by the neurosurgeon if the pin holder has been applied before the turn. Other team members support the feet and the torso during the turn. Care must be taken to protect the eyes and the airway, keep the body in alignment, and avoid injury to unsupported extremities. After the turn, the gurney is removed. The chest rolls may be repositioned to permit adequate respiratory movement. A roll or bolster may be placed under the pelvis to decrease pressure on the abdomen. Female breasts and male genitals should be free from compression. The lower legs are elevated on pillows and the toes are free from pressure. Pedal pulses are checked after positioning. A safety strap is placed over the thighs. The arms are secured at the patient's sides using the lift sheet, and a warming blanket is placed over the patient.

Creation and Maintenance of the Sterile Field

After the patient is positioned, the surgical preparation is done. The entire head may be shaved or only the posterior skull and neck. The preparation should extend from the midparietal area over the occiput to the posterior neck, including the upper shoulders. Care should be taken to avoid getting the preparation solution in the eyes or ears.

The draping process begins with a marking pen to mark the incisional line before the landmarks are covered. Towels are applied and secured to the skin with staples, sutures, or towel clips. A craniotomy sheet is positioned with the fenestration over the incisional area and clipped to intravenous poles to create an area for the anesthetist to visualize the patient. When the patient is sitting, either the scrub nurse can raise the Mayo stand over the patient's head and stand on a high platform or the nurse may position it alongside the OR bed at a convenient working height. If the patient is prone, the Mayo stands are placed over the patient's torso.

When the patient is in a sitting position, the scrub nurse must be constantly alert to the potential for air embolism. If this occurs, an Asepto syringe of irrigation fluid and sloppy wet sponges should immediately be passed to the surgeon to occlude the site of air entry. The scrub nurse should have two Asepto syringes so that at least one can always be full with irrigating solution. If the entry site is in bone, the area is closed with bone wax (Temple and Katz, 1987).

Equipment and Supplies

Special equipment needed for the procedure includes the usual craniotomy instruments with self-retaining retractors, laser, microscope, ultrasound, and monopolar and bipolar cautery.

Drugs and Solutions

Oral steroid administration causes gastric irritation, so steroids are usually given with antacids and a histamine receptor antagonist (cimetidine, ranitidine hydrochloride). This drug regimen is usually continued after surgery.

One special consideration when operating on the posterior fossa is the need for continuous attention to the temperature of the saline used for irrigation. This irrigation must be body temperature or slightly above; cold irrigation on the brain stem could cause cardiac arrest.

Physiological Monitoring

The circulating nurse is always aware of the potential for air embolism when posterior fossa surgery is performed with the patient in the sitting position and ready to assist the anesthetist if this occurs. Monitoring of blood loss via suction and sponges is done in conjunction with the anesthetist.

Specimens and Cultures

Specimens generated by the procedure are tumor and perhaps CSF. The surgeon may take specimens from the periphery of the tumor bed, which are sent for frozen section examination to confirm that the margins are free from disease.

Physician's Orders

The patient with a brain tumor is not necessarily hospitalized before surgery unless symptoms are so severe that outpatient diagnostic testing and preoperative work-up are precluded. Preoperative care is based on the types of symptoms the patient has. Many patients receive dexamethasone to combat cerebral edema, phenytoin to prevent seizures, and a pain medication for headache.

Laboratory and Dragnostic Studies

Diagnostic studies to document neoplastic lesions of the posterior fossa include skull films, electroencephalogram, carotid angiogram, computed tomography scan, and magnetic resonance imaging.

Procedure

Incision and Exposure

After the patient is prepared and draped, an incision is made in the posterior midline. The skin bleeders are controlled, and the skin edges are retracted with self-retaining retractors such as Weitlaner and cerebellar retractors. The muscles are freed from the bone using a periosteal elevator and divided using the cautery. Several holes are drilled in the bone with the cranial perforator. After the dura has been dissected away from the bone edges using the dural separator, the opening in the bone is enlarged with rongeurs. No actual flap is removed in this procedure. Bone chips removed are generally not saved. The bone edges are sealed with bone wax. The dura is elevated with a hook and nicked with a knife. The dural incision is enlarged using a scissors and dural tack-up stitches are placed. Special care is needed during the opening phase to monitor the patient for air embolism because entrainment of air is most likely to occur as openings into the venous system are made. If this does occur, occlude the area with soaking wet sponges and copious irrigation.

Details

After the lesion is located, it is resected using suction, bipolar cautery, various dissectors, cup forceps, and possibly the carbon dioxide laser or ultrasonic aspirator. The tumor bed is irrigated to ensure that all bleeding points have been eliminated. At this time, wet cotton balls may be inserted into the tumor bed to achieve hemostasis through direct pressure. During the entire procedure, the assistant should retract the brain as gently as possible to avoid unnecessary damage to normal tissue, assist with hemostasis, and irrigate as necessary.

Closure

The dura is closed using 4–0 braided nylon suture. The muscle layer is approximated using 2–0 Vicryl, and the skin is closed with nylon suture or staples. Antibiotic ointment is applied to the incision, and a dressing of a nonadherent material such as Telfa or Adaptic covered by several layers of gauze is secured with tape. The patient remains anesthetized until she or he is returned to the supine position, either by lowering the head of the bed or by removing the head holder and turning the patient onto the intensive care unit bed. The perioperative nurse performs a postoperative evaluation of the patient's skin integrity at this time.

Postoperative Care

Postoperative orders involve the medications previously mentioned, possibly with the addition of antibiotic therapy and stool softeners. Regular neurological assessments, monitoring of vital signs, and intake and output measurements signal any early complications. Patients who have had a large tumor removed, particularly in the posterior fossa, are at risk for bleeding because of traction on dural vessels caused by a shift in brain tissue. For this reason, the bed should be kept flat in the early postoperative period (Savoy, 1984). The patient may be turned from side to side.

Potential Surgical Complications

Bleeding
Seizures
Fever
Cerebral edema
Hydrocephalus
Infection

INSERTION OF A SHUNT OR RESERVOIR

Definition

A shunt is indicated when a patient has hydrocephalus, which is a larger than normal volume of CSF within the cranium. The purpose of the shunt is to divert the excessive fluid from the cranium to another area where it can be reabsorbed. Hydrocephalus can result from an abnormally large production of fluid, failure of the reabsorption mechanism, or a blockage in the normal fluid pathways. The condition may be congenital or acquired.

Indications

The shunt itself takes the form of a ventricular tubing segment that is inserted into the lateral ventricle, a reservoir, and a distal tubing segment with valves that extends into the recipient body cavity. The reservoir is a small domed device that has connectors for the proximal and distal tubing segments. The reservoir is filled with CSF and may be punctured percutaneously to obtain fluid samples, to irrigate the system, and to inject dye or medication (Gruendemann and Meeker, 1987). When manual compression is applied, the reservoir also serves as a pump to flush fluid through the system. The reservoir may also be a valve. If this is not the case, the distal tubing contains one-way valves that open and allow fluid out when a specific pressure is reached. The surgeon selects the appropriate valve on the basis of individual patient requirements.

The distal catheter may terminate in the central venous system (ventriculoatrial), the thoracic cavity (ventriculopleural), or the ureter (ventriculoureteral). A Tokildson procedure is the insertion of a shunt between the ventricle and the cisterna magna. Lumbar peritoneal shunts may be performed when it is advisable to avoid the ventricle. The most common type of shunt is the ventriculoperitoneal, which is the example in this discussion. The shunt tubing usually has a radiopaque tip marking for x-ray verification of placement and may be reinforced with wound wire. The shunt components are made of silicone material.

An Ommaya reservoir is an implantable device used for repeated access and drug delivery to the central nervous system (Ommaya, 1984). It consists of a ventricular catheter and a dome-shaped reservoir that are made of silicone material. The Ommaya reservoir is implanted in patients who require frequent examination of CSF or patients with cancer who need to receive anticancer agents or analgesics directly into the central nervous system. This device is usually placed in the head but may be placed at the hip with a catheter extending subcutaneously into the spine.

The shunt, the reservoir, and the distal tubing are joined together with connectors. The connectors fit inside the tubing segments and are grooved circumferentially near each end. The grooves facilitate placement of ties of nonabsorbable suture that keep the segments from separating. If used on children, the distal tubing segment can be lengthened using connectors to keep it in the intended area of drainage as a child grows.

The patient who requires an Ommaya reservoir is usually referred to the neurosurgeon from another service. The neurosurgeon performs the procedure and further treatment is carried out by the referring physician.

The symptoms of adult patients with hydrocephalus differ from those of children. In the infant, hydrocephalus is manifested by an expanding head. The head increases in size because the bones are soft and the sutures are open. As the condition progresses, the fontanelles enlarge and become tense, and the scalp skin becomes shiny. Nystagmus or strabismus may be present. The eyes deviate downward, and the sclera is visible above the iris. This is known as the setting-sun sign. The infant becomes irritable, anorectic, and weak and has a high-pitched cry. Seizures may occur (Marlow and Redding, 1988).

A child with hydrocephalus has symptoms indicative of increased intracranial pressure: headache, vomiting, papilledema, ataxia, and drowsiness progressing to stupor.

An adult with hydrocephalus may have a mass or an inflammatory process that prevents normal circulation of the CSF. This is known as noncommunicating hydrocephalus. If the fluid pathways are intact but reabsorption of fluid by the arachnoid villi is not taking place, communicating hydrocephalus results. Both entities cause enlargement of the ventricles, with consequent compression of the brain tissue. The major symptoms of this problem are mental changes and disturbances in gait (Hickey, 1986).

Perioperative Nursing Implications

Anesthesia

For these procedures, patients are placed under general anesthesia. Occasionally, if the patient cannot tolerate general anesthesia and if he or she is able to cooperate during the procedure, the patient has only local anesthesia when receiving an Ommaya reservoir.

Position

The patient is supine, with the head slightly elevated and turned to the nonoperative side for a shunt. The head is straight for the placement of an Ommaya reservoir. A foam doughnut stabilizes the head in position. The arm on the operative side is tucked in at the patient's side. The opposite arm is placed on an arm board. Foam protectors are placed on the heels, and a small pillow under the knees eases strain on the back muscles. A restraint strap is placed across the thighs.

Creation and Maintenance of the Sterile Field

The shaved area is minimal. An area 3 to 4 inches in diameter is adequate for an Ommaya reservoir and the temporoparietal area for a shunt. The area prepared is the shaved area extending into the surrounding hair and the operative side of the neck and, because interim incisions may be required, the chest and the abdomen. Scalp hair may be excluded from the preparation area by isolating the shaved area using several plastic drapes with an adhesive edge.

Equipment and Supplies

The circulating nurse must ensure that all implantable materials required are available before the beginning of the procedure. Most shunt components are available presterilized from the manufacturer. If these items are not sterile, they should be sterilized according to the manufacturer's instructions and practices recommended by the Association of Operating Room Nurses (AORN, 1993). Proper documentation of any implanted materials according to hospital policy is also the responsibility of the circulating nurse.

The instruments for the procedure are a small neurosurgical dissecting set with a Hudson brace, a cranial perforator, ventricular needles, several syringes for irrigating and testing the shunt components, a shunt passer, and uterine dressing forceps to tunnel under the skin.

The scrub nurse must be aware of the special handling requirements of the silicone material. This material attracts particles of lint or starch and also absorbs body oils. When preparing the items for sterilization, never handle them with bare hands. Gloved hands must be free from glove powder. The implants should not be laid on linen or gauze but should always be kept in a basin.

Drugs and Solutions

Some surgeons like to soak and irrigate the reservoirs and catheters with an antibiotic solution before implantation. The circulator should prepare this solution as required.

Specimens and Cultures

This procedure usually yields CSF, which is sent for culture and cytological examination.

Physician's Orders

After the shunt and reservoir are implanted, the surgeon confirms placement via x-ray film. The circulator should confirm that radiography department personnel are aware of the need for x-ray films and notify them in time to be present when radiographs are required.

Laboratory and Diagnostic Studies

The easiest diagnostic study to perform to demonstrate enlarged ventricles is the CT scan. Other preoperative studies are routine chest radiography, electrocardiography, urinalysis, complete blood count, and electrolyte and clotting studies.

Procedure

Incision and Exposure

After the patient is prepared and draped, a U-shaped incision is made behind and above the mastoid process for a shunt or in the frontal area for an Ommaya reservoir. The nondominant side is used when possible. The small scalp flap is elevated using a periosteal elevator, and hemostasis of the scalp edges is performed. A burr hole craniotomy is made. The dura is incised, and the edges coagulated with bipolar cautery.

Details

A ventricular needle or the ventricular catheter with a stylet in place is introduced into the ventricle through the burr hole. If the needle is used, it is withdrawn and replaced with the catheter and stylet in the same track.

The reservoir is filled with saline and attached to the ventricular segment with a connector and tied securely. The distal tubing and valve are filled with saline and tested for proper function. A tunnel is made from the scalp flap under the skin to the distal site. Several incisions may need to be made depending on the relative size of the patient and the tunneling device. A uterine packing forceps or a special shunt passer is used for this procedure. The tubing is pulled through the tunnel. A small subcostal incision is made, and the catheter tip is inserted into the peritoneum and secured with a purse-string suture.

Closure

The incisions are closed, and a dressing is applied.

Postoperative Care

Postoperative care consists of monitoring of vital signs, neurological assessment, and care of the incisional lines. The surgeon may order pumping of the shunt. Postoperatively, if the size of the ventricles is reduced too rapidly, excessive traction on the meninges may cause tearing and consequent subdural bleeding. For this reason, excessive pumping of the shunt should be avoided and the head of the bed should be kept flat for 24 hours. Sutures are removed in 7 to 10 days. The time of discharge depends on accompanying medical problems.

Potential Surgical Complications

The potential complications of shunt insertion are displacement, shunt malfunction, and infection. Shunt revisions are not uncommon and are necessary because of shunt failure or growth of the child. One or more parts of the shunt may need to be replaced or the distal segment lengthened. Infection is treated with antibiotics. If this is not effective, the shunt is removed. Interim external drainage systems can be used until the infection resolves, and then another shunt is implanted.

LUMBAR LAMINECTOMY FOR HERNIATED DISK

Definition

This procedure is surgical removal of a herniated lumbar disk.

Indications

As an individual ages, changes in the spine occur that make it more vulnerable to injury. Loss of fluid content of the nucleus pulposus and weakening of the annulus fibrosus and the posterior longitudinal ligaments pro-

duce a situation in which the disk may herniate into the spinal canal when an unusual stress is placed on the spine (Hickey, 1986). Herniations occur most commonly in the lumbar spine and the cervical spine. Herniation in the less flexible thoracic spine is uncommon. Herniations may be caused by trauma (from lifting, falls, and sneezing) or degenerative diseases such as osteoarthritis and ankylosing spondylitis.

Herniation of the disk causes pain. The pain is due to pressure on the nerve root (Fig. 25–39). If pain relief is not achieved by conservative therapy (rest, use of a supportive garment, physical therapy, traction, medication), the herniation is removed surgically.

The patient who is scheduled for a laminectomy has usually been through a series of conservative treatments before being scheduled for surgery. The major symptom of lumbar disk disease is pain in the lower back, which may radiate down one or both legs. Normal posture is modified to compensate for the pathological alterations; normal lumbar lordosis is absent, and lumbar scoliosis occurs with spasms of the paravertebral muscles (Hickey, 1986). Because pain is often aggravated by movement, the patient moves stiffly, slowly, and cautiously. There may be some motor weakness on the affected side, numbness and paresthesias of the leg and foot, and diminished or absent reflexes in the knee and ankle. Lasègue maneuver (straight leg raising), Neri sign, Naffziger test, and Kernig sign are all positive.

There are several surgical options for the treatment of lumbar disk disease. In addition to the long-standing traditional approach of lumbar laminectomy with diskectomy, choices include microdiskectomy, percutaneous lumbar diskectomy, and chemonucleolysis. The lumbar laminectomy involves a midline incision over the lumbar spine (4–6 inches long) and removal of a vertebral lamina, ligamentum flavum, and disk material.

Microdiskectomy involves a 1-inch incision; the microscope is used for visualization and illumination of the anatomical structures, allowing a smaller incision and more precise dissection. Less tissue disruption results in less postoperative pain, quicker recovery, and earlier hospital discharge, usually within 2 days of surgery.

In percutaneous lumbar diskectomy, the surgeon inserts an automated probe through a cannula into the disk. The probe placement is verified intraoperatively by fluoroscopy. The disk is removed by the aspirating and cutting action of the probe. This procedure is done on an outpatient basis using local anesthesia. Recovery time is reduced because there is no disruption of bone, muscle, or ligament (Brooks, 1989).

Chemonucleolysis is a procedure in which an enzyme (chymopapain) is injected percutaneously into the disk. This reduces the size of the disk and therefore the encroachment onto the nerve roots. The procedure is performed in the OR under general anesthesia with fluoroscopy. There is the possibility of a major complication with this procedure, such as allergic reaction to the chymopapain, which may lead to anaphylactic shock. The advantage of chemonucleolysis is that it is a short procedure and the postoperative hospital stay is minimal. This procedure was widely advocated after the drug

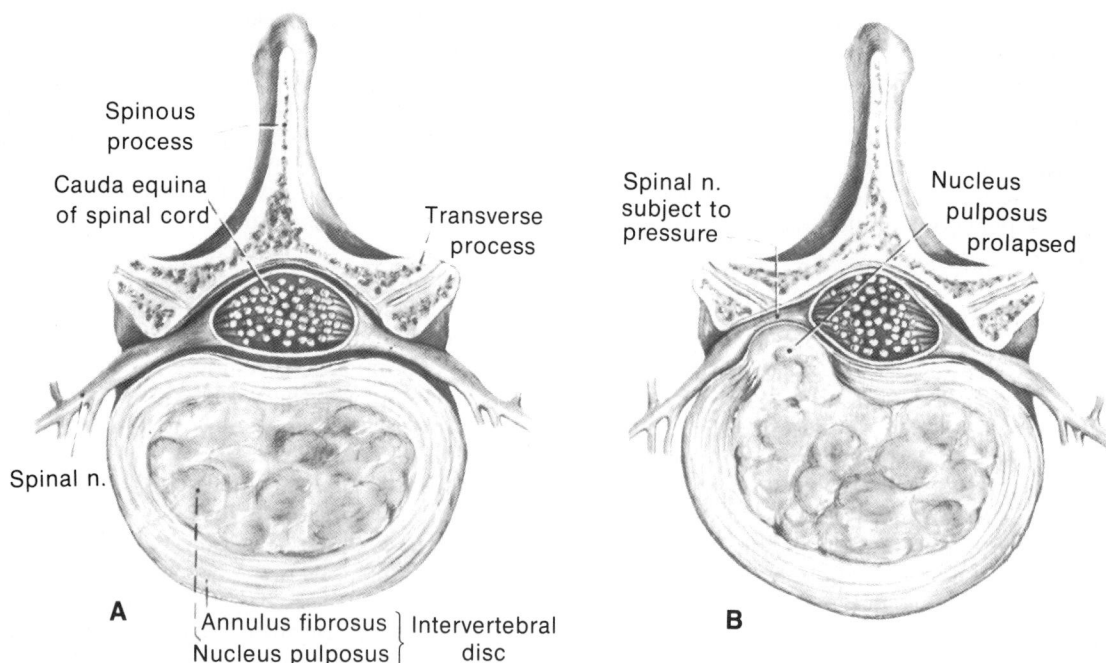

FIGURE 25–39. *A*, Normal relationship of the intervertebral disk to the spinal cord and nerve branches. *B*, Prolapsed nucleus pulposus impinging on the nerve. (From Jacob, S. W., Francone, C. A., Lossow, W. J. [1982]. *Structure and function in man* [5th ed.]. Philadelphia: W. B. Saunders.)

was approved for use in the United States. Further experience has diminished the enthusiasm for the procedure; several studies indicated a lower success rate for this procedure than for microdiskectomy (Maroon and Alba, 1985).

Lumbar disk surgery may be accompanied by spinal fusion if several levels are involved. Fusion is performed to provide stability of the area. A bone graft is taken from the iliac crest and placed between the vertebrae. Movement is limited to prevent injury to the spinal cord and nerve roots.

Perioperative Nursing Implications

Anesthesia

Lumbar laminectomy is performed under general anesthesia. The major anesthetic concern is that the necessary positioning not compromise the respiratory process. Blood loss from the procedure is usually minimal.

Position

Conventionally, the patient is prone when undergoing a lumbar laminectomy, and the torso is supported on chest rolls or a Wilson frame. Some surgeons prefer to position the patient in knee-chest position or the prone sitting position. The Wilson frame is an arch-shaped frame that supports the patient's torso on two longitudinal pads extending from the clavicle to the pelvis. The

frame serves the same purpose as chest rolls (i.e., to permit adequate expansion of the chest). The angle of the arch can be adjusted with a crank to provide optimal visualization of the surgical site. When placing the frame on the bed, the nurse should ensure that it is positioned so that the crank is extended over the side of the OR bed and is freely movable. The frame should be covered with cloth to protect the patient from direct contact with it. Each side of the frame must be covered separately to avoid a sling effect, which would compromise respiratory excursion.

In the absence of a frame, chest rolls are used. These may be commercially available rolls of foam or silicone gel material, or sheets or bath blankets may be rolled to an appropriate size and secured with tape. Any roll should extend from the level of the clavicle to the pelvis and be firm enough to elevate the patient's chest off the OR bed. The surgeon may wish to use another roll transversely under the pelvis, in addition to the chest supports. This helps to decrease pressure on the vena cava.

The nurse should also prepare the OR bed with a doughnut headrest for the head, foam padding for the knees, and pillows to go under the lower legs. Two padded arm boards are also needed. The patient is anesthetized on the transport gurney. Elastic leg wraps should be applied to cover the entire leg. This promotes venous return after the surgery. A Foley catheter is usually not necessary because this is a fairly short procedure. The eyes are protected with eye pads taped in place.

The surgical team then turns the patient onto the OR bed. The anesthetist controls the head and the airway.

At least one team member stands at each side and one at the feet. More help may be necessary for a large patient. At a signal from the anesthetist, the patient is turned slowly and smoothly. The stretcher is removed. The patient's arms are pronated on padded arm boards, with the elbows flexed and the lower arms parallel to the body. Care must be taken not to overextend the shoulder. The pillows under the lower legs are adjusted to prevent plantar flexion of the feet, and the toes should be free from pressure. Pedal pulses should be palpated to ensure that knee flexion and leg wraps are not compromising arterial circulation. The head is turned to one side with a doughnut headrest, preventing pressure on the ear. Ensure that there is no pressure on the eyes. Check the breasts and the male genitalia to confirm that these areas are not compressed. A thermia blanket may be placed over the legs. A safety strap is secured over the upper thighs.

Creation and Maintenance of the Sterile Field

Before preparing the skin, the nurse may apply a plastic drape with an adhesive edge over the buttocks to isolate that area from the surgical site. Preparation includes the lumbar area and extends to the lower scapulae, to the gluteal fold, and laterally on the torso to the supporting devices.

After the patient is prepared, the scrub nurse hands the surgeon a folded towel to blot the area to be incised. A marking pen or scalpel is used to mark the incisional line while landmarks are still visible. The incisional line may be cross-hatched for ease of approximation at closure. A plastic incise drape may be used, followed by four towels to square off the incision area. These are secured with towel clips or staples. A fenestrated sheet or square draping is used next. The sheet is attached to intravenous poles at the head of the patient for access by the anesthetist. The Mayo stand is placed over the patient's legs.

Equipment and Supplies

Supplies needed for the procedure are laminectomy instruments, a marking pen, a self-retaining spinal retractor, curets, Cobb elevators, a plastic incise drape, Cottonoid sponges, Gelfoam, and bipolar and monopolar cautery. Some surgeons use a Taylor retractor with a roll bandage attached to the handle for retraction. The end of the bandage is dropped off the field and weighted with hanging weights used for traction. Power equipment is usually not needed for a laminectomy. If the laminectomy is to be accompanied by spinal fusion, additional bone instruments, straight and curved osteotomes, and gouges are needed.

During the procedure, the surgeon uses a variety of rongeurs and punches. Each time that material is removed, the surgeon holds out the instrument to be cleaned. The scrub nurse should be ready with a damp sponge to remove any debris from the instrument as the surgeon holds it. She or he must also be aware that some of this material is a specimen that needs to be removed from the sponge and placed in the appropriate container.

Specimens and Cultures

Specimens generated in this procedure are disk material and ligamentum flavum. Bone fragments removed are usually discarded.

Physician's Orders

The physician orders routine preoperative laboratory studies and perhaps medications for analgesia, muscle relaxation, and sedation.

Laboratory and Diagnostic Studies

Diagnostic tests to prove disk herniation are myelogram, CT scan, and magnetic resonance imaging scan (Fig. 25–40).

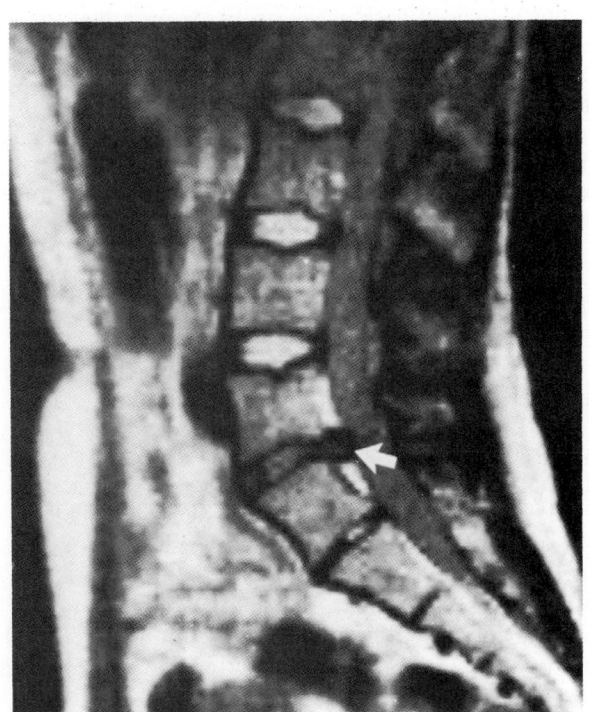

FIGURE 25–40. MRI scan demonstrating herniation of the L5-S1 disk *(arrow)*. (From Richardson, M. L., Gillespy, T., III, Olson, D. O., et al. [1986]. Magnetic resonance imaging of the musculoskeletal system. In F. A. Mettler, Jr., L. R. Muroff, M. V. Kulkarni [Eds.]. *Magnetic resonance imaging and spectroscopy.* New York: Churchill Livingstone. By permission.)

Procedure

Intraoperative radiographs should be anticipated for disk localization. A spinal needle is inserted into the disk space, and a lateral radiograph is taken. The x-ray cassette is either suspended on a Mayo stand with adhesive tape and positioned at the side of the patient outside the sterile field or placed in a sterile cassette cover and propped along the patient's side within the sterile field. The radiograph confirms that the surgeon is dissecting at the correct level.

Incision and Exposure

After the patient is prepared and draped, the incision is made in the midline vertically. Finger pressure on gauze sponges provides hemostasis while cauterization of vessels is performed. Cutting current is used with the electrosurgical pencil to incise fascia and muscle. The muscles are dissected from the lamina and spinous processes and packed back by pushing opened gauze sponges around the bony structures with Cobb elevators. When hemostasis is achieved, the sponges are removed and a self-retaining retractor is placed.

Details

Rongeurs are used to remove lamina, the ligamentum flavum is incised with a No. 15 blade on a No. 7 knife handle, and a window is created. Cottonoid strips are placed into this incision for protection and hemostasis. The nerve root and dura are retracted. Hemostasis of epidural vessels is performed with bipolar coagulation. Disk rongeurs are used to remove disk material. The area is irrigated and hemostasis ensured. All sponges are removed and accounted for.

Closure

The wound is closed in layers, and a pressure dressing is applied.

Postoperative Care

Postoperatively, the patient remains in bed for only a short time. Many patients ambulate during the first 24 hours after surgery, and early ambulation is a factor in reducing the length of hospital stay (Ende, 1986). The majority of patients are discharged within a week of the surgery.

Potential Surgical Complications

Pain
Numbness
Impaired muscle function
Incontinence
Impotence
Urinary retention
CSF leak

PERIPHERAL NERVE REPAIR

Definition

Surgical repair of a damaged or injured peripheral nerve is performed to restore function to the area affected by an injured nerve. This is done by either anastomosing a transected nerve or by resecting a damaged nerve segment.

Indications

Most nerve injuries in civilian situations are caused by glass or sharp knives. Of these injuries, 95% are at or distal to the wrist (Smith, 1986). For this reason, the procedure described below is repair of a transected nerve of the wrist.

The patient with a nerve injury generally has a primary repair if the wound is clean. In the case of a dirty, ragged wound, the surgeon may choose to débride and close the wound with nerve repair as a delayed secondary procedure.

Symptoms of nerve injury are sensory and motor deficits distal to the injury. When a primary repair of an injured nerve has not been performed, evidence of nerve function can be determined by the usual neurological examination, including testing for motor ability, abnormal movements, reflexes, light touch pinprick, and temperature differential. More detailed testing of nerve function may be carried out by nerve stimulation, electromyography, and evoked nerve action potentials.

These procedures may be done on an outpatient or same-day admission basis with minimal preoperative testing indicated.

Related Surgical Procedures

Other types of peripheral nerve surgery similar to nerve repair are

neurectomy (resection of a nerve)
neurolysis (freeing a nerve from entrapment and compression); carpal tunnel release is the most common
excision of neuroma (removal of a tumor from the nerve)
nerve transposition (repositioning a nerve, most frequently the ulnar nerve, affected by pressure and entrapment that causes a palsy)

Perioperative Nursing Implications

Anesthesia

This procedure may be performed under general or regional anesthesia. Regional anesthesia takes the form of an axillary block or a Bier block. A pneumatic tourniquet is usually used to control bleeding at the operative site, and in the case of a Bier block, a double cuff is required. The cuffs are inflated alternately during the procedure so that the patient can tolerate the cuff pressure with less discomfort. The tourniquet also keeps the anesthetic agent in the extremity. The cuff size should be appropriate to the size of the limb in length and width, the width of the cuff being approximately equal to the diameter of the extremity. The area under the cuff should be wrapped with cast padding. Position the cuff as high on the extremity as possible, and secure it with the connectors for the tubing on the outside of the limb. Do not attempt to twist or shift the cuff after it has been placed. If it is not in the correct position, remove and reapply it. The function of the pressure regulator should be tested before the procedure. The nurse also monitors and documents tourniquet pressure inflation time and deflation time.

Position

The patient is positioned supine with the arm extended on an arm table. The bed may be flexed slightly for patient comfort under regional anesthesia. A restraint strap is placed over the upper thighs. The unaffected arm is extended on a padded arm board.

Creation and Maintenance of the Sterile Field

The skin preparation should include the hand and arm circumferentially up to the tourniquet cuff. A liberal extent of preparation is necessary because a long incision may be necessary to dissect enough nerve length for a tension-free repair. The arm can be elevated on a bolster or limb elevator placed under the shoulder during the preparation.

After draping, the circulator positions the microscope and provides sitting stools for the surgical team members.

After the patient has been prepared, the arm is elevated while drapes are placed over the arm table. At least one layer of drapes should be impervious. A towel folded lengthwise is placed around the tourniquet and clipped in place. The arm is covered with a sterile stockinet, which may be secured with a roller bandage. The arm is lowered onto the arm table, and the patient is covered with sterile drapes. The drapes should be secured around the upper arm in such a way as to avoid exposing an unsterile area as the arm is manipulated.

During the procedure, the scrub nurse sits either opposite the surgeon if there is no assistant or at the end of the arm table. The microscope stands on the unaffected side of the patient with the objective portion of the microscope over the field.

As with any microsurgical procedure, the scrub nurse should pay careful attention to the surgeon's need to return instruments and receive instruments in the position for use without looking away from the field.

Equipment and Supplies

The circulator should provide impervious draping material to drape the arm table, an Esmarch bandage to exsanguinate the limb, and a stockinet drape to cover the limb. A microscope or loupes and microsurgical instruments, a small dissecting set, sterile razor blades, bipolar and monopolar electrosurgical units, a sterile tongue blade, a marking pen, a nerve stimulator, small self-retaining retractors, 8–0 or 10–0 nylon suture for nerve repair, and 5–0 nylon for wound closure are used. Casting material is needed at the end of the procedure.

Procedure

Incision and Exposure

When the patient has been prepared and draped, the arm is elevated into a straight vertical position, and an Esmarch bandage is applied circumferentially from the distal to the proximal end of the arm. The arm remains in this position until the pneumatic tourniquet is inflated. The pressure used depends on the patient's blood pressure, the patient's age, and the size of the limb and should be determined by the surgeon. The usual pressure on an average adult arm is 300 mm Hg (Association of Operating Room Nurses, 1989). The circulating nurse should alert the surgeon after the tourniquet has been inflated for 1 hour.

The incision is made longitudinally over the area of nerve injury. Usually, the wound is explored to locate the nerve endings, which tend to retract after transection. The nerve may have to be dissected for a substantial distance to mobilize adequate length for a tension-free repair.

Details

When a primary repair is performed, the transected ends of the nerve are inspected for damage and resected as necessary. In a secondary repair, the nerve endings are located and fixed to one another with lateral sutures to prevent rotation. The proximal and distal stumps are placed on a moistened tongue blade and sectioned serially with a razor blade until good fascicular structure is identified under magnification. Traction on the lateral sutures by the assistant during this process provides stability to the nerve endings. The fascicular bundles are then aligned to facilitate good return of function after healing and regeneration of tissue. Smith (1986) recommended an epineural repair with fascicular alignment of digital nerves and fascicular bundle repair followed by epineural suturing for larger nerves. Suture used for the nerve repair is 8–0 or 10–0 nylon.

Closure

The soft tissue and skin are closed and a dressing applied to the wound. The arm is immobilized in a cast or splint in a position that avoids tension on the area of anastomosis.

Postoperative Care

Rehabilitation after injury begins as soon as the cast is removed. Disuse of the extremity results in pain and poor future function. Physical therapy, regular exercise, strengthening activity, and dynamic splinting are used to restore all possible function to the injured arm.

Bibliography

Alspach, J. G., Williams, S. M. (1985). *Core curriculum for critical care nursing* (3rd ed.). Philadelphia: W. B. Saunders.

American Association of Neuroscience Nurses. (1980). *Core curriculum for neurosurgical nursing in the operating room.* Park Ridge, IL: American Association of Neuroscience Nurses, 1992.

Association of Operating Room Nurses. (1993). *Standards and recommended practices for perioperative nursing.* Denver, CO.

Brooks, B. J. (1989). Percutaneous lumbar discectomy. *AORN Journal, 49,* 1332–1344.

Ende, R. M. (1986). The significance of selected variables in laminectomy length of stay. *Journal of Neuroscience Nursing, 18*(3), 150–152.

Gary, R. A. (1983). Caring for patients with cerebral aneurysms. *AORN Journal, 37,* 631–642.

Gruendemann, B. J., Meeker, M. H. (1987). *Alexander's care of the patient in surgery* (8th ed.). St. Louis: C. V. Mosby.

Hickey, J. V. (1986). *The clinical practice of neurological and neurosurgical nursing* (2nd ed.). Philadelphia: J. B. Lippincott.

Houston, C. S., Murphy-Irwin, K. (1986). Intraoperative ultrasound of the brain and spinal cord. *Perioperative Nursing Quarterly, 2*(1), 59–70.

Koch, F., Poisson, C. (1989). Targeting cerebral tumors. *AORN Journal, 49,* 740–757.

Marlow, D. R., Redding, B. A. (1988). *Textbook of pediatric nursing* (6th ed.). Philadelphia: W. B. Saunders.

Maroon, J. C., Alba, A. (1985). Microdiscectomy versus chemonucleolysis. Neurosurgery, *16(5),* 644–649.

Ommaya, A. K. Implantable devices for chronic access and drug delivery to the central nervous system. *Cancer Drug Delivery, 1*(2), 169–179.

Savoy, S. M. (1984). The craniotomy patient: identifying the patient's neurological status. *AORN Journal, 40,* 716–724.

Smith, J. W. (1986). Peripheral nerve surgery—Retrospective and contemporary techniques. *Clinics in Plastic Surgery, 13,* 249–254.

Temple, A. P. (1984). Stereotaxic surgery. *AORN Journal, 40,* 543–550.

Temple, A. P., Katz, J. (1987). Air embolism. *AORN Journal, 45,* 387–402.

Walker, M. L. (1983). Using lasers in neurosurgery. *AORN Journal, 38,* 238–241.

Youmans, J. R. (Ed.). (1982). *Neurological surgery* (2nd ed.). Philadelphia: W. B. Saunders.

CHAPTER 26

Urological Surgery

Carolyn Grous and Marc Cendron

DEFINITION

Urology is the surgical specialty that investigates and manages diseases of the urological system in both males and females. Included are diseases and malformations of the adrenal glands, kidneys, ureters, bladder, and male genitalia (penis, urethra, prostate gland, and scrotum). Urology offers a broad spectrum of treatment modalities, which include open surgery, endoscopic procedures, laser therapy, and lithotripsy (literally meaning the breaking up of stones).

The history of urological surgery goes back to antiquity: Illustrated and written documents describe such procedures. Circumcision is present in Egyptian hiero-glyphs. Lithotomy (Greek for "cutting for stone") was practiced by specialists; Hippocrates, however, admonished, "I will not cut for stone, even for patients in whom the disease is manifest but leave that to crafts men who are skilled therein" (Hippocratic Oath, 430 B.C.). Since that time, urological surgery has progressed. It now encompasses a wide spectrum of diseases and procedures from surgery for trauma to the genitourinary system to cancer therapy. Many congenital abnormalities affect the urinary tract and are amenable to surgical management. The past 20 years have also brought about dramatic changes in the approach to stone disease with the advent of equipment such as the extracorporeal shock wave lithotriptor. Furthermore, the urologist is called on to manage and treat complications involving the bladder and the ureters, which may result from standard surgical procedures on adjacent organs (e.g., colon or uterus).

A team approach is essential in carrying out urological surgery. The perioperative nursing team plays a major role in the preoperative, intraoperative, and postoperative care of the patient undergoing a urological surgical procedure. Preoperative assessment and planning are carried out by the perioperative nurse for each patient. Intraoperatively, nurses intervene to act as patient advocates during the procedure. Furthermore, as members of the perioperative nursing team, nurses are involved in the preparation and operation of sophisticated equipment such as lasers, ureteroscopes, and lithotripsy instruments, as well as direct patient care. Postoperatively, evaluation and education are performed by the perioperative nurse to provide a total patient care framework.

This chapter introduces urological surgery by describing its salient features as it pertains to the perioperative nursing team. Elements of anatomy and surgical methods are presented. A discussion of the perioperative management and care of the patient undergoing urological surgery focuses on the role of the nursing staff. A description of various surgical procedures and urological instruments is provided. Potential complications of each procedure are reviewed.

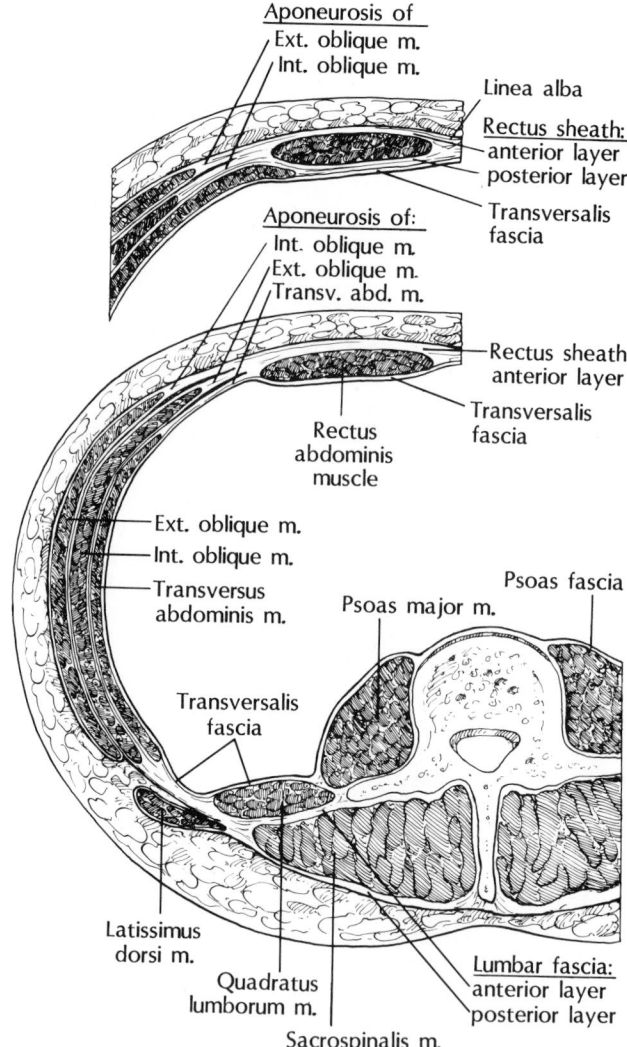

FIGURE 26–1. Cross-section in the lumbar region showing the lamina of the lumbar (lumbodorsal) fascia and the musculature and fusion of the anterior abdominal below the arcuate line. *Inset*, Composition of the rectus sheath above the arcuate line. (Original drawing by Christine Young.) (From Gillenwater, J. Y., Grayhack, J. T., Howards, S. S., Duckett, J. W. [Eds.]. [1987]. *Adult and pediatric urology* [p. 5]. Chicago: Mosby-Year Book.)

ANATOMY

Abdominal Wall

Surgery on the urinary tract necessitates incisions through the abdominal wall musculature. The abdominal wall, which extends from the rib cage to the bony pelvis, can be divided into anterior, anterolateral, and postero-lateral walls (Fig. 26–1).

Two paired, segmented muscles, surrounded by fascial layers, form the anterior abdominal wall: the rectus abdominis muscles (Fig. 26–2). They extend from the pubic crest to fifth, sixth, and seventh ribs, where they insert. These muscles are surrounded by a fibrous envelope, the rectus sheath. This sheath represents the continuation of the fascial layers from the anterolateral

abdominal wall. In the midline, the rectus muscles are separated by a dense fibrous tissue known as the *linea alba* (the white line). Inferiorly, between the umbilicus and the pubic bone, on which it inserts, can be found a small triangular muscle, the pyramidal muscle.

The flank is made up of strong muscles. The external oblique, internal oblique, and transversus abdominis form the anterolateral abdominal wall (see Fig. 26–2). The fibers of each muscle course in a different direction to provide strength and support to an area of the body where there is a great deal of mass and little skeletal support, except for the spine. At the inferior aspect of the anterolateral abdominal wall, in the inguinal area, exists a communication between the abdominal cavity and the inguinal canal, the internal ring. This represents an area of potential weakness through which hernias

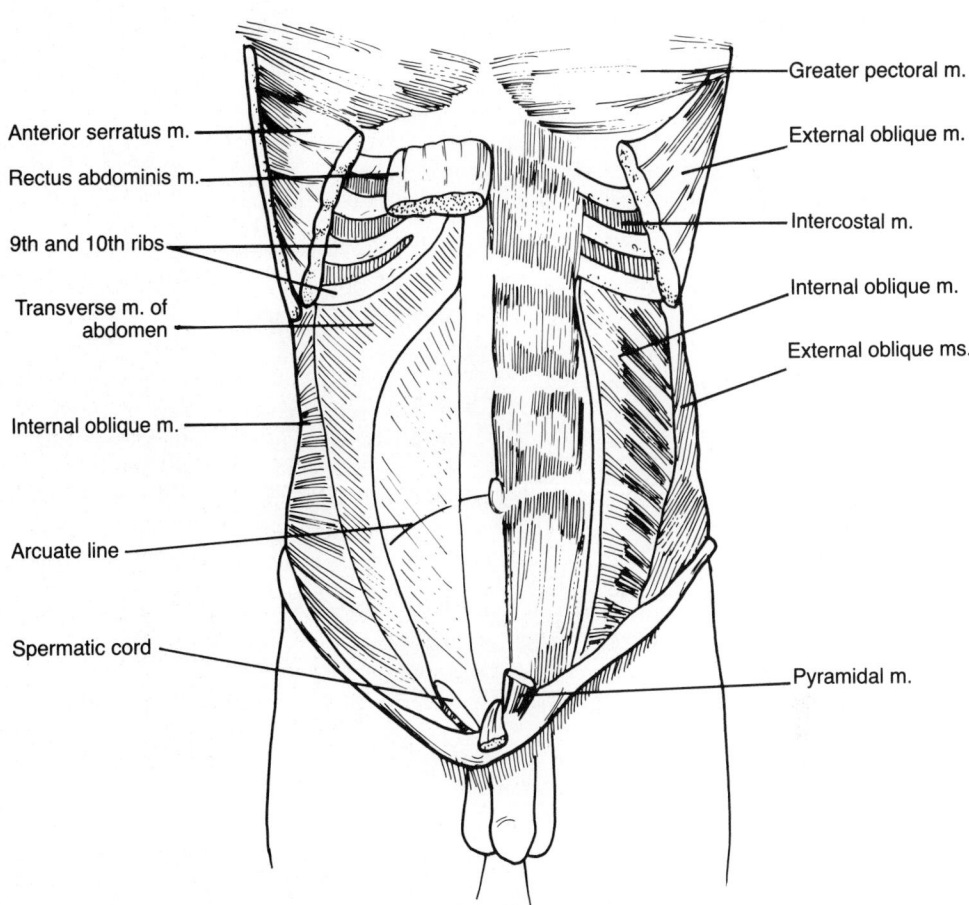

Greater pectoral m.

External oblique m.

Intercostal m.

Internal oblique m.

External oblique ms.

Pyramidal m.

Anterior serratus m.

Rectus abdominis m.

9th and 10th ribs

Transverse m. of abdomen

Internal oblique m.

Arcuate line

Spermatic cord

FIGURE 26–2. Layers of the anterior abdominal wall.

may develop. The spermatic cord in the male and the round ligament in the female course through the internal ring. The posterolateral abdominal wall can be divided into three muscle groups: deep, superficial, and intermediate. The superficial group comprises the external oblique muscle and latissimus dorsi muscle. In the intermediate group are the serratus posterior inferior, internal oblique, and sacrospinal muscles. In the deep group are the transversus abdominis, quadratus lumborum, and psoas muscles (Fig. 26–3).

After the retroperitoneum has been entered through an incision in the abdominal wall, access to the kidneys, ureters, and adrenal gland is possible by reflecting the peritoneal contents with or without entering the peritoneum (Fig. 26–4).

Kidneys

Both kidneys lie in the retroperitoneum on either side of the spine and great vessels (Fig. 26–5). They are surrounded by dense fat and are bean shaped, measuring approximately 12 cm in length by 7 cm in width and 3 cm in thickness. Each kidney weighs 150 g in the average adult man and 135 g in the woman. The lateral border of the kidney is convex. Near the center of the medial aspect of each kidney is a shallow depression, the renal

hilum, through which pass the renal artery, vein, nerves, and lymphatics, and the renal pelvis. The central part of the kidney, the renal sinus, is occupied by the major urine-collecting system, the renal pelvis, which branches out into two or three major calyces. These, in turn, branch out into minor calyces. Between the minor calyces are the renal papillae, which are projections of medullary renal tissue. There is a wide variation in the anatomy of the pelvis and the calyces.

The kidney itself is covered by a fibroelastic capsule, which extends over the kidney into the renal sinus to merge with the ends of the calyces. The capsule itself is penetrated by a number of small capsular vessels. The renal tissue is divided into medulla and cortex (Fig. 26–6). When the kidney is cut open and bivalved, one can observe that the medulla is composed of striated groups of tissue called the *renal pyramid*. The tops of the pyramids actually form the renal papilla. The striations of the renal pyramids represent the linear arrangement of the renal tubules. The cortex has a more granular appearance. The microanatomy of the kidney is beyond the scope of this discussion, and the interested reader should refer to a standard textbook of nephrology.

In 70% of individuals, there are single left and right renal arteries. Both arise from the aorta, the right renal artery being higher than the left. Before entering the hilum of the kidney, the renal artery usually divides into

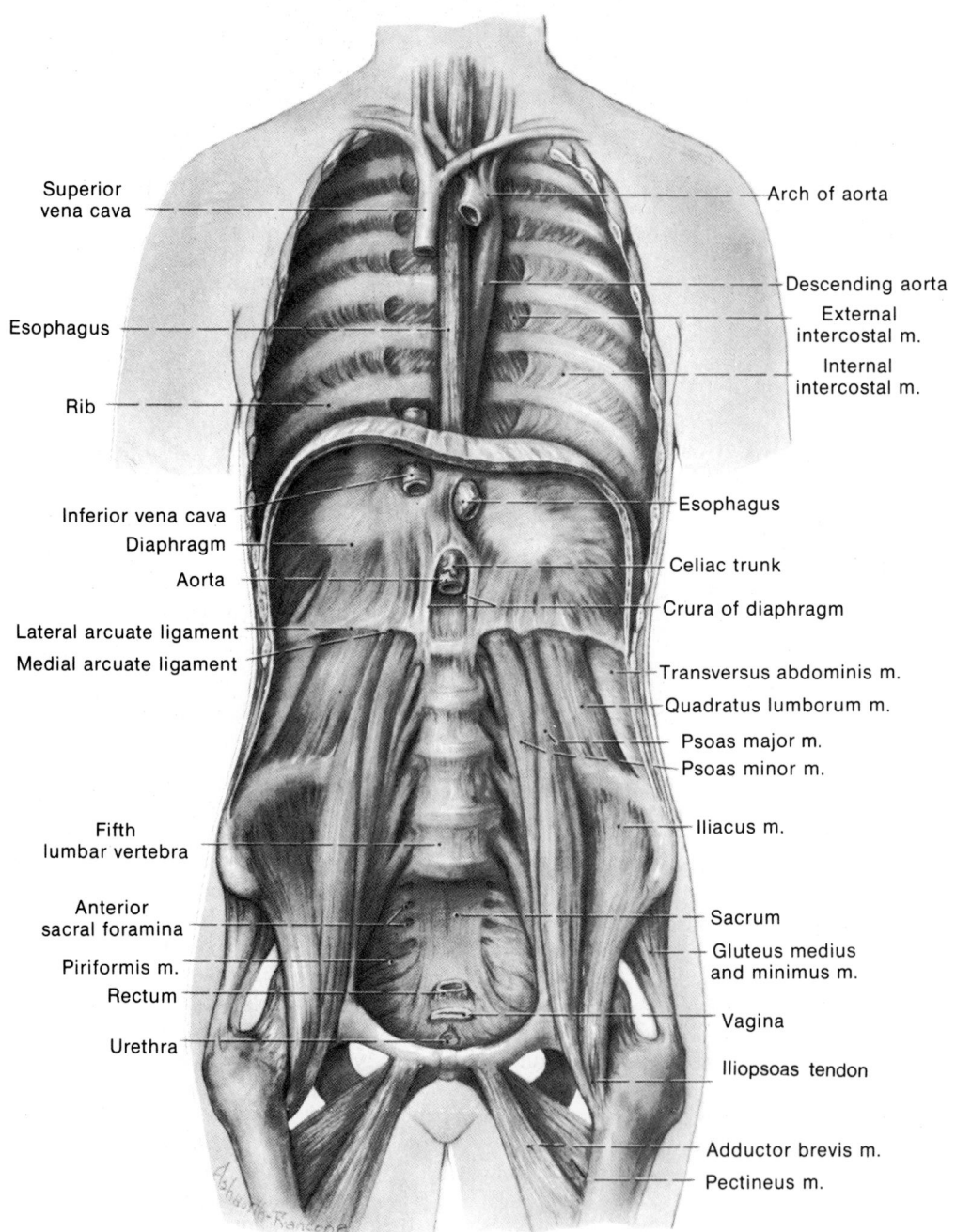

Superior vena cava

Esophagus

Rib

Inferior vena cava

Diaphragm

Aorta

Lateral arcuate ligament

Medial arcuate ligament

Fifth lumbar vertebra

Anterior sacral foramina

Piriformis m.

Rectum

Urethra

Arch of aorta

Descending aorta

External intercostal m.

Internal intercostal m.

Esophagus

Celiac trunk

Crura of diaphragm

Transversus abdominis m.

Quadratus lumborum m.

Psoas major m.

Psoas minor m.

Iliacus m.

Sacrum

Gluteus medius and minimus m.

Vagina

Iliopsoas tendon

Adductor brevis m.

Pectineus m.

FIGURE 26–3. Cross section showing extension of the iliolumbar abscess: perinephric and psoas abscesses. (From Jacob, S. W., Francone, C. A. [1989]. *Elements of anatomy and physiology* [2nd ed.]. Philadelphia: W. B. Saunders, Fig. 5–24.)

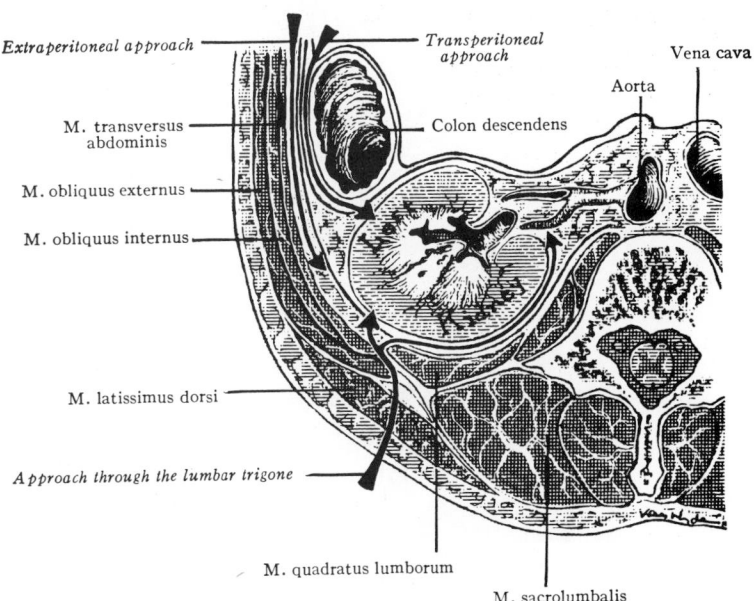

Extraperitoneal approach

Transperitoneal approach

Vena cava

Aorta

M. transversus abdominis

Colon descendens

M. obliquus externus

M. obliquus internus

M. latissimus dorsi

Approach through the lumbar trigone

M. quadratus lumborum

M. sacrolumbalis

FIGURE 26–4. Cross section showing the paths of approach to the left kidney. (From McVay, C. B. [1984]. *Anson & McVay surgical anatomy* [6th ed.]. Philadelphia: W. B. Saunders, Fig. IV–260.)

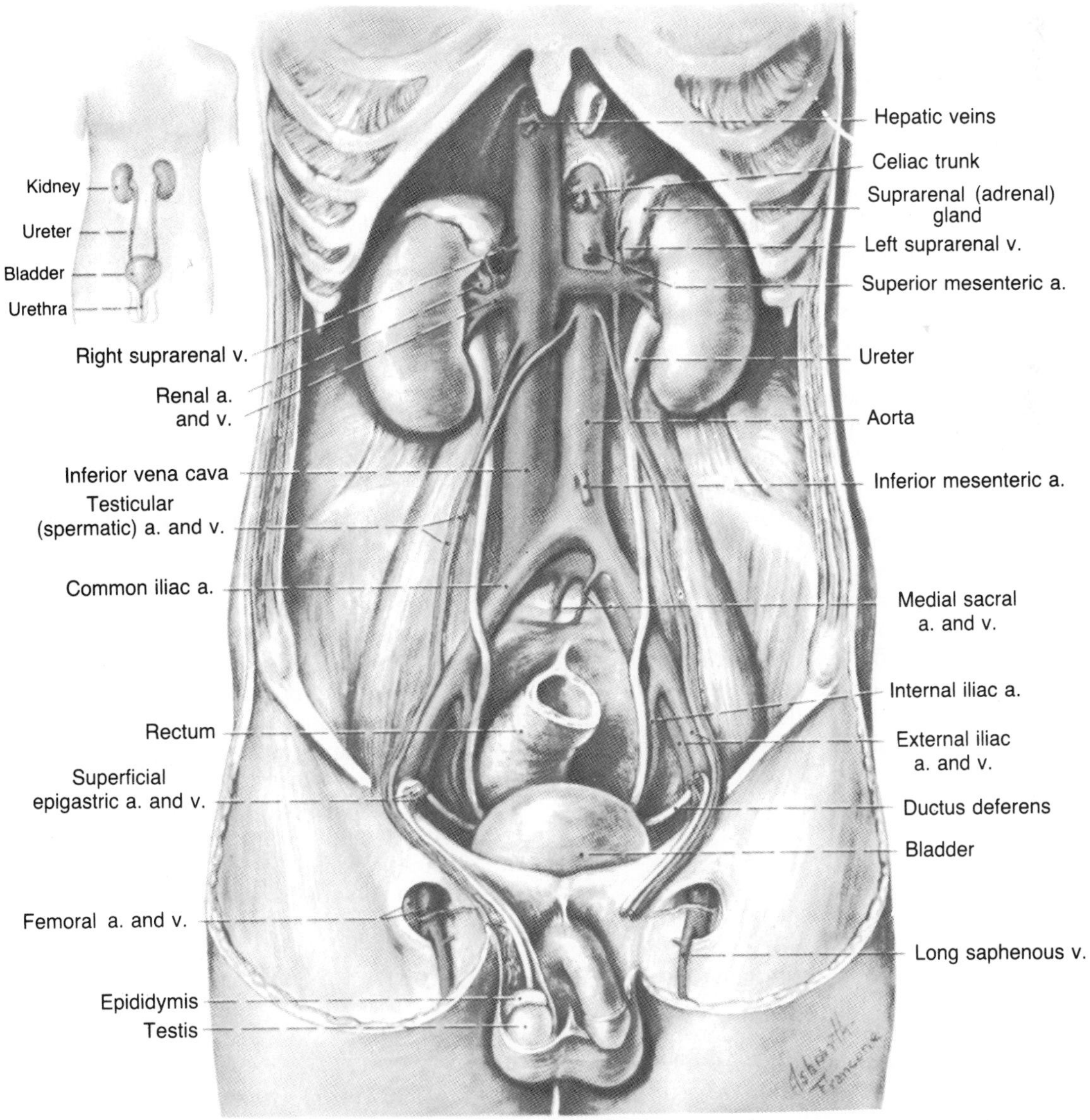

Kidney

Ureter

Bladder

Urethra

Right suprarenal v.

Renal a. and v.

Inferior vena cava

Testicular (spermatic) a. and v.

Common iliac a.

Rectum

Superficial epigastric a. and v.

Femoral a. and v.

Epididymis

Testis

Hepatic veins

Celiac trunk

Suprarenal (adrenal) gland

Left suprarenal v.

Superior mesenteric a.

Ureter

Aorta

Inferior mesenteric a.

Medial sacral a. and v.

Internal iliac a.

External iliac a. and v.

Ductus deferens

Bladder

Long saphenous v.

FIGURE 26–5. Posterior abdominal wall showing the relationship of the urinary system, genital system, and great vessels. (From Jacob, S. W., Francone, C. A., Lossow, W. J. [1982]. *Structure and function in man* [5th ed.]. Philadelphia: W. B. Saunders, Fig. 15–1.)

575

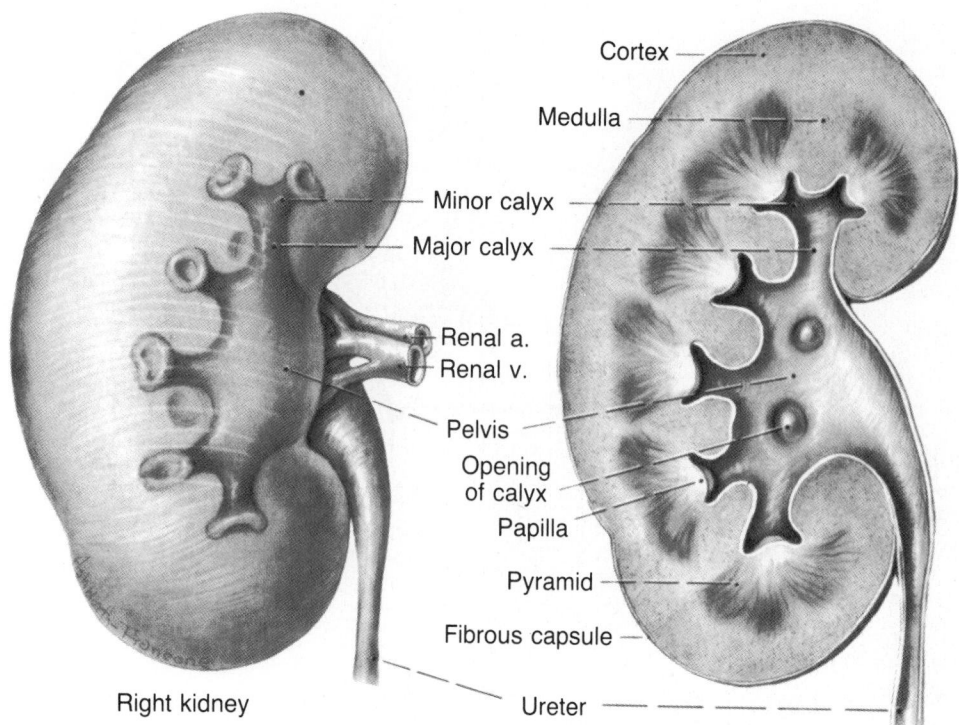

Cortex
Medulla
Minor calyx
Major calyx
Renal a.
Renal v.
Pelvis
Opening of calyx
Papilla
Pyramid
Fibrous capsule
Right kidney
Ureter

FIGURE 26–6. Entire and sagittal views showing the relation of calyces to the kidney as a whole. (From Jacob, S. W., Francone, C. A., Lossow, W. J. [1982]. *Structure and function in man* [5th ed.]. Philadelphia: W. B. Saunders, Fig. 15–3.)

anterior and posterior divisions. Again, some variation in the anatomy may be found, with some patients having two or more arteries supplying one kidney. Within the kidney, the arteries further branch into interlobar, or arcuate and interlobar, arteries. A single vein drains the kidney into the inferior vena cava. The renal vein is situated anterior to the artery. On the left side, there are two veins draining into the renal vein, one from the adrenal and one from the gonad.

Surrounding the kidney and adrenal gland is a thick layer of fat known as *perinephric fat*, which in turn is covered by a layer of connective tissue, Gerota fascia. More fatty tissue is found outside Gerota fascia, further helping to cushion the kidney.

Several major organs are in close proximity to the kidneys. The right lobe of the liver, the descending duodenum, and the hepatic flexure of the colon are adjacent to the right kidney, and on the left, the stomach, the spleen, the splenic flexure of the colon, the pancreas, and the small intestine are close to the kidney (see Fig. 26–6).

Adrenal Gland

An adrenal gland lies on top of each kidney (see Fig. 26–5). As mentioned above, they are embedded in the perinephric fat and appear as thin, bright yellow structures. The right adrenal is triangular, whereas the left one has an elongated shape. The blood supply to the adrenal is composed of three small arteries. The lower portion of the adrenal gland is supplied by an artery coming from the renal artery. The middle portion is supplied by a branch from the aorta, and the upper

portion gets a branch from the phrenic artery. The adrenal gland is drained by a single vein, which empties on the right into the renal artery and on the left into the vena cava.

Ureters

The urine produced by the kidney is collected into the calyces, which coalesce to form major calyces. These in turn drain into the renal pelvis. The pelvis opens into the ureter at the ureteropelvic junction. The ureter courses down to the bladder in the retroperitoneum (Fig. 26–7) and enters the bladder on its posterior aspect at the ureterovesical junction. Much like the small intestine, the ureter is a hollow, muscular tube that uses peristalsis to propel urine toward the bladder. Along its course, the ureter is in close relationship with several organs of importance: on the right, the duodenum, the body of the pancreas, the ascending colon, the iliac vessels; and on the left, the tail of the pancreas, the descending colon, and the iliac vessels. In the pelvis, the ureter is in close proximity to the vas deferens and the seminal vesicles in the male, and the ovaries, the uterus, and the vagina in the female.

Bladder

The bladder (see Fig. 26–7) is a hollow, muscular organ that rests anteriorly in the pelvis and is contained in a layer of retroperitoneal tissue (fat and connective tissue). Its role is storing urine, and its shape changes as it fills. The bulk of the bladder is formed by the

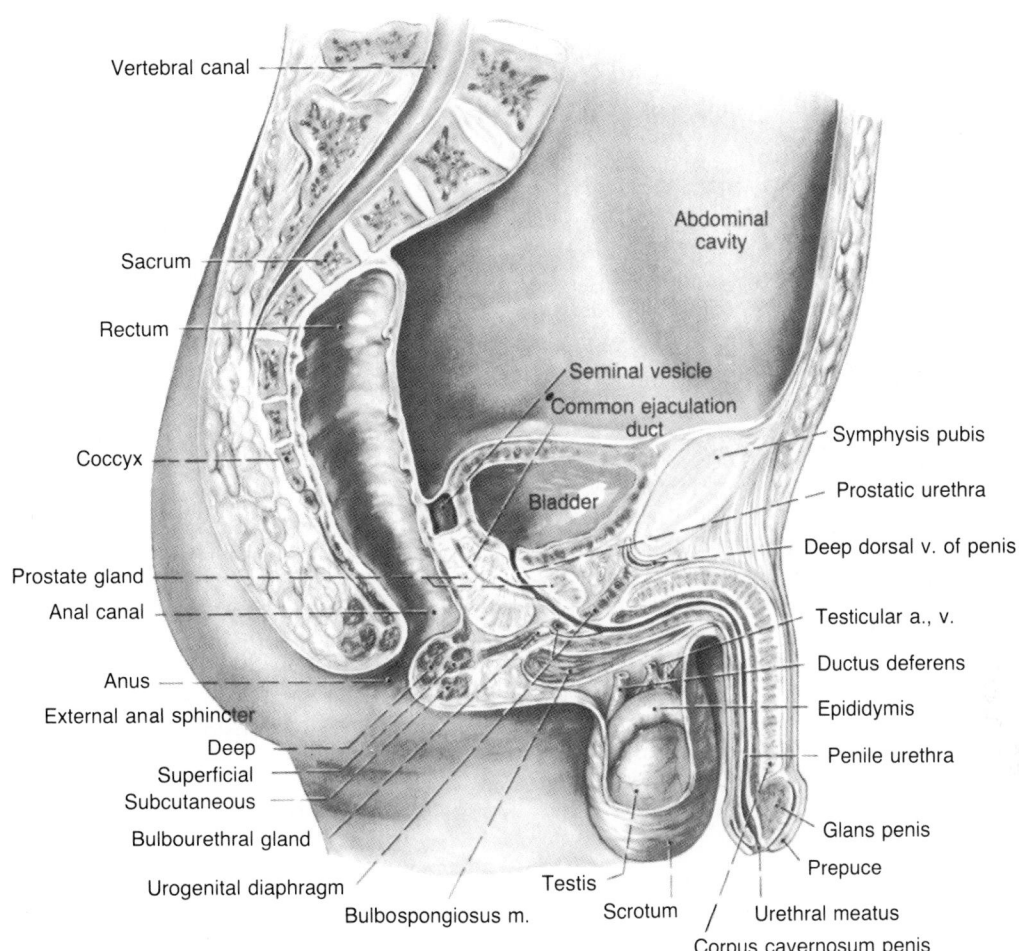

FIGURE 26–7. Midsagittal section of the male pelvis and external genitalia. (From Jacob, S. W., Francone, C. A., Lossow, W. J. [1982]. *Structure and function in man* [5th ed.]. Philadelphia: W. B. Saunders, Fig. 14–3.)

detrusor muscle. Anatomically, the bladder can be described as having two lateral walls, a posterior wall, and a dome. At the base of the bladder, a triangular area can be seen, the trigone. The angles of the triangle are formed by each of the ureteral orifices and the bladder neck. The dome of the bladder is in contact with the peritoneum.

The blood supply to the bladder arises from branches of the internal iliac artery, the superior and inferior vesical arteries, and a number of smaller vessels. Venous drainage occurs through several venous plexuses, which drain into the internal iliac vein. These vessels are found in the lateral and posterior ligaments of the bladder, which are located deep in the pelvis.

Urethra

The urethra extends from the bladder neck to the urinary meatus. In the female, the urethra is short (3–4 cm) and runs through the layers of the perineum anterior to the vagina. Muscular sphincter mechanisms that ensure urinary continence surround the proximal part of the urethra. The male urethra is substantially longer and can be divided into two segments as it extends from the bladder neck to the tip of the penis. The posterior, or membranous, urethra traverses the urogenital diaphragm and is surrounded proximally to the bladder by the prostate gland and by the muscle fibers of the urethral sphincter. The anterior urethra extends from the urogenital diaphragm to the urethral meatus. It can be divided into three parts: bulbar, penile, and glanular urethra. The anterior urethra is surrounded by the erectile tissues of the penis. Several structures can be identified within the urethra: the striated sphincter, the verumontanum with the openings of the ejaculatory ducts, and the lobes of the prostate gland.

Male Genital System

The male genital system is composed of the prostate gland, the seminal vesicles, the vas deferens, the epididymis, and the testes (see Fig. 26–7). The penis and scrotum are discussed separately. The prostate gland lies at the base of the bladder and can be examined only by digital rectal examination. It is roughly the size of a chestnut, and it encircles the urethra. The prostate gland has been thought to be composed of several lobes, which are not readily apparent on examination. In the older man, the prostate enlarges by growth of adenomatous tissue (nonmalignant) in the lateral and anterior lobes. Prostatic cancer is believed to arise in the posterior lobes. The prostate is covered by a dense capsule, and it is fixed to the pelvic floor by investments of parietal fascia and by the endopelvic fascia. The blood supply to the prostate comes from a branch of the inferior vesical artery. The dorsal vein of the penis drains into the plexus of veins (the plexus of Santorini) on the anterior aspect of the prostate. Venous drainage of the prostate occurs via hypogastric veins.

To better understand the anatomy of the male genital system, one can follow the passage of the sperm from the testis to the urethra. After spermatozoa are formed in the testis, they are moved to the epididymis, which is a structure lying alongside and on top of the testis. The epididymis is formed by the convolution of the epididymal duct, which stores sperm. The next structure encountered is the vas deferens, which courses from the scrotum to the prostate through the inguinal canals and the pelvis, posteriorly and then medially. The vas deferens passes between the ureters and the posterior aspect of the bladder. The seminal vesicles are paired structures sitting at the back of the bladder that communicate with the vas deferens. The vas ends at the ejaculatory duct, which opens into the urethra on either side of the verumontanum.

Penis

The penis is composed of erectile tissue organized in three distinct cylindrical bodies: two corpora cavernosa and one corpus spongiosum through which courses the urethra. Each corpus is enclosed in a thick fascia, the *tunica albuginea corporis spongiosi.* Surrounding this fascia is a fibrous envelope known as Buck's fascia. The corpora end in the glans penis, which is covered by the prepuce. The meatus of the urethra is found at the tip of the glans.

Scrotum

The scrotum contains both testicles in separate pouches. The scrotal skin covers the dartos muscles, which in turn cover three thin fascial layers derived from the abdominal wall. The testis measures 4.5 cm in length, 3 cm in width, and 2 cm in thickness and is covered by dense fascial covering called the *tunica albuginea testis.* The mass of the testis is made up of coiled up seminiferous tubules, where spermatozoa are made. Blood supply to the testis is provided by spermatic vessels that arise from the aorta on the right and the renal artery on the left and course down in the retroperitoneum parallel to the ureters, and through the inguinal canal, in the spermatic cord to the testes.

TABLE 26–1. NONHYDRAULIC PENILE PROSTHESES
Semirigid
Small-Carrion
Hinged
Flexi-Rod II
Malleable
AMS Malleable 600
Jonas Silicon-Silver
Mentor Malleable
Positionable
DuraPhase
Mechanically activated
OmniPhase

INSERTION OF PENILE PROSTHESIS

The first implantation of a prosthesis for male erectile dysfunction was performed in 1936 when Borgoras implanted a rib in the penis to provide rigidity (Goodwin and Scott, 1952). Since that time, nonreactive compounds have been developed and prosthetic urological surgery has grown considerably.

Definition

Penile prostheses currently available for implantation are divided into two categories: rigid and semirigid devices and inflatable prostheses (Tables 26–1 and 26–2). The rigid and semirigid devices are made of two malleable rods. Each rod is composed of silicone elastomer with a metal or alloy core (Fig. 26–8). When the devices are placed within the penis, a permanent degree of rigidity is provided to allow vaginal penetration and sexual intercourse.

The inflatable penile prosthesis is more complex and is composed of several parts, which are a reservoir placed in the abdomen extraperitoneally, a pump placed in the scrotum, connecting tubing, and paired cylinders placed within the corporal bodies. A hydraulic mechanism allows the filling of the paired cylinders, which impart tumescence and rigidity to the penis. Newer inflatable models consist of only the corporal cylinders containing the fluid and a hydraulic system. These

TABLE 26–2. HYDRAULIC PENILE PROSTHESES
One piece
AMS Hydroflex
Flexi-Flate
Two piece
GFS Inflatable
Uni-Flate 1000
Three piece
AMS 700CX
Mentor Inflatable

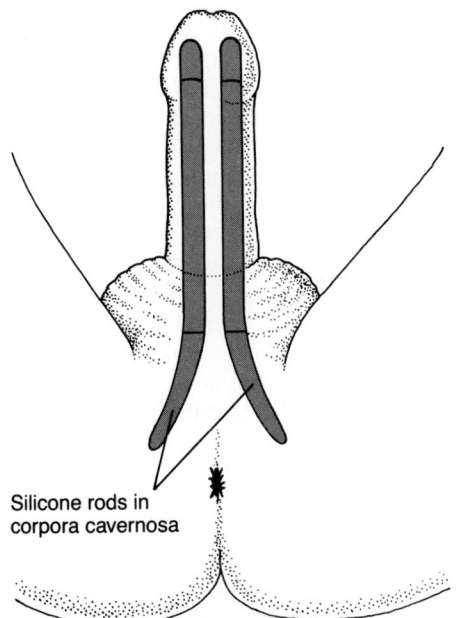

Semirigid penile prostheses consist of rods inserted into the corpora cavernosa via a perineal or dorsal penile incision. The penis remains in a constant state of semierection.

Silicone rods in corpora cavernosa

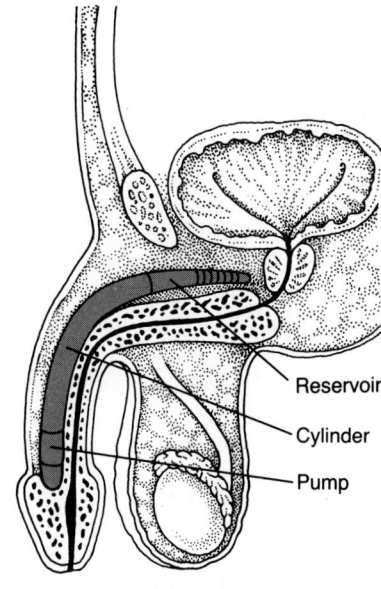

Reservoir

Cylinder

Pump

Self-contained penile prostheses consist of a pump, a cylinder, and a reservoir, all in a single unit. The client squeezes the pump just below the head of the penis to fill the cylinder and achieve erection.

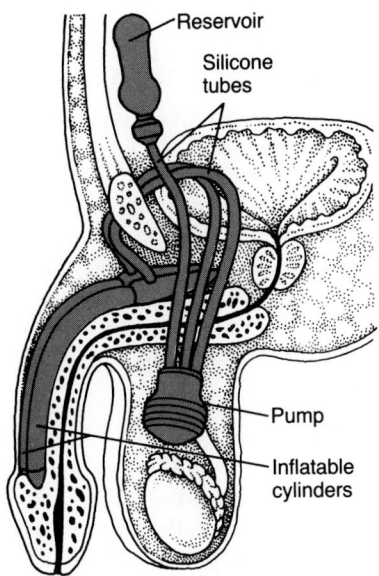

Reservoir

Silicone tubes

Pump

Inflatable cylinders

Inflatable penile prostheses consist of two hollow silicone cylinders, an abdominal reservoir, and a scrotal pump. The client squeezes the pump to fill the cylinders and achieve erection.

FIGURE 26–8. Penile prostheses. (From Ignatavicius, D. D., Bayne, M. V. [1991]. *Medical-surgical nursing: a nursing process approach*. Philadelphia: W. B. Saunders, Fig. 55–8.)

devices enable both an erect and a flaccid state and may be activated on demand by the patient.

Indications

Indications for the insertion of a penile prosthesis include organic impotence not amenable to medical treatment and psychogenic impotence in which conventional therapy has failed. Patients who wish to undergo placement of a penile prosthesis must undergo an extensive medical and psychiatric evaluation. They should be informed that normal erectile tissue is destroyed at the time of surgery to place the corporal rods or cylinder and that they will never be able to attain a normal erection. However, it should be stressed that, in most cases, placement of a prosthesis does not affect sensation, ejaculation, or orgasm.

Related Surgical Procedures

Similar to the placement of the penile prosthesis is the insertion of the artificial genitourinary sphincter, which is placed around the urethra in selected cases of urinary incontinence. Components used in the making of the sphincter are a reservoir, a pump, connecting tubing, and a cuff that is placed around the urethra. This cuff can be operated to open or close via the pump that is placed in the male scrotum or in the labia majora of the female.

Perioperative Nursing Implications

Anesthesia

Insertion of a penile prosthesis can be performed under general or regional anesthesia. If the patient is awake during the procedure, the circulating nurse must make sure that conversation is kept to a minimum and is relevant to the procedure at hand. Transfusions are not generally required.

Position

Positioning of the patient depends on the surgical approach to be used. If a suprapubic incision is planned, the patient is in the supine position. If a perineal approach is planned, the patient should be placed in the low lithotomy position. The reader should refer to Chapter 12 for routine requirements for the supine and low lithotomy positions.

Creation and Maintenance of the Sterile Field

As for the insertion of any prosthetic device, an extensive skin preparation is performed for this proce- dure. Depending on the surgeon's preference, the patient may be shaved from the umbilicus to the midthigh. This area is then scrubbed with brushes and a suitable antiseptic solution for 10 minutes, following standard surgical preparation guidelines. The circulating nurse must make sure that side towels are used in any area where pooling of the preparation solution could occur. These towels are removed before the patient is draped. A plastic, adhesive drape should be provided to the scrub nurse for the draping procedure. If the patient is awake, the circulating nurse should make sure that a screen is set up with an unsterile drape so that the patient does not watch the preparation and the procedure.

In creating a sterile field, the scrub nurse uses a plastic adhesive drape to isolate the rectal area from the field when the patient is in the low lithotomy position. Other draping requirements for the supine and low lithotomy positions are routine. To avoid contact of the prosthetic devices with lint, most manufacturers suggest the use of a plastic disposable Mayo stand cover to provide a surface for working with the prosthesis. The cover is placed on the Mayo stand so that the plastic surface is on top of the stand. In setting up, the scrub nurse places all prosthetic components on this Mayo stand, and it is reserved for manipulation of the components during the procedure. All components are usually submerged in an antibiotic solution.

Equipment and Supplies

Equipment and supplies for the procedure are gathered in advance by the circulating nurse.

2 plastic Mayo stand covers
3 No. 10 blades
2 No. 15 blades
2 packages of large laparotomy sponges
2 packages of E-tape sponges
2 20-ml syringes
1 Asepto bulb syringe
2 Yankauer suction tips with tubing
1 electrocautery pencil
1 basin set
1 skin marker
1 needle counter
1 pair of light handles or light glove covers
1 7-mm Jackson-Pratt drain
1 16 Fr. Foley catheter with a 5-ml balloon
1 2–0-polypropylene (Prolene) on a cutting needle
4 packages 2–0 polyglactin 910 (Vicryl) or control release on a No. 6 needle
plastic adhesive drape
Drape packs appropriate for patient position
1 soft tissue dissection set
1 penile prosthesis set

A writing surface and marker should be available to the circulating nurse to record the measurements made by the surgeon. The circulator is asked to record the right and left, and distal and proximal, figures. From these measurements, the surgeon calculates the size of prosthesis that is inserted. The circulating nurse should also have available all components of the type of the prosthesis to be used. As a general precaution, two of each component should be available in case of inadvertent contamination or problems.

Components of the malleable penile prosthesis usually include a pair of cylinders and a complete set of paired rear tip extenders (1, 2, and 3 cm). Components of the inflatable penile prosthesis usually include

1 inflate-deflate pump
1 reservoir
3 pairs of rear tip extenders (1, 2, and 3 cm)
1 preparation package, which includes blunt needles, Keith needles, and tubing
1 connector package (can be tie or sutureless)
1 pair of expandable cylinders

Before the start of surgery, the scrub nurse needs to prepare the manufacturer's recommended solutions. In addition, the scrub nurse should perform recommended preparation of the components (e.g., filling and extracting air) according to the manufacturer's guidelines.

During the tissue dissection, the scrub nurse carries out normal role requirements. As the corpora are dilated, the scrub nurse should announce the size of the dilator as it is handed to the surgeon. The dilators should be kept in order so that the scrub nurse can easily move forward or backward in the sequence. In addition, the scrub nurse should also be familiar with the loading of the Furlow instrument so that the cylinder can be loaded and ready for insertion by the surgeon.

Drugs and Solutions

In addition to this equipment, the drugs and solutions necessary for the penile prosthesis procedure include

Sterile water for irrigation
Sterile saline for irrigation
Contrast media such as diatrizoate meglumine, diatrizoate sodium, diatrizoate meglumine 30% (Urovist Cysto)
Neomycin and polymixin B (Neosporin GU irrigant).

Physiological Monitoring

During the procedure, the circulating nurse weighs all sponges and records all blood loss and irrigation. Urine is not routinely emptied from the bladder during this procedure.

Specimens and Cultures

There are no routine specimens and/or cultures for this procedure. If the patient is having a prosthesis removed for infection, the circulator sends several cultures for microbiological examination.

Physician's Orders, Laboratory and Diagnostic Studies

Patients with erectile dysfunction may have either psychological problems or systemic diseases known to affect erectile capability. These include vascular disease (e.g., arteriosclerosis), neurological disease (e.g., multiple sclerosis), and endocrine or metabolic diseases (e.g., diabetes mellitus). These patients, therefore, need a presurgical evaluation that includes a chest x-ray film, a complete set of laboratory data, and an electrocardiogram (ECG). Other diagnostic studies may include penile ultrasonography, probe Doppler analysis of the penile vasculature, and nocturnal penile tumescence studies. These studies help to document erectile dysfunction and provide the indications for surgical management.

Procedure

Incision and Exposure

Several surgical approaches can be used to insert penile prostheses (Table 26–3). In the early years of penile prosthetic surgery, the devices were introduced through a dorsal midline penile incision (Fig. 26–9) with the patient in the supine position. A subcoronal approach was also used (Fig. 26–10). More recently, a perineal approach has been advocated with the patient in the low lithotomy position (Fig. 26–11). Before surgery the patient has been instructed to take one or more chlorhexidine gluconate (Hibiclens) or povidone-iodine (Betadine) showers. Parenteral antibiotics are administered preoperatively.

The incision is brought sharply down to the corpora carvernosa, which are easily recognized by the white tunica albuginea. The tunica is then opened longitudinally for 3 to 4 cm. The intracorporal space containing the erectile tissue is then dilated with Hegar dilators proximal to the ischial tuberosity and distal to the end of the corpora cavernosa at the glans. The space is then copiously irrigated with antibiotic solution, and a prosthesis of the appropriate size is inserted after careful measurement of the corporal space. The procedure is repeated for the opposite side.

Details

Components of the inflatable penile prosthesis can be placed either through an incision extending from the

TABLE 26–3. INCISIONS FOR PENILE PROSTHESIS INSERTION
Dorsal subcoronal
Dorsal penile midline
Ventral penile midline
Penoscrotal
Infrapubic
Perineal

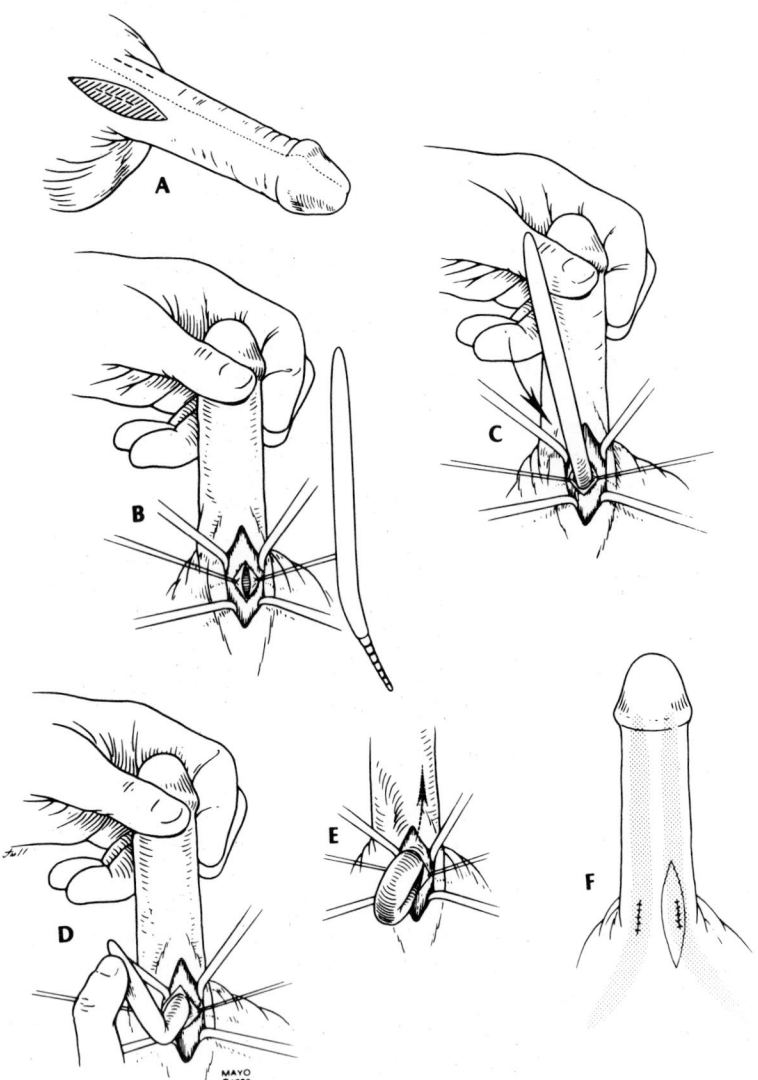

FIGURE 26–9. Penile shaft approach for placement of a penile prosthesis. (From Glenn, J. T. [Ed.]. [1983]. *Urologic surgery* [p. 840]. Philadelphia: J. B. Lippincott.)

base of the penis over the pubis or through a small scrotal or penoscrotal incision with the patient in the supine position and a urethral catheter inserted. An inflatable prosthesis necessitates placement of the reservoir in the paravesical space, medial to the epigastric vessels. The pump is placed in a subdartos scrotal pouch on the right for the right-handed patient or on the left for left-handed patients. Pump, reservoir, and penile cylinders are connected by tubing, which has been cut at an appropriate length and placed in such a way that it neither kinks nor is under tension. Before closure, the operative field is irrigated with copious amounts of antibiotic solution. Systemic antibiotics should be used. Figures 26–12 and 26–13 show examples of complicated implantations of inflatable penile prostheses.

Closure

Closure is done using absorbable suture material in several layers.

Postoperative Care

Postoperative care is relatively simple. Patients may have the urethral catheter removed on the first postoperative day. Ice should be applied to the groin to prevent excessive swelling. Parenteral antibiotics should be administered for at least 24 hours, and patients should be discharged on a regimen of oral antibiotics for at least 7 days. Inflatable prostheses should not be activated or used for at least a month. The patients should be instructed to watch for any signs of local infection.

Potential Surgical Complications

The risk of infection is the primary potential complication. If the prosthesis becomes infected, it must be removed and antibiotics administered. Late complications include severe pain from an inappropriately sized prosthesis, skin or urethral erosion, urinary retention, skin necrosis from increased local pressure, and me-

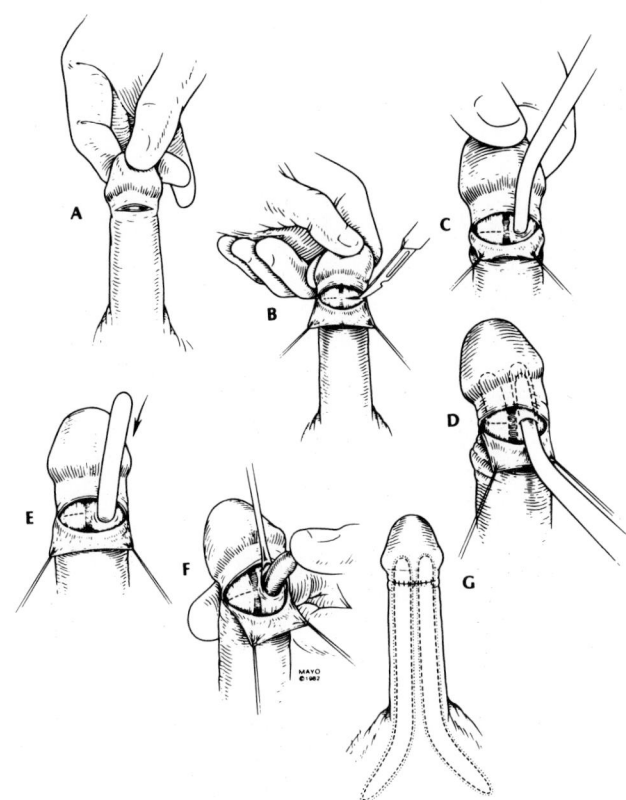

FIGURE 26–10. Subcoronal incision for the insertion of a semirigid penile prosthesis. (From Glenn, J. T. [Ed.]. [1983]. *Urologic surgery* [p. 841]. Philadelphia: J. B. Lippincott.)

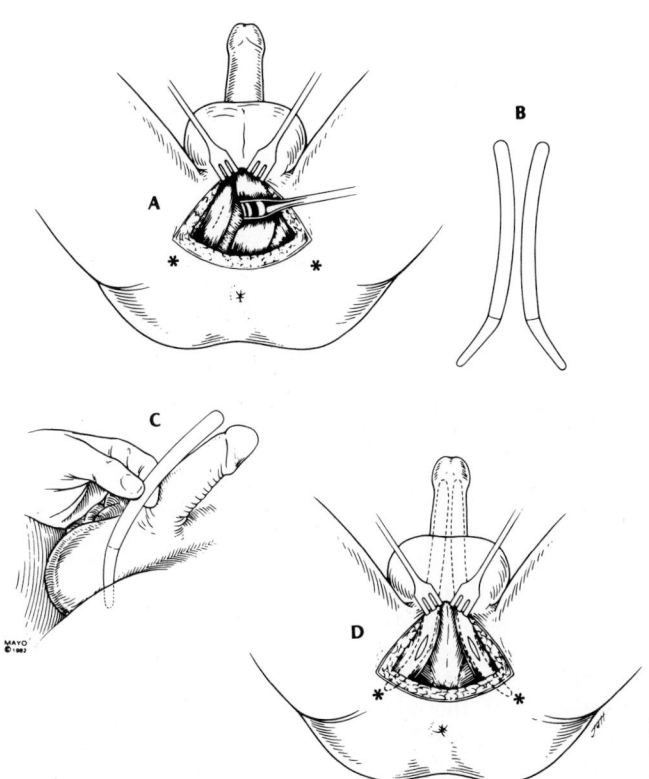

FIGURE 26–11. Perineal incision for the insertion of a penile prosthesis. (From Glenn, J. T. [Ed.]. [1983]. *Urologic surgery* [p. 839]. Philadelphia: J. B. Lippincott.)

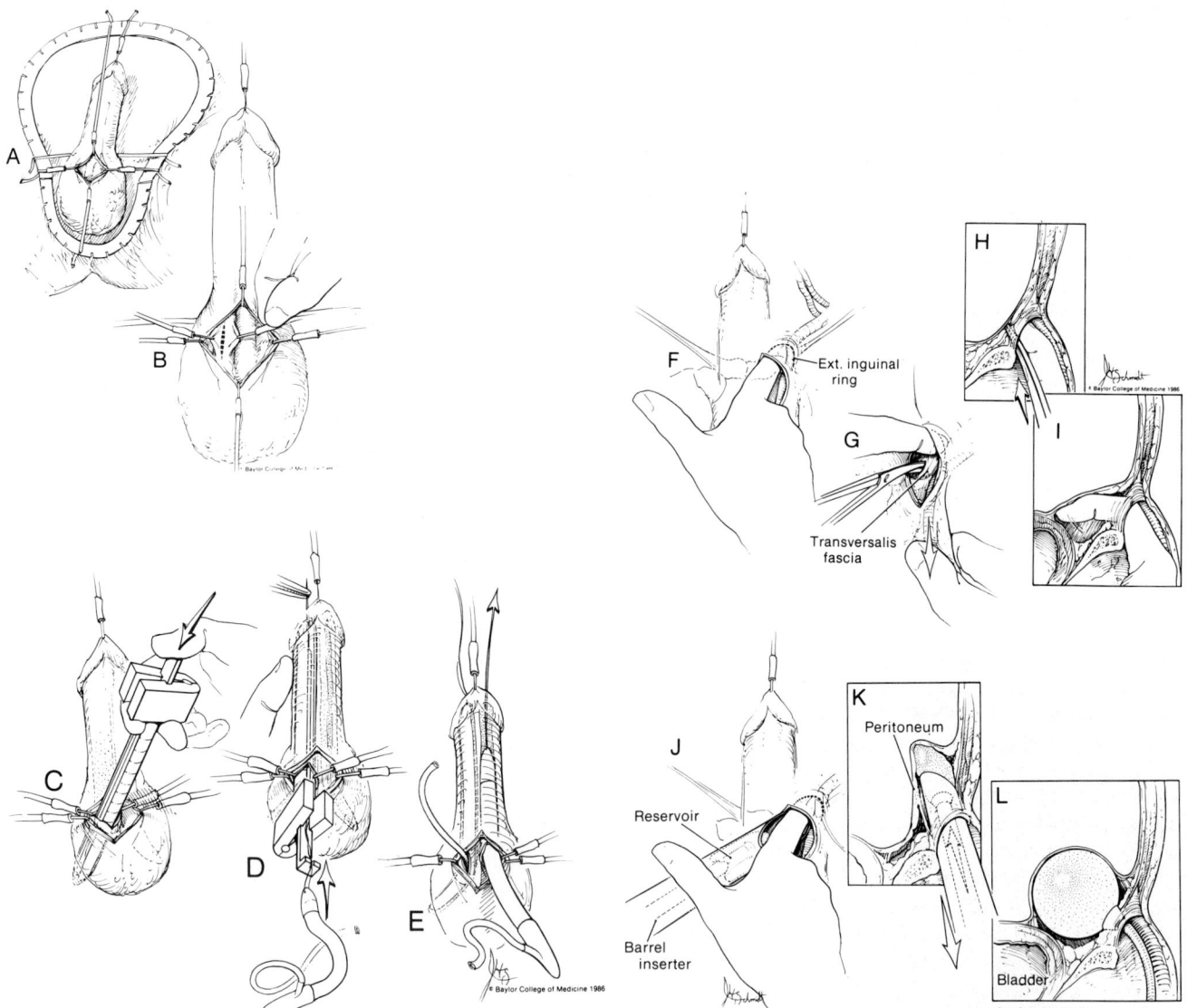

FIGURE 26–12. *A*, Penoscrotal incision. *B*, A 2-cm longitudinal corporeal incision. *C*, The proximal corpora is dilated and measured with a Dilamezinsert. *D*, The distal corpora is dilated and measured with a Dilamezinsert, and a needle threaded with a cylinder is advanced through the corpora. *E*, The properly sized cylinder is pulled into the appropriate position inside the corpora. *F* to *I*, Implantation of the reservoir into a paravesical space is accomplished by first palpating the external inguinal ring and bluntly perforating the transversalis fascia. The Metzenbaum scissors is positioned perpendicular to the transversalis fascia and is used only to initiate the dissection with a spreading action. *J*, The lip of the barrel reservoir inserter is advanced under digital guidance through the defect created in the transversalis fascia. *K*, The obturator of the barrel inserter with the attached reservoir is advanced into the paravesical space. *L*, The inflated reservoir is in the paravesical space.

chanical failure in the case of an inflatable prosthesis. Over time, a fairly high incidence of mechanical failure has been noted with these devices. Most problems are due to cylinder leak, tubing kinks, and aneurysmal dilation of the corpora. Erosion of the reservoir into the bladder and large bowel has also been reported. Because of such complications, there should be extended and careful follow-up for patients with penile prostheses.

CIRCUMCISION

Definition

Circumcision is the surgical removal of the foreskin, or prepuce.

Indications

The practice of circumcision goes back to antiquity. It can be a religious rite for newborn babies and young boys but is not a surgical necessity, except in certain rare specific instances when the foreskin cannot be retracted easily (phimosis), when the foreskin cannot be brought back over the glans (paraphimosis), or when infection develops posthitis or balanoposthitis. Circumcision of the newborn has been the focus of controversy. It is one of the most commonly performed surgical procedures in the United States, despite the American Academy of Pediatrics statement that "there is no absolute medical indication for routine circumcision of the newborn" (Thompson et al., 1975). Circumcision in the adult is performed for phimosis, paraphimosis, and balanitis.

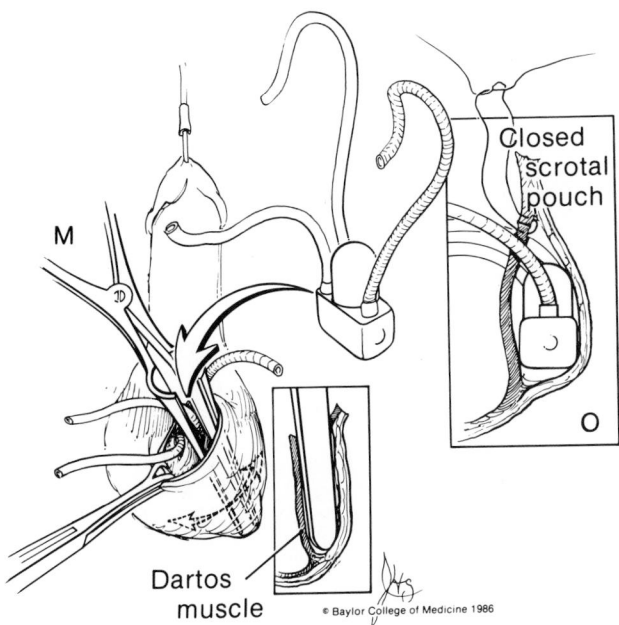

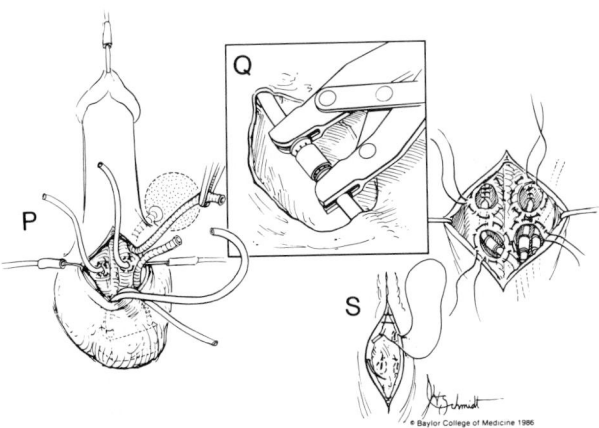

FIGURE 26–12 *Continued M* and *N*, An extended nasal speculum is used to create a subcutaneous predartos pouch for the pump. *O*, The pump tubing is tracked through the dartos muscle, and the opening of the scrotal pump pouch is closed with a pursestring suture of 3–0 plain catgut. *P* and *Q*, The tubes from the various components are aligned, and connections are accomplished using Quick-Connect–type connectors. *R* and *S*, The incision is closed in multiple layers. (From Fishman, I. J. [1987]. Complicated implantations of inflatable penile prostheses. *Urologic Clinics of North America, 14*, 217–239.)

Perioperative Nursing Implications

Anesthesia

In most patients, circumcision is performed under local anesthesia.

Position

Patients are placed in the supine position. Infants may be placed on a restraining device, which keeps the legs and arms from moving into the operative field.

Creation and Maintenance of the Sterile Field

In adult and infants, the penis is prepared with a povidone-iodine solution. No preoperative shave is performed. The penis is draped into the sterile field.

Because most circumcisions are performed under local anesthesia, care should be taken not to cover the face of the awake patient during the creation of the sterile field. The scrub nurse should have the local anesthesia ready for injection by the surgeon when she or he asks for it to avoid anxiety on the patient's part while waiting for the anticipated injection. No special supplies are required.

Equipment and Supplies

Patient drapes
1 electrosurgical pencil
1 suction tubing

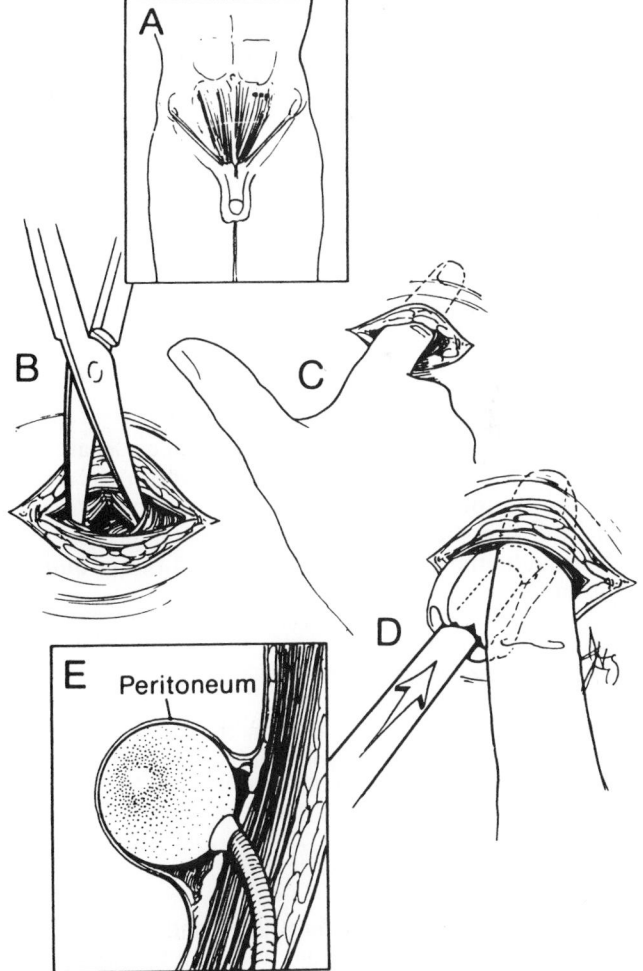

FIGURE 26–13. *A*, Transverse paramedian lower abdominal incision. *B*, The rectus muscle fibers are split. *C*, The preperitoneal, submuscular space is developed. *D*, The reservoir is advanced into this space. *E*, The reservoir is inflated, creating its own space. (From Fishman I. J. [1987]. Complicated implantations of inflatable penile prostheses. *Urologic Clinics of North America, 14*, 217–239.)

1 package of Raytek (4 × 8 inch) sponges
1 No. 15 blade
1 local syringe
1 basin set
1 plastic tray or minor dissecting set
1 No. 25, ⅝-inch needle
1 package of 3–0 or 5–0 chromic catgut ties
5–0 chromic catgut swedge
Petrolatum (Vaseline) gauze
Marking pen

Drugs and Solutions

Sterile saline for irrigation
Neomycin and polymixin B (Neosporin GU irrigant)
Local anesthetic (according to the surgeon's request)

Physiological Monitoring

Physiological monitoring of the patient includes all of the guidelines for the care of patients receiving local anesthesia if an anesthesiologist is not part of the procedure. During circumcision, sponges may be weighed or blood loss may be estimated. Urinary catheterization is not routinely performed.

Specimens and Cultures

Cultures are not usually required, and the surgical specimen is the foreskin, or prepuce. This specimen should be processed according to hospital policy.

Procedure

The procedure can be performed under local, regional, or general anesthesia. Most newborn circumcisions are performed by the obstetrician or pediatrician using a device such as the Plasti bell or Gomco clamp. In the adult, the procedure is performed on an outpatient basis.

Incision and Exposure

Two incisions are made: one on the outer skin, and one approximately 3 mm from the corona of the glans (Fig. 26–14).

Details

Small vessels are electrocoagulated and ligated. The subcutaneous tissue is then removed with the scissors.

Closure

Both skin edges are reapproximated using either running or interrupted 5–0 chromic catgut. A light dressing may be applied.

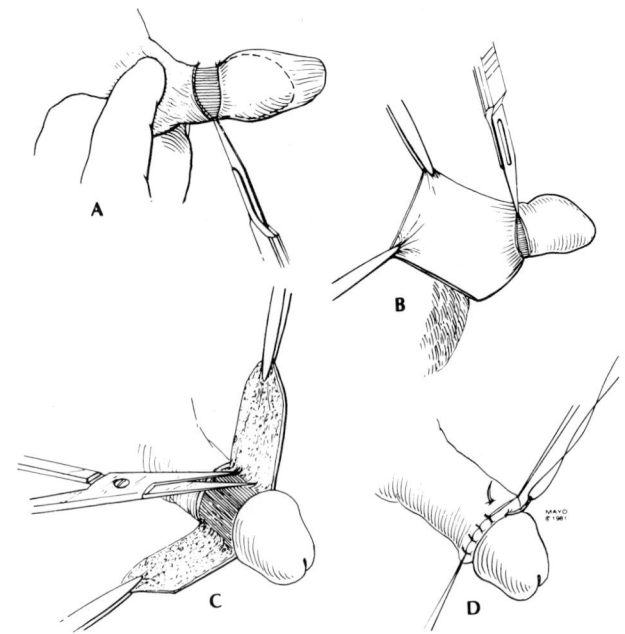

FIGURE 26–14. Sleeve resection technique of circumcision. *A,* The coronal junction on the skin is outlined and incised circumferentially following the V of the frenulum on the ventral surface. *B,* The foreskin is retracted, the adhesions are thoroughly broken, and a circumferential incision is made in the mucosal skin just proximal to the coronal sulcus. *C,* The sleeve of the skin between the two incisions is excised. *D,* The skin edges are reapproximated, giving a good cosmetic result. (From Glenn, J. T. [Ed.]. [1983]. *Urologic surgery* [p. 801]. Philadelphia: J. B. Lippincott.)

Postoperative Care

The suture line may be covered with petrolatum gauze to prevent adherence to underwear or bedclothes. Patients should be instructed not to rub or wash the penis vigorously for at least a week.

Potential Surgical Complications

Immediate complications of circumcision include hemorrhage, removal of insufficient or excessive foreskin, infection, urinary retention (from too tight a bandage), and meatitis. Long-term complications include meatal stenosis, skin breakdown, and urethrocutaneous fistula.

SURGERY OF THE TESTICLE

Orchiectomy

Definition

Orchiectomy, or orchidectomy, is the term used to refer to the surgical removal of testicles.

Indications

There are several reasons to remove testicles. In the pediatric population, testicles may be removed if, at the time of surgery, they are found to be atrophic or nonviable (e.g., as a consequence of prolonged ischemia from torsion). A testis may also be removed if it harbors a tumor with a malignant potential. This is mostly the case in the young adult population in which the incidence of testicular cancer is highest. In the older patient population, testicles may be removed either because of tumor or as part of the treatment of prostatic cancer. Growth of adenocarcinoma of the prostate has been found to be hormonally dependent. By removing the testes, the source of male hormones, one can palliate the progression of advanced prostate cancer.

Orchiectomy can be either unilateral or bilateral and either simple or radical. Bilateral orchiectomy is reserved for patients with prostate cancer who require endocrine control of their malignancy. Indications for unilateral orchiectomy are testicular maldevelopment when the testis is not believed to be worth salvage, testicular trauma when the testicle is thought to be nonviable because of the extent of the damage, prolonged testicular torsion with irreversible ischemic changes, severe infection with the presence of testicular abscess, and testicular malignancy. In radical orchiectomy for testicular malignancy, the cord and surrounding fat are removed as far up as the internal ring. This necessitates an inguinal approach. The incision is the same as for inguinal herniorrhaphy. Simple orchiectomy refers to the removal of the testis, the cord structures being divided at any level. The epididymis is usually removed with the testis. Simple orchiectomy can be performed through either an inguinal or a scrotal approach.

Vasectomy

Definition

Vasectomy is a surgical form of contraception. Ligation and division of the vas deferens is performed through a small incision in the upper scrotum. The procedure can be done under local or general anesthesia and does not necessitate admission to the hospital.

Indications

Any male patient wishing to be provided with a reliable method of birth control is a candidate for vasectomy.

Hydrocelectomy

Definition

Hydroceles are collections of fluid around the testicle. The fluid is usually contained between the tunica albu-

ginea and the tunica vaginalis (Fig. 26–15). There are two categories of hydroceles: congenital and acquired. *Congenital* hydroceles are seen in the male pediatric population. A persistent communication between the peritoneum and the scrotum allows fluid to accumulate around the testis (Fig. 26–16). In most male babies, this communication closes by age 2 years, but in 1 to 4% it persists, usually in association with an inguinal hernia. In the adult, *acquired* hydrocele frequently develops because of a local inflammatory process such as infection of the testis or epididymis. Tumor and trauma are also known to cause the development of a hydrocele. A *spermatocele* is a similar accumulation of fluid located not around the testis but above the testis (Fig. 26–17).

Indications

Surgery is different for congenital hydrocele than for acquired hydrocele. The purpose of hydrocele surgery in the pediatric population is to alleviate the communication between the peritoneum and the scrotum and to fix the inguinal hernia. In the adult population, surgery is elective and its goal is to remove the pocket of accumulated fluid. The approaches are therefore quite different and are described separately. Indications for surgery in the adult include pain secondary to the size of the hydrocele, unacceptable scrotal appearance, and the patient's request for removal of the hydrocele.

In the child, a history of waxing and waning scrotal swelling localized to one or both sides is typical. The swelling is usually asymptomatic, but some redness of the scrotal skin may appear. The swelling may become considerable and alarming to the parents. The adult patient has a persistent, nonpainful swelling around the testis, which may become quite cumbersome because of its size. A history of trauma or of epididymitis may be elicited.

On physical examination, the testis itself may be hard to palpate because of the surrounding fluid. If a light is placed against the testis, it transilluminates. In the child, the cord is thickened, a feature referred to as the silk glove sign.

Related Surgical Procedures

Similar and related procedures include orchiopexy (testicular fixation), testicular biopsy, and insertion of testicular prosthesis. Orchiopexy is performed through an inguinal incision in cases of maldescent or through a scrotal incision for cases of torsion. Testicular torsion is a urological emergency, and surgery should be performed for suspected testicular torsion with minimal delay. Fixation of the testis can be done by either placing the testicle in a dartos pouch made under the scrotal skin in cases of maldescent or by fixing the testes in

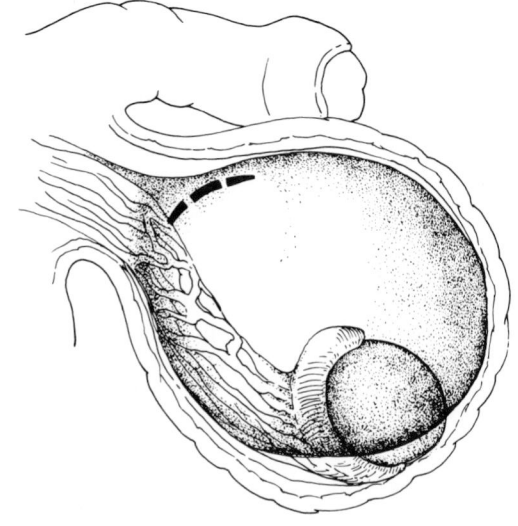

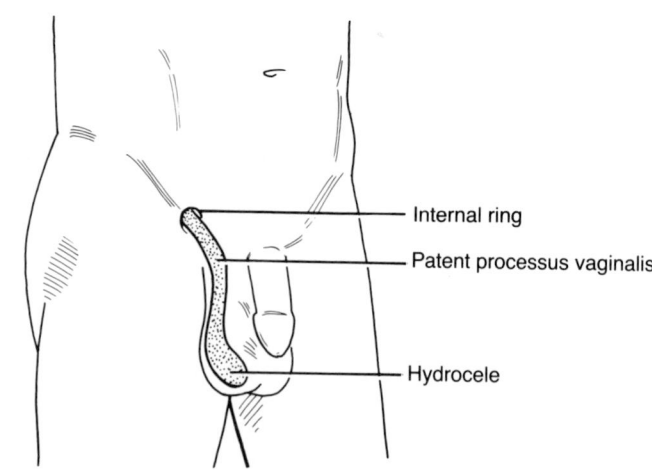

FIGURE 26–16. Communicating hydrocele.

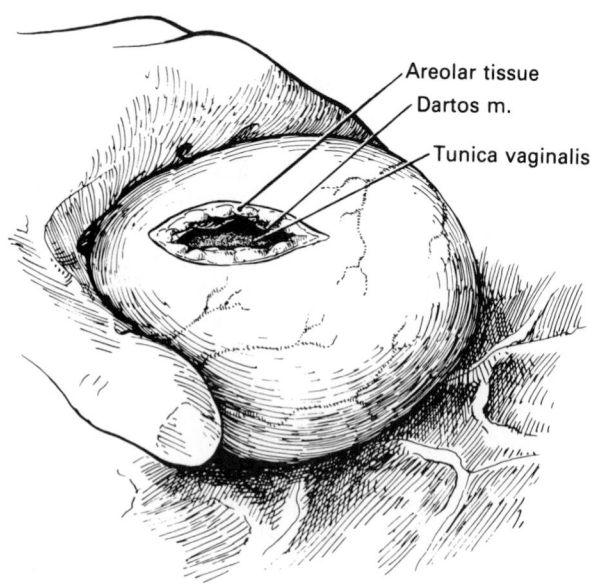

FIGURE 26–15. Hydrocele. (From McDougal, W. S. [Ed.]. 1986. *Operative surgery: Urology* [4th ed.] [p. 677]. Stoneham, MA: Butterworth.)

Perioperative Nursing Implications

Anesthesia

Surgery of the testicle and scrotum may be performed under local, regional, or general anesthesia. Routine nursing care of these patients is practiced. Blood loss is usually insignificant. Most patients are extremely apprehensive before surgery. Helping to reassure and comfort the patient before and during the anesthesia may be necessary.

Position

Patients are placed in the supine position. No special positioning equipment is required. If the patient is awake, make sure that he is in a comfortable position before draping.

place using three or four tacking stitches in the scrotal cavity. Indications for testicular biopsy include evaluation for male infertility.

A testicular prosthesis may be placed in the scrotum when the testis is congenitally absent or has been surgically removed. It is standard practice to place the prosthesis some time after the initial surgery (usually after a 3-month wait). Principles of prosthetic surgery should be applied. Meticulous care is paramount in preventing infection. Perioperative antibiotics should be administered and copious antibiotic irrigation of the surgical field should be done. Testicular prostheses are placed through an inguinal incision (see discussion of the procedure for orchiectomy below).

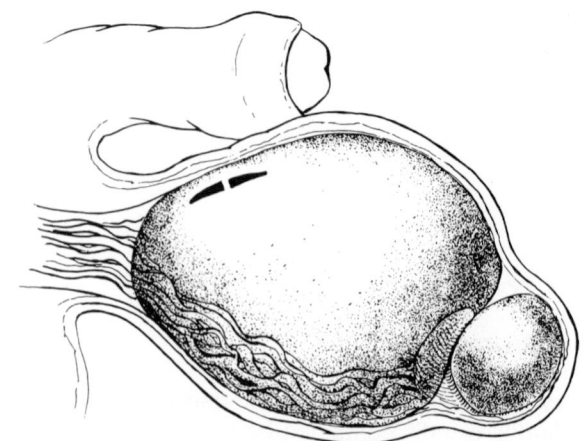

FIGURE 26–17. Spermatocele. (From McDougal, W. S. [Ed.]. 1986. *Operative surgery: Urology* [p. 681]. Stoneham, MA: Butterworth.)

Creation and Maintenance of the Sterile Field

During patient preparation, the patient's abdomen from the umbilicus to the upper thigh, including the scrotal area, is shaved on the side of the procedure. If the procedure is bilateral, both sides are shaved. The same area is then painted with a povidone-iodine solution. The circulating nurse may be required to assist in the preparation so that the entire scrotal area can be covered. If the patient is awake, a drape should be placed as a barrier to prevent him from watching the shave, preparation, and/or surgery. Drip towels should be placed by the circulator in areas where the preparation solution could pool. They should be removed after the preparation and before the draping of the patient. In creating the sterile field, the penis is usually not included in the operative field.

Equipment and Supplies

The scrub nurse must be prepared for an inguinal or scrotal approach. In addition, to the soft tissue dissection set, a Weitlaner self-retaining retractor should be available. During the procedure, the spermatic cord is isolated and secured by sliding a Penrose drain around it. The small Penrose drain may also be used at the end of the procedure for drainage of the wound.

The circulating nurse should gather the following supplies and equipment for the procedure:

Patient drape packs
1 basin set
1 suction tubing
1 electrocautery pencil
1 needle counter
1 skin marker
1 pair of light handles or light gloves
1 package of pushers (Kittner)
2 No. 10 blades
1 No. 15 blade
1 No. 11 blade
1 small Penrose drain
1 package of Raytek 4 × 8 inch sponges
1 package of large laparotomy sponges
1 package of E-tape sponges
1 minor dissection set
Self-retaining (Weitlaner) retractor
3–0 chromic swedge
4–0 chromic swedge
3–0 chromic ties
3–0 silk ties
0 chromic ties
3–0 Vicryl swedge
0 chromic swedge
1 scrotal support (have small, medium, and large available)
2 Kling wraps—for possible pressure dressing
Elastic bandage (Elastoplast)—for possible pressure dressing
1 package of fluff dressings
1 ice bag—to be filled before the patient goes to the postanesthesia care unit
Local syringe and needle—if necessary
Sterile testicular prosthesis—two of each size (youth, adult average, and adult large, if indicated)

Drugs and Solutions

The circulating nurse should also have sterile saline for irrigation, neomycin and polymixin B (Neosporin GU irrigant), and a local anesthetic (if necessary) available. He or she also needs to fill the ice bag for use during transport of the patient to the postanesthesia care unit.

Physiological Monitoring

With pediatric patients, all sponges are weighed. In addition, the circulating nurse records blood loss and irrigation. The bladder is not usually emptied during these procedures.

Specimens and Cultures

Cultures are not routinely performed during these procedures, unless an infection is present or suspected. The specimens in each procedure are:

Simple orchiectomy: testicle, epididymis, and spermatic cord
Radical orchiectomy: testicle, epididymis, spermatic cord, and surrounding fat
Bilateral orchiectomy: both testicles
Testicular biopsy: biopsy specimen of the testicle
Hydrocelectomy: redundant sac from the hydrocele
Vasectomy: segment of vas deferens

Physician's Orders, Laboratory and Diagnostic Studies

With ultrasonography, a precise diagnosis can be obtained. Routine preoperative laboratory studies are obtained.

Procedure

Procedure for Orchiectomy

Orchiectomy may be performed under general, spinal, or local anesthesia, and most patients are admitted for same-day surgery. No preoperative preparation or antibiotics are necessary. Diagnostic studies are limited to routine studies, except that serum markers are obtained if testicular cancer is present. These include alpha-fetoprotein and chorionic gonadotropin–beta subunit.

These markers are elevated in certain specific types of germ cell tumors of the testis and have an important role in monitoring the management of these patients.

Inguinal Approach

Incision and Exposure

Both inguinal and scrotal approaches are described. The inguinal approach is performed by making an incision parallel to the inguinal ligament, two fingerbreadths above and extending just above the pubic tubercle to the midinguinal point. The incision is brought down through subcutaneous tissue and fat to the fascia of the external oblique muscle. The fatty covering of the fascia is cleared away to expose the external inguinal ring. The fascia is then opened from the external ring up to the internal ring. The spermatic cord is then exposed lying in the inguinal canal. It is then dissected carefully and freed up. Care is paid to two small sensory nerves that course in close proximity to the cord, the iliohypogastric and ilioinguinal nerves.

Details

The testicle can then be brought into the field by traction. The lower pole of the testicle is attached to the scrotum by remnants of the gubernaculum. These are tied and divided using absorbable sutures (3–0 Vicryl). The cord can then be clamped, ligated, and divided using absorbable sutures (1–0 chromic catgut) at the level of the internal ring, and the testis is removed.

Closure

After inspection for hemostasis, the fascia of the external oblique is closed using absorbable suture material (4–0 and 3–0 chromic catgut). Care should be given to inspection of the scrotal cavity where hematomas may form. If an incipient hematoma is noted, drainage of the scrotum may be accomplished with a small Penrose drain. The skin should be closed with an absorbable suture (4–0 chromic catgut), using a subcuticular stitch for cosmetic purposes.

Scrotal Approach

Incision and Exposure

Simple orchiectomy may be performed through a scrotal incision. The skin of the scrotum is put under stretch and a longitudinal incision is made through the layer of the scrotum. The last layer is the tunica vaginalis. After this layer is opened, the glistening white covering of the testis is observed and a small amount of fluid can be found.

Details

The cord structures are identified above the upper pole of the testis. Clamping, ligation, and division of the cord is done.

Closure

The scrotum is closed in two layers using absorbable suture after careful inspection for hemostasis. Again, drainage of the scrotum can be accomplished by the use of a small Penrose drain. The skin is closed with a chromic catgut (4–0) using an interrupted stitch.

Procedure for Vasectomy

Incision and Exposure

The procedure is usually carried out under local anesthesia (1 or 2% lidocaine). An incision is made either on each side of the scrotum or along the median raphe. The vas deferens must be palpated before the incision is made, separated from the surrounding tissue, and then firmly held in place.

Details

After the skin incision is made, the vas is dissected free over 1 to 2 cm and then divided. A 1-cm segment is removed, and both ends are occluded using small metal clips. Needlepoint cautery can be used to fulgurate the vasal lumen in order to prevent recanalization. Closure is carried out in two layers. The skin can be closed using a subcutaneous stitch.

Postoperative Care

A compression dressing is placed around the scrotum, and the patient should be instructed to wear a scrotal support for 7 to 10 days. Ice should be applied to the groin area for 24 to 36 hours.

The patient must be told that he should consider himself fertile until the result of a semen analysis is obtained 6 to 8 weeks after surgery. Other forms of contraception must be used until then. The procedure is reversible, but fertility can be expected in only 30 to 40% of cases by reanastomosis of the vas (vasovasostomy).

Procedure for Hydrocelectomy

Surgery is usually done on an outpatient basis.

Incision and Exposure

Pediatric hydrocele is treated similarly to pediatric hernias. Preparation and incision are made over the inguinal area. Dissection is aimed at mobilizing the cord and the hydrocele. The principles of pediatric hydrocelectomy are to interrupt the communication between the peritoneum and the scrotum by ligating and dividing the processus vaginalis.

Several techniques are used to treat adult hydrocele surgically. A transverse midscrotal incision is used (Fig. 26–18).

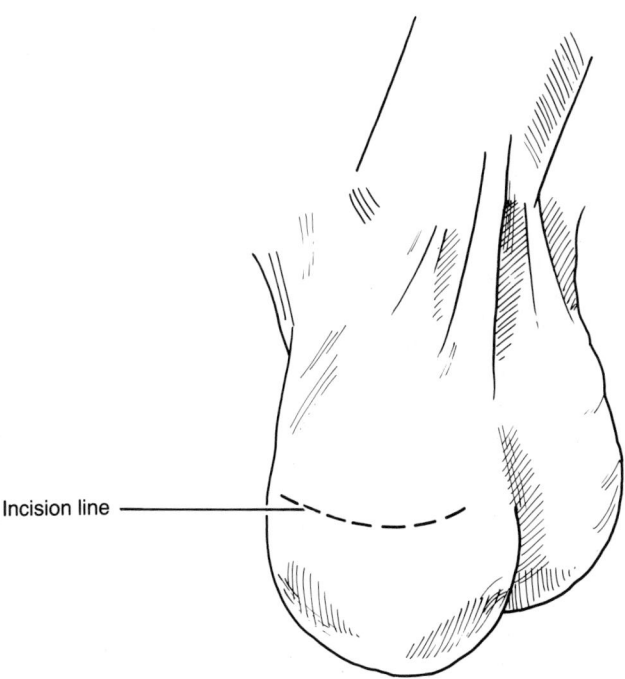

Incision line

FIGURE 26–18. Transverse midscrotal incision.

Details

The testicle and hydrocele can be delivered into the field. The hydrocele can then be opened, and the redundant sac may be removed, leaving a 5- to 10-mm rim of tissue. Hemostasis is carried out, and the edge of sac is oversewn with 4–0 absorbable suture in a continuous locked fashion. The cut edges of the hydrocele sac can also be brought in back of the testis and oversewn to each other. Other techniques have been developed to allow drainage of the fluid. These include "window" procedures and reposition of the hydrocele sac around the testis.

Closure

Closure of the scrotal incision is done in two layers using absorbable catgut (4–0, 5–0). The deep layer is closed with a running stitch, and the skin layer should be closed in interrupted fashion. Placement of a Penrose drain is recommended for cases in which hematoma may develop. Wound infection and scrotal abscess occur rarely. Hydroceles may recur and reoperation may be indicated. Hydrocele recurrence is due to inadequate dissection of the hydrocele sac, allowing reaccumulation of fluid within it.

Postoperative Care

Postoperative care for surgery of the testicle should include the application of an ice pack to the scrotum for at least 12 hours to minimize swelling and pain. The patient should be instructed to wear an athletic support and limit activities. Patients are sent home with a prescription for pain medication (a mild narcotic such as codeine) and are seen 1 week after surgery.

Potential Surgical Complications

Surgical complications include hematomas and infection. These complications can be prevented by achieving proper hemostasis and by observing careful sterile techniques. Long-term complications occur rarely. A small number of patients describe chronic local pain that may be due to nerve injury to the ilioinguinal or iliohypogastric nerves.

HYPOSPADIAS REPAIR

Definition

Hypospadias is a congenital anomaly of the penis in which the opening of the urethra is found on the ventral surface of the penis. This abnormality is believed to result from incomplete embryological development of the distal urethra. Hypospadias is found in 1 of 300 live male births, which corresponds to approximately 6200 new cases a year. The cause of hypospadias is unknown (Fig. 26–19). Ventral curvature of the penis is frequently found in patients with hypospadias and is due to fibrous tissue bands. It is called *chordee*. Undescended testis and inguinal hernias may be found in association with hypospadias.

Epispadias is a congenital abnormality of the penis in which the meatus is located on the dorsum of the penis. This condition is rare. Some patients with more severe forms of hypospadias may have ambiguous genitalia and require further evaluation to rule out an intersex condition. Anatomically, the penis of the patient with hypospadias demonstrates an anomalous meatus; dorsal hooded foreskin, which is deficient on the ventral aspect of the penis; and frequently some degree of curvature.

The patient has usually been diagnosed at birth. Associated abnormalities (undescended testicle and inguinal hernia) should be noted. Parents provide additional information regarding the child's health and immunization status. A significant amount of parental anxiety is usually readily apparent, and the nursing staff plays a major role in alleviating both parental and infant anxiety.

Indications

The main goal of hypospadias repair is to reconstruct a straight penis with a meatus placed as close as possible to the tip of the glans, allowing for straight voiding and good cosmesis. There are five major maneuvers involved in this surgical repair:

1. Meatoplasty and glansplasty, which are repositioning of the meatus and fashioning of the glans

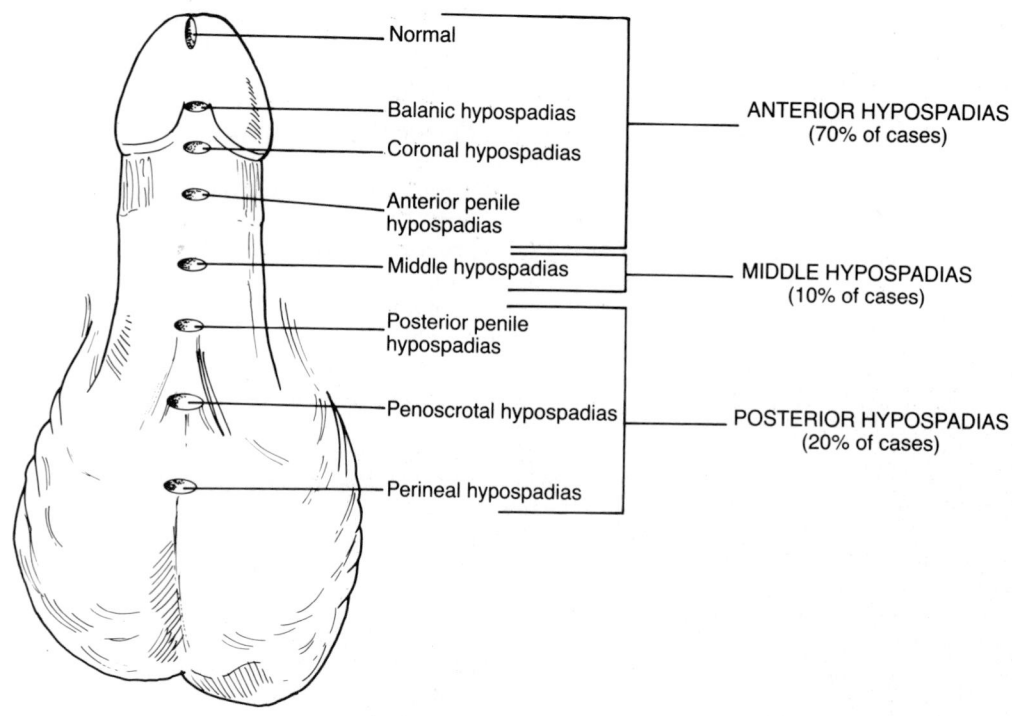

FIGURE 26–19. Classification of hypospadias.

2. Removal of the ventral curvature (chordee) or orthoplasty
3. Urethroplasty (reconstruction of the urethra), if needed, when a deficiency in urethral length coexists
4. Cosmetic skin rearrangement over the shaft of the penis
5. Scrotoplasty (reconstruction of the scrotum), as needed

Correction of hypospadias necessitates significant surgical skills and should be performed by surgeons experienced in the various techniques. Determining the type of technique to use depends on the location and the degree of chordee. The current trend is to perform hypospadias surgery in one stage and at a young age (between ages 6 months and 2 years). Because of improvements in anesthesia technique, the procedure can be performed on an outpatient basis.

Indications for surgery, therefore, are any anomaly in the position of the urethral meatus in a baby boy who has been diagnosed as having hypospadias.

Related Surgical Procedures

Related surgical procedures are circumcision and meatoplasty. The latter procedure involves creating a larger urethral opening.

Perioperative Nursing Implications

Anesthesia

Hypospadias repair is usually performed under general anesthesia. Children may be anxious when coming to the operating room (OR). Care must be taken to make the child as comfortable as possible and to allay his anxiety.

Position

The patient is placed in the supine position with the legs in a frog-leg position. The legs should be padded so that they are supported in this position rather than suspended over the OR bed. Careful application of the safety strap above the operative area is necessary. The OR should be warmed before the child is brought in. A warming blanket may also be necessary to prevent intraoperative heat loss from the child's body.

Creation and Maintenance of the Sterile Field

The skin is prepared with a povidone-iodine solution from umbilicus to midthigh to include the entire genitalia. Drip towels should be placed where pooling of the preparation solution can occur. These should be removed after the preparation and before the draping of the patient. During the preparation, the foreskin should be fully retracted and all smegma removed. The circulating nurse must make sure that the electrosurgical grounding pad is placed and positioned appropriately for the size and muscle mass of the child. The lower back, buttocks, and thigh are preferred areas for placement.

A sterile field is created around the genital area of the child. The scrub nurse must remember that the patient's legs will be spread apart and bent in a frog-leg position. Care must be taken to prevent the surgical team from leaning on the bent legs or chest when they are covered by the sterile drape.

The draped Mayo stand can be placed over the feet of the patient, providing a convenient work surface for the scrub nurse. The scrub nurse should have a sterile catheter and collection device available for emptying of the bladder during the procedure. He or she must also prepare injectable solutions, such as the saline used for artificial erection. Care must be taken while handling the smaller suture used for hypospadias repair. Use of a magnetic pad below the operative area, between the scrub nurse and the surgeon, is helpful in catching stray needles.

Equipment and Supplies

Equipment and supplies for the hypospadias repair are gathered in advance by the circulating nurse and vary according to the type of procedure to be performed.

Basic supplies include

Patient drape
Thyroid sheet (fenestrated drape)
Adhesive towel drapes
Suction tubing
5- and 10-ml syringes
8 Fr. feeding tube (16 inch)
Basin set
Electrocautery pencil
Bugbée cord and electrode
Needle and blade counter
Light handles or light glove covers
Marking pen
Hypospadias set
4 × 8 or 4 × 4 inch Raytek sponges
Butterfly tubing infusion set
18- and 30-gauge hypodermic needles
Tourniquet or rubber bands
Urethral stent (6 Fr. Silastic tubing)
Suprapubic catheter
Microsurgery instruments as requested by the surgeon (e.g., Castroviejo needle holders, 0.5 forceps, and fine mosquito clamp).
Bougies à boule
Suture
     5–0 Prolene C–1
     6–0 chromic C–1
     7–0 chromic 1745G
     6–0 PDS TF
     7–0 Vicryl J–566
     6–0 Vicryl F–1
     6–0 polyglycolic acid (Dexon) T–30
     6–0 Prolene C–1
Xeroform gauze
Prosthetic foam dressing
Diaper

Drugs and Solutions

Medications and solutions include lidocaine (Xylocaine) 1% with 1:100,000 epinephrine, sterile saline solution for injection, neomycin and polymixin B (Neosporine GU irrigant), and sterile saline for irrigation.

Physiological Monitoring

Urine is emptied from the bladder after the area has been prepared and draped. The circulating nurse should record this urine output as well as other urine output during the procedure.

Sponge and bottle blood loss is measured carefully because of the ease with which children can deplete circulating blood volume with small amounts of blood loss. Transfusion may be necessary if significant loss of circulating blood volume occurs. The circulating nurse should follow hospital procedures for the identification and matching of blood.

Specimens and Cultures

The urine emptied from the bladder initially is sent for culture. Specimens may include redundant foreskin from the repair. This should be fixed according to hospital policy and sent as a routine specimen.

Physician's Orders, Laboratory and Diagnostic Studies

Perioperative orders will include routine laboratory testing (complete blood count [CBC], electrolyte values, and clotting variables) and no food after midnight on the day before surgery.

Procedure

At the time of surgery, the surgeon performs an artificial erection test by injecting sterile saline into the corpora of the penis, which has had a tourniquet placed at its base to evaluate the degree of penile curvature (chordee).

Meatal Advancement and Glanuloplasty

For patients with minimal chordee and a meatus located anteriorly, surgery is recommended to alleviate urinary stream deflection, abnormal appearing foreskin, and unaesthetic meatus (Fig. 26–20). The procedure is done on an outpatient basis, and no urinary catheter is left in place after the procedure.

Incision and Exposure

The surgeon places a holding stitch of 2–0 Prolene through the glans, performs a circumcision incision below the corona, and frees up the shaft from its overlying skin.

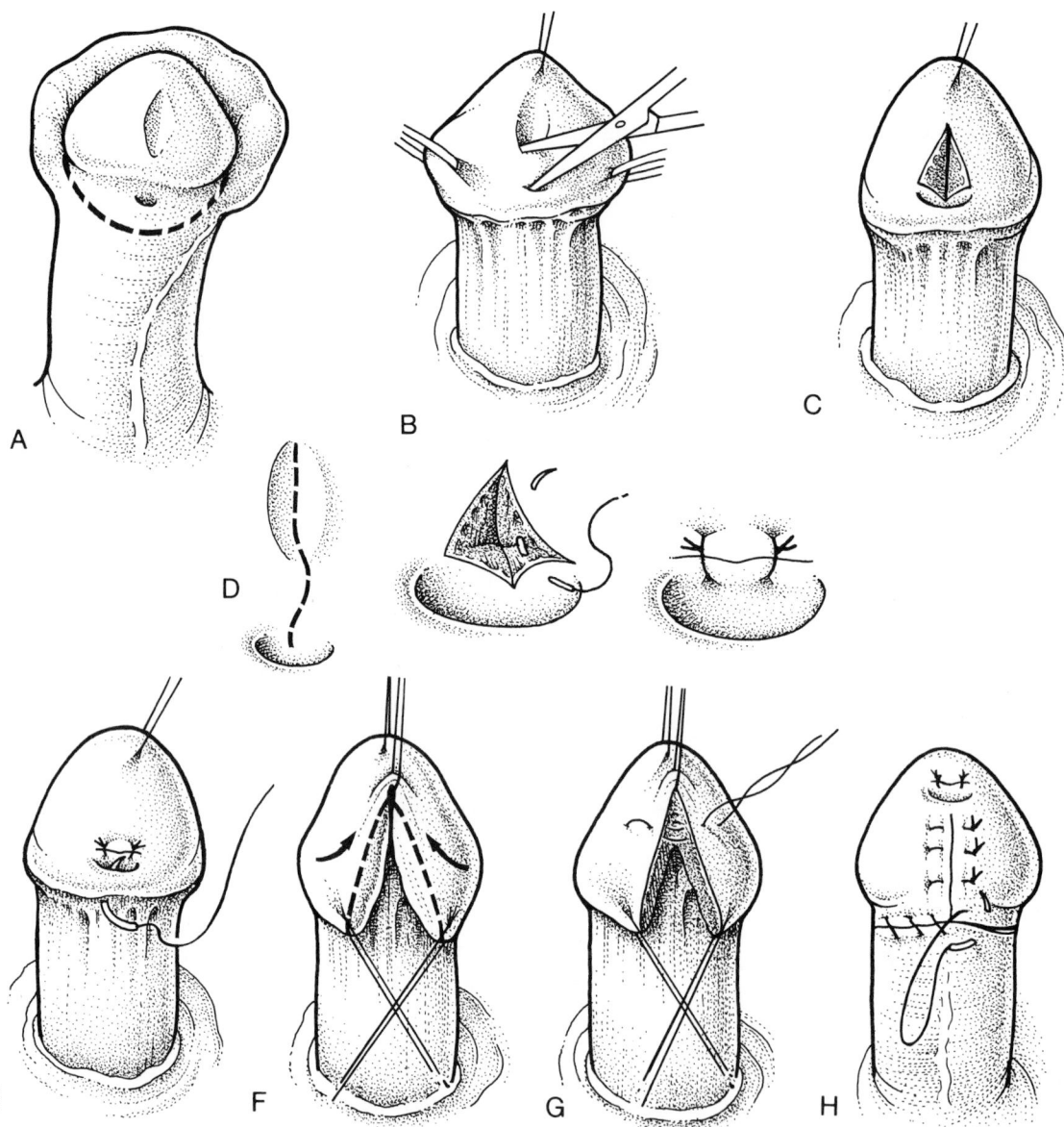

FIGURE 26–20. MAGPI (meatal advancement and glanuloplasty) procedure. *A*, Subcoronal hypospadias. *B* and *C*, A circumferential incision has been made sparing the underlying urethra, and a longitudinal incision in the glanular groove is demonstrated. *D*, The longitudinal glanular groove incision is closed transversely. *E* and *F*, A traction suture in the midline ventral meatus is drawn toward the tip of the glans. *G*, Mattress sutures are placed in the glans to approximate the epithelium. *H*, The penile skin is reapproximated to the coronal margin. (From Blandy, J. P. [1988]. In A. R. Mundy [Ed.], *Current operative surgery: Urology*. Philadelphia: Ballière Tindall.)

Details

A dorsal meatotomy on the ventral aspect of the glans is done and the meatus is advanced to the tip of the penis by placing absorbable 6–0 stitches transversely. The wings of the glans are then brought back in the midline and the glans is reshaped conically (5–0 chromic catgut stitches).

Closure

The redundant foreskin is removed and the penile skin is reapproximated to the coronal margin using 6–0 or 7–0 chromic catgut. A petrolatum gauze dressing is applied.

Perimeatus-based Flap (Mathieu Procedure)

If the meatus is not adequate for a meatal advancement and glanuloplasty procedure because it is too far from the tip of the glans or abnormal and there is minimal chordee, a meatus-based flap is used (Fig. 26–21).

Incision and Exposure

The surgeon makes parallel lines along the glanular groove and then a subcoronal incision.

Details

A skin flap is raised from the skin overlying the urethra and is brought over to be sutured on the edges of the glanular groove (5–0 or 6–0 Vicryl).

Closure

The wings of the glans are brought over to the midline, and the skin is then reapproximated using 5–0 or 6–0 chromic catgut. A small (6–8 Fr.) Silastic catheter is left in place for 7 to 10 days, sewn into place. Either foam dressing or a single layer of mesh nonadherent dressing may be applied and left in place for 3 to 5 days.

Onlay Island Flap

When the meatus is placed too proximally (middle or posterior hypospadias) or if the ventral skin is not suitable for a meatus-based flap, the preputial skin may be used to form the missing wall of the urethra (Fig. 26–22).

Incision and Exposure

The penile shaft is dissected from its skin covering. The skin flap is then taken from the inner surface of the foreskin, having been measured to provide adequate length and width.

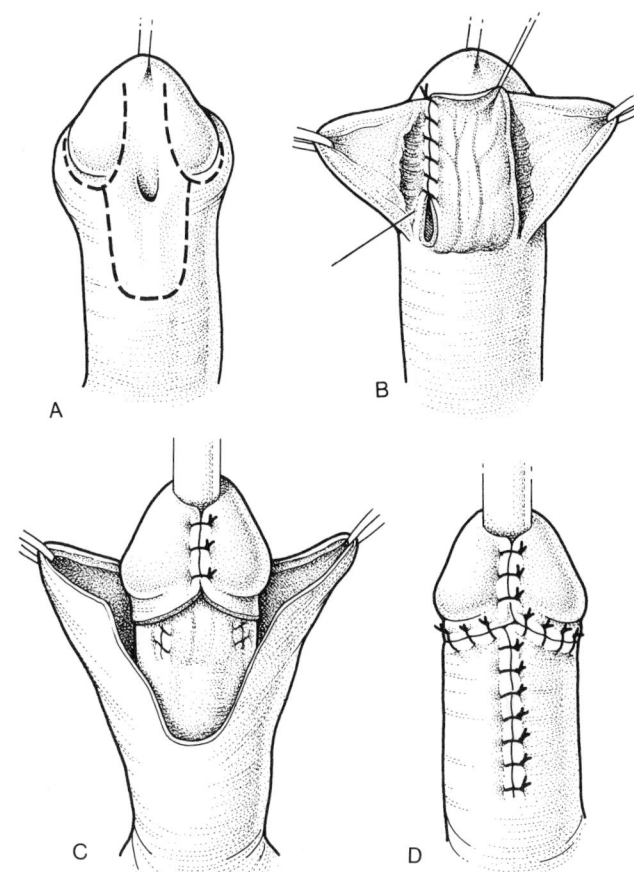

FIGURE 26–21. Mathieu procedure. *A*, The circumferential coronal incision as well as the distal ventral glans strip and perimeatus-based flap is outlined. *B*, The perimeatus-based flap is rotated distally and sutured to the preserved ventral glanular epithelial strip. *C*, The glanular wings are approximated in the midline. *D*, The penile skin is sutured to the coronal margin and drawn together in the midline. (From Blandy, J. P. [1988]. In A. R. Mundy [Ed.], *Current operative surgery: Urology.* Philadelphia: Ballière Tindall.)

Details

Care is taken to preserve the vascular blood supply to the skin flap, which is then transposed to the ventral surface of the penis and sutured onto the urethral plate using 6–0 Vicryl. A 6 Fr. urethral stent is placed for 7 to 10 days to allow for urinary drainage. Alternatively, urinary drainage may be accomplished by using a 10 Fr. suprapubic tube secured and left in place for 10 days.

Closure

The excessive preputial skin is removed, and the skin is reapproximated using 6–0 chromic catgut. A nonadherent mesh dressing or foam dressing is applied.

Tube Grafts

For more extensive reconstruction of the urethra, a tube graft may be fashioned from preputial skin (Fig. 26–23). Free grafts may also be used. Skin from the inner upper arm or lateral margins of the superior edge of the iliac crest is harvested, defatted, and fashioned

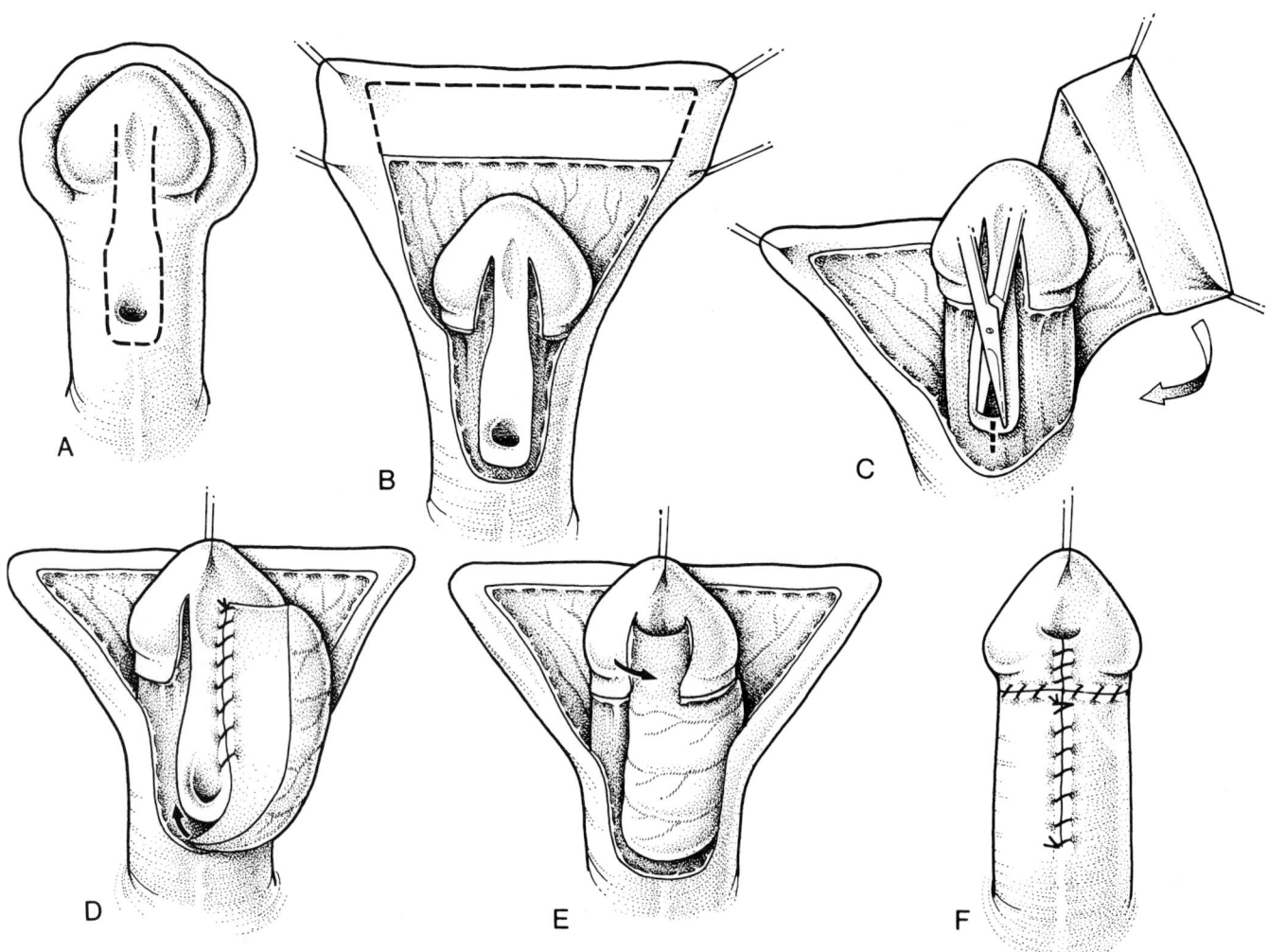

FIGURE 26–22. Island onlay flap. *A*, Spared ventral strip of urethral plate. *B*, Longitudinal strip outlined on the inner aspect of the foreskin. *C*, This strip is being rotated ventrally on its own separate vascular pedicle. *D* and *E*, The foreskin strip is sutured to the ventral strip to form the neourethra. *F*, Penile skin is reapproximated. (From Blandy, J. P. [1988]. In A. R. Mundy [Ed.], *Current operative surgery: Urology.* Philadelphia: Ballière Tindall.)

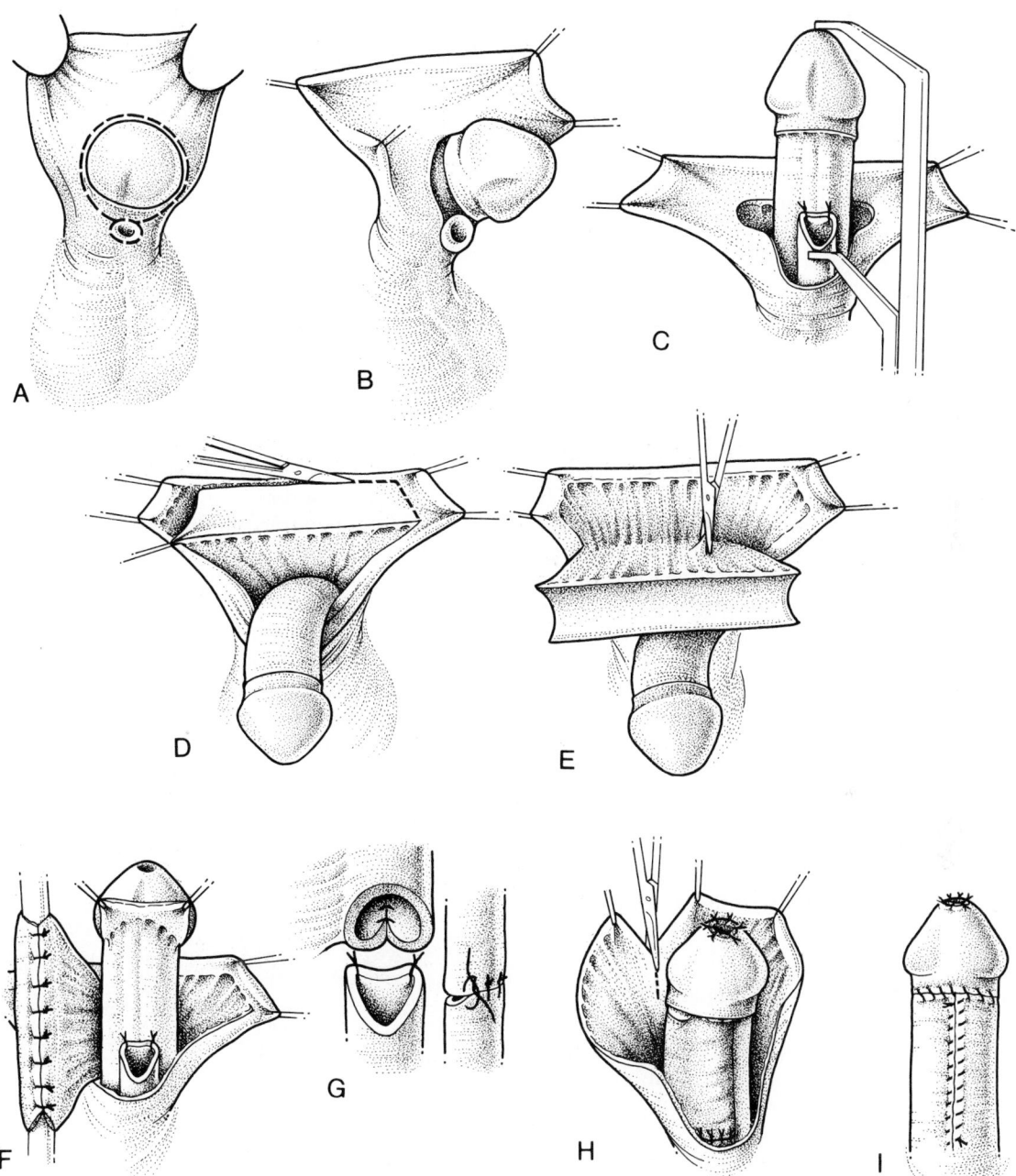

FIGURE 26–23. Transverse preputial island flap. *A*, Incisions are outlined. *B*, Early skin mobilization. *C*, Chordee tissue is excised and the urethra has been spatulated and sutured to the tunica albuginea. Neourethral length is measured. *D*, The inner aspect of the foreskin has a rectangle outline and is incised. *E*, The vascular pedicle to the inner foreskin is separated from the penile skin. *F*, The preputial rectangle is tubularized and brought to the ventrum. The glans channel is made. *G*, The proximal anastomosis is demonstrated. *H*, The neourethra has been brought through the glans channel and sutured to the tip of the glans. The penile skin is incised in the dorsal midline. *I*, The penile skin is approximated to the coronal margin and closed in the midline as well. (From Blandy, J. P. [1988]. In A. R. Mundy [Ed.], *Current operative surgery: Urology*. Philadelphia: Ballière Tindall.)

into a tube using 6–0 Vicryl running suture. They should be non–hair bearing. The bladder mucosa and the buccal mucosa may serve as a substitute for a large deficiency in the urethra.

Postoperative Care

The patient is awakened and returned to the recovery room. After he is sufficiently recovered, he is taken to his parents and is encouraged to drink liberally. He should void at least once before discharge. The dressing usually falls off within 24 hours or should be removed at the time of the first bath.

The parents are instructed in the care of the dressing and of the catheter. The parents should be told to encourage fluid intake to ensure continual flushing of the urinary tract to prevent infection.

Monitoring of urine output is important. Drainage of the catheter into diapers is easy but requires a minimum of hygiene, and parents should clean the meatus and the catheter after bowel movements. For the older patient, the catheter is attached to a ureteral drainage bag. The patients with an indwelling catheter should be sent home on a regimen of oral antibiotic suppression.

Patients who have undergone a meatal advancement and glanuloplasty procedure can be discharged on the same day, and the trend is to send most patients who have a more complex surgical repair home within the first 24 hours after surgery. The patients are seen 7 to 10 days after the procedure for removal of the urethral catheter. Dressings are removed with the child in a warm bath. No medications should be applied to the incision. Gentle cleansing with warm water and hydrogen peroxide can be performed. The child should be monitored for fever, chills, flank pain, and foul-smelling or cloudy urine, which are indicative of a urinary tract infection, and/or an unusual swelling or redness as well as purulence around the incision, indicating a wound infection.

Potential Surgical Complications

Blood loss is usually minimal, but in the young infant, it should be monitored closely, as the penis is a well-vascularized organ and may bleed significantly, leading to anemia and postoperative hematoma. Hematoma formation may seriously compromise a delicate repair. Wound infection is rare and can be prevented with a minimum of hygiene. Long-term complications include urethral strictures and urethrocutaneous fistula, which have been reported in approximately 10 to 15% of cases. These complications necessitate further surgical repair.

SURGERY OF THE KIDNEY

Definition

Surgery of the kidney is performed for infection, stone disease, cancer, and trauma.

Indications

Patients with infections of the kidney exhibit signs and symptoms related to infection. Flank pain, fever, chills, and pyuria may be present. The patient may report the presence of hematuria. Stone disease manifests with flank pain and hematuria; however, in this instance, the flank pain may be different in nature. It usually is severe, intermittent (colicky), and deep seated. Signs and symptoms of infection may coexist with the presence of renal stones. Patients who harbor a renal tumor may be completely asymptomatic, except for painless hematuria (Table 26–4). Patients may have experienced blunt or penetrating injuries, which necessitate a full evaluation, including computed tomographic (CT) scan, intravenous urogram (IVU), and anteriogram to plan therapeutic management.

Surgery of the kidney can be divided into five general categories according to its indication.

1. Simple nephrectomy for nonfunctional renal units resulting from obstructive uropathy, severe infection, injuries to the kidney, and congenitally nonfunctional kidneys
2. Radical nephrectomy for renal cancer
3. Partial nephrectomy for injuries limited to one pole of the kidney, for segmental parenchymal disease, or for tumors confined to a solitary kidney
4. Nephroureterectomy for transitional cell carcinoma of the renal pelvis. The approach in these cases is similar to a simple nephrectomy. The entire ureter and cuff, however, of bladder are removed during nephroureterectomy.
5. Open surgical procedures on the kidney, such as anatrophic lithotomy in which the kidney is opened up to remove stones. Such cases have become extremely rare with the advent of endoscopic surgical technique and are not discussed here.

TABLE 26–4. PRESENTING FINDINGS IN RENAL CELL CARCINOMA PATIENTS

Finding	Occurrence (%)
Hematuria	50–60
Elevated erythrocyte sedimentation rate	50–60
Abdominal mass	24–45
Anemia	21–41
Flank pain	35–40
Hypertension	22–38
Weight loss	28–36
Pyrexia	7–17
Hepatic dysfunction	10–15
Classic triad (hematuria, abdominal mass, flank pain)	7–10
Hypercalcemia	3–6
Erythrocytosis	3–4
Varicocele	2–3

From Gillenwater, J. Y., Grayhack, J. T., Howard, S. S., Duckett, J. W. (1987). *Adult and pediatric urology* (p. 521). Chicago: Mosby-Year Book. Data from Skinner, D. G., Colvin, R. B, Vermillion, C. D., et al. (1971). Diagnosis and management of renal cell carcinoma. *Cancer, 28,* 1165; Chisholm, G. D. (1974). Nephrogenic ridge tumors and their syndromes. *Ann NY Acad Sci, 230,* 402; Fallon, B. (1985). Renal parenchymal tumors. B: Clinical and diagnostic features. In D. A. Culp, S. A. Loening (Eds.), *Genitourinary oncology.* Philadelphia: Lea & Febiger.

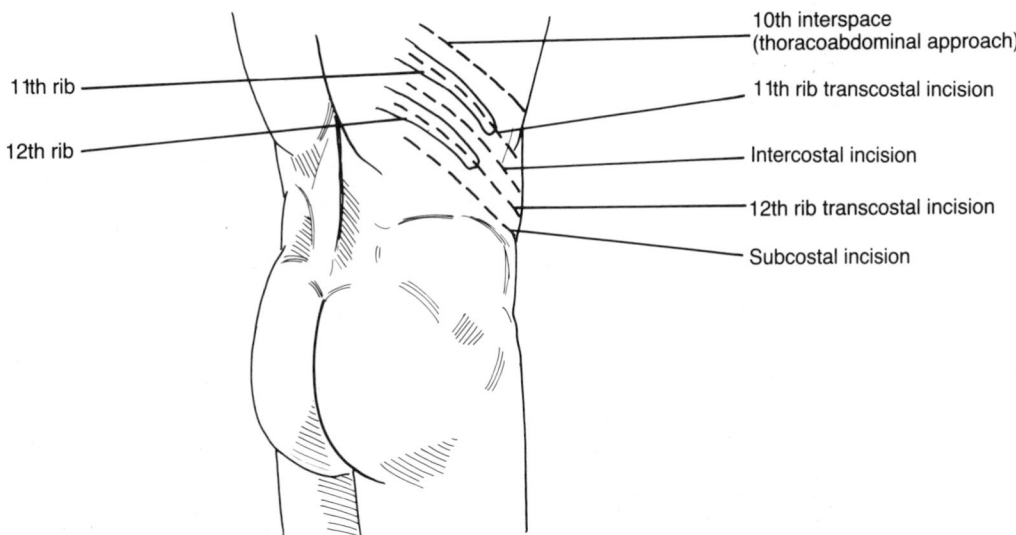

FIGURE 26–24. Flank incisions.

6. Surgery on the renal pelvis or proximal ureter to relieve a ureteropelvic junction obstruction. Obstruction to the flow of urine from the renal pelvis may be caused by a congenital narrowing of the most proximal portion of the ureter or by crossing vessels that press on the ureter. This procedure is more common in children.

Surgical Approaches to the Kidney

The flank approach avoids entering the peritoneal cavity. The incision may be transcostal, intercostal, or subcostal (Fig. 26–24).

The abdominal approach uses either a midline or a paramedian incision. Anterior subcostal or chevron incisions are used infrequently (Fig. 26–25).

The posterior lumbotomy approach uses an incision made in the back with the patient in the prone or lateral position (Fig. 26–26).

The thoracoabdominal approach is through the chest. The pleura may or may not be opened. A transcostal or intercostal incision may be used (see Fig. 26–24).

The operative team for urological surgery should be familiar with each approach as each necessitates specific patient positioning and instruments.

Related Surgical Procedures

A related surgical procedure is surgery on the adrenal gland, which entails a similar flank approach to the retroperitoneum.

Perioperative Nursing Implications

Anesthesia

Surgery of the kidney is performed under general anesthesia. This may be supplemented with an intercostal nerve block using bupivacaine hydrochloride with epinephrine. Blood is usually typed and cross-matched before surgery in case a transfusion is needed. The

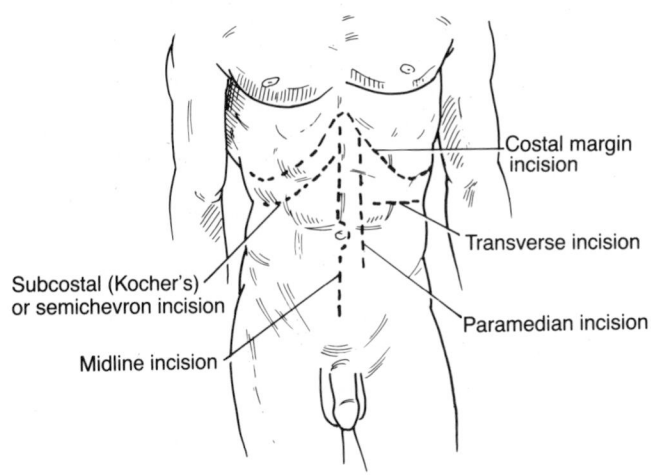

FIGURE 26–25. Anterior approaches to the kidney.

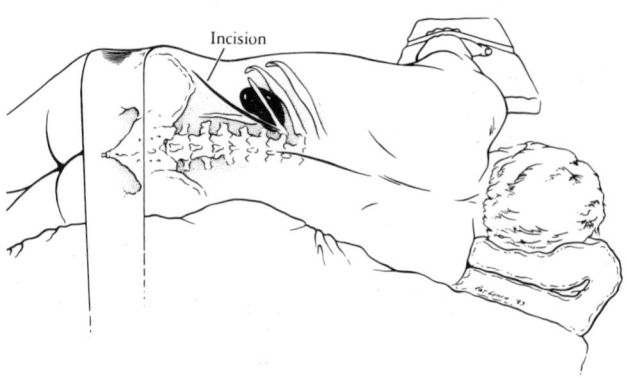

FIGURE 26–26. Posterior lumbotomy incision. (From Walsh, P. C., Gittes, A. D., Perlmutter, R. F., Stamey, T. A. [Eds.]. [1986]. *Campbell's urology* [5th ed.] [p. 2423]. Philadelphia: W. B. Saunders.)

circulating nurse and the anesthesiologist should follow hospital policy regarding blood administration.

Position

When the patient is placed on his or her side, special consideration is given to the ventilation of both lungs. Breath sounds are checked carefully after the patient is positioned, and adjustments are made in the patient's position or the placement of endotracheal tube as needed.

During the procedure, the anesthesiologist needs to know if the pleura is entered or a tear is suspected.

Proper positioning of patients for kidney surgery helps to ensure the best possible exposure of the operative field. Before surgery, the circulating nurse should have the following equipment ready in the OR:

3 pillows
3 sandbags
Sequential compression stockings
2 inch tape
Double arm board or a substitute arm-holding device
Axillary roll
Foam padding (e.g., eggcrate padding)

Placing the patient in the flank position is a unique experience for every patient. Some patients require more supportive equipment than others to secure them in the correct position and prevent injury. Only after the positioning begins are the surgeon, the anesthesiologist, and the nurse able to work out the best position for the patient. Therefore, it is imperative that the circulating nurse have all positioning equipment in the room before positioning begins. The circulating nurse should document on the nursing record the patient's position and positional aids in place.

When positioning the patient for the flank approach (Fig. 26–27), the tip of the 12th rib should lie on the kidney bar. If the OR bed flexes, the tip of the patient's iliac crest should be placed just below the break in the OR bed. One or two pillows are placed between the patient's legs, with the bottom leg flexed at a 90-degree angle and the top leg straight. Sandbags or beanbags

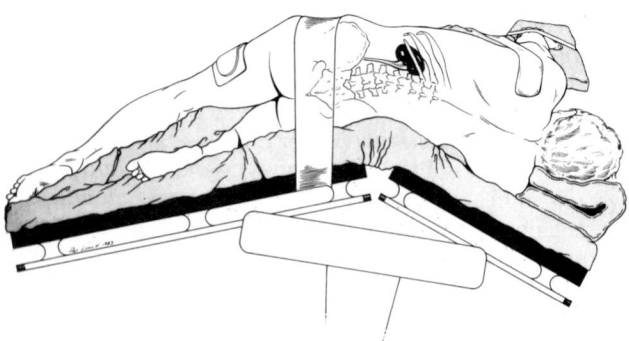

FIGURE 26–27. Patient position for flank surgery. (From Novick, A. C., & Streem, S. B. [1992]. Surgery of the kidney. In P. C. Walsh, A. B. Retik, T. A. Stamey, E. D. Vaughan, Jr. [Eds.], *Campbell's urology* [6th ed.] [p. 2419]. Philadelphia: W. B. Saunders.)

may be used to stabilize the patient. An axillary roll is placed under the patient's axilla to prevent injury to the nerves and vessels of the contralateral arm. The ipsilateral arm is supported. The OR bed is then flexed, placing the patient's flank muscles under tension. The patient is secured in place with 2-inch adhesive tape placed from one side of the OR bed to the other over the greater trochanter. Similarly, adhesive tape is placed over the superior chest wall. Certain patients may not tolerate this position because of spine disease or decreased cardiopulmonary function. They should not be placed in the flank position but rather in the supine position to permit an abdominal approach.

The patient is in the lateral position or prone position for the posterior lumbotomy incision with the OR bed slightly flexed. Positioning for an anterior subcostal incision is different. The patient is in the supine position with his or her arm brought anteriorly and superiorly. A sandbag or roll may be placed under the flank on the side of the incision. The legs may be crossed as shown in Figure 26–27.

Because the patient is placed on his or her side, other guidelines for this position should be considered by the circulating nurse.

Insert the Foley catheter before turning the patient, but wait to secure the drainage tubing and bag until the positioning is completed. Thus, proper drainage can be ensured.
Place sequential compression stockings on the patient before turning.
Do not place the electrosurgical grounding pad on the patient until after positioning is completed. This helps to avoid poor contact owing to pad manipulation during the positioning of the patient.

Creation and Maintenance of the Sterile Field

Patient preparation varies according to the position of the patient. If the patient is in the supine position, the area from the nipple line to the midthigh is shaved and prepared with a povidone-iodine solution. Draping is carried out in the routine fashion for this position.

When the patient is on his or her side, the entire back, flank, and abdomen on the operative side are shaved and prepared with a povidone-iodine solution. Side towels should be placed by the circulator to avoid pooling of the preparation solution. These should be removed after the preparation and before the draping is started.

When draping the patient who has been positioned on one side, care must be taken to secure the drapes in place to create the sterile field. The scrub nurse should provide skin clips or suture to fix the drapes to the skin. At the end of the procedure, the scrub nurse should remind the surgeon to remove the clips or sutures in the drapes before the patient begins to wake up.

The Mayo stand is placed over the patient's legs. The scrub nurse should be careful to avoid contact of the

Mayo stand with the patient as the OR bed is raised and lowered.

Equipment and Supplies

The following equipment and supplies should be gathered in advance by the circulating nurse. Depending on the exact procedure to be done, all of the equipment may not be necessary:

Basin set
Patient and table drapes
Mayo stand cover
2 suction tubings
Electrosurgical pencil, extension tip, and cleaner
Balfour retractor with malleable blades
Extra deep and elephant Deaver retractors
1 long instrument pack
1 laparotomy set
1 vascular set
1 nephrectomy set
1 brown bag
1 skin marker
3 packages of large laparotomy sponges
2 packages of E-tape sponges
1 package of 4 × 8 inch sponges
Pushers (Kittner)
Needle counter
Large and medium hemoclips
1 magnetic pad
50-ml syringe
Bladder irrigation kit
Asepto syringe
Foley catheter and drainage bag (size according to the surgeon's request)
Vessel loops
Hernia tape
Nos. 10, 11, and 15 blades
1–0 and 2–0 chromic ties
1–0, 2–0, and 3–0 silk ties
No. 1, 1–0, 2–0, and 3–0 chromic swedge (on a taper needle)
5–0 and 4–0 chromic swedge (RB–1 needle)
Skin staples
Sterile light handles or light glove covers
No. 1 or 1–0 Vicryl on a CT needle
Plastic intestinal bag
No. 8 Fr. or No. 10 Fr. red rubber catheter
Drains—Penrose or No. 10 Jackson-Pratt (according to the surgeon's preference)
10-ml syringe
25-gauge 1½-inch needle
Sterile ice
Ureteral catheters (according to the surgeon's preference)
Chest tube (according to the surgeon's preference)
Pleur-Evac set

The scrub nurse should have the following equipment ready for the surgeon's use:

An extra-long instrument pack and electrosurgical tip should be used in deep cavities.
Raytek 4 × 8 inch sponges may be rolled and folded and placed on the end of a ring forceps for blunt dissection.
A No. 8 or 10 Fr. red rubber catheter is used if the pleura has been entered. The catheter is placed through the hole and air aspirated as the pleura is closed. If the pleura cannot be closed satisfactorily, a chest tube is used.
Ureteral catheters may be used if the ureter is in danger of injury or if it has been opened.
A sterile magnetic pad can be placed over the patient's hips to help control the loss of instruments and needles, especially if the patient is in the flank position.
A local syringe and needle should be available for injection of local anesthetic in the intercostal area during closure.
The sterile ice may be used during partial nephrectomy. When used, the sterile ice is placed in a sterile intestinal bag and then placed around the kidney to decrease blood flow before the incision into the kidney.

Drugs and Solutions

Sterile saline for irrigation
Sterile water for irrigation
Neomycin and polymixin B (Neosporin GU irrigant)
Hemostatic agents (according to the surgeon's choice), such as microfibrillar collagen hemostat (Avitene), oxidized regenerated cellulose (Surgicel), and absorbable gelatin sponge (Gelfoam)
Dexon or Vicryl mesh, for partial nephrectomy
Local anesthesia, usually bupivacaine hydrochloride with epinephrine, for local intercostal injection before the end of surgery, during closure

Physiological Monitoring

Rapid blood loss can occur during surgery of the kidney. The circulating nurse should keep a current record of sponge and bottle blood loss as well as the volume of irrigation fluids used. The circulating nurse assists the anesthesiologist in the monitoring of urine output via the urine collection system.

Specimens and Cultures

Cultures are performed when infection is present or suspected. Specimens in kidney surgery can include all of the following:

Kidney (right or left)
Kidney and ureter

Perinephric fat
Kidney, adrenal gland, perinephric fat, and Gerota fascia en bloc
Upper or lower pole of the kidney
Stones

Each specimen should be handled according to hospital policy (e.g., fresh, fixed, and frozen section).

Physician's Orders, Laboratory and Diagnostic Studies

Preoperative evaluation of the patient undergoing surgery on the kidney should include functional studies of the kidney (either IVU or radioisotopic renal scan) to ensure adequate function in the contralateral kidney and an anatomical study (IVU, retrograde pyelogram, ultrasound, CT scan, magnetic resonance imaging scan, and/or arteriogram).

The patient being prepared for elective surgery may be placed on a modified bowel preparation (clear liquids, enemas, and administration of magnesium citrate on the day before surgery). Preoperative teaching, breathing exercises, and incentive spirometry should be initiated. One dose of parenteral broad-spectrum antibiotic should be given before initiating surgery. Routine laboratory studies (blood urea nitrogen, creatinine, and electrolyte determinations, CBC, platelets, prothrombin time, partial thromboplastin time, chest x-ray film, and ECG) are obtained and checked. Blood should be available in the blood bank (1 to 2 U of packed red blood cells). Patients with suspected pulmonary disease should undergo pulmonary function studies and blood gas analysis to help plan the surgical approach. There is a slightly higher rate of complications in flank incision (10%) as compared with anterior incisions (5%).

Patients found to have a urinary tract infection should be treated with the appropriate intravenous antibiotic therapy for at least 48 hours preoperatively. Certain severe infections may warrant immediate surgical therapy, and in such cases, broad-spectrum intravenous antibiotic therapy should be initiated with minimal delay.

Preoperative teaching should include a full explanation of the procedure. The patient should be reassured and told that he or she can live a normal life after a nephrectomy, provided there is good function in the remaining kidney. This kidney actually increases its function to compensate for the loss of the other kidney.

Procedure

Some basic surgical principles must be adhered to for surgery on the kidney. The incision and approach must be planned according to the anatomy of the patient and to the nature of his or her disease. Preoperative evaluation (IVU, CT scan, arteriogram, ultrasound, and magnetic resonance imaging scan) helps to define the anatomy and the extent of the disease and should be

available for review. Given the position of the kidney in the retroperitoneum, exposure should be adequate to provide access and control of the renal vascular pedicle.

Simple Nephrectomy

Simple nephrectomy is performed for pyonephrosis, chronic pyelonephritis with extensive destruction of the kidney, renal abscess not amenable to percutaneous drainage, congenitally malformed and nonfunctional kidney (e.g., polycystic kidney disease), and severe renal damage from trauma.

Incision and Exposure

Depending on the position of the kidney, either a subcostal 11th or 12th rib or anterior 12th rib incision is made (Fig. 26–28). The layers of the abdominal wall are sharply traversed, with care being taken to achieving hemostasis and to noting the location of nerves, especially the 12th thoracic intercostal nerve (which lies between the transversus abdominis muscle and the internal oblique muscle). The retroperitoneum is entered and the peritoneum is reflected medially. If the peritoneum is inadvertently opened, it can be closed with 3–0 chromic catgut suture. Gerota fascia is then identified. A self-retaining (Balfour or Finochietto) retractor may be placed to improve exposure.

Details

Gerota fascia is incised, and the perinephric fat is bluntly dissected from the capsule of the kidney. The kidney is then mobilized by freeing it from its fatty surroundings. The lower pole is first mobilized. The ureter is identified, clamped, and divided using metallic clips. The kidney can be retracted, and the hilum is

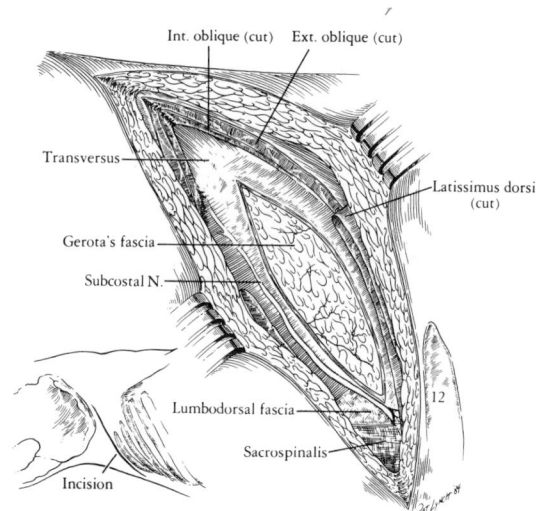

FIGURE 26–28. Subcostal incision. (From Novick, A. C., Streem, S. B. [1992]. Surgery of the kidney. In P. C. Walsh, A. B. Retik, T. A. Stamey, E. D. Vaughan, Jr. [Eds.], *Campbell's urology* [6th ed.] [p. 2422]. Philadelphia: W. B. Saunders.)

identified. Accessory vessels to the kidney should be kept in mind, and when found, they should be clamped, ligated, and divided. The main artery and vein are then identified, dissected, and mobilized. First the artery and then the vein is doubly clamped; ligated with heavy, free ties; and divided. A set of vascular instruments should be available if difficulties are encountered in controlling bleeding from either the vein or the artery. The kidney is then removed from the field. In case of severe infection, monofilament suture or absorbable suture should be used.

Closure

After removal of the kidney, the renal fossa is inspected carefully for any signs of bleeding, and hemostasis should be established. The incision is then closed and the renal fossa can be drained by a Penrose drain. Closure in three layers is standard, using running Vicryl sutures for the deep layers and interrupted suture for the external oblique layer. Skin is reapproximated using skin clips.

Posterior Lumbotomy

A posterior lumbotomy approach may be used (Fig. 26–29). It may lessen postoperative pain and respiratory compromise and allows a rapid approach to the renal artery. However, dissection of the kidney is harder. This approach is excellent for an open renal biopsy. Simple nephrectomy for injury may be performed through a transabdominal approach at the time of exploratory laparotomy. It offers the advantage of easy access and control of the renal vessels. The same principles of dissection, mobilization, and control of the renal vasculature should be adhered to.

Nephroureterectomy

Nephroureterectomy is used to remove transitional cell carcinoma involving the renal collecting system. The kidney and entire ureter with a cuff of bladder are removed en bloc. The approach for nephroureterectomy is also similar to that for a simple nephrectomy; however, a second incision or a larger incision is usually needed to obtain access to the distal ureter and its insertion into the bladder (Fig. 26–30). A modified Gibson incision is usually used in these cases. A cuff of bladder is removed and surgery on the bladder follows the same principles as those used for open prostatectomy.

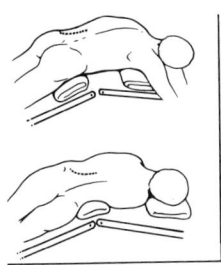

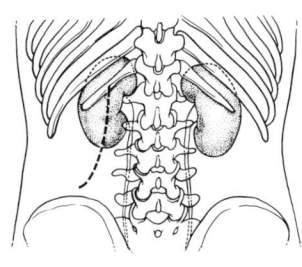

FIGURE 26–29. Patient position and incision site for posterior lumbotomy. (From Walsh, P. C., Retik, A. B., Stamey, T. A., Vaughan, E. D. [1992]. *Campbell's urology* [6th ed.]. Philadelphia: W. B. Saunders, Fig. 65–15.)

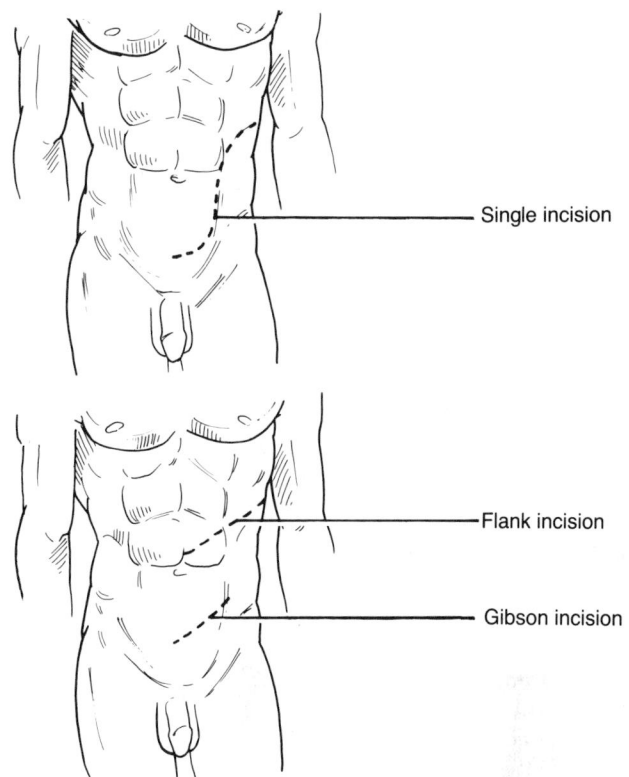

FIGURE 26–30. Incisions for nephroureterectomy.

Radical Nephrectomy

The indication for radical nephrectomy is renal cell carcinoma. The goal of the operation is to remove en bloc kidney, adrenal gland, all the perinephric fat, and Gerota fascia (Fig. 26–31).

Incision and Exposure

Several approaches can be used: thoracoabdominal, flank, or transabdominal. The thoracoabdominal and transcostal approaches are described. The thoracoabdominal approach provides excellent access to renal vessels, the aorta, the inferior vena cava, and the kidney (Fig. 26–32). The pleura may or may not be entered, depending on which rib or intercostal space is entered. The choice of level of incision depends again on the position of the kidney. The patient is positioned in similar fashion as for a flank incision with more of a posterior tilt (the patient's body is at a 45-degree angle to the OR bed and the pelvis is at 15–20 degrees). A transcostal incision is made right over the 9th or 10th rib, is brought down to the rib, and extends anteriorly

604 ■ CLINICAL APPLICATIONS

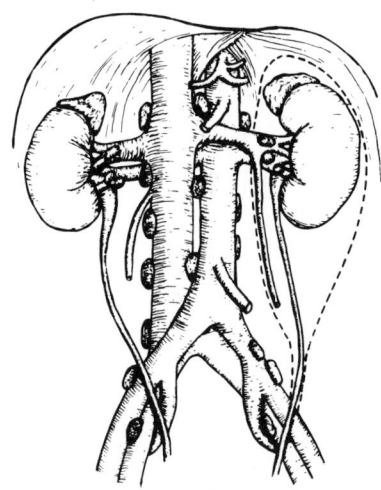

FIGURE 26–31. Boundaries of a left radical nephrectomy. Dotted line represents both the surgical margin and Gerota fascia. (From Gillenwater, J. Y., Grayhack, J. T., Howards, S. S., Duckett, J. W. [Eds.]. [1987]. *Adult and pediatric urology* [p. 529]. Chicago: Year Book Medical.)

to the lateral border of the rectus abdominis muscle (Fig. 26–33*A*). Rib resection is then carried out. This technique provides wider exposure.

Details

Using a periosteal (Alexander) elevator, the rib is dissected up on its anterior surface (Fig. 26–33*B*). A Doyen periosteal elevator is passed behind the rib, which is then freed up from the periosteum. The rib is transected as far back as possible with a rib cutter. Attention is then turned to dissecting the lower fibers of the diaphragm. The pleura is likewise dissected. The retroperitoneum is entered and the peritoneum is incised and opened. A self-retaining (Finochietto) retractor is placed on the right side.

The liver overlies the kidney and should be retracted upward by a wide Deaver retractor. The liver should be packed with a moistened laparotomy pad before the retractor is placed. The colon is then mobilized and reflected medially by incising the avascular white line. The duodenum is likewise mobilized and reflected medially, giving access to the renal hilum, which is then dissected carefully. The renal vein and, posterior to it, the renal artery are mobilized, dissected out, ligated, and divided. Extreme care should be given not to injure any adjacent structures.

The dissection is then carried out toward the liver along the vena cava, into which the adrenal vein drains. The vein, after being identified and mobilized, is ligated and divided. The lower pole of the kidney and the surrounding perinephric fat can then be freed up, and the ureter is identified. After the ureter is identified, it can be dissected toward the bladder and then doubly ligated with hemoclips and divided. The upper pole is then mobilized. Adrenal vessels should be clipped and divided. Blunt and sharp dissection are used, and hemoclips are applied to ensure hemostasis. After the upper

pole is freed, the kidney is removed from the field and sent to the pathology department. The renal fossa is inspected for bleeding and hemostasis is ensured. The wound is irrigated.

Closure

The pleura is closed, and if necessary, a chest tube is placed. The flank incision is closed in three layers as described above with 1 or 1–0 Vicryl suture material. No drains are placed.

Left Radical Nephrectomy

A left radical nephrectomy is different insofar as the anatomy of the renal vein is concerned: the adrenal vein and the gonadal vein drain into it. The descending colon is dissected and reflected medially from Gerota fascia. The great vessels are identified and the left renal vein is dissected in front of the aorta. Both the gonadal vein and the adrenal vein are identified, dissected out, ligated, and divided. The renal artery is then localized and freed from its surrounding tissue. The artery and then the vein are further mobilized, ligated, and divided using heavy silk stitches (2–0 silk). The vein is divided close to the aorta. The rest of the dissection and mobilization of the kidney follow as for the right side. Attention should be given to the left gastroepiploic

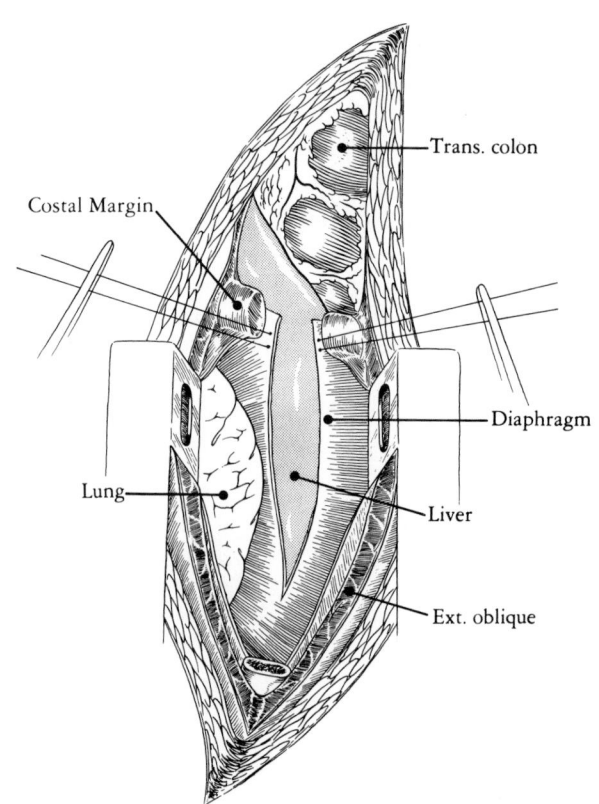

FIGURE 26–32. Right thoracoabdominal incision. (From Walsh, P. C., Gittes, A. D., Perlmutter, R. F., Stamey, T. A. [Eds.]. [1986]. *Campbell's urology* [5th ed.] [p. 2423]. Philadelphia: W. B. Saunders.)

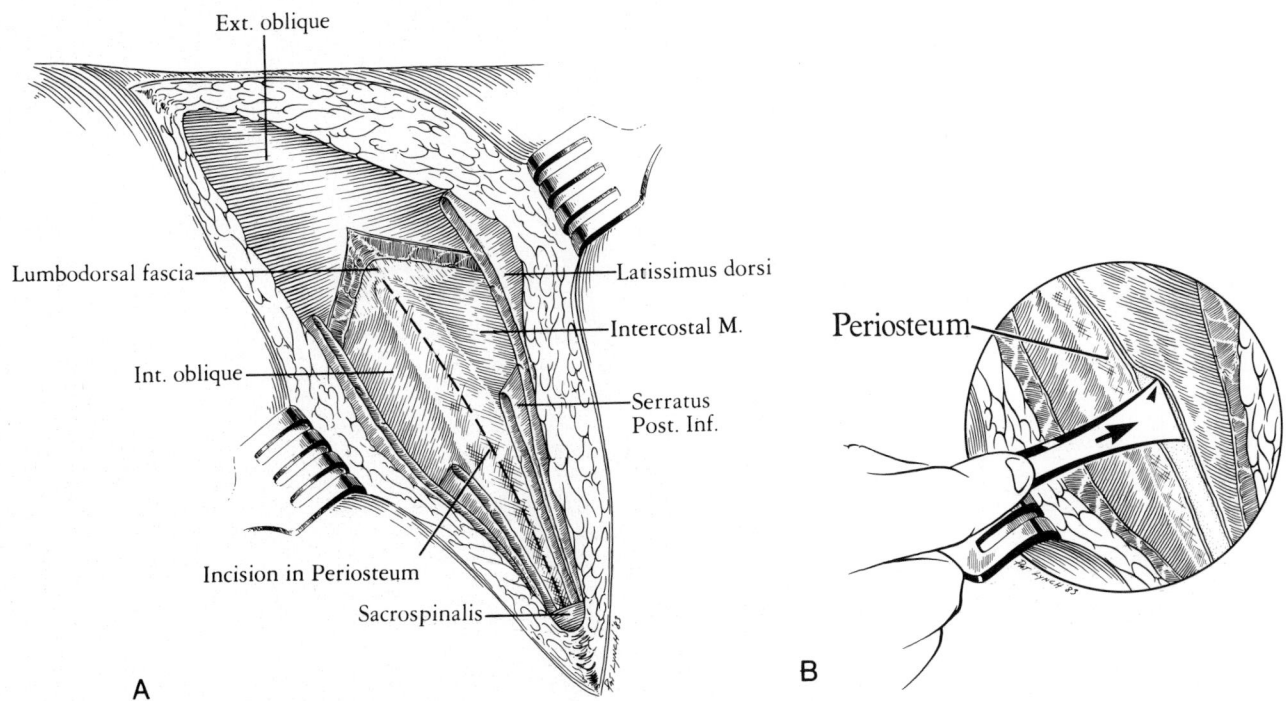

Ext. oblique

Lumbodorsal fascia

Int. oblique

Incision in Periosteum

Sacrospinalis

Latissimus dorsi

Intercostal M.

Serratus Post. Inf.

A

Periosteum

B

FIGURE 26–33. *A*, Left transcostal incision. *B*, The periosteum is reflected off the upper surface of the rib. Note that the periosteal elevator is moved distally or downward on the upper edge of the rib against the direction of the intercostal muscle fibers. (From Novick, A. C., Streem, S. B. [1992]. Surgery of the kidney. In P. C. Walsh, A. B. Retik, T. A. Stamey, E. D. Vaughan, Jr. [Eds.], *Campbell's urology* [6th ed.] [p. 2421]. Philadelphia: W. B. Saunders.)

artery and short gastric vessels, which may be ligated during mobilization of the upper pole of the kidney. Careful handling of the spleen and descending colon should be ensured.

Partial Nephrectomy

Incision and Exposure

The approach to a partial nephrectomy is similar to that for the simple nephrectomy.

Details

After the kidney is mobilized and freed up from its fatty surrounding, the tumor or injury should be identified in either the upper or the lower pole. If the lesion is clearly confined to either pole, partial nephrectomy can be carried out. The renal hilum is dissected out, and the vessels should be mobilized to provide good control of renal vasculature (Fig. 26–34). A moistened umbilical tape is then placed around the kidney proximal to the hilum and cinched down to occlude intrarenal circulation (alternatively, a Rumel clamp may be used).

The renal capsule is incised, and the renal parenchyma is incised with the handle of a scalpel. The cut edge of the kidney is inspected for vessels, and these are sutured using 4–0 chromic catgut placed in a figure of eight. The umbilical tape or clamp may be released to identify vessels that have not been sutured. The collecting system is closed with a running 5–0 or 4–0 chromic catgut stitch.

Closure

The edges of the renal capsule are then brought back together using the interrupted mattress sutures of 2–0 chromic catgut. Care should be taken not to tear the friable parenchyma. Perinephric fat may be brought back over the closed capsule to provide extra tamponade. The kidney is then placed back into the gutter, and the incision is closed. One or two Penrose drains should be placed around the kidney and should be removed 2 to 5 days after surgery.

Nephroureterectomy

Incision and Exposure

A flank incision extended to the lower abdomen, or a second incision (Gibson incision or transplant incision) should be used. The approach to the kidney is similar to that for a simple nephrectomy. The exposure to the distal ureter and bladder is the same as for renal transplantation. Closure is no different than for nephrectomy or renal transplantation. No drains are placed.

Postoperative Care

Postoperative orders include intravenous administration of antibiotics for a short course (two or three doses), strict monitoring of vital signs and urine output, and breathing exercises with incentive spirometry. Patients should not be fed until flatus is passed. If patients

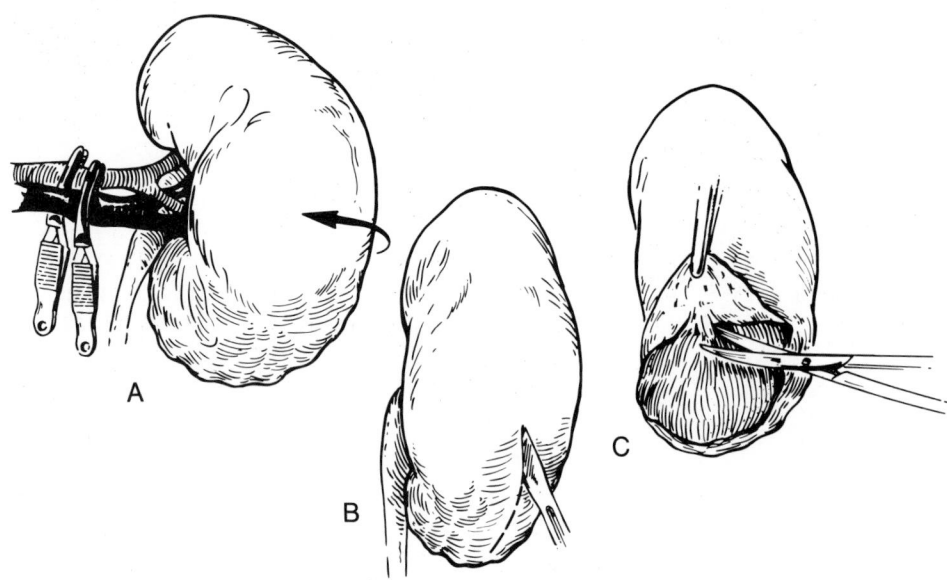

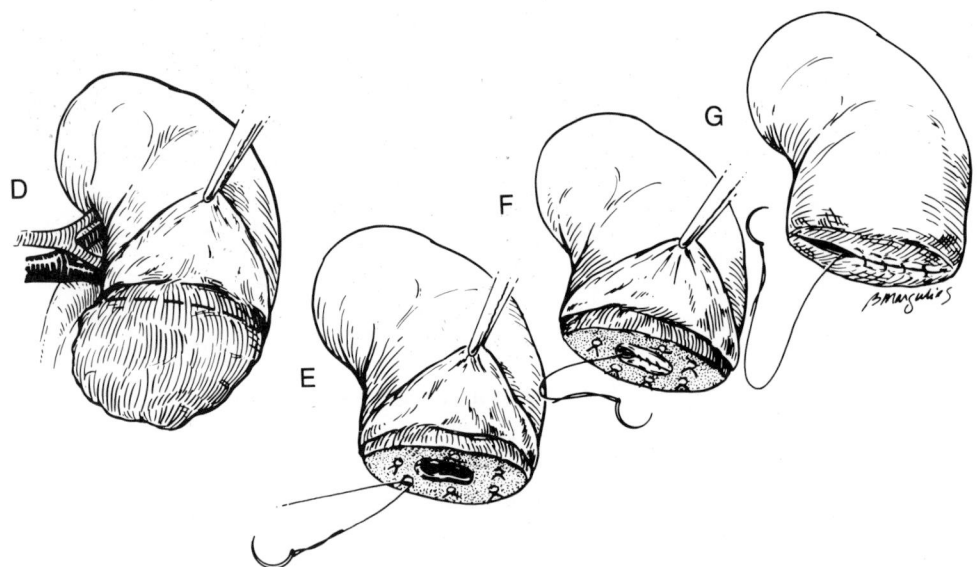

FIGURE 26–34. Partial nephrectomy. (From Glenn, J. T. [Ed.]. [1985]. *Urologic surgery* [p. 92]. Philadelphia: J. B. Lippincott.)

TABLE 26–5. POTENTIAL COMPLICATIONS OF NEPHRECTOMY

Operative	Postoperative
Hemorrhage or shock	Wound
Pleural or pulmonary complications	Dehiscence
Cardiovascular complications	Infection
Visceral injury	Hernia
	Gastrointestinal
	Ileus
	Fistula
	Pulmonary
	Pneumothorax
	Pneumonia
	Atelectasis
	Cardiovascular
	Myocardial infarction
	Congestive failure
	Thrombophlebitis
	Pulmonary embolism
	Cerebrovascular accident
	Shock secondary to blood loss, septicemia
	Renal functional impairment

experience nausea and vomiting, a nasogastric tube should be placed. The Foley catheter is left in place for 24 hours and then removed. Narcotics should be administered liberally to allow the patient to breathe freely. A chest x-ray film is helpful to document or rule out pneumothorax caused by entry into the pleura. If the pneumothorax is significant (greater than 15–20%), a chest tube should be inserted. The sequential compression device should be left in place for 2 to 3 days. The patient may be out of bed on the first postoperative day and should ambulate. Intravenous fluids are administered until the patient is able to resume normal oral fluid intake. Sutures or skin clips may be removed 5 to 7 days postoperatively.

Potential Surgical Complications
(Table 26–5)

Intraoperative complications are described above. There can be significant bleeding and injury to adjacent organs during renal surgery. Both can be avoided by controlling the renal vasculature and by using careful technique. Postoperative complications include infections, prolonged ileus, pneumonia, wound dehiscence, and herniation. Some patients may experience varying degrees of intercostal neuralgia, which usually resolves during several months. Mortality is reported as less than 1%. Increased mortality rates are noted in patients with renal failure, azotemia, or infections.

SURGERY OF THE PROSTATE

Surgery on the prostate is performed for benign prostatic hyperplasia. A prostatectomy is performed when the gland is configured in such a way that it is not amenable to transurethral resection.

Open Prostatectomy

Definition

The typical patient with symptoms of bladder outlet obstruction is older than 50 years of age. The physical examination is usually unrevealing, except in the rare cases when patients have urinary retention and are found to have an easily palpable bladder on examination of the abdomen. The rectal examination may help in assessing prostatic size as well as in ruling out a prostatic nodule or induration indicative of a possible malignancy.

Operative options are considered for benign prostatic hyperplasia when symptoms of bladder outlet obstruction become significant to the patient. These include urinary frequency, urgency, decreased stream, straining to void, dribbling nocturia, and ultimately urinary retention. Even though most men experience some degree of benign prostatic hyperplasia, only 10% of all men require an operation to relieve symptoms of bladder outlet obstruction. The goal of surgery is therefore to alleviate the symptoms and prevent further consequences of chronic outlet obstruction, such as progressive renal failure, recurrent urinary tract infections because of urine stasis, and development of bladder stones. Surgery on the prostate for benign disease can be either open or closed. Open surgery refers to procedures done through an incision that extends down to the prostatic tissue. Closed surgery refers to transurethral resection carried out through a cystoscope.

Indications

Indications for open prostatectomy are limited to significant bladder outlet obstruction, urodynamic evaluation consistent with bladder obstruction (high bladder pressure and low urinary flow), a large prostate not amenable to transurethral resection, and the presence of large bladder stones. At cystoscopy, the prostate may appear to extend into the bladder, obscuring the ureteral orifices.

Related Surgical Procedures

Related procedures include radical prostatectomy for prostatic cancer. In other related procedures to remove bladder stones and to reimplant the ureters, a similar transvesical approach is used. Several approaches to the prostate are possible: suprapubic, transvesical, retropubic, and perineal. Only the suprapubic approach will be described.

Perioperative Nursing Implications

Anesthesia

Open prostatectomy is usually performed under general anesthesia. Occasionally, continuous epidural anesthesia is used alone or as an adjunct to the general anesthesia. Blood is typed and cross-matched for all patients for possible transfusion in the OR. The circulating nurse should follow hospital policy when assisting in blood administration.

Position

The patient undergoing suprapubic or radical retropubic prostatectomy is placed in the supine position. A small roll or sandbag is placed under the patient's sacrum. The OR bed is placed in a slight Trendelenburg position. Pneumatic compression stockings should be placed by the circulator during patient positioning. If the surgeon also requires the table to be flexed to accentuate the patient's position, make sure that the patient's pelvic area is over the break in the bed. In addition, if indicated, a 28 or 30 Fr. red rubber catheter may be placed in the rectum at this time and hooked to straight drainage. The electrosurgical grounding pad should be placed at this point, avoiding the area to be prepared.

Creation and Maintenance of the Sterile Field

In creating a sterile field, the patient is shaved from umbilicus to midthigh. A preparation of povidone-iodine covering the same area is done for 5 minutes. The circulating nurse should place drip towels where the potential for pooling of preparation solution exists. These are removed after the preparation, before the draping. Because the penis is prepared into the field, the circulating nurse may need to assist the surgeon to ensure adequate preparation of the area. A sterile towel is placed under the penis after the preparation.

In creating the sterile field, the scrub nurse should anticipate the need for skin clips or sutures to secure the drapes. During the prostatectomy, the scrub nurse should keep the following in mind:

A Foley catheter is inserted, using sterile technique, at the start of the procedure.

Urine is drained at intervals from the clamped catheter and must be measured.

A bladder irrigation kit should be available for instillation of fluid into the bladder.

The prostate specimen is removed, as well as the top of the Foley catheter. Another 30-ml catheter should be available for use.

During the reanastomosis of the urethra and bladder, free needles as well as swedges are used.

Extralong instruments, electrocautery extension tip, and so on may be needed.

Equipment and Supplies

The following equipment and supplies should be available for open prostatectomy:

Patient and table drapes
Laparotomy set
Vascular set
Prostatectomy set
Basin set
2 suction tubings
Foley irrigation set
Large laparotomy sponges
E-tape sponges
4 × 8 inch Raytek sponges
Vessel loops
Pushers (Kittner)
Electrosurgical pencil with tip extender
Nos. 10, 11, and 15 blades
Light handles
Needle counter
Marking pen
Brown bag
30-ml balloon Silastic Foley catheter (according to the surgeon's preference)
28 or 30 Fr. red rubber catheter (rectal tube)
Extradeep and elephant Deaver pack
Long instrument pack
Balfour malleable blades
Spleen roll
Straight drainage bag
Silastic Malecot catheter (for suprapubic tube according to the surgeon's preference)
Penrose or Jackson-Pratt drains (according to the surgeon's preference)
Magnetic pad
Ureteral catheter
2–0 chromic ties and swedges (SH, UR–5, UR–6, MH, CT)
1–0 chromic ties and swedges (SH and CT–1)
No. 1 chromic swedge
No. 1 Vicryl swedge
Plastic button
1 Ethilon suture
Hernia tape
3–0 silk on Keith straight needle
2–0 silk ties and swedges
1–0 silk ties
No. 2140–2 free needles (Kelly intestinal)
3–0 silk ties
Skin staples

Drugs and Solutions

Drugs and solutions delivered by the circulating nurse include

normal saline for irrigation (warm)
neomycin and polymixin B (Neosporin GU irrigant)
lubricant (K-Y jelly)

Physiological Monitoring

During the procedure, the circulating nurse maintains accurate blood loss records, including sponge and bottle blood loss and irrigation. Urine drained onto the field via the sterile catheter must also be measured and recorded.

Specimens and Cultures

Cultures are not routinely performed during prosta-tectomy unless an infection is suspected. Specimens include

prostate gland with surrounding tissue
pelvic lymph nodes for frozen section examination
    (for radical prostatectomy only)

Physician's Orders, Laboratory and Diagnostic Studies

Before surgery, the patient undergoes routine labo-ratory assessment (CBC, platelet count, electrolyte panel, blood urea nitrogen and creatinine measure-ments), ECG, chest x-ray film, and an evaluation of the upper urinary tract by either ultrasound or IVU. At least 4 U of blood should be available in the blood bank before surgery.

The patient recieves a Fleet enema the night before surgery, as well as a perineal, genitalia, and lower abdomen povidone-iodine preparation. Preoperatively, parenteral antibiotics can be administered.

Procedure

The patient is placed in the supine position. The lower abdomen, genitalia, and perineum are prepared with povidone-iodine. The penis is included in the field.

Incision and Exposure

An infraumbilical incision is made in the midline to the fascia, which is sharply incised, with care being given not to enter the bladder prematurely (Fig. 26–35). The peritoneum is identified and reflected toward the pa-tient's head, and the bladder is dissected from its lateral attachments by blunt dissection.

The bladder is filled with 200 to 300 ml of saline and then opened. A self-retainely (Balfour) retractor is then

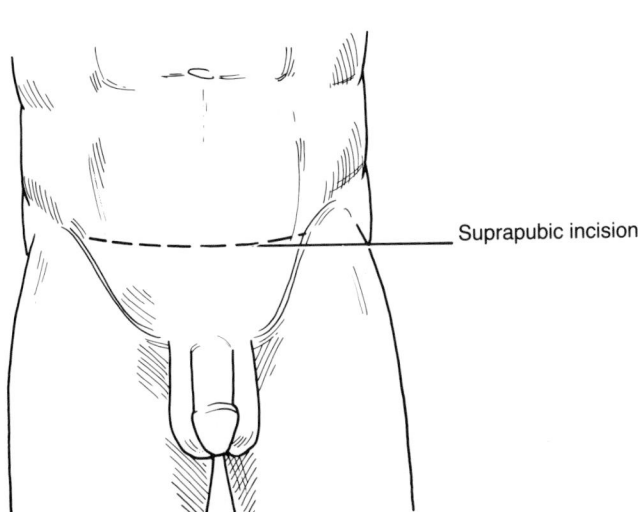

FIGURE 26–35. Suprapubic incision.

Suprapubic incision

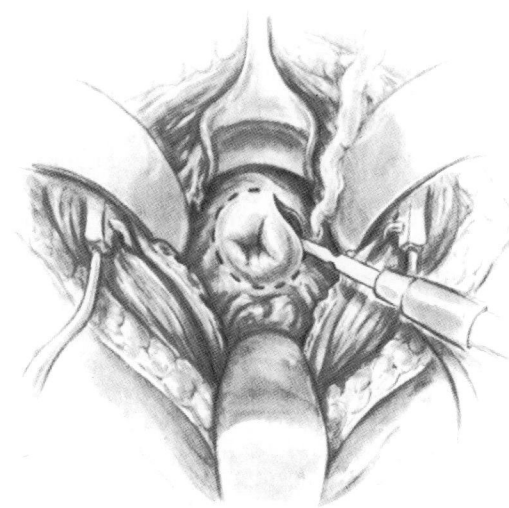

FIGURE 26–36. Circumferential bladder neck incision before transvesical enucleation of a prostatic adenoma. The bladder neck is most easily exposed by the placement of small Deaver and malleable retractors laterally and a medium Deaver superiorly. The trigone and ureteral orifices should have been exposed and kept from harm's way. The incision through the mucosa overlying the bladder neck is best established with electrosurgical instruments. (From O'Conor, V. J., Jr. [1979]. Suprapubic and retropubic prostatectomy. In J. H. Harri-son, R. F. Gittes, A. D. Perlmutter, et al. [Eds.], *Campbell's urology* [4th ed.] [p. 2305]. Philadelphia: W. B. Saunders.)

placed and the dome of the bladder is packed with several moist sponges. The ureteral orifices are identi-fied, and if they are hard to identify, ureteral stents (5 Fr.) are placed. With electrocautery, a cicumferential incision is made below the bladder neck (Fig. 26–36).

Details

Blunt dissection is then carried out to shell out the prostatic adenoma. After the adenoma is removed, there may be fairly brisk bleeding, and the prostatic fossa is packed with a warm laparotomy pad or spleen roll, which is left in place for at least 5 minutes. The fossa is then reinspected and 1–0 chromic catgut stitches may be placed at 5 and 7 o'clock positions. A Foley catheter is placed and the balloon is inflated with 60 to 100 ml of fluid. Traction on the Foley catheter helps tamponade bleeding from the prostatic fossa.

Closure

The bladder is then closed in two layers with either chromic or Vicryl absorbable suture material. A Malecot catheter is placed as a suprapubic catheter. Drainage of the perivesical space may be accomplished by either Jackson-Pratt drains or Penrose drains. The fascia is then closed using nonabsorbable suture. Subcutaneous and skin closure are performed in the standard fashion.

Postoperative Care

After surgery, the patient should be given parenteral antibiotics for 24 to 48 hours and kept well hydrated.

The urine output should be monitored carefully. The Foley catheter and suprapubic tube should be checked periodically to ensure patency and irrigated gently to dislodge any clots. Drainage from the wound should be monitored. CBC and electrolytes should be checked for at least 2 days postoperatively. The drains can be removed on day 3 or 4 if the drainage is scant. The suprapubic tube may be removed 5 to 7 days after surgery. A cystogram may help to ascertain that the bladder is well closed and does not leak before removing the Foley catheter, which is done a day or two later.

Potential Surgical Complications

Intraoperative bleeding may be significant, and all patients should be warned that they may need a transfusion. The risk of mortality from open prostatectomy is close to 1%, slightly more than for transurethral resection. Retrograde ejaculation is an anticipated occurrence after prostatectomy. Stricture disease and bladder contracture may occur later, causing recurrent voiding symptoms. Incontinence may result from prostatectomy in approximately 1% of patients. Impotence has been reported in 5 to 46% of patients. Potential injuries to intraabdominal organs should be avoided. A persistent bladder leak may necessitate prolonged bladder drainage.

Radical Retropubic Prostatectomy (Nerve Sparing)

Definition

This procedure involves removal of the entire prostate gland including the prostatic urethra, the seminal vesicles, and vas deferens with subsequent reconstruction of the bladder neck and proximal urethra.

Indications

Radical retropubic prostatectomy is believed to be the most effective form of treatment for patients younger than age 70 years with prostatic cancer limited to the prostatic capsule.

On physical examination, the only notable feature is a palpable nodule or induration on rectal examination, usually picked up on routine examination. The history is unremarkable.

Perioperative Nursing Implications

Anesthesia

Radical retropubic prostatectomy is performed under general anesthesia with continuous epidural anesthesia as an adjunct. The continuous epidural catheter may later be used for postoperative pain control. Blood is typed and cross-matched for all patients. The circulating nurse assists in blood administration according to hospital policy.

Position

The patient is placed in the same position as for a suprapubic prostatectomy.

Creation and Maintenance of the Sterile Field

The patient is prepared and draped as for a suprapubic prostatectomy. The sterile field is also maintained in a similar fashion.

Equipment and Supplies

The same instruments used for suprapubic prostatectomy should be available.

Drugs and Solutions

Drugs and solutions delivered by the circulating nurse include

normal saline for irrigation (warm)
Neomycin and polymixin B (Neosporin GU irrigant)
lubricant (K-Y jelly)
indigo carmine (administered by the anesthesiologist to observe urine flow)

Physiological Monitoring

Physiological monitoring is similar to that done during the suprapubic prostatectomy. In this procedure, rapid, large-volume blood loss can occur when the surgeons are working on the dorsal venous complex. Both the scrub nurse and the circulator should be aware of this potential and be prepared.

Specimens and Cultures

During lymph node dissection, right and left obturator lymph node packets specimens are sent to the pathology lab for frozen section examination and diagnosis. Extension of prostate cancer into the lymph nodes contraindicates radical retropubic prostatectomy.

The radical prostatectomy specimen consists of the entire prostate gland including the prostatic urethra, the seminal vesicles, and the vas deferens.

Physician's Orders, Laboratory and Diagnostic Studies

Before surgery, the patient should undergo prostatic specific antigen determination, cystoscopy and needle biopsy of the prostate, bone scan, chest x-ray film, IVU, and CT and/or MRI scan to rule out any spread of the tumor. A delay of 5 to 6 weeks between the time of needle biopsy of the prostate and surgery is recommended. As for the suprapubic prostatectomy, blood loss may be significant and the patient should have at least 4 U of banked blood available.

Procedure

Incision and Exposure

The bladder is approached in a manner similar to that described above. Before radical prostatectomy, a bilateral staging pelvic lymphadenectomy is carried out. This may be done laparoscopically. The lymph node packets lying in an area limited anteriorly by the external vein, inferiorly by the pelvic side wall, and posteriorly by the obturator nerve up to the bifurcation of the great vessels are then removed on the right then on the left (Fig. 26–37). The lymph nodes are sent for frozen section examination. If the lymph nodes do not contain tumor, attention is then turned to the prostatectomy.

Details

With the Balfour self-retaining retractor in place, the bladder is retracted toward the abdomen. A Foley catheter has been inserted into the bladder. The anterior

surface of the prostate is revealed and the endopelvic fascia can be identified and incised (Fig. 26–38). The dorsal venous complex and puboprostatic ligaments are then ligated and divided. The urethra is palpated and dissected from the rectum using a right-angled clamp. The urethra is cut, revealing the Foley catheter, which is also cut and its bladder end grasped (Figs. 26–39 and 26–40). This then allows the prostate to be lifted up, and further dissection of the posterior aspect of the prostate is carried out to reveal the lateral pedicles. These pedicles contain the neurovascular bundles which should be preserved to decrease the risk of postoperative impotence. The lateral pedicles are then divided using hemoclips (Fig. 26–41). Further posterior dissection is necessary to remove the seminal vesicle and divide the vas deferens; the specimen is then removed.

Closure

The bladder is brought down to the urethra, and a Foley catheter (24 Fr. 30-cc balloon) is placed in the bladder. The bladder is anastomosed to the urethra using interrupted sutures (Fig. 26–42). Drains are placed on either side of the bladder (either Penrose or closed suction devices), and closure is accomplished in a man-

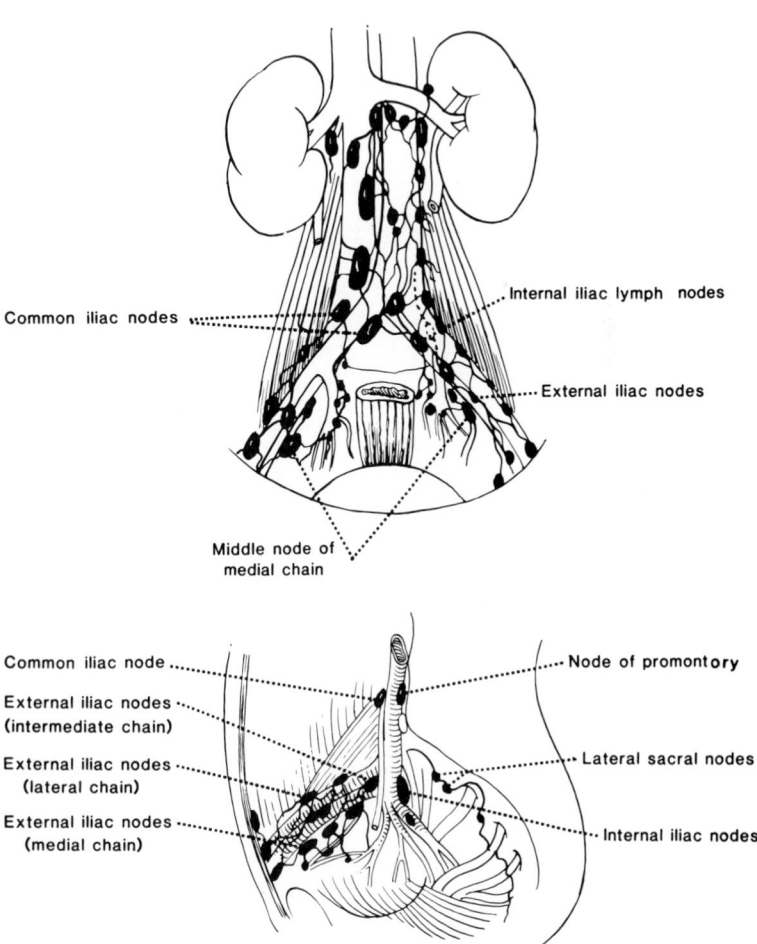

FIGURE 26–37. Lymph node anatomy of the pelvis. (From Walsh, P. C., Gittes, A. D., Perlmutter, R. F., Stamey, T. A. [Eds.]. [1986]. *Campbell's urology* [5th ed.] [p. 2650]. Philadelphia: W. B. Saunders.)

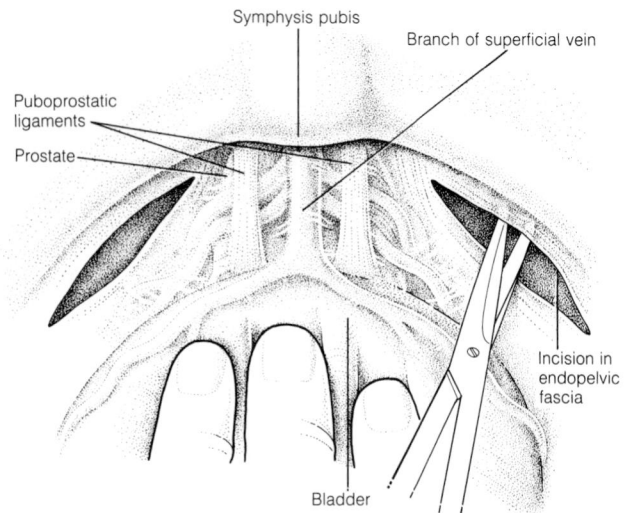

FIGURE 26–38. Incision of the endopelvic fascia. (From Walsh, P. C. [1988]. Radical retropubic prostatectomy: An anatomical approach with preservation of sexual function. In A. R. Mundy [Ed.], *Current operative surgery: Urology* [p. 40]. Philadelphia: Ballière Tindall.)

ner similar to that used for suprapubic prostatectomy. Postoperatively, the Foley catheter is left in place for 3 weeks to allow the urethrovesical anastomosis to heal.

Postoperative Care

Patients are admitted to the intensive care unit the first night after surgery for close monitoring.

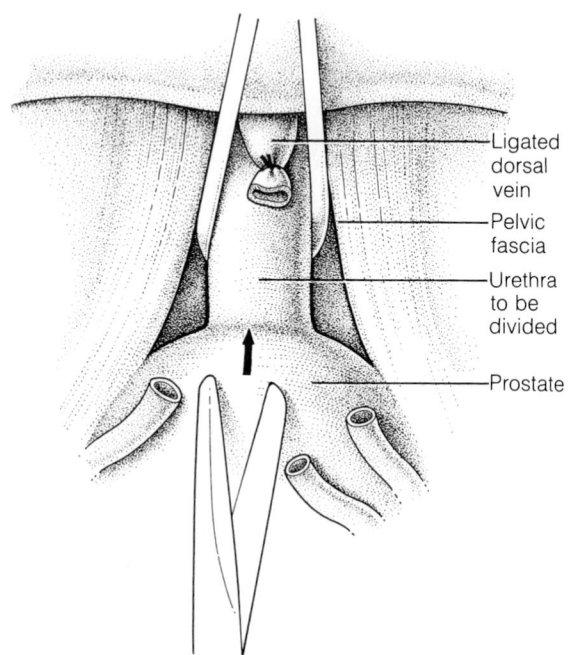

FIGURE 26–39. Transection of the urethra. (From Walsh, P. C. [1988]. Radical retropubic prostatectomy: An anatomical approach with preservation of sexual function. In A. R. Mundy [Ed.], *Current operative surgery: Urology* [p. 43]. Philadelphia: Ballière Tindall.)

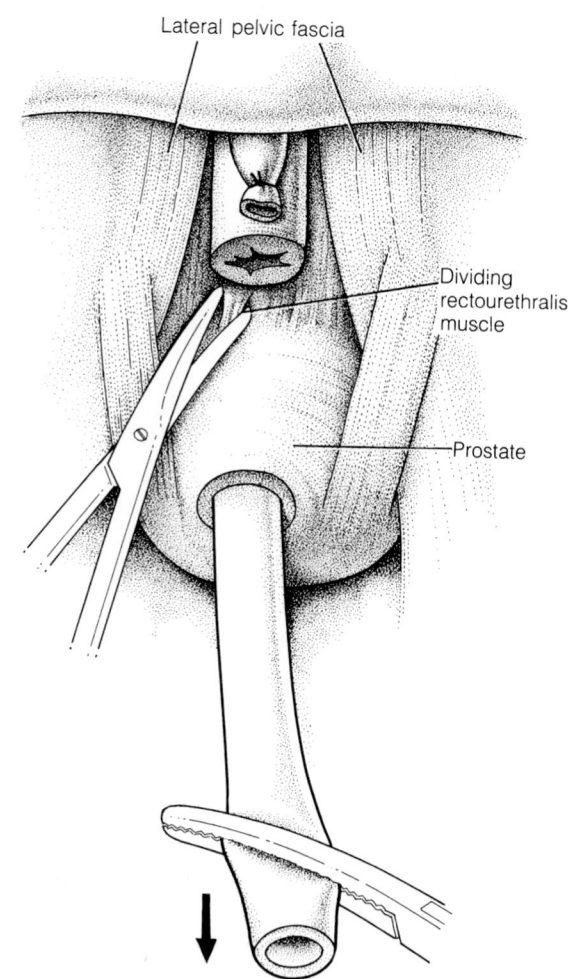

FIGURE 26–40. Posterior dissection of the prostate. (From Walsh, P. C. [1988]. Radical retropubic prostatectomy: An anatomical approach with preservation of sexual function. In A. R. Mundy [Ed.], *Current operative surgery: Urology* [pp. 43–44]. Philadelphia: Ballière Tindall.)

Nursing care focuses on measures to prevent thromboembolic sequelae, such as the use of knee-high antiembolism stockings, pneumatic or sequential compression stockings, and a footboard.

Respiratory care via incentive spirometry is provided every 4 hours while the patient is awake. Also, patients are ambulated the day after surgery.

Postoperative pain control is accomplished by a number of alternatives, such as an epidural catheter that can be injected by an anesthesiologist or the patient-controlled pump. Also used are intramuscular and oral pain medications, as well as patient-controlled intravenous pain medication.

The Foley catheter functions as a stent, bridging the urethral bladder neck anastomosis. The nurse must monitor the patency and functioning of the Foley catheter at all times.

The nurse is also responsible for strict intake and output measurements and for maintaining the Foley catheter in straight drainage. Minimal manipulation of the Foley is necessary to avoid aggravation of the anastomosis. Irrigation, if done at all, is usually done by the physician.

Additional postoperative orders are as follows:

Vital signs every hour for 8 hours, every 2 hours for the next 8 hours, then every 4 hours

Jackson-Pratt drain that is connected to bulb suction, which is reconstituted every shift

Nothing by mouth until the patient expels flatus

Nothing per rectum

Intravenous 5% dextrose in half-normal saline solution with 10 mEp/L of potassium chloride at 125 to 150 ml/hr

Medications:

Narcotic morphine sulfate or meperidine

Antibiotics for 48 hours

Antacids

Laboratory studies:

CBC and platelet count

Electrolytes, blood urea nitrogen, and creatinine determinations for 3 days postoperatively

Potential Surgical Complications

Intraoperative complications include hemorrhage and injury to nerve structures and to the rectum, which may be entered inadvertently. Rectal injury can be closed in two layers, provided that the patient has received a bowel preparation postoperatively.

Thrombophlebitis and pulmonary emboli are seen as early postoperative complications and can be minimized by the use of sequential compression devices and early ambulation. Disruption of the urethrovesical anastomosis may occur most often, leading to permanent

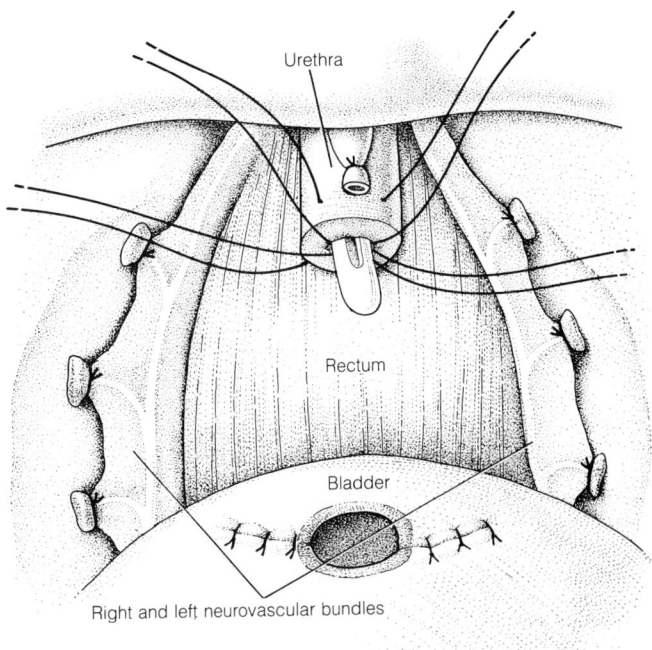

FIGURE 26–42. Anastomosis of the bladder to the urethra after removal of the prostate. (From Walsh, P. C. [1988]. Radical retropubic prostatectomy: An anatomical approach with preservation of sexual function. In A. R. Mundy [Ed.], *Current operative surgery: Urology* [p. 51]. Philadelphia: Ballière Tindall.)

incontinence and urine leak. This can be prevented by keeping the Foley catheter in place for the adequate length of time. Late postoperative complications include urinary bladder incontinence (5%) and impotence (at least 30%).

RADICAL CYSTECTOMY AND DIVERSION

Definition

Removal of the bladder is usually performed for invasive bladder cancer. Certain rare conditions, however, may also lead to removal of the bladder: intractable bleeding from hemorrhagic cystitis, pyocystis (chronically infected bladder), severe painful symptoms from interstitial cystitis, and severe cases of neurogenic bladder. *Simple* cystectomy refers to removal of the bladder only. *Radical* cystectomy is recommended for cancer therapy and includes removal of the iliac and obturator lymph node packets. In the male, the bladder, the peritoneum covering the bladder, the ureteral stumps, the seminal vesicles, the prostate, and a small part of the membranous urethra are removed (Fig. 26–43). In the female, the uterus, the anterior vaginal wall, the ovaries, the fallopian tubes, and the entire urethra are excised (Fig. 26–44). In addition, a procedure to divert the stream of urine is performed. Since the 1950s, the standard of care has been the Bricker ileal loop diversion. A large number of authors have described

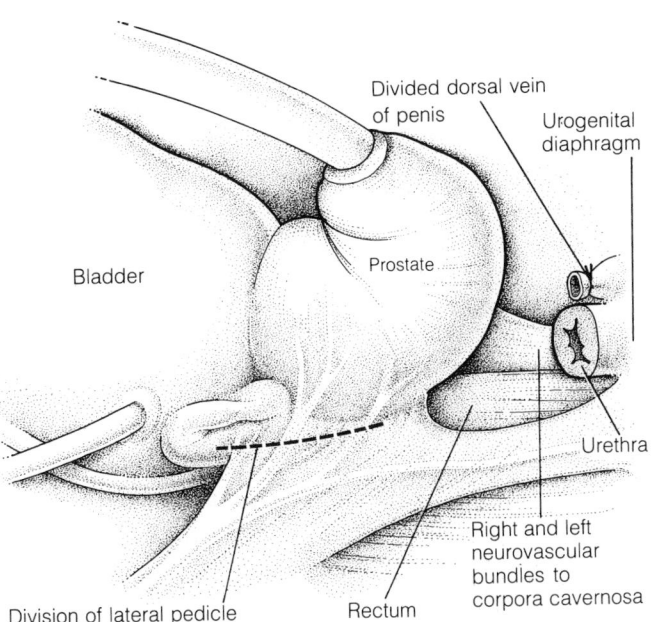

FIGURE 26–41. Division of the lateral pedicles. (From Walsh, P. C. [1988]. Radical retropubic prostatectomy: An anatomical approach with preservation of sexual function. In A. R. Mundy [Ed.], *Current operative surgery: Urology* [p. 46]. Philadelphia: Ballière Tindall.)

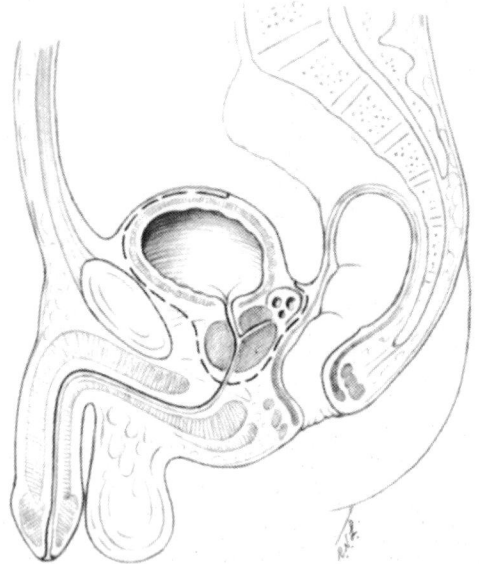

FIGURE 26–43. Simple cystectomy in the male means removal of the bladder with a portion of the overlying pelvic peritoneum, the ureteral stumps, the prostate, the seminal vesicles, and a portion of the membranous urethra. (From Richardson, J. R. [1986]. Simple and radical cystectomy. In W. S. McDougal [Ed.], *Operative surgery: Urology* [4th ed.] [p. 349]. Stoneham, MA: Butterworth.)

various techniques aimed at creating a continent urinary reservoir (DeKernion et al., 1991). Other techniques of diversion include colon conduit, ureterosigmoid diversion, and cutaneous ureterostomy.

Indications

Bladder cancer is usually found in patients older than age 50 and only rarely in younger patients. There are approximately 40,000 new cases a year with more than 70% of these occurring in a superficial form. The male-to-female ratio is 3:1. Gross or microscopic hematuria is present in 85% of cases. Patients may also note bladder irritability with increased frequency of urination, dysuria, and urgency. The diagnosis is made at cystoscopy when biopsy and transurethral resection of the lesion is carried out. The physical examination is usually unrevealing.

A general indication for radical cystectomy is transitional cell carcinoma of the bladder, which is invasive into the detrusor muscle. Diagnosis is confirmed by microscopic examination of bladder biopsy material obtained during cystoscopy. If the tumor extends into the urethra, urethrectomy should also be done.

Related Surgical Procedures

Partial cystectomy may be performed in selected patients, thus preserving voiding function. Several other surgical procedures, including open bladder surgery for stone disease, prostatectomy, and ureteral reimplantation employ a similar approach to the bladder.

Perioperative Nursing Implications

Anesthesia

Patients undergoing a radical cystectomy and diversion procedure are given a general anesthetic. Continuous epidural infusion may be used to supplement the general anesthetic as well as to help control postoperative pain. Blood is typed and cross-matched for possible transfusion. If an autologous blood supply has been arranged, these units should be administered first. The circulating nurse should follow hospital policy while assisting the anesthesiologist with blood transfusion. The circulating nurse may need to locate a blood warmer or a pressure bag for transfusion.

Position

Patients are placed in the supine position with a small roll under the sacrum. If urethrectomy is planned, the patient is placed in the relaxed lithotomy position. Owing to the length of the procedure, an eggcrate mattress is usually placed on the OR bed before the patient arrives. If the low lithotomy position is used, the patient's feet must be supported in the stirrups. Allen stirrups are recommended. In addition, make sure that routine precautions used with the lithotomy position are followed. A 28 to 30 Fr. red rubber catheter is inserted to act as a rectal tube. Thigh-high antiembolism or pneumatic compression stockings should be placed on the patient before the preparation begins.

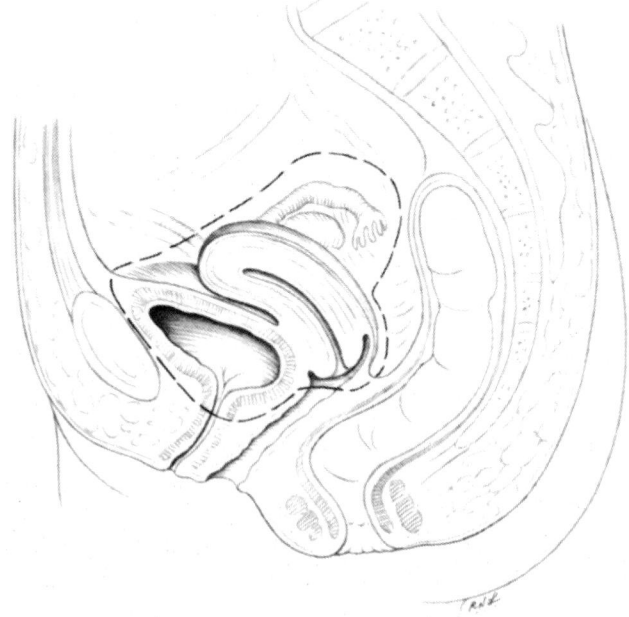

FIGURE 26–44. In the female patient, the uterus, ovaries, Fallopian tubes, and a portion of the vaginal vault and urethra are included in the surgical specimen. (From Richardson, J. R. [1986]. Simple and radical cystectomy. In W. S. McDougal [Ed.], *Operative surgery: Urology* [4th ed.] [p. 349]. Stoneham, MA: Butterworth.)

Creation and Maintenance of the Sterile Field

The patient is shaved from the nipple line to the midthigh. A povidone-iodine preparation is performed over the same area, including the penis in men and the perineum and vagina in women. Side towels should be placed by the circulator to avoid collection of preparation solution against the skin. These should be removed after the preparation is performed but before the patient is draped.

Creation and maintenance of the sterile field is challenging for the scrub nurse. Leg drapes must be used if the patient is in the low lithotomy position. Skin staples or sutures may be used to keep drapes in place. When the patient is in the lithotomy position, the Mayo stand can usually be brought between the legs and placed over one leg. Care must be taken to avoid leaning on the patient's legs by the members of the surgical team. Some surgeons need to work between the open legs during the procedure. Because the surgeons usually sit down, care must be taken to avoid contamination of other areas owing to changes in the height of the sterile field. If the Bookwalter self-retaining retractor is used, the pieces should be kept together on one small table so that the retractor can be moved from side to side of the operative field during placement of the retractor pieces.

The scrub nurse should have enough extra cartridges for the reusable disposable stapling device as requested by the surgeon.

During insertion and positioning of the single-J diversion stents, mineral oil should be provided to lubricate the end of the guidewire before insertion into the stent. The guidewire should remain on the back table in case the stents need to be reinserted or adjusted.

Equipment and Supplies

Patient and table drapes
Leg drapes (for lithotomy position)
Basin set
Laparotomy set
Vascular set
Gastric and bowel pack
Long instrument pack
Bookwalter self-retaining retractor
Malleable bladder blades for Balfour retractor (if used)
Army-Navy retractor
Curved mosquito
Reusable, disposable stapling devices
P-Linear Cutting Reloading Unit
Large laparotomy sponges
E-tape sponges
4 × 8 inch Raytek sponges
Electrosurgical pencil, cleaner, and extender tip
Suction tubing
Skin marker
Brown bag
Sterile light handles or light glove covers
Vessel loops
Webster cannula
24 Fr. Silastic Foley catheter with 30-ml balloon
Nos. 10, 11, and 15 blades
Pushers (Kittner)
50-ml and Asepto syringe
Large and medium hemoclips
Needle counter
1–0 and 2–0 chromic ties
3–0, 2–0, and 1–0 silk ties
No. 1, 3–0, 2–0, and 1–0 chromic swedge
4–0 and 5–0 chromic swedge (RB-1 needle)
1–0 Vicryl swedge (taper needle)
3–0 Vicryl swedge (taper needle)
Skin staples
3–0 silk swedge (CR-SH needle)
4–0 silk swedge (SH needle)
2 Mayo No. 3 taper-free needles
Retention sutures with bolsters
No. 28 or 30 Fr. red rubber rectal tube anchor with 3–0 silk on a Keith needle
Urostomy pouch with a skin barrier wafer (as ordered by the enterostomal therapist)
2 single-J diversion stents
3-ml syringe
Babcock sponges
1000 Steri-Drape (towel drape)
Small Allis clamps
Closed suction drains (e.g., Jackson-Pratt if the surgeon requests)
Gastrostomy tube (if the surgeon requests)

Drugs and Solutions

Sterile lubricant
Sterile mineral oil
Sterile normal saline for irrigation
Neomycin and polymixin B (Neosporin GU irrigant)

Physiological Monitoring

Blood loss during the radical cystectomy and diversion can be sudden and severe. The circulating nurse must provide current records of sponge and bottle blood loss, irrigation, and urine output. The circulator should also assist the anesthesiologist in the estimation of blood and urine volume on the surgical drapes.

Specimens and Cultures

Cultures are not usually indicated in this procedure, unless an infection is suspected. Specimens include

right and left distal ureter for frozen section examination
right and left iliac and obturator lymph node packets for routine processing

appendix

for males: bladder, peritoneum covering the bladder, ureteral stumps, seminal vesicles, prostate, and small amount of the membranous urethra

for female: bladder, uterus, anterior vaginal wall, ovaries, fallopian tubes, and entire urethra

Physician's Orders

Admittance 2 days before surgery

Diagnosis of bladder cancer

Vital signs every shift

Clear liquid diet; nothing-by-mouth status after midnight the night before surgery

Intravenous 5% dextrose in half-normal saline with 10 mEq/L of potassium chloride at 100 ml/hour

Incentive spirometry teaching

Enterostomal therapy consultation

Magnesium citrate, ½ bottle in the morning and in the afternoon 2 days before surgery and ½ bottle 1 day before surgery

Fleet enemas in the morning and in the afternoon 2 days before surgery

Tap water enemas until the return is clear in the morning and in the afternoon 1 day before surgery

Abdominal and genital povidone-iodine preparation at half strength 1 day before surgery and vaginal povidone-iodine douche for females

Erythromycin 1 g orally at 1 PM, 2 PM, 9 PM, and neomycin base, 1 g orally at 1 PM, 2 PM, and 9 PM, 1 day before surgery

Parenteral antibiotics before surgery

Vitamin K, 1 mg twice prior to surgery; alternatively, GoLYTELY preparation 1 day before surgery

Laboratory and Diagnostic Studies

Before undergoing cystectomy and diversion, the patient undergoes routine laboratory evaluation (as described for prostatectomy), chest x-ray film, ECG, bone scan, IVU, and CT scan. A standard mechanical bowel preparation is started 3 days before surgery. Preoperative incentive spirometry should be taught. The enterostomal therapist marks the location of the urinary stoma before the operation, and the patient should be familar with ostomy care and appliances.

Procedure

Incision and Exposure

A midline abdominal incision is made from the upper abdomen to the pelvis, around the umbilicus and at least 4 to 5 cm away from the medial aspect of the stomal site (Fig. 26–45). The peritoneal cavity is entered, and abdominal and pelvic exploration is carried out. The self-retaining retractor is placed (Balfour or Buckwalter, preferably the latter), and the intestines are packed superiorly with moist towels.

Details

The peritoneum overlying the ureters on either side is opened, and the ureters are dissected out, doubly ligated, with surgical clips, and divided. The proximal ends of the ureters are sent for frozen section examination to ensure that they are free of tumor. The ureters are left clamped to allow them to dilate. This facilitates the anastomosis between the bowel and the ureter. A tunnel is then made in the mesentery of the sigmoid colon so that the left ureter can be brought over to the right side.

Pelvic lymph node dissection is carried out on both sides; both obturator and iliac packets are taken. At the end of the dissection, the lateral pelvic walls and vessels should be free of any lymphatic tissue.

The bladder is dissected from the pelvic wall. In the female, dissection of the female genital organs is carried out. The ovarian and uterine vessels are ligated and divided. With a povidone-iodine–soaked sponge in the vagina, the vaginal cuff is removed and oversewn with a 1–0 chromic running stitch. The lateral pedicles containing blood supply and lymphatic drainage to the bladder are then identified.

Division of the lateral pedicles of the bladder is then performed posteriorly. Anteriorly, in the male, a maneuver similar to that for the radical suprapubic prostatectomy is used to divide the endopelvic fascia, the dorsal venous complex, and the urethra. In the female, the entire urethra is grasped at the bladder neck, dissected to the vulva, and removed with the bladder. Care is then taken to dissect the posterior aspect of the bladder, avoiding any injury to the rectosigmoid.

After removal of the bladder, the pelvis is packed with moist laparotomy pads. Appendectomy is performed in a standard fashion. An ileal conduit is constructed.

A loop of ileum is selected and measured to be approximately 15 cm in length, and the mesenteric vascular pedicle is prepared. The ileum is divided either between two clamps or with a GIA autostapling device. The conduit is placed in an inframesenteric position, and the ileum is reanastomosed. The mesenteric defect is closed (Fig. 26–46). The ureters are then anastomosed to the ileal loop. The ureters may be attached to the proximal end of the loop or directed into the loop by making small circular openings in the distal part of the loop (Figs. 26–47 and 26–48). Ureteroileal anastomosis is then performed using interrupted stitches of 4–0 chromic catgut. Before completing the anastomosis, ureteral stents (single-J 6 Fr.) are placed up to the kidney and brought through the stoma. Having completed the ureteroileal anastomosis, a circular incision in the abdominal wall is made at the site of the stoma (Fig. 26–49). Subcutaneous fatty tissue is removed, and a cruciate incision is made in the fascia. The ileal loop is then brought through the anterior abdominal wall and a stoma is fashioned (Fig. 26–50).

The pelvis is then carefully reinspected and hemostasis is established. Urine output from the ureteral stents should be carefully monitored, and the stents can be

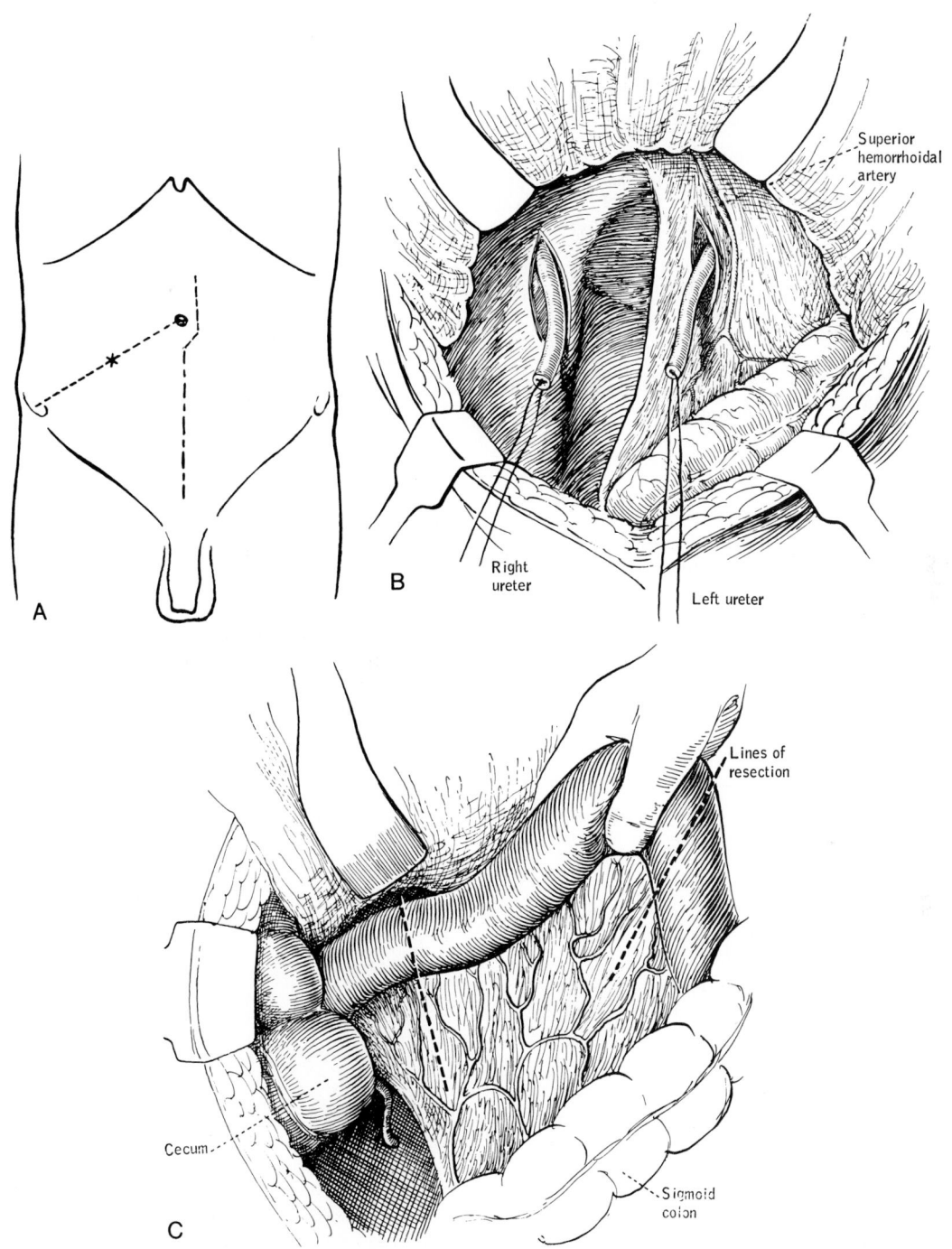

FIGURE 26–45. Major steps of an operation for ileal conduit, urinary diversion. *A*, Location of the ileal stoma. *B*, Ureters freed. The left ureter is brought under the base of the mesosigmoid. *C*, Location of the ileal segment. (From Cordonnier, J. J., [1963]. In M. F., Campbell [Ed.], *Urology* [2nd ed.]. Philadelphia: W. B. Saunders.)

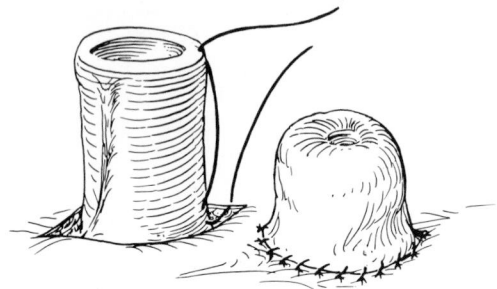

FIGURE 26–46. Method of stomal maturation to create a protruding "nipple" stoma. The suture should incorporate the subcuticular portion of the skin and the serosa of the loop at the level of the skin with the muscularis and mucosa of the distal end of the segment. (From Richie, J. P., Skinner, D. G. [1986]. Ureterointestinal diversion. In P. C. Walsh, R. F. Gittes, A. D. Perlmutter, T. A. Stamey [Eds.], *Campbell's urology* [5th ed.] [p. 2611]. Philadelphia: W. B. Saunders.)

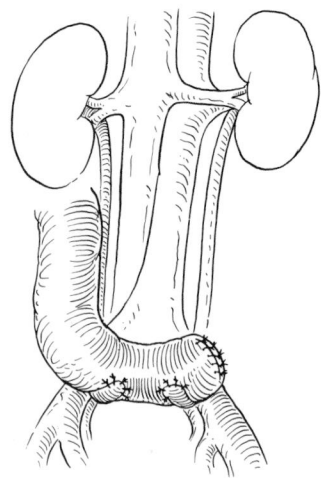

FIGURE 26–48. Bricker method of ureteral placement for ileal loop cutaneous diversion. (From Richie, J. P., Skinner, D. G. [1986]. Ureterointestinal diversion. In P. C. Walsh, R. F. Gittes, A. D. Perlmutter, T. A. Stamey [Eds.], *Campbell's urology* [p. 2605]. Philadelphia: W. B. Saunders.)

irrigated to ensure patency. The abdominal contents are reinspected and replaced in an anatomical position.

Closure

The ileal loop is placed in such a way that neither loop nor ureter is kinked. Drains are then placed in the pelvis and close to the ureteroileal anastomosis. The anterior abdominal wall is closed in a standard fashion. Skin staples are used to reapproximate the skin. Some surgeons recommend placement of a gastrostomy tube before closure.

Postoperative Care

After surgery, the patient is awakened and taken to the intensive care unit for at least a 24-hour observation period. During that time, careful monitoring of urine output and vigorous fluid replacement may be necessary to keep up with third spacing (loss of fluid from the intravascular space into the soft tissues and the abdominal cavity). Early ambulation and vigorous pulmonary toilet should prevent postoperative pulmonary complications. Postoperative orders include the following:

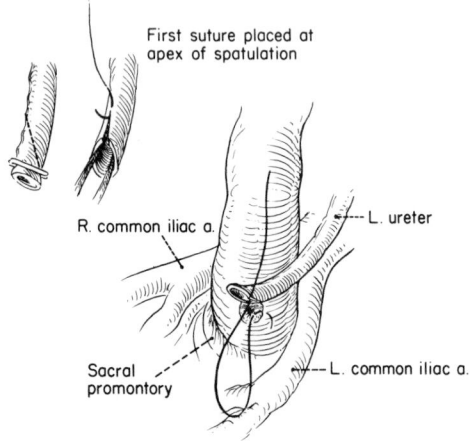

FIGURE 26–47. Left ureteroileal anastomosis. Note the medial spatulation of the ureter with placement of the first suture at the apex of the spatulation. A traction suture should be placed through the distal lateral margin of the ureter for traction, and care must be taken not to injure the ureter by mechanical manipulation of forceps. Correct placement of the sutures in the ileum should include the lateral edge of mucosa with a generous portion of the muscularis and serosa. This essentially telescopes the ureteroileal anastomosis into the ileum and takes tension off the direct mucosa-to-mucosa anastomosis. (From Richie, J. P., Skinner, D. G. [1986]. Ureterointestinal diversion. In P. C. Walsh, R. F. Gittes, A. D. Perlmutter, T. A. Stamey [Eds.], *Campbell's urology* [p. 2609]. Philadelphia: W. B. Saunders.)

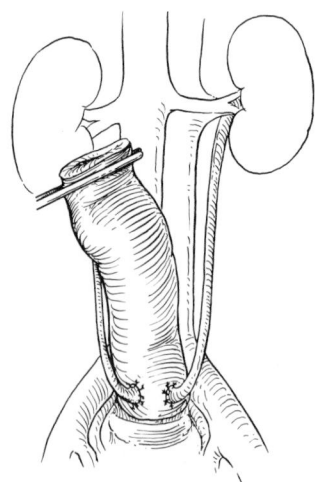

FIGURE 26–49. Leadbetter technique of ileal loop diversion. Note that the base of the ileal loop is sutured to the sacral promontory or to the fibrous tissue at the aortic bifurcation. The ureters are anastomosed end-to-side, either at the same level or staggered, according to the individual's anatomical characteristics. (From Richie, J. P., Skinner, D. G. [1986]. Ureterointestinal diversion. In P. C. Walsh, R. F. Gittes, A. D. Perlmutter, T. A. Stamey [Eds.], *Campbell's urology* [p. 2606]. Philadelphia: W. B. Saunders.)

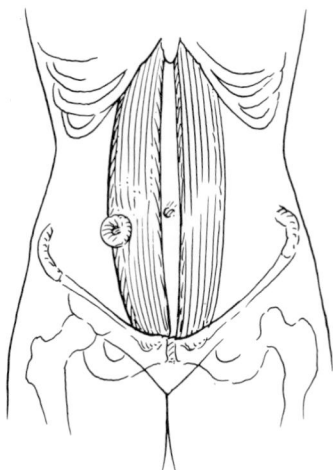

FIGURE 26–50. Correct placement of the stoma. The loop should be brought through the rectus muscle and the optimal placement determined before surgery with the patient placed in the supine, standing, and sitting positions. Care must be taken not to place the stoma too close to the umbilicus or bony protuberances, or in a skin fold. (From Richie, J. P., Skinner, D. G. [1986]. Ureterointestinal diversion. In P. C. Walsh, R. F. Gittes, A. D. Perlmutter, T. A. Stamey [Eds.], *Campbell's urology* [p. 2606]. Philadelphia: W. B. Saunders.)

Admit to the surgical intensive care unit.
Ascertain that the patient's condition is stable.
Obtain vital signs every hour for 12 hours, then every 2 hours for 12 hours, and then every 4 hours.
Strictly monitor intake and output.
Continue ECG and arterial catheter monitoring.
Connect the nasogastric tube to low intermittent suction.
Connect the gastrostomy tube to gravity drainage.
Connect the Hemovac to suction.
Perform chest physiotherapy and incentive spirometry every 2 hours while the patient is awake.
Maintain intermittent compression devices at all times.
Administer postoperative narcotics.
Administer antibiotics intravenously for 24 to 48 hours.
Give antacids.

Skin staples are removed on day 7 postoperatively. The ureteral stents are left in place for 2 to 3 weeks. The patient is usually discharged 10 to 15 days postoperatively.

Potential Surgical Complications

Immediate postoperative complications of radical surgery on the bladder are those encountered with any extensive procedure that also involves bowel surgery. Patients require large amounts of fluid to keep up with losses and third spacing. Blood loss may also be significant. Postoperatively, every measure to prevent pulmonary complications and deep venous thrombosis and/or pulmonary embolism should be taken. Early ureteroileal anastomosis disruption may occur and necessitates reoperation. Small-bowel obstruction may develop from adhesions formed in the peritoneal cavity.

Parastomal hernia results from a fascial defect at the level of the stoma. Revision may be required, if the loop does not drain properly.

Late complications include ureteroileal stenosis, which leads to obstruction of the flow of urine from the kidney to the ileal conduit. Metabolic disturbance may also develop in the form of metabolic acidosis.

Most complications from the procedure are related to the ileal loop diversion. Close patient follow-up and monitoring is therefore mandatory.

ENDOSCOPY

Direct observation of the entire urinary tract is possible with the use of refined endoscopic techniques. In the past, the cystoscope allowed examination of the bladder and the urethra. At present, the upper urinary tract can be visualized through ureteroscopy (rigid or flexible) and percutaneous nephroscopy. Furthermore, biopsy and resection of suspicious lesions as well as stone extraction and resection of the prostate can be performed endoscopically. The various endoscopic techniques, their applications, and the equipment used to carry them out are described.

Cystoscopy

Definition

Cystoscopic evaluation provides insight into the patient's urological condition. It is primarily a diagnostic tool.

Indications

Patients with hematuria (gross or microscopic), voiding dysfunction, recurrent infection, stone disease, and fistulas should undergo cystoscopy. The procedure may be done under local anesthesia on an outpatient basis.

Related Surgical Procedures

Related surgical procedures include urethroscopy and ureteroscopy.

Perioperative Nursing Implications

Cystoscopic equipment as all other endoscopic equipment is composed of a light source, sterile irrigation fluid (water or saline for cystoscopy), a working sheath, an obturator, and a set of optical lenses (0, 30, 70, and 120 degrees). The lenses are made up of a fiberoptic bundle that conveys light from the light source to the tip of the cystoscope. The light bundles are angulated at the tip of the cystoscope to direct light into the field of vision. A variety of fiberoptic cystoscopes are available. Video attachments are also available for use as teaching aids.

Bridges and deflector mechanisms permit the introduction and passage of ureteral stents. Through these components, electrosurgical devices (Bugbee electrode) and electrohydraulic lithotrite electrodes may be introduced. Cold cup biopsy forceps may also be passed through the sheath to biopsy urethral or bladder lesions. Flexible cystoscopes are available for patients who cannot be placed in the lithotomy position or cannot tolerate rigid cystoscopy.

Urine may be sent at the time of cystoscopy for culture, and bladder washings may be obtained for cytological examination. Associated diagnostic studies such as IVU or renal ultrasound should be available for review.

Procedure

During the procedure, the cystoscope is carefully advanced under direct vision. Examination of the urethra, the prostate in the male, and the bladder is carried out. Suspicious lesions should be biopsied with the cold cup biopsy forceps. Areas of bleeding may be fulgurated using the Bugbee electrode. Imaging of the ureters and upper collecting system may be performed by retrograde injection of contrast material using bulb-tipped catheters. Ureteral catheters may also be placed at the time of cystoscopy.

Postoperative Care

Postoperatively, the patient should be instructed to increase his or her fluid intake for 24 to 48 hours and warned of possible symptoms such as urgency, frequency, and burning on urination. Gross hematuria can be expected. The patient should be given a prescription for oral antibiotics to be taken for 3 to 5 days. If the patient is unable to void or experiences fevers and chills, he or she should report immediately to the physician.

Transurethral Resection

Transurethral Resection of the Prostate

Definition

Resection for benign prostatic hypertrophy may be accomplished endoscopically if the prostate gland is of moderate size and if it does not extend into the bladder, obscuring the ureteral orifices. Resectoscopes are similar to cystoscopes but include additional components. There are different types of resectoscopes: McCarthy, Nesbit, Iglesias, Baumrucker, and continuous flow resectoscopes. Elements of the resectoscopes are obturator, sheath, working element, cutting loops, and lens. Isotonic nonhemolytic and nonelectrolyte irrigation fluid (1.5% glycine solution) provides a clear visualization during the procedure.

Indications

Indications for transurethral resection of the prostate are similar to those for suprapubic prostatectomy.

Related Surgical Procedures

Related surgical procedures include transurethral resection of bladder tumors, endoscopic extraction of bladder tumors, and endoscopic resection of urethral strictures and posterior urethral valves.

Perioperative Nursing Implications/ Procedure

The surgeon should check the equipment with the nurse and may elect to dilate the urethra using sounds. Cystoscopy may be performed before resection. The resectoscope sheath and obturator are then lubricated generously and passed into the urethra and then to the bladder. The working element with lens and cutting loop is then inserted. Light cord, irrigation tubing, and electrosurgical cord are connected. Current setting for cutting and cautery should be set and the patient grounded by the circulating nurse. The surgeon controls the delivery of current via a foot pedal. Resection of the prostate is then carried out. Landmarks for resection are the ureteral orifices and the verumontanum. Careful monitoring of bladder filling by irrigation fluid should be performed to prevent overdistention and possible bladder rupture. The enlarged lobes of the prostate are removed piecemeal, leaving the capsule intact. Bleeding vessels are cauterized with cutting loops. Blood clots and prostatic chips are then removed by manual irrigation of the bladder using either an Ellik evacuator or a Toomey syringe, placed on the resectoscope sheath. The prostatic chips are sent to the pathology department for microscopic examination.

After evacuation of the bladder, the prosatic fossa is reinspected carefully for bleeding points and residual chips. These should be removed. The resectoscope sheath is then removed and a Foley catheter is inserted (two or three way, 22 or 24 Fr., with 30-ml balloon). Traction on the Foley catheter helps tamponade persistent venous ooze from the prostatic fossa. Isotonic saline solution for continuous bladder irrigation may be started, and the Foley catheter is attached to a 2000-ml drainage system. If continuous bladder irrigation is used, careful monitoring of the system is mandatory.

Postoperative Care

Postoperative observation includes monitoring of urine output, mental status, and abdominal girth. Routine laboratory evaluation should be obtained for at least 2 days (CBC, electrolyte, blood urea nitrogen, and creatinine determinations). The bladder irrigation may be discontinued when the urine is clear or light rose-colored and the Foley catheter is removed 48 hours postoperatively.

Transurethral Resection of Bladder Tumor

Transitional cell carcinoma of the urinary tract covers a broad spectrum from superficial lesions to aggressive, invasive tumors. It is also ubiquitous but most frequently found in the bladder. It is also known to recur and therefore necessitates careful follow-up.

Perioperative Nursing Implications

At the time of evaluation for bladder tumor, panendoscopy of the urethra and bladder is carried out. Random biopsy specimens of the bladder and bladder washings for cytological examination are obtained. Preoperatively, radiological imaging of the entire urinary tract should be performed. Tumors that are found to invade into the muscle layer of the bladder are treated with radical cystectomy. At the time of transurethral resection, bladder tumor, adjacent mucosa, and a portion of the bladder wall are removed to evaluate the extent of invasion by the tumor.

Procedure

The setup, instruments, and procedure are similar to those for transurethral resection of the prostate. A retrograde pyelogram may be performed at the same time. Sterile water or normal saline may be used for irrigation fluid. Electrocautery is used to ensure hemostasis after resection of the tumor. A large Foley catheter (22 or 24 Fr.) is left in place postoperatively for 24 to 48 hours.

Superficial bladder tumors may be treated with the neodymium:yttrium-aluminum-garnet laser. The laser beam is transmitted through a flexible glass fiber passed through the cystoscope sheath. Bladder tumors are cauterized by pulses of laser beam. There is minimal bleeding associated with the procedure and the operating time is short. No catheter drainage of the bladder is necessary, and the procedure can be done on an outpatient basis.

Postoperative Care

Postoperative care in patients having undergone transurethral resection of bladder tumor is similar to that after transurethral resection of the prostate. Bladder irrigation is not used.

Ureteroscopy

Definition

Transurethral endoscopic evaluation of the upper urinary tract is an addition to the urological procedures. The procedure, using a long, narrow, rigid or flexible endoscope, enables access to the upper urinary tract: ureter, pelvis, and calyces. Because it entails the use of biopsy forceps, baskets, and laser attachment, ureteroscopy is both a diagnostic tool and a therapeutic instrument.

Indications

Indications for ureteroscopy are shown on Table 26–6.

TABLE 26–6. INDICATIONS FOR URETEROSCOPY

Evaluation and Treatment of Urothelial Tumors

Direct visualization
Biopsy
Selective cytological evaluation
Electrocoagulation
Resection
Laser photocoagulation
Follow-up

Evaluation and Treatment of Ureteral Obstruction

Examination and localization of stones and ureteral strictures
Guidewire placement
Ureteral dilation
Stone disintegration and/or retrieval
Internal ureterotomy
Stent placement

Evaluation and Treatment of Upper Urinary Tract Bleeding

Localization of bleeding sites
Diagnosis
Treatment

Foreign Body Retrieval

Displaced or fragmented ureteral stents
Extraction of broken instrument parts

Related Surgical Procedures

Related surgical procedures include any endoscopic procedure.

Physician's Orders, Laboratory and Diagnostic Studies

Typical admissions orders include routine laboratory evaluation as described above. Preoperative and postoperative intravenous antibiotics are recommended because of pyelorenal backflow of urine and irrigation fluid during the procedure.

Postoperatively, urine output monitoring is important. Most patients have ureteral stents left in place, and careful measuring of the urine production must be carried out. Irrigation of the stent may be necessary to alleviate obstruction by either clot or stone fragments. Most patients experience pain similar to that of renal colic and bladder spasm. Analgesics must therefore be administered for 24 to 48 hours after the procedure.

Stent removal may be performed as early as 48 hours postoperatively. Further radiological studies may be carried out before removal of the ureteral stents.

Procedure

Ureteroscopy necessitates cystoscopic examination. In the female, the cystoscope sheath may be left in place. In the male, the sheath is removed. The ureteral orifice is identified, and a cone-tipped retrograde ureterogram with preinjection and postinjection films is taken to identify the course of the ureter. A floppy-tipped guidewire is then passed up the ureter to the pelvis under fluoroscopic guidance. The lower ureter is then dilated by either using bougies (up to 16 Fr.) or balloon dilator. The ureteroscope is then passed into the bladder, through the ureteral orifice, and carefully advanced up the ureter to the pelvis along the guidewire.

Identification, biopsy, and treatment of papillary tumors may then be carried out. Stones, the most common indication for ureteroscopy, can be extracted using a basket or three-pronged grabber or disintegrated with ultrasonic equipment or an electrohydraulic lithotripter. Because none of the stone-extracting instruments work all the time, a wide variety of accessories should be available during the procedure.

After diagnosis and treatment has been achieved, a retrograde study of the ureter and pelvis should be done to check the integrity of the upper urinary tract. A ureteral stent is then left in place after removal of the ureteroscope. Foley catheter drainage of the bladder is carried out for 24 to 48 hours.

Postoperative Care

Postoperative care for ureteroscopy is similar to that for percutaneous endoscopy.

Percutaneous Endoscopy of the Renal Pelvis (Percutaneous Nephroscopy)

Definition

Percutaneous puncture of the urinary collecting system has become possible with the development of fluoroscopy and nephrostomy tube drainage. The basic principle is to obtain access to the collecting system under x-ray guidance and place a tube into it, which is then used as a track. The track can be dilated to allow the passage of a nephroscope. The nephroscope permits visualization of the collecting system. Stones may be fragmented and extracted under direct vision.

Indications

The principal indication for percutaneous nephroscopy is stone removal. Nephroscopy may also be employed to diagnose and treat urothelial tumors not accessible by ureteroscopy.

Perioperative Nursing Implications

The large majority of patients have staghorn calculi (large infectious stones that take up most of the collecting system). The patient may therefore have a history of urinary tract infection. Flank pain and recurrent urinary tract infection are common presenting symptoms.

The patient undergoes radiological evaluation and placement of a nephrostomy tube in the radiology suite.

X-ray films must be available for review. Routine preoperative evaluation should be carried out. Preoperative parenteral antibiotic therapy is mandatory and the patient should have blood available in the blood bank. Urine must be sent for culture to identify possible pathogens.

Procedure

With the patient in the prone position under epidural or general anesthesia, and under fluoroscopic guidance, a wire is advanced through the nephrostomy tube down the ureter to the bladder. The nephrostomy tube is then removed and the track is dilated with Teflon dilators (12 to 30 Fr.). A working sheath is passed over the largest dilator and the nephroscope is inserted through the sheath. Examination of the collecting system is carried out. Stones may be extracted directly, if they are small enough to be grasped and passed through the sheath, or they are fragmented using the ultrasonic probe. A flexible nephroscope may be used to gain access to the calyces. After extraction or disintegration of the stones, the collecting system is reinspected and contrast material is injected to ensure the integrity of the system. A larger nephrostomy tube (22 Fr. Malecot) is placed via the working sheath, which is then removed. The nephrostomy tube is sewn into place and a sterile dressing is applied.

The patient keeps the nephrostomy tube in place for approximately 2 weeks, at which time it is removed after x-ray evaluation of the collecting system. Similarly, the nephroscope can be used to diagnose urothelial tumor of the collecting system in selected patients. Laser photocoagulation may be used to treat these cancerous lesions.

Postoperative Care

Postoperative orders are similar to those for ureteroscopy. Urine output should be monitored carefully and parenteral antibiotics administered for at least 48 hours. Laboratory studies include CBC and electrolyte, blood urea nitrogen, and creatinine determinations.

Perioperative Nursing Implications

Anesthesia

Endoscopic procedures can be performed under general, regional, or local anesthesia. During general or regional anesthesia, the circulating nurse should assist the anesthesiologist in any way possible. If an anesthesiologist is not present during the local endoscopic examination, the circulating nurse should follow hospital policy and Association of Operating Room Nurses Recommended Practice on the Care of Patients Receiving Local Anesthesia (AORN, 1983). These patients are not routinely typed and cross-matched for blood transfusion.

Position

Positioning requirements vary according to the type of procedure being performed. In each of these positions, routine precautions (Table 26–7) for positioning should be followed (refer to Chapter 12).

When positioning the patient, the circulator must consider whether the image intensifier will be used during the procedure. The patient must be positioned on the OR bed so that the area in question is clear of any object that would interfere with the image picture of the patient's body part. A special endoscopy table is manufactured by a few companies. This table offers many advantages in the positioning of patients and the use of radiological studies.

Creation and Maintenance of the Sterile Field

Shaving is not usually performed for endoscopic procedures. The preparation is usually done with a povidone-iodine solution, encompassing the appropriate area (see Table 26–7).

During many endoscopic procedures, a scrub nurse may not be required after the instruments are set up and the patient is prepared and draped. Of supreme importance during the draping is the creation of a dry environment to avoid strike through contamination. Sterile, adherent, impervious drapes should be used to proved a barrier when draping the patient. In addition, impervious gowns should be worn by the surgical team. Protective eyewear and boots are also recommended. If the rectum is to be isolated from the surgical area, an impervious transurethral resection (TUR) drape should be used.

All endoscopic equipment such as telescopes, sheaths, obturators, and bridges are delicate instruments. The scrub nurse should use care when handling these items and instruct the surgical team in this routine as necessary.

Equipment and Supplies

Equipment and supplies used during an endoscopic examination also vary according to the procedure. The circulator should have the following equipment available before the start of the procedure:

Cystoscopy

Transurethral resection drape pack
Cystoscopy set
Transurethral resection Y tubing
Irrigation fluid (3000-ml bags)
Silastic Foley catheter (size by the surgeon's choice)
Preparation set
Raytek 4 × 8 inch sponges

Retrocath insertion

Ureteral catheter (according to the surgeon's preference)
Ureteral drainage bag
Catheter deflecting mechanism

Ureteroscopy

Transurethral resection drape pack
Cystoscopy set
Transurethral resection Y tubing
Raytek 4 × 8 inch sponges
Preparation set
Irrigation fluid (3000-ml bags)
Silastic Foley catheter
Angled ureteroscope
Impervious plastic drapes
Bulb or Asepto syringe
20-ml syringe
Guidewires
Ureteral catheters
Ureteral drainage bag
Stone baskets
9.5 ureteroscope
Flexible ureteroscope
Ultrasound probe

Percutaneous Nephroscopy

Patient drape
Table drape
Impervious drapes
Plastic set
Percutaneous nephrolithotomy tray

TABLE 26–7. POSITION AND PREPARATION OF PATIENTS UNDERGOING ENDOSCOPIC PROCEDURES

Procedure	Position	Area Prepared	Irrigation Solution
Cystoscopy	Lithotomy	Perineum, genitalia, and lower abdomen	Water or saline
Transurethral resection of the prostate	Lithotomy	Perineum, genitalia, and lower abdomen	Glycine
Transurethral resection of the bladder	Lithotomy	Perineum, genitalia, and lower abdomen	Water or saline
Ureteroscopy	Lithotomy	Perineum, genitalia, and lower abdomen	Water or saline
Percutaneous nephrolithotomy	Prone*	Nephrostomy†	Saline

*Pillows under chest, hips, and legs.
†Tube site and surrounding area.

Ultrasonic probe
Transurethral resection Y tubing
Raytek 4 × 8 inch sponges
Suction tubing
1 No. 10 blade
1 2–0 Prolene suture (cutting needle)
Bulb syringe
20-ml syringe
Malecot catheter (20, 24, 28, or 32 Fr. according to the surgeon's preference)
Urine drain bag

Transurethral Resection of the Prostate and Bladder

Transurethral resection drape
Transurethral resection flow pouch system and extension set
Iglesias resectoscope set
Transurethral resection basin
Irrigation fluid
20-ml syringe
Transurethral resection drape
Silastic Foley catheter and 30-ml balloon (size according to the surgeon's preference)
Preparation set
Raytek 4 × 8 inch sponges

Drugs and Solutions

Drugs and solutions are important to endoscopic examination. The continuous, uninterrupted flow of the desired irrigation solution allows surgeons good visualization of the area (see Table 26–7). In addition, during resection of tissue or stone dissolution, the irrigation provides a timely removal of debris. Listed below are the drugs and solutions used for urological endoscopic procedures:

Normosol solution for bladder washings and urinary tract washings
Iothalamate meglumine for contrast visualization via x-ray film or image
Sterile water for irrigation
Sterile saline solution for irrigation
Glycine solution
Lubricant K-Y jelly
Lidocaine uroject for local procedures

Physiological Monitoring

Blood loss is not usually severe during endoscopic procedures but, because of the nature of endoscopy, blood loss estimation is more difficult. Blood is washed out with the irrigation fluid and usually flows into a drain of some type. Screens can be used to catch stones, tissue, and so on, but do not filter smaller particles.

Specimens and Cultures

Routine bladder washings and/or right and left ureteral washings are sent for cytological examination and routine culture and sensitivity testing. Specimens may include

stone fragments
bladder chips
prostate chips
bladder biopsy specimen
prostate biopsy specimen
kidney or ureter biopsy specimen

Laboratory Studies

Before a patient undergoes endoscopy of the upper urinary tract (either ureteroscopy or percutaneous nephroscopy), routine preoperative laboratory tests are required. Urinalysis and urine culture are mandatory.

Postoperative Care

After an endoscopic procedure, the patient will have an indwelling ureteral catheter or stent. The stent will be placed in the renal collecting system and exit through either the skin or the bladder and urethra. Careful monitoring of urine output through various catheters and stents is required. Postoperative orders include the following:

Admit to the floor
Ascertain that the patient's condition is stable
Obtain vital signs every 4 hours
Strictly monitor intake and output (output should be recorded for each drainage device)
Call physician if there is any evidence of drainage device occlusion
Administer antibiotics intravenously for 48 hours
Administer postoperative narcotics

Potential Surgical Complications

Cystoscopy and Transurethral Resection

Potential complications from cystoscopy include injuries to the urethra and to the bladder. Incontinence, erectile dysfunction, retrograde ejaculation, and persistent voiding symptoms are potential complications of transurethral resection of the prostate. Some patients may experience post-TUR syndrome caused by dilutional hyponatremia and experience the sudden onset of tachycardia, hypotension, tachypnea, and mental status changes. This is a life-threatening situation, and therapy is aimed at rapid correction of the electrolyte imbalance.

Ureteroscopy

Ureteral perforation and disruption, urinary extravasation, instrument breakage, bleeding, and infection can occur. The principal long-term complication of ureteroscopy is the development of ureteral strictures.

Percutaneous Nephroscopy

The most significant immediate complications are infection or sepsis and hemorrhage. Extravasation of contrast material outside the collecting system can also be seen but is usually not a problem, provided there is adequate drainage of the collecting system. Injury of adjacent structure is possible but rare. Approximately 5% of patients experience a pleural effusion, which resolves spontaneously over time.

Bibliography

American Medical Systems. (1985). *AMS operating room manual.* Minnetonka, MN.

Association of Operating Room Nurses. (1993). *Standards and recommended practice for perioperative nursing.* Denver.

Benson, G. S. (1987). The penis, sexual function and dysfunction. In J. Y. Gillenwater, J. T. Grayhack, S. S. Howards, J. W. Duckett (Eds.), *Adult and pediatric urology.* Chicago: Mosby-Year Book.

Brogna, L., Lakasawski, M. (1986). The continent urostomy. *American Journal of Nursing, 86*(2), 160–163.

Clayman, R. V., Bagley, D. H. (1987). In J. Y. Gillenwater, J. T. Grayhack, S. S. Howards, J. W. Duckett (Eds.), *Adult and pediatric urology.* Chicago: Mosby-Year Book.

Clemente, D. (1981). *Anatomy—A regional atlas of the human body* (2nd ed.). Baltimore: Urban & Schwarzenberg.

Crafts, R. C. (1979). *Textbook of human anatomy* (2nd ed.). New York: Wiley.

Cubler, A. J., Whalen-Myers, M. A. (1985). Ureteroscopy—Using endoscopes for ureterolithotripsy. *AORN Journal, 42,* 853–858.

DeKernion, J. B., Stenzl, A., Mukamel, I. (1991). Urinary diversion and continent reservoir. In J. Y. Gillenwater, J. T. Grayhack, S. S. Howards, J. W. Duckett (Eds.), *Adult and pediatric urology.* Chicago: Mosby-Year Book.

Duckett, F. W. (1987). Hypospadias. In J. Y. Gillenwater, J. T. Grayhack, S. S. Howards, J. W. Duckett (Eds.), *Adult and pediatric urology.* Chicago: Mosby-Year Book.

Freiha, F. S. (1991). Open bladder surgery. In P. C. Walsh, A. B. Retik, T. A. Stamey, E. D. Vaughan (Eds.), *Campbell's urology* (6th ed.). Philadelphia: W. B. Saunders.

Goodwin, W. E., Scott, W. W. (1952). Phalloplasty. *Journal of Urology, 68,* 903–908.

Gordon, M. (1987). *Manual of nursing diagnosis: 1986–1987.* New York: McGraw-Hill.

Gray, M. (1980). Myology. In P. L. Williams, J. R. Warwick (Eds.), *Gray's anatomy* (36th British ed.). Philadelphia: W. B. Saunders.

Grayhack, J. T. (1983). Nephrectomy. In J. T. Glenn (Ed.), *Urologic surgery.* Philadelphia: J. B. Lippincott.

Grayhack, J. T., Kozlowski, J. M. (1991). Benign prostatic hyperplasia. In J. Y. Gillenwater, J. T. Grayhack, S. S. Howards, J. W. Duckett (Eds.), *Adult and pediatric urology.* Chicago: Mosby-Year Book.

Green, L. F. Transurethral surgery (1986). In P. C. Walsh, R. F. Gittes, A. D. Perlmutter, T. A. Stamey (Eds.), *Campbell's urology* (5th ed.). Philadelphia: W. B. Saunders.

Herman, J. R. (1983). *Handbook of urology.* New York: Harper & Row.

Hippocrates, Hippocratic Oath, 430 B.C.

Kaye, K. W., Goldberg, M. E. (1982). Applied anatomy of the kidney and ureters. *Urologic Clinics of North America, 9,* 3–13.

La Fallette, S. S. (1987). Radical retropubic prostatectomy. *AORN Journal, 45,* 57–71.

Loening, S. A. (1985). The prostate. In D. A. Culp, B. Fallon, S. A. M. Loening (Eds.), *Surgical urology* (5th ed.). Chicago: Year Book Medical.

Lowler, P. E. (1984). Benign prostatic hyperplasia. *AORN Journal, 40,* 745–750.

Lyon, E. S., Huttman, J. L., Bagley, D. M. (1989). Ureteroscopy and ureteropyeloscopy. In E. D. Whitehead (Ed.), *Current operative urology.* J. B. Lippincott.

Macky, W. (1986). Transvesical prostatectomy. In W. S. McDougal (Ed.), *Operative surgery: Urology* (4th ed.). Stoneham, MA: Butterworth.

Martinez-Pinero, J. A. (1986). Ileal conduit diversion. In W. S. McDougal (Ed.), *Operative surgery: Urology* (4th ed.). Stoneham, MA: Butterworth.

Mayo, M. E., Longe, P. H. (1991). Percutaneous approach to urologic surgery. In J. Y. Gillenwater, J. T. Grayhack, S. S. Howards, J. W. Duckett (Eds.), *Adult and pediatric urology.* Chicago: Mosby-Year Book.

McConnel, E. A., Zimmerman, M. G. (1983). *Care of patients with urologic problems.* Philadelphia: J. B. Lippincott.

McVay, C. B. (1984). *McVay and Anson surgical anatomy* (6th ed.). Philadelphia: W. B. Saunders.

Novick, A. C., Streem, S. B. (1991). Surgery of the kidney. In P. C. Walsh, A. B. Retik, T. A. Stamey, E. D. Vaughan (Eds.), *Campbell's urology* (5th ed.). Philadelphia: W. B. Saunders.

Orihuela E., Smith A. D. (1988). Percutaneous treatment of transitional cell carcinoma of the upper urinary tract. *Urologic Clinics of North America, 15,* 425–431.

Pansadoro, V. (1983). The posterior lumbotomy. *Urologic Clinics of North America, 10,* 573.

Pavolowski, J. (1984). Percutaneous nephrolithotripsy: A nurse care plan. *AORN Journal, 39,* 779–781.

Pavolowski, J. (1986). Intraoperative nursing responsibilities during percutaneous surgery. *AUAA Journal, 6,* 7.

Petillo, M. H. (1987). The patient with a urinary stoma—nursing management and patient education. *Nursing Clinics of North America, 22,* 263–279.

Richardson, J. R. (1986). Simple and radical cystectomy. In W. S. McDougal (Ed.), *Operative surgery: Urology* (4th ed.). Stoneham, MA: Butterworth.

Richie, J. P., Skinne, D. G. (1986). Ureterointestinal diversion. In P. C. Walsh, R. F. Gittes, A. D. Perlmutter, T. A. Stamey (Eds.), *Campbell's urology* (5th ed.). Philadelphia: W. B. Saunders.

Robson, C. J. (1983). Radical nephrectomy. In J. T. Glenn (Ed.), *Urologic surgery.* Philadelphia: J. B. Lippincott.

Robson, C. J. (1986). Radical nephrectomy. In W. S. McDougal (Ed.), *Operative surgery: Urology* (4th ed.). Stoneham, MA: Butterworth.

Rohner, J. J. (1986). Simple nephrectomy. In W. S. McDougal (Ed.), *Operative surgery: Urology* (4th ed.). Stoneham, MA: Butterworth.

Sant, J. P. (1986). Artificial urinary sphincter—Restoring continence. *AORN Journal, 43,* 866–875.

Smith, M. D. (1988). Endourology update. *Urologic Clinics of North America, 15.*

Stone, L. (1984). Percutaneous nephrolithotripsy. *AORN Journal, 39,* 773–779.

Thompson, H. C., King, L. R., Knox, E., et al. (1975). Ad Hoc Task force on circumcision report. *Pediatrics, 560,* 610.

Walsh, P. C. (1988). Radical retropubic prostatectomy: An anatomical approach with preservation of sexual function in current operative surgery. In A. R. Mundy (Ed.), *Urology.* Philadelphia: Baillière Tindall.

Walsh, P. C. (1991). Retropubic prostatectomy for benign and malignant diseases. In F. F. Marshall (Ed.), *Operative urology.* Philadelphia: W. B. Saunders.

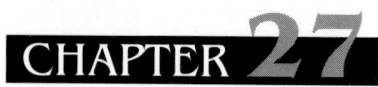

CHAPTER 27

Orthopedic Surgery

Barbara Jeane Kalman

DEFINITION

The term *orthopedic* has been adopted from the Greek words: *orthos*, meaning straight and *pais*, meaning child. The specialty of orthopedic surgery has an extremely broad scope. The subject matter concerns the deformities, diseases, and injuries of bones and joints and of their related structures, which include tendons, ligaments, muscles, and nerves. The emphasis of orthopedic surgery is placed equally on the prevention and the correction of a deformity or disability and not just on surgical intervention.

ANATOMY

The musculoskeletal system is made up of bones, joints between bones, muscles, tendons, ligaments, and cartilage. As a whole, it is responsible for body shape and support, protection of internal organs, and locomotion.

Bones

The skeletal system is composed of 206 bones, which compose the supportive framework of the body and its appendages (Fig. 27–1).

The internal and external structures of bone are shown in Figure 27–2. Bone forms by the process of *ossification* through either a membranous or a cartilaginous phase. The bone formed by membranous ossification is spongy or cancellous. It is normally found in flat, irregular, and short bones and in the epiphysis of the long bones. The process begins with the secretion of an intercellular substance composed of calcium salts by cells called *osteoblasts*. This deposit of calcium salts is known as *calcification*. Osteoblasts surrounded by the matrix of calcium salts form a network of trabeculae, which become entrapped and fuse. The trapped cells are termed *osteocytes*. The trabeculae of cancellous bone never fuse and the remaining spaces become filled with bone marrow. The fibrous membrane that surrounds the growing bone mass forms the periosteum.

The second type of ossification is cartilaginous, referring to bone formation within hyaline cartilage. It is also known as endochondral ossification and occurs in the diaphysis, or shaft, of long bones. The bone that is formed is compact and replaces the cartilaginous model. Along with a change in pH, the deposit of calcium salts begins the calcification of cartilage. Osteoblasts are produced and begin to form an outer surface bone around the middiaphysis. Blood vessels along with osteoblasts arise from the newly formed periosteum into cavities of the diaphysis. These spaces will become the marrow cavity. The epiphyseal ends of the bone eventually derive their blood supply from the transformed periosteum. As the ossification proceeds, the cartilaginous model grows in length at the epiphyseal ends. The area between the diaphysis and the epiphysis remains cartilaginous until early adulthood to allow an increase in bone length.

Bones formed by endochondral and membranous ossification remodel themselves continuously, with the destruction of old bone and the formation of new bone (Fig. 27–3). This remodeling and replacement vary in different parts of the body, depending on body needs and injury.

Grossly, bones are classified according to their shape: short, long, flat, and irregular. Long bones are those of the limbs (e.g., femur and humerus) and are longer than they are wide. Bones of the ankle and wrist are classified as short and are about equal in length and width. Examples of flat and irregular bones are the ribs and the vertebral column, respectively.

Joints

The junction between the articular surfaces of two or more bones is termed a *joint* (Fig. 27–4). Movable joints are the fulcrums for movement. These areas are further classified according to the degree of movement at the articulation. The immovable, or fibrous, joints are those in which the joint cavity is absent and the primitive joint plate develops into a fibrous tissue. If the amount of tissue is minimal, it is known as a *suture*, as in the flat bones of the skull. Articulations with larger amounts of fibrous tissue are called *syndesmoses*. The tibiofibular joint is an example. The second type of joint is the slightly movable, or cartilaginous. Cartilage grows between the articular surfaces of the bones and is eventually replaced by bone, as in the epiphyseal plate, or remains throughout life, as seen between vertebral bodies. Synovial joints are freely movable and are surrounded by a protective capsule of connective tissue. A membrane lines the joint cavity on all but the articular surfaces and is called *synovium*. Synovium secretes a fluid rich in mucins, which owing to its viscosity and lubricating quality, reduces friction on the articulating surfaces. There are six types of synovial joints:

1. *Hinge*: movement in only one axis at right angles to the bones (e.g., elbow)
2. *Gliding*: small and flat surfaces, with one sliding over the other (e.g., vertebrae)
3. *Pivot*: movement around a single axis (e.g., first cervical vertebra on the process of the second)
4. *Saddle*: movement in two directions at right angles to each other
5. *Condyloid*: also biaxial (e.g., wrist)
6. *Ball and socket*: movement in many axes with a common center (e.g., shoulder and hip)

Muscles

Bones and joints are not capable of movement by themselves but rely on the contraction of muscles (Fig. 27–5). The muscular system is made up of voluntary

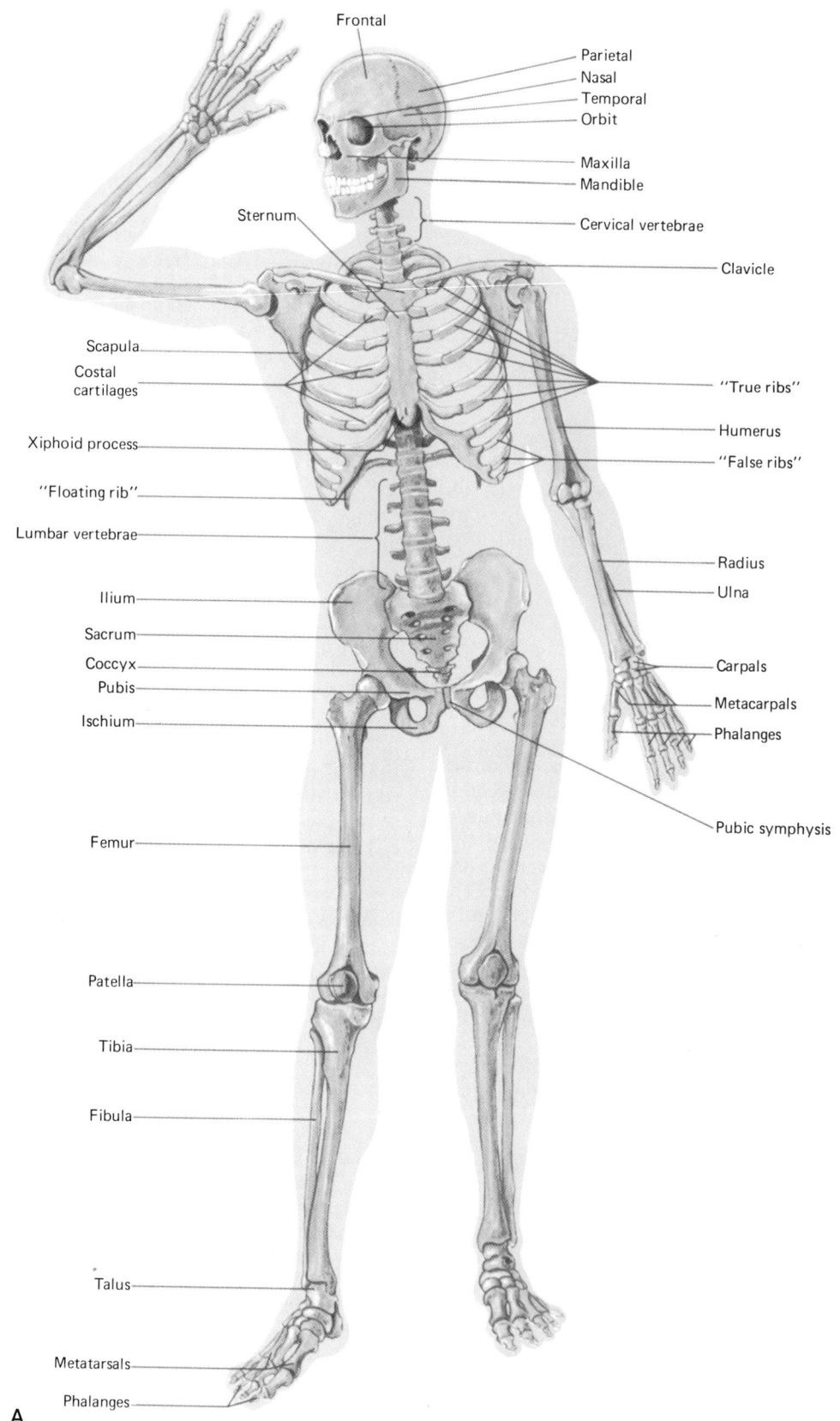

FIGURE 27–1. *A,* Anterior view of the skeleton. *B,* Posterior view of the skeleton. (From Solomon, E. P., Davis, P. W. [1983]. *Human anatomy and physiology* [pp. 156, 157]. Philadelphia: Saunders College.)

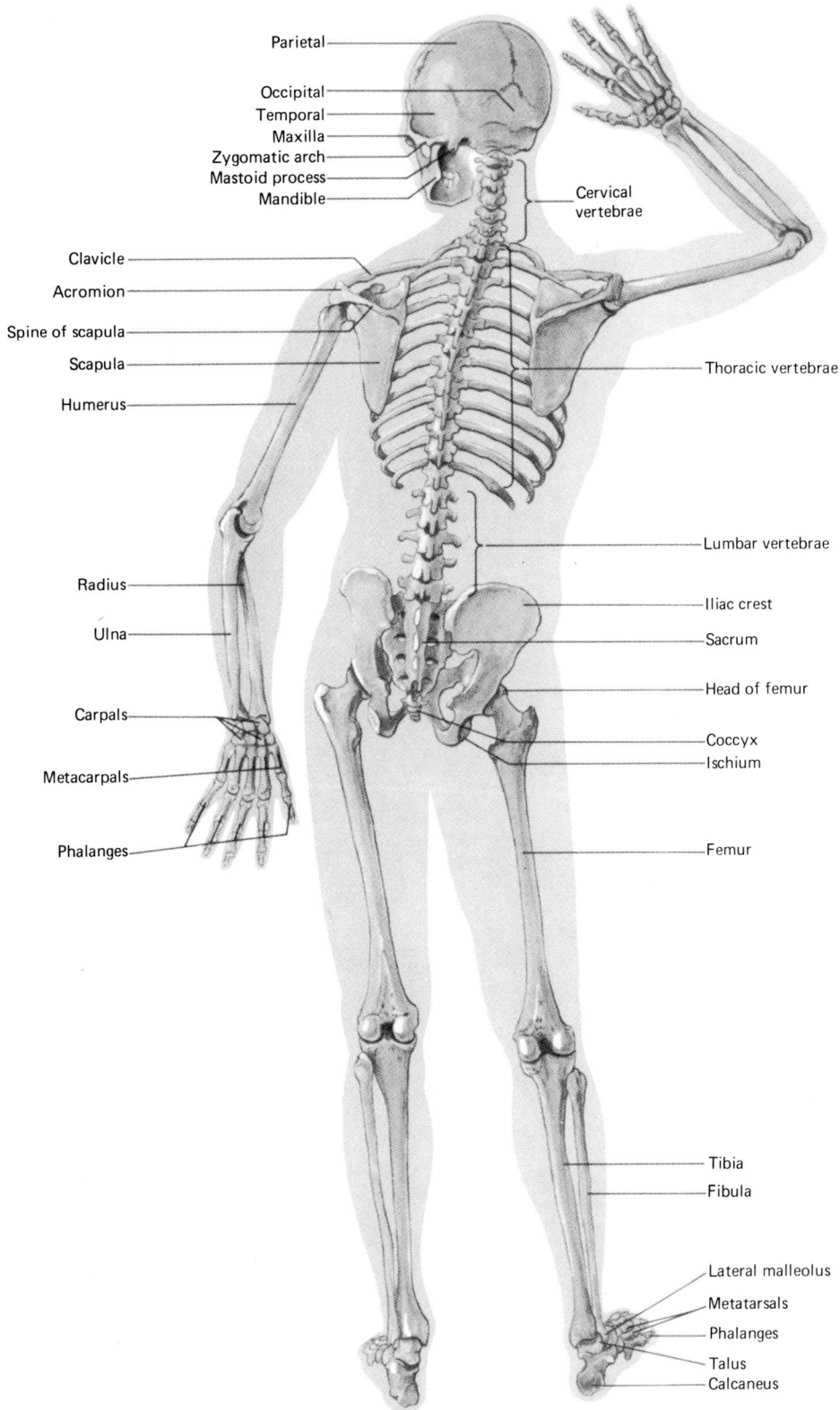

Parietal
Occipital
Temporal
Maxilla
Zygomatic arch
Mastoid process
Mandible
Cervical vertebrae
Clavicle
Acromion
Spine of scapula
Scapula
Humerus
Thoracic vertebrae
Lumbar vertebrae
Radius
Ulna
Iliac crest
Sacrum
Head of femur
Carpals
Coccyx
Ischium
Metacarpals
Phalanges
Femur
Tibia
Fibula
Lateral malleolus
Metatarsals
Phalanges
Talus
Calcaneus

B

FIGURE 27–1 *Continued*

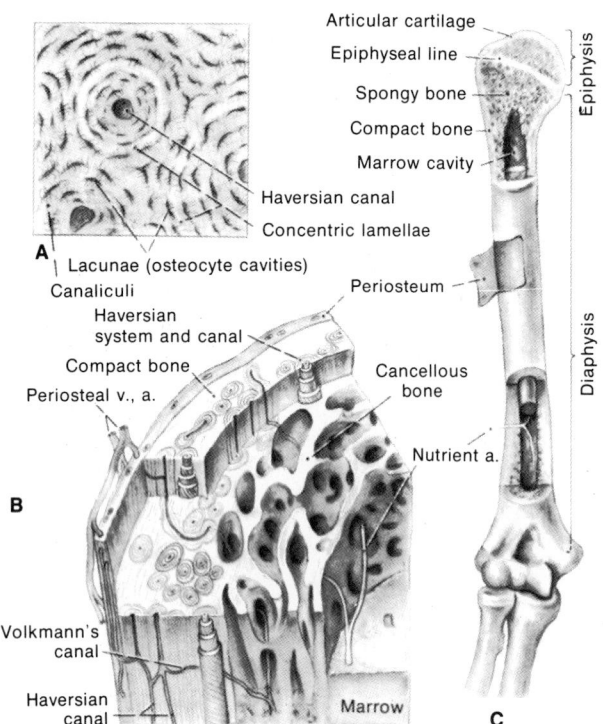

FIGURE 27–2. Cross section of a long bone showing internal and external structures. (From Jacob, S., Francone, C., Lossow, W. J. [1982]. *Structure and function in man* [5th ed.] [p. 109]. Philadelphia, W. B. Saunders.)

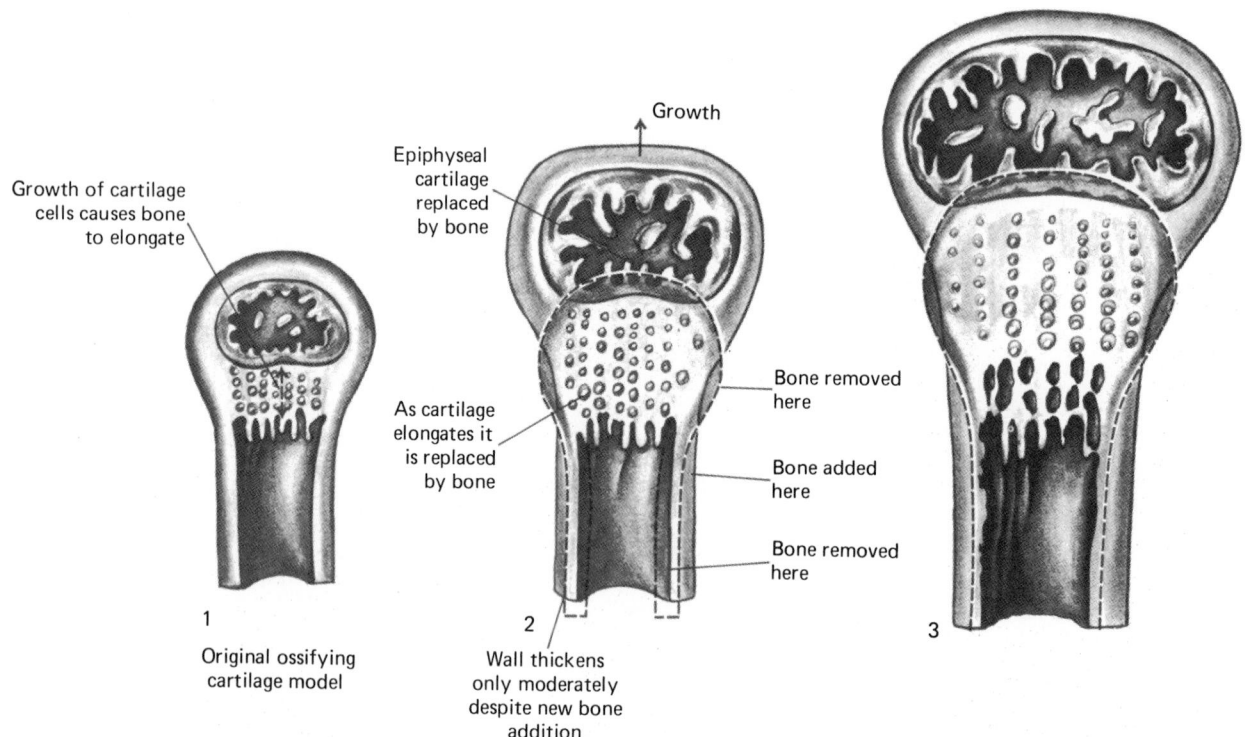

FIGURE 27–3. Bone remodeling associated with growth. (From Solomon, E. P., Davis, P. W. [1983]. *Human anatomy and physiology* [p. 136]. Philadelphia: Saunders College.)

skeletal muscles, visceral muscle (also called smooth muscle), connective tissue, blood vessels, nerves, and lymphatics. Skeletal muscles provide stability to articulations and maintain the posture of the body. Skeletal muscle cells are enclosed in a membrane called the *sarcolemma* (Fig. 27–6). Elongated cells, or muscle fibers, which contain thin and thick fibrils, constitute the body of skeletal muscle. Thin myofibrils are composed of the protein actin and the thick myofibrils of the protein myosin. These cylindrical fibrils produce a faint longitudinal striation. The elongation of the cells makes skeletal muscle efficient at producing a shortening when contracted.

The contractile elements, sarcomeres, in a voluntary skeletal muscle differ in arrangement from those in cardiac or smooth muscle. When a muscle contracts, the thin actin filaments slide between the myosin filaments. This change in their relationship, and not a shortening of the filaments, is the explanation of muscle contraction.

Skeletal muscles respond rapidly to stimuli but fatigue more readily than smooth muscle. They are under the control of the voluntary nervous system and therefore respond to the will of the individual. Muscles consist of two parts: the muscle fibers, or belly, and the tendons. Tendons are the fibrous connective tissue that attaches to the skeleton. The end that remains stationary is the origin, and the end that attaches to the more movable part is the insertion. Sometimes, the origin of a muscle attaches directly to the periosteum, whereas the insertion is usually tendinous. Skeletal muscles are held together by connective tissue called the *epimysium*, which divides the muscle into bundles, or fasciculi. The tissue surrounding the fasciculi is the *perimysium*. The *endomysium* is the connective tissue that extends and surrounds each muscle fiber (see Fig. 27–6).

Muscle shapes vary according to their function. They may be long, short, broad, narrow, or irregular. Muscle fibers also vary in arrangement, relating directly to the strength of a muscle. Muscle function depends on a good vascular supply and sufficient innervation from the spinal or cranial nerves. Contraction of skeletal muscles may be one of several types:

Isometric: an increase in tension without movement or change in muscle length, with the ends remaining fixed

Isotonic: same tension but changing length

Twitch: a momentary, spasmodic response to a single stimulus followed by relaxation

Tonic: a longer lasting contraction than twitches, produced by multiple impulses and without relaxation between; tautness without movement

Fibrillation: a sustained twitching of fibers

Convulsions: involuntary, violent tetanic contraction of muscle groups

Terms used to describe the effect of muscle contractions on the joints of the body in the anatomical position are as follows (Fig. 27–7):

Flexion: a decrease in the angle between two bones (e.g., bending knee)

Extension: an increase in the angle between two bones (e.g., straightening leg at the knee)

Abduction: movement away from the midline (e.g., left arm from side)

Adduction: movement toward the body

Rotation: movement of a bone around an axis, either its own or that of another bone; medial or lateral rotation

Supination: lateral rotation of the forearm; palm up

Pronation: medial rotation of the forearm; palm down

Eversion: outward rotation of the foot; sole outward

Inversion: inward rotation of the foot; sole inward

Circumduction: flexion, extension, abduction, adduction, and rotation

Vertebral Column

The *vertebral column* protects the spinal cord and forms the flexible longitudinal axis of the skeleton (Fig. 27–8). It is composed of a series of bones called *vertebrae*. Between each vertebra are pads of fibrocartilage, or *intervertebral disks*. The vertebral column is also the point of attachment of many skeletal muscles of the back and supports the head. The spinal cord passes through the vertebral canal, which is formed by the vertebrae. Impulses to and from the spinal cord, via spinal nerves, pass through openings *(intervertebral foramina)* between adjacent vertebrae.

Thirty-three vertebrae constitute the vertebral column. They are classified according to the regions of the body they occupy: 7 cervical, 12 thoracic, 5 lumbar, 5 sacral, and 4 coccygeal. Each vertebra is divided into two parts that together form the vertebral foramen. The body, or the anterior portion, is the thickest part. Its surfaces are flattened and rough, which allows attachment to the intervertebral disk. Anteriorly, the body has a few small foramina, which enable the passage of nutrient vessels. Posteriorly, irregular apertures for the channel of the basivertebral veins from the body of the vertebra are present.

The vertebral arch consists of two pedicles and two laminae, from which emerge seven processes (Fig. 27–9). The pedicles are short, thick structures that appear from the posterolateral sides of the body. Posteriorly and medially from the pedicle ends are the broad, flat laminae that join in the midline. The spinous process is the projection posteriorly and inferiorly from the point of junction of the laminae. On each side where the laminae and pedicles meet is the transverse process, which extends laterally. The spinous and transverse processes provide the attachment of muscles and ligaments.

The vertebral bodies are the weight-bearing structures of the vertebrae. As the vertebral column descends, each vertebra has to carry more weight. To accommodate, the bodies become more massive and the intervertebral disks increase in size and thickness. The vertebral canal differs only slightly in size, and the spinal cord remains approximately the same size throughout. Where the spinal cord increases slightly in diameter, the vertebral foramina also enlarge.

Text continued on page 639

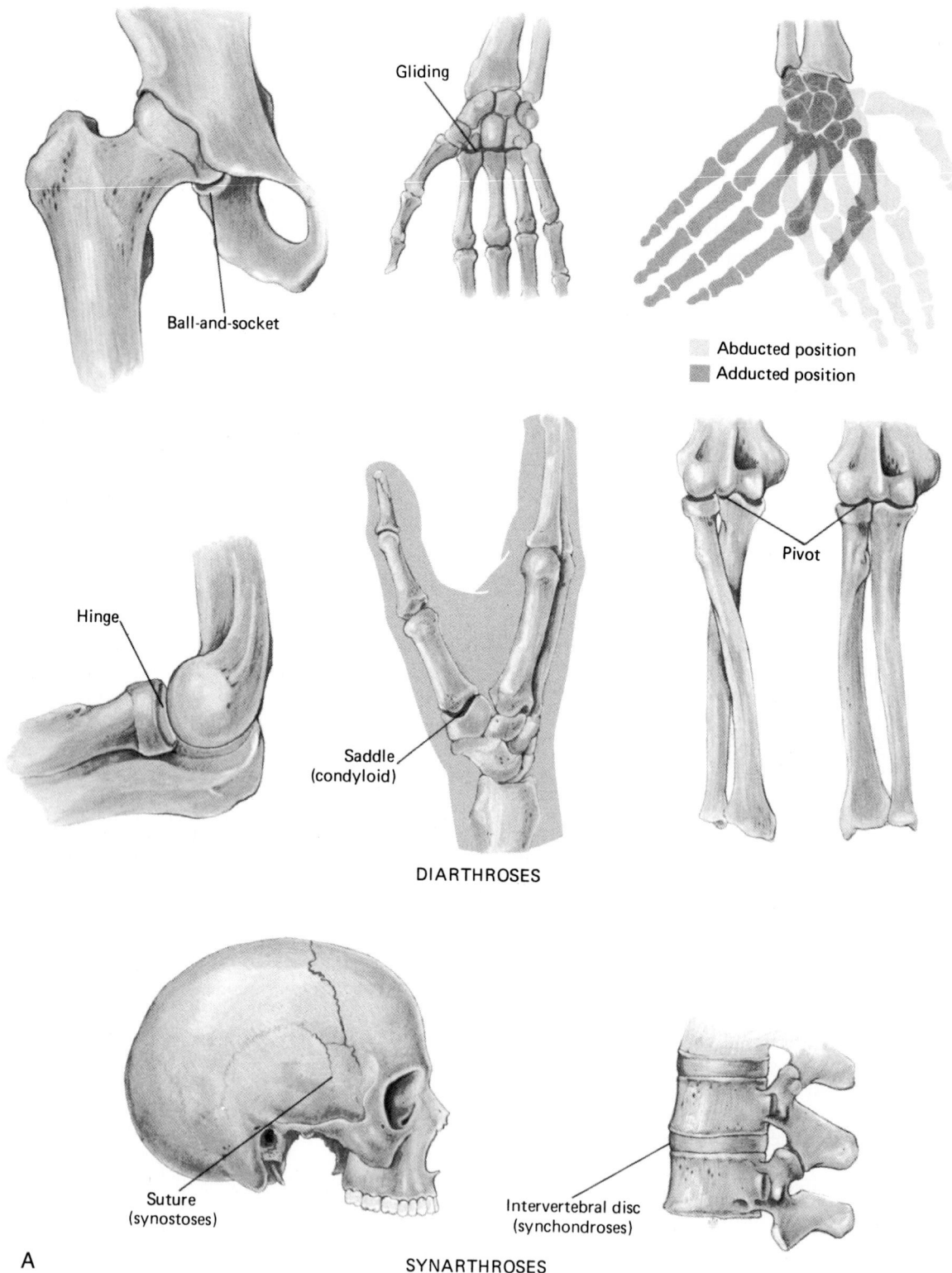

Gliding

Ball-and-socket

Abducted position
Adducted position

Hinge

Saddle
(condyloid)

Pivot

DIARTHROSES

Suture
(synostoses)

Intervertebral disc
(synchondroses)

A

SYNARTHROSES

FIGURE 27–4. *A,* Kinds of joints.

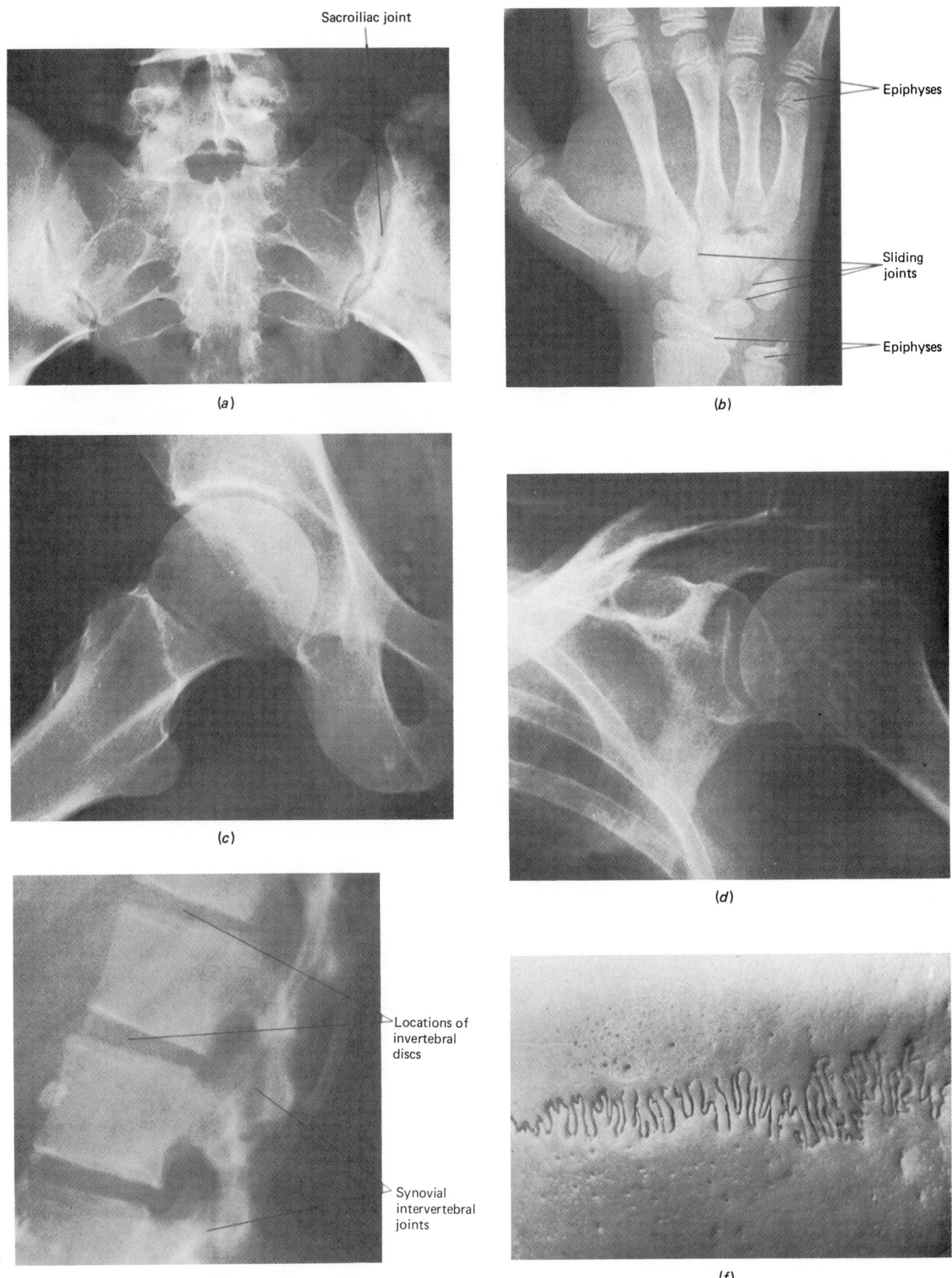

FIGURE 27–4 *Continued B,* Representative joints. *(a)* Sacroiliac joint. *(b)* Gliding joints. *(c)* Ball-and-socket hip joint. *(d)* Ball-and-socket shoulder joint. *(e)* Intervertebral joints. *(f)* A skull suture. (From Solomon, E. P., Davis, P. W. [1983]. *Human anatomy and physiology* (pp. 148, 151). Philadelphia: Saunders College.)

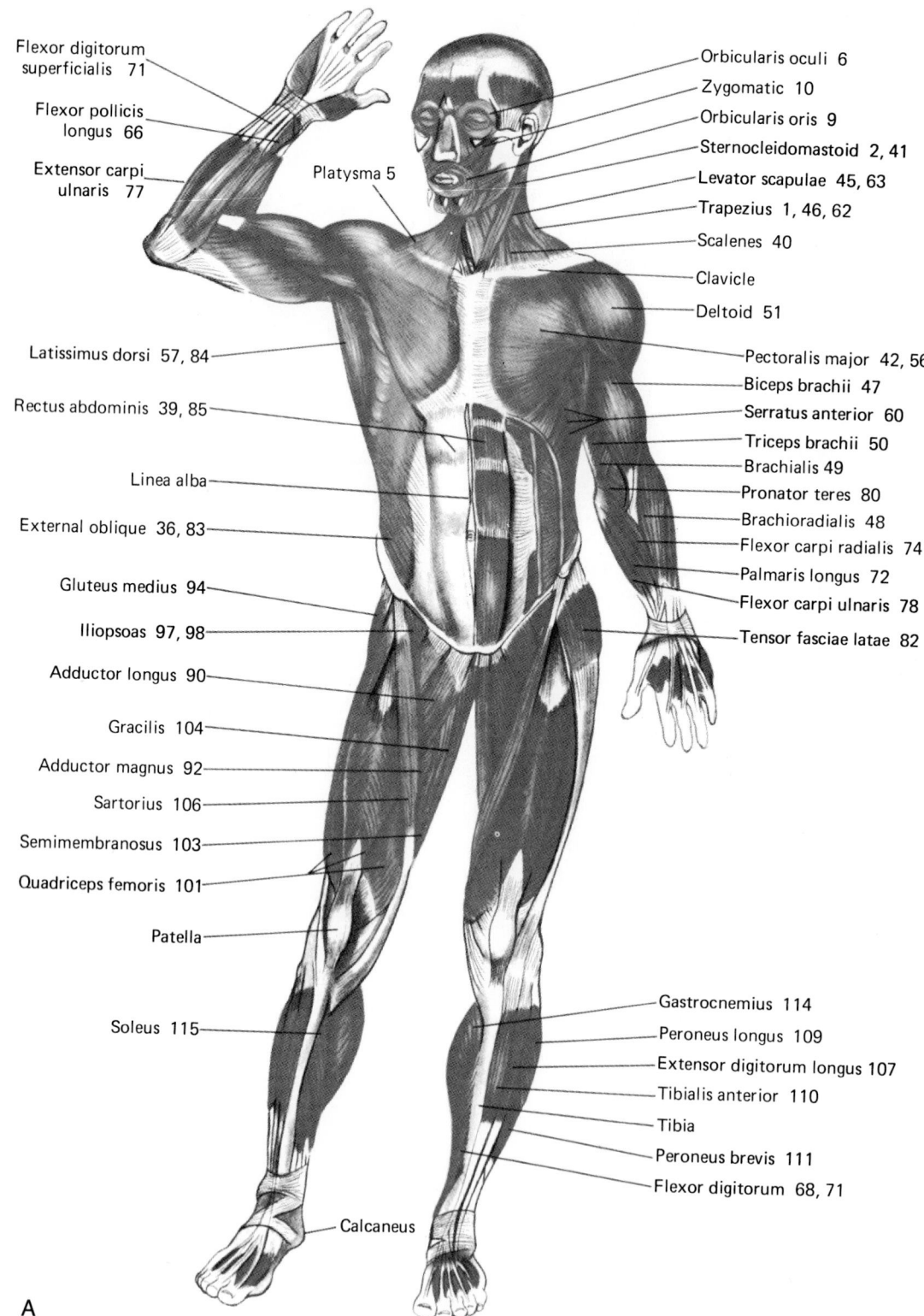

Flexor digitorum superficialis 71
Flexor pollicis longus 66
Extensor carpi ulnaris 77
Platysma 5
Latissimus dorsi 57, 84
Rectus abdominis 39, 85
Linea alba
External oblique 36, 83
Gluteus medius 94
Iliopsoas 97, 98
Adductor longus 90
Gracilis 104
Adductor magnus 92
Sartorius 106
Semimembranosus 103
Quadriceps femoris 101
Patella
Soleus 115
Calcaneus

Orbicularis oculi 6
Zygomatic 10
Orbicularis oris 9
Sternocleidomastoid 2, 41
Levator scapulae 45, 63
Trapezius 1, 46, 62
Scalenes 40
Clavicle
Deltoid 51
Pectoralis major 42, 56
Biceps brachii 47
Serratus anterior 60
Triceps brachii 50
Brachialis 49
Pronator teres 80
Brachioradialis 48
Flexor carpi radialis 74
Palmaris longus 72
Flexor carpi ulnaris 78
Tensor fasciae latae 82

Gastrocnemius 114
Peroneus longus 109
Extensor digitorum longus 107
Tibialis anterior 110
Tibia
Peroneus brevis 111
Flexor digitorum 68, 71

A

FIGURE 27–5. *A*, Anterior superficial muscles.

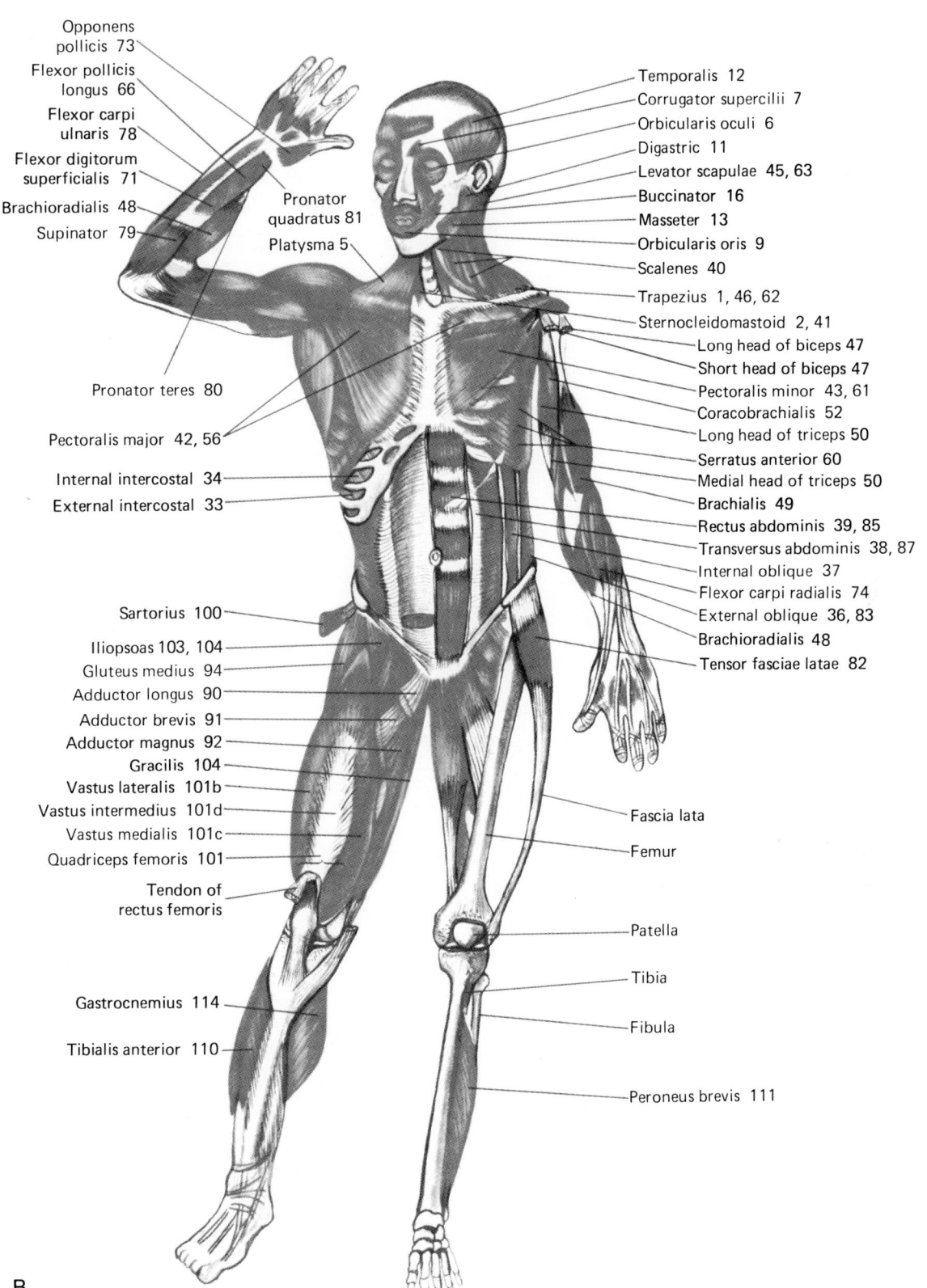

Opponens pollicis 73
Flexor pollicis longus 66
Flexor carpi ulnaris 78
Flexor digitorum superficialis 71
Brachioradialis 48
Supinator 79
Pronator quadratus 81
Platysma 5
Pronator teres 80
Pectoralis major 42, 56
Internal intercostal 34
External intercostal 33

Temporalis 12
Corrugator supercilii 7
Orbicularis oculi 6
Digastric 11
Levator scapulae 45, 63
Buccinator 16
Masseter 13
Orbicularis oris 9
Scalenes 40
Trapezius 1, 46, 62
Sternocleidomastoid 2, 41
Long head of biceps 47
Short head of biceps 47
Pectoralis minor 43, 61
Coracobrachialis 52
Long head of triceps 50
Serratus anterior 60
Medial head of triceps 50
Brachialis 49
Rectus abdominis 39, 85
Transversus abdominis 38, 87
Internal oblique 37
Flexor carpi radialis 74
External oblique 36, 83
Brachioradialis 48
Tensor fasciae latae 82

Sartorius 100
Iliopsoas 103, 104
Gluteus medius 94
Adductor longus 90
Adductor brevis 91
Adductor magnus 92
Gracilis 104
Vastus lateralis 101b
Vastus intermedius 101d
Vastus medialis 101c
Quadriceps femoris 101
Tendon of rectus femoris

Fascia lata
Femur

Patella

Tibia

Fibula

Peroneus brevis 111

Gastrocnemius 114
Tibialis anterior 110

B

FIGURE 27–5 *Continued B*, Anterior deep muscles.

Illustration continued on following page

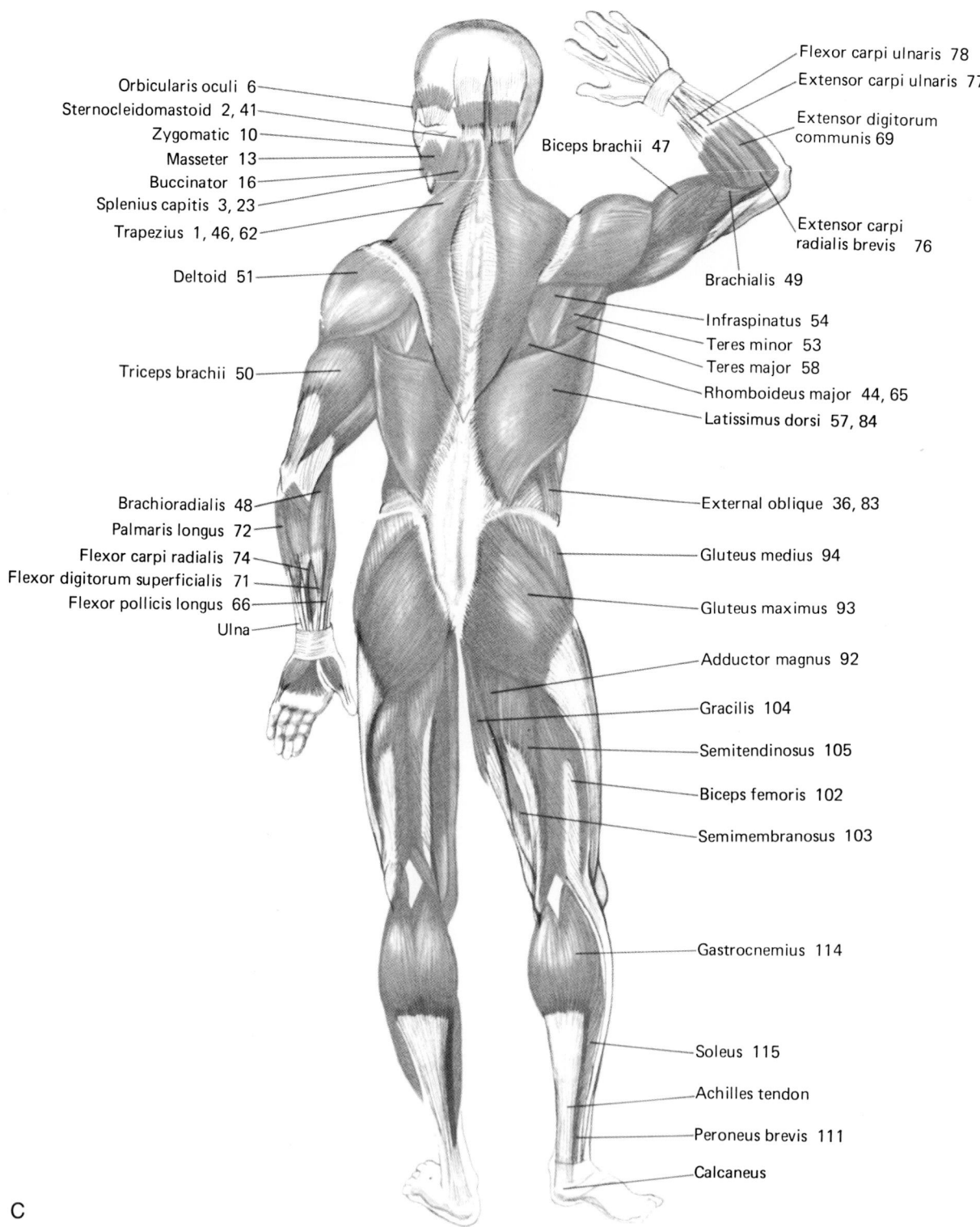

Orbicularis oculi 6
Sternocleidomastoid 2, 41
Zygomatic 10
Masseter 13
Buccinator 16
Splenius capitis 3, 23
Trapezius 1, 46, 62

Deltoid 51

Triceps brachii 50

Brachioradialis 48
Palmaris longus 72
Flexor carpi radialis 74
Flexor digitorum superficialis 71
Flexor pollicis longus 66
Ulna

Flexor carpi ulnaris 78
Extensor carpi ulnaris 77
Extensor digitorum communis 69

Biceps brachii 47

Extensor carpi radialis brevis 76

Brachialis 49

Infraspinatus 54
Teres minor 53
Teres major 58
Rhomboideus major 44, 65
Latissimus dorsi 57, 84

External oblique 36, 83

Gluteus medius 94

Gluteus maximus 93

Adductor magnus 92

Gracilis 104

Semitendinosus 105

Biceps femoris 102

Semimembranosus 103

Gastrocnemius 114

Soleus 115

Achilles tendon

Peroneus brevis 111

Calcaneus

C

FIGURE 27–5 *Continued C,* Posterior superficial muscles.

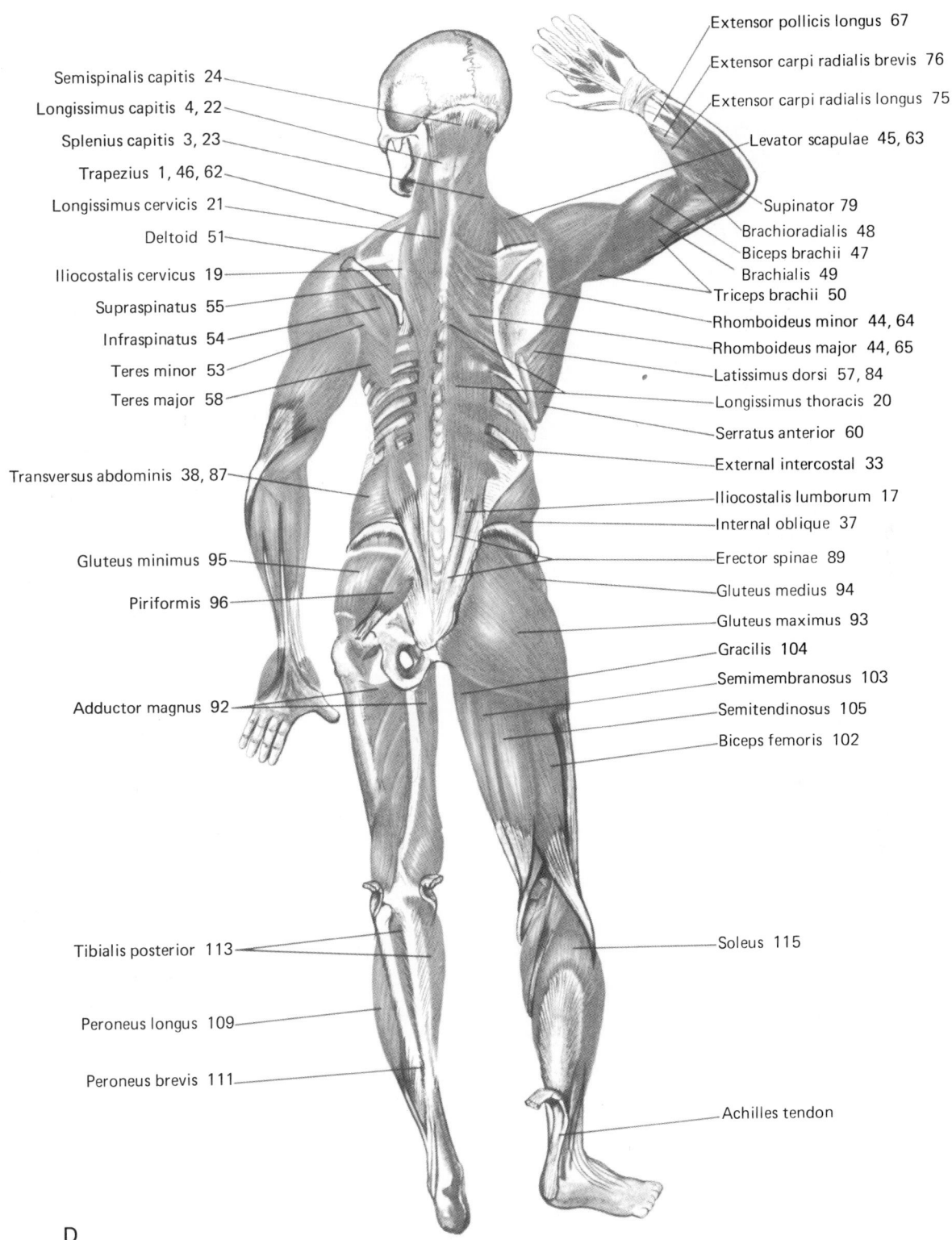

Semispinalis capitis 24
Longissimus capitis 4, 22
Splenius capitis 3, 23
Trapezius 1, 46, 62
Longissimus cervicis 21
Deltoid 51
Iliocostalis cervicus 19
Supraspinatus 55
Infraspinatus 54
Teres minor 53
Teres major 58
Transversus abdominis 38, 87
Gluteus minimus 95
Piriformis 96
Adductor magnus 92
Tibialis posterior 113
Peroneus longus 109
Peroneus brevis 111

Extensor pollicis longus 67
Extensor carpi radialis brevis 76
Extensor carpi radialis longus 75
Levator scapulae 45, 63
Supinator 79
Brachioradialis 48
Biceps brachii 47
Brachialis 49
Triceps brachii 50
Rhomboideus minor 44, 64
Rhomboideus major 44, 65
Latissimus dorsi 57, 84
Longissimus thoracis 20
Serratus anterior 60
External intercostal 33
Iliocostalis lumborum 17
Internal oblique 37
Erector spinae 89
Gluteus medius 94
Gluteus maximus 93
Gracilis 104
Semimembranosus 103
Semitendinosus 105
Biceps femoris 102
Soleus 115
Achilles tendon

D

FIGURE 27–5 *Continued D,* Posterior deep muscles. (From Solomon, E. P., Davis, P. W. [1983]. *Human anatomy and physiology* (pp. 212–215). Philadelphia: Saunders College.)

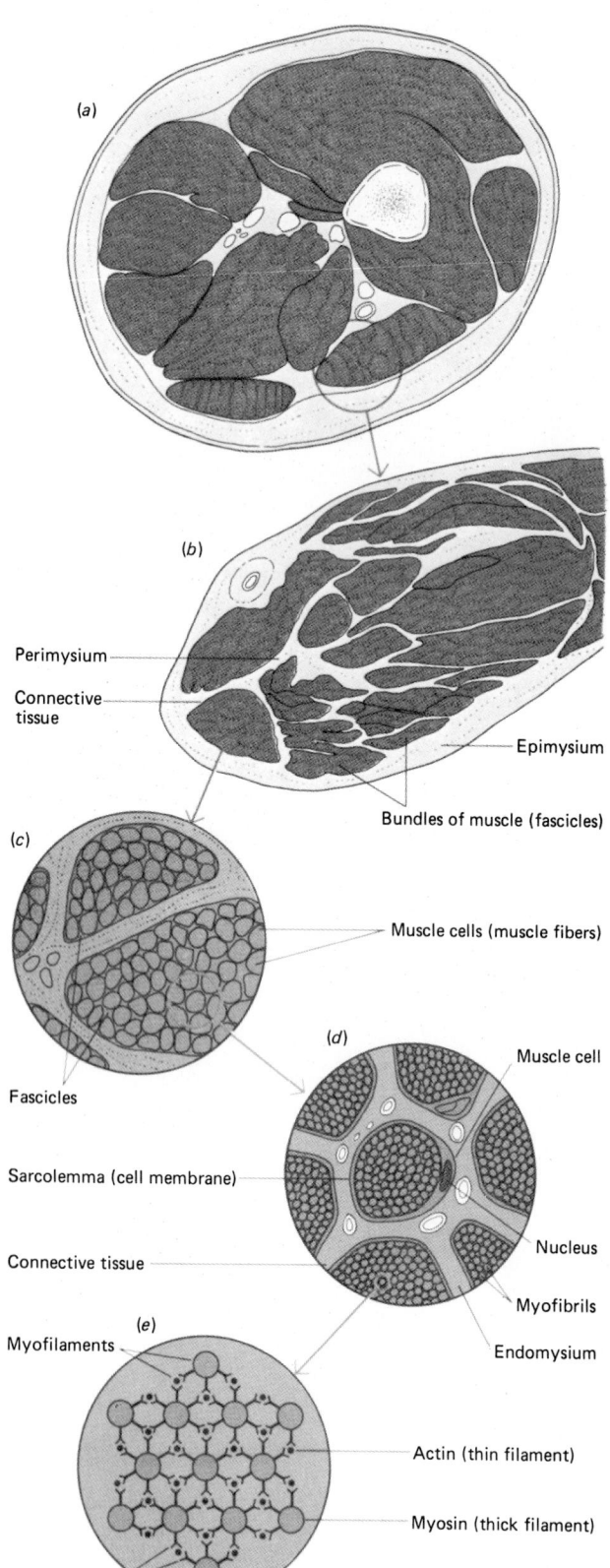

(a)

(b)

Perimysium

Connective tissue

Epimysium

Bundles of muscle (fascicles)

(c)

Muscle cells (muscle fibers)

Fascicles

(d)

Muscle cell

Sarcolemma (cell membrane)

Nucleus

Connective tissue

Myofibrils

(e)

Endomysium

Myofilaments

Actin (thin filament)

Myosin (thick filament)

Cross bridges

FIGURE 27–6. Cross section of the thigh dissected into smaller and smaller parts. *(a)* Section through the entire thigh. *(b)* A single muscle. *(c)* and *(d)* Microscopic views of the muscle. *(e)* Arrangement of the contractile filaments. (From Solomon, E. P., Davis, P. W. [1983]. *Human anatomy and physiology* [p. 192]. Philadelphia: Saunders College.)

When viewed anteriorly or posteriorly, the vertebral column appears almost straight, except for a slight lateral curve to the right. The lateral view shows four normal curves: cervical, thoracic, lumbar, and sacral. Abnormal column curves are not uncommon. An abnormal curvature laterally is called a *scoliosis*, excessive thoracic curve posteriorly is a *kyphosis*, and a lumbar curve is called *lordosis*. Spinal ligaments bind together and strengthen the vertebral column and also limit its movement. There are anterior, posterior, and lateral ligaments that run the length of the vertebral column and connect the bodies of adjacent vertebrae. Restraining ligaments are present between vertebral arches and adjacent spinous processes are connected by interspinous ligaments. Supraspinous ligaments adjoin over a group of spinous processes.

Shoulder and Upper Extremity

The *shoulder girdle* is the point of attachment of the upper extremity to the axial skeleton (Fig. 27–10). There is no articulation of the shoulder to the vertebral column. The anterior girdle is formed by the clavicle, which communicates anteriorly and in the midline with the sternum and laterally with the acromion process of the scapula. The latter attachment forms the acromioclavicular joint. The scapula forms the posterior part of the shoulder girdle. Below the acromion, the glenoid forms an articulation with the humeral head. This joint, surrounded by a loose capsule, is a ball-and-socket joint that allows considerable motion. The coracoid process, which is at the lateral end of the superior border anteriorly, provides muscular attachment.

The *humerus*, which is the longest and largest bone of the upper extremity, has many distinct landmarks: greater and lesser tuberosities, anatomical neck, and the surgical neck, which is the site of most humeral fractures (Fig. 27–11). The upper surface of the greater tuberosity is the area of insertion of the tendons of the rotator cuff. The supraspinous, infraspinous, and teres minor tendons compose the rotator cuff. The distal portion of the humerus articulates laterally with the radius and medially with the ulna at the olecranon.

The *radius* and *ulna* are the bones that form the forearm (Fig. 27–12). The radius rotates around the ulna, which is medial. The proximal end, or head, articulates with the distal end of the humerus. The biceps tendon attaches to a tuberosity below the radial head. Distally, the radius divides into two articular surfaces. The distal surface communicates with the carpal bones of the wrist, and the medial side with the distal end of the ulna.

Wrist and Hand

The *wrist*, or carpus, and *hand* consist of three parts: the carpals, or wrist bones; the metacarpals, or bones of the palm; and the phalanges, or bones of the digits (Fig. 27–13). The wrist is composed of two transverse rows of the eight carpal bones. Each carpal bone has several smooth articular surfaces for contact with adjacent bones and coarse surfaces for the attachment of ligaments. There are no tendinous or muscular attachments to the wrist bones. Consequently, movement of the carpal bones is accomplished by the tendons that insert into the metacarpals and phalanges. There are five metacarpal bones, whose heads form the knuckles. The distal articulation is with its proper phalanx, and proximally, they articulate with the distal carpal bones. The phalanges consist of 14 bones in each hand. There are three bones in each finger and only two in each thumb.

Pelvic Girdle and Femur

The pelvic girdle's function is to support and stabilize the lower extremities and protect underlying organs. The *pelvic girdle* is formed by two hip bones, which join anteriorly at the pubic symphysis, and posteriorly each attaches to the sacrum laterally (Fig. 27–14). Each hip bone is the fusion of three other bones: the ilium, the ischium, and the pubis. The sacrum, the coccyx, and both hip bones form the pelvis. The pelvis is further divided into the greater, or false, pelvis, which is the flaring posterior portion, and the lesser, or true pelvis, which lies below the brim. The ilium is the large upper flaring portion of the hip bone. The iliac crest is the superior border of the ilium and ends anteriorly and posteriorly in superior iliac spines. Muscles of the abdominal wall attach beneath on the inferior iliac spines. Gluteal muscles attach on the outer surface of the ilium. The ischium is the lowest and strongest part of the hip bone. At the point of the lateral fusion of the ilium, the ischium, and the pubis is the acetabulum. This area is a socket into which the head of the femur fits.

The rounded smooth head of the femur extends superiorly and medially and articulates with the hip bone at the acetabulum. This union forms the hip joint (Fig. 27–15). The hip joint is a ball-and-socket joint and is surrounded by a capsule, ligaments, and muscles. The acetabulum is deep in the anteroposterior direction and deepened by a fibrocartilaginous rim called the *glenoid labrum*. This rim provides stability of the position of the head of the femur. The capsule is a strong, thick extension from the acetabulum to the intertrochanteric line of the femur. This capsule is weakened in areas posteriorly and inferiorly. The iliofemoral ligament strengthens the hip joint anteriorly, and the pubofemoral and ischiofemoral ligaments reinforce anteriorly and posteriorly. Intracapsularly, the ligamentum teres loosely attaches the femoral head to the acetabulum and channels vasculature to the head of the femur.

The *femur*, not unlike the humerus, has distinguishing markings. The proximal end consists of the femoral head and neck, the upper shaft, and the greater and lesser trochanters (Fig. 27–16). The greater trochanter is the insertion point of the abductor and short rotator muscles. The distal femur ends in two condyles, which articulate with the tibial condyles. Anteriorly, the fem-

Text continued on page 649

Although the movements of which the body is capable are almost infinitely varied, they can be classified into a surprisingly few basic categories. Even the schooled movements of a ballerina or a gymnast are combinations of these basic movements.

Specific terms are used to describe these basic movement categories. Try to touch the more medial of the two creases in your palm with the tip of your thumb (Fig. 7-1). This action is called **flexion**. Now straighten your thumb out as far as it will go. This is **extension**. (Some persons can hyperextend the thumb. This can be done only if the joint capsule is loose enough to permit the partial dislocation of the metacarpophalangeal joint.) Now place your hand on a table, palm up and fingers straight. Move your thumb directly alongside your index finger. This is called **adduction**. Now move your thumb laterally away from your index finger. This

movement is **abduction**, the opposite of adduction. Now grasp a small object between your thumb and index finger. This is **opposition**, which involves rotation in addition to adduction. Each of these movements of the thumb is produced by a different combination of muscles. The total range of movements of which the thumb is capable is made possible by the interaction of several muscles contracting at the same time, as in twiddling (circumducting) the thumbs, for example.

With respect to the body as a whole, flexion and extension are movements carried out in an anteroposterior plane, whereas abduction and adduction are lateral-medial movements. Generally (but not always) flexion and abduction move a part away from the anatomic position (Chapter 1), while extension and adduction return the part to the anatomic position.

Flexion The bending of a joint; usually a movement that reduces the angle that two movably articulated bones make with each other. When one crouches, the knees are flexed.

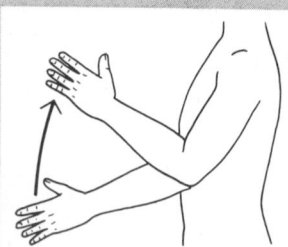

Circumduction A combination of movements that makes a body part describe a circle.

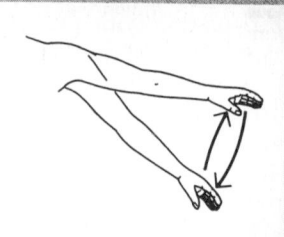

Extension The opposite of flexion. It increases the angle between two movably articulated bones, usually to a 180-degree maximum. If the angle of extension exceeds 180 degrees (as is possible when throwing back the head), this action is termed **hyperextension**.

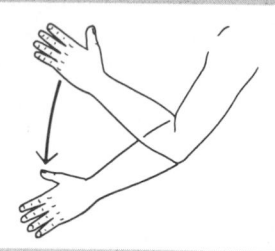

Rotation The pivoting of a body part around its axis, as in shaking the head. No rotation of any body part is complete (i.e., 360 degrees).

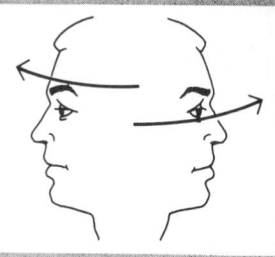

FIGURE 27–7. Types of body movements. (From Solomon, E. P., Davis, P. W. [1983]. *Human anatomy and physiology* [pp. 149–150]. Philadelphia: Saunders College.)

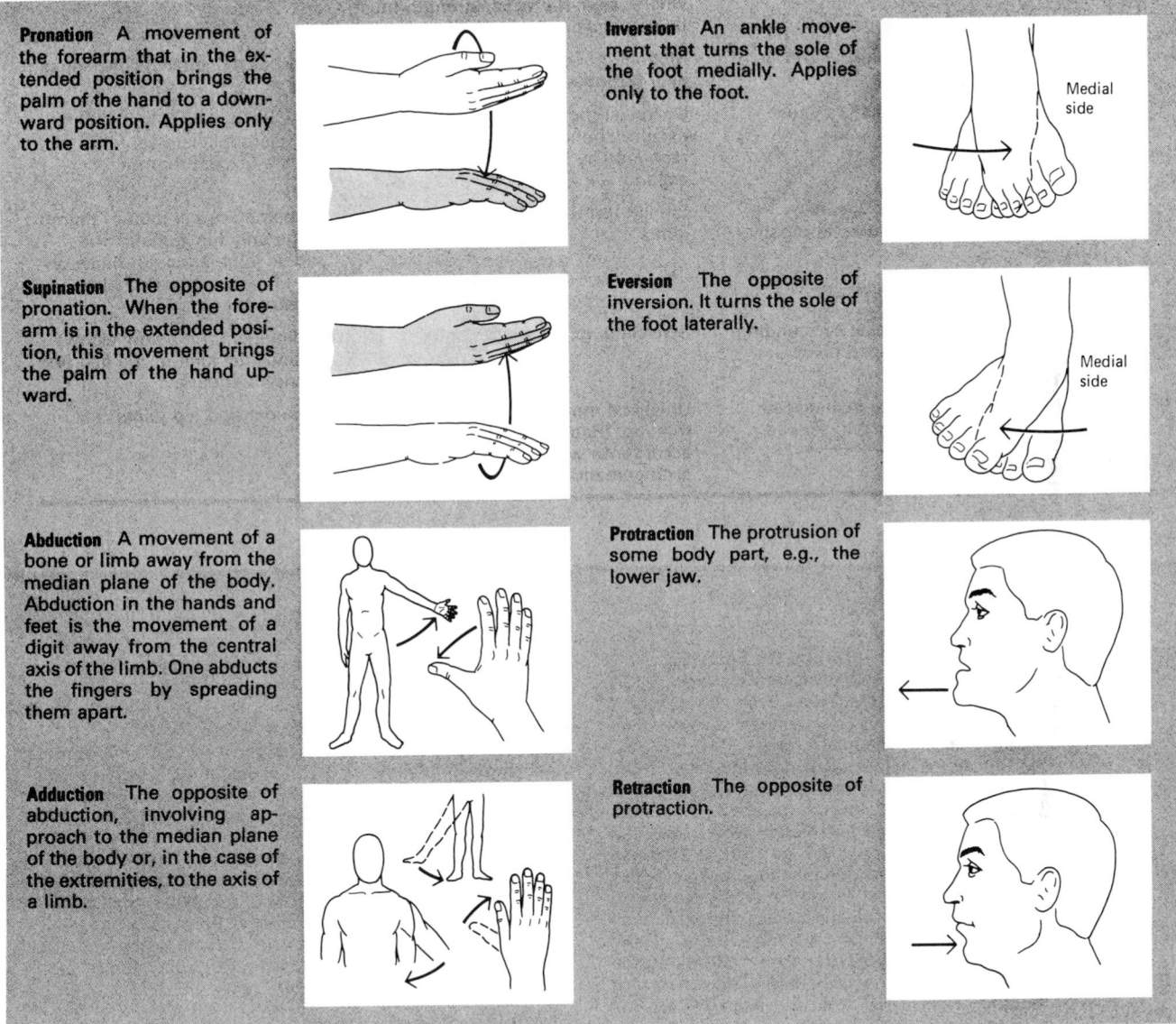

Pronation A movement of the forearm that in the extended position brings the palm of the hand to a downward position. Applies only to the arm.

Supination The opposite of pronation. When the forearm is in the extended position, this movement brings the palm of the hand upward.

Abduction A movement of a bone or limb away from the median plane of the body. Abduction in the hands and feet is the movement of a digit away from the central axis of the limb. One abducts the fingers by spreading them apart.

Adduction The opposite of abduction, involving approach to the median plane of the body or, in the case of the extremities, to the axis of a limb.

Inversion An ankle movement that turns the sole of the foot medially. Applies only to the foot.

Medial side

Eversion The opposite of inversion. It turns the sole of the foot laterally.

Medial side

Protraction The protrusion of some body part, e.g., the lower jaw.

Retraction The opposite of protraction.

FIGURE 27–7 *Continued*

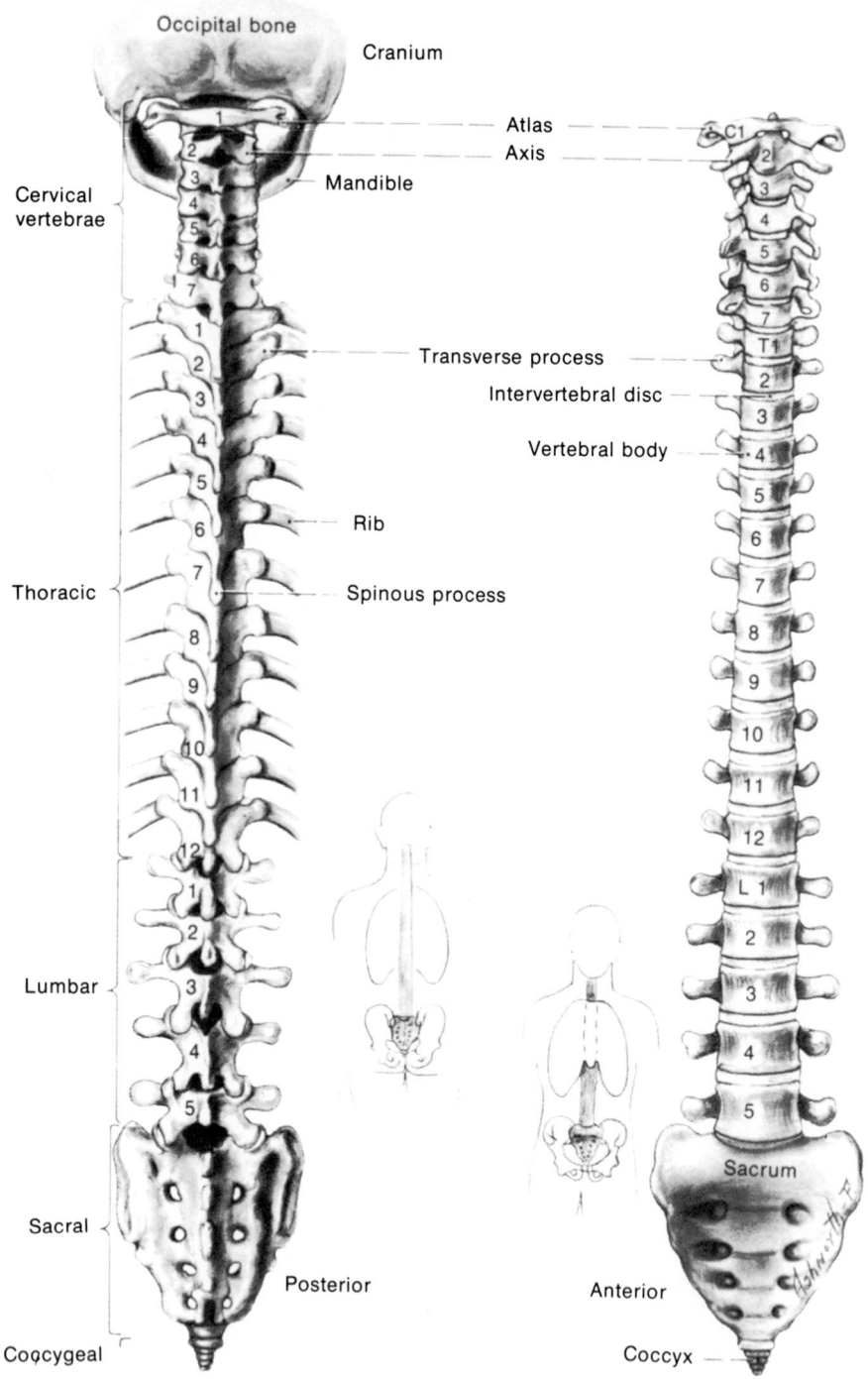

Occipital bone

Cranium

Atlas

Axis

Mandible

Cervical vertebrae

Transverse process

Intervertebral disc

Vertebral body

Rib

Spinous process

Thoracic

Lumbar

Sacral

Posterior

Anterior

Coccygeal

Sacrum

Coccyx

FIGURE 27–8. The vertebral column. (From Jacob, S., Francone, C., Lossow, W. J. [1982]. *Structure and function in man* (5th ed.) (p. 132). Philadelphia: W. B. Saunders.)

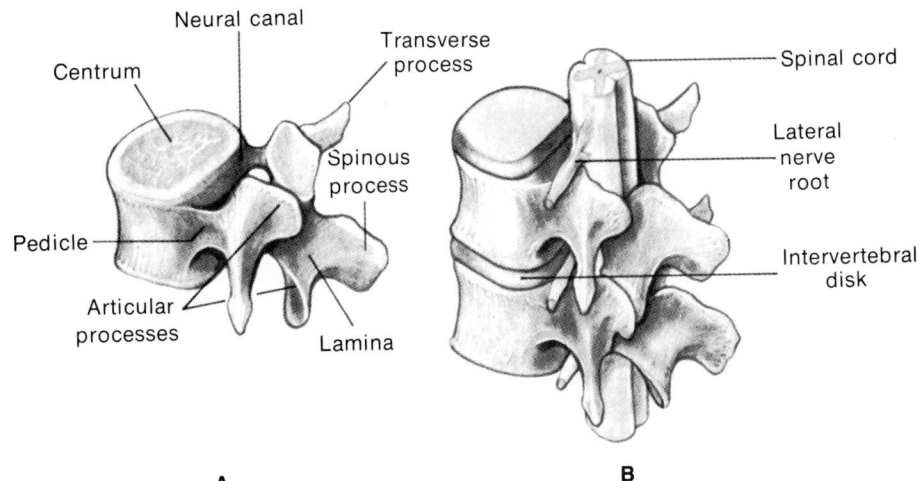

FIGURE 27–9. *A*, Diagonal view from the top of a typical vertebra. *B*, Two vertebrae held in position by an intervertebral disk to show the position of the spinal cord and its peripheral nerves. (From Anderson, P. D. [1976]. *Clinical anatomy and physiology for allied health sciences* [p. 68]. Philadelphia: W. B. Saunders.)

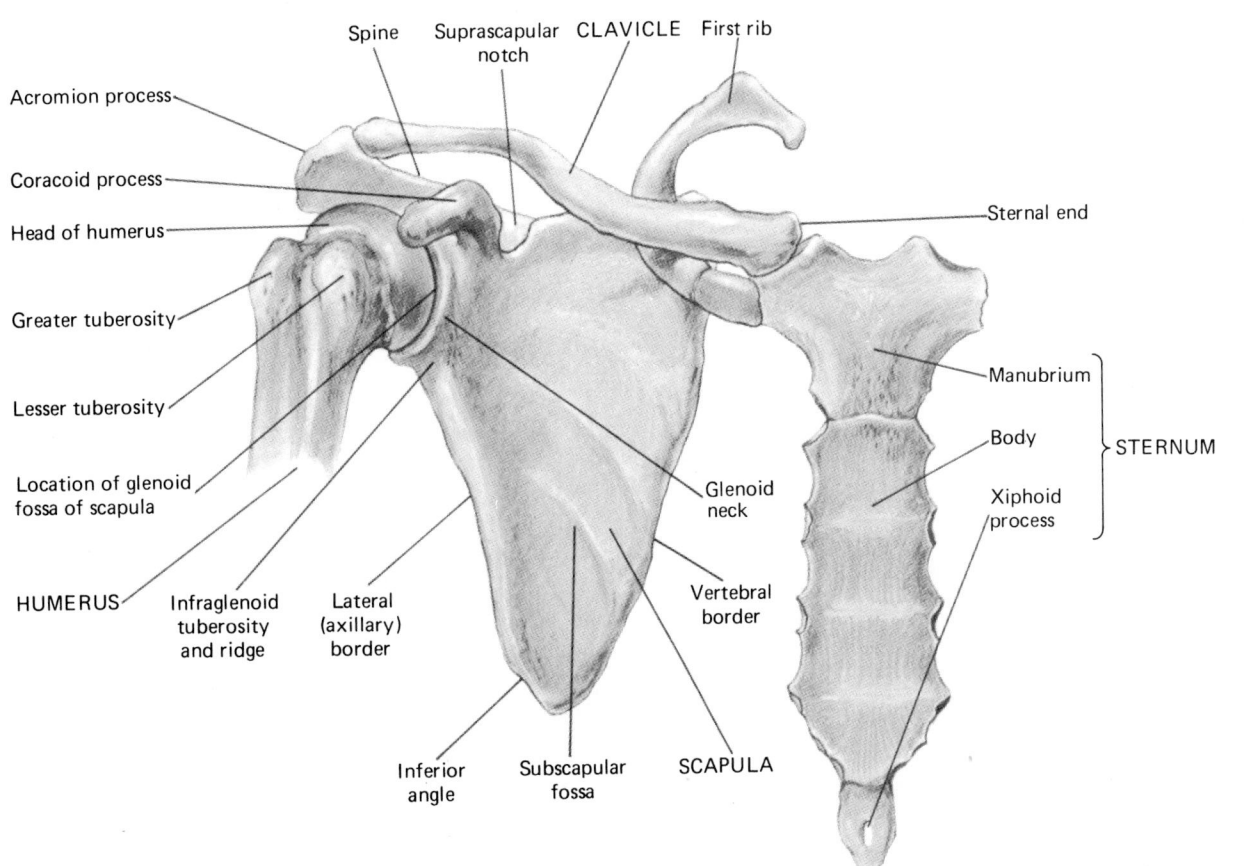

FIGURE 27–10. Anterior view of the scapula, sternum, and shoulder girdle. (From Solomon, E. P., Davis, P. W. [1983]. *Human anatomy and physiology* (p. 174). Philadelphia: Saunders College.)

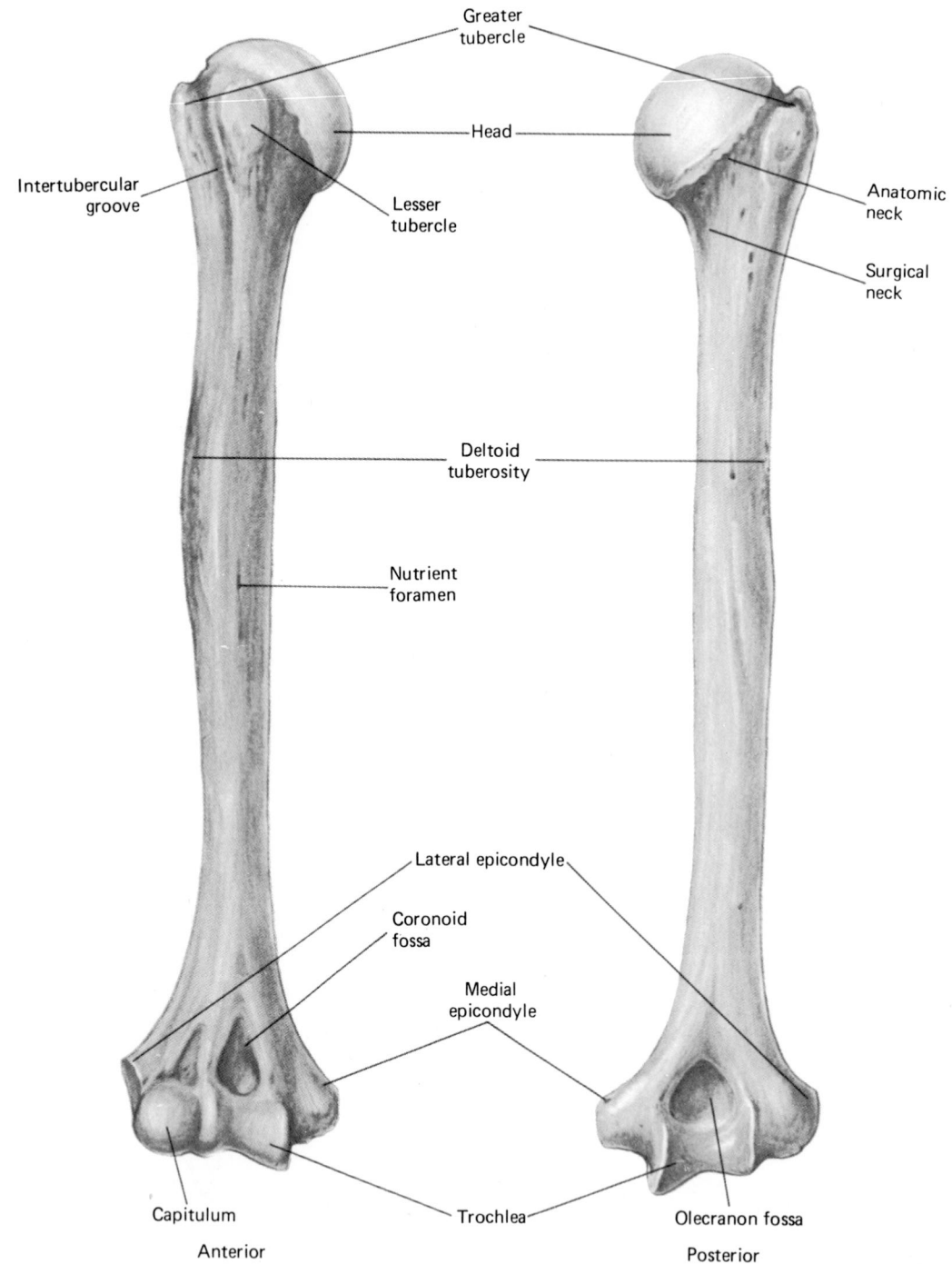

FIGURE 27–11. The right humerus. (From Solomon, E. P., Davis, P. W. [1983]. *Human anatomy and physiology* [p. 176]. Philadelphia: Saunders College.)

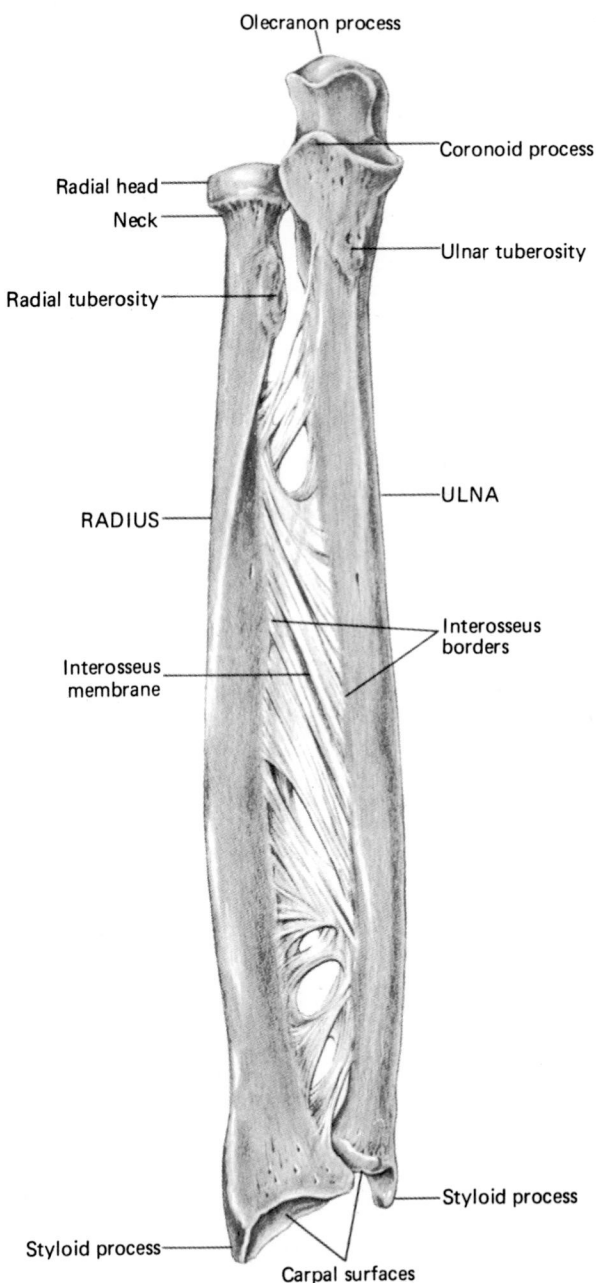

FIGURE 27–12. Anterior view of the bones of the right forearm. (From Solomon, E. P., Davis, W. P. [1983]. *Human anatomy and physiology* [p. 177]. Philadelphia: Saunders College.)

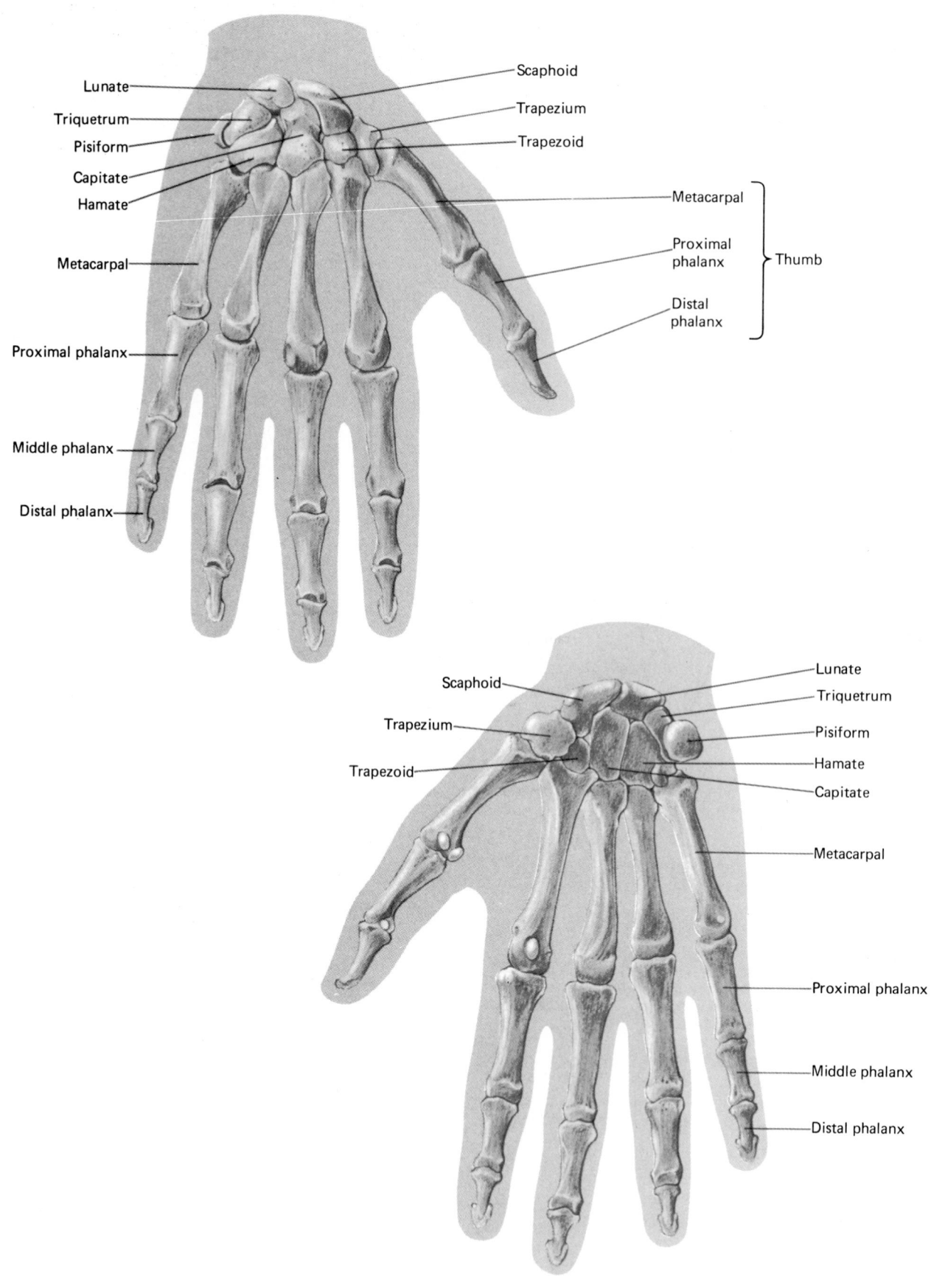

FIGURE 27–13. The bones of the wrist and hand. (From Solomon, E. P., Davis, W. P. [1983]. *Human anatomy and physiology* (p. 178). Philadelphia: Saunders College.)

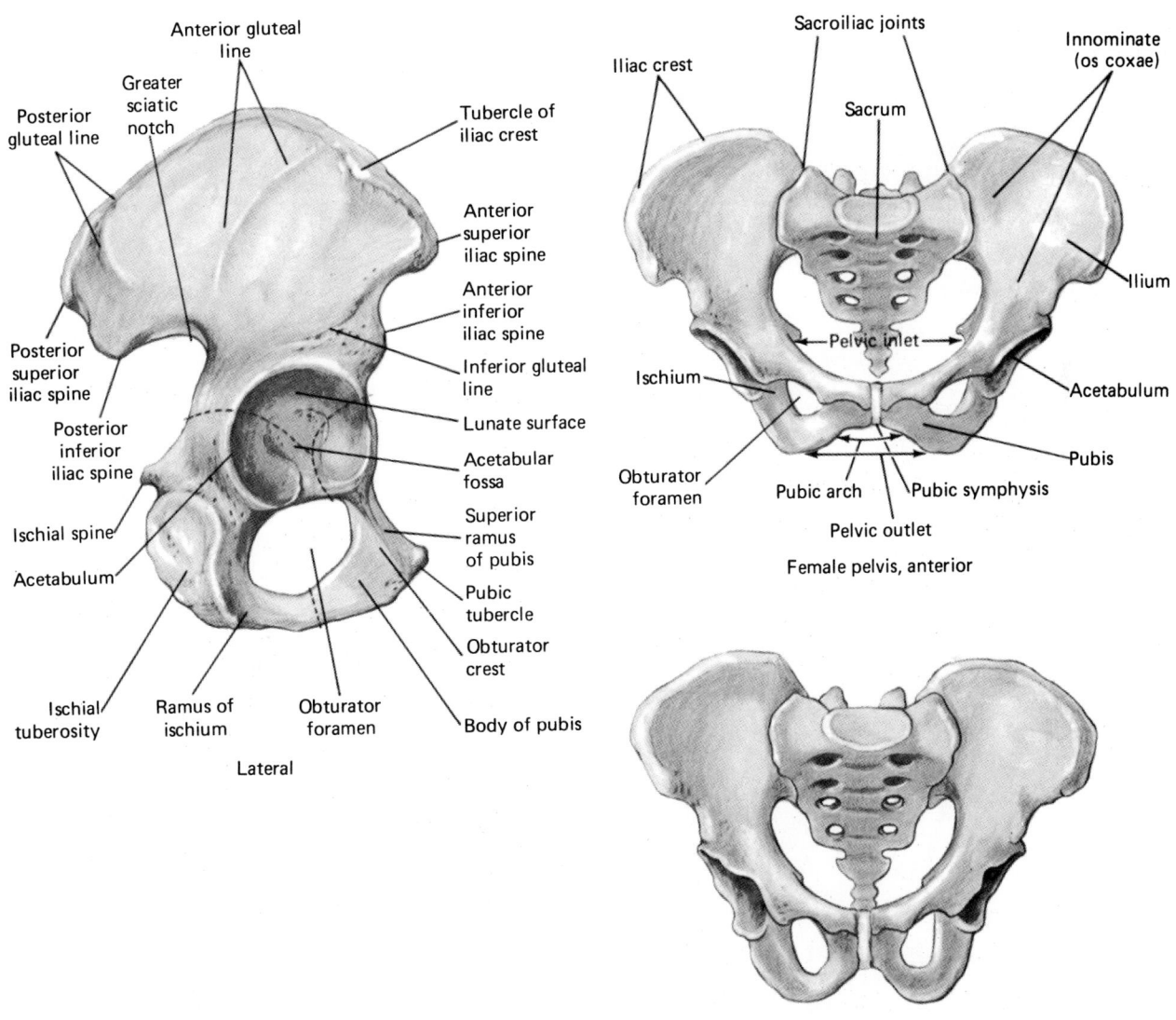

Lateral

Female pelvis, anterior

Male pelvis, anterior

FIGURE 27–14. The pelvis. (From Solomon, E. P., Davis, W. P. [1983]. *Human anatomy and physiology* [p. 181]. Philadelphia: Saunders College.)

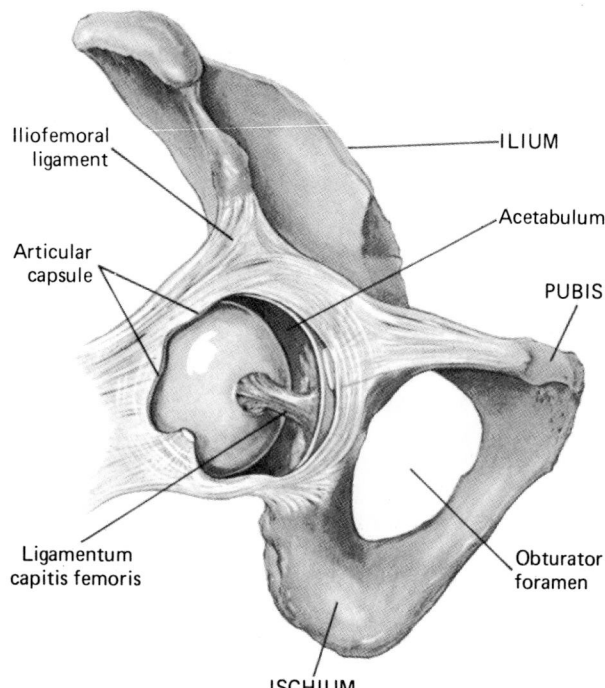

Iliofemoral ligament

Articular capsule

Ligamentum capitis femoris

ILIUM

Acetabulum

PUBIS

Obturator foramen

ISCHIUM

FIGURE 27–15. The right hip joint. (From Solomon, E. P., Davis, W. P. [1983]. *Human anatomy and physiology* [p. 183]. Philadelphia: Saunders College.)

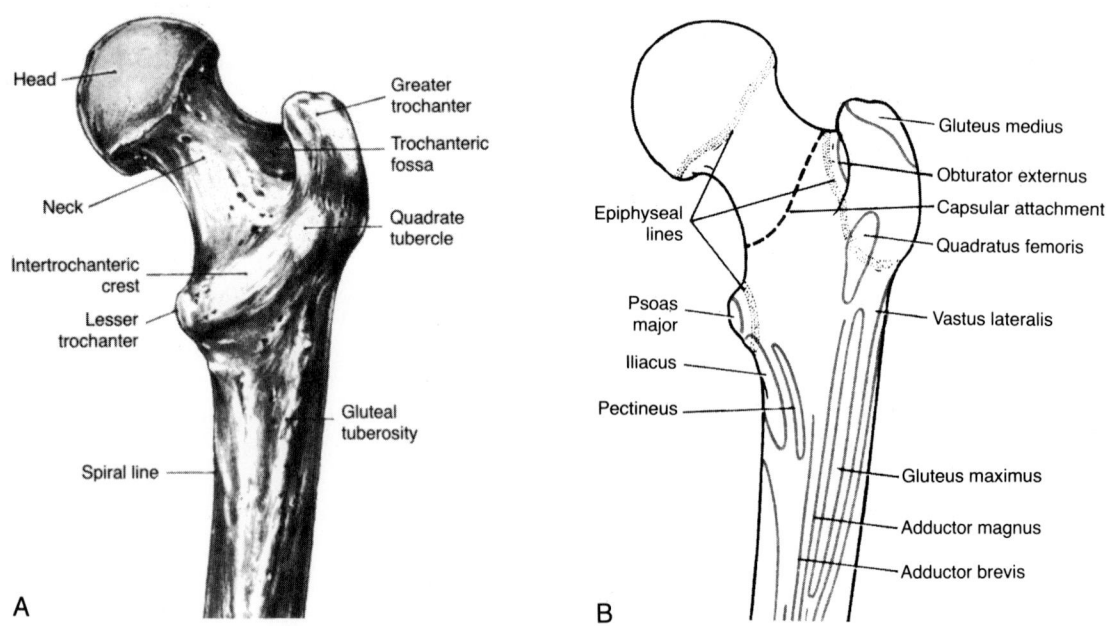

Head

Neck

Intertrochanteric crest

Lesser trochanter

Spiral line

Greater trochanter

Trochanteric fossa

Quadrate tubercle

Gluteal tuberosity

A

Epiphyseal lines

Psoas major

Iliacus

Pectineus

Gluteus medius

Obturator externus

Capsular attachment

Quadratus femoris

Vastus lateralis

Gluteus maximus

Adductor magnus

Adductor brevis

B

FIGURE 27–16. *A*, Posterior aspect of the proximal right femur. *B*, Attachments and epiphyseal lines. (From Williams, P. L., Warwick, R. [1980]. Gray's anatomy [36th ed.] [p. 394]. New York: Churchill Livingstone.)

oral condyles are separated by a smooth depression called the *intercondylar groove*. This groove is the articular surface for the patella. The posterior condyles project slightly, and the space between them forms a deep fossa, the intercondylar fossa. The femoral shaft bows and directs the distal end of the femur more medially.

Knee Joint and Lower Extremity

The intercondylar fossa of the femur receives the intercondylar eminence of the tibia when in flexion. The articulating condylar surfaces of the tibia form two facets, which are deepened by cartilages into fossae to accept the distal femoral condyles. The *patella*, or kneecap, is a triangular bone found anteriorly in the intercondylar groove of the distal femur. The patella does not articulate with the tibia at any point, but the posterior surface communicates with the femur. It is held in position by ligaments and muscles and united with the patellar tendon on its anterior surface.

The *knee joint* consists of all the above mentioned articulations (Fig. 27–17). The bones that form the knee joint are connected by extraarticular and intraarticular structures (Fig. 27–18). Extraarticular attachments are the collateral ligaments, the quadriceps muscle, and the capsule. The structures provide support for the knee

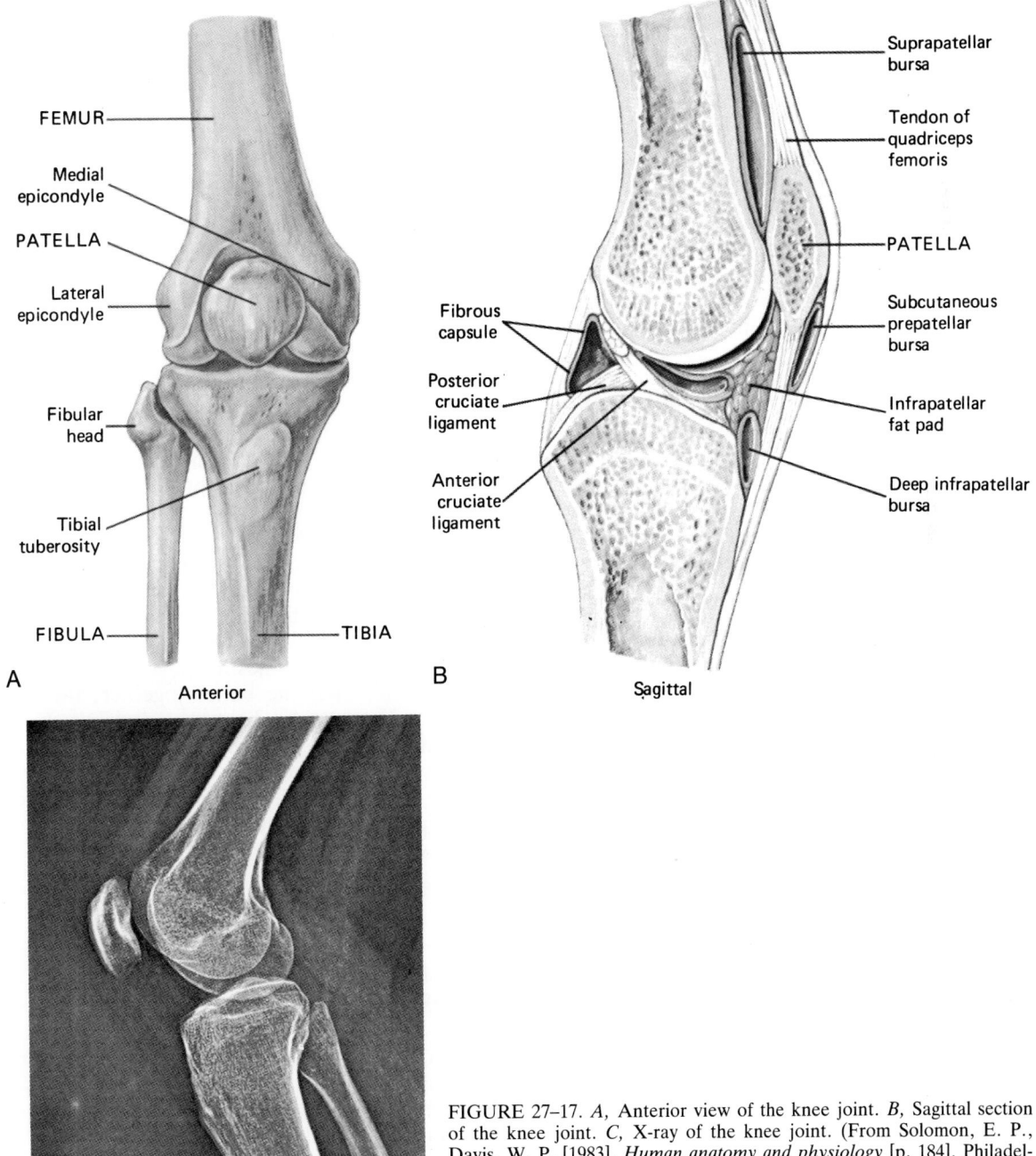

FIGURE 27–17. *A,* Anterior view of the knee joint. *B,* Sagittal section of the knee joint. *C,* X-ray of the knee joint. (From Solomon, E. P., Davis, W. P. [1983]. *Human anatomy and physiology* [p. 184]. Philadelphia: Saunders College.)

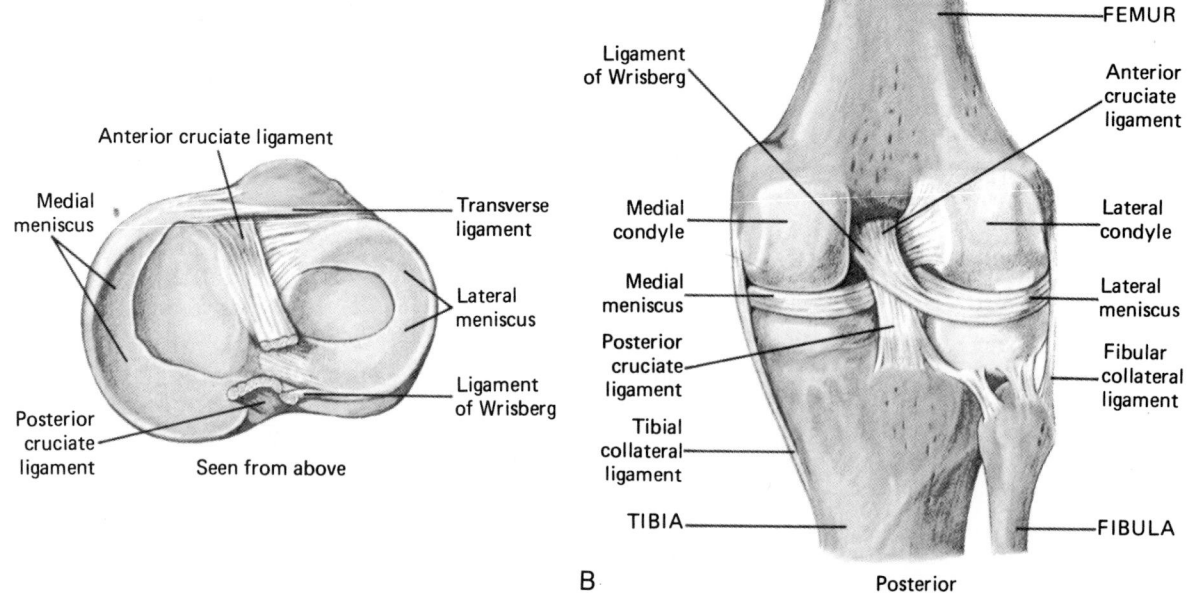

FIGURE 27–18. *A*, Superior view of the knee joint and cartilages. *B*, Posterior view of the entire joint. (From Solomon, E. P., Davis, W. P. [1983]. *Human anatomy and physiology* [p. 184]. Philadelphia: Saunders College.)

joint medially, laterally, and anteriorly, respectively. Anteroposterior support is provided by the anterior and posterior cruciate ligaments, which are intraarticular. The knee joint is a diarthrotic joint that allows flexion and extension but also some glide as the joint approaches complete extension.

Between the articular surfaces of the femur and the tibia are two disks, or menisci. These medial and lateral semilunar cartilages provide lateral support to the weight-bearing joint. Each meniscus is attached to the capsule, with the ends attached to the upper articular surface of the tibia. The inside of the joint capsule is lined with a membrane, synovium, that secretes a synovial fluid. The synovial fluid bathes the menisci and prevents extreme wear and tear. Often, injuries to ligaments or menisci cause an inflammatory response and an increase in the production of the synovial fluid.

The *tibia*, the larger medially placed bone, articulates proximally with the fibula and the femur and distally with the talus and the fibula (Fig. 27–19). The smooth, concave, medial and lateral condyles articulate with the femoral condyles and are separated by an intercondylar eminence that projects upward. The intercondylar fossa is anterior and posterior to the eminence. The fibula is the long, narrow bone running laterally to the tibia. Its expanded proximal head articulates with the tibia. Distally, it extends to the lateral malleolus and articulates with the talus.

Ankle Joint and Foot (Fig. 27–20)

The hinge joint formed by the lower end of the tibia and its malleolus and the malleolus of the fibula is called the *ankle joint*. The joint is surrounded by a capsule and connected by ligaments, which extend from the malleoli to the calcaneus and navicular bones.

The bones of the foot include 7 tarsal bones, 5 metatarsal bones, and 14 phalanges. The *talus* is an irregularly shaped bone that fits into a mortise formed by the malleoli and articulates with the calcaneus and navicular bones. The *calcaneus* is the heel bone and provides support to the talus. The posterior surface of the calcaneus is the attachment site of the Achilles tendon. The talus bone accepts all the body weight and transfers a large portion to the calcaneus and a portion to the anterior tarsal bones. There are five metatarsal bones, which lie anterior to the tarsals. The metatarsals articulate proximally with the cuneiforms and distally with the corresponding phalanges.

The foot bones are arranged lengthwise and crosswise to form supportive arches. Because of the ligaments and tendons that bind the bones together, the arches are elastic and not rigid. The arches distribute weight over the entire foot, provide rigidity and strength to the foot as a lever, provide a protective area for the vessels and nerves of the sole of the foot, and absorb shock. The arches are supported by several tendons, ligaments, and muscles.

SPECIAL INSTRUMENTS, SUPPLIES, AND EQUIPMENT

A variety of special accessories, in addition to routine operating equipment, are required in orthopedic suites. Equipment, instruments, and supplies may vary from hospital to hospital.

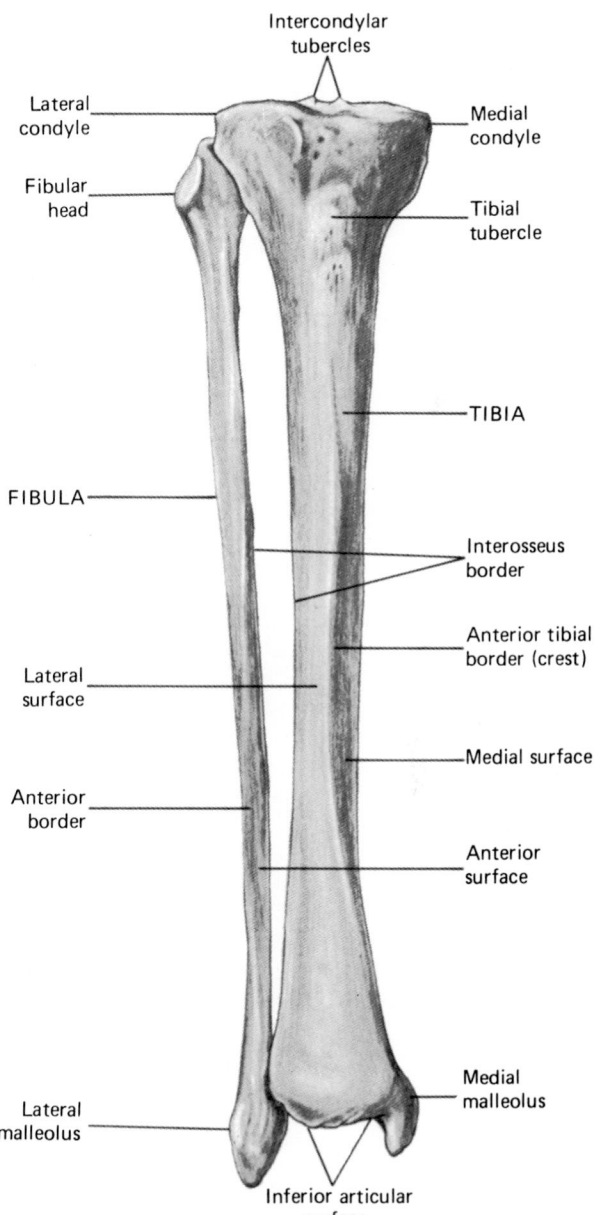

Intercondylar
tubercles

Lateral
condyle

Medial
condyle

Fibular
head

Tibial
tubercle

TIBIA

FIBULA

Interosseus
border

Anterior tibial
border (crest)

Lateral
surface

Medial surface

Anterior
border

Anterior
surface

Medial
malleolus

Lateral
malleolus

Inferior articular
surface

FIGURE 27–19. Anterior view of the bones of the right shank. (From Solomon, E. P., Davis, W. P. [1983]. *Human anatomy and physiology* [p. 183]. Philadelphia: Saunders College.)

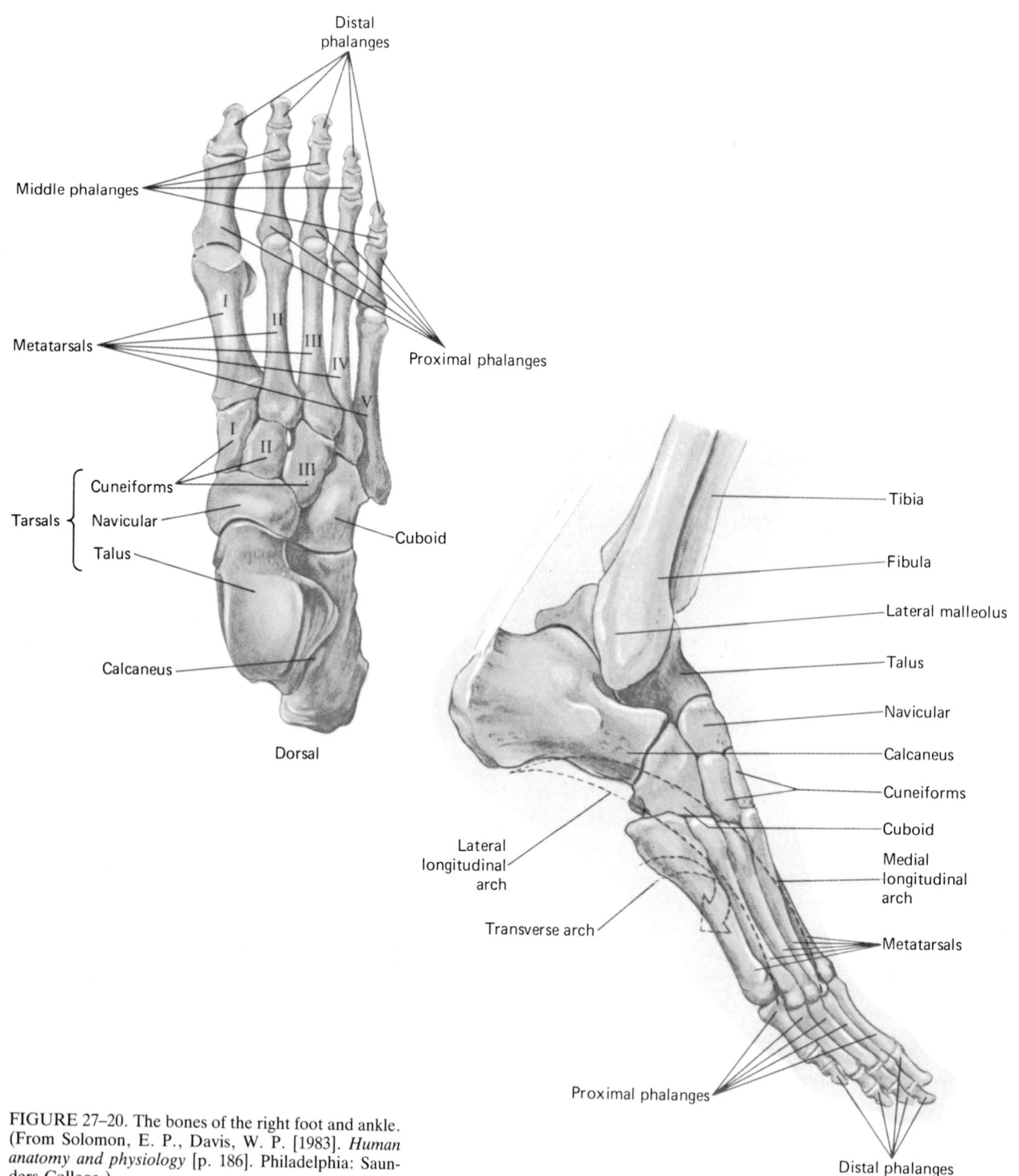

Distal phalanges

Middle phalanges

Metatarsals

Proximal phalanges

I
II
III
IV
V

I
II
III

Tarsals {
Cuneiforms
Navicular
Talus

Cuboid

Calcaneus

Dorsal

Tibia

Fibula

Lateral malleolus

Talus

Navicular

Calcaneus

Cuneiforms

Cuboid

Medial longitudinal arch

Metatarsals

Lateral longitudinal arch

Transverse arch

Proximal phalanges

Distal phalanges

Lateral

FIGURE 27–20. The bones of the right foot and ankle. (From Solomon, E. P., Davis, W. P. [1983]. *Human anatomy and physiology* [p. 186]. Philadelphia: Saunders College.)

Fracture Table

The fracture table (Fig. 27–21) is used for a variety of orthopedic procedures for several reasons:

- The design allows traction to be released, maintained, or increased as necessary on the operative extremity.
- Rotation of the extremity during the procedure can be adjusted.
- Anteroposterior (AP) and lateral x-ray films can be taken during the procedure without disruption of the extremity.
- Easy application of body cast and hip spicas is possible.
- Additional personnel to hold the extremity are not necessary.

Perioperative Nursing Implications

The patient is in a supine position (Fig. 27–21*A*), with the pelvis supported by a supplementary table top, which is translucent to x-rays and incorporates a slot for the introduction of film cassettes. The feet are wrapped in 4-inch Webril bandage before placement in leather boot attachments. Traction is achieved by the stabilization of the pelvis against the vertical perineal post. Proper position is obtained when the well-padded perineal post is in contact with the perineum but is not exerting excessive pressure on the ischial tuberosities or genitalia. Both arms are placed across the patient's chest or one is extended on a padded arm board for transfusion purposes. The ipsilateral arm must be flexed and adducted as far as possible on the chest to avoid contusion of the elbow or ulnar nerve by the image intensifier and to allow unobstructed access to the operative site. Padding is placed under the elbow and under the strap used to secure the arm in position. Radial pulse checks should be obtained to confirm that the arm has not been secured too tightly. Body supports are necessary when lateral tilting of the table top is needed to obtain greater exposure of the operative site. The degree of abduction of the legs depends on the surgeon's wishes but must be adequate to allow the positioning of the lateral x-ray machine. If a calf rest is used, it should be positioned distal to the fibular head to avoid pressure on the peroneal nerve.

When the patient is in the lateral position, he or she is held on the fracture table by a well-padded radiolucent post placed ventrally in the area of the anterosuperior iliac spine (Fig. 27–21*B*). An additional padded post placed between the upper and lower thighs completes the stabilization. The genitalia are protected from injury caused by pressure from the post. A pad should be placed caudad to the dependent axilla. The arms are gently secured on a padded double arm board. The uninjured leg is placed on a padded board or in a leg holder.

Tourniquets

Many orthopedic operations performed on the extremities are carried out in a bloodless field under a

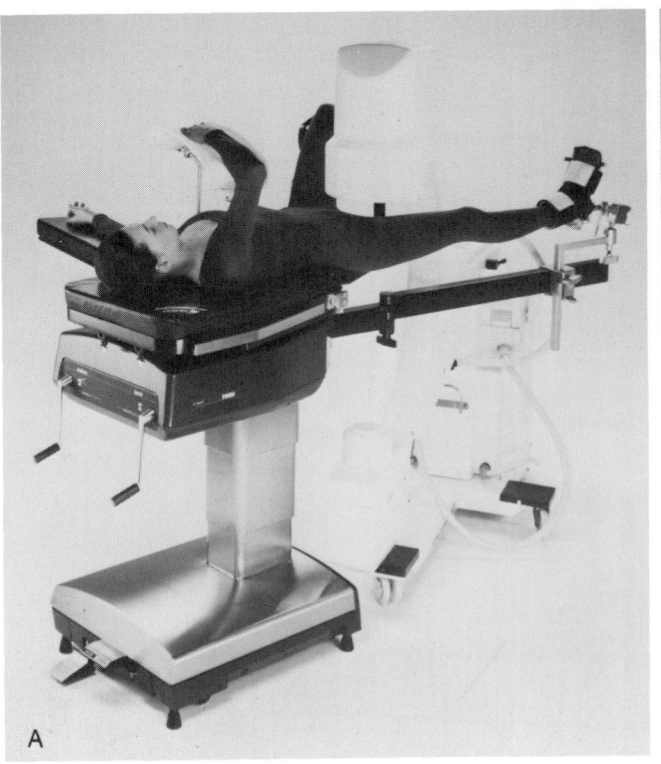
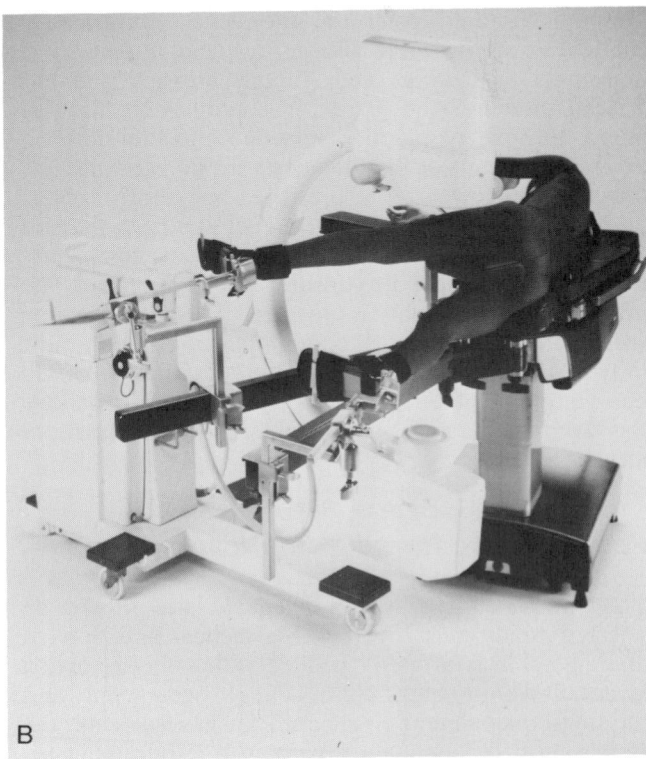

FIGURE 27–21. *A*, A patient supine on a fracture table. *B*, A patient lateral on a fracture table. (Courtesy of AMSCO Healthcare, Pittsburgh, PA.)

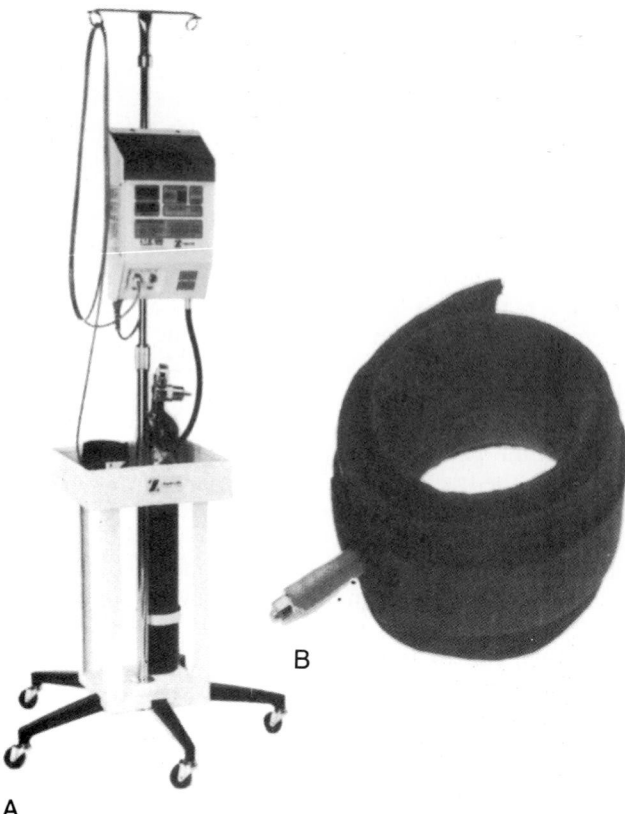

A

B

FIGURE 27–22. *A,* A.T.S. 500 Tourniquet System. *B,* A.T.S. 500 Tourniquet Cuff. (Courtesy of Zimmer, Inc., Warsaw, IN.)

pneumatic tourniquet (Fig. 27–22*A*). A properly applied tourniquet should compress the vessels sufficiently, enough to stop arterial blood flow and no more. If tourniquet pressure exceeds venous pressure and not arterial pressure, the extremity continues to fill with blood; the exit of blood is impeded and therefore an excessive amount of blood collects in the extremity. A tourniquet below arterial pressure, but above venous pressure, is worse than no tourniquet at all. At the end of the procedure, the tourniquet may be completely loosened and removed to ensure venous drainage. The use of excessive pressure is unnecessary, and irreversible ischemia and nerve damage are potential risks. In most instances, this means the application of a pressure of 50 mm Hg greater than systolic pressure. Pressures above this level may be necessary to compensate for muscle or fat.

Perioperative Nursing Implications

A cuff (Fig. 27–22*B*) of adequate size should be selected (ends must overlay 2–3 inches) and applied after the skin is properly padded with smooth applied layers of Webril (Fig. 27–23). The nitrogen supply and the tourniquet should be checked for gas leaks and the supply must be adequate to sustain the tourniquet for at least 2½ hours. The tourniquet is to be placed as high as possible on the extremity (Fig. 27–24). Caution

is taken not to pinch the skin folds or genitalia. The connecting hose should lead away from the patient so as not to get kinked or loosened and for easy access. The tourniquet should be inflated as rapidly as possible (for reasons described above), with the extremity elevated. The extremity, while elevated, may be wrapped distally to proximally with a 4- or 6-inch elastic (Ace) wrap or Esmarch rubber bandage to exsanguinate the limb. Cleansing solution must not be allowed to pool under the cuff. An extra layer of Webril applied around the edge of the cuff, and taken off after area is prepared, may prevent any skin burns.

Accurate tourniquet times must be recorded and maintained as part of the nursing record. Surgeons should be informed of the tourniquet time at hourly intervals. Tourniquets are usually released every 2 hours for several minutes. Original settings should be checked at intervals during the procedure.

Spinal Frames and Positioning Devices

Most orthopedic operations are performed with the patient in the supine position. To operate on a patient in the prone position, however, it is necessary to use special positioning devices that allow proper respiratory exchange and permit flexion at the operative site. Most surgeons favor a particular set of equipment while performing spine operations. The following are some available choices.

With Morgan disk pads, the pelvis is flexed at 90 degrees to maximize exposure of the operative site.

A Wilson convex frame provides adjustable flexion of the lumbosacral spine without flexion of the OR bed.

An Andrews spinal table is used for exposure of a large number of vertebrae for spinal fusions (Fig. 27–25).

Chest rolls are custom made or made by rolling and taping sheets or large foam pads together. They are used when flexion is not necessary.

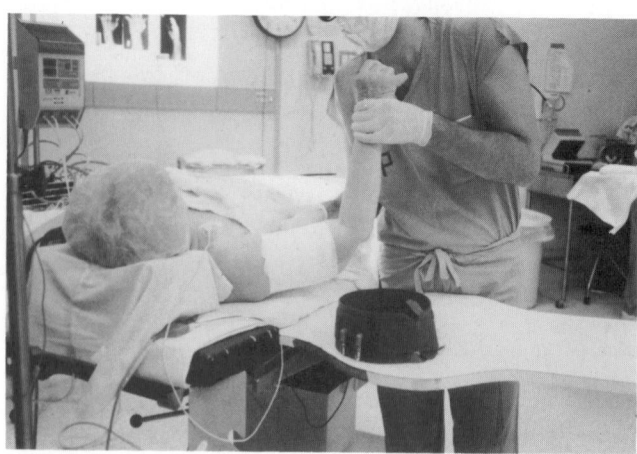

FIGURE 27–23. The appropriate tourniquet is made ready, and Webril is applied to the arm before the tourniquet.

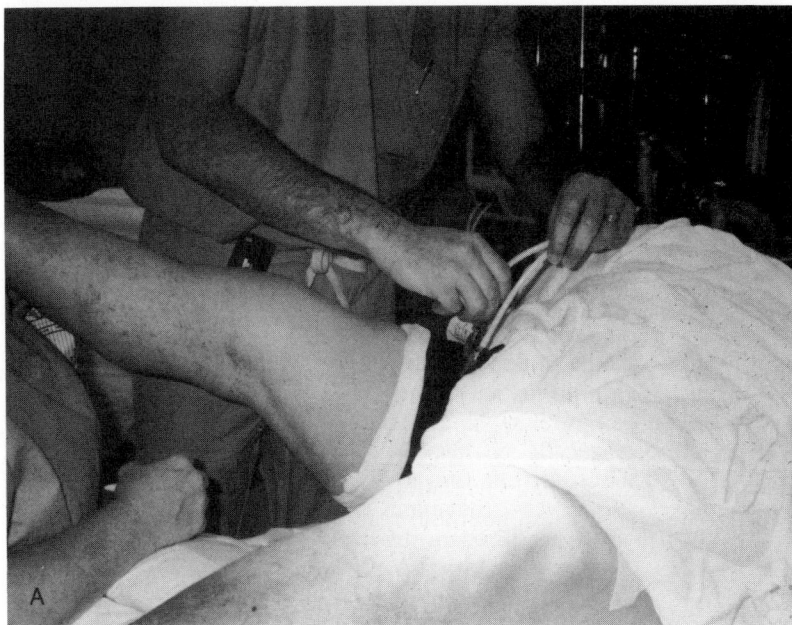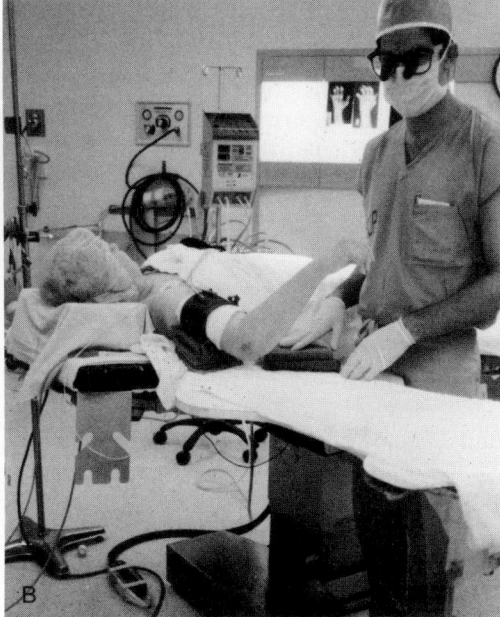

FIGURE 27–24. *A*, Application of the tourniquet around the thigh. *B*, Position of the arm in the tourniquet and on the arm rest of the hand table.

Perioperative Nursing Implications

Soft bolsters (Fig. 27–26) are placed under both sides from just distal to the axillae to the iliac crests. No pressure should be exerted on the axilla. This position allows the abdomen to hang free, improves respiration, and decreases operative bleeding caused by pressure on the vena cava. Bolsters should be padded or covered. Pads are placed under the knees and the dorsa of the feet to protect the toes from pressure.

Arms are abducted to slightly less than 90 degrees and placed on padded arm boards or at the patient's sides to avoid brachial plexus injury. For additional security, adhesive strapping may be placed round the

thorax and table top. Caution is taken not to impede respiratory excursion. A small pad may be placed under the symphysis to avoid undue pressure.

The patient's weight should be adjusted to avoid pressure on the knees. The patient's head is positioned on a small pillow, doughnut, or padded head support. Caution is taken to protect the airway. Frequent checks of the eyes for any signs of pressure are made throughout the procedure.

Bone Cement

Bone cement (methyl methacrylate) is often used to hold a metal or synthetic prosthesis in place. Because

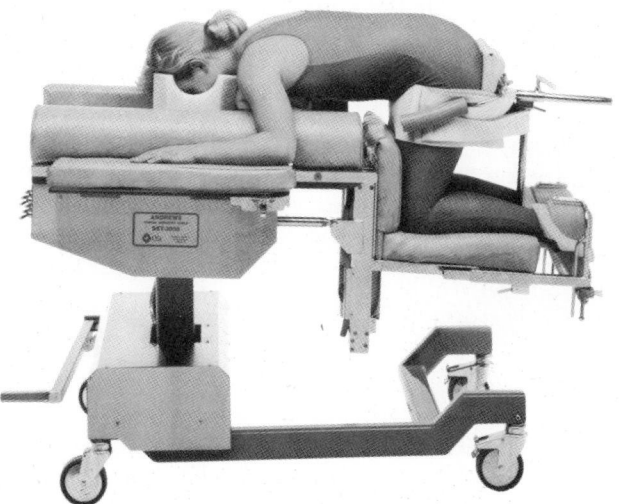

FIGURE 27–25. The Andrews SST-3000 Spinal Surgery Table. (Courtesy of Orthopedic Systems, Inc., Hayward, CA.)

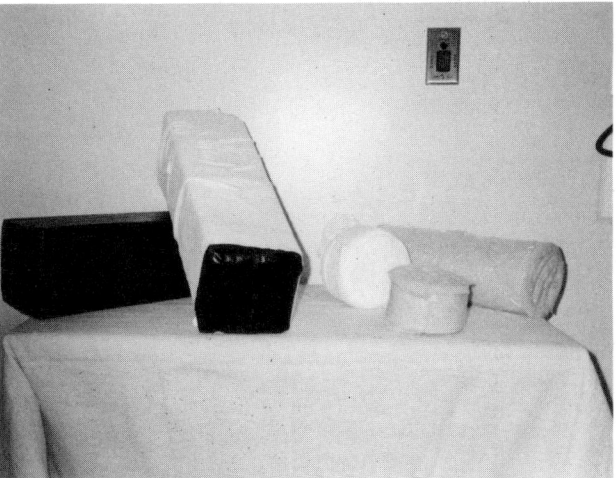

FIGURE 27–26. Positioners, pads, and rolls used to position the patient.

the fumes from the cement are toxic to the respiratory system, closed mixing units equipped with suction should be used whenever possible. In addition, many orthopedic surgical teams don a second pair of gloves to prevent the fumes from permeating and irritating the skin.

The methyl methacrylate is formed by two components, one a liquid and the other a powder. The powder is placed in the mixing unit and the liquid is added in accordance with the surgeon's directive. At least 3 minutes of continuous mixing is necessary to prepare the cement (the time varies with the humidity and temperature of the air).

Manually operated insertion cartridges and devices are frequently used in total joint replacements (Fig. 27–27A). The bone cement is transferred from the mixing unit (Fig. 27–27B) to the cement guns (Fig. 27–27C) while it is still pourable. The cement can be placed in a centrifuge to increase the fatigue strength and provide a homogeneous mixture.

Perioperative Nursing Implications

The initial time of preparation is noted, and the surgeon is kept informed of the consistency of the remaining mixture. Additional gloves should be made readily available to the surgical team and donned if adherent cement is present. Proper evacuation of fumes from the mixing unit is accomplished by the use of a suction device. The operative site and surgical field should be free from any loose particles of bone cement. The potential benefits are weighed against possible hazards of the use during pregnancy or by women of childbearing years. Soft contact lenses that are permeable should not be worn in the presence of methyl methacrylate. Specific training is necessary to be thoroughly familiar with the properties, handling characteristics, and application of the cement.

Power Equipment

The use of all powered surgical instruments in the OR eliminates the need for many hand-operated tools,

thereby reducing operating time. Fingertip control allows the surgeon to control speed and power instantly. Power tools, whether air or electrically powered, can be used in a variety of ways, including drilling the bone, cutting the bone, shaping the joint, and inserting screws. Figure 27–28 shows examples of power instruments.

Perioperative Nursing Implications

It is important to be familiar with the proper use of power equipment. Knowledge of the manufacturer's recommended cleaning, lubricating, and sterilizing instructions is essential. Routine maintenance of power equipment should be performed.

Power equipment can generate heat, which can damage bone cells and normal tissue, and must be carefully controlled. Irrigation of the surgical site may decrease generated heat and contain debris.

Specific Orthopedic Instruments

In addition to the basic instruments needed on all cases, the following instruments are needed for orthopedic surgery:

Elevators (Fig. 27–29) are necessary to strip the periosteum and to expose the bone.

Retractors (Fig. 27–30) are contoured to fit around a bone or a joint when placed in proper position and are designed so that muscles are neither cut nor torn.

Rongeurs (Fig. 27–31) remove soft tissue directly around the bone, cut into the bone, smooth jagged edges, and remove small portions of bone.

Osteotomes or chisels (Fig. 27–32) are used for cutting the bone. The chisel has a tapered side, which is required when a finer, straighter cut is desired.

Bone clamps (Fig. 27–33) are used to grasp a fragmented bone and hold it in place until a fixating device can be applied.

Curets (see Fig. 27–32) are used for scraping, shaping, and removing bone, particularly cancellous.

Text continued on page 665

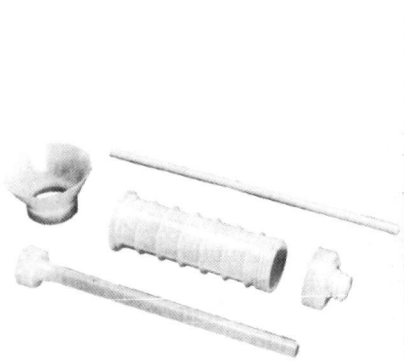
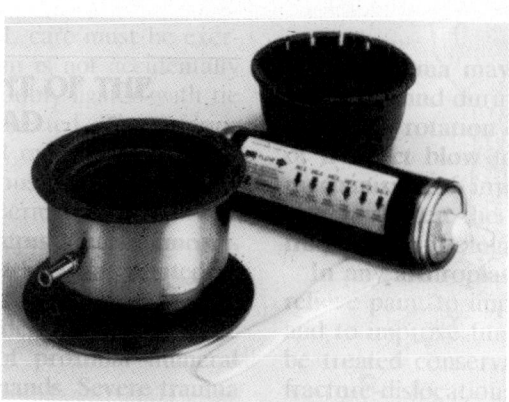
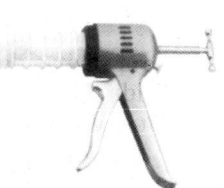

A   B   C

FIGURE 27–27. *A,* Cartridge Kit for the Bone Cement Injector. *B,* Monomer Fume Evacuating System. *C,* Miller Bone Cement Injector. (Courtesy of Zimmer, Inc., Warsaw, IN.)

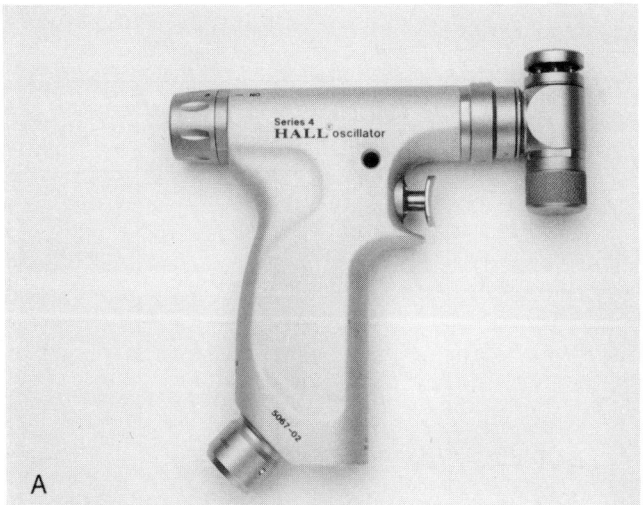

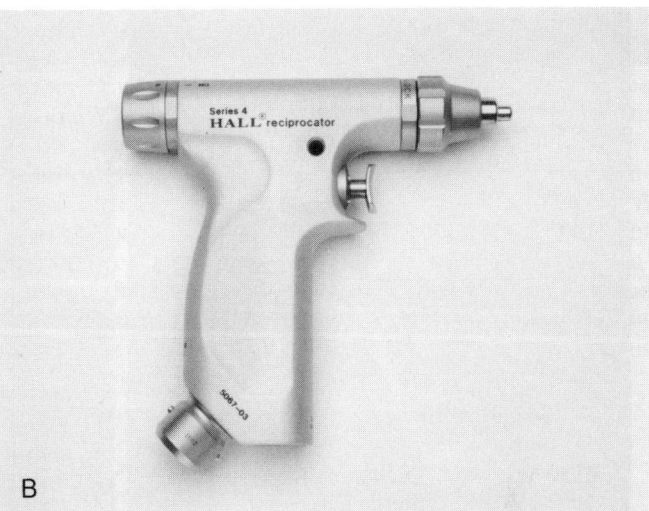

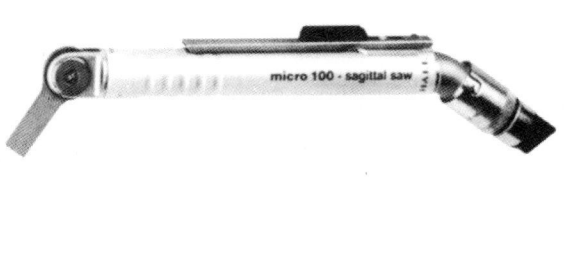

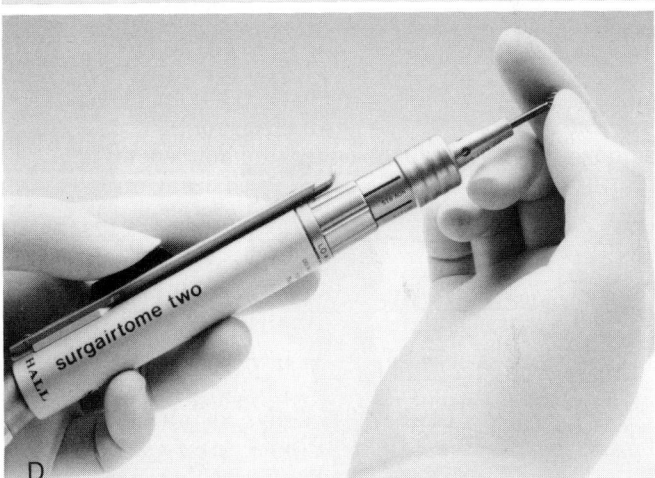

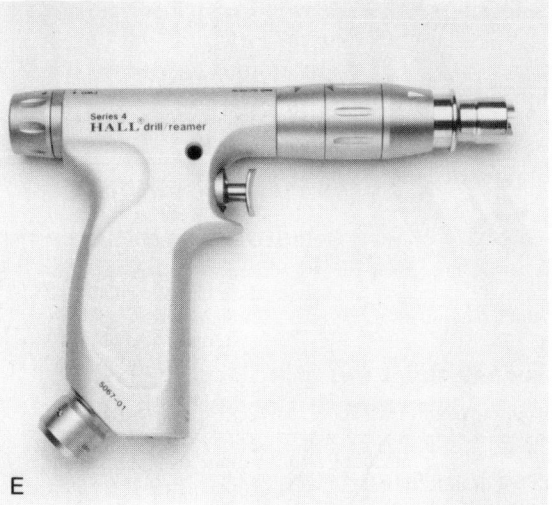

FIGURE 27–28. *A*, Hall Series 4 Oscillating Saw. *B*, Hall Series 4 Reciprocating Saw. *C*, Micro 100 Sagittal Saw. *D*, Hall Surgairtome Two. *E*, Hall Series 4 Drill/Reamer.

Illustration continued on following page

Cat. No.	Description	Blade Width cm	Maximum Cutting Depth cm	Thickness mm	Teeth per cm	Qty.
5052-50	Oscillating Blade	5.1	6.35	0.6	7	1
5052-250	Sterile Disposable	5.1	6.35	0.6	7	5/box
5052-51*	Oscillating Blade	3.2	6.35	0.6	7	1
5052-251*	Sterile Disposable	3.2	6.35	0.6	7	5/box
5052-52	Oscillating Blade	1.25	6.35	0.6	7	1
5052-252	Sterile Disposable	1.25	6.35	0.6	7	5/box
5052-53	Oscillating Blade	1.9	6.35	0.6	7	1
5052-253	Sterile Disposable	1.9	6.35	0.6	7	5/box

Blades not shown actual size

F

FIGURE 27–28 *Continued F,* Hall Series 4 assorted oscillating blades.

Straight Sagittal Saw Blades

Cat. No.	Description	Blade Width cm	Maximum Cutting Depth cm	Thickness mm	Teeth per cm	Quantity
5053-38	Fine Tooth Sagittal	0.95	2.55	0.4	14	1
5053-238	Sterile Disposable	0.95	2.55	0.4	14	5/box
5053-39	Fine Tooth Sagittal	0.45	2.55	0.4	14	1
5053-239	Sterile Disposable	0.45	2.55	0.4	14	5/box
5053-40	Fine Tooth Sagittal	0.95	4.1	0.4	14	1
5053-240	Sterile Disposable	0.95	4.1	0.4	14	5/box
5053-41	Fine Tooth Sagittal	0.6	3.4	0.4	14	1
5053-241	Sterile Disposable	0.6	3.4	0.4	14	5/box
5053-42	Fine Tooth Sagittal	0.4	3.4	0.4	14	1
5053-242	Sterile Disposable	0.4	3.4	0.4	14	5/box

Blades not shown actual size

G

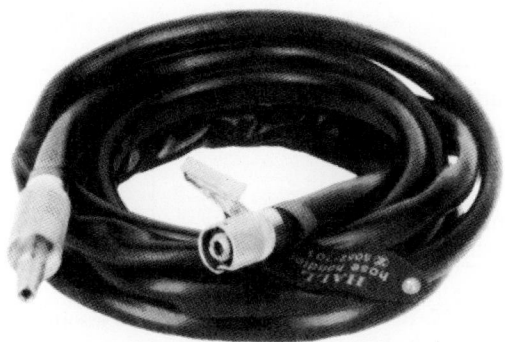

H

FIGURE 27–28 *Continued G,* Hall Microsagittal blades. *H,* Universal hoses.

Illustration continued on following page

Cat. No.	Bur Type	Head Material	Head Diameter mm	Cutting Length cm	Quantity
5092-103	Sterile Side Cutting, Tapered	Carbide	1.7	1.2	1
5092-203	Sterile Side Cutting, Tapered	Carbide	1.7	1.2	5/box
5092-104	Sterile Side Cutting, Straight	Carbide	1.5	0.75	1
5092-204	Sterile Side Cutting, Straight	Carbide	1.5	0.75	5/box
5092-106	Sterile Side Cutting, Tapered	Carbide	2.0	0.75	1
5092-206	Sterile Side Cutting, Tapered	Carbide	2.0	0.75	5/box
5092-114	Sterile Side Cutting, Tapered	Carbide	2.0	1.9	1
5092-214	Sterile Side Cutting, Tapered	Carbide	2.0	1.9	5/box
5092-120	Sterile Round Cutting	Carbide	1.0		1
5092-220	Sterile Round Cutting	Carbide	1.0		5/box
5092-122	Sterile Round Cutting	Carbide	1.5		1
5092-222	Sterile Round Cutting	Carbide	1.5		5/box
5092-124	Sterile Round Cutting	Carbide	2.0		1
5092-224	Sterile Round Cutting	Carbide	2.0		5/box
5092-126	Sterile Round Cutting	Carbide	3.0		1
5092-226	Sterile Round Cutting	Carbide	3.0		5/box
5092-128	Sterile Round Cutting	Carbide	4.0		1
5092-228	Sterile Round Cutting	Carbide	4.0		5/box
5092-130	Sterile Round Cutting	Carbide	5.0		1
5092-230	Sterile Round Cutting	Carbide	5.0		5/box
5092-132	Sterile Round Cutting	Carbide	6.5		1
5092-232	Sterile Round Cutting	Carbide	6.5		5/box

Burs not shown actual size

FIGURE 27–28 *Continued I*, Surgairtome Two assorted burs.

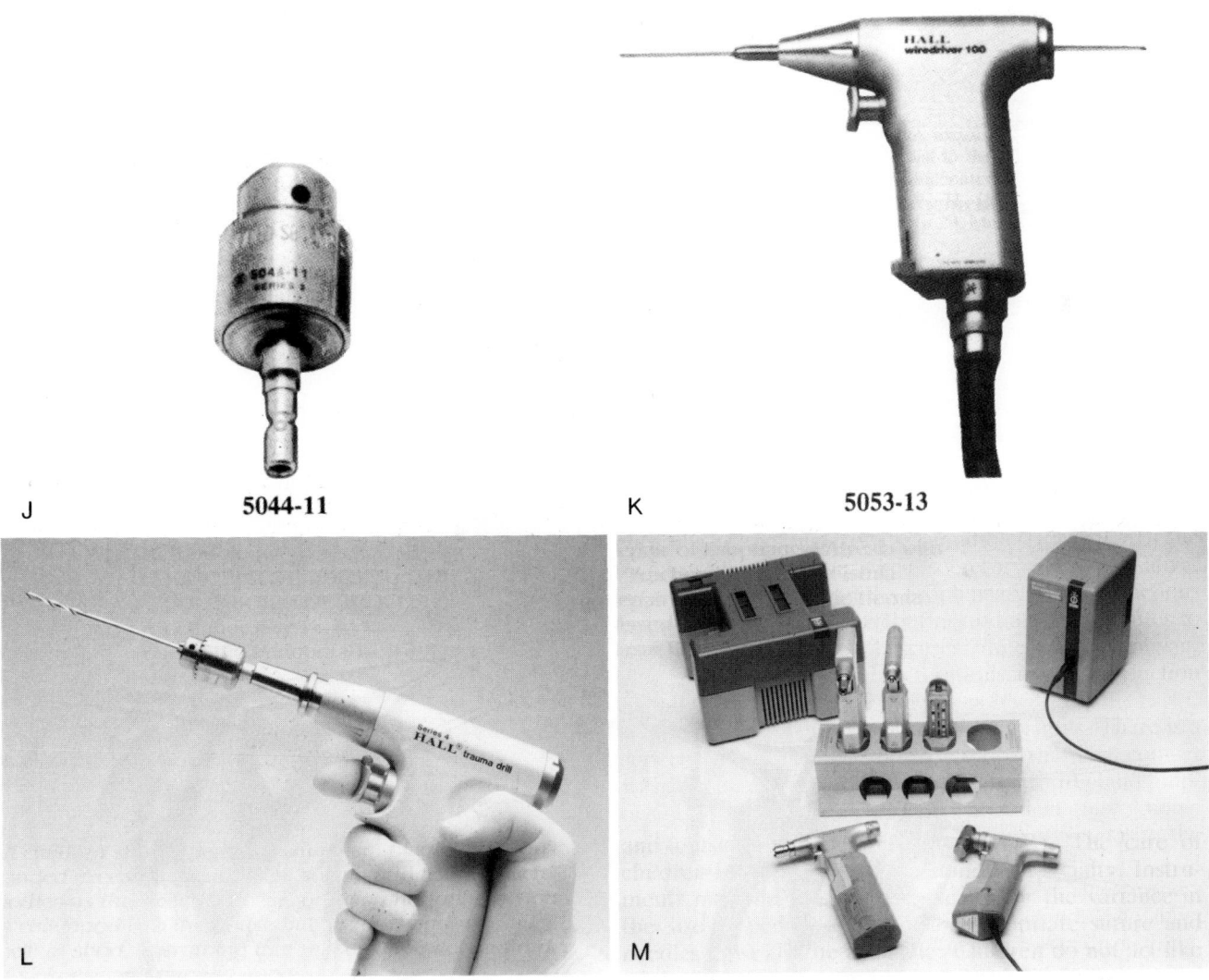

J **5044-11**   K **5053-13**

L   M

FIGURE 27–28 *Continued J,* Series 3 and 4¼" Jacobs Chuck Adaptor. *K,* Hall Wiredriver 100. *L,* Series 4 Hall Trauma Drill. *M,* Hall Surgical portable battery system. (Courtesy of Hall Surgical, Carpinteria, CA.)

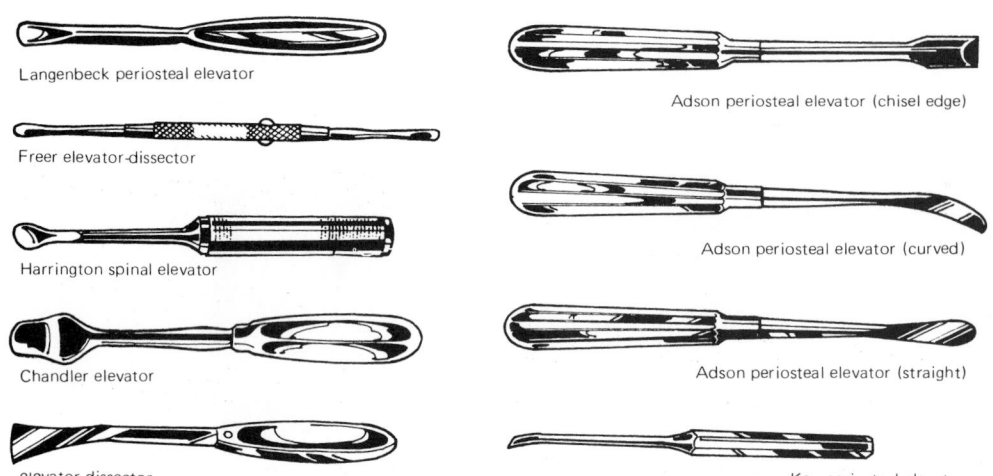

Langenbeck periosteal elevator

Freer elevator-dissector

Harrington spinal elevator

Chandler elevator

elevator-dissector

Adson periosteal elevator (chisel edge)

Adson periosteal elevator (curved)

Adson periosteal elevator (straight)

Key periosteal elevator

FIGURE 27–29. Elevators. (Courtesy of Zimmer, Inc., Warsaw, IN.)

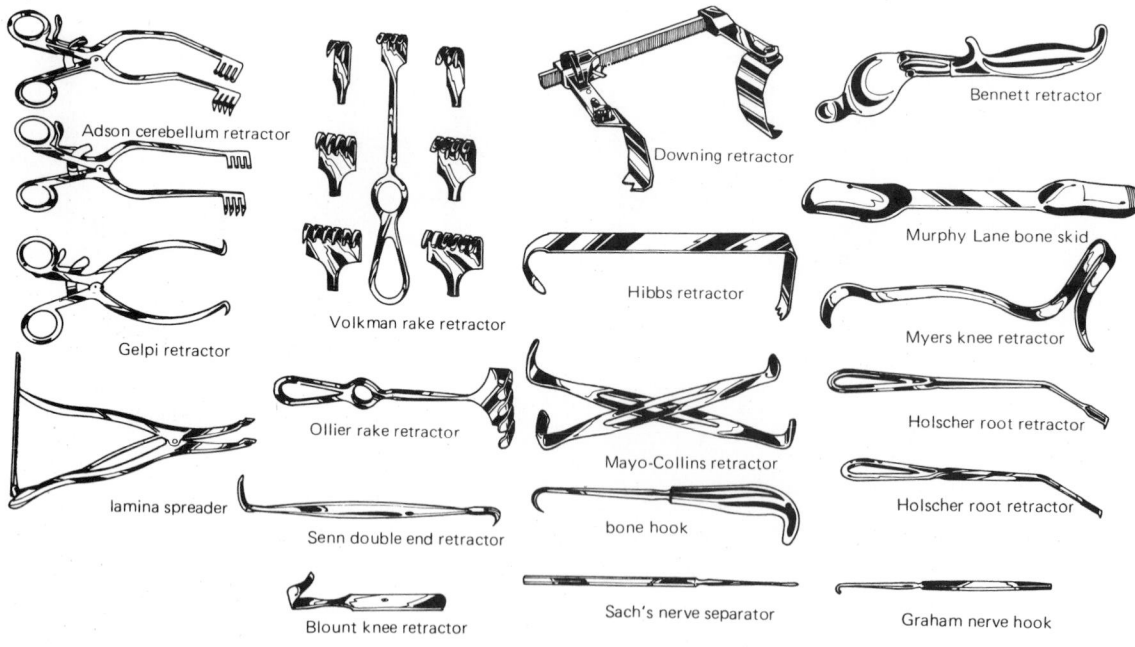

Adson cerebellum retractor

Gelpi retractor

Volkman rake retractor

lamina spreader

Ollier rake retractor

Senn double end retractor

Blount knee retractor

Downing retractor

Hibbs retractor

Mayo-Collins retractor

bone hook

Sach's nerve separator

Bennett retractor

Murphy Lane bone skid

Myers knee retractor

Holscher root retractor

Holscher root retractor

Graham nerve hook

FIGURE 27–30. Assorted retractors. (Courtesy of Zimmer, Inc., Warsaw, IN.)

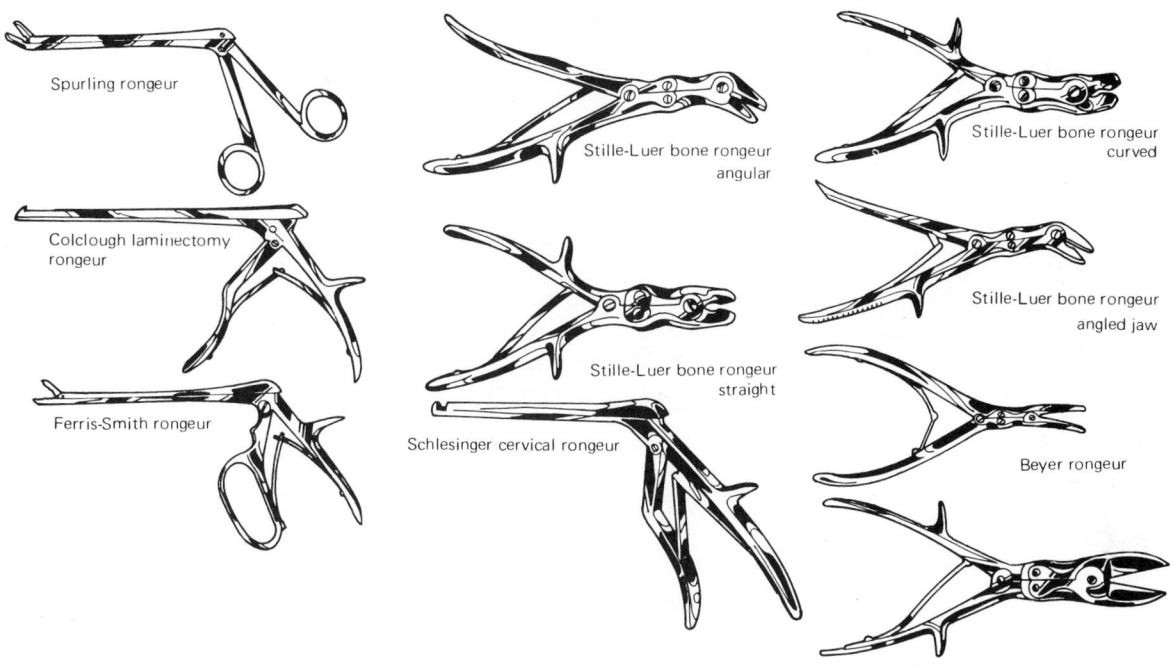

FIGURE 27–31. Rongeurs. (Courtesy of Zimmer, Inc., Warsaw, IN.)

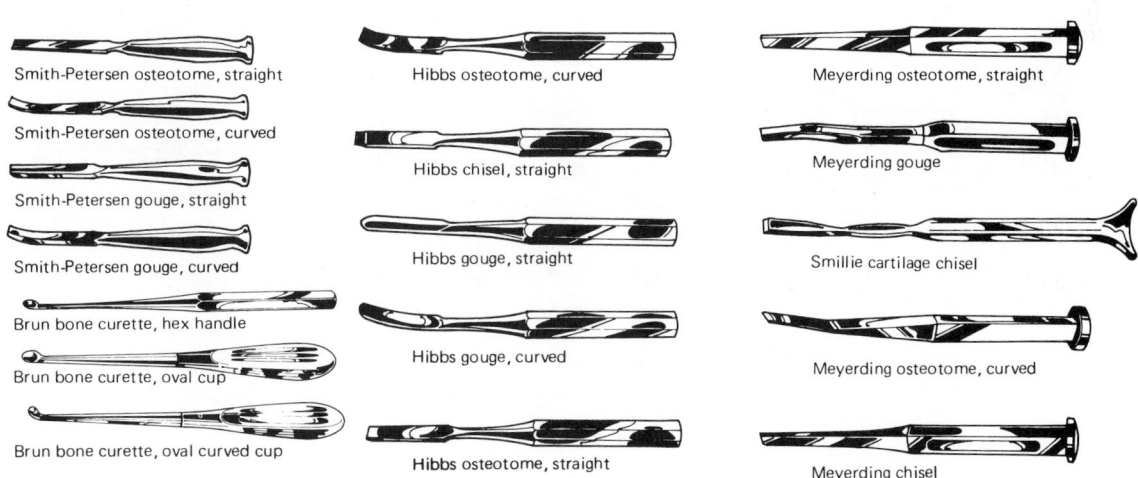

FIGURE 27–32. Osteotomes, curets, and gouges. (Courtesy of Zimmer, Inc., Warsaw, IN.)

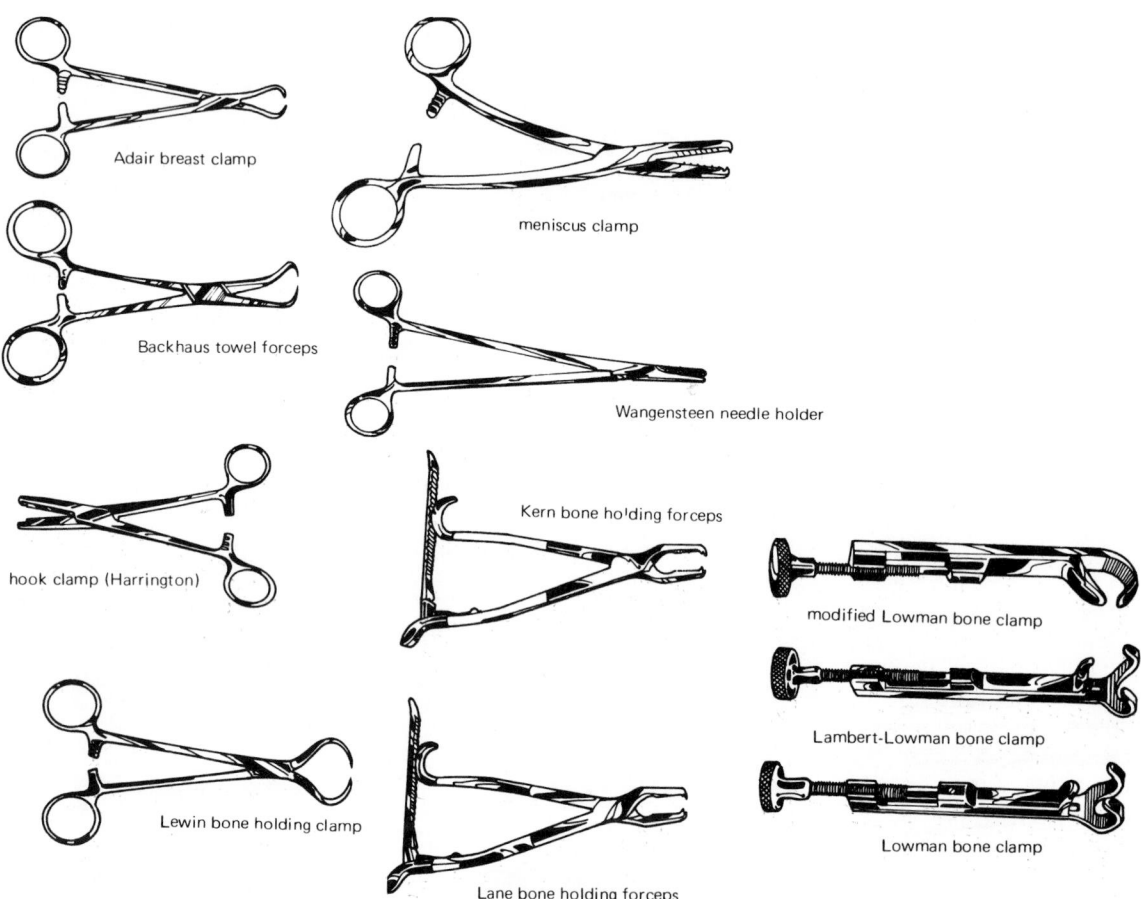

FIGURE 27–33. Bone clamps. (Courtesy of Zimmer, Inc., Warsaw, IN.)

Perioperative Nursing Implications

It is important to be familiar with the proper use of instruments and to perform routine maintenance.

Arthroscopic and Video Equipment

It is now possible to achieve improved visualization and enhanced cutting capabilities in arthroscopic surgery. Instruments are designed for the surgeon to see clearly and sharply and with powerful illumination any pathological lesion that needs surgical correction.

An arthroscope with sheaths is a fiberoptic instrument that allows direct visualization of a joint. Owing to the delicate nature of the arthroscope, a sheath is needed to house the scope during the operative procedure. Sharp and blunt trocars are used to insert the sheath into the joint.

Arthroscopes are manufactured in a variety of diameters (1.7–4 mm) and lens angles (0–120 degrees) to provide different views of the joint. The 30-degree arthroscope is the most common choice for the knee joint. Arthroscopy sheaths are usually 0.5 mm larger in diameter than and are the same length as the arthroscope. Irrigation valves on the sheath may be used for water inflow or suction. Each sheath also has a locking mechanism to secure it to the arthroscope.

The irrigating system is necessary for arthroscopic surgery and includes 2000- to 3000-ml bags of normal saline. The function of the irrigation is to remove the joint fluid, improve visualization, and distend the knee. The irrigating system should be maintained at a height of 6 to 8 feet above the surgical field to improve the pressure that maintains distention and hence visualization. Arthroscopy irrigation pumps are available. Settings of pressure and height are dialed in and maintained throughout the surgical procedure.

Lighting equipment is composed of a light source and a light cable. The arthroscopist must have a high-intensity light to visualize the posterior portion of a joint. The light cable transmits that light through fiber glass strands to the arthroscope. The strands are susceptible to breakage, when the cable is bent, and cannot be repaired. Each arthroscope has a different type of light cable connector; however, manufacturers make attachments for other arthroscopes. The light source can be adjusted to change the light intensity being transmitted.

Camera equipment (a video camera) is necessary for transmitting the image from the arthroscope to the video monitor. Video monitoring allows the assistant to view the procedure and anticipate the needs of the surgeon. The image viewed is magnified and makes visualization easier.

Computer chip cameras have replaced the tube cameras in arthroscopic surgery. They were designed to give a high resolution and attach directly to the arthroscope. These small, solid-state cameras may be soaked, thereby eliminating the need for covering the camera with a sterile drape.

Other equipment used in arthroscopic surgery is shown in Figure 27–34.

Perioperative Nursing Implications

Arthroscopy is an instrument- and equipment-dependent procedure. Failure of a video system or an irrigation system can disrupt a procedure. Proper care and storage of equipment is vital to the proper functioning of the equipment. Arthroscopes should be handled separately; a scratch on the lens may distort the image viewed. All instruments and equipment should be examined before and after each use. Refer to the manufacturer's guidelines for individual standards and recommended policies regarding sterilization, maintenance, and function.

ARTHROSCOPY OF THE KNEE

Definition

Diagnostic arthroscopy is the direct visualization of the interior of a joint through a specially designed fiberoptic instrument called an arthroscope. Since the advent of this technology, the ability to accurately diagnose joint injuries has dramatically increased.

Surgical arthroscopy is performed to repair cruciate or meniscal tears, obtain biopsy specimens, and visualize and remove loose bodies. With the advent of this procedure, the need for the arthrotomy (the surgical cutting into a joint) has decreased. When successful, the operative arthroscopy has many advantages over the standard arthrotomy procedures. Included are a significantly shorter hospital stay, a lower risk of operative complications, and a more rapid return to normal activities.

Indications

Arthroscopy is useful in detecting anterior cruciate ligament or meniscal tears, articular cartilage damage, or synovial defects. However, visualization of the posterior cruciate ligament, the posterior capsule, and the inferior or most anterior aspects of the menisci is not as good.

Related Surgical Procedures

Occasionally, arthrotomy may be necessary if the task cannot be completed through the arthroscope.

Perioperative Nursing Implications

Anesthesia

General or spinal anesthesia is generally used. General anesthesia is preferable, whether the procedure is

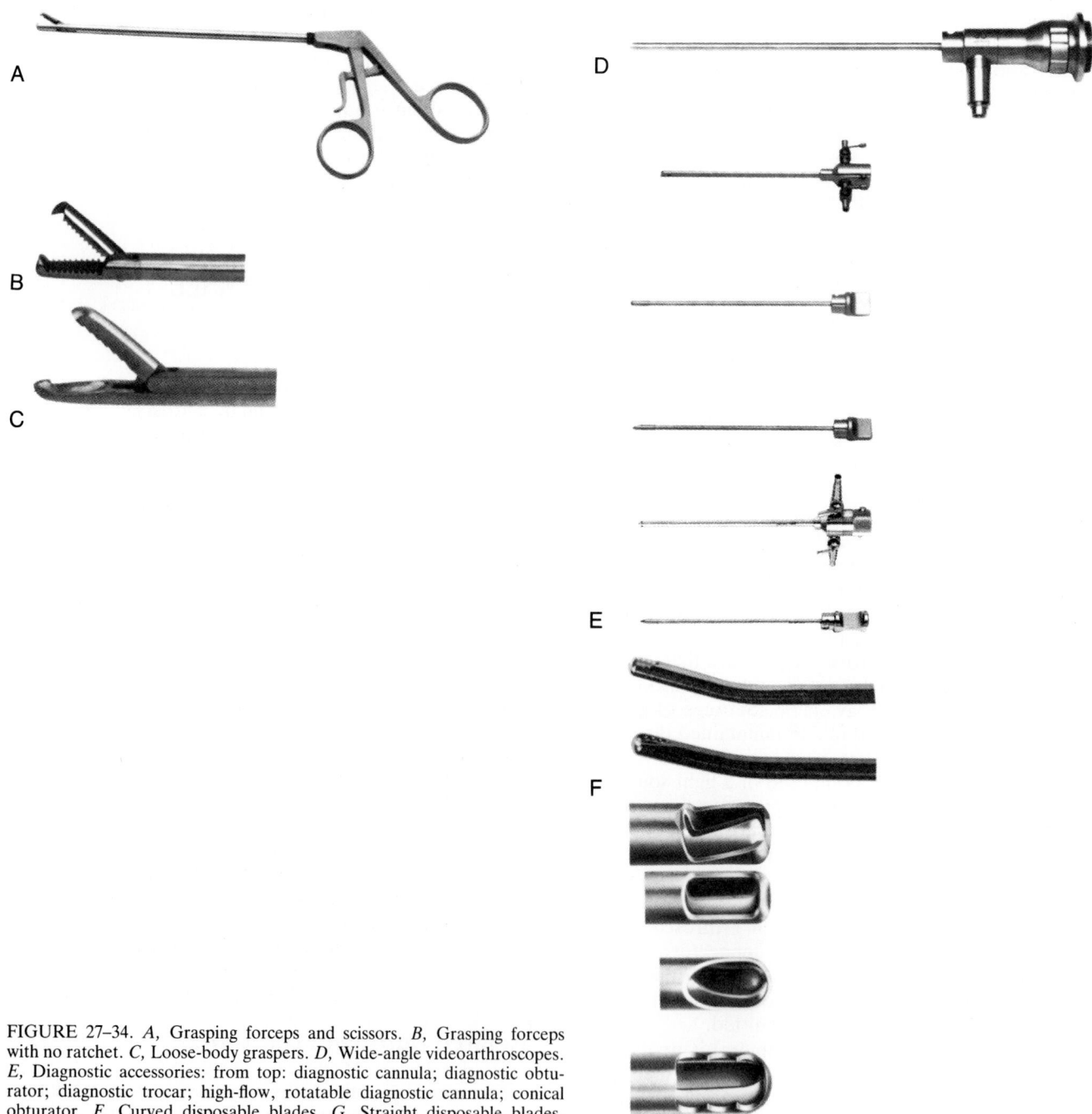

FIGURE 27–34. *A*, Grasping forceps and scissors. *B*, Grasping forceps with no ratchet. *C*, Loose-body graspers. *D*, Wide-angle videoarthroscopes. *E*, Diagnostic accessories: from top: diagnostic cannula; diagnostic obturator; diagnostic trocar; high-flow, rotatable diagnostic cannula; conical obturator. *F*, Curved disposable blades. *G*, Straight disposable blades. (Courtesy of Smith & Nephew Dyonics, Andover, MA.)

done on an inpatient or an outpatient basis. Local infiltration may result in undue discomfort from the tourniquet or leg holder during a prolonged procedure and even an inadequate examination. Some surgeons may use an intraarticular injection of lidocaine to distend the knee and minimize bleeding.

Position

The patient is placed in the supine position (Fig. 27–35). The head is in line with the body. Both arms may be extended on padded arm boards with the palms down. Brachial plexus injury may occur if extension of the arm is greater than 90 degrees. The arm on the operative side may be positioned at the side and tucked under the draw sheet, with the fingers and elbows close to the body. A safety strap is placed loosely across the abdomen, preventing any restriction of respiratory excursion. Additional knee holders may be attached to the OR bed for more specific positioning. Caution is used to avoid team members' inadvertently leaning on the patient. Vulnerable pressure points that may require additional padding include the occiput, scapula, olecranon, sacrum, ischeal tuberosity, and calcaneus. The eyes should be protected from corneal abrasions or irritation by use of an eye patch. The operative extremity is placed in a foot-holding device, which elevates and supports the extremity during the skin preparation (Fig. 27–36).

A tourniquet is then applied to the operative extremity, following the technique and procedures mentioned above (refer to the discussion of equipment). The tourniquet settings are made and confirmed by the operating surgeon.

Creation and Maintenance of the Sterile Field

One of three methods is used to remove the hair from the operative site: electrical clipping, using depilatory, and shaving. A wet shave is preferable and should be done as near the operative time as possible. With the

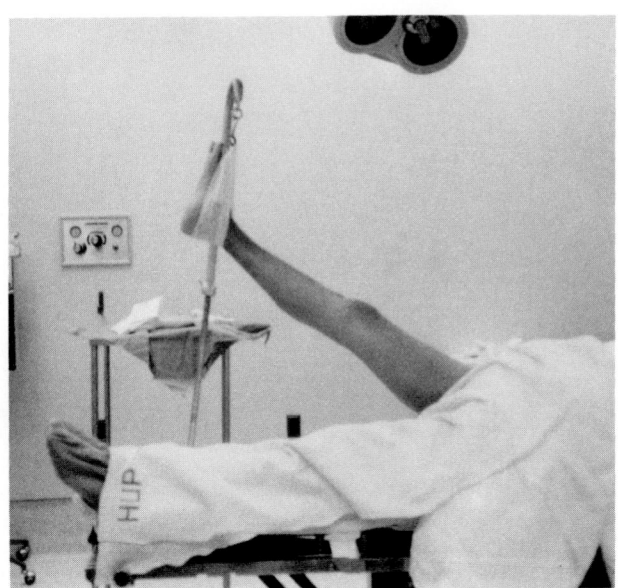

FIGURE 27–36. The patient's leg in a foot-holder.

operative limb in the prep holder, the skin is removed circumferentially 2 inches above and below the knee. An unsterile drape is placed under every operative limb and removed by the circulating nurse after the preparation to prevent pooling of prep solution. The surgical limb is scrubbed, again circumferentially, with an antimicrobial scrub extending the length of the leg, from ankle to midthigh, for 5 minutes (Fig. 27–37A). The area is then blotted dry with sterile towels.

The entire area is then painted with an antimicrobial solution and allowed to dry (Fig. 27–37B). The area around the incision may then be painted with isopropyl alcohol if a plastic adhesive drape is to be utilized. A sterile drape is placed first over the foot of the OR table to protect sterile surgeons' gowns from contamination. The foot is removed from the holder by the circulating nurse while the surgical assistant holds the operative limb with a sterile towel. A sterile stockinet is applied and telescoped down the entire leg (Fig. 27–38). Stockinets may be secured around the foot and ankle with a sterile bandage or wrap. A large drape is then used to cover the nonoperative limb.

A hinged impervious sheet is placed under the operative leg on the sterile field formed by the first drape, and the drape is unfolded to the sides and over the end of the OR table (Fig. 27–39A). The paper backing is removed, and the tails are secured around the top of the limb and the stockinet. A large drape is placed over the upper part of the patient, followed by another large drape. A final large drape is placed over the impervious sheet and secured to the upper sheets around the top of the limb with towel clips (Fig. 27–39B). Custom drape packs are available and, if used, may necessitate alternative methods of draping. The stockinet is then fenestrated, and if required, the plastic adhesive drape is applied to the incisional area. It is important that the drapes are secured to withstand any manipulation during the surgical procedure.

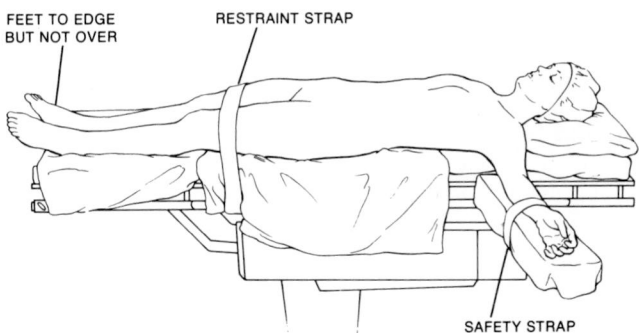

FEET TO EDGE BUT NOT OVER

RESTRAINT STRAP

SAFETY STRAP

FIGURE 27–35. The patient is in the supine position with the arms extended. (From Fuller, J. [1981]. *Surgical technology: Principles and practice* [2nd ed.] [p. 70]. Philadelphia: W. B. Saunders.)

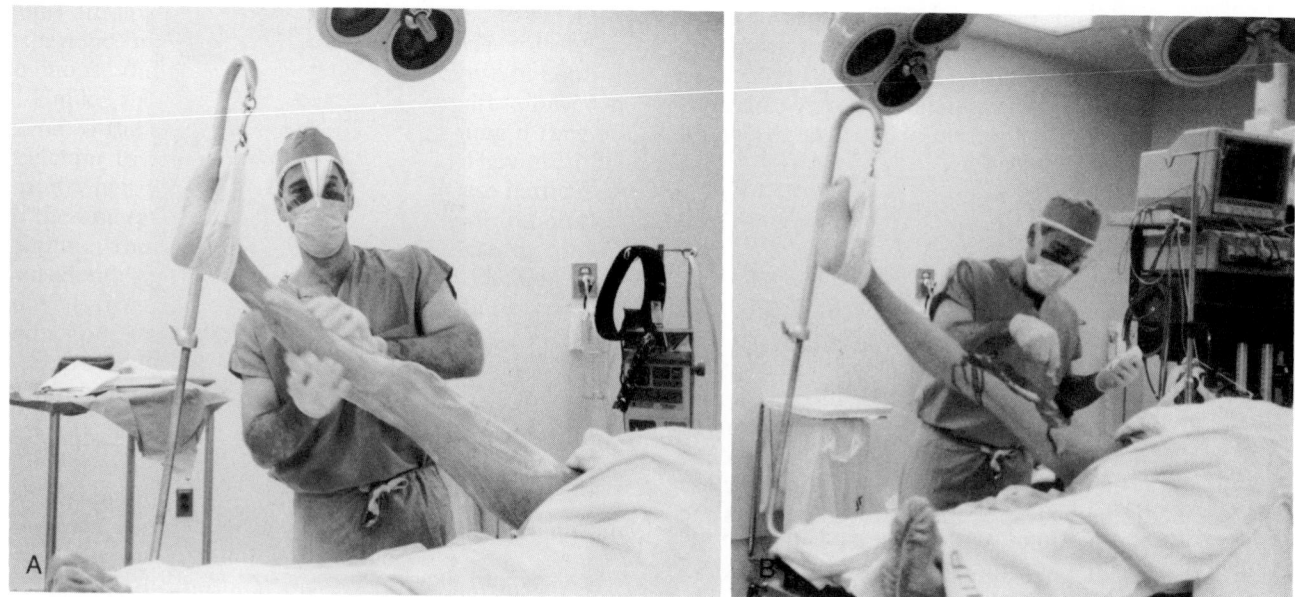

FIGURE 27–37. *A,* In preparation for arthroscopy, the leg is scrubbed with an antimicrobial solution. *B,* The area is then painted with an antimicrobial solution.

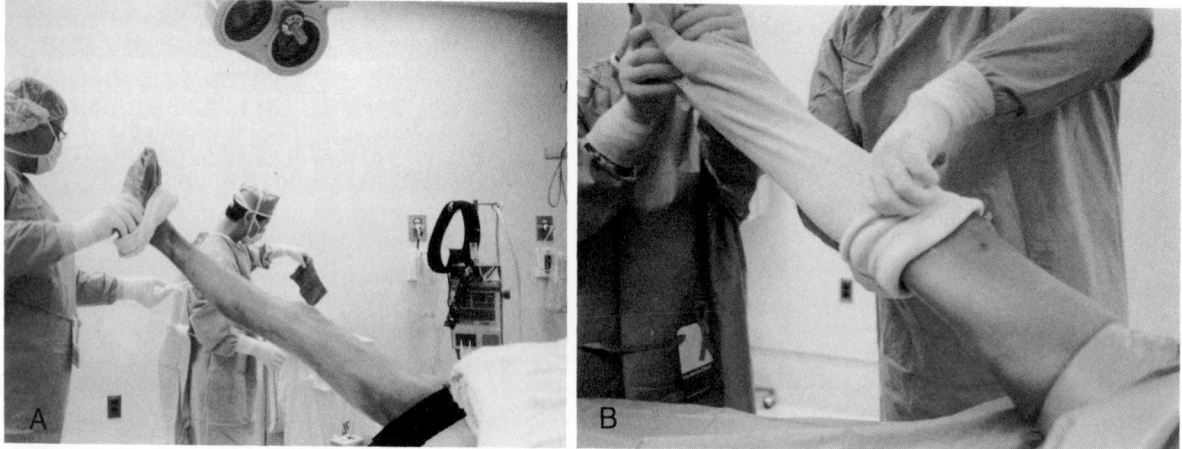

FIGURE 27–38. *A,* A stockinet or towel is held on the patient's foot during draping. *B,* A second sterile stockinet is applied and telescoped down the patient's leg.

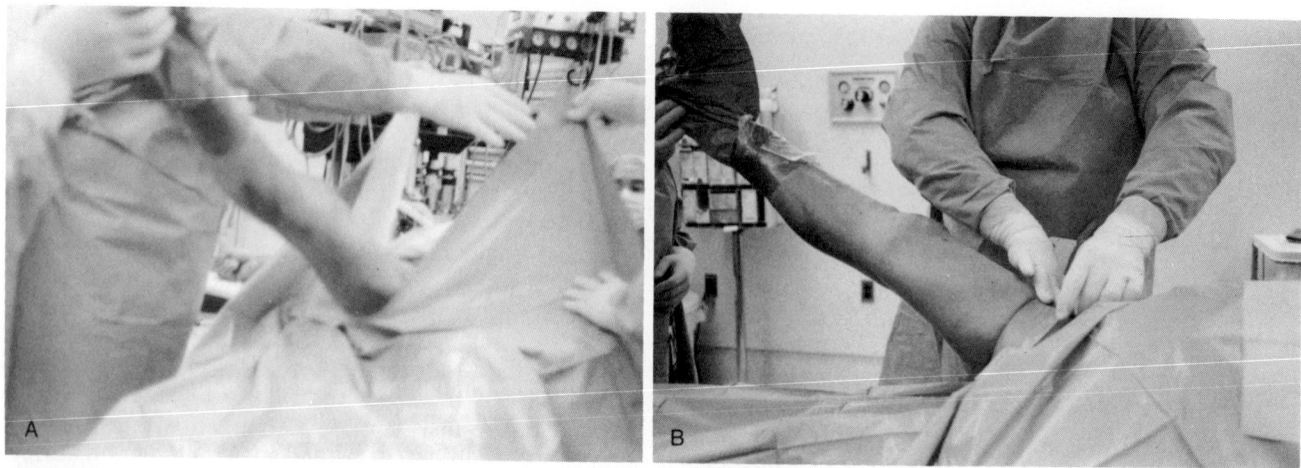

FIGURE 27–39. *A,* A hinged impervious sheet is placed around the top of the patient's thigh. *B,* The hinged impervious sheet is closed around the upper thigh.

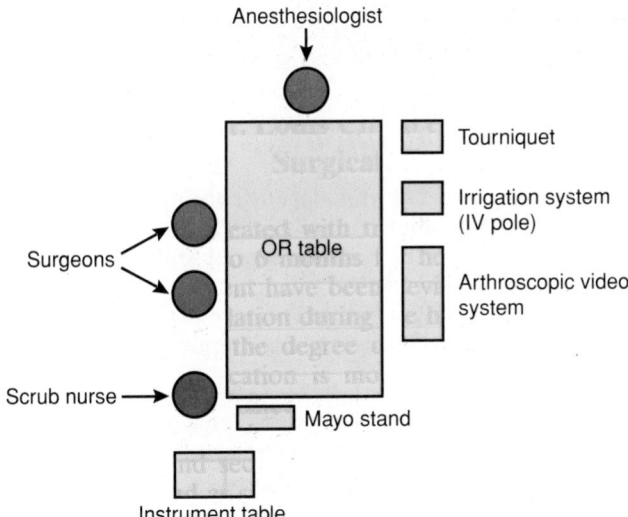

FIGURE 27–40. Operating room set-up for right-knee arthroscopy. The set-up would be reversed for left-knee arthroscopy.

The creation of the sterile field is achieved with the assistance of the scrub nurse. Arthroscopy provides some unique challenges to the scrub nurse. As instruments and the arthroscope are switched from portal to portal, irrigation fluid spills frequently throughout the case. Movement of the joint from full flexion to full extension disrupts the sterile field and is anticipated by the scrub nurse during the draping.

Equipment and Supplies

4–0 Vicryl (cutting needle)
18-gauge, 3½-inch spinal needle
2 No. 11 blades
4 × 8 inch radiopaque sponges
Skin marker
Egress cannula
Inflow tubing
6 3-L bags of normal saline
Kling bandages
Ioban Steri-Drape
Steri-Strips
25-gauge, ⅝-inch needle
25-gauge, 1½-inch needle
Lidocaine 1%, 30 ml
Lidocaine 1% with 1:100,000 epinephrine, 30 ml
2 60-ml Luer-Lok syringes
2 20-ml Luer-Lok syringes
Suction tubing
Assorted arthroscopic surgical blades (according to the surgeon's preference)
Skin preparation tray
Povidone-iodine (Betadine) solution
2 povidone-iodine preparation brushes
Alcohol (according to the surgeon's preference)
2 4 × 4 inch prep or dressing sponges

The tourniquet controls are positioned on the operative side and are easily accessible to the anesthesiologist and the circulating nurse (Fig. 27–40). The tourniquet hose is positioned to prevent any kinking. The identification number of the specific tourniquet is recorded on the patient's chart. After the patient is draped, the circulating nurse positions the arthroscopy video equipment on the nonoperative side in line with the visual field of the operating surgeon.

The circulating nurse then positions the irrigating fluid system on the nonoperative side at the head of the table. Tubing and solution bags should not be in direct view to avoid distracting the surgical team or interfering with visualization of the video monitor (Fig. 27–41).

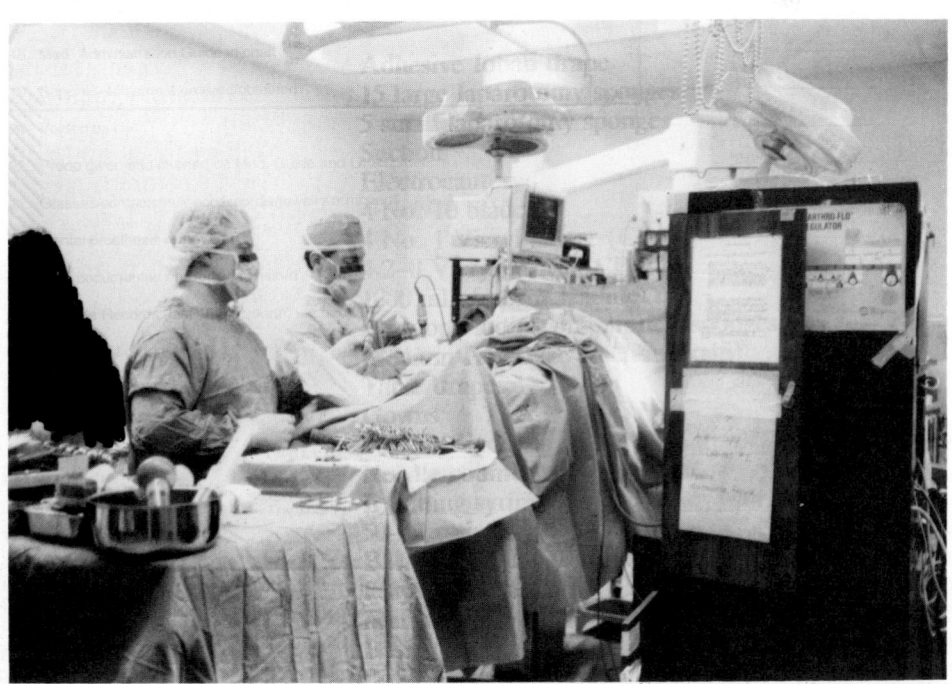

FIGURE 27–41. The surgical team in position to perform arthroscopy.

2 6-inch Webril bandages
2 6-inch elastic (Ace) bandages
Preparation razor
Impervious stockinet
Hinged impervious sheet
500 ml of normal saline
6-inch Esmarch bandage
Fiberoptic light cable and source
Video camera and control unit
Adjustable intravenous (IV) pole
Arthroscopic surgical system
  Shaver
  Abrader
Lateral knee post (arthroscopic leg holder)
Television monitor
Prep leg holder
Tourniquet and cuff

Instruments

Suture scissors
Smillie knife
Meniscus clamp
Bandage scissors
6 hemostats
2 Z-retractors
Anterior knee retractor
Small Weitlaner retractor
Adson forceps with teeth
Tissue forceps with teeth
2 Senn retractors
4 mosquito clamps
4 Allis clamps
2 needle holders
6 towel clips
No. 12 Frazier suction
Arthroscope with sheaths
Light cable
Nos. 3 and 7 knife handles
Dandy nerve hook
Metzenbaum scissors
2 Army-Navy retractors
Arthroscopic instruments
  Suction punch
  Basket forceps
  Scissors
Intraarticular shaver

Physiological Monitoring

Intraoperative nursing care of the arthroscopy patient focuses on patient support before the induction of anesthesia and protection of the patient's musculoskeletal, skin, and peripheral vascular systems. A patient having surgery under local anesthesia must be monitored carefully for reactions. Pressure points should be periodically assessed and monitored throughout the procedure. The area beneath the tourniquet should be examined before the application and after the removal of the cuff and documented accordingly. Tourniquet pressure settings and time should be closely monitored and verbalized to the surgeon every 30 minutes.

Specimens and Cultures

Specimens and cultures vary according to individual pathological examination findings. Routinely, an excised portion of a meniscus is removed and sent for definitive studies. Other diagnostic studies that may be required are anaerobic or aerobic cultures or a cell count of synovial fluid in the presence of a septic joint.

Drugs and Solutions

Depending upon the type of anesthesia, additional local infiltration is often required. Commonly used is lidocaine 1% with 1:100,000 epinephrine. Adjustments and calculations of the solution by the circulating nurse may be needed if it is not premixed by the supplier.

Physician's Orders

Patients are usually admitted the day of the surgery and have the following tests performed on an outpatient basis:

Hematology profile, including
  White blood cell count
  Red blood cell count
  Hemoglobin
  Hematocrit
  Mean cell volume
  Differential cell count
  Platelet count
AP and lateral roentgenograms
Magnetic resonance imaging
Urinalysis
Chest x-ray film (for patients older than age 40)
Electrocardiogram (ECG) (for patients older than age 40)
Nothing-by-mouth status (NPO) after midnight the night before surgery

Laboratory and Diagnostic Studies

Complete blood count (CBC) with differential cell count
Urinalysis
Radiography
  Four-view films are necessary for a complete evaluation.
  Loose bodies and fractures of the patella, distal femur, and proximal tibia can be identified.
  Chondromalacia patella can be diagnosed.
Magnetic resonance imaging
  The above-mentioned meniscal and ligamentous tears may be identified.
  Soft tissue injury can be detected.

Procedure

Incision and Exposure

Knee arthroscopy may be performed with or without tourniquet control. If a tourniquet is used, the operative extremity is either elevated 10 minutes before inflation or evacuated with a 6-inch Esmarch bandage.

Usually, arthroscopy begins with an incision in the anterior superior lateral quadrant or medial aspect of the suprapatellar pouch. A stab incision, made with a No. 11 blade, is followed by the insertion of a cannula and a sharp trocar. After the periarticular tissue and joint capsule are pierced, a blunt trocar replaces the first trocar. The blunt trocar permits entry through the synovium without any damage to the articular surfaces. Any effusion may be removed at this time and possibly sent to the laboratory. The blunt trocar is exchanged for the arthroscope. With the knee in full extension, the irrigating system is attached and opened to distend the knee.

Additional stab wound incisions are made horizontally just above the joint line, again with a No. 11 blade. At this point, there are three portals into the knee joint.

Details

Light cables are connected to the arthroscope, and irrigation from the inflow tubing continues. The arthroscopy equipment (camera monitor, light source, arthroplasty unit and foot pedal, and printer) is brought into the field by the circulating nurse and arranged for efficient use. All electrically powered units are turned on after cables are connected.

The arthroscope is then directed into the medial compartment for initial examination. The medial joint surfaces, synovium, menisci, and anterior cruciate ligament are thoroughly examined. A blunt probe is manipulated through the third portal. For adequate visualization, the soft tissue can be manipulated closer to the arthroscope with the use of the blunt probe. The probe may be exchanged with the motorized intraarticular shaver if débridement of meniscal tears or lesions is documented. After the evaluation of the medial compartment, the arthroscope is replaced by the blunt probe, and inspection of the lateral compartment is performed in a similar manner. The undersurface of the patella and the suprapatellar pouch is visualized by inserting the arthroscope through the infrapatella lateral portal. The intraarticular shaver may be inserted into the infrapatella medial portal for débridement of lesions. Instruments may be repositioned so all aspects of the patella are visualized. The burr is used to cut through the subchondral bone to a depth of 1 mm.

During an arthroscopy, manipulation of the knee is required to bring all of the recesses into view. Thorough evaluation of the medial compartment might necessitate a valgus force on the knee with external rotation of the tibia. A varus stress is applied with internal rotation of the tibia while the lateral compartment is being evaluated. The most difficult area to examine is the posterior compartment of the knee. The posterior cruciate may be seen via a posterolateral or posteromedial portal.

Removal of a loose body is accomplished with arthroscopic grasping forceps. The visualization of a loose body sometimes presents a problem to the arthroscopist. Ballottement of the popliteal and suprapatellar compartment may facilitate the search for a loose body.

Multiple cutting tools may be utilized during a single procedure. They include knives, basket forceps, scissors, motorized burrs, and punches.

Closure

The small stab incisions are closed with a running 4-0 Vicryl suture on a cutting needle followed by application of Steri-Strip bandages. The area is covered with dry, sterile dressings and wrapped with a compression dressing (6-inch Webril followed by 6-inch Ace bandages).

Postoperative Care

Diet is given as tolerated.

Activity is gradually increased as it is comfortable; excessive use should be avoided for 48 hours.

Elevation of leg while sitting or lying down for 7 days is encouraged.

Activity should be decreased if swelling increases.

Quadricep strengthening exercises (straight leg lifts) should be performed.

Elevation and ice pack application should be instituted for 72 hours.

Rest and elevation are suggested for pain; if pain does not subside, the patient should take prescribed pain medication and not return to normal activity.

The patient should not forcefully bend the knee until given permission by the surgeon.

The patient may drive a car as soon as pain and swelling have subsided enough to allow good mobility.

The dressing may be removed in 48 hours and an adhesive bandage (Band-Aid) is applied for several days.

Do not apply any cream or lotion to incisions.

The patient may shower 48 hours postoperatively. Bathing or soaking should be avoided for 4 days.

The patient should contact the surgeon if any of the following occur: fever greater than 101°F, increased pain not relieved by pain medication prescribed, and redness or swelling in the calf.

Schedule a return visit 7 days postoperatively.

Potential Surgical Complications

Knee effusion: a painfully tense effusion that frequently develops during the first few postoperative days and may be relieved by aspiration of the knee joint

Infection: a complication that is extremely uncommon but should be considered if erythema, excessive pain with motion, and fever are present

Thrombophlebitis and pulmonary embolus: rare occurrences that are treated with anticoagulants

Neuropraxia: a condition due to prolonged use of the tourniquet during the procedure, which is managed by observation until symptoms resolve

Hemarthrosis: an occasional complication that is usually associated with cutting of vascularized tissue within the knee and that may necessitate aspiration if it does not resolve

Decreased range of motion: a complication due to hemarthrosis and subsequent adhesive capsulitis that may necessitate manipulation of the knee joint

---

BUNIONECTOMY

Definition

A deformity characterized by lateral angulation of the metatarsophalangeal joint of the great toe, with enlargement and the development of a bursa, is termed a *hallux valgus* (Fig. 27–42*A*). This constitutes a bunion (Fig. 27–42*B*). There is medial rotation of the great toe on its long axis and the extensor tendon of the long toe is displaced laterally. Hallux valgus is more frequently seen in females and there appears to be a familial tendency. Poorly fitting shoes, degenerative arthritic changes, flat feet, and a wedging of bone causing a medial angulation of the first metatarsal are known contributory causes. The pain of hallux valgus may be due to traumatic arthritis, pressure on the digital nerves, and compression and inflammation of the overlying bursa. Atrophy of the articular cartilage may occur and become extensive.

Indications

Surgical intervention is considered for the relief of symptoms and not for cosmetic reasons.

Related Surgical Procedures

There are numerous procedures to correct a hallux valgus deformity. Other deformities, such as hammertoes or corns, may also be associated with the bunion and may necessitate correction. In addition to the excision of the exostosis, various procedures may also utilize partial resection of the first metatarsal head (Mayo procedure), partial resection of the first proximal phalanx (Keller procedure), tendon transfer to lateral portion of the first metatarsal (McBride procedure), or osteotomy of the first metatarsal (Mitchell procedure).

Perioperative Nursing Implications

Anesthesia

General or spinal anesthesia is generally used.

Position

The patient is placed in the supine position as discussed previously for arthroscopy of the knee.

Creation and Maintenance of the Sterile Field

The operative extremity should be placed in a preparation holder to allow access to the ankle and foot (Fig. 27–43*A*). The tourniquet is then applied to the extremity. The area is scrubbed in the routine orthopedic fashion and painted with an antimicrobial solution (Fig. 27–43*B*). The area included is the foot, the ankle, and the entire leg below the knee, including the area between the toes. The operative extremity is draped in the same fashion as for arthroscopic surgery of the knee, but the stockinet and drapes are taken to just below the knee (Fig. 27–43*C*).

The tourniquet controls are placed on the nonoperative side (Fig. 27–44), where they are easily accessible to the circulating nurse and the anesthesiologist. Caution is taken to prevent any kinking of the tourniquet hose.

Equipment and Supplies

Basin set
Tourniquet and cuff
Power microsagittal saw and blade
6 No. 15 Blades
2 No. 1 Vicryl on a cutting needle (CP–2)
2 2–0 Vicryl on a cutting needle (CP–2)
4–0 Prolene on a cutting needle
Skin marker
4 × 8 inch radiopaque sponges
Kling bandage
Ioban Steri-Drape
Steri-Strips
Impervious stockinet
Irrigation syringe
Suction tubing
Skin preparation tray
Nitrogen power source
Drape pack
Povidone-iodine solution
2 povidone-iodine preparation brushes
Alcohol (according to the surgeon's preference)
Hinged impervious sheet
4-inch Webril
4 × 4 inch preparation or dressing sponges
4-inch Ace bandage

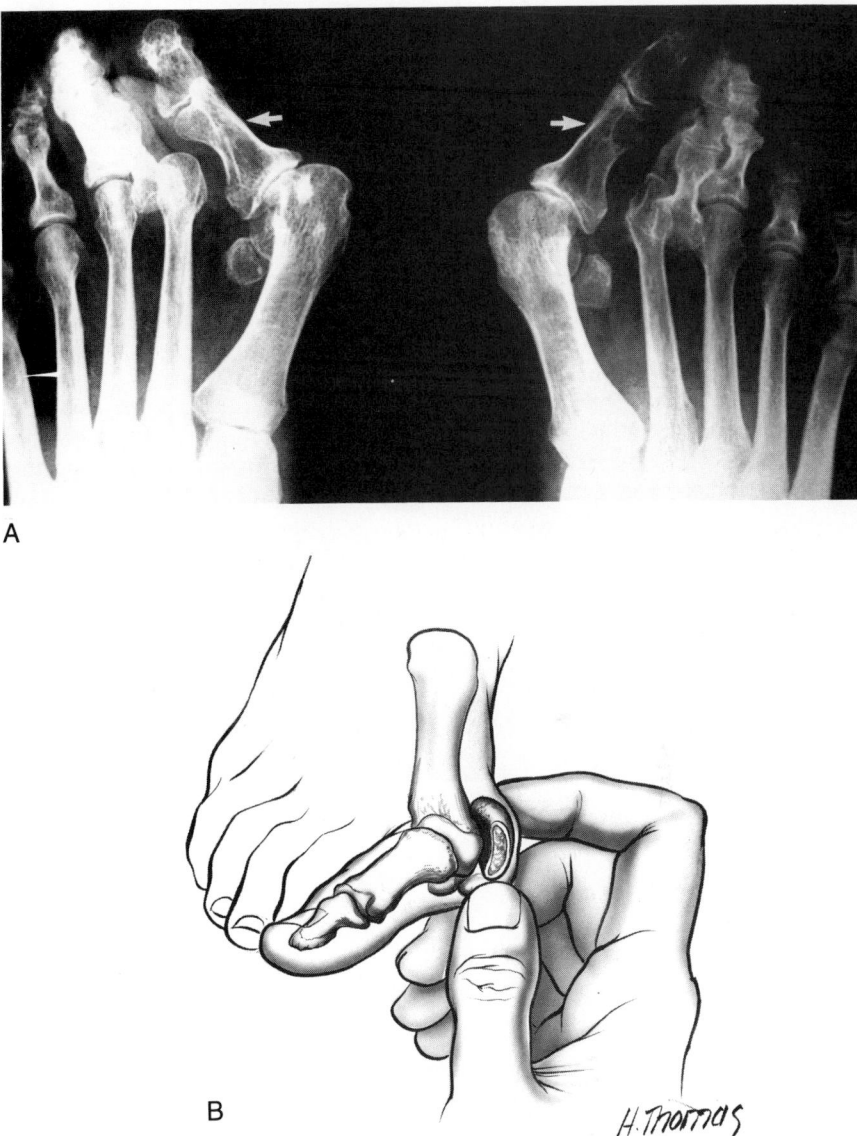

A

B

H. Thomas

FIGURE 27–42. *A,* X-rays of advanced hallux valgus. Note the medial rotation of the hallux *(arrows)*, narrowing of the first MTP joint, dislocation of the second MTP joint, and the sesamoids in the intermetatarsal space. *B,* Illustration of a bunion. (From Jahss, M. [1991]. *Disorders of the foot and ankle: Medical and surgical management* [2nd ed.] [pp. 948, 60]. Philadelphia: W. B. Saunders.)

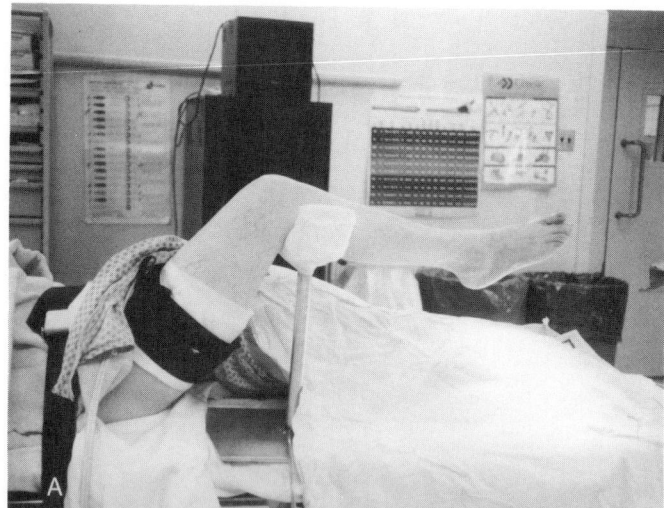

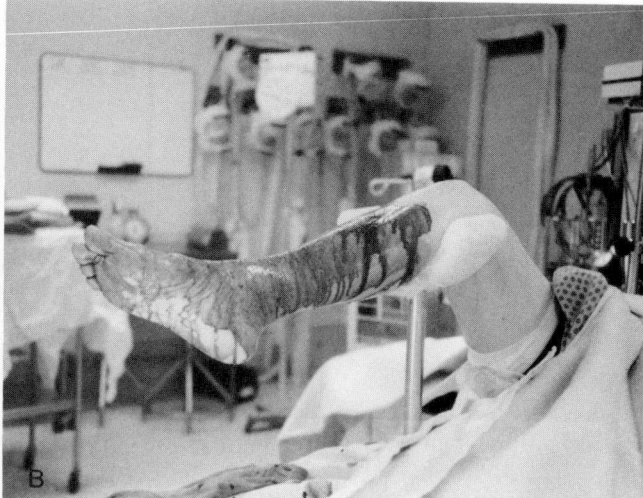

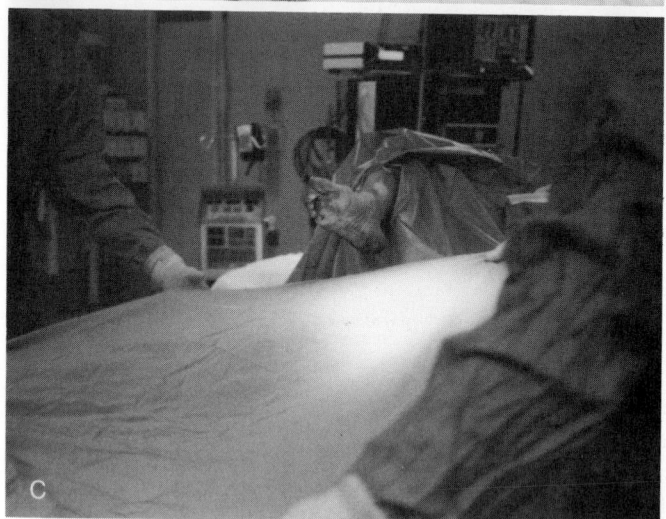

FIGURE 27–43. *A,* Position of the foot in the holder prior to bunionectomy. *B,* The operative area is painted with an antimicrobial solution. *C,* Draping of the area prior to bunionectomy.

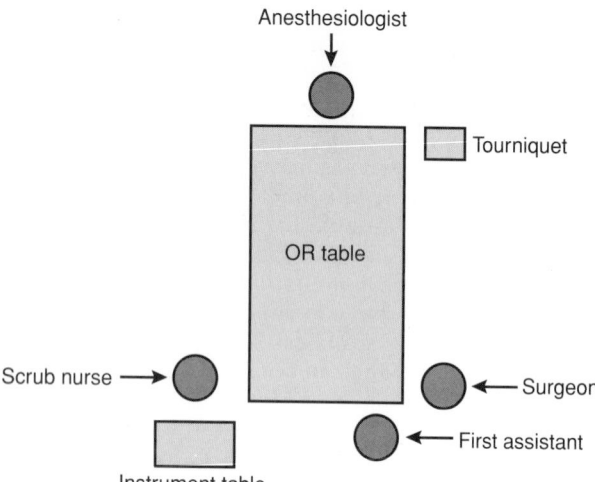

FIGURE 27–44. Operating room set-up for left bunionectomy. The set-up would be reversed for right bunionectomy.

4 0.065 Kirschner wires
Power wire driver
Electrocautery
1500 ml of normal saline
Bacitracin, 50,000 U
Polymyxin, 500,000 U
500 ml of normal saline
Prep leg holder
6-inch Esmarch bandage
Casting material

Instruments

2 No. 3 knife handles
Metzenbaum scissors
2 Senn retractors
Small bone rongeur (double action)
4 mosquito clamps
4 Allis clamps
4 Kocher clamps
2 tissue forceps with teeth
2 Adson forceps with teeth
6 towel clips
Heiss retractor
2 needle holders
Suture scissors
Bunion retractors
Small curet
Key periosteal elevator
Freer periosteal elevator
Assorted drill bits and drill
Mallet
¼-inch osteotome (hand osteotome)
½-inch osteotome (hand osteotome)
Microsagittal power saw and blade
No. 12 Frazier suction
2 sponge-holding forceps
2 ribbon retractors
Pin cutter
Bandage scissors
Hand drill and key

Drugs and Solutions

An irrigating solution of 500,000 U of polymyxin and 50,000 U of bacitracin in 1500 ml of normal saline is routinely used before closure in most orthopedic procedures.

Physiological Monitoring

The same principles of intraoperative nursing care apply to all surgical patients. Pressure points and tourniquet pressure and times are closely monitored and documented. With the deflation of any tourniquet, blood loss is calculated on the basis of suction collection and weighing of sponges. Neurovascular status is checked after any extremity procedure and documented.

Specimens and Cultures

Routine pathological testing is performed on the resected portion of the metatarsal head or proximal phalanx, depending on which type of correction is performed.

Physician's Orders

The patient is usually admitted the day of surgery, and preoperative testing is performed on an outpatient basis.

Chest x-ray film
ECG
AP and lateral x-ray films of bilateral feet, weight-bearing
Hematology profile
Urinalysis
NPO status after midnight

Laboratory and Diagnostic Studies

For laboratory studies, refer to the discussion of arthroscopy of the knee. AP and lateral x-ray films document a valgus deformity of the great toe at the metatarsophalangeal joint (the base of the proximal phalanx is subluxed laterally), the presence of a medial exostosis on the first metatarsal head, and a varus deformity of the first metatarsal.

Procedure

Incision and Exposure

An incision is made with a No. 15 blade over the dorsomedial aspect of the metatarsal head, giving access to the exostosis. Retraction is minimal owing to the prominent metatarsal head. Additional exposure may be achieved with Senn retractors placed dorsomedially and dorsolaterally to the exostosis. The bursa is excised and retracted with the Senn retractors (Fig. 27–45).

The incision is curved over the metatarsophalangeal joint dorsally. Caution is taken to avoid the extensor hallucis longus tendon. It is then curved back along the medial aspect of the shaft of the first metatarsal, continuing 2 to 3 cm from the metatarsophalangeal joint.

The deep fascia is incised with a No. 15 blade, keeping in line with the incision and then followed down to the dorsomedial aspect of the metatarsophalangeal joint. The dorsal digital branch of the medial cutaneous nerve along with the skin flap is retracted laterally with a small right-angled retractor. The joint capsule is incised, leaving the proximal end attached to the proximal phalanx.

Details (Keller Procedure) (Fig. 27–46)

The periosteum of the proximal phalanx and first metatarsal is incised with a No. 15 blade. The covering

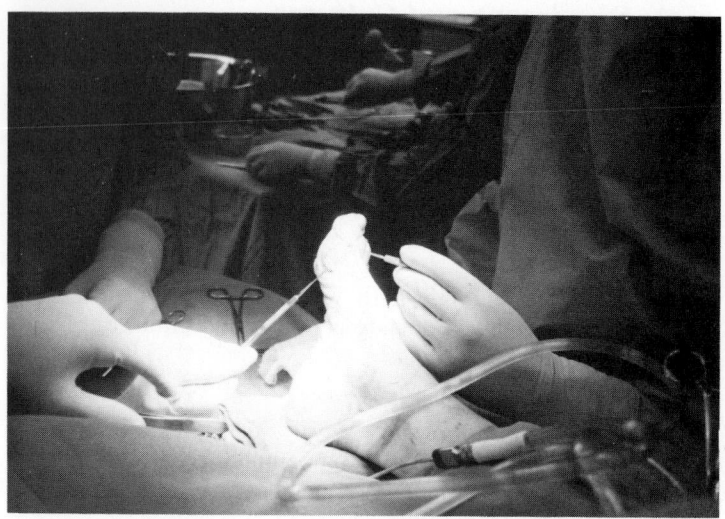

FIGURE 27–45. Incision and exposure of the bunion.

is removed from the bone by a Key periosteal elevator. Again, caution is taken to preserve the flexor hallucis longus on the plantar surface of the proximal phalanx. Small bunion retractors are inserted on each side of the midphalanx and act as bone levers.

The proximal half of the proximal phalanx is then cleanly resected across the middle of the shaft with a ¼-inch hand osteotome and a small sharp-pointed bone cutter (Fig. 27–47). The cut surface of the distal fragment is examined for projecting bone spurs. Any remaining, uncut bone is removed with a small bone rongeur. Small Metzenbaum scissors dissect any bursa from the underlying bone on the medial side. The exostosis is removed with the ¼-inch hand osteotome. Fixation is achieved with the insertion of a 0.062 Kirschner wire through the proximal phalanx and the first metatarsal with a power drill or wire driver (Fig. 27–48).

Closure

The tourniquet is deflated and hemostasis is achieved with an electrocautery unit or hemostats. The wound is copiously irrigated with an antibiotic solution. The capsule is revised with a continuous 2–0 chromic suture to promote stability of the soft tissues and great toe. The skin is closed with an interrupted 4–0 nylon suture. The incision is covered with dry, sterile gauze dressings, with attention to the area between the great and second toes. A bandage of 4-inch Webril followed by a posterior plaster splint is applied. The toe is splinted in 5 degrees of flexion and slight varus position.

Postoperative Care

Diet as tolerated when taken by mouth
Bed rest for 48 hours
Out of bed as tolerated with crutches in 48 hours
Vital signs every 2 hours 4 times and then 4 times per day

Neurovascular checks every 2 hours for 24 hours
Elevation of the operative extremity
Application of ice packs for 24 hours
Foot cradle at foot of bed
IV fluids until oral intake is instituted, then heparin lock
Antibiotic coverage for 7 days
Cough and deep breathing every 2 hours when the patient is awake
Administration of analgesics as necessary
Physical therapy consultation; crutch walking, walking boot cast
Discharge instructions
  Discharge in 3 to 10 days, depending on the ability to ambulate
  Appointment in 10 days; removal of sutures
  Maintenance of nutritional status and fluid volume
  No bathing until the sutures are removed
  Elevation of the foot while lying or sitting
  Elevation of the foot if increased pain or swelling occur until the symptoms subside
  Use of a bunion shoe for 6 weeks
  No high-heeled shoes until the physician approves
  Observation for signs of infection: redness, warmth, point tenderness, swelling, drainage
  Report of any paresthesias or numbness of the great toe
  Encouragement of straight leg raises and active ankle range-of-motion exercises
  Kirschner wire removal in 4 to 6 weeks

Potential Surgical Complications

Recurrence of deformity is a risk and may redevelop or occur at any point postoperatively.
Hallux varus deformity is due to overcorrection of the valgus deformity and may create a new deformity that necessitates correction.
Necrosis of the wound edges occurs because the skin on the medial aspect of the metatarsophalangeal joint is thinner and may not heal as well, and the

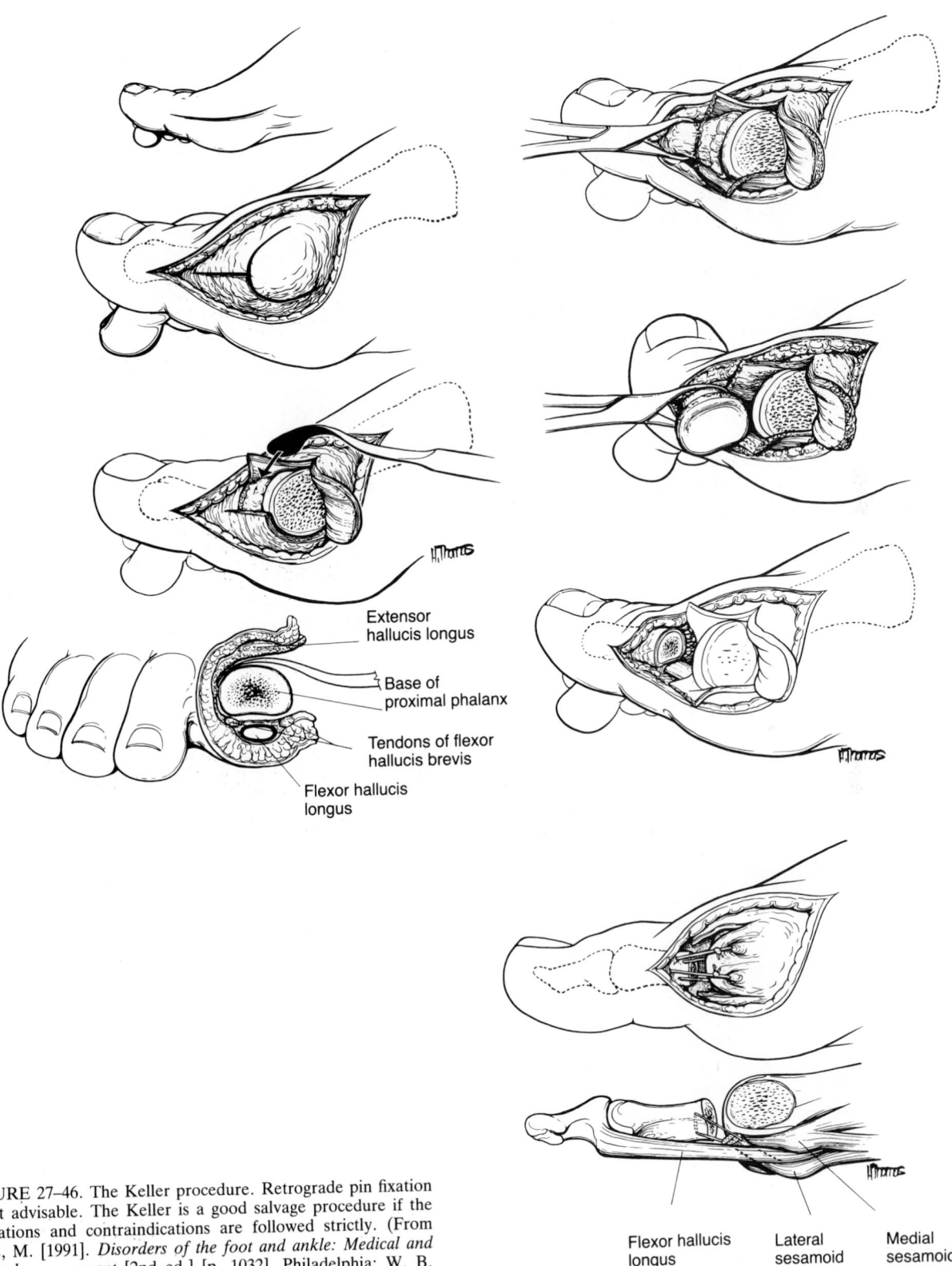

Extensor
hallucis longus

Base of
proximal phalanx

Tendons of flexor
hallucis brevis

Flexor hallucis
longus

Flexor hallucis
longus   Lateral
              sesamoid   Medial
                               sesamoid

FIGURE 27–46. The Keller procedure. Retrograde pin fixation is not advisable. The Keller is a good salvage procedure if the indications and contraindications are followed strictly. (From Jahss, M. [1991]. *Disorders of the foot and ankle: Medical and surgical management* [2nd ed.] [p. 1032]. Philadelphia: W. B. Saunders.)

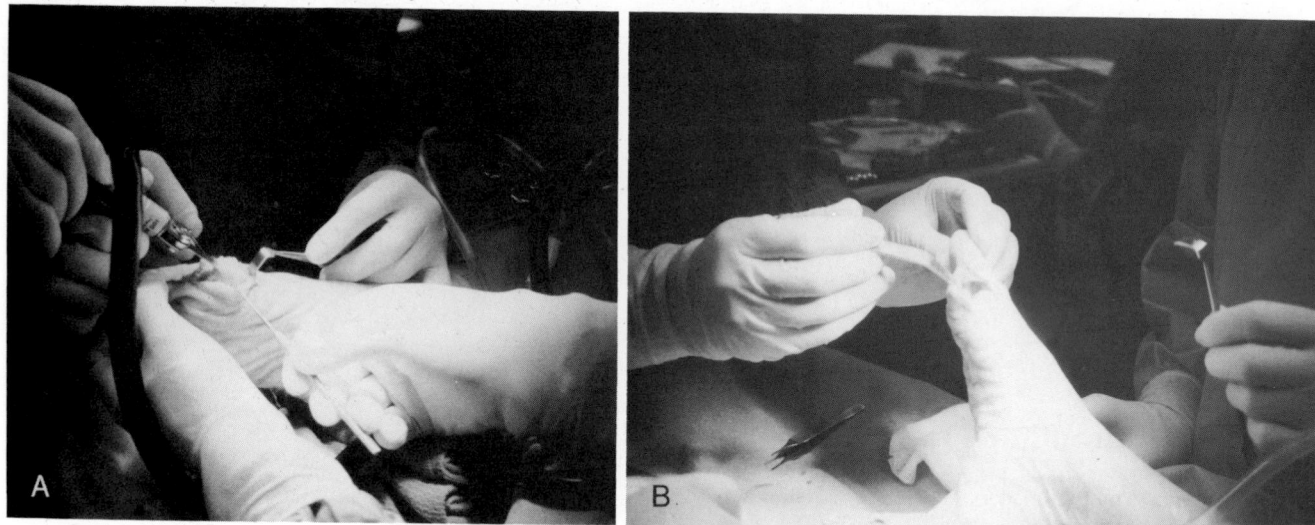

FIGURE 27–47. *A*, Resection of the bone in bunionectomy. *B*, Alignment of the bone after resection.

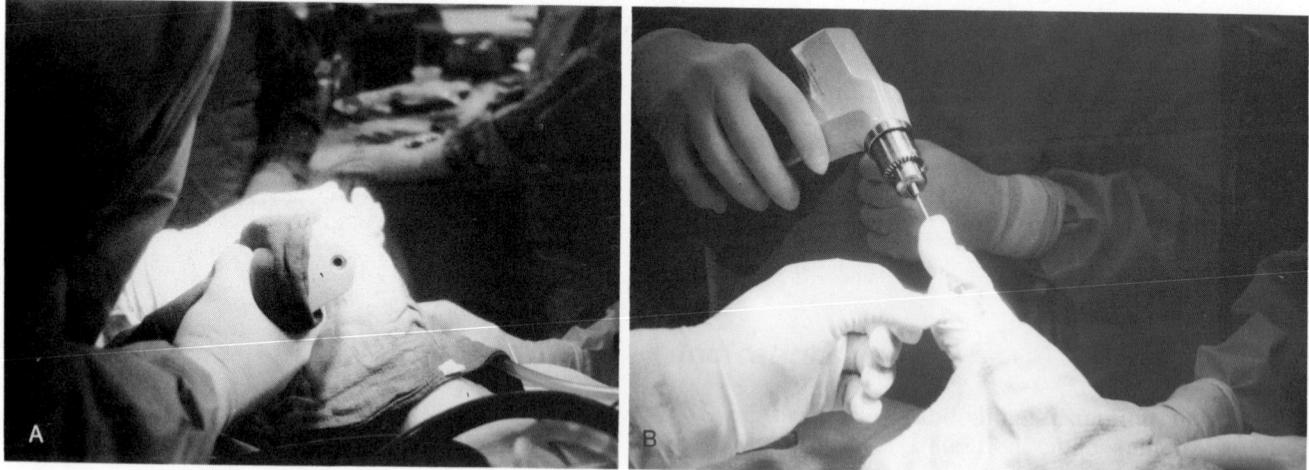

FIGURE 27–48. *A*, Insertion pin used in bunionectomy. *B*, Insertion of the K-wire during bunionectomy.

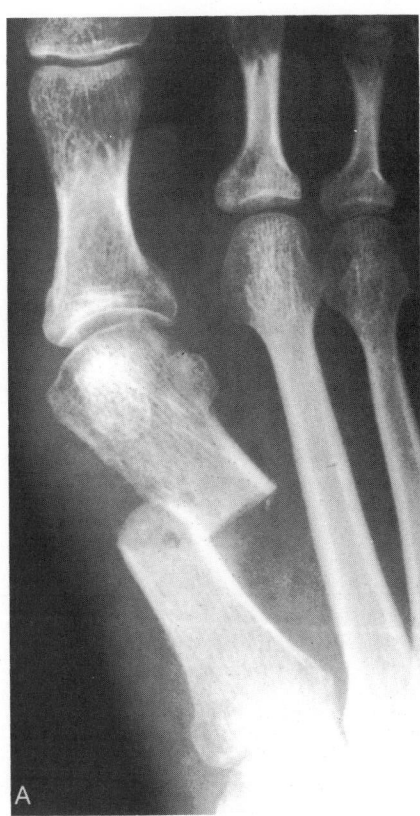
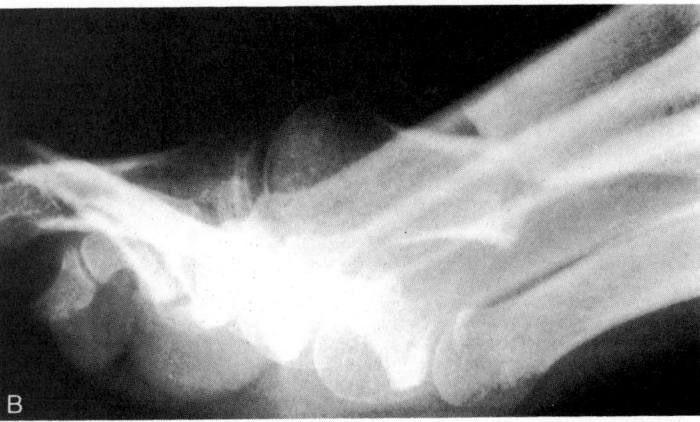

FIGURE 27–49. *A,* Anteroposterior view of a standard Mitchell operation. The osteotomy is too proximal. The chromic suture tore early postoperatively. Note the poor fragment contact and the medial angulation of the head fragment, which increases the metatarsus prima varus. *B,* Lateral view. Note the poor bone contact and the head tilt upward, which drastically reduces weight bearing. The osteotomy united, but with weight-bearing transfer. (From Jahss, M. [1991]. *Disorders of the foot and ankle: Medical and surgical management* [2nd ed.] [p. 979]. Philadelphia: W. B. Saunders.)

bursa may have been inflamed and complicated the procedure.

Numbness or paresthesias are due to transection of the medial dorsal cutaneous nerve during incision and may persist for up to a year. If the nerves are severed or neuromas form, further treatment is necessary.

Limitation of motion of the metatarsophalangeal joint may be caused by excessive capsular tightening during reconstruction, fibrous tissue formation, scarring of extensor hallucis longus

Nonunion or avascular necrosis of osteotomy

Infection

Other complications are shown in Figure 27–49.

EXCISION OF A GANGLION

Definition

A *ganglion* is a cystic swelling overlying a joint or a tendon sheath. One large cyst usually develops and is either unilocular or multilocular. Multiple small accessory cysts usually lie adjacent to the large cyst. The ganglion consists of a dense fibrous capsule surrounding a thick, sticky, clear odorless fluid. The cystic fluid has the consistency of soft jelly. There usually is no apparent communication with the joint or tendon, but invariably the cyst is bound to those structures by dense tissue.

Two theories explain why ganglia develop. One is that the dense collagenous tissue of the wrist degenerates and leads to the formation of multiple small cysts containing mucin. Small cysts may, over time, coalesce into one large cyst. The other theory postulates a deficit in the joint capsule or tendon sheath, permitting a protrusion of synovial tissue. The communicating channel between the protruding tissue and the joint becomes obliterated, and a cyst remains as a pedicle or adhesion. Additional cysts may be formed if the defect in the capsule or sheath persists.

A ganglion occurs most frequently about the wrist but may appear adjacent to the wrist. The usual location, at the wrist, is the dorsum between the long extensor of the thumb and the extensor to the index finger. It may be traced down to the articulation between the lunate and the scaphoid. When the ganglion is over the volar aspect of the wrist, it usually appears between the brachioradialis and the flexor carpi radialis tendons. In the palm of the hand, it develops from the deep pulley of the finger flexors over the metacarpal heads.

Indications

Ganglion excision is indicated for persistent discomfort that does not respond to medical treatment and when the ganglion interferes with activities of daily living.

Related Surgical Procedures

A ganglion of the wrist may be treated by both nonoperative and operative procedures. Nonoperative procedures include the following:

1. Aspirating the cyst fluid with a 21-gauge needle and injecting the remaining tissue with a steroid or a sclerosing agent
2. Rupturing the cyst by means of an external force
3. Using roentgenographic therapy, a 1.5-erythema dose repeated in 1 month

Frequently, however, nonoperative methods are unsuccessful and surgical excision is required.

Perioperative Nursing Implications

Anesthesia

The procedure can be performed under regional or general anesthesia.

Position

The patient is placed in the supine position. The operative arm is extended on a hand table, preventing extension of greater than 90 degrees. The nonoperative arm is extended on a padded arm board with the palm down. A safety strap is placed 2 inches above the knees, making sure that the patient's legs are uncrossed. The head is in anatomical alignment with the body and may be gently turned away from the operative side during the preparation of the surgical field. Vulnerable pressure points (occiput, scapula, olecranon, sacrum, ischeal tuberosity, and calcaneus) may be protected with additional padding, especially if the patient is under regional anesthesia.

The knees may be flexed on a pillow or the table adjusted to put the body in a more anatomically neutral position. This is helpful in the patient undergoing regional anesthesia. Conscious humans, lying supine and motionless, maintain normal distribution of tissue perfusion for only about 1 hour. If enforced immobility continues, increasing discomfort and restlessness (necessitating sedation) may occur.

The operative arm is raised on an arm support or bolster positioned under the upper arm. The appropriate-sized tourniquet is applied high on the upper arm after the procedures outlined above are accomplished.

Creation and Maintenance of the Sterile Field

With the arm elevated, the hair is removed circumferentially to the midforearm. The skin preparation is then performed from the hand, including all fingers, to just above the elbow. The end of the hand table is covered first to protect the front of the sterile surgical

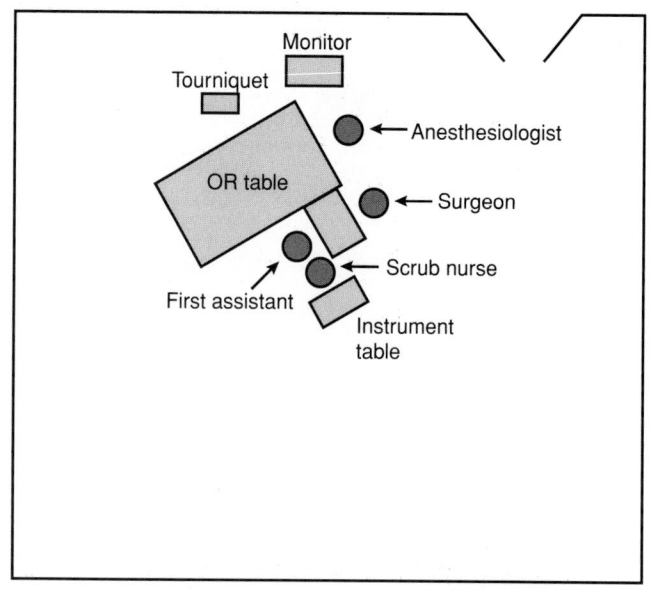

FIGURE 27–50. Operating room set-up for right ganglion excision. The set-up would be reversed for left ganglion excision.

gowns. A sterile stockinet is then placed over the hand; the arm is held suspended and the arm support removed. The stockinet is telescoped to above the elbow, and a large sterile drape is used to cover the hand table and is taken to, and fastened around, the arm at the end of the stockinet. The hinged impervious sheet is placed under the operative arm on the sterile field and secured around the top of the limb and stockinet. A final down sheet is placed, followed by two large drapes covering the patient's body. The arm drapes and body drapes are then secured to each other, around the upper arm, with towel clips. The stockinet is then fenestrated and, if required, may be loosely secured on the upper forearm with a sterile bandage or wrap.

The OR bed is positioned, accommodating the hand table and the operating surgeons but maintaining the sterile boundary between the anesthesia equipment and personnel. Figure 27–50 shows the operating room set-up.

Equipment and Supplies

Tourniquet and cuff
4 No. 15 blades
Impervious stockinet
Irrigating syringe
1500 ml of normal saline
Electrocautery (bipolar cord and tip)
Skin marker
4 × 8 inch radiopaque sponges
Kling bandage
Suction tubing
Skin preparation tray
2 3–0 Vicryl on a cutting needle
2 4–0 nylon on a cutting needle

Povidone-iodine solution
2 povidone-iodine preparation brushes
4-inch Webril bandage
2 4 × 4 inch preparation dressing sponges
Bacitracin, 50,000 U
Polymyxin, 500,000 U
Hand table
2 3–0 silk on a cutting needle
500 ml of normal saline
Drape packs
Basin set
4-inch Esmarch bandage
Casting material
5–0 chromic on a cutting needle
Impervious hinge sheet

Instruments

2 No. 3 knife handles
Tenotomy scissors
Metzenbaum scissors
Suture scissors
Bandage scissors
Small double-action rongeur
4 mosquito clamps
4 Allis clamps
4 Kocher clamps
2 tissue forceps with teeth
4-inch Esmarch bandage
2 Adson forceps with teeth
4 towel clips
2 Heiss retractors
2 needle holders
Freer periosteal elevator
2 sponge-holding forceps
Bipolar cautery cord and tip
2 Senn retractors
No. 12 Frazier suction
2 3-prong sharp rake retractors
Key periosteal elevator
6 hemostats

Drugs and Solutions

The routine antibiotic irrigation of bacitracin, 50,000 U, and polymyxin, 500,000 U, in 500 ml of normal saline is used before closure.

Physiological Monitoring

Refer to the discussion of bunionectomy.

Specimens and Cultures

The ganglion sheath is routinely sent to the pathology laboratory for definitive testing. A synovectomy might be performed and synovial tissue sent to the pathology or the rheumatology department.

Physician's Orders

Chest x-ray film
ECG (for patients older than 40 years)
Hematology profile
Urinalysis
AP and lateral x-ray films of the wrist and hand (bilaterally)
NPO status after midnight

Laboratory and Diagnostic Studies

For laboratory studies, refer to the discussion of arthroscopy of the knee. X-ray films may reveal calcification in the tendon or sheath.

Procedure

Incision and Exposure (Dorsal Approach)

The operative extremity is exsanguinated with an elastic bandage and the tourniquet is inflated accordingly. With the forearm pronated, a longitudinal incision is made on the dorsal aspect of the wrist with a No. 15 blade. The incision extends across the wrist joint midway between the radial and ulnar styloids, beginning 3 cm proximal and 5 cm distal to the wrist joint. The skin is retracted on both sides with the aid of skin hooks. A No. 3–0 silk suture on a cutting needle can also be placed on each side as a traction stitch. The subcutaneous fat is incised, in line with the skin incision, with small Metzenbaum scissors. The extensor retinaculum is exposed. The retinaculum over the extensor carpi radialis longus and brevis is incised with a No. 15 blade. This is the compartment on the radial side of Lister tubercle.

The sharp dissection is carried out in the same fashion on the ulnar edge of the cut retinaculum. The extensor retinaculum should be preserved. The tendons are mobilized and lifted from their beds in an ulnar and radial direction. The underlying radius and joint capsule are exposed. The incision is taken down to the retinaculum before the ulnar and radial flaps are elevated to protect the radial nerve in the subcutaneous fat.

Details

The joint capsule is incised longitudinally with a No. 15 blade. The dissection continues subcapsularly on the radial and ulnar sides of the radius, thus exposing the entire distal end of the radius and carpal bones. As long as the dissection (at the level of wrist) remains subperiosteal, the radial artery remains protected. The tendons on both sides of Lister tubercle are carefully inspected for any ganglion or satellite lesions. The cysts are released from tendon attachment with small Metzenbaum scissors. The cysts are then carefully dissected from their base. A large cuff of joint capsule tissue is also removed to prevent recurrence. The tendons at the level of Lister tubercle are retracted with small right-angled retractors, and the wrist joint and capsule are thoroughly inspected for any smaller cysts. Any defects in the joint capsule or tendon sheaths are repaired with a running 5–0 chromic suture on a cutting needle.

Closure

The wound is copiously irrigated with the routine antibiotic irrigation. The joint capsule is closed using a continuous 5–0 chromic suture on a cutting needle. The subcutaneous tissue is then irrigated and closed with a 3–0 Vicryl interrupted suture on a cutting needle. The skin is closed with an interrupted 4–0 nylon suture on a cutting needle.

The incision is covered with dry, sterile gauze dressings. Bandage of 4-inch Webril followed by a neutral volar splint is then applied. The tourniquet is deflated after compression is achieved by the Webril. The patient's arm is positioned in a sling for additional support and comfort.

Postoperative Care

Diet as tolerated when taken by mouth
Out of bed as tolerated
Application of ice packs for 24 hours
Elevation of the operative extremity
Vital signs every 2 hours 4 times then four times daily
Neurovascular checks every 2 hours for 24 hours
Administration of analgesics per doctor's orders
Antibiotic coverage for 7 days
Cough and deep breathing every 2 hours while the patient is awake
Discharge instructions
   Observation for signs of infection: redness, warmth, point tenderness, swelling, drainage
   Report of any paresthesias
   No bathing until the sutures are removed
   Appointment in 10 days
   Discharge usually the same day
   Maintenance of nutritional status and fluid volume
   Elevation of the extremity for 72 hours or if increased pain or swelling occurs
   Splint removal in 3 weeks
   Active range-of-motion exercises after the cast is removed

Potential Surgical Complications

Limitation of motion may be caused by excessive capsular tightening during reconstruction, fibrous tissue formation, and scarring of extensor tendons.
Neuromas may be caused by scarring of the radial nerve.

Recurrence is due to a remaining defect in the capsule or the tendon sheath or a remaining cyst.
Infection may be due to underlying systemic inflammatory condition and is always a surgical risk.

SILASTIC WRIST JOINT IMPLANT

Definition

A Silastic wrist implant is utilized in patients with arthritic or traumatic disabilities that have resulted in wrist instability. The instability may be due to subluxation, severe deviation of the wrist, stiffness, or fusion of the wrist in a nonfunctional position.

Indications

The goals of the procedure are to provide stability, restore motion, and relieve pain.

Related Surgical Procedures

A resection of the distal ulna is done to relieve pain and restore wrist motion. It is indicated in cases of malunion or nonunion after a Colles fracture (a fracture of the distal radius with volar angulation and a dorsal displacement of the distal fragment), pain and disability due to radioulnar arthritis, and dislocation or subluxation of the ulna. A Silastic ulnar head implant may be necessary in rheumatoid, degenerative, or traumatic arthritis. Carpal bone implants (carpal lunate, carpal scaphoid, and carpal trapezium) have significantly improved motion and reduced pain in the wrist for patients with numerous pathological conditions.

Perioperative Nursing Implications

Anesthesia

General anesthesia is preferable, but regional anesthesia can also be administered.

Position

The patient's position is the same as for an excision of a ganglion. The same safety measures are also followed.

Creation and Maintenance of the Sterile Field

The arm is positioned, prepared, and draped in the same fashion as for excision of ganglion.

Equipment and Supplies

Drape packs
Tourniquet and cuff
Hand table
6 No. 15 blades
Impervious stockinet
Impervious hinged sheet
Irrigating syringe
1500 ml of normal saline
Bipolar cautery cord and tip
Skin marker
2 4 × 8 inch radiopaque sponges
Kling bandage
Suction tubing
4-inch Esmarch bandage
Basin set
Skin preparation tray
Povidone-iodine solution
2 povidone-iodine preparation brushes
4-inch Webril bandage
2 4 × 4 inch preparation or dressing sponges
Bacitracin, 50,000 U
Polymyxin, 500,000 U
500 ml of normal saline
2 3–0 silk suture on a cutting needle
2 3–0 Vicryl suture on a cutting needle
4–0 nylon suture on a cutting needle
Small microsagittal saw and blade
Silastic trial sizers and implants
Power microdrill
Medium pineapple burr
Pulsatile lavage
Casting material
Nitrogen power source

Instruments

The following are required in addition to equipment for the excision of a ganglion:

Bone curets (assorted)
Nitrogen power source
2 Army-Navy retractors
¼-inch osteotome (hand osteotome)
⅛-inch osteotome (hand osteotome)
2 bunion retractors
2 ribbon retractors
Senn retractors
Key periosteal elevator
Mallet

Drugs and Solutions

The Silastic component is soaked in the antibiotic solution that is used for irrigation before implanting. The incision is copiously irrigated before the implant insertion and again before closure.

Physiological Monitoring

Refer to the discussion of the excision of a ganglion.

Specimens and Cultures

The resected bone from the distal radius is sent to the pathology laboratory for definitive studies. A portion of the distal radius may be used as an allograft if there is severe bone loss.

Physician's Orders

Physical therapy or occupational therapy consultation
Vital signs every 4 hours
Chemistry and hematology profile
Urinalysis
Chest x-ray film
ECG
Out of bed as tolerated
Diet as tolerated
AP and lateral x-ray films of both forearms, including the hands

Laboratory and Diagnostic Studies

Refer to the discussion of the excision of a ganglion.

Procedure

Incision and Exposure

The operative extremity is elevated and exsanguinated with an elastic bandage; the tourniquet is then inflated accordingly. A straight, longitudinal incision is made over the dorsum of the wrist with a No. 15 blade. It extends from the middle of the third metacarpal proximally for 12 cm. The skin is retracted on both sides of the incision using skin hooks or a 3–0 silk traction stitch. The skin and subcutaneous tissue are elevated from the underlying fascia and retinaculum with small Metzenbaum scissors.

The retinaculum is incised longitudinally with a No. 15 blade and elevated medially and laterally. The extensor pollicis longus is freed with the scissors and retracted laterally with a small right-angled retractor. The retinaculum is elevated from the radial side of the wrist with the small Metzenbaum scissors and dissected to subperiosteal bone. Care is taken not to injure the extensor tendons during dissection. The distal ulna is exposed subperiosteally with a Freer elevator. A rim of the dorsal radioulnar capsule remains attached to the radius.

Details

The distal 1 cm of the radius is excised with a microsagittal saw. The radius is elevated and exposed with the aid of a ribbon (bunion) retractor. Dissection around the scaphoid, carpal lunate, capitate, and triquetrum is performed with a No. 15 blade. The scaphoid and carpal lunate bones are elevated and removed with a Freer periosteal elevator and a No. 15 blade. The proximal third of the capitate and the medial portion of the triquetrum are excised with a microsagittal saw and a ¼-inch osteotome.

The intramedullary canal of the radius is prepared with the appropriate reamer for the power microdrill. The remaining portion of the capitate and the intramedullary canal of the third metacarpal are also reamed accordingly. The trial implant is fitted into the radial canal and through the capitate into the third metacarpal canal. Soft tissues may be released, with a No. 15 blade, volarly to allow easy dorsiflexion if necessary. The wrist is moved through passive range of motion. When proper ligament balance and tension are achieved, the wrist is copiously irrigated with an antibiotic solution. The distal portion of the ulna may or may not be excised and fitted with a Silastic ulnar head implant. The extensor tendons may be shortened or transferred as necessary for stabilization.

The implant is soaked in a basin of antibiotic irrigation and handled only with a smooth tissue forceps. The implant is positioned into the radial canal first. Dorsiflexion of the wrist assists in the insertion of the distal end of the implant into the metacarpal canal. The wrist once again is moved through passive range of motion and irrigated.

Closure

The capsular tissues are repaired with an interrupted 4–0 Vicryl suture. The subcutaneous tissue is irrigated and closed with an interrupted 3-0 Vicryl suture. The skin is closed with an interrupted 4-0 nylon suture.

The incision is covered with dry sterile gauze dressings. A 4-inch Webril bandage and then a long arm compression dressing are applied. The wrist is maintained in a neutral position.

Postoperative Care

X-ray films in the recovery room
Physical therapy and occupational therapy
Neurovascular checks every 2 hours for 24 hours
Antibiotic coverage
Administration of analgesics as needed
Diet as tolerated
Out of bed as tolerated
CBC with differential cell count; panel 7 in the morning after surgery
Deep venous thrombosis (DVT) prophylaxis
Discharge instructions
    Application of a short arm cast in 3 to 5 days for 2 to 4 weeks
    Active range-of-motion exercises after cast removal
    Suture removal in 5 to 7 days
    Discharge in 5 to 7 days

Potential Surgical Complications

Limitation of motion may be caused by excessive capsular tightening during reconstruction, scarring of extensor tendons, and malalignment of a component.
Infection is always a surgical risk.
Breakage or dislocation of the implant may be due to malalignment of a component or excessive range of motion.

OPEN REDUCTION AND INTERNAL FIXATION OF THE FRACTURED ULNA

Definition

Fixation by plates is used frequently in fractures of the shafts of the ulna, which must unite with perfect apposition and alignment if normal function is to be restored. A fracture should be described with regard to its location in the bone (metaphyseal, diaphyseal, or epiphyseal) (Fig. 27–51). It should also be described with regard to its rotation, angulation, and displacement. These fractures generally occur as result of a fall on an outstretched arm, but there is usually a component of direct force as well. Fractures of the ulna alone are rare, but fractures of both the ulna and the radius can occur at any age.

There is often angulation and shortening, causing a deformity because of problems that are special to the forearm. Muscle groups that pull at oblique angles between the radius and the ulna tend to malalign the fracture ends and cause the deformity. The type of deformity depends on the level of the fracture. If closed fractures are left displaced, they lead to not only a deformity but also a limitation of rotation of the forearm. There is also the risk of ischemic damage to the forearm muscles, leading to severe loss of function of the hand.

Indications

Open reduction is a method in which the fracture site is surgically opened and the fragments united into correct anatomical position. Most commonly used for internal fixation are intramedullary nails and compression plates. The latter are most suitable for fractures of the ulna. Applied to the bone cortex, and with proper techniques, substantial compression can be applied to the fracture site.

Related Surgical Procedures

Many transverse fractures of the forearm heal satisfactorily by closed reduction and application of a plaster

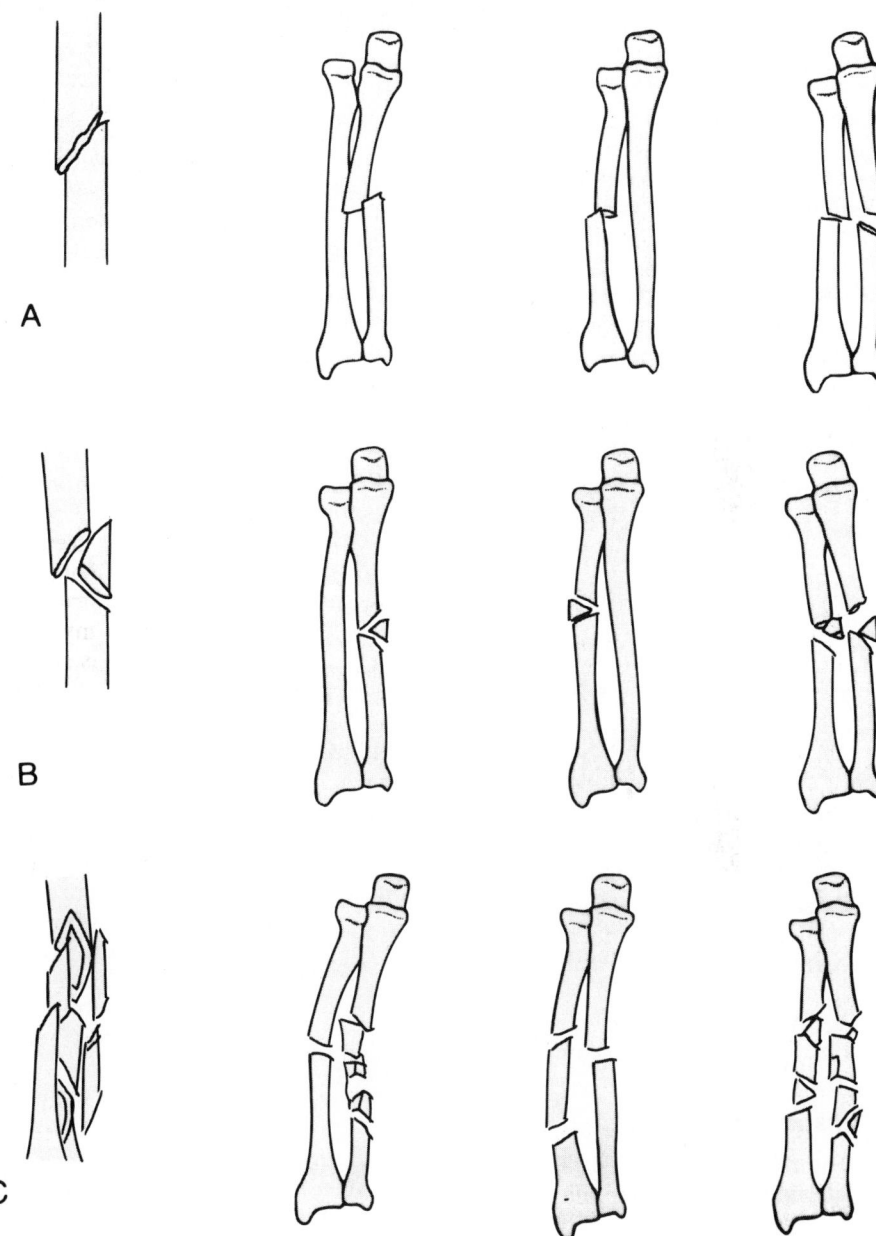

FIGURE 27–51. The classification for diaphyseal forearm fractures recommended by the AO/ASIF. *A,* Simple fracture: ulna (radius intact); radius (ulna intact) and both bones. *B,* Wedge fracture: ulna (radius intact); radius (ulna intact); and one bone (other simple/wedge fracture). *C,* Complex fracture: ulna (radius intact/simple/wedge); radius (ulna intact/simple/wedge); and both bones. (From Browner, B., Levine, A., Jupiter, J., Trafton, P. [1992]. *Skeletal trauma* [p. 1098]. Philadelphia: W. B. Saunders.)

cast. With more complex fractures, open reduction may be necessary. In general, internal fixation is not used initially in the treatment of open fractures of the forearm. The wound is usually first treated by irrigation and débridement. After the wound is healed, surgery may be done to insert an appropriate internal fixation device (e.g., a compression plate, and an intramedullary rod) or an external fixation device may be applied.

Perioperative Nursing Implications

Anesthesia

General anesthesia is preferable, but a regional anesthetic may be utilized.

Position

The patient's position is the same as for an excision of a ganglion. The same safety measures are also followed.

Creation and Maintenance of the Sterile Field

Refer to the discussion of the excision of a ganglion.

Equipment and Supplies

The following are used in addition to supplies for a Silastic wrist joint implant:

Power drill
2 2–0 Vicryl sutures (CP–2)
4-inch roll of casting material
Pulsatile lavage system
3000-ml bags of normal saline
X-ray cassette cover or image intensifier cover
Arm sling
X-ray machine, cassettes, and covers
Fixation device (e.g., compression plates and screws)

Instruments

The following are used in addition to instruments for a Silastic wrist joint implant.

Assorted bone clamps
  Lowman
  Lambotte
  Bone cutter (double action)
  ½-inch osteotome
  2 medium Weitlaner retractors
  2 four-prong rakes (sharp)
  Cobb periosteal elevator
  6 Kelly clamps
  Plate benders
Appropriate drills, and taps for use with the fixation device

Drugs and Solutions

For an open wound, the area is copiously irrigated with the routine antibiotic irrigation via a pulsatile lavage system. Any debris, bone fragments, and/or fracture hematoma particles must be removed before the reduction of bone ends and again before closure.

Physiological Monitoring

Neurovascular status in the affected arm should be assessed every 15 minutes. The potential for a neurovascular deficit related to soft tissue swelling and trauma to the bone should be of great concern.

In addition to tourniquet times and pressures, blood loss should be measured, documented, and verbalized to the surgeons and the anesthesiologist.

Specimens and Cultures

Any resected or fragmented bone that is not utilized as an allograft is delivered to the pathology laboratory for conclusive testing.

Physician's Orders

Chest x-ray film
ECG (for patients older than 40 years)
Hematology profile
Urinalysis
AP and lateral x-ray films of both bones of the forearm, including the wrist and elbow joints
Neurovascular checks every 2 hours
Type and screen 2 units of packed cells
NPO status; IV administration of fluids
Immobilization of the extremity
Application of ice packs
Elevation of the extremity
Analgesics as needed
DVT prophylaxis
Physical therapy and occupational therapy consultation

Laboratory and Diagnostic Studies

AP and lateral x-ray films to confirm the fracture diagnosis
Hemoglobin level and hematocrit, which may be lower if there is excessive bleeding or trauma to the extremity

Procedure

Incision and Exposure

With the patient supine on the OR bed, place the operative extremity on an arm board. Exsanguination of the limb is achieved either by elevation or by application of an Esmarch bandage.

The forearm is fully pronated to expose the subcutaneous border of the ulna. A linear, longitudinal incision with a No. 15 blade is made over the fracture site (Fig. 27–52). The length of the incision depends on the amount of bone that is to be exposed. Deep fascia is incised along the same line as the skin incision distally. Exposure is achieved with the use of Army-Navy retractors. Dissection is carried down to the subcutaneous border of the ulna. The periosteum is incised longitudinally over the ulna using a Cobb periosteal elevator and the incision is continued around the bone to reveal the flexor and extensor aspects.

The ulnar nerve and the ulnar artery are preserved if the flexor carpi ulnaris is stripped from the ulna subperiosteally. If the dissection strays into the substance of the muscle, the nerve may be damaged.

The fracture site is irrigated with an antibiotic solution, and both ends are carefully cleaned with a small curet.

Details (Fig. 27–53)

Apposition and alignment of the fracture must be perfect if normal function is to be restored. The reduction is achieved and maintained with the aid of a Lowman or a Lambotte bone clamp. A plate is chosen and contoured with the plate benders. The length of the plate should ensure that a minimum hold of six good cortices is possible on either side of the fracture line. One side of the plate is drilled through the hole nearest the fracture site in a neutral position through both cortices. A drill guide for the plate is used to ensure accurate direction of the drill bit. The hole is measured to the opposite cortex with a depth guage. While the nurse is retrieving the appropriate screw, the hole is tapped to accept the screw. The screw is then inserted.

For the first hole on the opposite side of the fracture line, the load guide is used. This offsets the drill hole to move the bone by 1 mm in a compressive action. The arrow on the drill guide must be pointing toward the fracture site. The same procedure follows as described above. When the desired compression is achieved, the

neutral guide is used in the remaining holes. Figure 27–54 shows radiographs of a fracture following fixation.

Any bone loss at the fracture site should be filled using autogenous cancellous bone graft to strengthen the fixation.

The wound is again copiously irrigated with an antibiotic solution.

Closure

Fascia is closed with an interrupted 2–0 Vicryl suture on a cutting needle. Skin closure is achieved with an interrupted 4–0 nylon suture.

Sterile gauze dressings and then a 4-inch Webril bandage are applied. A posterior plaster splint is applied.

Postoperative Care

X-ray films in the recovery room
Out of bed as tolerated
Diet as tolerated
Incentive spirometry every 2 hours while the patient is awake
Antibiotic coverage for 7 days
Administration of analgesics as needed
DVT prophylaxis
Occupational therapy consultation
CBC with differential count; panel 7 on the morning after surgery and in 2 days
Suture removal in 2 weeks
Cast application with the elbow at 90 degrees in 2 weeks for 10 weeks

Potential Surgical Complications

Infection
Neurovascular compromise may be due to pressure on nerves and vessels or the pressure of a splint or cast
Decreased mobility may be due to the immobility imposed by a splint or cast

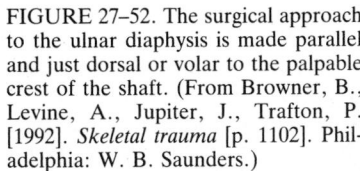

FIGURE 27–52. The surgical approach to the ulnar diaphysis is made parallel and just dorsal or volar to the palpable crest of the shaft. (From Browner, B., Levine, A., Jupiter, J., Trafton, P. [1992]. *Skeletal trauma* [p. 1102]. Philadelphia: W. B. Saunders.)

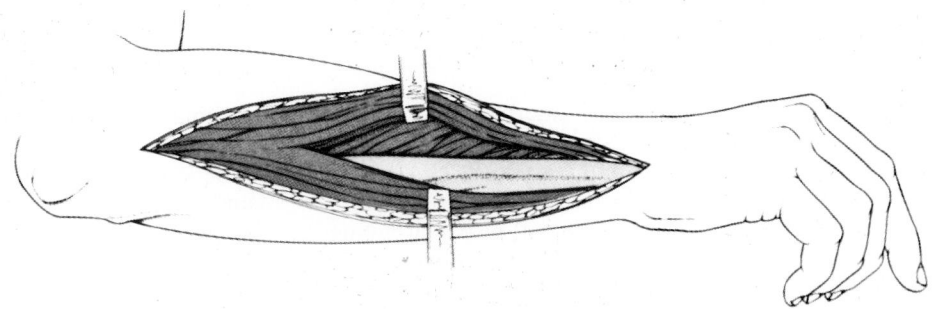

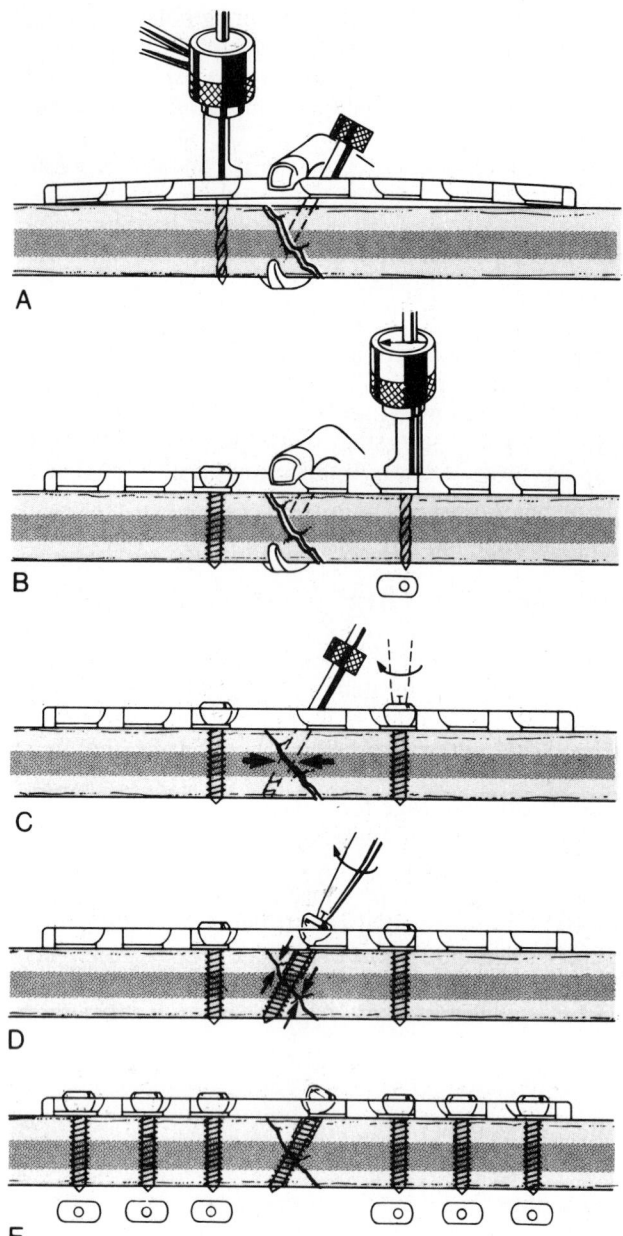

FIGURE 27–53. Technique of applying a dynamic compression plate to an oblique forearm shaft fracture. *A,* The plate is precontoured to sit 1 mm off the shaft over the fracture site. The fracture is reduced, the plate is held with a clamp, and a screw is applied in a neutral mode in the fragment, which has its obliquity facing away from the plate. *B,* The gliding hole for an interfragmentary lag screw through the plate is then drilled. *C,* A screw is applied in the "load" or compression position in the opposite fragment, which will allow this fragment to be "pulled into" the plate when compression is applied. *D* and *E,* The interfragmentary lag screw is then placed through the plate by drilling the far cortex with the appropriate drill and placing an appropriate length of screw, and the remainder of the screws are applied through the plate. (From Browner, B., Levine, A., Jupiter, J., Trafton, P. [1992]. *Skeletal trauma* (p. 1106). Philadelphia: W. B. Saunders.)

PROSTHETIC REPLACEMENT OF THE FRACTURED HUMERAL HEAD

Definition

Fractures of the proximal humerus are not uncommon, especially in the elderly. They are accounted to be the most common humeral fracture. The reason for the increase in incidence in the elderly is osteoporosis. The most common mechanism of proximal humeral fractures is a fall on outstretched hands. Severe trauma does not necessarily play a significant role; the distance may be from standing height or less. In younger individuals, the resulting fracture is often more serious, and

severe trauma may be the cause. The position of the arm and hand during the initial injury is a major factor. Excessive rotation of the arm in the abducted position or a direct blow to the side of the shoulder are also mechanisms of injury. Metastatic disease may significantly weaken the bone, and with minimal activity or trauma, a pathological fracture may occur.

In any arthroplastic procedure, the objectives are to relieve pain, to improve mobility, to maintain stability, and to improve function. Some proximal fractures may be treated conservatively; some displaced fractures or fracture-dislocations may necessitate more invasive therapy. Malunion and nonunion of fractures may shatter the balance of forces across the shoulder girdle and thus lead to an impingement.

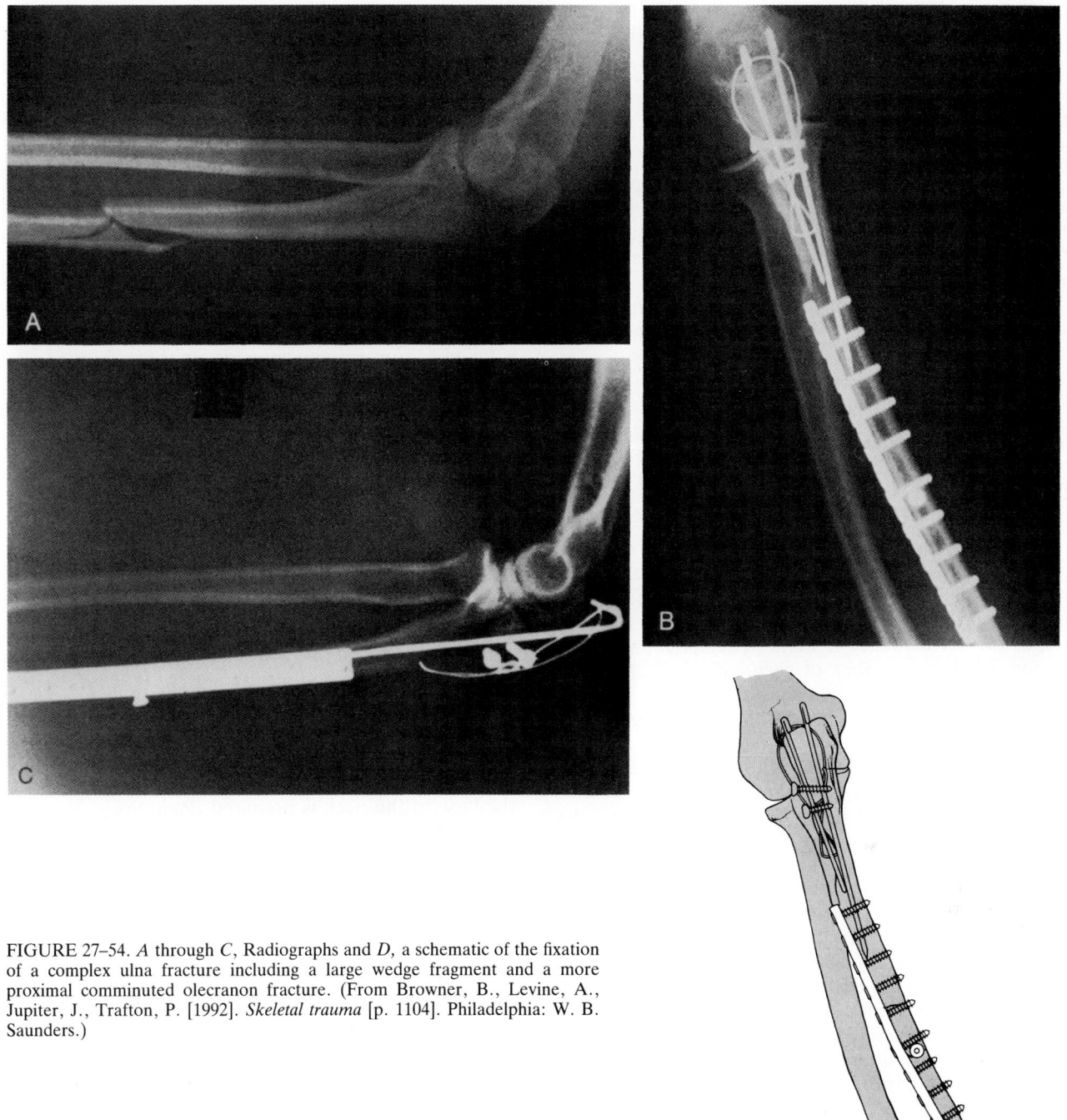

FIGURE 27–54. *A* through *C*, Radiographs and *D*, a schematic of the fixation of a complex ulna fracture including a large wedge fragment and a more proximal comminuted olecranon fracture. (From Browner, B., Levine, A., Jupiter, J., Trafton, P. [1992]. *Skeletal trauma* [p. 1104]. Philadelphia: W. B. Saunders.)

An understanding of the classification system for fractures of the proximal humerus is necessary to initiate proper management. The Neer classification, which is commonly used, identifies the four major fragments of the proximal humerus and their relationship to each other:

Grade I: less than 5 mm
Grade II: to one third the width of the shaft
Grade III: to two thirds the width of the shaft
Grade IV: greater than two thirds the width of the shaft, including total displacement

Indications

A humeral head prosthesis may be indicated for a fracture of the anatomical neck if internal fixation is not feasible. For other selected cases of osteoporotic three-part fractures, head-splitting fractures, and four-part fracture-dislocations, a prosthesis is generally the rule.

Related Surgical Procedures

Numerous techniques and devices have been proposed to treat proximal humeral fractures. The choice depends on several factors: the type of fracture, the quality of the bone and soft tissue, and the age and reliability of the patient.

Alternative methods of fixation include intramedullary nails, plates and screws, staples, wire, and suture material.

Perioperative Nursing Implications

Anesthesia

A large population of patients scheduled for shoulder surgery have numerous medical conditions. Rheumatoid arthritis frequently damages other joints; these patients need support and protection during anesthesia to avoid pain or further damage. General or regional anesthesia is considered. A number of regional anesthetic techniques may be used for shoulder surgery.

Shoulder replacement is facilitated by the use of an acrylic methyl methacrylate cement. A number of problems have been reported immediately after the insertion of the cement. Hypotension and cardiac arrest have been reported after inserting acrylic cement into the femur. It has been proposed that the liquid monomer produced a reduction in peripheral vascular resistance, which caused the cardiopulmonary changes. Embolization of fat and bone marrow to the lungs may result from high intermedullary pressures. Oxygen desaturation has also been documented after cement application. Venting the medullary cavity during prosthetic insertion can reduce the incidence of these side effects.

Findings of these studies are not confirmed to the use of bone cement in shoulder replacements. Because cement application can be potentially life threatening, all possible precautions should be taken during application of the cement:

maintenance of normal volume status and blood pressure before cementing

supplemental oxygen in awake patients or high inspired oxygen pressure in a patient receiving general anesthesia

communication between the surgeon and the anesthesiologist

monitoring of oxygen saturation

meticulous lavage to eliminate intramedullary contents

venting of the medullary cavity during prosthetic insertion

Position

The patient lies supine and is positioned closer to the side of the OR bed of the operative shoulder (Fig. 27–55). The lateral aspect of the head should be in line with the lateral aspect of the OR bed. The affected shoulder is raised forward on a padded sandbag placed beneath the scapula. All patient safety and comfort measures are maintained. The table is flexed 45 degrees at the waist and 30 degrees at the knees. A patient safety strap is secured across the patient's knees to prevent sliding. The patient's head is placed in a padded doughnut-shaped headrest. The patient's head and chest are securely positioned with additional straps. Caution is taken to prevent any pressure on the patient's face or malalignment of the cervical spine. A pillow is placed under the patient's knees to reduce back strain during the procedure. The unoperated arm is protected and secured at the patient's side.

Creation and Maintenance of the Sterile Field

The operative site is shaved, avoiding any bony prominences. The areas included are the upper arm from the elbow to the midsternum, including the axilla and the midback. With the patient's arm suspended in a finger trap positioning device, the skin is prepared in the routine orthopedic fashion. The affected extremity from the wrist to the superior aspect of the shoulder area to the base of the neck is prepared. Posteriorly, the shoulder, including the lateral aspect of the scapula, and the anterior and lateral chest wall to the nipple line are included. The arm is held with a sterile towel while the circulating nurse removes the finger traps. An impervious stockinet is placed over the hand and telescoped to above the elbow. The sterile area is squared off with sterile towels held in place with towel clips. A drape sheet is placed under the operative extremity and unfolded over the patient's torso and lower body. A second drape sheet is taken cephalad and fastened to create a barrier between anesthesia personnel and the surgical team. A hinged impervious sheet is placed beneath the operative arm and secured around the area of the skin preparation. An additional layer of drapes is placed as described above and fastened with towel clips. The skin is covered with an adhesive drape, with careful attention to the axilla. The stockinet may be secured with a Kling bandage.

Caution is taken to prevent any pooling of povidone-iodine solution beneath the patient. The patient's face and hairline may be protected by the use of plastic adherent towels.

The OR bed is positioned as for procedures performed on the upper extremity.

The Mayo stand is positioned across the patient's feet and the instrument table beside the scrub nurse (Fig.

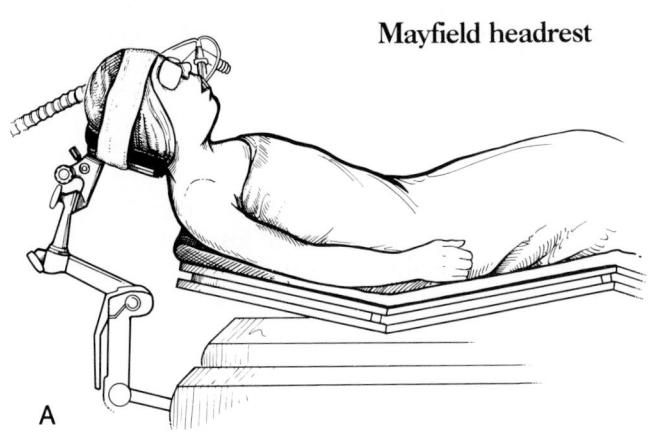

Mayfield headrest

A

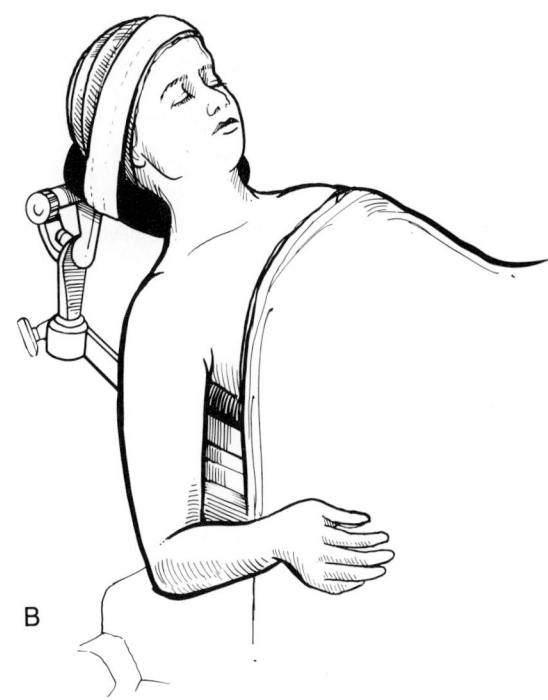

B

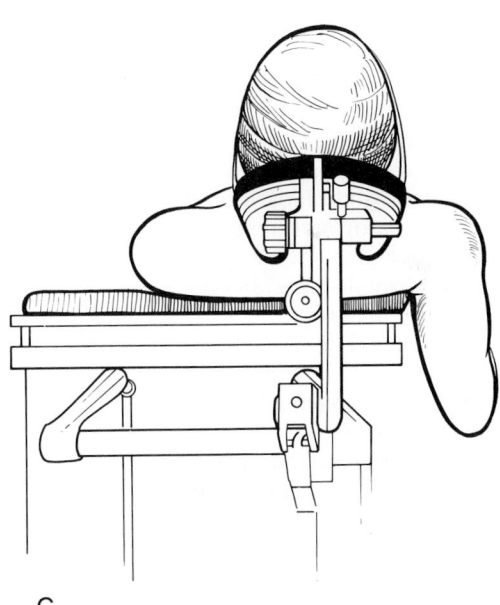

C

FIGURE 27–55. Position of the patient for prosthetic replacement of the fractured humeral head. *A,* The patient is placed in a semi-Fowler position on the operating table. *B* and *C,* The standard headrest portion of the table is removed and replaced with a Mayfield headrest, and the patient is positioned so that the involved shoulder extends over the top corner of the table. The patient's head is secured with tape. (From Global Total Shoulder Arthroplasty System [1991]. p. 4. Courtesy of DePuy, Inc., Warsaw, IN.)

27–56). An additional sterile Mayo stand may be positioned under the operative extremity for added support.

Equipment and Supplies

6 No. 10 blades
Impervious stockinet
Impervious hinged sheet
Irrigating syringe
1500 ml of normal saline

Electrocautery
Skin marker
1 package of 4 × 8 inch radiopaque sponges
Kling bandage
2 suction tubings
Povidone-iodine solution
Skin preparation tray
Povidone-iodine preparation brushes
2 4 × 4 inch preparation dressing sponges
Basin set
Drape packs

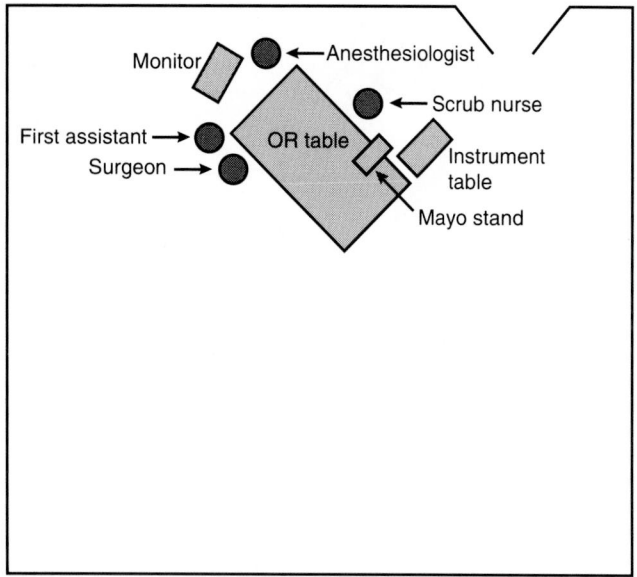

FIGURE 27–56. Operating room set-up for prosthetic replacement of the fractured right humeral head. The set-up would be reversed for replacement of a fractured left humeral head.

Pulsatile lavage and tips
Arm sling
3 1–0 Vicryl suture (CP–1)
3 2–0 Vicryl suture (CP–1)
4–0 Vicryl suture
1 package of large laparotomy sponges
2 packages of small laparotomy sponges
Cement restrictor and insertor
Cement gun
500 ml of normal saline
2 bacitracin, 50,000 U
2 polymyxin, 500,000 U
Adhesive drape
2 polymethyl methacrylate
Mixing bowls
2 impervious Mayo stand covers
Right-angled tip (for cement gun)

Instruments

Required in addition to equipment for a Silastic wrist implant are

trial prosthesis and reamers
2 polymethyl methacrylate and mixing bowl
Cobb periosteal elevator
2 medium Weitlaner retractors
large double-action rongeur
2 Crile forceps
suction drain
2 dull Hohmann retractors
Fukuda retractor
bone hook

Drugs and Solutions

The routine antibiotic solution is administered via a pressurized pulsatile lavage system. The mixture prepared by the circulating nurse is as follows: two doses of bacitracin, 50,000 U, and 2 doses of polymyxin, 500,000 U, in a 3000-ml normal saline solution. The incision might be infiltrated with lidocaine 1% with 1:100,000 Epinephrine to aid in hemostasis.

Physiological Monitoring

In addition to the measures in the discussion of anesthesia, calculation of blood loss is performed carefully throughout the surgical procedure. Sponges are weighed and suction devices are measured and recorded.

Specimens and Cultures

The humeral head is sent to the pathology department for a definitive diagnosis.

Physician's Orders

Shoulder x-ray films: AP, axillary lateral, and Grashey views (patient at 15-degree angle to the beam)
Urinalysis
Blood type and screen
CBC
ECG
Chest x-ray film
Coagulation profile
Occupational therapy and physical therapy consultation
Immobilization of extremity
NPO status after midnight
DVT prophylaxis
Administration of analgesics as needed
Bed rest
Vital signs every 4 hours

Laboratory and Diagnostic Studies

The Grashey view shows the thickness and integrity of the articular surfaces of the shoulder joint. X-ray films confirm the diagnosis and assist in preoperative planning.

Procedure

Incision and Exposure

Beginning over the distal clavicle, an anterior skin incision is made with a No. 10 blade approximately 1½

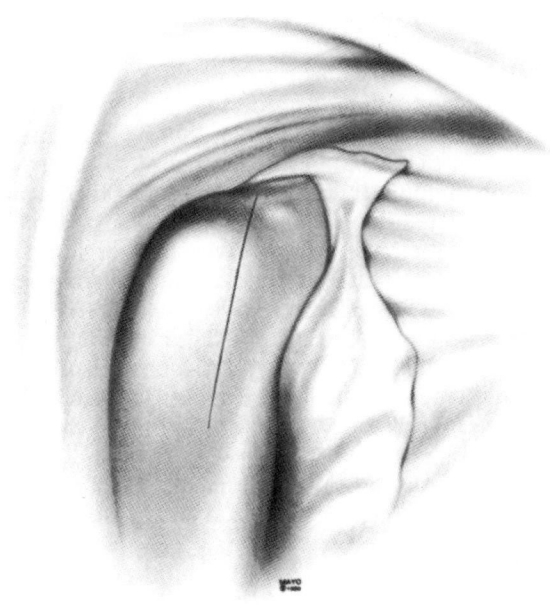

FIGURE 27–57. The anterior skin incision begins over the distal clavicle, approximately 1.5 cm medial to the acromioclavicular joint. It extends distally, slightly lateral to the anterior portion of the deltoid muscle insertion. (From Cofield, R. H. [1991]. *The Cofield Total Shoulder System: Surgical technique* [p. 3]. Memphis: Smith & Nephew Richards.)

cm medial to the acromioclavicular joint. The incision is extended distally and slightly laterally to the coracoid process, ending 1½ cm medial to the deltoid insertion (Fig. 27–57). The skin edges are freed from the underlying deep fascia and held apart by small rake retractors.

The deep fascia is incised (with a No. 15 blade), in line with the skin incision and the cut edges retracted to identify the deltopectoral groove. The pectoralis

major and deltoid muscles are separated with small Metzenbaum scissors. The cephalic vein is identified and retracted medially along with the pectoralis major muscle (Fig. 27–58A). The medial portion of the deltoid muscle is separated from the clavicle over a distance of 2 to 3 cm. This is performed by Metzenbaum scissors after the muscle has been separated from the underlying tissues. A small rim of muscle should be left attached

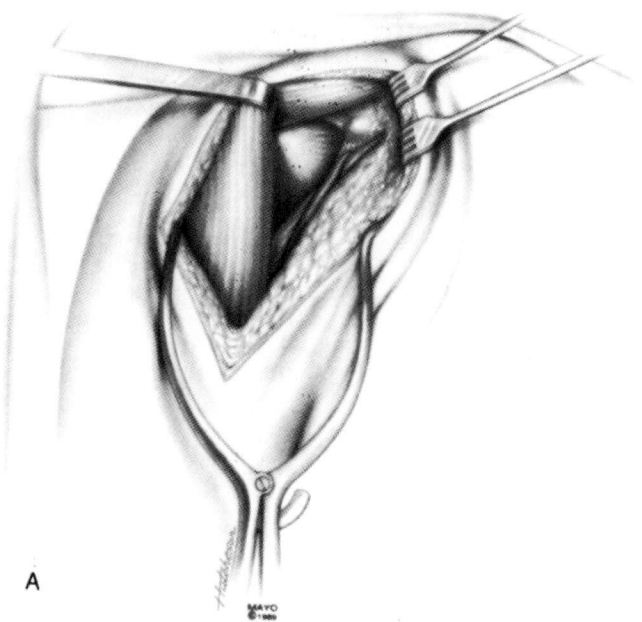

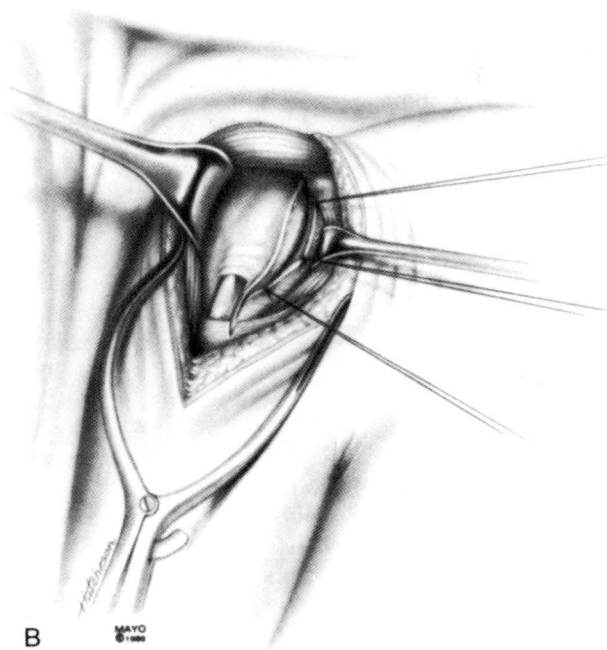

FIGURE 27–58. *A,* The deltoid branch of the thoracoacromial axis, which lies deep to the deeper layer of the pectoralis major–deltoid investing fascia, is cauterized. The surgeon allows full development of the delto-pectoral interval. *B,* The distal portion of the rotator cuff incision courses inferiorly and slightly laterally, incising the distal 1 cm of the subscapularis from its attachment to the humerus along with the underlying shoulder capsule. (From Cofield, R. H. [1991]. *The Cofield Total Shoulder System: Surgical technique* [pp. 3, 5]. Memphis: Smith & Nephew Richards.)

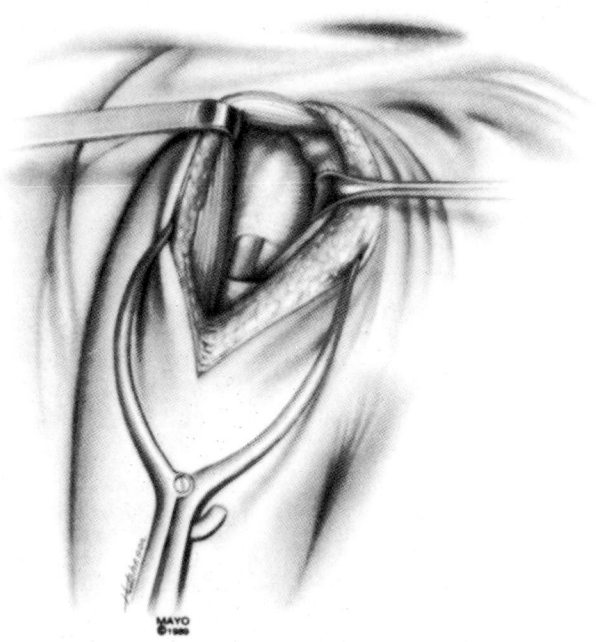

FIGURE 27–59. A large Richardson retractor is placed along the lateral aspect of the humeral head, the deltoid muscle is retracted laterally, and a small knee retractor placed beneath the conjoint tendon retracts it medially. (From Cofield, R. H. [1991].) *The Cofield Total Shoulder System: Surgical technique* [p. 4]. Memphis: Smith & Nephew Richards.

to the bone to aid reconstruction at the end of the operation.

The pectoralis major and the deltoid are separated widely with a blunt Weitlaner retractor to reveal the coracoid process and coracobrachialis and biceps muscles. The coracoid process is stripped of soft tissue with a Cobb elevator, and the distal portion is separated with a ¼-inch straight osteotome. The fascia surrounding the biceps muscle is divided with Metzenbaum scissors. The muscle origin is marked distally to the coracoid and the muscles reflected distally with the attached fragment.

Caution is taken to protect the musculocutaneous nerves, which enter the deep surface of the conjoined muscles (Fig. 27–58*B*).

The inferior and superior borders of the subscapularis muscle are defined by the stretch of the muscle on lateral rotation of the humerus. The borders are freed from the surrounding tissue with Metzenbaum scissors, and the lateral tendinous portion is divided. A small right-angled retractor is placed over the tendon. All branches of the cephalic vein are cauterized from the deltoid muscle. The subscapularis muscle belly is retracted with holding sutures of No. 1 Vicryl suture inserted proximally. The subscapularis is divided proximal to its insertion into the humerus. Another retraction stitch may be placed to retract the distal portion of the muscle laterally.

The anterior aspect of the shoulder capsule is exposed and incised vertically with a No. 15 blade. Retraction of the flaps of the capsule with small Kelly-Richardson retractors exposes the head of the humerus and the anterior rim of the glenoid fossa (Fig. 27–59).

Details

The Kelly-Richardson retractors are removed, and a Cobb elevator is placed in the shoulder joint (Fig. 27–60). The humerus is extended and placed in external rotation. The shoulder joint is dislocated, and the humeral head is slid anteriorly. The humeral head is cleared of all osteophytes for better visualization of the shoulder joint. With the elbow flexed at 90 degrees, the forearm is aimed at the operating surgeon's midline and the humerus is externally rotated 30 to 35 degrees.

With a ½ inch straight osteotome, the surgeon marks the osteotomy cut downward and medially from the superolateral point of the humeral head. The cut is continued distally and medially 45 degrees to the axis of the humerus with a microsagittal saw. The head is removed with an osteotome and a large towel clip if

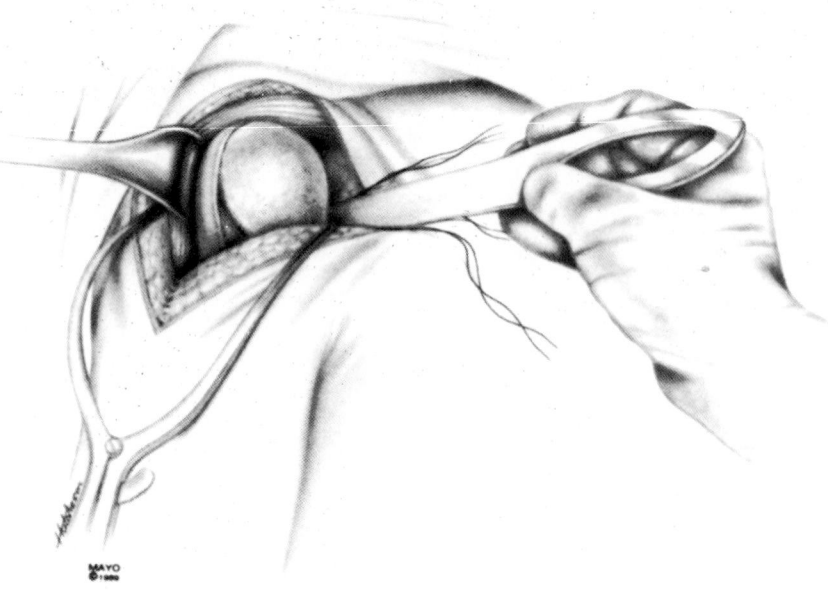

FIGURE 27–60. A large elevator is placed within the shoulder joint, and the humerus is externally rotated and slightly extended. The humeral head slides forward on the elevator, dislocating the shoulder joint anteriorly. (From Cofield, R. H. [1991]. *The Cofield Total Shoulder System: Surgical technique* [p. 5]. Memphis: Smith & Nephew Richards.)

necessary. All remaining osteophytes around the circumference of the proximal humerus are trimmed.

The humeral reamer is placed ½ cm posterior to the bicipital groove and 1 cm medial to the lateral edge of the cut osteotomy surface (Fig. 27–61). The appropriate trial humeral component is seated until the base of the prosthesis touches the osteotomized humeral surface. The rotation of the trial component can be adjusted, and trial reduction is performed.

The trial component is removed, and the intramedullary canal is irrigated with a pulsatile lavage of antibiotic irrigation. An intramedullary cement restrictor is inserted and the canal is thoroughly dried. The humerus is levered slightly laterally with a Cobb elevator and exposure of the proximal humerus achieved with Kelly-Richardson retractors. Methyl methacrylate is injected into the humeral canal with a cement gun, and the humeral component of the correct size is impacted into position. Excess cement is removed with a Cobb elevator or curet from around the prosthesis. When the cement has set, any apparent or potentially loosened fragments of cement are removed. The wound is irrigated again and the humeral component is reduced to the glenoid.

Closure

The horizontal and vertical limbs of the subscapularis incision are closed with an interrupted No. 1 Vicryl suture on a cutting needle. A suction drain is placed in the distal aspect of the subdeltoid space. The deltopectoral interval and subcutaneous tissues are closed with an interrupted 2–0 Vicryl suture on a cutting needle. The skin is closed with a subcuticular 4–0 Vicryl suture.

Dry, sterile gauze dressings are applied followed by a shoulder immobilizer.

Postoperative Care

Coughing and deep breathing every 2 hours while the patient is awake
Antibiotic coverage
Application of ice packs for 72 hours
Administration of analgesics as needed
CBC, prothrombin time, partial thromboplastin time the morning after surgery, and in 5 days
X-ray films in the recovery room
Neurovascular checks every 2 hours for 24 hours
Out of bed as tolerated
Diet as tolerated
DVT prophylaxis
Use of a shoulder immobilizer for 1 week then at night for 4 weeks
Active exercises of the hand in 24 hours
Passive motion of the shoulder in 36 hours; pendulum exercises
Isometric exercises in 1 week
Discharge in 10 days

Potential Surgical Complications

Infection is always a surgical risk.
Loosening may be due to surgical technique or improper bone stock.

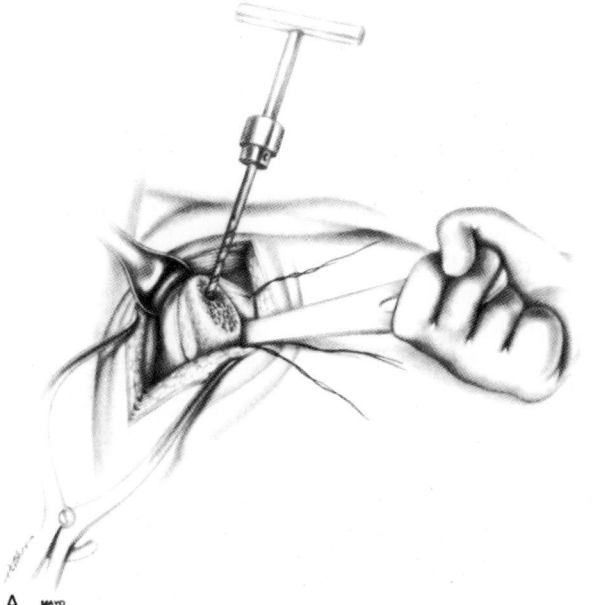
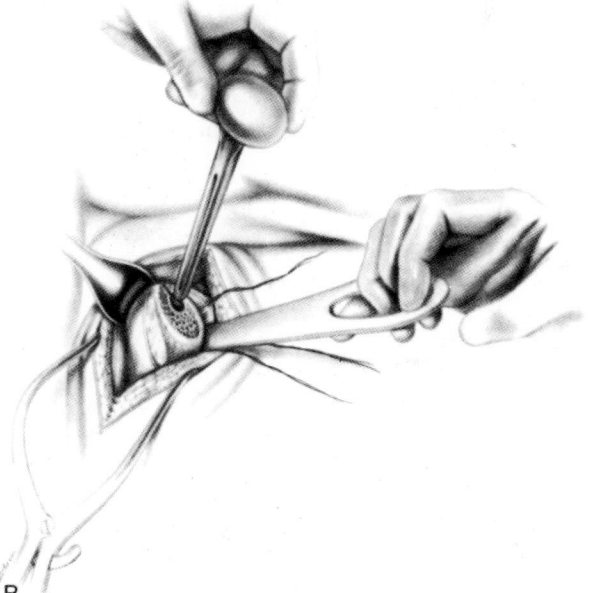

FIGURE 27–61. *A,* The small humeral reamer is directed from the pilot hole distally into the humeral diaphysis. The hole is enlarged as needed with the medium, large, or extra-large humeral reamer, as required by the size of the medullary canal. *B,* The trial humeral component is seated and its rotation adjusted so that the prosthetic's undersurface parallels the cut surface of the osteotomy. The trial prosthesis is removed, and using a small rongeur, a slot is made to accept its lateral fin. (From Cofield, R. H. [1991]. *The Cofield Total Shoulder System: Surgical technique* [p. 10]. Memphis: Smith & Nephew Richards.)

Some loss of motion or strength may be due to improper component size, overcorrection of muscular reconstruction, or instability of the shoulder joint

OPEN REDUCTION AND INTERNAL FIXATION OF THE HIP

Definition

Fracture of the hip refers to a fracture of the proximal one third of the femur that extends up to 5 cm below the lesser trochanter. It occurs most commonly through the neck or the intertrochanteric region of the femur, but it is also seen in the subtrochanteric region (Fig. 27–62). Hip fractures are classified as either intracapsular or extracapsular. *Intracapsular* fractures occur within the hip joint capsule. They are as follows: capital (fractures of the femoral head), subcapital (fractures just below the head of the femur), and transcervical (fractures of the neck of the femur). *Extracapsular* fractures are outside of the joint capsule through the femur's greater or lesser trochanter, in the intertrochanteric area, or in the subtrochanteric location.

Indications

Treatment of hip fracture consists of realigning the fragments by either closed or open methods, followed by the operative insertion of a internal fixation device (Fig. 27–63).

Related Surgical Procedures

The choice of procedure in the treatment of a hip fracture depends primarily on the type of fracture and secondarily on the patient's general physical condition, the length of the time since the fracture was sustained, and the surgeon's preference and judgment.

The following is a list of possible surgical interventions for the various intracapsular and extracapsular fractures.

Capital and Subcapital. The principles of treatment are prosthetic head replacement for fractures that are severly comminuted or severely displaced for a prolonged period. Closed reduction and pinning are appropriate for fractures relatively nondisplaced or impacted and can be reduced adequately.

Transcervical. Same as for capital and subcapital.

Intertrochanteric. Intertrochanteric fractures heal readily in traction (8–12 weeks). However, this prolonged bed rest increases the patient's risk of complications. Thus, the preferred method of treatment is open reduction and internal fixation using a sliding screw and slide plate.

Perioperative Nursing Implications

Anesthesia

Surgery is performed most frequently under general anesthesia because the patient's position on the fracture table for a prolonged period of time can be uncomfortable. However, epidural anesthesia can be used for patients with compromised pulmonary function. If the fracture is produced by severe trauma, there may be extensive bleeding into the soft tissue. Because of the relative abundance of the blood supply in the cancellous segment of the femur, an intertrochanteric fracture is a severe injury. Because of the high incidence of complications (blood loss, shock, fat embolism, pulmonary embolism and pneumonia), blood loss, vital signs, oxygen saturation, ECGs, pulmonary status, and urine output are carefully monitored intraoperatively and postoperatively.

Position

The patient is positioned on the fracture table (Fig. 27–64; see Perioperative Nursing Implications for fracture table use). The affected limb is held in slight medial rotation, so that the patella is directed about 15 degrees inwards. The sound limb is abducted almost fully and locked in this position by clamping the appropriate swivel surface of the table. The injured limb is abducted about 30 degrees and locked in this position. The arm on the operative side is padded and taped across the patient's chest to allow easy movement of the x-ray C-arm.

The mobile x-ray image intensifier is moved into position between the abducted lower extremities. The tube should be placed close up against the inner side of the sound knee and directed horizontally toward the neck of the femur on the injured side.

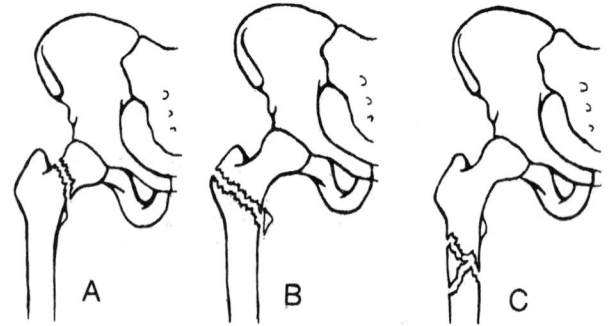

FIGURE 27–62. Types of hip fractures. *A*, Femoral neck fracture. *B*, Intertrochanteric fracture. *C*, Subtrochanteric fracture. (From Zuidema, G. D., Rutherford, R. B., Ballinger, W. F. [1985]. *The management of trauma* [4th ed.] [p. 678]. Philadelphia: W. B. Saunders.)

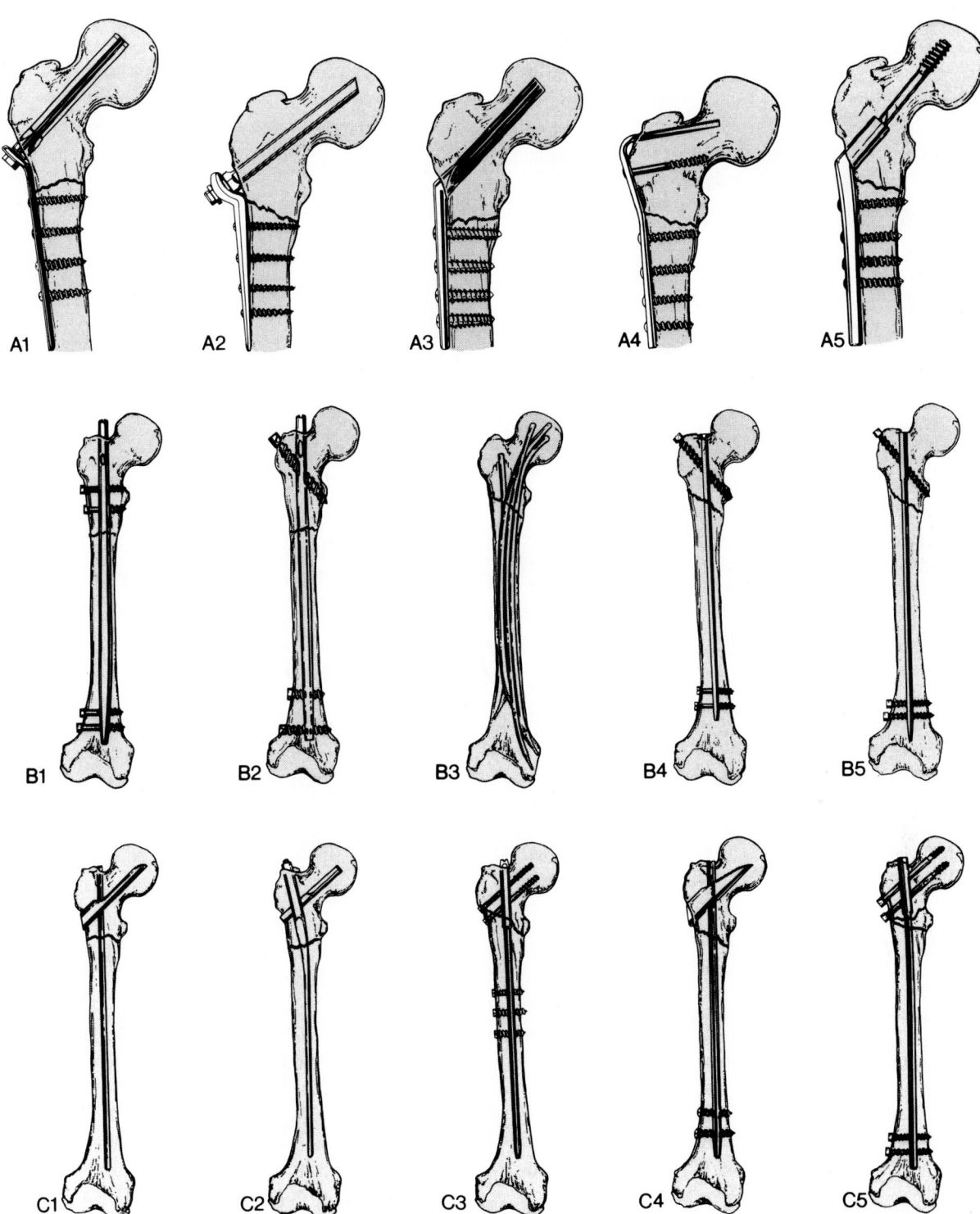

FIGURE 27–63. *A*, Evolution of plate design. (1) Thornton device. (2) McLaughlin nail plate. (3) Jewett nail plate. (4) AO blade plate. (5) Richards hip compression screw. *B*, Centromedullary and condylocephalic devices. (1) Küntscher interlocking screws and detensor. (2) Klemm-Schellmann device with diagonal proximal locking screw. (3) Ender condylocephalic devices. (4) Grosse-Kempf interlocking device. (5) Russell-Taylor closed section interlocking femoral nail. *C*, Cephalomedullary implants with proximal fragment stabilization by internal fixation into the femoral head and neck. (1) Küntscher Y nail, (2) Zickle device, (3) Huckstep nail, (4) Williams Y nail, (5) Russell-Taylor reconstruction interlocking nail. (From Browner, B., Levine, A., Jupiter, J., Trafton, P. [1992]. *Skeletal trauma* [p. 1495]. Philadelphia: W. B. Saunders.) Redrawn from Calandruccio, R. A. Chairman, AAOS Committee on the History of Orthopaedic Surgery. *Internal fixation devices for fractures of the proximal femur.* Exhibit at the 55th Annual Meeting, Atlanta. February 4–9, 1988.)

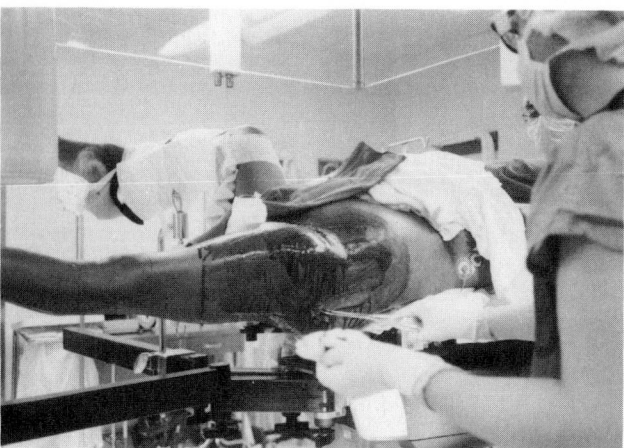

FIGURE 27–64. Preparation of the extremity for femoral rod insertion.

Creation and Maintenance of the Sterile Field

The OR lights must be positioned to ensure adequate lighting on the operative limb. The fracture table should be centered in the room to allow the surgical team and equipment to be located on the operative side (Fig. 27–65).

The area from above the iliac crest to the knee is shaved and prepared in the routine manner as described above. The leg need not be painted circumferentially, but as medially and posteriorly as possible.

The clear plastic Redi-Drape is applied in the following manner: Remove the paper backing from the adhesive portion. Center the adhesive portion over the incisional area and apply. Fan fold open the drape and fold the upper portion over a shower curtain pole.

Equipment and Supplies

3 No. 10 blades
3 packages of large laparotomy sponges
Marking pen
Needle counter
3 No. 1 Vicryl sutures (CP-1)
3 2–0 Vicryl sutures (CP-2)
Skin staples
Basin set
Bacitracin, 50,000 U
Polymyxin, 500,000 U
Redi-Drape (clear plastic drape)
Suction tubing
Irrigating syringe
100 ml of normal saline
Electrocautery
Povidone-iodine solution
Povidone-iodine preparation sponges
2 4 × 4 inch drip or dressing sponges
Medium Hemovac (suction drain)

Instruments

2 Lowman bone clamps
2 Cobb periosteal elevators
6 Kelly clamps
6 Curved hemostats
2 Weitlaner retractors
2 Beckman retractors
2 Bennett retractors
Assorted curets
2 Ferris Smith forceps
2 Adson forceps
No. 10 knife handle
Small and large rongeurs
Mallet
Bone hook
Yankauer suction tip
Mayo scissors
Bandage scissors
Suture scissors
3 needle holders
4 Kocher clamps
2 sponge sticks
Power drill
Double-action bone cutter
Appropriate hip compression system, drill bits, and implants

Drugs and Solutions

The routine antibiotic irrigation is used.

Physiological Monitoring

Refer to the discussion of anesthesia.

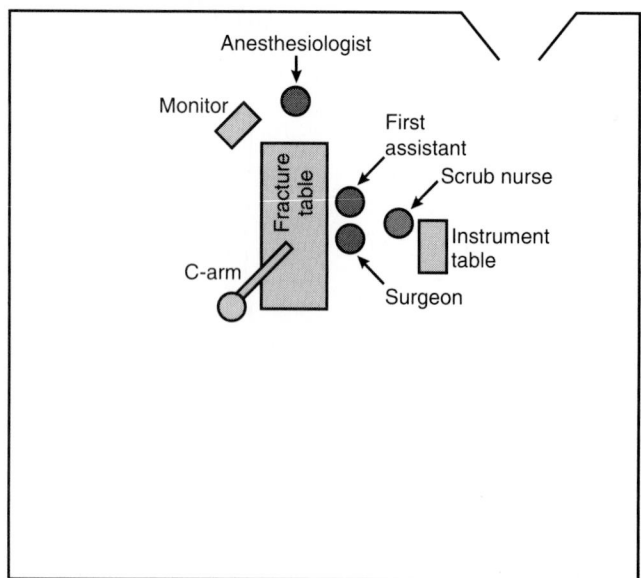

FIGURE 27–65. Operating room set-up for open reduction and internal fixation of the left hip. The set-up would be reversed for the right hip.

Specimens and Cultures

A bone sampling may be sent to the pathology laboratory if there is suspicion of a pathological fracture without any evidence of traumatic injury.

Physician's Orders

Vital signs every 4 hours
Bed rest
NPO status after midnight
Physical therapy and occupational therapy consultation
Administration of analgesics as needed
Prophylactic antibiotics
Hematology profile
Foley catheter connected to gravity drainage
DVT prophylaxis
ECG
Chest x-ray film
Typing and cross-matching of blood
AP and lateral hip x-ray films
Urinalysis

Laboratory and Diagnostic Studies

Obtain a hematology profile. Decreased hemoglobin level or hematocrit is noted if there is excessive bleeding. X-ray films confirm the presence and type of fracture.

Procedure

Incision and Exposure

The incision is made on the lateral aspect of the hip, extending from the greater trochanter distally, with a No. 10 blade. The length of the incision depends on the length of the implant. Weitlaner retractors are placed under the subcutaneous fat. The fascia lata is split in the direction of the incision distally with Mayo scissors. Proximally, the slit is extended upward into the tensor fascia lata muscle again with Mayo scissors. Beckman retractors can now replace the Weitlaner retractors. The deeper muscle layer, the vastus lateralis, is retracted anteriorly with a Bennett retractor. Any remaining muscle fibers overlying the lateral aspect of the femur are divided by a vertical cut straight onto the bone with Mayo scissors. The periosteum is stripped over a length of about 7 to 10 cm from the base of the greater trochanter downward with a Cobb elevator.

Details (Intertrochanteric Fractures)

With traction applied to the operative extremity, a guide pin is inserted under image intensification by means of a power drill. The level of insertion varies with the angle of the plate used. The lesser trochanter

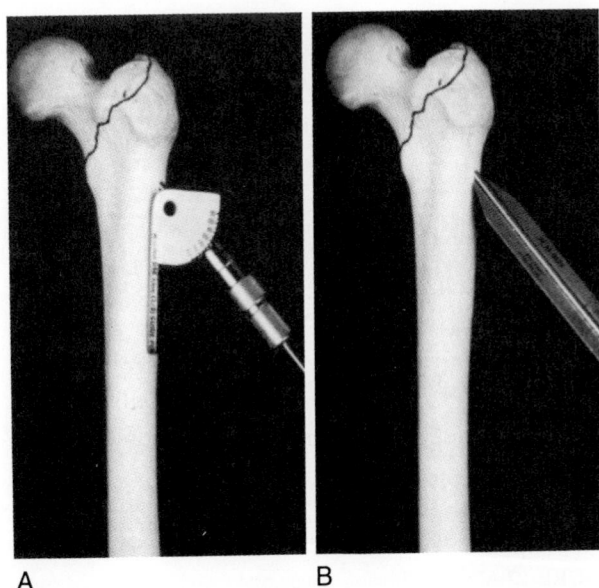

A   B

FIGURE 27–66. *A,* The guide pin can be inserted freely and the angle verified with an adjustable angle guide. *B,* The length of the guide pin within the femur can be confirmed with a direct measuring gauge and adjusted according to the specific circumstances. (From *Richards Classic hip screw and supracondylar plate: Surgical technique* [1991] [p. 4]. Memphis: Smith & Nephew Richards.)

helps to verify the point of entry: The guide pin enters just opposite the tip of the lesser trochanter for a 135-degree angle plate (Fig. 27–66*A*), and 2 cm lower for a 150-degree angle plate. The guidewire position is checked by means of AP and lateral views. Ideal pin position is slightly inferior to the center of the femoral head on the view and slightly posterior on the lateral view. The depth of the guide pin should be within a distance of 1 cm of the articular surface of the femoral head. This length should be confirmed with a direct measuring gauge (Fig. 27–66*B*). An additional stabilization pin may be inserted at the time, if necessary, parallel to the guide pin.

The length of the guide pin is measured, and the reamer is prepared accordingly. The lag screw is determined by the direct measuring gauge. This measurement permits 5 mm of compression.

The reamer is then adjusted and slid over the guidewire and driven on through the femoral neck into the head (Fig. 27–67). Penetration of the reamer should be checked radiographically.

Assemble the appropriate plate and lag screw into the insertion wrench. The entire assembly is then placed over the guidewire and introduced into the channel (Fig. 27–68).

The lag screw is driven past the fracture site (Fig. 27–69*A*), and its depth checked periodically radiographically and with a depth gauge (Fig. 27–69*B*) in both planes. The insertion wrench is removed, and the plate is impacted over the lag screw. The plate is attached to the femur with Lowman bone clamp and the guidewire removed.

Some traction can be released, and manual impaction of the fracture fragments can be performed if necessary.

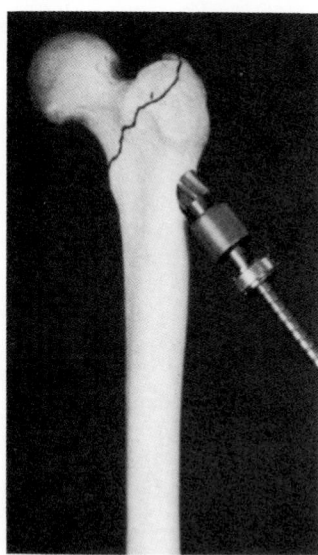

FIGURE 27–67. The surgeon reams osteoporotic bone and around areas of comminution. A rongeur can be used to enlarge the opening. Reaming is continued until the depth stop reaches the lateral cortex. (From *Richards Classic hip screw and supracondylar plate: Surgical technique* [1991] [p. 5]. Memphis: Smith & Nephew Richards.)

The screws of the side plate are inserted using the same technique discussed for open reduction and internal fixation of the fractured ulna. The compression screw is engaged into the end of the lag screw and tightened judiciously. It is important not to overtighten the screw, lest the threads of the lag screw pull through the bone.

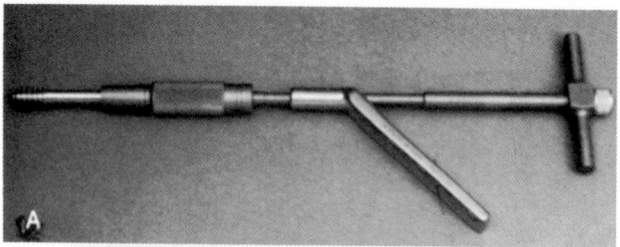

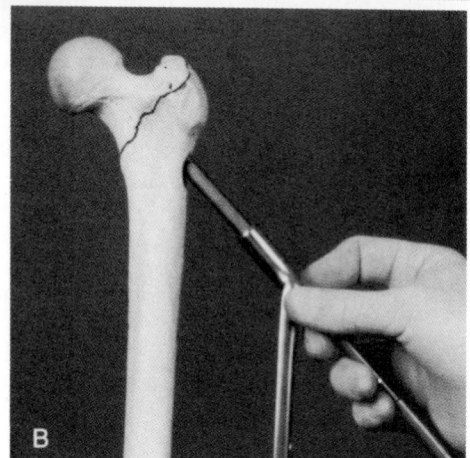

FIGURE 27–68. *A,* The wrench stabilizer is screwed tightly into the distal end of the lag screw until a firm connection is obtained, and the centering sleeve is slipped onto the wrench. *B,* After the screw's position is verified, the centering sleeve is removed and the sideplate is advanced onto the lag screw. (From *Richards Classic hip screw and supracondylar plate: Surgical technique* [1991] [p. 6]. Memphis: Smith & Nephew Richards.)

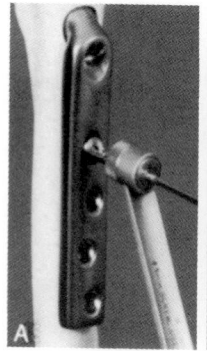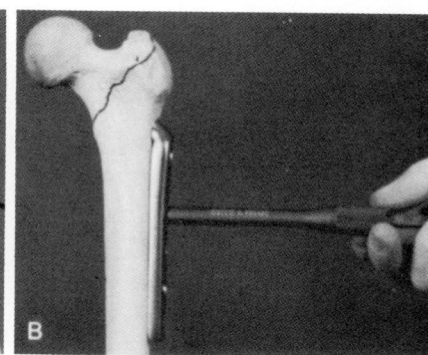

FIGURE 27–69. *A,* A drill guide is used for drilling the screw holes. *B,* The length of the cortical screws is ascertained with a depth gauge. (From *Richards Classic hip screw and supracondylar plate: Surgical technique* [1991] [p. 7]. Memphis: Smith & Nephew Richards.)

Closure

Closure of the vastus lateralis muscle and the fascia lata is done is layers with No. 1 Vicryl suture on a cutting needle. A wound suction device is placed between these layers. Subcutaneous fat is closed with 2–0 Vicryl suture on a cutting needle. Skin is approximated with staples. Dry gauze dressings are applied.

Postoperative Care

Vital signs every 4 hours
Neurovascular checks every 2 hours
Administration of analgesics as needed
Administration of antibiotics
DVT prophylaxis
Out of bed as tolerated the next day
X-ray films in recovery and the morning after surgery
Panel 7 after surgery and the next morning
Incentive spirometry every 2 hours
Discharge in 10 to 14 days with a cane or walker

Potential Surgical Complications

Fat embolism complicates fracture of the long bone.
Breakage of fixation device is due to additional injury or poor bone stock.
Pin penetration into the acetabulum is due to improper technique or poor bone stock.
Infection is always a potential surgical complication.

OPEN REDUCTION AND INTERNAL FIXATION OF THE FEMUR WITH AN INTRAMEDULLARY ROD

Definition

The femur is the largest bone in the body. The fractures seen in this location are due to high-velocity and high-energy accidents. Consequently, these fractures frequently are associated with other fractures or other internal injuries. The femur also heals slowly.

Indications

If a patient is treated with traction alone, it would take as long as 4 to 6 months for healing. Therefore, methods of treatment have been devised in an attempt to get earlier ambulation during the healing period.

Classification of the degree of comminution of the fracture and its location is most important. Femoral fractures can be classified as open or closed. Those that are open necessitate immediate operative débridement, stabilization, and secondary closure. The fracture can also be classified as simple, comminuted, or segmental. The anatomical locations of femoral shaft fractures are divided in subtrochanteric, midshaft, and distal shaft. Each area lends itself to specific types of treatment.

Open intramedullary nailing of the femur involves inserting a nail after reduction and surgical exposure of the fracture. Intramedullary fixation is the treatment of choice of closed uncomminuted and severely comminuted fractures through the midshaft. Subtrochanteric fractures can also be treated with interlocking intranail medullary fixation devices (Fig. 27–70).

Related Surgical Procedures

Closed intramedullary nailing is a method to nail shaft fractures without exposing the fracture site. The fracture

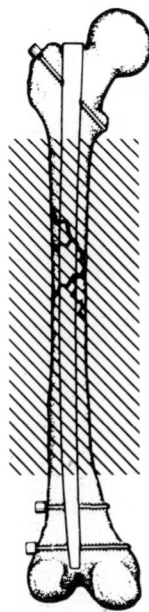

FIGURE 27–70. Fractures situated in the shaded area can be fixed with a Russell-Taylor femoral or Delta femoral interlocking nail. (From Russell, T. A., Taylor, J. C., LaVelle, D. G. [1991]. *Russell-Taylor femoral nail system: Surgical technique* [p. 14]. Memphis: Smith & Nephew Richards.)

site may be manipulated to get the nail across the fracture, but the fracture site is never opened.

Perioperative Nursing Implications

Anesthesia

The same principles apply as for a open reduction and internal fixation of the hip.

Position

The patient is placed on the fracture table in the supine (Fig. 27–71A) or in the lateral decubitus (Fig. 27–71B) position. The foot of the affected extremity is placed in the traction boot with 15 degrees of internal rotation. The fractured side is placed in 15 to 30 degrees of hip flexion with the unaffected side in neutral position. Safety and positioning were discussed above.

Creation and Maintenance of the Sterile Field

The thigh is shaved and prepared from the iliac crest to the knee circumferentially. Posteriorly, the buttocks are also shaved and circumferentially prepared. The routine orthopedic preparation is followed.

Sterile drapes are placed distally and proximally to the prepared area and secured with skin staples. A large adhesive povidone-iodine drape is placed over the prepared area. The thigh is covered circumferentially with the adhesive drape.

Equipment and Supplies

Adhesive Ioban drape
15 large laparotomy sponges
5 small laparotomy sponges
Suction
Electrocautery
4 No. 10 blades
4 No. 1 Vicryl suture (CP–1)
4 2–0 Vicryl suture (CP–1)
1000 ml of normal saline
Povidone-iodine preparation sponges
Medium Hemovac (suction drain)
Table drapes
Gowns
Patient drapes
Needle counter
Irrigating syringe
50-ml syringe
Bacitracin, 50,000 U
Polymyxin, 500,000 U
Marking pen
Basin Set
Povidone-iodine solution

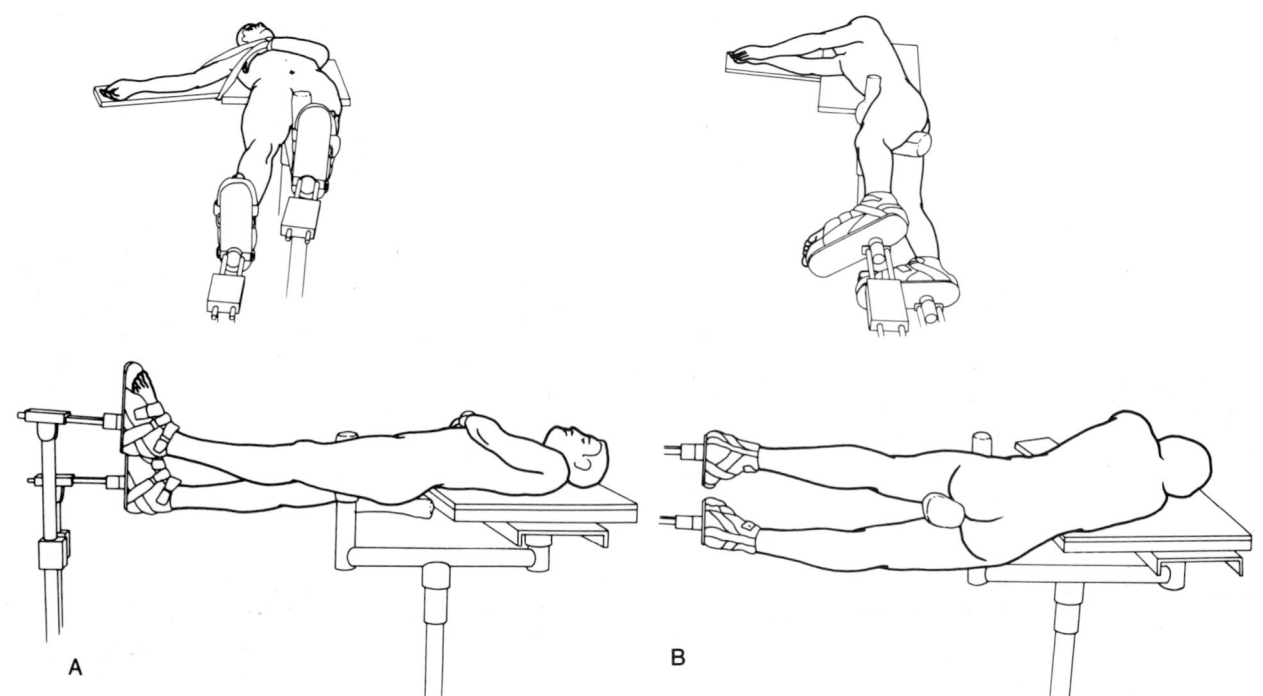

FIGURE 27–71. *A,* Patient in the supine position, with the trunk and affected extremity adducted. *B,* Patient in the lateral decubitus position. (From Russell, T. A., Taylor, J. C., LaVelle, D. G. [1991]. *Russell-Taylor femoral nail system: Surgical technique* [pp. 14, 15]. Memphis: Smith & Nephew Richards.)

4 × 4 inch preparation or dressing sponge
Heavy pliers
Assorted osteotomes
Tissue protector
Appropriate intramedullary fixture devices and instruments: reamers, drills, drill guides, impactors, guidewires
Flexible intramedullary reamers
Curved awl

Drugs and Solutions

The routine antibiotic irrigation is used.

Physiological Monitoring

The same principles apply as for open reduction and internal fixation of the hip.

Specimens and Cultures

Refer to the discussion of open reduction and internal fixation of the hip.

Physician's Orders

NPO status after midnight
Bed rest with immobilization

Chest x-ray film
ECG
Urinalysis
Physical therapy and occupational therapy consultation
DVT prophylaxis
Typing and cross-matching of 4 units of blood
Administration of analgesics as needed
AP and lateral x-ray films
Vital signs every 4 hours
Neurovascular checks every 2 hours
Hematology profile
Antibiotic coverage

Laboratory and Diagnostic Studies

Refer to the discussion of open reduction and internal fixation of the hip.

Procedure

Incision and Exposure

With a No. 10 blade, a longitudinal incision on the posterolateral aspect of the thigh is made (Fig. 27–72). The distal part of the incision is on the lateral femoral epicondyle and continues proximally along the posterior portion of the femoral shaft. The exact length of the incision depends on the degree of comminution of the fracture. Weitlaner retractors are positioned to retract

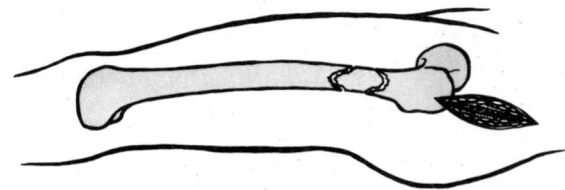

FIGURE 27-72. Skin incision for the standard Russell-Taylor femoral nail. (From Browner, B., Levine, A., Jupiter, J., Trafton, P. [1992]. *Skeletal trauma* [p. 1509]. Philadelphia: W. B. Saunders.)

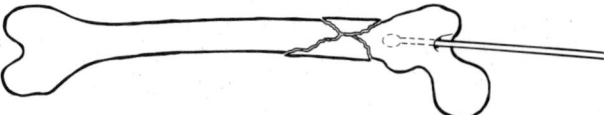

FIGURE 27-74. For the unreamed technique, sounds can be used to determine the diameter of the canal and proper nail size prior to insertion of the nail. (From Russell, T. A., Taylor, J. C., LaVelle, D. G. [1991]. *Russell-Taylor femoral nail system: Surgical technique* [p. 17]. Memphis: Smith & Nephew Richards.)

the subcutaneous fat layer. The deep fascia is incised with a No. 10 blade in line with its fibers and the skin incision. The femoral and sciatic nerves are in the internerve plane between the vastus lateralis and the hamstring muscles. Caution is taken to identify and maintain these structures.

The vastus lateralis is followed posteriorly to the lateral intermuscular septum (which covers the hamstring muscle). The muscle is reflected anteriorly with a Beckman retractor, and dissection between muscle and septum is performed with Mayo scissors. Ligation or cauterization of the branches of the perforating arteries is accomplished to gain hemostasis.

The dissection is continued until the femur is exposed. The periosteum is incised longitudinally and stripped off the muscles covering the femur with a Cobb periosteal elevator.

Details

After the fracture site is exposed, the bone ends are cleared so that reduction is accurate. The proximal fragment is reduced to the distal fragment using an internal fracture alignment device. When perfect reduction has been secured by manipulation and application of traction, the fracture is held together with Lowman bone-holding forceps.

An oblique incision 2 cm distal to the proximal tip of the greater trochanter is made with a No. 10 blade and continued proximally and medially for 8 to 10 cm. Weitlaner retractors are positioned, and the fascia of the gluteus maximus is incised with a No. 10 blade in

line with the skin incision. The gluteus maximus is divided in line with its fibers with Mayo scissors. Weitlaner retractors are removed and replaced with Beckman retractors for deeper exposure.

The trochanteric fossa is palpated, and a curved awl is introduced manually in line with the femoral shaft (Fig. 27-73). This step is verified with AP and lateral x-ray films. The entry portal can be further enlarged with the awl. A tapered T-handle reamer is inserted and the metaphyseal canal enlarged.

A ball-tipped guidewire is introduced to the level of the fracture (Fig. 27-74). The ball tip is to facilitate retrieval of a reamer head should it break off. The position of the wire is checked with the intensifier because the wire may take a false course. A skin protector is placed over the proximal skin edges during reaming and insertion of the nail.

Flexible reamers of graded sizes are passed over the guidewire in order of increasing diameter. Reaming should begin with the smallest diameter, and only moderate pressure should be applied on the power tool. The process is repeated until the canal has been enlarged to the desired size (Fig. 27-75). AP and lateral views are periodically checked during the reaming process. Manufacturer's recommendations as to overreaming the canal for proper nail size must be investigated.

Systems vary as to nail diameter and stated size. Most manufacturers recommend reaming of 1 to 1½ mm greater than the desired diameter for midshaft fractures.

A flexible, cannulated exchange tube is passed over the ball-tipped guidewire to maintain reduction when the wire is removed. A nail guidewire is then inserted and the medullary tube removed.

The correct length of the nail is determined from the known length of the guidewire within the bone. A nail length gauge can determine the correct nail size (Fig. 27-76). The nail should be allowed to penetrate to within 2 to 3 cm of the lower articular surface of the femur, but not as far for fractures above midshaft. The

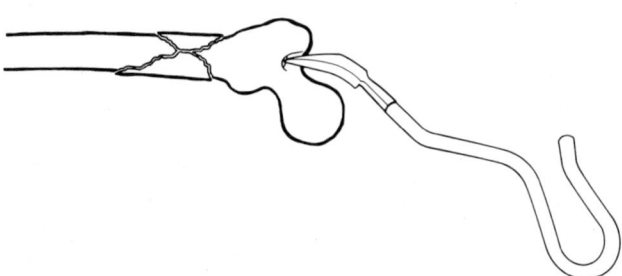

FIGURE 27-73. A curved awl can be introduced at the trochanteric fossa, usually with the straight portion parallel to the floor and in line with the femoral shaft. (From Russell, T. A., Taylor, J. C., LaVelle, D. G. [1991]. *Russell-Taylor femoral nail system: Surgical technique* [p. 17]. Memphis: Smith & Nephew Richards.)

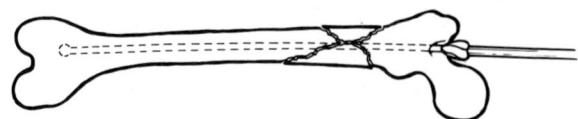

FIGURE 27-75. The entire femur should be reamed until the desired diameter is achieved. (From Russell, T. A., Taylor, J. C., LaVelle, D. G. [1991]. *Russell-Taylor femoral nail system: Surgical technique* [p. 20]. Memphis: Smith & Nephew Richards.)

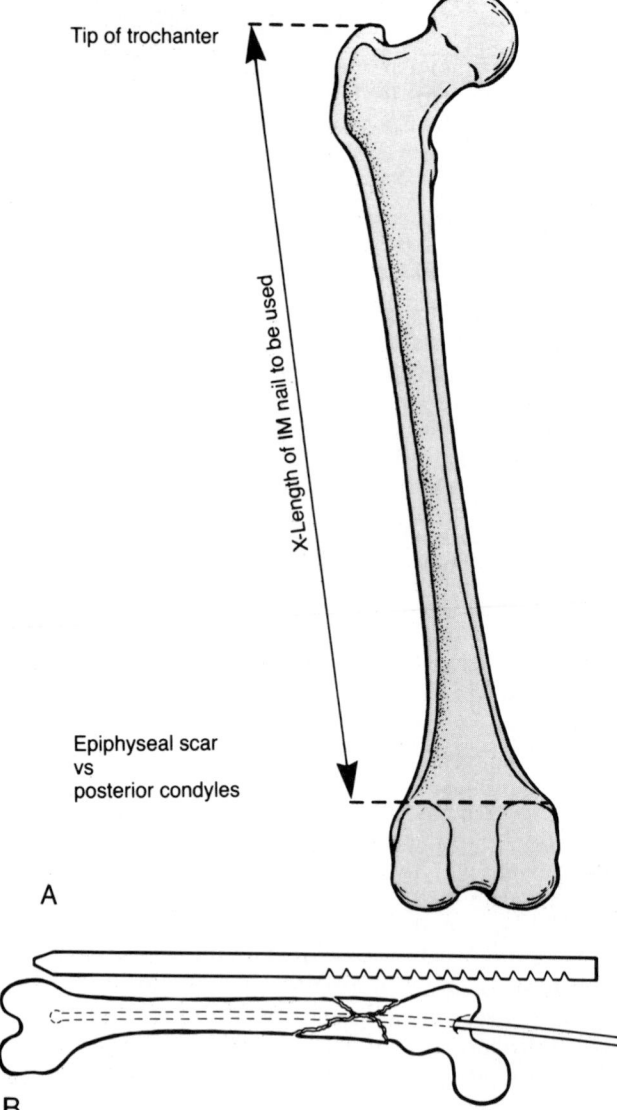

Tip of trochanter

X-Length of IM nail to be used

Epiphyseal scar
vs
posterior condyles

A

B

FIGURE 27–76. *A*, Reproducible points on the proximal and distal femur. (From Browner, B., Levine, A., Jupiter, J., Trafton, P. [1990]. *Skeletal trauma* [p. 1612]. Philadelphia: W. B. Saunders.) *B*, The nail length gauge is positioned anterior to the femur to determine the correct nail size. (From Russell, T. A., Taylor, J. C., LaVelle, D. G. [1991]. *Russell-Taylor femoral nail system: Surgical technique* [p. 20]. Memphis: Smith & Nephew Richards.)

type and size of the nail is also dependent on patient characteristics and fracture classification.

The scrub nurse attaches the appropriate nail on the nail insertion device. The nail is placed so that its curvature matches that of the femur: horizontally when the patient is in the lateral decubitus position. With the use of the correct handle to control rotation, the surgeon inserts the nail (Fig. 27–77). The nail guidewire is removed after the nail has entered the distal fragment by several centimeters. Figure 27–78 shows the technique for using the standard Russell-Taylor femoral nail.

Repeated observations with the image intensifier show if distraction is occurring and will allow preventive measures to be taken. The nail should be felt to drive

on with each blow. With the length of the nail calculated correctly, when hammered into its optimal position the head of the nail should have disappeared within the bone just at the point of entry.

Stable fractures of the isthmus may be treated by means of the conventional unlocked method. Fractures proximal to the isthmus necessitate a proximal locking screw, whereas more distal fractures should be locked with one or two distal screws. All unstable fractures should be locked distally and proximally, thereby maintaining length and preventing rotation.

Closure

Refer to the discussion of open reduction and internal fixation of the hip.

Postoperative Care

Vital signs every 4 hours
Neurovascular checks every 2 hours
Administration of analgesics as needed
Administration of antibiotic coverage
DVT prophylxis
X-ray film in the recovery room and in the morning after surgery
Diet as tolerated
Ambulation as soon as possible if the fracture site is stable
Panel 7 in the morning after surgery for 2 days
Incentive spirometry
Discharge in 7 to 10 days
Quadriceps setting and plantar flexion and dorsiflexion exercises immediately postoperatively

Potential Surgical Complications

Infection
Nonunion can be caused by a nail that is too small; a fracture too proximal or distal in the shaft; or a nail

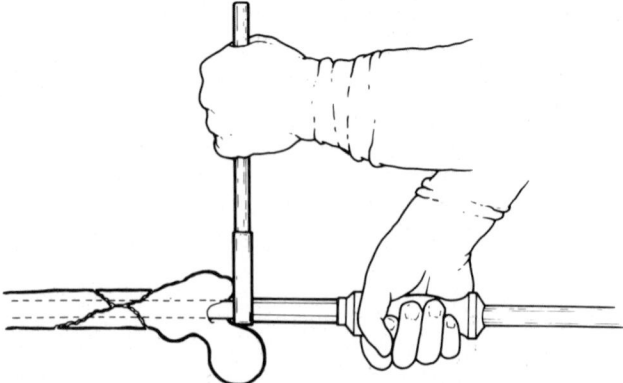

FIGURE 27–77. The nail is driven so that the proximal drill guide is flush with the tip of the greater trochanter. (From Russell, T. A., Taylor, J. C., LaVelle, D. G. [1991]. *Russell-Taylor femoral nail system: Surgical technique* [p. 22]. Memphis: Smith & Nephew Richards.)

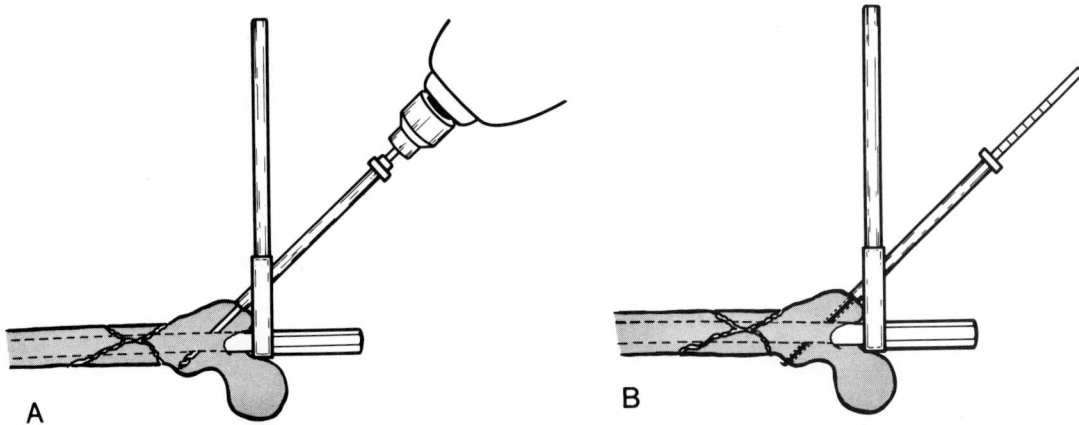

FIGURE 27–78. Technique for the standard Russell-Taylor femoral nail. *A*, Predrilling for the proximal screw. *B*, Determination of the length of the proximal screw. (From Browner, B., Levine, A., Jupiter, J., Trafton, P. [1990]. *Skeletal trauma* [p. 1509]. Philadelphia: W. B. Saunders.)

that cannot completely fill the canal and control rotation.

Fat embolism is always a potential complication when there is a fracture of a long bone, especially associated with intramedullary nail insertion.

Peroneal nerve injury may be due to externally applied pressure from splints or traction devices.

Loss of fixation and migration of the nail are due to failure to accomplish fixation.

TOTAL HIP ARTHROPLASTY

Definition

An *arthoplasty* is the surgical reformation of a joint. In a total arthroplasty, both the articulating surfaces of the hip joint are replaced. The hip replaced by an acetabular component made of high-density polyethylene and a femoral component made of metal. Implant placement may be with or without bone cement; however, the implant material must have a precise finish and placement.

Indications

The primary goals of a total hip arthroplasty are to relieve pain and to increase mobility and stability of the joint.

The indications for total hip arthroplasty are

severe primary rheumatoid arthritis
osteoarthritis
inactive inflammatory arthritis
ankylosing spondylitis
congenital dysplasia
traumatic arthritis
osteonecrosis
failed femoral osteotomy
bilateral oseoarthritis

Related Surgical Procedures

Three common types of hip arthroplasty are the cup or mold arthroplasty, the total hip arthroplasty, and the total hip surface replacement arthroplasty.

In a cup arthroplasty, the acetabulum and the head of the femur are reamed down to an untraumatized surface, and an appropriate-sized metal cup is fitted over the head of the femur. This procedure has been replaced by the other two. The total hip surface replacement arthroplasty consists of reaming out the acetabulum and implanting an acetabular cup while the femoral head is only reamed down to accept a metal femoral cup.

Perioperative Nursing Implications

Anesthesia

Surgery is performed under general or spinal anesthesia. Some orthopedic surgeons insist on transient hypotensive anesthesia during the cementing phase of the procedure. The anesthesiologist may be willing to do this by pharmacological means.

Blood loss during the entire procedure must be well controlled, and if possible, circulating blood volume should be maintained throughout the operation. The same anesthetic and nursing interventions apply as for the replacement of the proximal humerus during the cementing stage.

Position

The anesthetized patient is rolled onto his or her side with the operative hip up (Fig. 27–79A and B). The pelvic and lumbar area is firmly stabilized anteriorly and posteriorly with padded positioners attached to the OR bed (Fig. 27–79C). Care is taken not to restrict normal respiratory excursion. The anterior positioner should be tightened to allow the insertion of a hand between the positioner and the patient's abdomen.

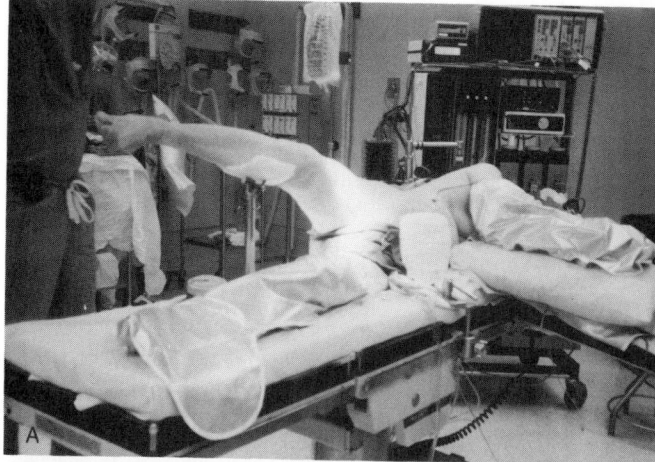
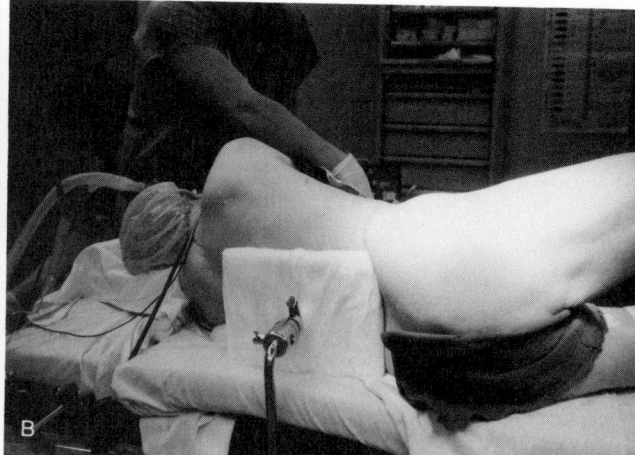
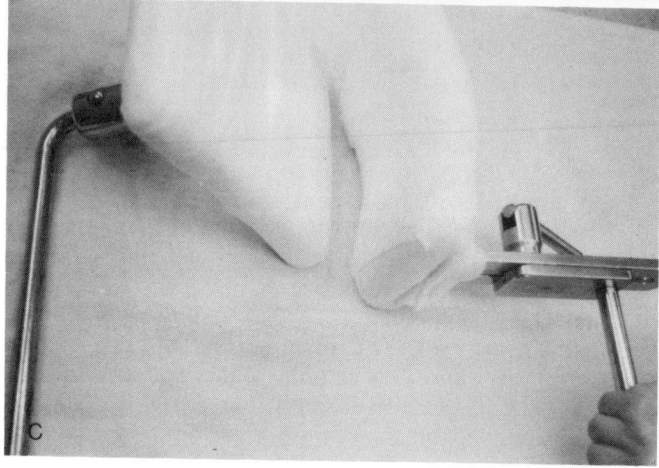

FIGURE 27–79. *A*, Anterior and *B*, Posterior views of patient positioned laterally for total hip arthroplasty. *C*, Lateral hip arthroplasty positioners.

The patient's arms are positioned on a well-padded double arm board and secured with straps or tape. A soft chest roll is position under the upper thorax.

Safety measures as discussed above are followed for all pressure point areas.

Creation and Maintenance of the Sterile Field

With the patient secured safely in the lateral position, the operative extremity is placed in a preparation holder and abducted. A unsterile hinged sheet is placed between the legs and covering the perineum. The hinges are taken over the gluteal fold posteriorly and to the groin anteriorly. The extremity is shaved and prepared from below the rib cage, including the buttocks posteriorly, to midcalf circumferentially. The gluteal fold and the groin are painted last to avoid contamination.

With the patient in the lateral position and the affected extremity abducted in the leg holder, the limb is held by an assistant with a sterile towel while the circulating nurse removes the holder from the ankle.

A sterile drape sheet is placed over the foot of the OR bed while an impervious stockinet is telescoped over the foot to above the knee. The towels holding the extremity are then discarded. A sterile drape sheet is placed over the down extremity to the groin. A sterile impervious hinged sheet is placed directly over the previously placed hinged sheet. Another drape is placed over the hinged sheet and fastened with towel clips. A sterile drape sheet is placed over the patient's upper torso to the level of the waist (prepared area). A second sheet follows in a similar fashion. Side sheets are placed and fastened beneath the affected extremity, in the groin area, and around the prepared area and clipped together at the top. Sterile adhesive drapes are taken around the thigh and knee circumferentially. A second adhesive drape is taken over the incision site and under the groin. Special attention is taken to seal the groin area carefully during the draping procedure. The stockinet may be fastened with a sterile Kling bandage.

Figure 27–80 shows the operating room set-up for a total hip arthroplasty.

Equipment and Supplies

2 suction tubings
15 large laparotomy sponges
15 small laparotomy sponges
Electrocautery
Bulb syringe
6 No. 10 blades

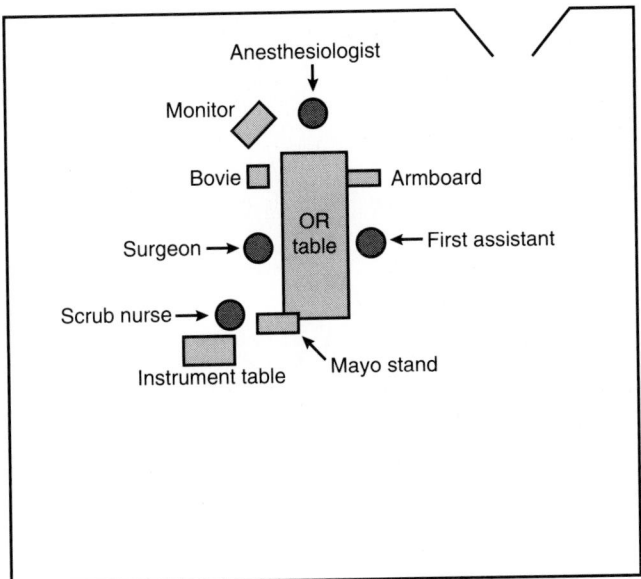

FIGURE 27–80. Operating room set-up for total hip arthroplasty of the right hip. The set-up would be reversed for the left hip.

60-ml syringe
Pulsatile lavage and tips
Suction drain
Skin marker
4 No. 1 Vicryl sutures (CP–1)
4 2–0 Vicryl sutures (CP–1)
Alcohol
Cement gun cartridges
Lavage irrigation tips
Long straight shower head
Impervious stockinet
2 adhesive drapes
Kling bandage
Impervious hinged sheet
3000 ml of normal saline
Bacitracin, 50,000 U
Polymyxin, 500,000 U
Methyl methacrylate
Cement mixing bowls
Skin staples
4 × 4 preparation or dressing sponges
Povidone-iodine scrub brushes
Mayo stand cover
Intramedullary brush
Disposable Yankauer suction tips

Instruments

Charnley hip retractor
2 Beckman retractors
2 Weitlaner retractors
2 Ferris Smith forceps
2 Adson forceps
2 No. 3 knife handles with teeth
2 No. 3 long knife handles

10 Kelly clamps
6 Kocher clamps
10 curved hemostats
8 towel clips
4 Allis clamps
4 Mayo-Hegar needle holders
Yankauer suction tip
9-inch long smooth forceps
Suture scissors
Mayo scissors
Canal finders
Mallet
Assorted curets
Assorted straight and curved osteotomes
Large double-action rongeur
Small double-action rongeur
Cobb elevator
Impervious hinged sheet
4 sponge sticks
Bone hook
Ligamentum teres knife
Power saw: reciprocating or oscillating
Saw blade
Long Frazier suction tip
Bandage scissors
Long Metzenbaum scissors
Assorted curved curets
Acetabular positioner
Femoral impactor
Acetabular trials
Femoral trials
Femoral broaches
Acetabular reamers
Appropriate screws and drill bits
Power reamer drills
Femoral neck elevator
6-mm drill bit
8-mm drill bit
Box osteotome

Drugs and Solutions

Refer to the discussion of prosthetic replacement of the proximal humerus.

Physiological Monitoring

See the discussion of anesthesia.

Specimen and Cultures

Routinely, a portion of the joint capsule and the femoral head are sent to the pathology department for definitive studies. Specimens might be sent to the rheumotology department for investigational purposes. Cultures are taken if indicated.

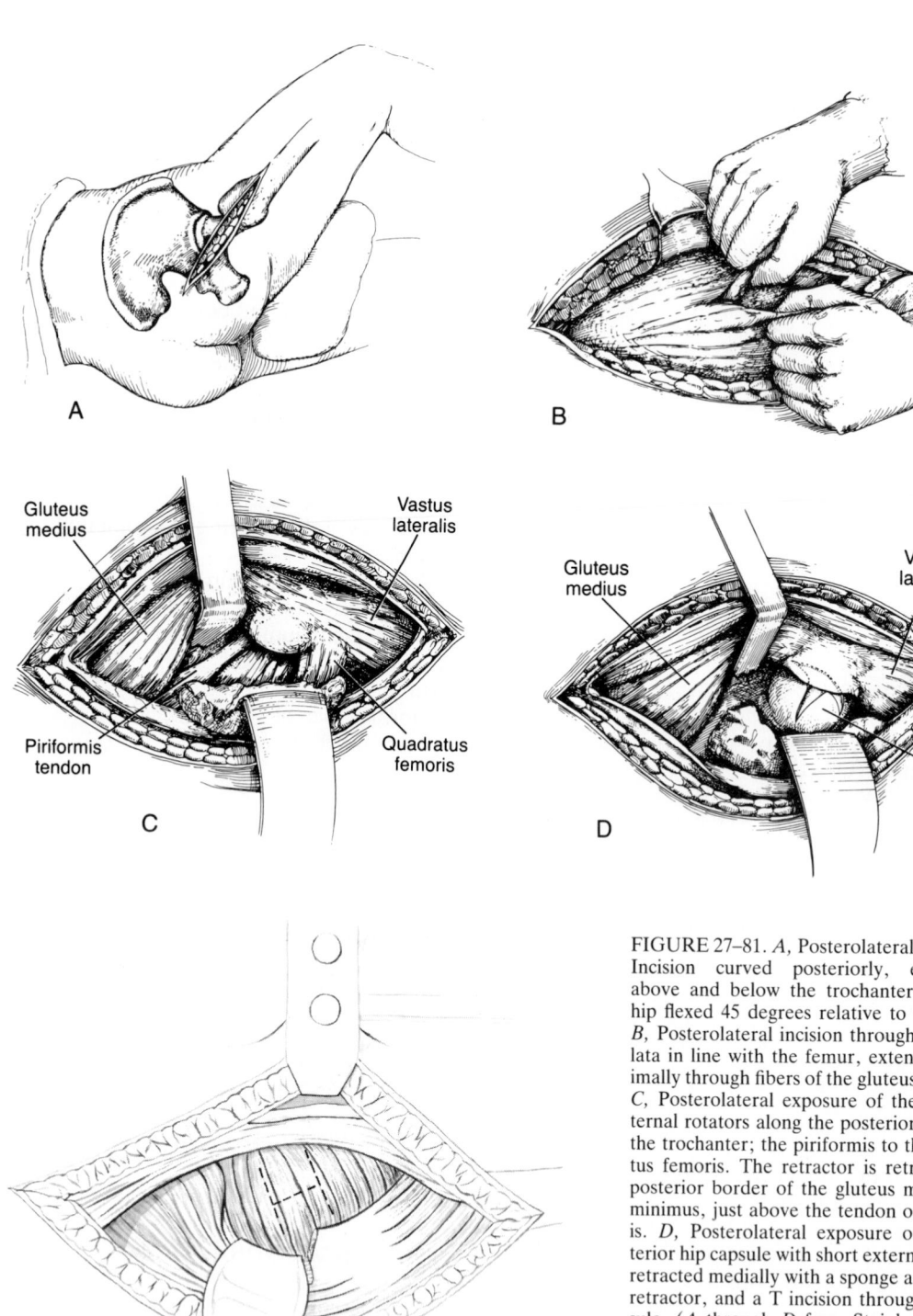

A

B

Gluteus
medius

Vastus
lateralis

Piriformis
tendon

Quadratus
femoris

C

Gluteus
medius

Vastus
lateralis

Posterior
hip
capsule

D

E

MORAN

FIGURE 27–81. *A*, Posterolateral approach. Incision curved posteriorly, equidistant above and below the trochanter, with the hip flexed 45 degrees relative to the pelvis. *B*, Posterolateral incision through the fascia lata in line with the femur, extending proximally through fibers of the gluteus maximus. *C*, Posterolateral exposure of the short external rotators along the posterior border of the trochanter; the piriformis to the quadratus femoris. The retractor is retracting the posterior border of the gluteus medius and minimus, just above the tendon of piriformis. *D*, Posterolateral exposure of the posterior hip capsule with short external rotators retracted medially with a sponge and Deaver retractor, and a T incision through the capsule. (*A* through *D* from Steinberg, M. E. [1991]. *The hip and its disorders* [p. 96]. Philadelphia, W. B. Saunders.) *E*, Exposure of the anterior hip joint capsule and capsulotomy. (From Petty, W. [1991]. *Total joint replacement* [p. 216]. Philadelphia: W. B. Saunders.)

Physician's Orders

NPO status after midnight
Activity as tolerated
Diet as tolerated
AP and lateral x-ray films (bilaterally)
Antibiotic prophylaxis
DVT prophylaxis
Typing and cross-matching 4 units of blood
Transport to the OR in a bed with an overhead frame and trapeze
ECG
Chest x-ray film
Urinalysis
Hematology profile
Physical therapy and occupational therapy consultation

Laboratory and Diagnostic Studies

X-ray films confirm the diagnosis and help in preoperative planning.

Procedure

Incision and Exposure

The proximal, anterior, and posterior margins of the greater trochanter are identified by palpation. The skin incision is made with a No. 10 blade just below the most prominent part of the greater trochanter, toward the greater sciatic notch (Fig. 27–81). Subcutaneous fat is incised with another No. 10 blade and retracted with Weitlaner retractors. The incision is extended posteriorly to expose the gluteus maximus fascia. The fascia lata, just below the most prominent portion, is incised with a No. 10 blade. Beckman retractors may now replace the Weitlaner retractors. Hemostasis is maintained with the electrocautery unit.

The gluteus maximus muscle is bluntly divided with Mayo scissors along the line of its fibers. The bursal tissue over the greater trochanter is excised with the Mayo scissors. The posterior aspect of the hip is exposed and the gluteus maximus tendon is released.

Details

The thigh is internally rotated and a Hohmann retractor is placed under the border of the gluteus medius and over the gluteus minimus. The Hohmann retractor is retracted anterosuperiorly, and the piriform and the insertions of the short external rotator muscles are identified. The external rotators are cut with the electrocautery unit. The Hohmann retractor is repositioned at the lesser trochanter and the inferior aspect of the hip capsule. Internal rotation of the hip followed by the

release of the piriform tendon at its femoral insertion improves exposure of the joint.

A No. 1 Vicryl suture is placed on the ends of the cut external rotators for later identification and reattachment. The detached rim of the external rotators is peeled off the hip capsule toward the posterior rim of the acetabulum.

A longitudinal incision is made in the superior hip capsule as far anteriorly as possible from the acetabular rim to the greater trochanter with a No. 10 blade on a long handle. The capsule along the rim of the acetabulum is further incised.

The hip is flexed and adducted with a bone hook placed around the femoral neck (Fig. 27–82). The femoral head is lifted out of the acetabulum during longitudinal traction and internal hip rotation. If intact, the ligamentum teres is cut with a teres knife or a No. 10 blade. After dislocation, the tibia is placed in a vertical position with the foot pointed upward and the hip in flexion, adduction, and internal rotation. The femur is pushed posteriorly and upward by the first assistant.

The femoral neck elevator is placed under the neck to expose the area completely. The neck is resected 1.5 to 2 cm above the beginning of the lesser trochanter with a reciprocating or oscillating saw (Fig. 27–83). The cut stops at the greater trochanter and then is resected vertically to meet the horizontal cut. The femur is internally rotated and the neck is elevated with a bone hook. The capsulectomy is completed all around with a No. 10 blade on a long handle to provide an excellent

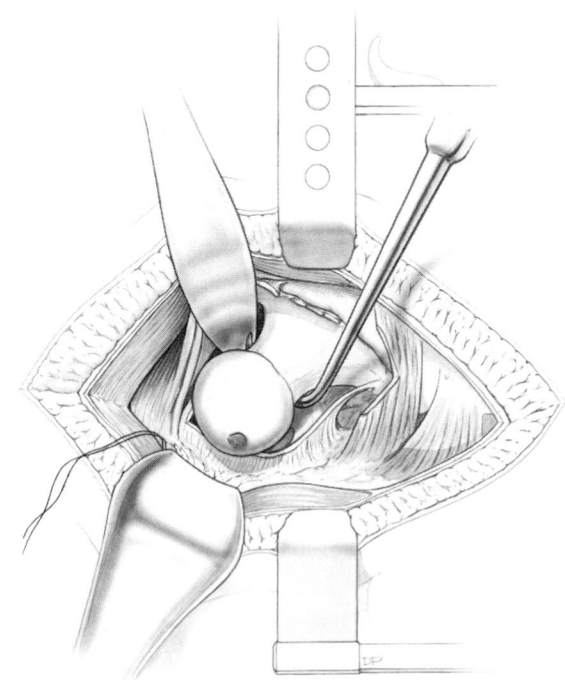

FIGURE 27–82. The hip joint is dislocated posteriorly by flexion, adduction, and internal rotation. A bone hook may be helpful in completing the dislocation. (From Petty, W. [1991]. *Total joint replacement* [p. 224]. Philadelphia: W. B. Saunders.)

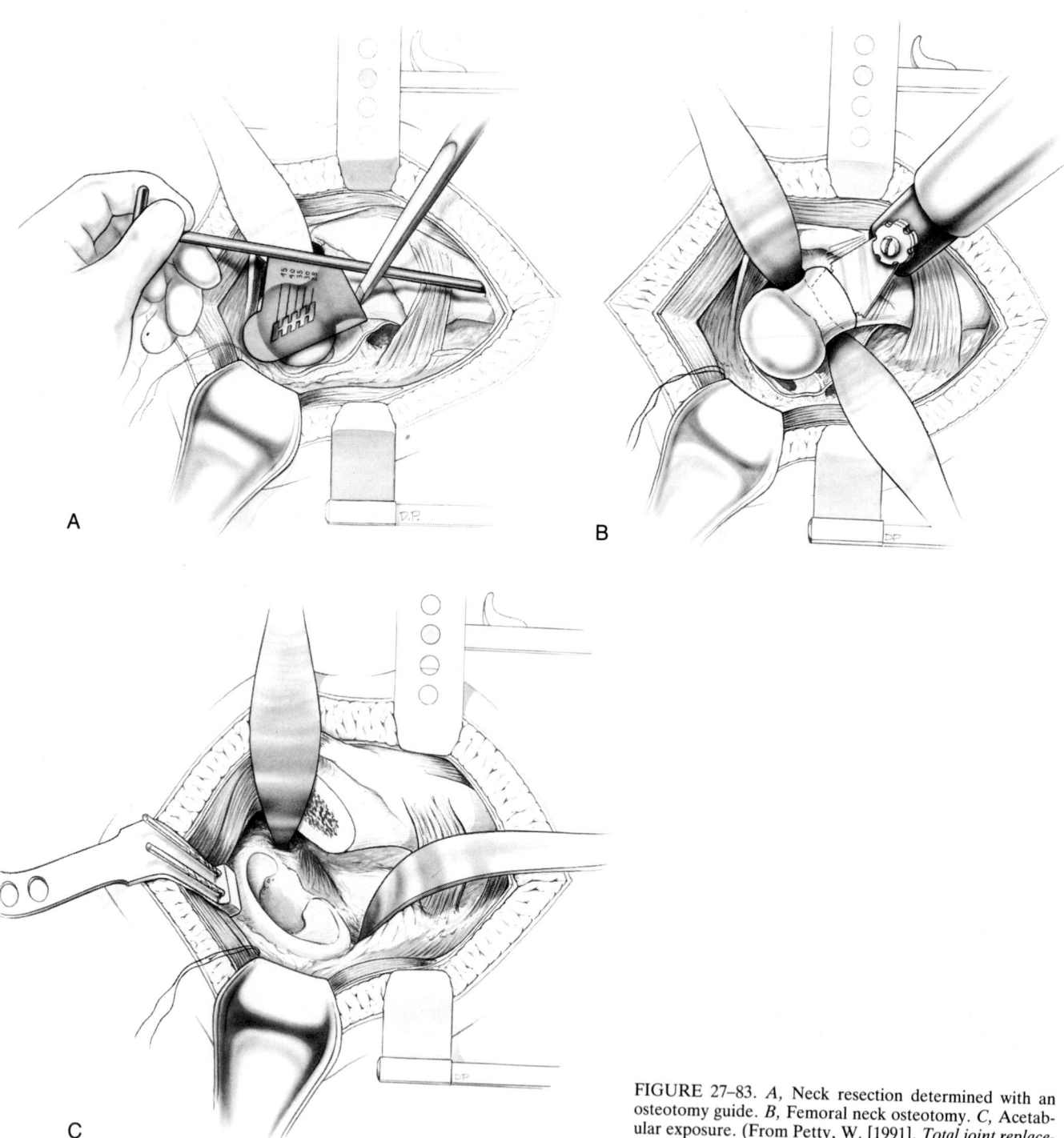

FIGURE 27–83. *A*, Neck resection determined with an osteotomy guide. *B*, Femoral neck osteotomy. *C*, Acetabular exposure. (From Petty, W. [1991]. *Total joint replacement* [pp. 246, 249]. Philadelphia: W. B. Saunders.)

A

B

C

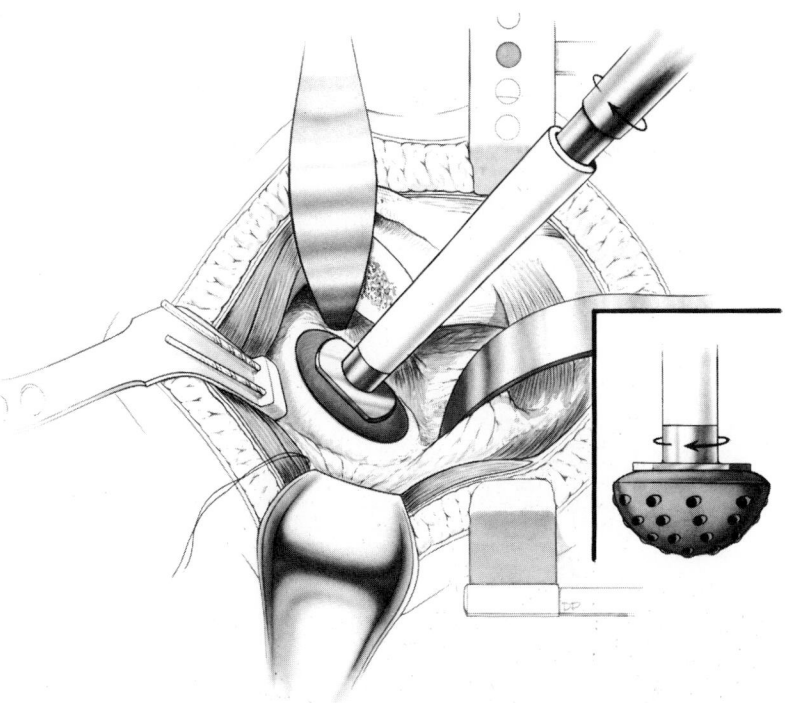

FIGURE 27–84. Acetabular reaming. (From Petty, W. [1991]. *Total joint replacement* [p. 250]. Philadelphia: W. B. Saunders.)

view of the acetabulum. Soft tissue or osteophytes should be cleaned from the acetabular fovea.

A Hohmann retractor is placed under the remaining neck with the tip up over the anterior margin of the acetabulum into the pelvis. The acetabulum is reamed in a concentric manner with a power reamer starting with the smallest size (Fig. 27–84). Manufacturer's rec-

ommendations vary with regards to final reamer size and specific components (cemented and noncemented).

The reamer should be directed medially, and over-reaming should be avoided. Anchor holes are created in the acetabulum to enhance cement fixation (Fig. 27–85). They are made with a long 6- or 8-mm drill bit and are undercut with a curved curet. When proper size and

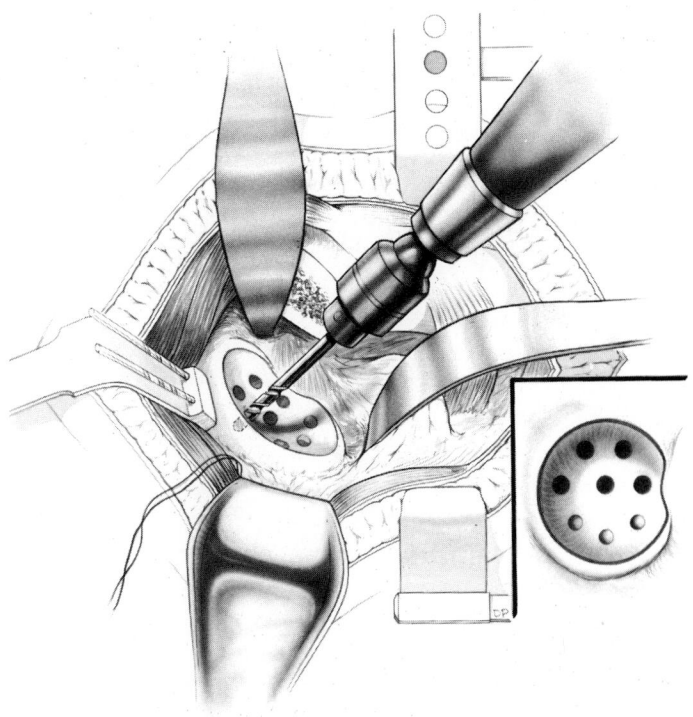

FIGURE 27–85. Cement fixation holes in the acetabulum. (From Petty, W. [1991]. *Total joint replacement* [p. 251]. Philadelphia: W. B. Saunders.)

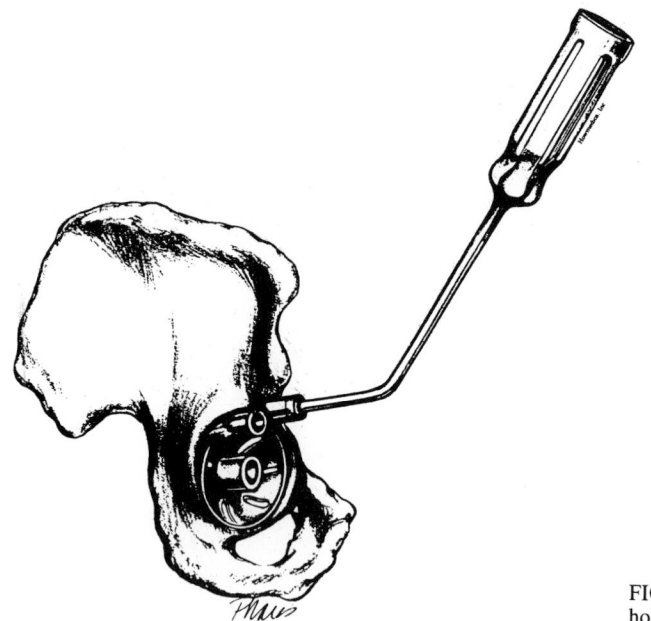

FIGURE 27–86. A drill guide designed for accurate placement of a hole for a socket peg. (Courtesy of Howmedica, Inc.)

position of the cup have been established, the acetabulum is irrigated with a pulsatile antibiotic lavage. Reamed bone debris and blood are removed to open the interstices of cancellous bone. Bleeding should be stopped with an electrocautery.

The proper acetabular component (cemented or porous) is presented to the table by the circulating nurse.

The appropriate postioner and impactor are readied, along with drill guides (Fig. 27–86) and drill bits for a noncemented component.

The methyl methacrylate is prepared as discussed above and injected into the acetabulum via a cement gun. The cement may be manually impacted, or an acetabular cement compressor may be used. When the

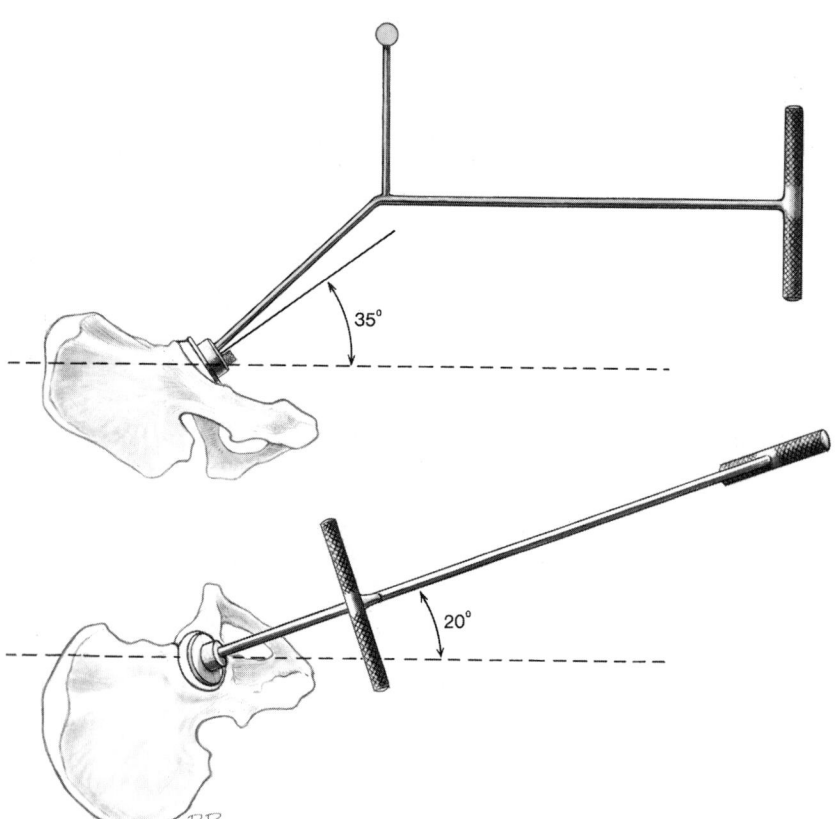

FIGURE 27–87. Acetabular component positioning. (From Petty, W. [1991]. *Total joint replacement* [p. 252]. Philadelphia: W. B. Saunders.)

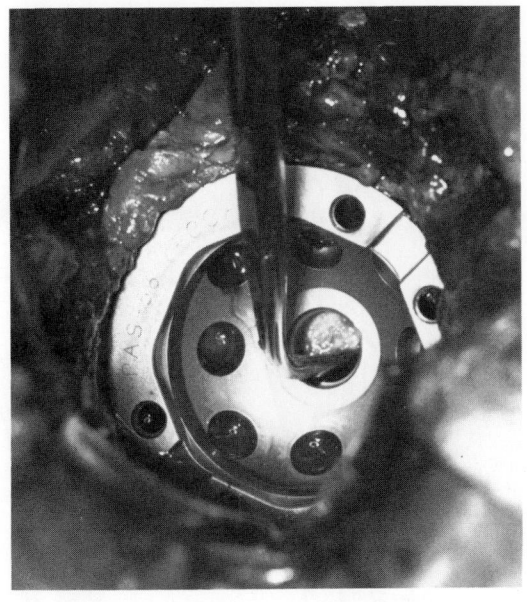

A

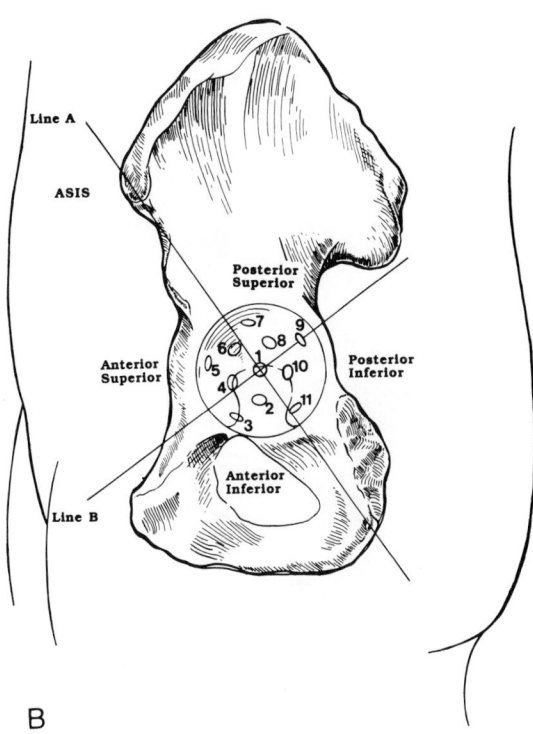

B

FIGURE 27–88. *A*, The screw holes and the central hole allow evaluation of prosthesis-bone apposition. (From Petty, W. [1991]. *Total joint replacement* [p. 262]. Philadelphia: W. B. Saunders.) *B*, Quadrant system for determination of safer screw placement in acetabular prostheses. (From Wasielewski, R. C., Cooperstein, L. A., Kruger, M. P., and Rubash, H. E. [1991]. Acetabular anatomy and the transacetabular fixation of screws in total hip arthroplasty. *Journal of Bone and Joint Surgery 72A,* 504.)

cement can be handled, the selected acetabular component is pushed into the cement of the acetabulum. The excessive cement is trimmed with a curet from the rim of the acetabulum. When the position is satisfactory (Fig. 27–87), the positioner is removed and replaced by an impactor until there is complete cure of the cement. The area is then again copiously irrigated to remove any loosened cement.

For a porous-coated acetabular component, the implant is inserted and impacted at the desired inclination. Screw holes are drilled through the holes in the component to avoid penetration of the inner cortex of the pelvis or the sciatic notch (Fig. 27–88). A drill guide is used when drilling, and the length is measured with the appropriate depth gauge. The selected screw is inserted and fully seated within the screw hole. The permanent polyethylene liner is then impacted into the acetabular shell.

The initial preparation of the femur is started with a hollow box chisel (Fig. 27–89), starting in the middle of the longitudinal axis of the femoral neck, and directed parallel with the femoral neck. The canal is entered with a tapered reamer (Fig. 27–90*A*) or a flexible reamer (Fig. 27–90*B*). The femoral canal is further prepared with a series of broaches (Fig. 27–91), which correspond to the size of the final implant. In general, start with the smallest broach and increase sizes until cortical bone is reached. If the prosthesis has a collar, an oscillating saw is used to adjust the collar against the medial aspect of the femoral neck cortex (Fig. 27–92). A trial femoral head and neck are then placed on the final broach and a trial reduction is performed (Fig. 27–93).

When the surgeon is satisfied with the preparation, the trials are removed and the canal prepared in the same manner as the acetabulum. A cement restrictor is inserted in the final component to be cemented. The

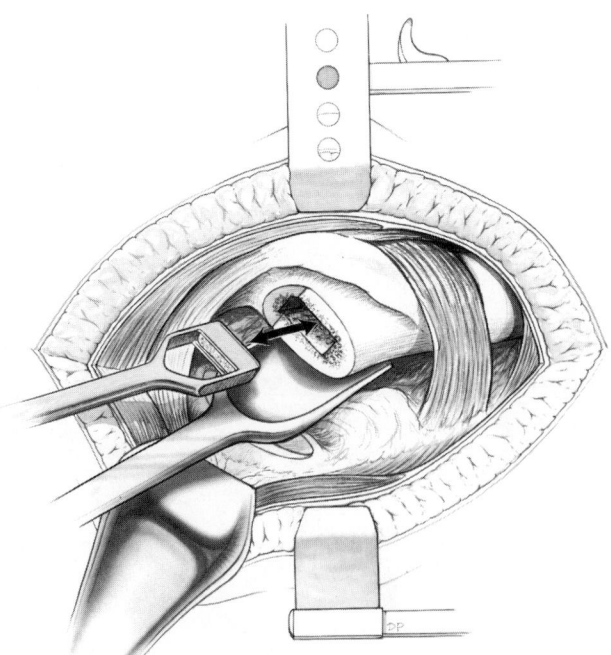

FIGURE 27–89. Lateralization of the entry point into the femoral canal with a box osteotome. (From Petty, W. [1991]. *Total joint replacement* [p. 253]. Philadelphia: W. B. Saunders.)

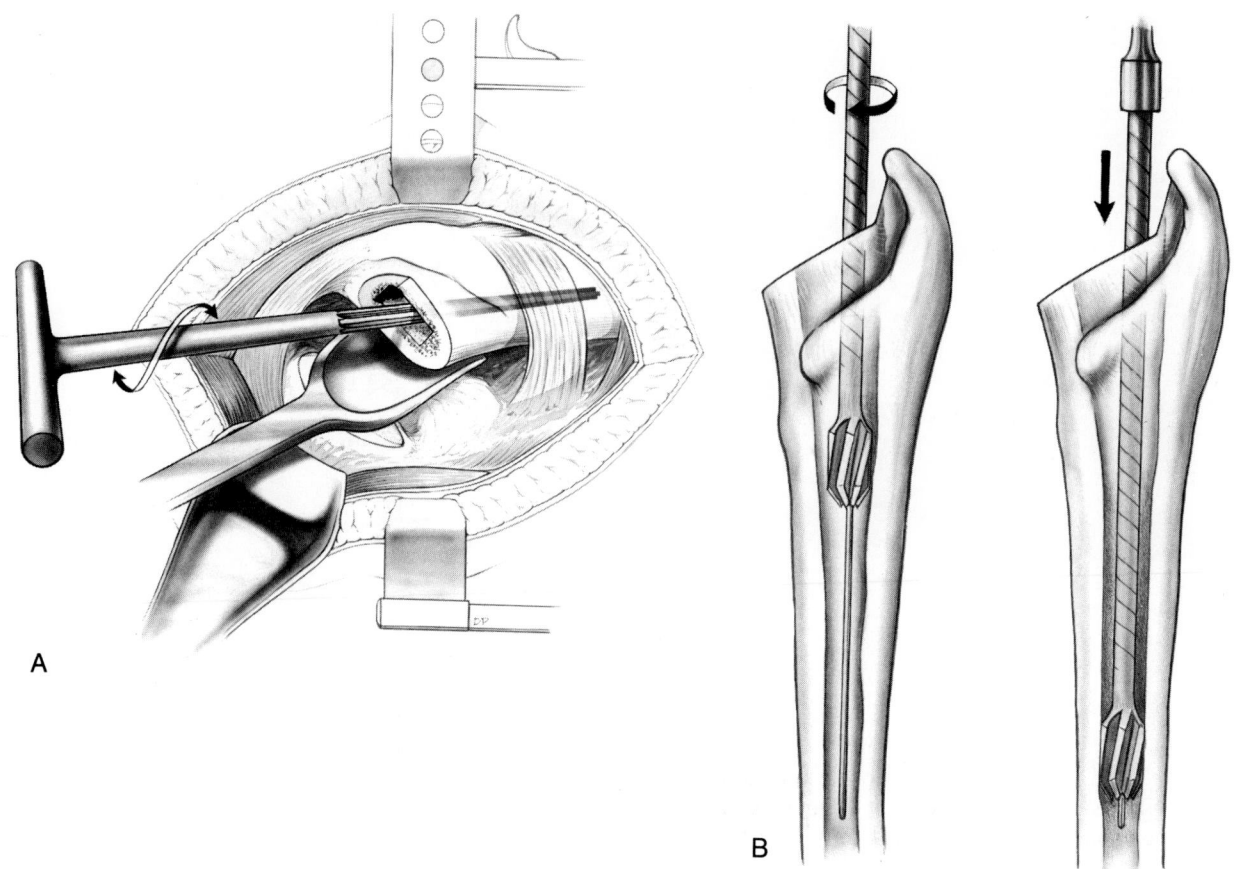

FIGURE 27–90. *A*, Entry into the femoral canal with a tapered reamer. *B*, Flexible reaming of the intramedullary canal. (From Petty, W. [1991]. *Total joint replacement* [pp. 253, 254]. Philadelphia: W. B. Saunders.)

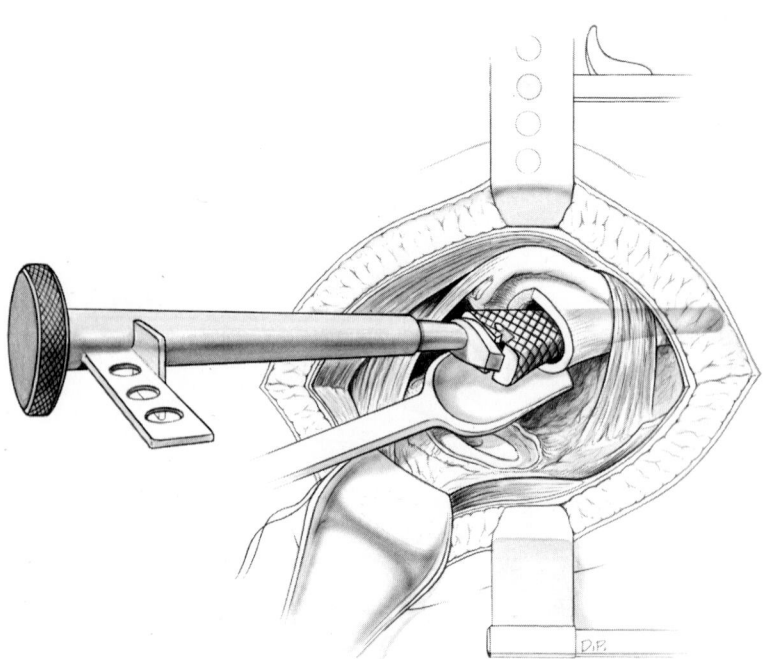

FIGURE 27–91. Broaching the proximal femur. (From Petty, W. [1991]. *Total joint replacement* [p. 254]. Philadelphia: W. B. Saunders.)

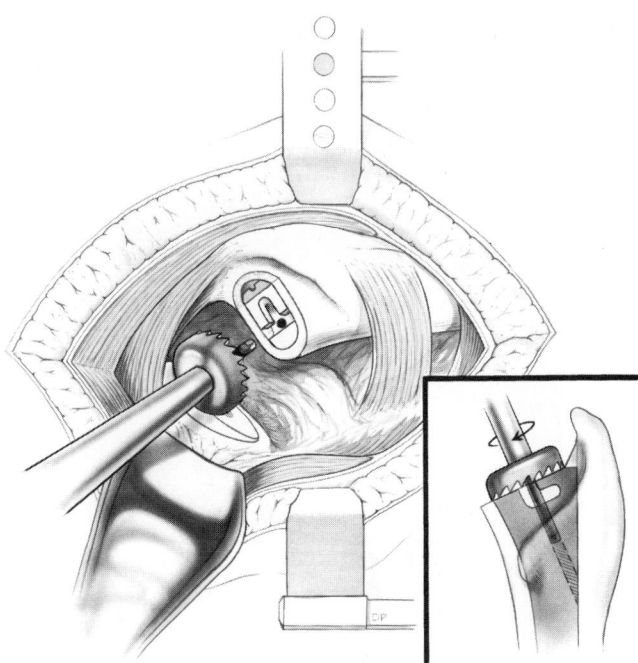

FIGURE 27–92. Preparation of the femoral neck for improved collar contact. (From Petty, W. [1991]. *Total joint replacement* [p. 255]. Philadelphia: W. B. Saunders.)

selected femoral prosthesis is delivered onto the field and cement preparation begins again. The cement is injected into the canal via a long nozzle on the cement gun, starting distally at the cement plug (Fig. 27–94). The prosthesis is then inserted and impacted (Fig. 27–95). Cement is trimmed from around the stem collar, and gentle pressure is maintained until the cement is completely hardened.

The selected femoral head implant is placed onto the femoral component and impacted. The hip is reduced (Fig. 27–96) and placed through a range-of-motion test.

The wound is copiously irrigated with the pulsatile lavage. Any loose pieces of cement or potentially loose pieces are removed.

Closure

The previously placed sutures are identified and reattached to the greater trochanter. A suction drain is placed in the hip joint. The fascia lata is closed with interrupted No. 1 Vicryl suture, and a second suction

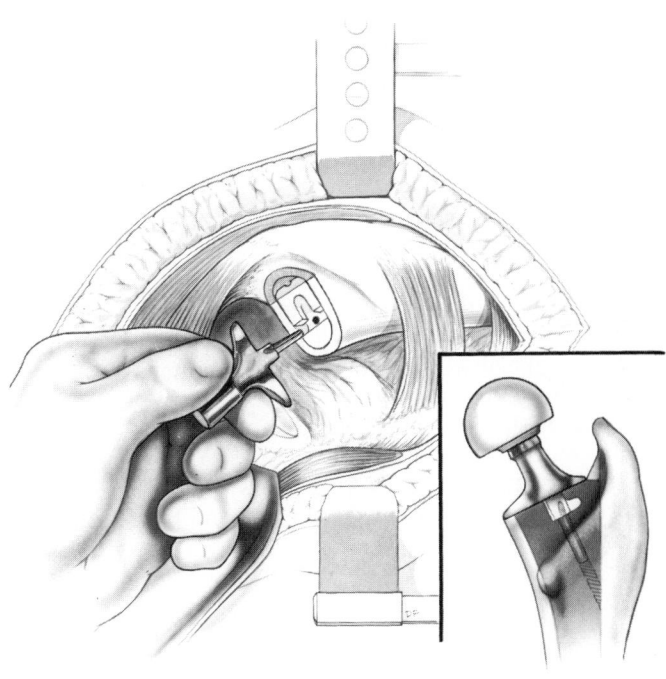

FIGURE 27–93. Placement of the trial neck and head. (From Petty, W. [1991]. *Total joint replacement* [p. 255]. Philadelphia: W. B. Saunders.)

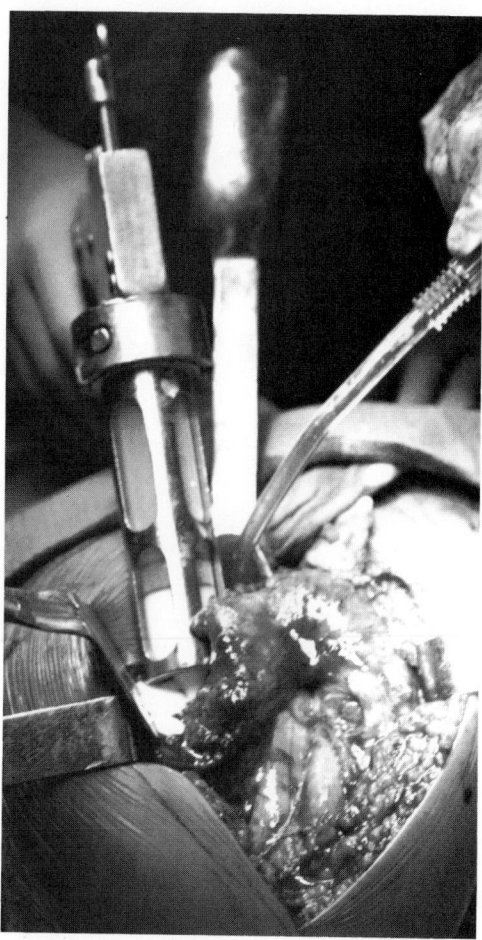

FIGURE 27–94. Cement placed in the femoral canal with a syringe. (From Petty, W. [1991]. *Total joint replacement* [p. 258]. Philadelphia: W. B. Saunders.)

drain is placed. The gluteus maximus is also closed with an interrupted No. 1 Vicryl suture.

The subcutaneous fat is closed with interrupted 2–0 Vicryl sutures. Skin is approximated with skin staples. Sterile, dry gauze dressings are applied. A hip abduction brace is applied immediately postoperatively.

Postoperative Care

Bed rest overnight with an abduction brace
Out of bed with physical therapy the morning after surgery
50% weight bearing for 6 weeks with crutches
X-ray film in 6 weeks
Abductor strengthening exercises
Vital signs every 4 hours
Neurovascular checks every 2 hours
Portable x-ray in the recovery room and the morning after surgery
Elevated toilet seat
Hip chair

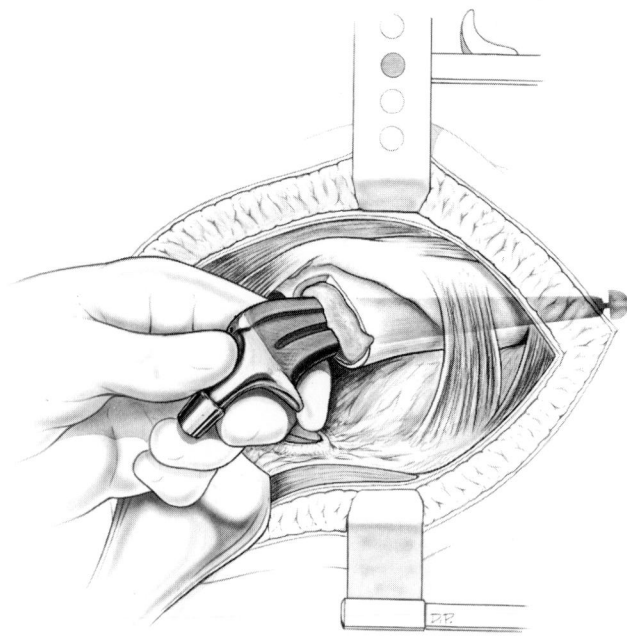

FIGURE 27–95. Femoral stem insertion. (From Petty, W. [1991]. *Total joint replacement* [p. 259]. Philadelphia: W. B. Saunders.)

CBC, prothrombin time, and partial thromboplastin time the morning after surgery and in 5 days
DVT prophylaxis
Administration of analgesics as needed
Antibiotic coverage
Urinalysis and culture and sensitivity in 5 days
Discharge in 10 days

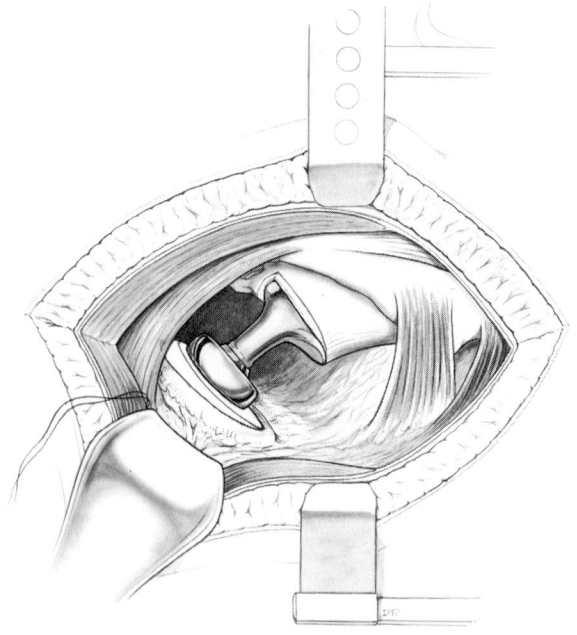

FIGURE 27–96. Final reduction. (From Petty, W. [1991]. *Total joint replacement* [p. 261]. Philadelphia: W. B. Saunders.)

Potential Surgical Complications

Infection

Hip dislocation is due to excessive flexion and internal rotation.

Prosthesis loosening is due to infection, fracture, dislocation, and migration of implants.

Thrombophlebitis is possibly due to preoperative screening radionuclide scans.

Bibliography

Allison, J., & Reeverts, R. (1985). Ceramic hip arthroplasty: Procedures and nursing care. *AORN Journal, 42,* 862–871.

Atkinson, L., & Kohn, M. (1986). *Introduction of Operative Room Technique.* New York: McGraw-Hill.

Bartell, L. (1985). Bunionectomies. *Orthopaedic Nursing, 4*(1), 21–28.

Berger, M. (1984). Bunions: An overview. *Orthopaedic Nursing, 3*(5), 17–22.

Crawford Adams, J. (1985). *Standard Orthopaedic Operations* (3rd ed.). New York: Churchill Livingston.

Cusack, M., & Forlic, D. (1986). Shoulder orthroplasty. Implications for nursing care. *AORN Journal, 44,* 198–211.

Foelman, V. (1988). Nursing care concerns in total shoulder replacement. *Orthopaedic Nursing, 7*(3), 29–31.

Groah, L. (1990). *Operating room nursing* (2nd ed.). Norwalk, CT: Appleton-Century-Crofts.

Gruebee Lee, D. (1983). *Disorders of the hip.* Philadelphia: J. B. Lippincott.

Gruendeman, J. (1987). *Alexander's Care of the Patient in Surgery* (8th ed.). St. Louis: C. V. Mosby.

Hoppenfeld, S. (1984). *Surgical approaches in orthopaedics.* Philadelphia: J. B. Lippincott.

Lubin, M., & Walker, H. K. (Eds.). *Medical management of the surgical patient* (2nd ed.). Stoneham, MA: Butterworths.

Martin, J. (1987). *Positioning in anesthesia and surgery* (2nd ed.). Philadelphia: J. B. Lippincott.

McConnell, E. (1987). *Clinical considerations in perioperative nursing.* Philadelphia: J. B. Lippincott.

Mulvey, T. (1988). Anatomy and pathology of the shoulder complex. *Orthopaedic Nursing, 7*(3), 23–28.

O'Bryan Doheny, M., (1985). Porous coated femoral prosthesis. Concepts and care considerations. *Orthopaedic Nursing, 4*(1), 43–45.

Rodringo, J. (1986). *Orthopaedic surgery: Basic science and clinical science.* Boston: Little, Brown.

Rothrock, J. (1987). *The RN first assistant: An expanded perioperative nursing role.* Philadelphia: J. B. Lippincott.

Schoen, D. (1986). *The nursing process in orthopaedics.* Norwalk, CT: Appleton-Century-Crofts.

Sennwald, G. (1987). *The wrist.* New York: Springer-Verlag.

Urbanski, P. (1984). The orthopaedic patient. *AORN Journal, 40,* 707–711

CHAPTER 28

Gynecological Surgery

Dietra A. Evans

DEFINITION

Gynecological surgery refers to all surgical procedures that involve the female reproductive organs, particularly those situated in the pelvis and perineum. From a surgical perspective, the structures include the uterus, the cervix, the ovaries, the fallopian tubes, the vagina, and the vulva.

ANATOMY

External Genitalia

The *external genitalia* consist of the mons pubis (veneris), the clitoris, the labia majora and minora, the hymen, Bartholin glands, and the orifice of the vagina (Fig. 28–1). Collectively, the external genitalia are referred to as the *vulva*.

The *mons pubis* is an area of fatty tissue and coarse skin that lies over the symphysis pubis. After puberty, this area is covered with hair.

The *clitoris* is an erectile structure; it is located beneath the anterior commissure and is partially hidden by the anterior ends of the labia minora. It is analogous to the corpora cavernosa in the male.

The *labia majora* are long folds of skin filled with subcutaneous fat that run downward and backward from the mons pubis. The labia majora are homologous to the scrotum of the male embryologically. The *labia minora* are two delicate folds of fat-free, hairless skin. They lie between the labia majora, and their lateral surfaces are in contact with the smooth surfaces of the labia majora. They enclose the vestibule of the vagina and lie on each side of the vaginal orifice.

The *hymen* is a thin mucous membrane that usually covers the entrance of the vagina in young females. The membrane remains intact until coitus but its presence is not reliable as a test of virginity.

Analogous to Cowper glands in the male, *Bartholin glands* lie on either side of the vagina and behind the hymen. They secrete mucus or lubricant at the time of coitus.

Internal Genitalia

The internal genitalia include the vagina, the uterus and its ligaments, the ovaries, and the fallopian tubes (Figs. 28–2 and 28–3).

Vagina

The *vagina* is a muscular membranous tube that forms the passageway between the uterus and the vulva. It lies posterior to the urinary bladder and anterior to the rectum. The vagina has four walls: two lateral and one each anterior and posterior. Its anterior wall is in contact with the cervix, the base of the bladder, the terminal parts of the ureters, and the urethra. Its posterior wall is connected to the rectum. The vagina consists of three layers: an internal mucous lining, a muscular coat, and between the two, an erectile layer of tissue. During pregnancy, the muscular coat increases, and the mucous coat allows for dilation of the birth canal during labor and birth. The vagina functions in the introduction of the penis during intercourse, the reception of the semen, the discharge of menstrual flow, and the delivery of a fetus during birth.

Uterus

The *uterus* is a hollow, thick-walled, pear-shaped muscular organ, which is approximately 2 inches deep and 3 inches long. It is composed of three layers: (1) the perimetrium, or outer layer; (2) the myometrium, or middle layer, which consists of smooth muscle; and (3) the endometrium, or inner layer, which outlines the hollow shell. During pregnancy, the uterus becomes extremely large. It returns to almost its original size approximately 3 months after delivery; this can be hastened by suckling. After menopause, the uterus always becomes smaller. The uterus consist of three areas: (1) the body, or upper portion; (2) the isthmus, or fundus; and (3) the cervix, which is the lower portion that is at the upper end of the vagina. Under normal conditions, the uterus is anteflexed, or bent forward, between the cervix and the body, but many women have retroflexed, or backward leanings, uteri (Fig. 28–4). The major function of the uterus is to contain and nourish the embryo and fetus from the time of fertilization to birth.

Uterine Ligaments

The uterus is suspended by eight ligaments: two broad, two round, two uterosacral, and two cardinal ligaments (Fig. 28–5).

The broad ligaments help to form a barrier extending across the pelvic cavity. These double folds of peritoneum hold the uterus in a normal position. Enclosed in the free edge of each broad ligament is a fallopian tube.

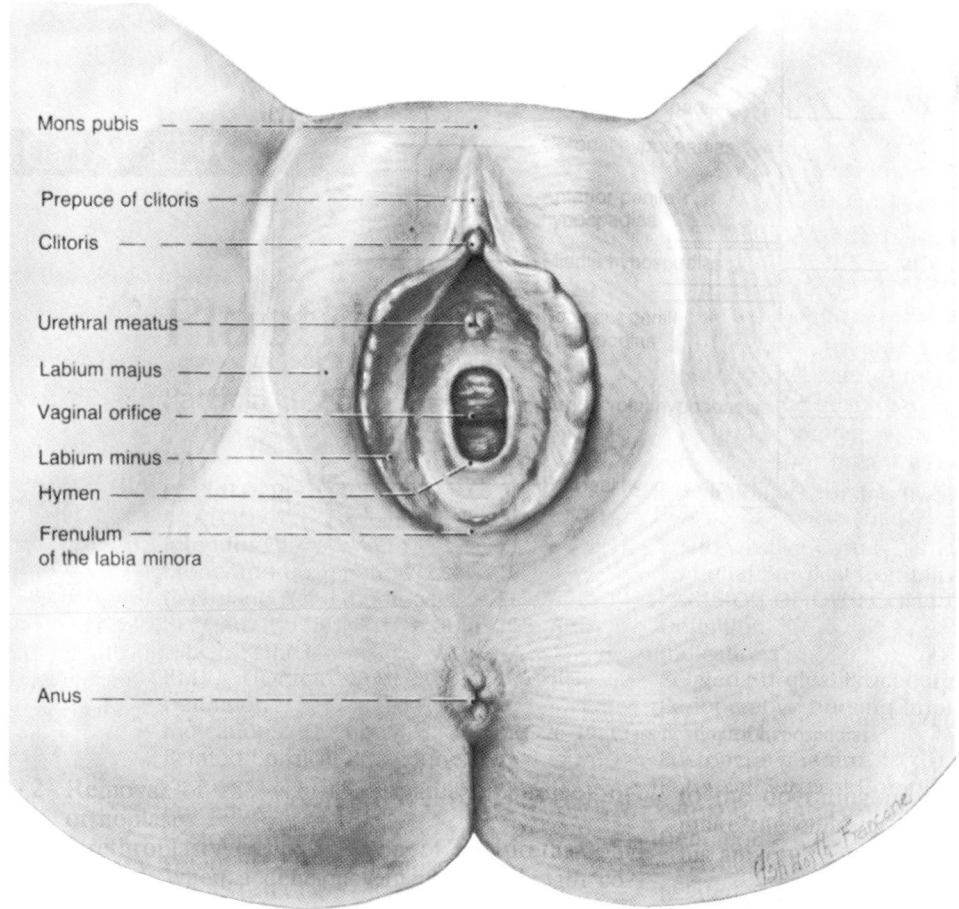

Mons pubis

Prepuce of clitoris

Clitoris

Urethral meatus

Labium majus

Vaginal orifice

Labium minus

Hymen

Frenulum
of the labia minora

Anus

FIGURE 28–1. Female external genitalia. (From Jacob, S., Francone, C., Lossow, W. J. [1982]. *Structure and function in man* [5th ed.] [p. 603]. Philadelphia: W. B. Saunders.

The round ligaments are two rounded bands continuous within the wall of the uterus. Each ligament runs between the layers of the broad ligament and across the pelvic wall. These ligaments help suspend the uterus anteriorly.

The uterosacral ligaments pass from the sides of the cervix toward the sacrum and deep in the pelvis to the peritoneum and superior to the levator ani muscle. The uterosacral ligaments are responsible for holding the uterus in its normal position in the pelvis.

The cardinal (MacKenrodt) ligaments help prevent prolapse of the uterus and consist of fibrous sheets that extend from the level of the isthmus to the lateral pelvic fascia (Fig. 28–6).

In addition to the eight ligaments, the uterus has peritoneal folds. They are posterior (rectouterine) and anterior (vesicouterine), with the posterior ligament behind the uterus forming a deep fold in the peritoneum and the anterior ligament forming a fold between the bladder and the uterus.

Ovaries

The *ovaries* are analogous to the testes in the male. Normally, two in number, the almond-shaped glands lie on either side of the uterus. Each ovary has an outer portion, called the *cortex*, consisting of connective tissue

and some smooth muscle. The cortex has many follicles. The inner portion of the ovary is called the *medulla* and is responsible for the vascularity of the gland. It consists of connective tissue containing nerves, blood, and lymphatic vessels. The ovary is responsible for the production of eggs (ova), and the two female hormones: estrogen and progesterone. These hormones are responsible for the maintenance and development of secondary sexual characteristics, the preparation of the uterus for pregnancy, and the development of the mammary glands.

The ovary has one ligament, the infundibulopelvic ligament, which contains the vessels and nerves of the ovary.

The blood supply of the ovary comes from the ovarian and uterine arteries.

Fallopian Tubes

The *fallopian tubes* are a pair of ducts about 4½ inches in length and ¼ inch in diameter. They connect the uterus to the ovary. They provide a means to transport the eggs from the ovary to the uterus. Each fallopian tube consists of an inner, a middle, and an outer layer. The inner mucosa consists of ciliated and nonciliated cells. The ciliated cells aid in the movement

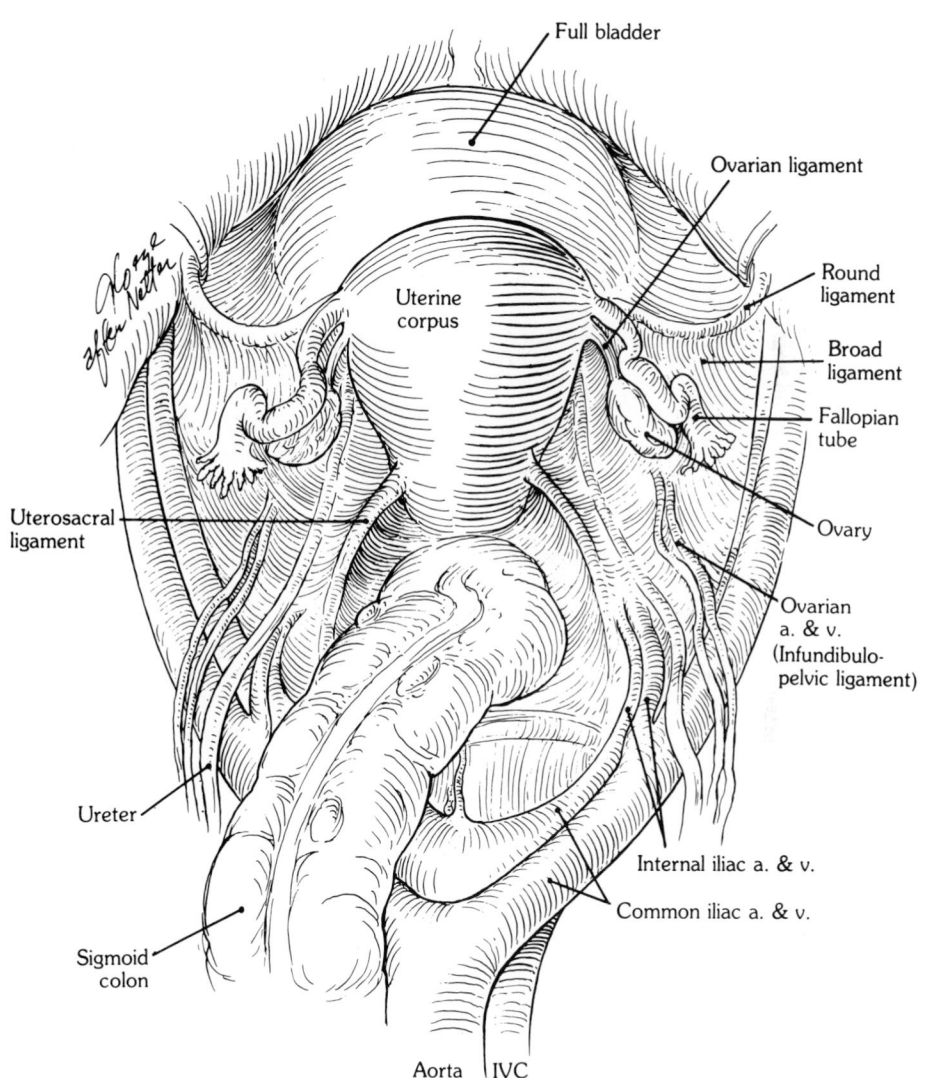

FIGURE 28–2. View of the organs in the female pelvis. (From Hacker, N. F., Moore, J. G. [1992]. *Essentials of obstetrics and gynecology* [2nd ed.]. Philadelphia: W. B. Saunders.)

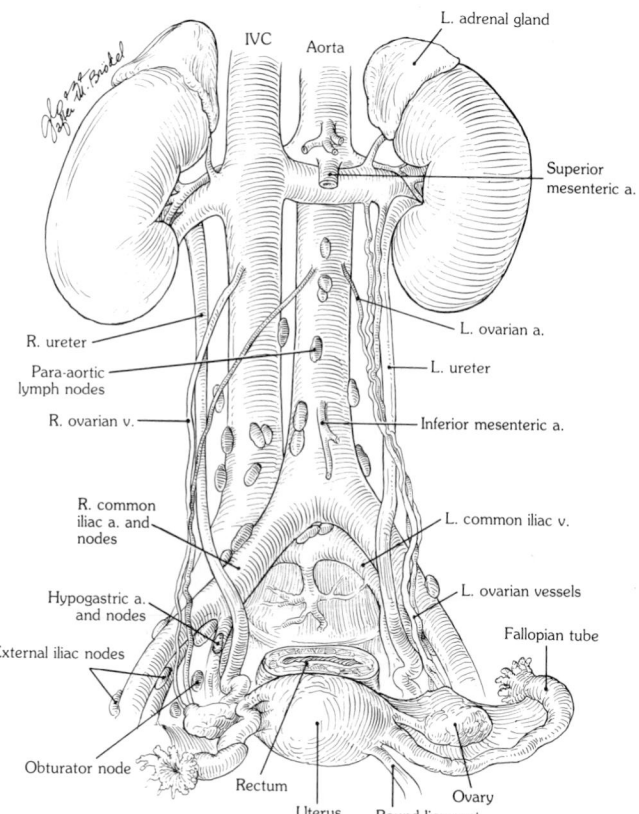

FIGURE 28–3. Lymphatic drainage of the female internal genital organs. (From Hacker, N. F., Moore, J. G. [1992]. *Essentials of obstetrics and gynecology* [2nd ed.]. Philadelphia: W. B. Saunders.)

of the ovum toward the uterus. The middle layer is muscular and consists of an inner circular and outer layer of smooth muscle. The serosa, or outer layer, is made up of connective tissue.

The fallopian tube itself is divided into four parts: (1) the infundibulum has a funnel-shaped distal end that opens into the abdomen; (2) the ampulla is the longest part of the fallopian tube, receives the oocyte from the infundibulum, and is the site where fertilization usually takes place; (3) the isthmus joins the horn of the uterus; and (4) the uterine part is the short segment that pierces the wall of the uterus.

The fallopian tubes lie in the free edges of the broad ligament of the uterus called the *mesosalpinx*.

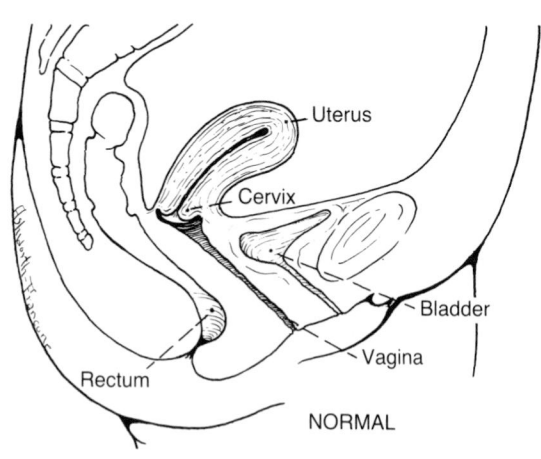

FIGURE 28–4. Normal and abnormal uterine positions. (From Jacob, S., Francone, C., Lossow, W. J. [1982]. *Structure and function in man* [5th ed.] [p. 606]. Philadelphia: W. B. Saunders.)

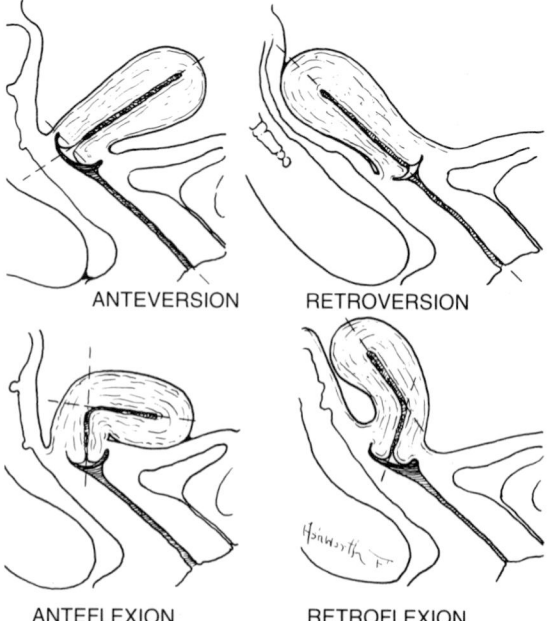

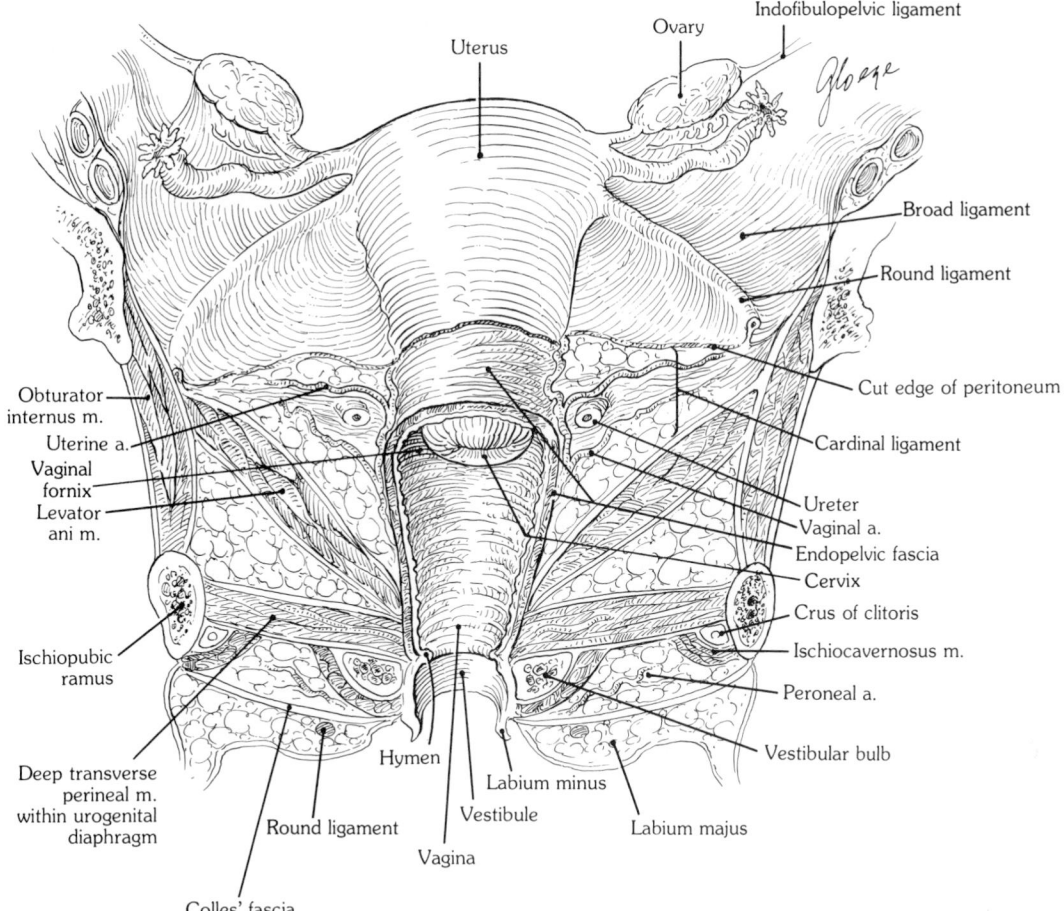

FIGURE 28–5. Coronal section of the pelvis at the level of the uterine isthmus and ischial spines, showing the ligaments supporting the uterus. (From Hacker, N. F., Moore, J. G. [1992]. *Essentials of obstetrics and gynecology* [2nd ed.]. Philadelphia: W. B. Saunders.)

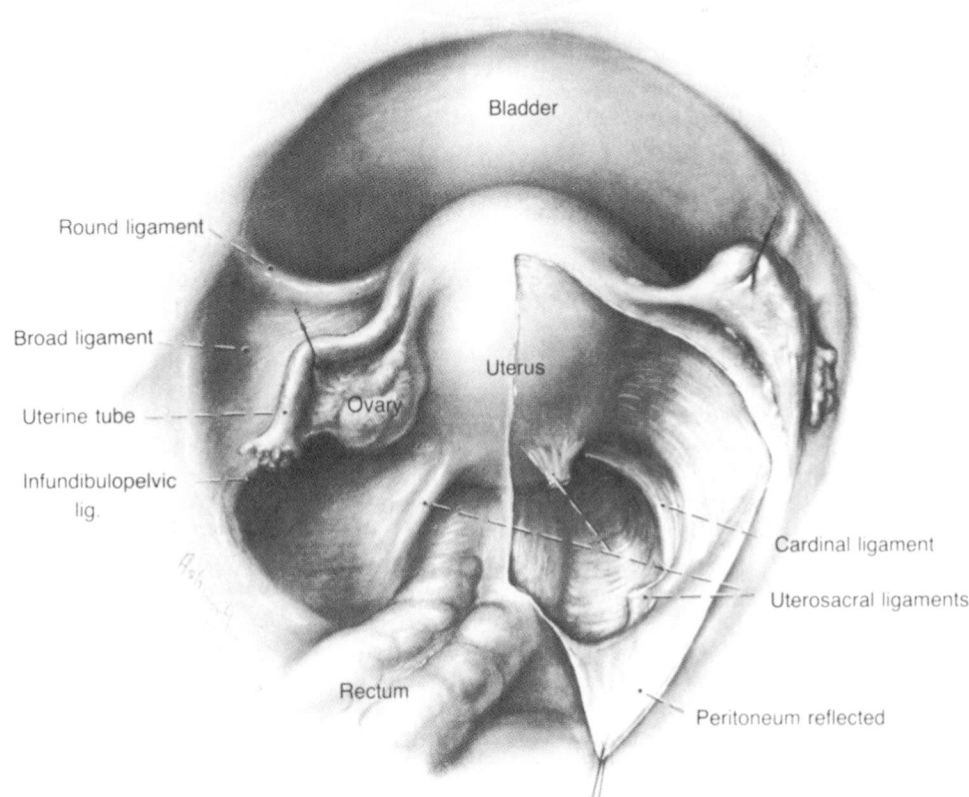

FIGURE 28–6. The uterus and ligaments as viewed from above. The peritoneum has been reflected back to show the cardinal ligament. (From Jacob, S., Francone, C., Lossow, W. J. [1982]. *Structure and function in man* [5th ed.] [p. 607]. Philadelphia: W. B. Saunders.)

723

SPECIAL INSTRUMENTS, SUPPLIES, AND EQUIPMENT

Electrosurgical Unit

All procedures to correct infertility use an electrocautery unit that has monopolar as well as bipolar capabilities (see Fig. 28–29). The current is usually set at 5.

Laser

Depending on the procedure, the use of the carbon dioxide, neodymium: yttrium-aluminum-garnet, and krypton lasers can be important. They can be used for treating vulvar and cervical lesions, as well as endometriosis and leiomyomas, and for accomplishing tubal reconstruction.

Shaw Scalpel

The Shaw scalpel is a precision instrument that can be used to open the abdomen. It achieves virtually a bloodless incision. Blades for the scalpel are of two sizes, Nos. 10 and 15. Usually, a No. 10 is used.

TUBOPLASTY

Definition

Tuboplasty is reconstructive surgery performed on the fallopian tubes to remove any obstruction, as a means to promote fertility and ultimately pregnancy.

Indications

Tuboplasty is indicated to correct any abnormality in the fallopian tubes.

Related Surgical Procedures

Tuboplasty is used to broadly describe a number of tubal procedures, such as

fimbrioplasty
salpingostomy
salpingolysis
tubal reanastomosis

Perioperative Nursing Implications

Anesthesia

Usually, these patients are not premedicated before arriving in the operating room (OR). Surgery is performed with general endotracheal anesthesia. Anesthesia is induced using a combination of drugs. Fentanyl is one of the narcotics commonly used. Inhalation agents include nitrous oxide, halothane, and enflurane.

Blood products are not needed during this surgery.

Position

The patient is placed in the dorsal recumbent (supine) position. The nurse extends both arms on arm boards, making sure that they are not abducted more than 90 degrees (Fig. 28–7). Safety straps are be applied to prevent the arms from dangling. The legs are not crossed, and the feet do not extend over the edge of the OR bed. The safety strap is placed above the knees. After the abdomen is opened, the patient is placed in the Trendelenburg position.

Creation and Maintenance of the Sterile Field

The shave for tuboplasty must start 3 inches above the nipple line and extend to the upper thighs. The skin is then prepared with a povidone-iodine (Betadine) solution. The grounding pad is placed on either thigh.

The patient is draped using basic laparotomy technique. The circulating nurse should be available to dispose of the paper backing from the impervious split sheet that is used in draping and assist the scrub nurse with the instrument tables. The Mayo stand is placed over the patient's feet, with the large instrument table to the scrub nurse's right. The square tables are placed behind the scrub nurse. The electrosurgical unit is placed at the right of the patient's head.

If the microscope is used during the procedure, it

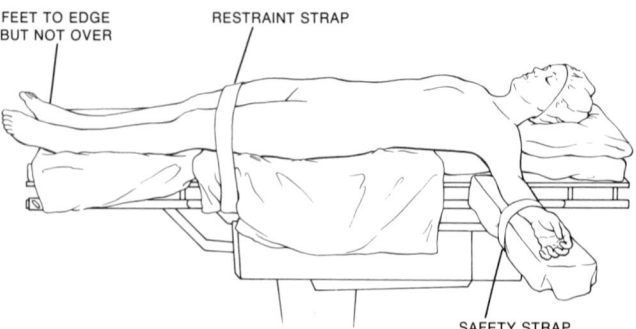

FIGURE 28–7. Supine position. (From Fuller, J. R. [1986]. *Surgical technology: Principles and practice* [2nd ed.]. Philadelphia: W. B. Saunders.)

must be draped by the scrub nurse. However, most surgeons prefer to use their own optical loupes.

The scrub nurse must wipe the microsurgical instruments after each use and keep irrigation fluid and dye available in 60-ml syringes.

Equipment and Supplies

Basic infertility set (Fig. 28–8)
  Strully and straight Lincoln scissors
  Skin hooks
  Vein, malleable, and shoehorn retractors
  7- and 10-inch diamond jaw forceps
  Curved and straight mosquito hemostats
  Short and long Williams clamps
  Buxton and Ziegler-Helman clamps
  Vascular and coronary needle holders
  Webster cannulas
  Lacrimal probes (various small sizes)
Microsurgical instruments (Fig. 28–9)
  Needle holders with and without ratchets
  Long, medium, and serrated scissors
  Toothed and smooth forceps
Impervious split sheet
2 sterile intravenous (IV) tubings
2 sterile stopcocks
2 microbipolar forceps
2 macrobipolar forceps
Electrosurgical unit with both monopolar and bipolar capabilities
Bipolar cord
Electrosurgical grounding pad
Electrosurgical pencil with fingertip control
3 60-ml syringes
19-gauge needle
Other basic laparotomy instruments
Suture of choice (polyglactin 910 [Vicryl])
Reanastomsis equipment
  2 No. 1 nylon double-armed sutures
  Suture boots
  Razor blade breaker and blades
  No. 22 Silastic tubing
Depending on the surgeon's preference, additional equipment
  Carbon dioxide laser
  Laser drape
  Smoke evacuator
  Microscope
  Microscope drape

Drugs and Solutions

During the procedure, several solutions are needed. Normal saline (0.9% sodium chloride), 1000 ml, with 5000 U of heparin added or lactated Ringer solution is used to moisten tissue. The solution is hung on an IV pole and is transported to the sterile field by way of sterile IV tubing that has been connected to a stopcock. Two 60-ml syringes are filled and a Webster cannula is attached to the tip.

Diluted indigo carmine is injected into the uterus with a 19-gauge needle to test for tubal patency (4 ml of indigo carmine in a 250-ml of normal saline).

In addition, a solution of 150-ml of normal saline with 25 mg of promethazine hydrochloride (Phenergan) and 4 mg of dexamethasone (Decadron) is mixed for instillation into the abdomen via the IV tubing, before the last subcutaneous stitches are sewn. Lactated Ringer solution may also be used, depending on the surgeon's preference. This solution helps in preventing pelvic adhesions.

Many surgeons now use a fine film of absorbable adhesion barrier, instead of the promethazine hydrochloride and dexamethasone mixture. This is placed over the fallopian tubes to prevent adhesions.

Wet sponges are used during the procedure; therefore, the circulating nurse should keep warm irrigation available.

Physiological Monitoring

The circulating nurse must catheterize the patient before the surgical preparation. A No. 14 Fr. Foley catheter is inserted into the bladder and attached to a urinary drainage bag. The tubing is positioned under the patient's knee to ensure urinary flow. The circulating nurse is responsible for measuring and recording the amount of blood loss and irrigating fluids used during the procedure. Blood loss is usually minimal.

Specimens and Cultures

Adhesions and a portion of the fallopian tubes are usually the only specimens resulting from this procedure. Specimens are sent to the pathology laboratory routinely, unless otherwise indicated.

Physician's Orders

The patient is instructed to have a Fleet enema and nothing to eat after 8:00 PM and nothing to drink after midnight the night before surgery. A shower is also encouraged.

Laboratory and Diagnostic Studies

The patient must have a complete blood count, (CBC), electrocardiogram (ECG), urinalysis, and electrolyte measurement. All test results should be within the normal range.

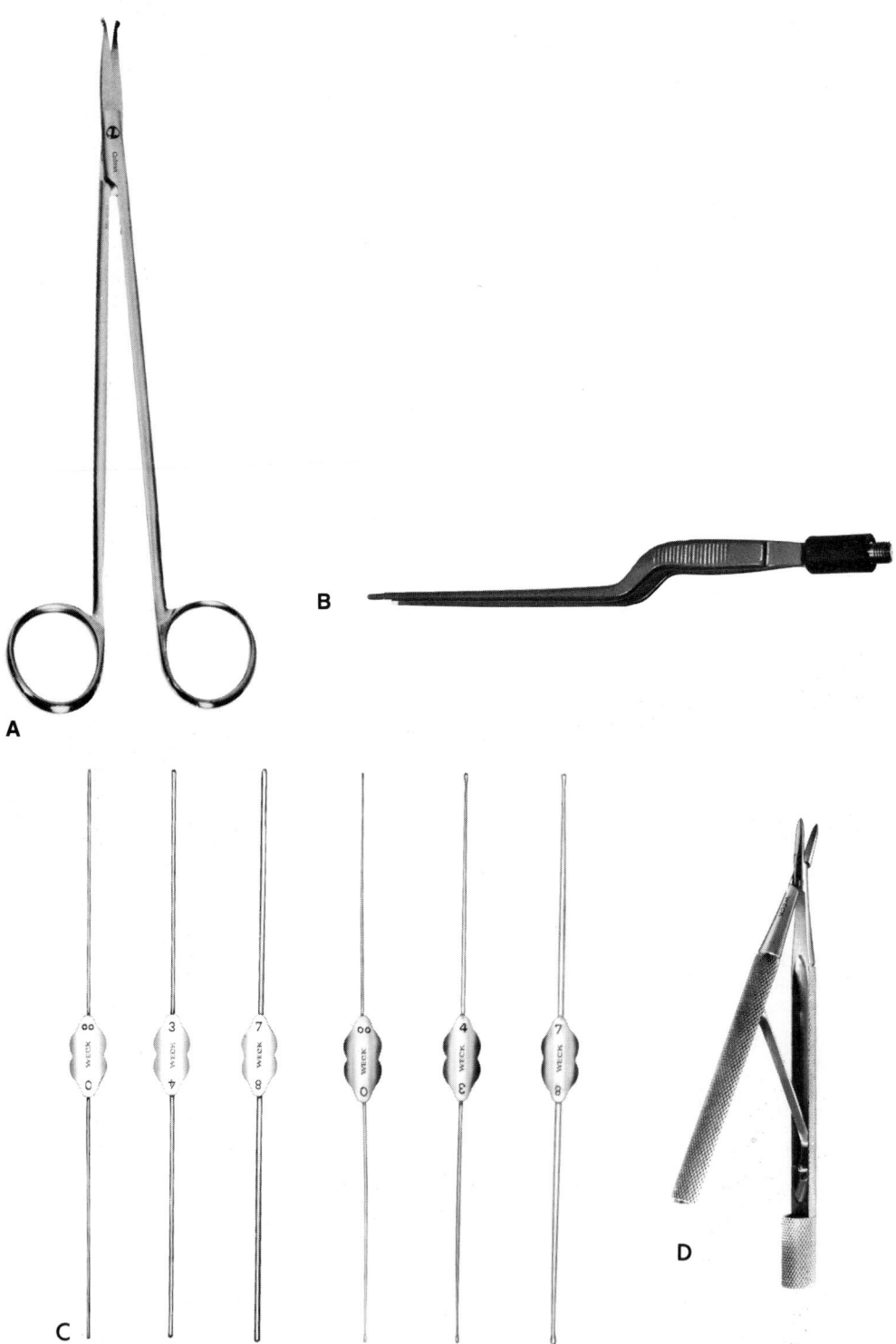

FIGURE 28–8. Neurosurgical instruments. *A*, Strully neurological scissors; *B*, bipolar forceps (Courtesy of Codman and Shurtleff, Inc., Randolph, MA); *C*, Bowman lacrimal probes; and *D*, razor blade breaker. (Courtesy of Edward Weck and Company, Inc.)

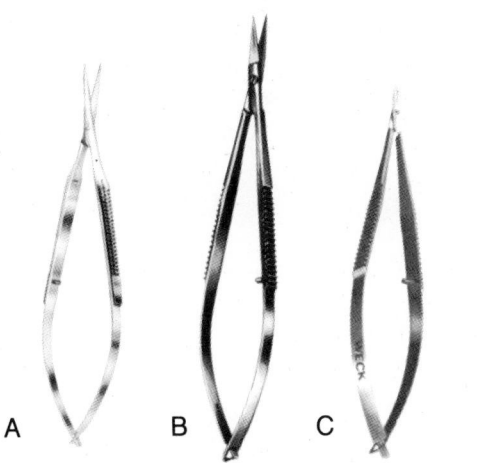

FIGURE 28–9. Scissors. *A,* Iris; *B,* fine stitch; and *C,* Castroviejo corneal, miniature. (Courtesy of Edward Weck and Company, Inc.)

Procedure

Incision and Exposure

The incision of choice is usually a Pfannenstiel incision (Fig. 28–10). It can be safely made parallel to the vessels and nerves and also leaves a less noticeable scar. A midline incision is used for patients with previous surgery to avoid a second scar.

An O'Connor-O'Sullivan retractor is the self-retaining retractor of choice. To control bleeders, 3–0 ties and suture ligatures, along with the electrocautery, are used.

The large intestines are packed out of the abdomen using large wet packs.

Details

If the obstruction is located in the proximal cornual area, the distal tube is reimplanted through the cornu into the uterine cavity, using 6–0 sutures.

Damage to the mucosa or fimbria that resulted in distal tubal obstruction necessitates opening that portion of tube. A 5–0 or 6–0 suture ligature is required.

Reversal of a previous sterilization procedure entails that the tube be reanastomosed, using a 7–0 double-armed suture.

Tubal adhesions necessitate the removal of those adhesions and are repaired with either 4–0 or 5–0 suture.

Closure

The abdomen is checked for any bleeding. All sponges are removed, and the abdomen is again irrigated with heparinized saline or lactated Ringer solution. The peritoneum is closed with a 1–0 Vicryl suture, followed by a 1–0 Vicryl suture for the muscular layer. A 3–0 Vicryl suture is next used for the subcutaneous fat. A 4–0 Vicryl suture on a cutting needle is used for sewing the skin. Before the last peritoneal stitches, the solution of promethazine hydrochloride and dexamethasone is instilled into the cavity.

Postoperative Care

The patient is taken to the postanesthesia care unit. Typical postoperative orders include

intake and output measurements
removal of the Foley catheter the morning after surgery, provided the urine is clear
measurement of vital signs
restriction to bed rest
intramuscular administration of pain medications, which when tolerated are continued by mouth
intake of clear liquids in the evening postoperatively, then a full diet as tolerated
administration of promethazine hydrochloride (steroid) and dexamethasone for nine doses
IV administration of potassium
administration of postoperative antibiotics per the surgeon's prescription

The hospital stay is usually no longer than 5 days.

Potential Surgical Complications

Infection
Pelvic adhesions
Hemorrhage

CERCLAGE

Definition

Cerclage is a procedure performed to prevent habitual abortion in patients who are prone to such an event. The procedure involves the suturing of the cervical os.

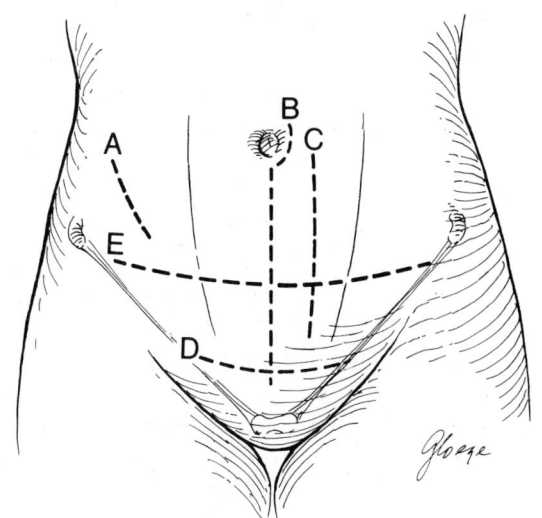

FIGURE 28–10. Abdominal wall incisions. *A,* McBurney; *B,* lower midline; *C,* left lower paramedian; *D,* Pfannenstiel or Cherny; and *E,* transverse. (From Hacker, N. F., Moore, J. G. [1992]. *Essentials of obstetrics and gynecology* [2nd ed.]. Philadelphia: W. B. Saunders.)

Indications

Cerclage is indicated for cervical incompetency, when a woman shows an inability to carry a pregnancy to term. Some causes are cervical trauma, exposure to diethylstilbestrol, prior conization of the cervix, and/or excessive muscular strain on the cervix.

Related Surgical Procedures

There are no related surgical procedures to cerclage.

Perioperative Nursing Implications

Anesthesia

Cerclage procedures are usually performed with general masked anesthesia. In some instances, epidural or spinal anesthesia may be used.

Position

The procedure is performed with the patient in the lithotomy position. The arms are extended on arm boards and safety straps are applied (Fig. 28–11).

Creation and Maintenance of the Sterile Field

A skin shave is not indicated for the procedure. Povidone-iodine solution is used for the surgical preparation, which should include the perineum and the

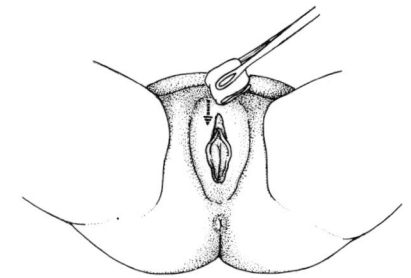

FIGURE 28–12. Vaginal preparation. (Reproduced by permission of Ethicon, Inc.)

internal vagina (Fig. 28–12). The internal preparation must be done gently to avoid any undue trauma to the cervix. A doubly folded sheet is placed as far under the buttocks as possible. Leg drapes are then applied, with an opened sheet placed low over the abdomen.

The surgeon sits during the procedure. The instrument table is placed closest to the surgeon's dominant arm.

Equipment and Supplies

Cerclage tray
  Several ring forceps
  Small narrow Deaver retractors
  Toothed and smooth forceps
  Needle holders
No. 5 polyester fiber suture and No. 3 Mayo taper needles
Stirrups and holders

The sutures are threaded on the No. 3 Mayo taper needle if the polyester fiber suture is used. The most important instruments used during the procedure are ring forceps and needle holders.

Drugs and Solutions

No drugs or solutions are used for this procedure.

Physiological Monitoring

No special monitoring is needed for this procedure. Blood loss is minimal.

Specimens and Cultures

This procedure has no specimens or cultures. A urine culture is taken rarely.

Physician's Orders

It is not necessary for the patient to be admitted the night before surgery. However, the patient should have

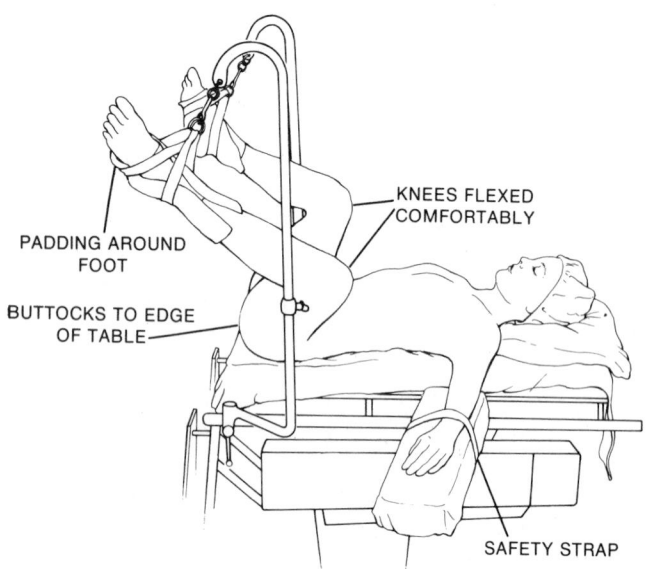

FIGURE 28–11. Lithotomy position. (From Fuller, J. R. [1986]. *Surgical technology: Principles and practice* [2nd ed.]. Philadelphia: W. B. Saunders.)

PADDING AROUND FOOT

KNEES FLEXED COMFORTABLY

BUTTOCKS TO EDGE OF TABLE

SAFETY STRAP

nothing by mouth (NPO) after midnight the evening before surgery. These patients should be first on the OR schedule.

Laboratory and Diagnostic Studies

No laboratory tests are necessary for this procedure. Owing to the nature of the problem, there are no tests that confirm cervical incompetency.

Procedure

Incision and Exposure

No incision is made for cerclage. Deaver retractors are used for exposure. A ring forceps is used to retract the cervix.

Details

The bladder is emptied using a metal catheter. The cervix is retracted, and a suture is placed at the junction of the vaginal mucosa and a portion of the cervical os (at the 12 o'clock position). A pursestring suture is placed in several bites around the cervix. Sutures are tied after they are all in place.

Closure

There is no closure for this procedure.

Postoperative Care

After a short stay in the postanesthesia care unit, the following are typical orders:

The patient is allowed toilet privileges but otherwise should be restricted to bed rest for 24 hours.
Vital signs are obtained every 4 hours with temperature monitored during the first 24 hours.
The nurse checks for cramping and any drainage from the vagina.
Indomethacin (Indocin) suppositories are given per the physician's prescription.

After the patient is discharged from the hospital, she should refrain from strenuous activity but have some form of physical exercise. The sutures are removed at 37 weeks.

Potential Surgical Complications

Infection
Premature labor

DILATION AND CURETTAGE

Definition

Dilation and curettage (D&C) involves the widening of the cervical os with a dilator; afterward, a sharp curet is used to scrape the endometrium. This procedure is instrumental in providing a definitive diagnosis and, in many instances, a cure for abnormal bleeding. D&C is the most common minor gynecological procedure performed.

Indications

D&C is performed for several reasons:

when the pain associated with menstruation suggests an abnormality of the uterus
when menstrual bleeding is abnormal, irregular, heavy, or postmenopausal
after an incomplete abortion has occurred

Related Surgical Procedures

Dilation and evacuation (D&E)
Uterine polypectomy

Perioperative Nursing Implications

Anesthesia

Although the procedure is most often performed with cervical block and sedation, a general anesthetic allows the surgeon to perform a better pelvic examination. Blood is usually not ordered for this procedure.

Position

The procedure is performed with the patient in the lithotomy position. The arms are extended on arm boards and safety straps are applied.

Creation and Maintenance of the Sterile Field

A skin shave is not necessary for this procedure. Povidone-iodine solution is used for the surgical preparation, which should include the perineum and the internal vagina. A doubly folded sheet is placed under the buttocks, with leg drapes applied next. Lastly, a open sheet is placed over the abdomen.

The surgeon sits for this procedure. The instrument table is placed closest to the surgeon's dominant arm.

Equipment and Supplies

D&C tray (Fig. 28–13)
  Narrow Deaver and Sims retractors
  Weighted and duckbill specula
  Dilators
  Tenacula
  Curets
  Polyp forceps
  Toothed and smooth forceps
Nonadherent dressing
Paracervical block tray and local anesthetic of choice
Lubricant
Foley catheter
Sitting stool

The instruments should be placed on the table from left to right, in the order that the surgeon will use them.

Drugs and Solutions

If the procedure is performed with a general anesthetic, no drugs are needed. However, if it is performed with sedation, local anesthetic is requested. Usually lidocaine 1% is used.

Physiological Monitoring

No special monitoring is needed for this procedure. Blood loss is usually minimal.

Specimens and Cultures

D&C usually has two specimens, labeled as endometrial and endocervical curettage specimens. Both specimens are sent to the pathology laboratory routinely.

Physician's Orders

It is not necessary for the patient to be admitted the night before surgery. However, the patient should have NPO orders. No special preparation is needed for this procedure.

Laboratory and Diagnostic Studies

Before admission, the patient's preoperative testing should include CBC, urinalysis, ECG, and electrolyte values. CBC may indicate a mild anemia; otherwise, results are within normal ranges.

Procedure

Incision and Exposure

No incision is needed for this procedure. A Sims retractor or weighted speculum is placed in the vagina for exposure.

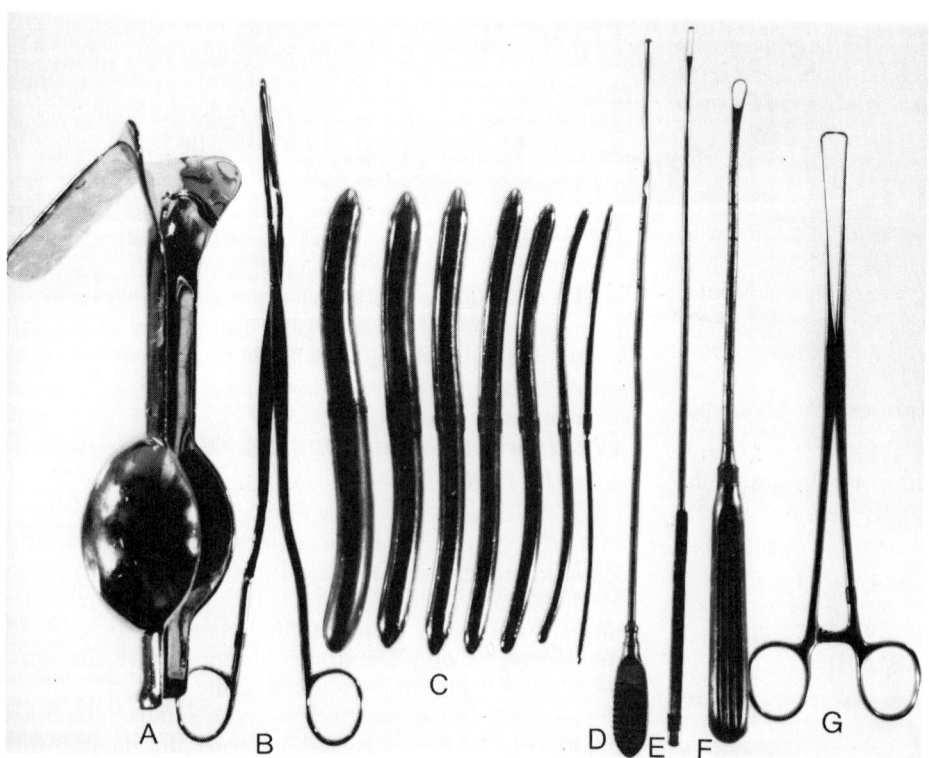

FIGURE 28–13. Instruments used for D&C. *A*, Weighted (Auvard) speculum; *B*, polyp forceps; *C*, Hegar dilators; *D*, uterine sound; *E*, Kevorkian curet for endocervical curettage; *F*, sharp uterine curette; and *G*, tenaculum. (From Hacker, N. F., Moore, J. G. [1992]. *Essentials of obstetrics and gynecology* [2nd ed.]. Philadelphia: W. B. Saunders.)

Details

A Foley catheter is used to empty the bladder and then removed. The lip of the anterior cervix is grasped with a tenaculum. A sound is carefully inserted into the endometrial cavity to determine the depth and direction of the uterus. Next, dilators are used to dilate the cervical os to at least 8 mm. A stone forceps is used to explore the cavity for polyps. A Tiemann curet is advanced into the fundus and moved back and forth until all of the endometrium is sampled. A nonadherent dressing is placed over the retractor to collect the curettage specimens. A smooth curet may also be used to obtain tissue.

Endocervical curettage specimens are obtained in the same fashion. The tenaculum is removed, and the site is checked for a cervical tear or any bleeding. If a tear or bleeder is discovered, pressure is applied or a 2–0 suture ligature is used for repair. The speculum is then removed.

Closure

No closure is needed.

Postoperative Care

The patient is taken to the postanesthesia care unit for a short time. Perineal pads are checked for heavy bleeding and clotting. Any cramping is also noted. The patient is discharged the same day.

The patient is instructed to take her temperature twice per day for 1 week and report to physician if it is more than 100°F. Acetaminophen (Tylenol) should be used for mild pain. Activity may be increased gradually during the first 24 hours.

Potential Surgical Complications

Bleeding
Infection
Uterine perforation

HYSTEROSCOPY

Definition

Hysteroscopy is the insertion of a fiberoptic scope into the vagina that aids in the visualization of the entire uterine cavity.

Indications

Hysteroscopy is performed for diagnostic and therapeutic purposes, including

infertility
suspected abnormal tissue
lysis of adhesions
uterine polyps
submucous myomas

Related Surgical Procedures

Like all endoscopic procedures, hysteroscopy employs the use of optics for visualization; otherwise, there are no related procedures.

Perioperative Nursing Implications

Anesthesia

The procedure is performed with general masked anesthesia or cervical block with sedation. Blood is not ordered for this patient.

Position

The patient is placed in the dorsal lithotomy position.

Creation and Maintenance of the Sterile Field

A skin shave is not needed for this procedure. Povidone-iodine solution is used for the preparation, which includes the perineum and the internal vagina. The patient is draped with a half sheet under the buttocks, leg drapes, and an open sheet across the abdomen. The instrument table should be to the surgeon's dominant side. The hysteroscopy insufflator should be on the side of the patient, close to the instrument table and so that the surgeon may see the pressure monitor for carbon dioxide flow rate.

The surgeon sits for the procedure.

Equipment and Supplies

Hysteroscope (Fig. 28–14)
Light cord
Light source
Hysteroscopy insufflator
Dilators
Foley catheter
Sponges
Possible D&C tray
If hysteroscopy fluid (Hyskon) is used, 60-ml syringes
IV extension tubing or cystoscopy tubing or IV pump and glycine

The hysterscopy equipment should be checked before its use to ensure that it is working properly.

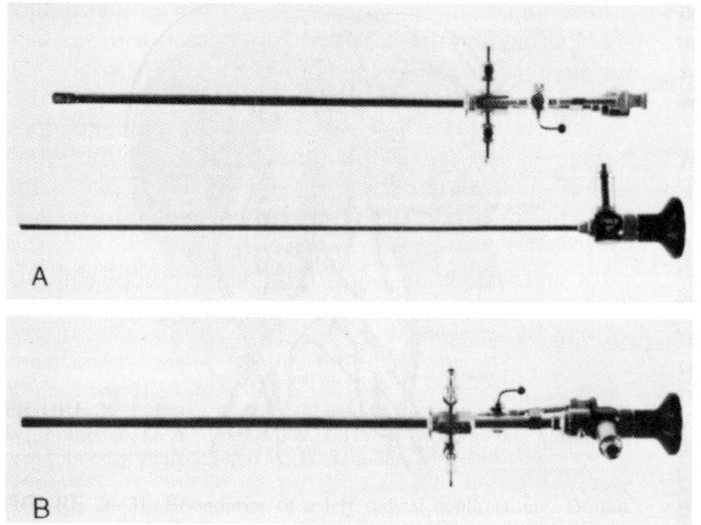

FIGURE 28–14. Storz operating hysteroscope: *A,* dismantled; *B,* assembled. (From Hacker, N. F., Moore, J. G. [1986]. *Essentials of obstetrics and gynecology.* [pp. 384–385]. Philadelphia: W. B. Saunders.)

Drugs and Solutions

Other than carbon dioxide, hysteroscopy fluid is the medium used by most surgeons. The circulating nurse should monitor and document the amount used.

Physiological Monitoring

No special monitoring is needed for this procedure. Blood loss is minimal. If hysteroscopy fluid is used, the amounts should be carefully monitored.

Specimens and Cultures

If the procedure is done in conjunction with D&C, curettage specimens are possible. Depending on the patient's history, a polyp or a submucous myoma may be obtained. All specimens are sent to the pathology laboratory routinely.

Physician's Orders

The patient is not admitted the night before surgery but is NPO after midnight. No special preparation is needed.

Laboratory and Diagnostic Studies

Preoperative testing includes CBC, ECG, urinalysis, and electrolyte determination. CBC may indicate a slight anemia.

Procedure

Incision and Exposure

No incision is made for this procedure. Exposure is obtained by a weighted speculum.

Details

The bladder is emptied with a Foley catheter, which is then removed. The cervix is dilated to accommodate the entrance of the hysterscope into the cervical os. Before the hysteroscope is inserted into the patient, the system should be checked:

Check the gas pressure.
Turn on the machine.
Close the insufflator switch.
Adjust the intrauterine pressure and carbon dioxide flow rate to zero.
Turn on the flow rate.
Adjust the flow rate with the insufflator to deliver 25 to 30 cc/minute.

After the system is checked, the cervix is grasped with a tenaculum. The hysteroscope is inserted into the cervical os after dilation. The carbon dioxide valve is opened on the hysteroscope, and it is advanced. The endometrial and endocervical cavities are explored, along with the fallopian tubes.

If hysteroscopy fluid is used during the procedure, it is introduced into the cavity by way of a 60-ml syringe.

Closure

There is no closure required.

Postoperative Care

The patient is not required to stay in the hospital overnight. Some vaginal discharge can be expected for a few day postoperatively. The patient should take her temperature for a week, with readings of more than 100°F reported to the surgeon.

Potential Surgical Complications

Intraoperative complications are rarely seen in hysteroscopy.

SUCTION CURETTAGE

Definition

Suction curettage (D&E) is the termination of a pregnancy by evacuating the products of conception with a suctioning device vaginally.

Indications

Suction curettage is performed to remove any remaining tissue that was not expelled during a missed or incomplete abortion. Termination may also be performed when there is a known fetal defect or when the mother's life is threatened.

Related Surgical Procedure

D&C

Perioperative Nursing Implications

Anesthesia

The procedure is performed with cervical block and sedation or general masked anesthesia. Depending on the nature of the procedure, blood may be ordered.

Position

D&E is done with the patient in the dorsal lithotomy position.

Creation and Maintenance of the Sterile Field

The patient is not shaved for this procedure. The perineum and the internal vagina must be prepared using povidone-iodine solution. The patient is draped in the usual fashion. The instrument table is placed closest to the surgeon's dominant arm. The suction machine is placed on the same side as the instrument table. The suction tubing is passed over the patient's leg and attached to the suctioning machine.

The surgeon sits during the procedure.

Equipment and Supplies

D&C tray
Paracervical block tray
Dilators
Suction machine (Fig. 28–15)
D&E suction tubing
Nos. 6 to 12 suction curets
Foley catheter

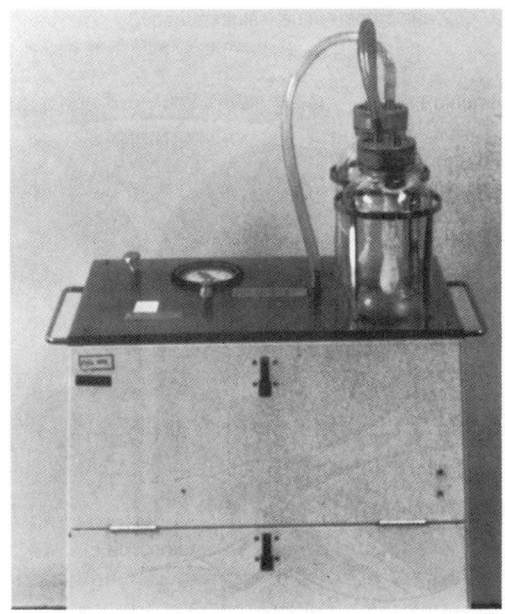

FIGURE 28–15. Suction apparatus used for therapeutic abortion. (From Fuller, J. R. [1986]. *Surgical technology: Principles and practice* [2nd ed.]. Philadelphia: W. B. Saunders.)

The scrub nurse should test the suction apparatus when it is attached to the suction machine, making sure that proper suction levels are attained. The circulating nurse turns the machine on when the surgeon is ready for suctioning.

Drugs and Solutions

If the procedure is performed with sedation, a local anesthetic is needed. Lidocaine 1% is the local anesthetic of choice. Oxytocin (Pitocin) may be added to the IV solution to contract the uterus.

Physiological Monitoring

No special monitoring is needed for a routine D&E; however, in some instances, blood loss may be excessive. Therefore, the circulating nurse should monitor blood loss and inform the anesthestist.

Specimens and Cultures

The specimen is sent routinely to the pathology laboratory, unless there is a question as to whether villi are present.

Physician's Orders

The patient is not required to stay the night preoperatively; however, she is NPO after midnight. No other orders are needed.

Laboratory and Diagnostic Studies

A Papanicolaou smear should be completed, and the results noted on the chart. CBC with a cross-match and type should be obtained. If the patient is Rh negative, she should receive immune globulin after abortion.

Procedure

Incision and Exposure

No incision or suture is needed for the procedure. A duckbill speculum is used for exposure.

Details

The bladder is emptied with a Foley catheter, which is then removed. After the cervix is exposed, it is grasped with a double-toothed tenaculum. A sound is passed through the cervix to check the length and direction of the cavity. Dilators, preferably Pratt dilators, are used to dilate the cervix to at least 6 mm to allow for the No. 6 curet. Suction tubing is applied to the curet, and the suction machine is turned on. The curet is rotated in a 360-degree arc and withdrawn slowly. It is reintroduced several times, making sure that all products are retrieved. Sponge forceps are introduced into the cavity as another means of making sure that all gestation tissue has been removed.

The specimen is collected in the gauge sack in the suction apparatus. When the procedure is completed, normal saline or sterile water is run through the tubing. This ensures that all tissue is collected in the gauge sack. The surgeon examines the tissue, and then it is placed in a specimen container.

Closure   .

No closure is required for this procedure.

Postoperative Care

Care is the same as that for the patient undergoing D&C. In addition, the patient is given ergonovine maleate (Ergotrate), 200 μg orally every 4 hours for six doses; this aids in contracting the uterus back to its normal size.

Potential Surgical Complications

Infection
Hemorrhage
Perforation of the uterus

CESAREAN SECTION

Definition

Cesarean section is a surgical procedure in which the infant is delivered through an abdominal incision rather than via the traditional vaginal delivery.

Indications

The indications to perform cesarean section are varied. The most common is dystocia, a failure to progress in labor. Other indications include

acute or chronic fetal distress
placenta previa
pelvic tumors
intrauterine infections
malpresentation
carcinoma of the cervix
failed induction of labor

Related Surgical Procedures

There are no related procedures.

Perioperative Nursing Implications

Anesthesia

The cesarean section can be performed under general, spinal, or epidural anesthesia. Usually, the procedure is performed with spinal or epidural anesthesia, which poses less hazard for the patient who has eaten or been in labor for a long period.

Position

The patient is placed in the dorsal recumbent (supine) position. To accommodate uteroplacental circulation, a 15-degree wedge should be placed under the patient's right hip.

Creation and Maintenance of the Sterile Field

The shave for cesarean section must include from 3 inches above the nipple line to the upper thighs, including the pubis. After the shave is completed, the area is prepared with povidone-iodine solution.

The circulating nurse assists with the instrument tables. The large instrument table is positioned on the scrub nurse's dominant side, and the square table with retractors is at the patient's foot. The patient should be draped using the usual laparotomy draping technique.

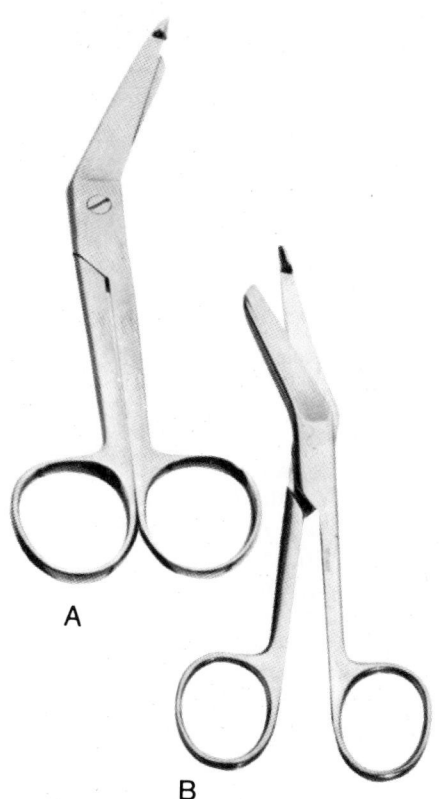

FIGURE 28–16. *A,* Lister bandage scissors; *B,* Episiotomy scissors. (Courtesy of Codman and Shurtleff, Inc., Randolph, MA.)

Equipment and Supplies

Cesarean section tray (Fig. 28–16)
Sterile blood tube
Bulb syringe
Irrigation syringe
Abdominal binder

The scrub nurse should use haste when the infant is removed from the uterus. Suction, clamps, and umbilical scissors should be available at once.

Drugs and Solutions

An antibiotic may be given.

Physiological Monitoring

A No. 14 Fr. Foley catheter is inserted by the circulating nurse, if it has not already been done. The tubing is attached and placed under the patient's knee to allow proper drainage. The circulation nurse is responsible for measuring and recording any unusual blood loss.

Specimens and Cultures

The placenta is sent to the pathology laboratory.

Physician's Orders

If the cesarean section is a scheduled procedure, the patient would have an NPO order the evening before surgery.

Laboratory and Diagnostic Studies

CBC, with cross-matching and typing for 2 U of blood, should be ordered. Urinalysis is also obtained.

Procedure

Incision and Exposure

Cesarean section may be performed with a midline or low transverse incision (Fig. 28–17). To prevent damage to the fetus, only hand-held retractors are used for exposure.

Details

A No. 22 or a No. 10 blade is used to open the abdomen. After the abdomen is opened, the vesicouterine fold is identified and opened, with a knife or forceps and heavy scissors. Moist sponges are placed on either side of the uterus to prevent blood or fluid from entering the peritoneal cavity. The bladder is dissected from the lower uterine segment with heavy scissors. The sac is opened, and the fetus is removed. The cord is doubly clamped with Kelly clamps and cut with cord scissors. The placenta is delivered manually. The surgeon then

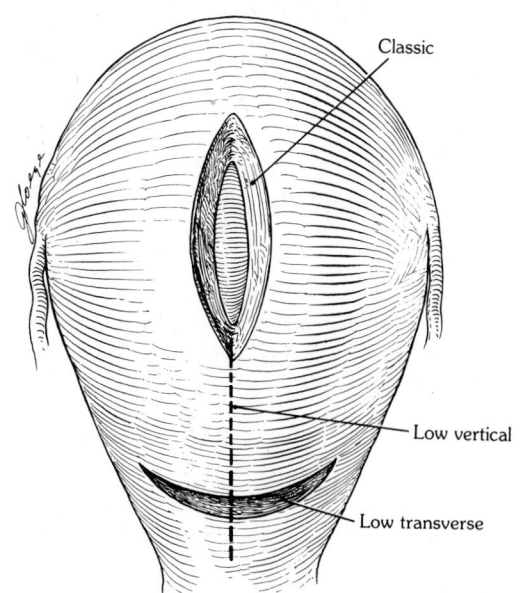

FIGURE 28–17. Types of cesarean section. (From Hacker, N. F., Moore, J. G. [1992]. *Essentials of obstetrics and gynecology* [2nd ed.]. Philadelphia: W. B. Saunders.)

controls any bleeding; the cavity is suctioned of any blood or placental parts.

Closure

Depending on the surgeon's preference, catgut or Vicryl suture may be used. The uterus is closed in two layers: the first layer with a continuous stitch and the next layer with an interrupted stitch. The serosa of the vesicouterine peritoneal fold is closed with a continuous stitch. Next the muscle is closed, then the subcutaneous layer, and finally the skin.

Postoperative Care

The Foley catheter is maintained for 24 hours.
Clear liquids are given, then a full diet as tolerated.
Vital signs are monitored until the patient is stable, then every 4 hours for 24 hours.
The fundus is assessed for height, tone, and location.
The type and amount of lochia and the presence of clots are assessed.
Dressings are checked for drainage.
Intake and output are assessed for 24 hours.
The Foley catheter is checked and then removed on postoperative day 1.
Bed rest is suggested.
Discuss infant feeding preference.
Check the breasts.
Provide discharge instructions.
The patient's length of hospital stay is usually 4 to 5 days.

Potential Surgical Complications

Infection
Intraoperative hemorrhage

VAGINAL HYSTERECTOMY

Definition

Vaginal hysterectomy is the removal of the uterus and cervix by way of the vagina rather than through an abdominal incision.

Indications

Vaginal hysterectomy is indicated and limited to benign disease or carcinoma in situ of the cervix. It should not be performed if the patient has extensive endometriosis, large uterine fibroids, invasive carcinoma, other suspected disease, or previous uterine suspension.

Perioperative Nursing Implications

Anesthesia

Refer to the discussion of tuboplasty.

Position

Refer to the discussion of cerclage.

Creation and Maintenance of the Sterile Field

A skin shave is not indicated for this procedure. Surgical preparation should include the perineum and the internal vagina. A doubly folded sheet is placed as far under the buttocks as possible. A second folded sheet is used to drape the rectum out of the sterile field. This is accomplished by using rubber tubing and two straight hemostats; the sheet is pulled and attached to each stirrup, and then the second folded sheet is placed over the rubber tubing. Leg drapes are then applied, with a large drape sheet over the abdomen.

The surgeon usually sits during this procedure. The scrub nurse should be positioned closest to the surgeon's dominant arm. The small square table is positioned to the right of the large table; this table holds all the retractors for the procedure. The grounding pad is placed on the patient's right upper thigh, with the machine near the patient's right arm. The circulating nurse assists the scrub nurse with the positioning of tables. A doubly folded plain sheet should be placed in the surgeon's lap. A sterile tray and magnetic pad may also be added to allow the surgeon to have available at all times some frequently used instruments.

Equipment and Supplies

Vaginal procedure tray (Figs. 28–18 and 28–19)
    4 double-toothed tenacula
    6 Heaney clamps
    2 Jacob tenacula
    2 curved Kocher clamps
    Vaginal and Metzenbaum scissors
    Toothed and smooth forceps, 8 inch
    Heaney and Mayo-Hegar needle holders
    Long and short weighted specula
    Heaney, Sweeney, and narrow Deaver retractors
Magnetic pad
Tray with Mayo cover
Foley catheter
Other basic supplies

A sterile tray in a Mayo cover allows the surgeon to keep some instruments (scissors, hemostats) close at hand.

A magnetic pad is used to prevent instruments that may be left on the field from falling to the floor.

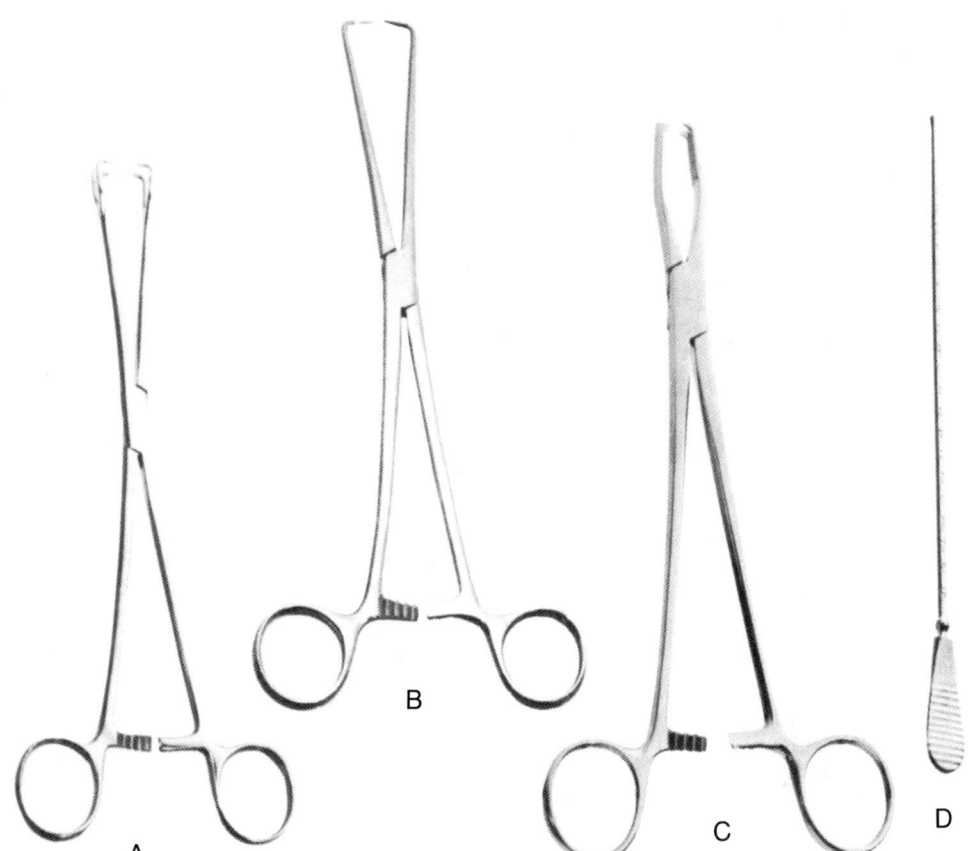

FIGURE 28–18. *A,* Schroeder vulsellum forceps; *B,* Schroeder tenaculum; *C,* Jacob tenaculum; and *D,* uterine sound. (Courtesy of Codman and Shurtleff, Inc., Randolph, MA.)

A

B

C

D

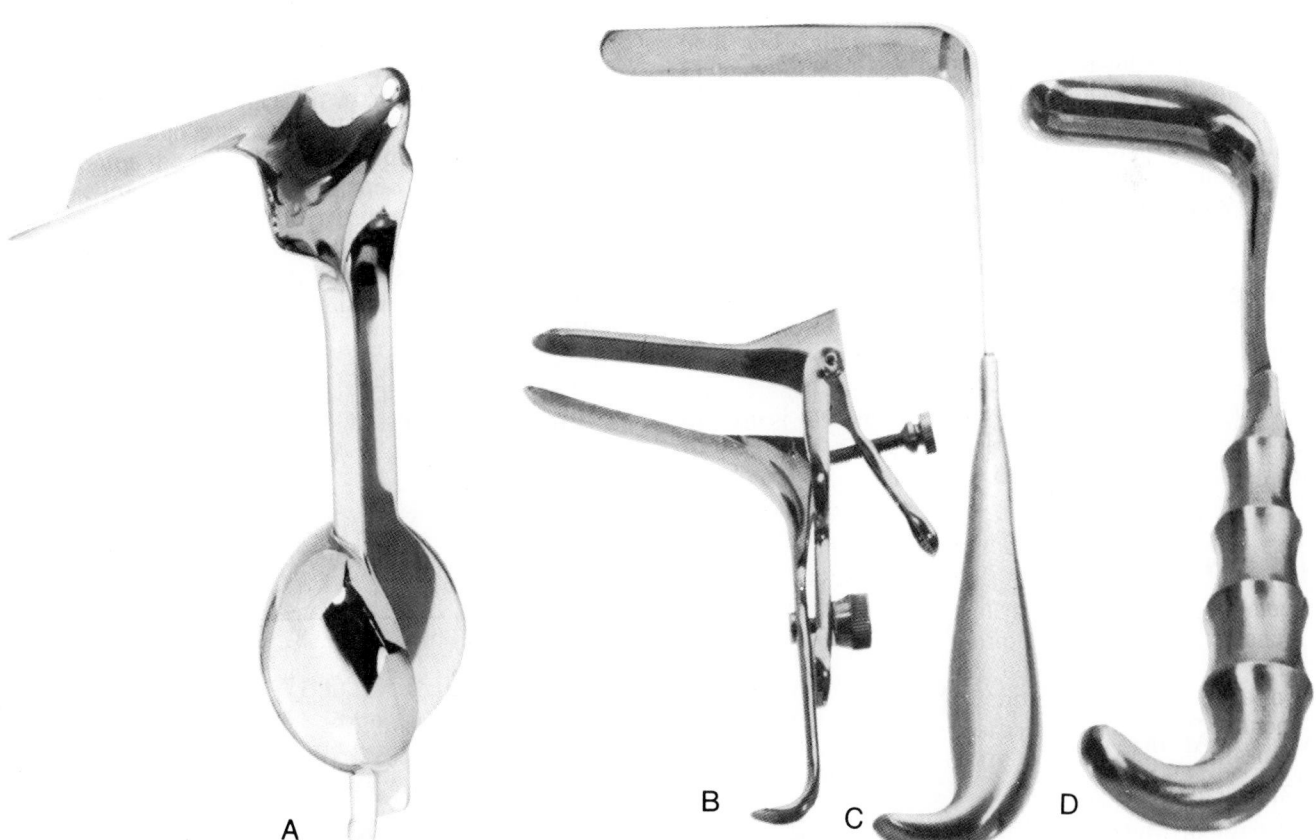

A

B

C

D

FIGURE 28–19. Obstetrical and gynecological instruments. *A,* Auvard weighted speculum; *B,* Graves vaginal speculum; *C,* Heaney retractor (lateral retractor); and *D,* Sims vaginal retractor. (Courtesy of Codman and Shurtleff, Inc., Randolph, MA.)

Drug and Solutions

Lidocaine 1% with 1:200,000 epinephrine is sometimes injected with a 10-ml syringe and tonsil needle attached. This aids in reducing bleeding.

Physiological Monitoring

The circulating nurse is responsible for accurately measuring and recording all blood loss.

Specimens and Cultures

The uterus and the cervix are routinely sent to the pathology laboratory. Fallopian tubes and ovaries may be included, if salpingo-oophorectomy is performed.

Physician's Orders

Admission and preoperative orders should include a Fleet enema the night before surgery, routine premedication, cross-matching and typing for 2 U of blood, NPO orders after midnight, and povidone-iodine douche. A shower is encouraged.

Laboratory and Diagnostic Studies

The patient must have CBC, ECG, urinalysis, chest x-ray film, and electrolyte determination. Results show normal white blood cell count, with the hemoglobin levels and hematocrit being low. If the hemoglobin level is less than 10 mg/ml, the surgeon may order a blood transfusion before surgery.

Procedure

Incision and Exposure

A weighted speculum or Sweeney retractor is used to achieve exposure anteriorly, with small Deaver or Heaney retractors used posteriorly.

Details

The patient undergoes straight catheterization with a Foley catheter at the start of the procedure. Retractors are positioned in the vagina. The cervix is grasped with a Jacob tenaculum to pull the uterus down into the vagina. At this point, if the surgeon believes it is necessary, the cervix is injected with lidocaine 1% with 1:200,000 epinephrine.

Heavy or Metzenbaum scissors and forceps are then used to cut around the cervix and into the peritoneum.

The bladder is freed from the uterus in front and the rectum in back.

The uterosacral ligaments are clamped with Heaney clamps, ligated with heavy suture, and then cut. Heaney clamps are next applied to the cardinal ligaments. After this is accomplished, the peritoneal cavity is entered and the uterine arteries are clamped, ligated, and cut. Again, heavy suture ligatures are used.

The fundus of the uterus is delivered from the abdomen. The round ligaments are clamped with Heaney clamps, ligated, and cut. The uterus is freed and removed from the vagina. To prevent prolapse, the cardinal ligaments are sutured to the superior angle of the vagina, with the uterosacral ligaments tied to prevent enterocele.

Closure

The vaginal cuff is closed with interrupted 2–0 catgut or 3–0 Vicryl suture. A Foley catheter is placed in the bladder at the end of the procedure. Occasionally, the vagina is packed with vaginal packing and antibiotic cream.

Postoperative Care

The patient is taken to the postanesthesia care unit for a short period of time. Postoperative orders may include

measurement of vital signs
restriction to bed rest
NPO status, then diet as tolerated
Foley catheter in place
intake and output monitored and recorded
IV administration of potassium
administration of pain medication as needed
administration of sleeping pills as needed
antibiotic regimen for 3 days
CBC on postoperative day 1

Potential Surgical Complications

Infection
Hemorrhage. There may be increased vaginal bleeding as compared with that after the abdominal procedure. Amounts should be recorded.

SKINNING VULVECTOMY

Definition

Skinning vulvectomy is the surgical removal of the entire vulva and can extend to the mons pubis, the gluteal and perisacral regions, and the anus.

Indications

Skinning vulvectomy is indicated for carcinoma in situ of the vulva in a younger woman (Table 28–1).

Related Surgical Procedures

Radical vulvectomy
Simple vulvectomy

Perioperative Nursing Implications

Anesthesia

Refer to the discussion of vaginal hysterectomy.

Position

The patient is placed in the lithotomy position.

Creation and Maintenance of the Sterile Field

Refer to the discussion of vaginal hysterectomy.

Equipment and Supplies

In addition to the instruments for vaginal hysterectomy, a skin graft tray and mesher should be available.

Drugs and Solutions

No drugs or solutions are needed for this procedure.

Physiological Monitoring

All sponges should be weighed, and bottled blood loss should be recorded at timely intervals. A Foley catheter is inserted at the end of the procedure.

Specimens and Cultures

The perivulvar tissue is sent to the pathology laboratory.

Physician's Orders

The evening before surgery, a tap water enema is ordered, along with a povidone-iodine shower. The enema is repeated in the morning before the patient goes to the OR.

The patient must have nothing to eat after 8 PM and nothing to drink after midnight the night before surgery. Sleeping pills are usually prescribed for comfort the night before surgery. Preoperative antibiotics and medications are given.

TABLE 28–1. STAGING OF VULVAR CARCINOMA

TNM Classification of Carcinoma of the Vulva

T Primary Tumor

Tis	Preinvasive carcinoma (carcinoma in situ)
T 1	Tumor confined to the vulva—2 cm or less in largest diameter
T 2	Tumor confined to the vulva—more than 2 cm in diameter
T 3	Tumor of any size with adjacent spread to the urethra and/or vagina and/or perineum and/or anus
T 4	Tumor of any size infiltrating the bladder mucosa and/or rectal mucosa, including the upper part of the urethral mucosa and/or fixed to the bone

N Regional Lymph Nodes

N 0	No nodes palpable
N 1	Nodes palpable in either groin, not enlarged, mobile (not clinically suspicious of neoplasm)
N 2	Nodes palpable in either one or both groins, enlarged, firm, and mobile (clinically suspicious of neoplasm)
N 3	Fixed or ulcerated nodes

M Distant Metastases

M 0	No clinical metastases
M 1a	Palpable deep pelvic lymph nodes
M 1b	Other distant metastases

FIGO* Staging of Carcinoma of the Vulva

Stage 0

Tis	Carcinoma in situ, intraepithelial carcinoma

Stage I

T1 N0 M0	Tumor confined to the vulva with a maximum
T1 N1 M0	diameter of 2 cm or less and no suspicious groin nodes

Stage II

T2 N0 M0	Tumor confined to the vulva with a diameter
T2 N1 M0	greater than 2 cm and no suspicious groin nodes

Stage III

T3 N0 M0	Tumor of any size with:
T3 N1 M0	(1) adjacent spread to the lower urethra, vagina, perineum, or anus, and/or
T3 N2 M0	(2) clinically suspicious lymph nodes in either
T1 N2 M0	groin
T2 N2 M0	

Stage IV

T4 N0 M0	Tumor of any size with:
T4 N1 M0	(1) infiltration of the mucosa of the bladder, rectum, or proximal urethra, and/or
T4 N2 M0	(2) Fixation to bone, and/or
All conditions containing N3 or M1a or M1b	(3) fixed or ulcerated nodes in either groin, and/or (4) distant metastases

*International Federation of Gynecology and Obstetrics.

Laboratory and Diagnostic Studies

CBC, platelet count with differential, prothrombin time, partial thromboplastin time, panel 4 (sodium, potassium, carbon dioxide, and creatine), ECG, urinalysis, and chest x-ray film are ordered before surgery.

Procedure

Incision and Exposure

The skin to be removed should be outlined with a marking pen before making an actual incision. The incision is made only down to the dermis.

Details

A No. 10 knife blade is used for the incision. An Allis clamp is used to grasp the skin. The outlined skin is removed (Fig. 28–20), and hemostasis is obtained by applying pressure to the operative area. All remaining bleeders are cauterized with the electrosurgical cautery. A split-thickness skin graft is usually applied to the affected area. The graft is taken from the outer thigh area.

Closure

The skin graft is sewn into place with interrupted 3–0 nylon or silk suture.

Postoperative Care

After a short stay in the postanesthesia care unit, orders are as follows:

Intake and output monitored
Foley catheter in place
Administration of pain medications
Dressing checks
Antibiotic therapy regimen
Bed rest
Discharge dependent on the progress of healing

Potential Surgical Complications

Infection

RADICAL VULVECTOMY AND GROIN LYMPHADENECTOMY

Definition

Radical vulvectomy entails the removal of all vulvar tissue and may include the bladder, rectum, urethra, and vaginal and inguinal nodes.

Indications

Radical vulvectomy is indicated in patients with biopsy specimens of the vulvar area that show invasive squamous cell carcinoma (Fig. 28–21). It is also indicated in some cases if biopsy specimens show melanomas and/or basal cell carcinoma.

Related Surgical Procedures

Skinning vulvectomy
Total skinning vulvectomy

Perioperative Nursing Implications

Anesthesia

In many instances, these patients are premedicated before arriving in the OR. Surgery is performed with a general endotracheal anesthetic. The anesthesia is induced using a combination of drugs. Fentanyl is the narcotic of choice, with inhalation gases such as nitrous oxide, halothane, and enflurane as breathing agents. Blood may or may not be needed for this procedure; 3 U is always ordered.

Position

Depending on the surgeon's preference, the patient may be placed in the dorsal supine position for node dissection and then placed in the lithotomy position, or in the modified dorsal lithotomy position for both parts of the procedure.

Owing to the length of the procedure, eggcrate padding should be used for positioning in both surgical positions. This aids in preventing breakdown of the patient's skin. Elastic (Ace) wraps or antiembolism stockings should be applied to the patient's legs. The nurse extends both arms on arm boards, making sure that they are not abducted more than 180 degrees; safety straps are applied to prevent them from dangling.

Creation and Maintenance of the Sterile Field

The shave for radical vulvectomy should include the abdomen and the perineum (Fig. 28–22). Iodine solution is used to prepare the abdomen, the perineum, and the upper thigh area. The grounding pad may be placed on the upper arm or the lower thigh.

If the modified lithotomy position is selected for the procedure, the area is draped, with both the abdomen and the perineum exposed. The rectum is draped out of the sterile field by placing rubber tubing attached with a hemostat and stretching it around the other stirrup. A plain sheet is then placed over the tubing. If the patient is placed in the supine position and then placed in the

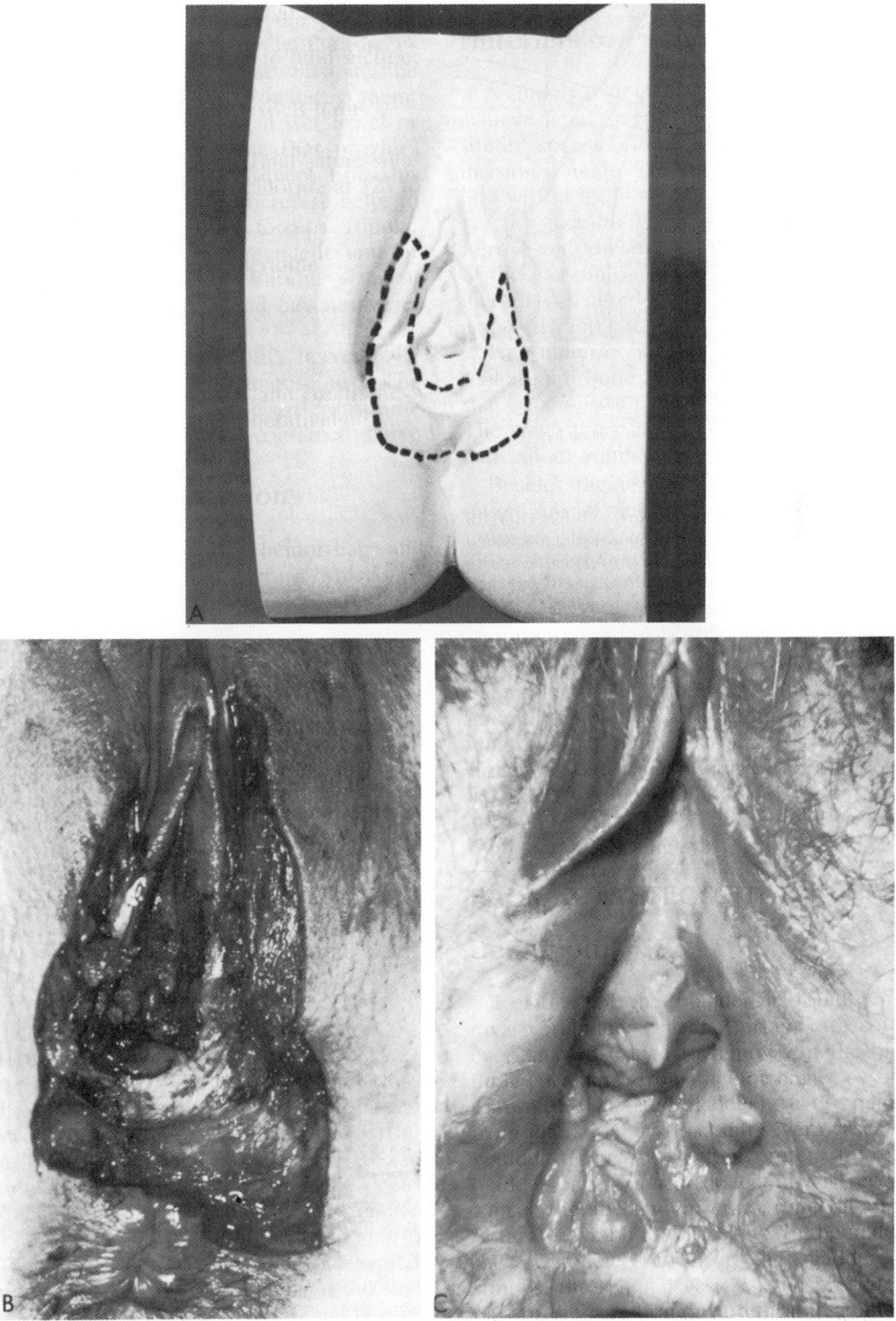

FIGURE 28–20. Partial vulvectomy. *A*, The incision encompasses all involved areas with an 8- to 10-mm margin but spares unaffected tissue. *B*, Dissection is shallow down to the underlying fat. *C*, The final result shows good cosmetic appearance. (From Friedrich, E. G., Jr. [1983]. *Vulvar disease* [2nd ed.]. Philadelphia: W. B. Saunders.)

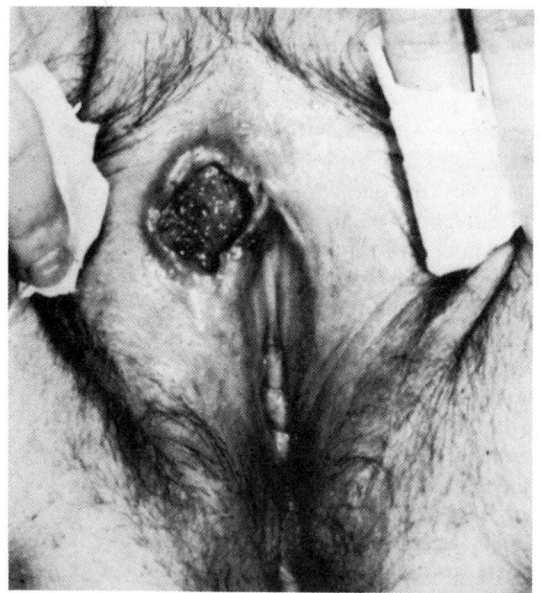

FIGURE 28–21. Carcinoma of the vulva. (Courtesy of Mr. C. P. Jones.)

lithotomy position, extra drapes should be available. The scrub nurse should make sure that the tables are not contaminated when the patient is repositioned. The instrument tables are placed closest to the scrub nurse's dominant arm. This position should accommodate either patient positioning.

Equipment and Supplies

Major gynecological set
Small retractors (Army-Navy retractors, skin hooks, Weitlaner retractors, and rakes)
Suture of preference
Large and medium hemoclips
Large wound drains

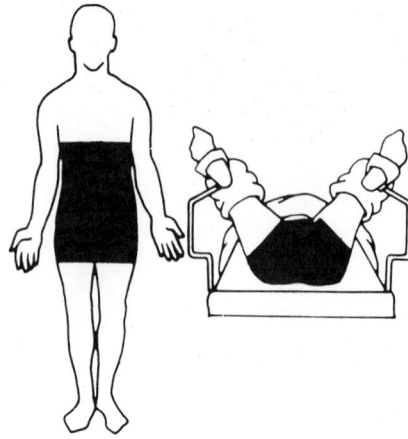

FIGURE 28–22. Preparation area for gynecological surgery. (From Fuller, J. R. [1986]. *Surgical technology: Principles and practice* [2nd ed.]. Philadelphia: W. B. Saunders. Copyright 1971, Ethicon, Somerville, NJ.)

Drugs and Solutions

No special drugs are used during this procedure. Saline or sterile water may be used for irrigation during node dissection.

Physiological Monitoring

Depending on the timing of the Foley catheter insertion, the circulating nurse may be responsible for its insertion. Blood loss must be accurately measured, along with any irrigating fluids used.

Specimens and Cultures

The Cloquet nodes are dissected and excised; these nodes are sent to the pathology laboratory for frozen section examination. If the results of the frozen section examination indicate carcinoma, the retroperitoneal nodes are then dissected. Other specimens include the vulva, which is sent to the pathology laboratory routinely.

Physician's Orders

The evening before surgery, a tap water enema is ordered, along with a povidone-iodine shower. The enema is repeated the morning of surgery. The patient must have NPO orders the evening before to surgery. Sleeping pills are prescribed. Preoperative antibiotics and medications are usually ordered.

Laboratory and Diagnostic Studies

Testing usually includes CBC, platelet count and differential, prothrombin time, partial thromboplastin time, panel 4 (sodium, potassium, carbon dioxide, and creatine), urinalysis, chest x-ray film, and ECG. All testing results may be within the normal limits.

Procedure

Incision and Exposure

A low Pfannenstiel incision is used and then extended to look like a rabbit's head (Fig. 28–23). A self-retaining retractor is rarely used for this procedure; hand-held retractors such as Deaver retractors are used and preferred. To control bleeders, 3–0 ties and suture ligatures are used, along with the electrocautery.

Details

The upper portion of the incision is made down to the fascia with a No. 10 knife blade. The femoral nerve,

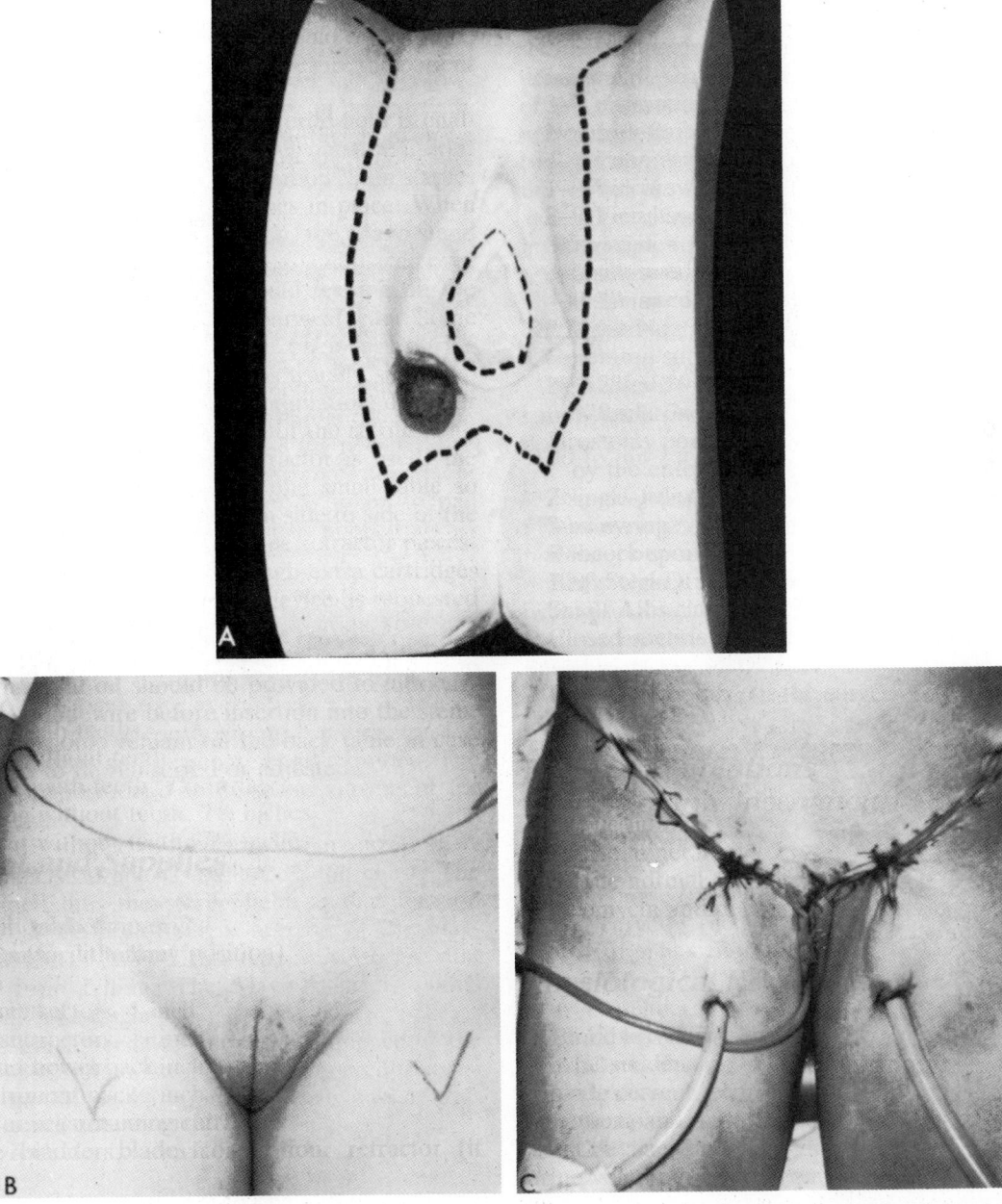

FIGURE 28–23. Radical vulvectomy. *A*, Outline of the incision includes the perineum. *B*, Landmarks for groin dissection incision are the iliac crests and the apexes of Hunter canal in legs. *C*, Postoperatively, a Way drainage system is in place. (From Friedrich, E. G., Jr. [1983]. *Vulvar disease* [2nd ed.]. Philadelphia: W. B. Saunders.)

artery, and vein in the femoral sheath are identified. The saphenous vein is next identified, doubly clamped, incised, and tied with silk suture. The Cloquet nodes are removed and sent for frozen section examination. As mentioned above, if the node results are abnormal, node dissection continues to include the deep pelvic nodes.

The procedure is continued, and the focus is on the vulva. The inguinal flaps are passed into the lower field. The pudendal artery and vein are clamped with Crile or Mixter clamps and tied with silk suture. Allis clamps are used to retract the area that is to be removed. The remainder of the incision is made. The incision is extended to include the lateral border of the labia majora and the vestibule around the meatus, to cross the posterior fourchette, and to continue on the other side.

With a No. 10 blade or Metzenbaum scissors and forceps, the dissection is made along the fascia until the perineal body is reached. The posterior vagina is elevated with an Allis clamp, and scissors are used to release the rectum.

Closure

A Foley catheter is reinserted into the bladder, if it was removed when the procedure focused on the vulva. Wound drains are placed in the groin bilaterally and sewn in place with 2–0 polypropylene (Prolene) suture (see Fig. 28–23C). The inguinal area and then the urethra, paravaginal area, and facsia are closed with the suture of choice. Next, the skin edges are closed, and surgery is completed.

Postoperative Care

The patient is taken to the postanesthesia care unit or the intensive care unit postoperatively. Routine orders are as follows:

Intake and output monitored
Foley catheter in place
Wound care (the edges should be kept dry)
Incision cleaned and packed
Antibiotic therapy regimen
Administration of medication for pain
Drains discontinued after 5 days
Discharge dependent on healing and/or wound breakdown

TOTAL ABDOMINAL HYSTERECTOMY WITH BILATERAL SALPINGO-OOPHORECTOMY

Definition

Total abdominal hysterectomy with bilateral salpingo-oophorectomy entails the removal of the uterus, the cervix, the fallopian tubes, and the ovaries through an abdominal incision.

Indications

Abdominal hysterectomy with bilateral salpingo-oophorectomy is performed for

endometriosis
uterine fibroids
premalignant or malignant conditions
obstretrical emergencies

The fallopian tubes are usually not affected by disease. However, they are included routinely to prevent future tubal carcinoma in postmenopausal women and those in their mid-40s.

Related Surgical Procedures

Simple abdominal hysterectomy
Vaginal hysterectomy
Radical hysterectomy

Perioperative Nursing Implications

Anesthesia

The procedure is performed with general endotracheal or spinal anesthesia. Two units of blood may be ordered for the patient. Refer to the discussion of tuboplasty.

Position

The patient is placed in the dorsal recumbent (supine) position. Refer to the discussion of tuboplasty.

Creation and Maintenance of the Sterile Field

The area is shaved and prepared (refer to the discussion of tuboplasty). To minimize contamination as the cervix is pulled up into the pelvis after the uterus is freed, the vagina must be prepared internally.

The preparation can be accomplished with the patient in either of two positions: the lithotomy position or the frog-leg position. The preparation should concentrate on the vagina itself. To accomplish this, sponge sticks (ring forceps) are used. After the preparation has been completed, a Foley catheter is inserted into the bladder and connected to a urinary drainage bag.

The grounding pad is placed on either thigh. The patient is draped using basic laparotomy technique. The circulating nurse should be available to dispose of the backing from the impervious split sheet used in draping the patient. The Mayo stand is placed over the patient's feet. The large instrument table is placed to the scrub nurse's dominant side, with square tables placed behind the scrub nurse. The electrosurgical unit is placed at the right side of the patient's head.

Equipment and Supplies

Gynecology major set (Fig. 28–24)
Double-toothed tenacula
Curved and straight Heaney clamps
Masterson clamps
Vaginal scissors
Medium uterine grasper
Somers clamp
60-ml syringe (if pelvic washing is to be obtained)
All other basic laparotomy instruments
Suture of choice

No. 1 catgut or Vicryl is used in abundance throughout the procedure. The scrub nurse should have them ready and on needle holders for the surgeon.

Drugs and Solutions

If washings are to be obtained, a 1000-ml bag of combined electrolyte solution (Normosol-R) with 5000 U of heparin is needed. Before the abdomen is closed, it is irrigated with warm sterile water or saline.

Physiological Monitoring

The circulating nurse must catheterize the patient before the surgical preparation is accomplished. A No. 14 Foley catheter is inserted into the bladder and attached to a urinary bag. The circulating nurse monitors and records blood loss and irrigating fluids during the procedure. In many instances, the surgeon prefers wet sponges after the abdomen is opened. Usually, 2 U of blood is requested for the procedure.

Specimens and Cultures

The uterus, the cervix, the ovaries, and the fallopian tubes are sent to the pathology laboratory. If after gross examination the surgeon believes that the specimen looks abnormal (ovaries), a frozen section examination may be requested.

Physician's Orders

Admission and preoperative orders should include a Fleet enema the night before surgery, routine premedication, cross-matching and typing for 2 U of blood, NPO orders after midnight before surgery, and povidone-iodine douche. A shower is encouraged.

Laboratory and Diagnostic Studies

The patient must have a CBC, ECG, urinalysis, chest x-ray film, and electrolyte determination. Results show normal white blood cell count, with hemoglobin level and hematocrit being low. If the hemoglobin level is less than 10 mg/ml, the surgeon may order a blood transfusion before surgery.

Procedure

Incision and Exposure

A midline or Pfannenstiel incision is used. An O'Connor-O'Sullivan retractor is the preferred. The bowel is packed off with warm wet sponges. Before introducing the retractor, the abdomen is explored. Bleeders are tied with 2–0 chromic, or 3–0 Vicryl ties and suture ligatures, along with the electrocautery.

Details (Fig. 28–25)

The round ligaments are identified and grasped with a Heaney or Kelly clamp close to the uterine cornu. The ligaments are ligated with heavy suture and cut. After both round ligaments are cut, the anterior leaf of the broad ligament is exposed and incised with Metzenbaum scissors. The anterior leaf is pushed forward and incised, making a hole in the broad ligament. The ureters are identified so that no injury can occur. Next, the infundibulopelvic portion of the broad ligament is clamped through the hole that was made previously. The ligament is divided, and the ovarian artery and vein are ligated.

The bladder is mobilized inferiorly with scissors and forceps, away from the cervix. The posterior leaf of the broad ligament is incised down to where the uterosacral ligament joins the cervix. Next, the uterine vessels are doubly clamped, ligated, and cut.

The peritoneum is dissected from the cervix posteriorly with scissors. The uterosacral ligaments are clamped, cut, and tied. The bladder base is cut away from the anterior vaginal wall. Next, the cardinal ligaments are clamped, cut, and sewn. Double-toothed tenacula are then placed across the vaginal angles, and the uterus is removed by incising the vagina below the cervix with a knife or scissors.

Closure

The abdomen is closed as described for tuboplasty.

Postoperative Care

The patient is taken to the postanesthesia care unit, with typical orders as follows:

Monitoring of vital signs
Restriction to bed rest

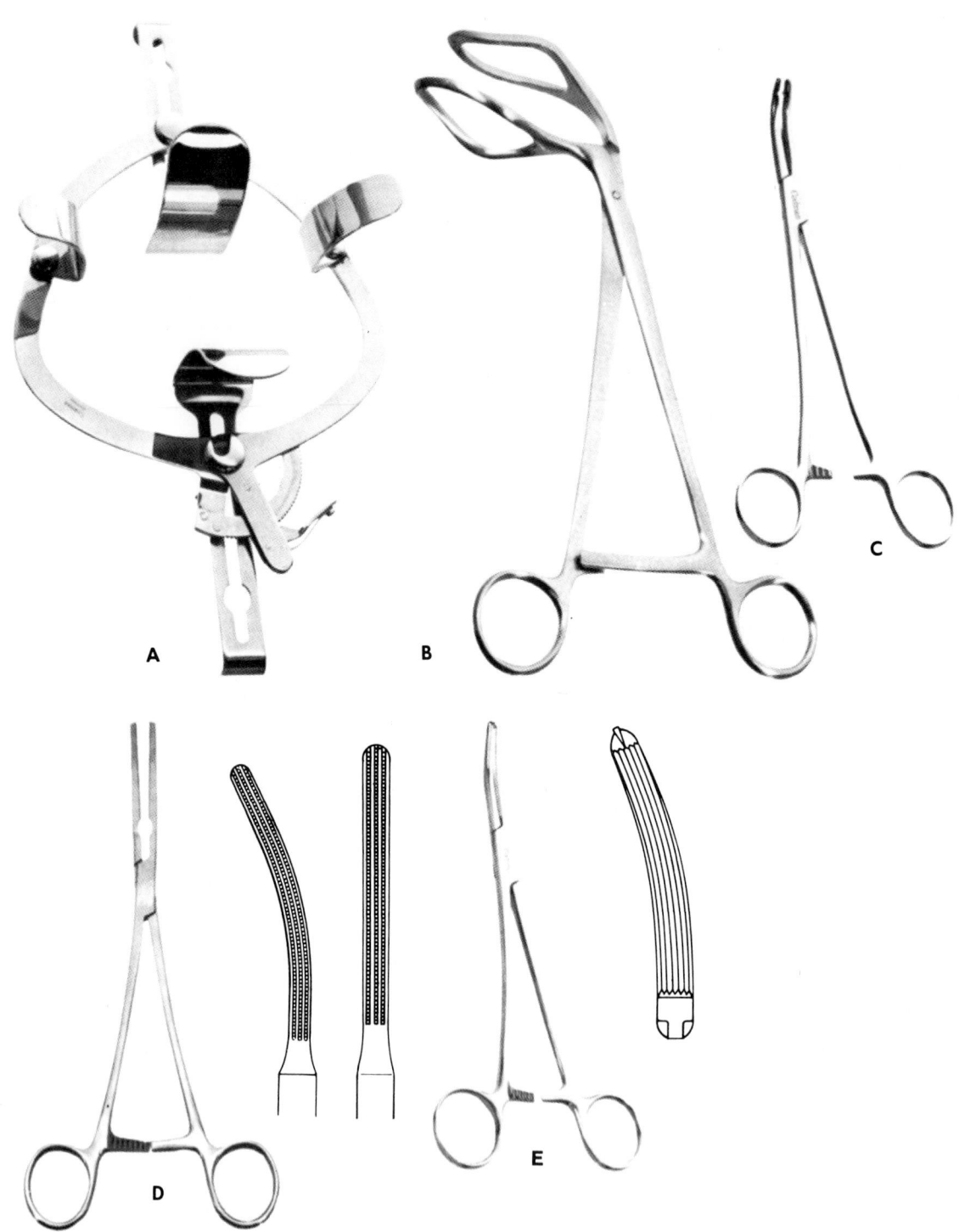

FIGURE 28–24. Hysterectomy instruments. *A,* O'Connor-O'Sullivan retractor; *B,* Somer uterine elevator (lemon squeezer); *C,* Heaney forceps; *D,* Masterson hysterectomy forceps; and *E,* long hysterectomy forceps. (Photographs courtesy of Codman & Shurtleff, Inc., Randolph, MA.)

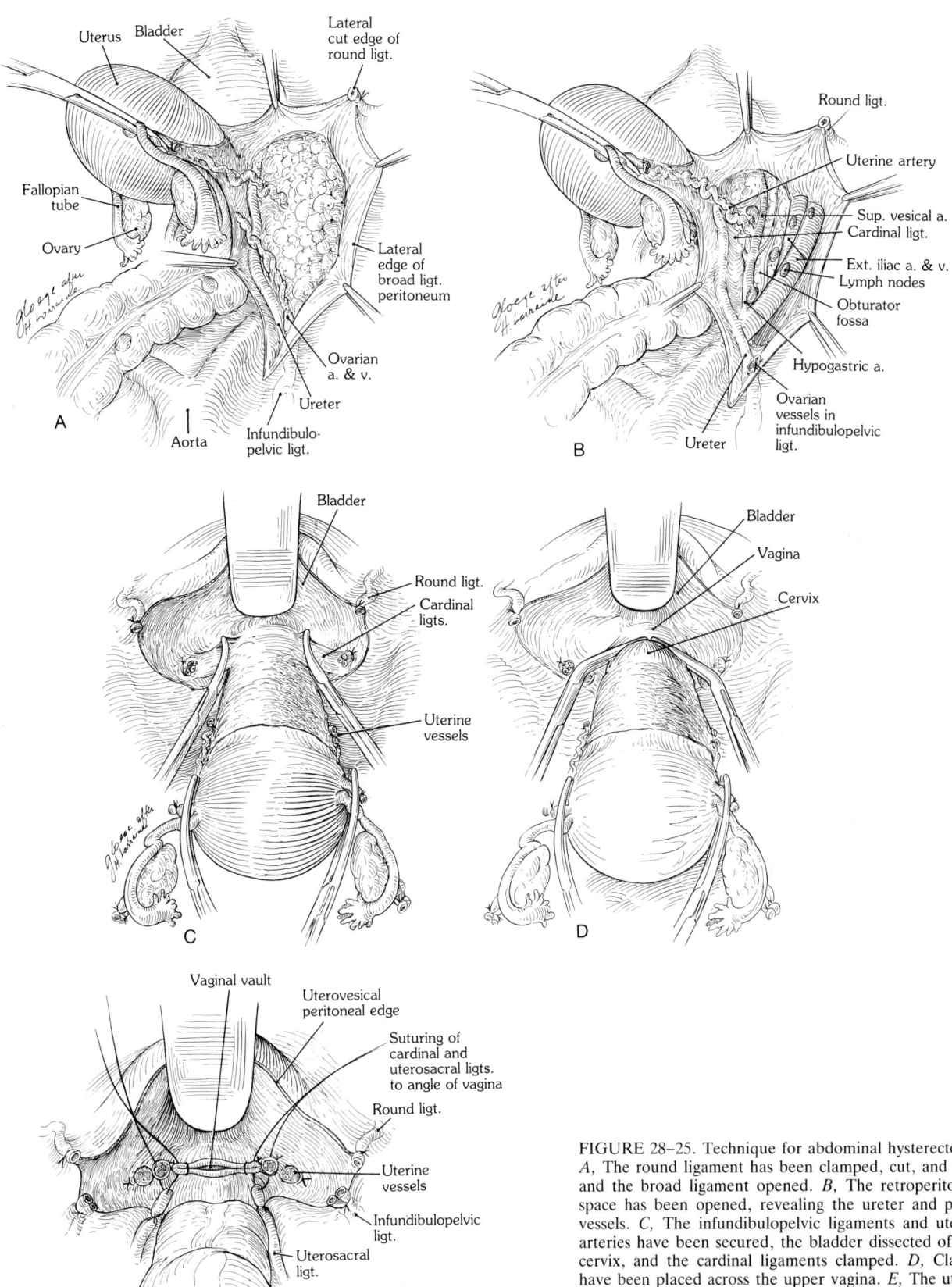

FIGURE 28–25. Technique for abdominal hysterectomy. *A,* The round ligament has been clamped, cut, and tied, and the broad ligament opened. *B,* The retroperitoneal space has been opened, revealing the ureter and pelvic vessels. *C,* The infundibulopelvic ligaments and uterine arteries have been secured, the bladder dissected off the cervix, and the cardinal ligaments clamped. *D,* Clamps have been placed across the upper vagina. *E,* The uterus has been removed. The vaginal vault is being closed. (From Hacker, N. F., Moore, J. G. [1986]. *Essentials of obstetrics and gynecology.* Philadelphia: W. B. Saunders.)

NPO status; diet as tolerated
Foley catheter in place
Monitoring of intake and output
Discharge usually in 5 to 7 days

LAPAROSCOPY

Definition

Laparoscopy is the visualization, examination, and/or observation of the peritoneal cavity by way of optics. The procedure may be diagnostic and/or therapeutic.

Indications

The indications for laparoscopy are numerous. It is used for but not limited to

diagnosis and treatment of endometriosis
assessment of infertility
diagnosis and treatment of ectopic pregnancy
assessment of the capability for tubal restoration
check for recurrence of ovarian cancer
check for suspected uterine perforation during D&E or D&C

Related Surgical Procedures

Laparoscopic cholecystectomy

Perioperative Nursing Implications

Anesthesia

These patients are usually admitted the day of surgery; therefore, no premedication is given. The procedure is performed with general endotracheal anesthesia. Blood products are not requested for this patient.

Position

The patient is placed in the modified lithotomy position. The patient's legs are angled to accommodate the surgeon when working in the abdomen; a 15-degree Trendelenburg position is used to displace the intestines from the abdomen to the diaphragm. The arms are extended on boards; they are not abducted more than 90 degrees.

Creation and Maintenance of the Sterile Field

An abdominal shave may or may not be indicated for this procedure. Povidone-iodine solution is used for the preparation, which should include the abdomen, the perineum, and the internal vagina. It is important that the umbilicus be concentrated on, because the instrument is inserted in it.

The patient is draped as follows: a half sheet is placed under the buttocks, next leg drapes are applied, a laparotomy sheet (preferably with a opening) is placed over the abdomen, and the arms are covered with opened plain sheets. If the procedure is a simple laparoscopy, no grounding pad is applied.

There are many different arrangements of equipment and surgical team members; one example is as follows: Depending on hospital's policy, two tables may be used during this procedure. If so, the vaginal and abdominal instruments are kept separate. A square table can accommodate the vaginal instruments, with a larger table for abdominal instruments. The surgeon is positioned to the patient's right, with the abdominal instrument table closest to the surgeon's dominant arm. The nonsterile television monitor, insufflator, and light source are on the patient's left in perfect view of the surgeon. The sterile assistant is positioned at the foot of the OR bed, managing the vaginal instruments. If another assistant is available, he or she is positioned on the patient's left. The circulating nurse is available to connect and manage the accessories being used in the procedure (e.g., camera).

The scrub nurse should check that

all trocars and sleeves have sealing caps with an adequate fit
the Verres needle is working properly
optics equipment is clear and provides good visualization

Depending on the hospital policy, the scrub nurse is or is not available after the actual procedure has begun.

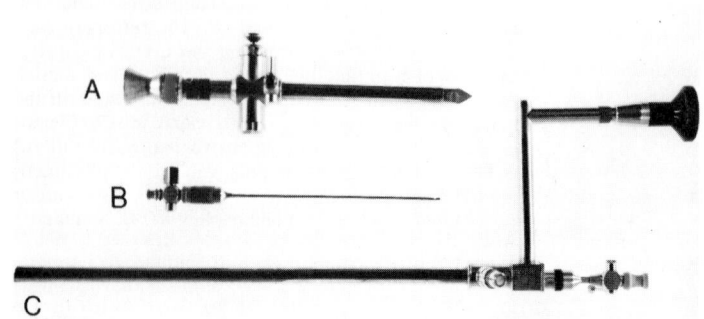

FIGURE 28–26. Instruments required for single puncture laparoscopy. *A,* Trocar and cannula; *B,* Verres needle; and *C,* Wolf laparoscope (10 mm). (From Hacker, N. F., Moore, J. G. [1986]. *Essentials of obstetrics and gynecology.* [pp. 384–385]. Philadelphia: W. B. Saunders.)

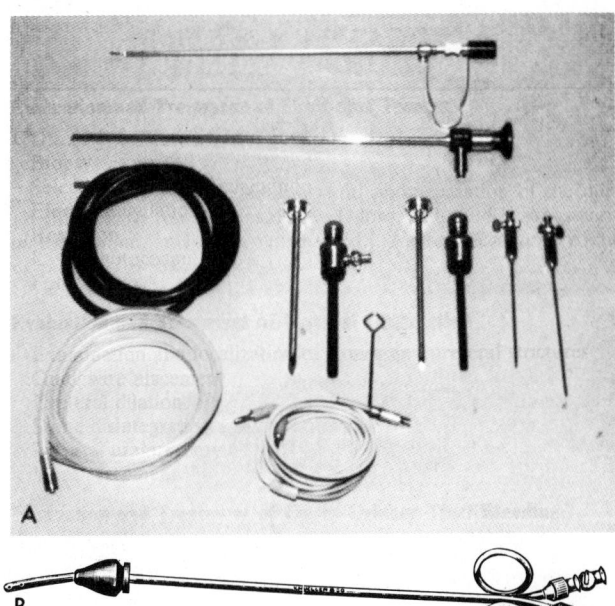

FIGURE 28–27. *A*, Laparoscope and accessories. *B*, Uterine manipulator. (Courtesy of V. Mueller, McGaw Park, IL.)

The scrub nurse may be available to assist the circulating nurse.

Equipment and Supplies

Laparoscopy set (Figs. 28–26 and 28–27)
    Laparoscope
    Verres needle
    Trocar and sleeve
    Fiberoptic light cord
    Insufflator tubing
    Probe
Light source

Gas insufflator (Fig. 28–28)
Camera equipment
No. 8 or 14 Fr. Foley catheter
No. 11 blade
Skin suture
Surgical sponges
Preparation tray
Adhesive bandage
Antibiotic ointment

Depending on the procedure, additional supplies

Laser
Laser instrumentation
Kleppinger forceps

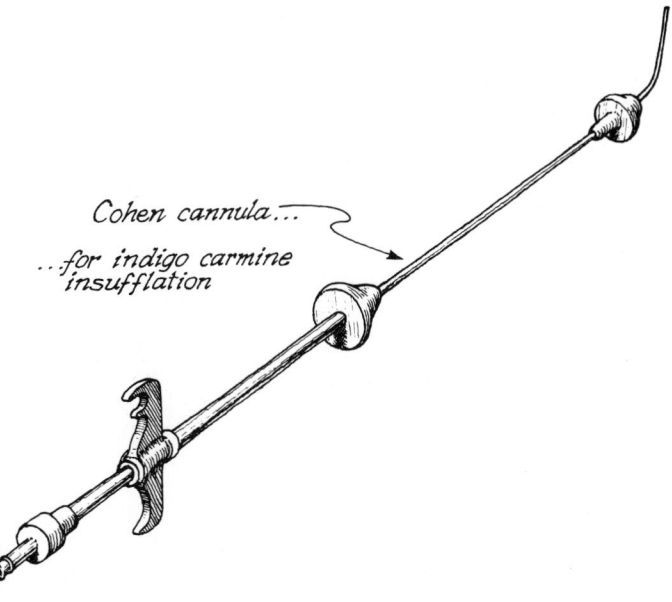

Cohen cannula...

...for indigo carmine insufflation

FIGURE 28–28. Uterine insufflator. (From Hulka, J. F. [1985]. *Textbook of laparoscopy*. Orlando, FL: Grune & Stratton.)

Matched generator and forceps

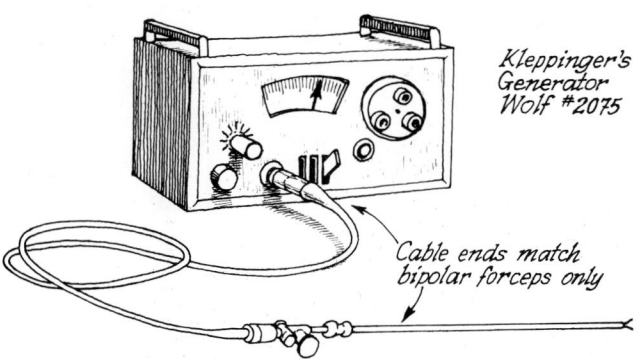

Kleppinger's Generator Wolf #2075

Cable ends match bipolar forceps only

FIGURE 28–29. Bipolar system. (From Hulka, J. F. [1985]. *Textbook of laparoscopy*. Orlando, FL: Grune & Stratton.)

Various sizes of trocars and sleeves
Aspiration or irrigator
Syringes
Sterile IV tubing
Electrosurgical unit (Fig. 28–29)
Various 3- and 5-mm bipolar and monopolar forceps, scissors, graspers, and electrical cords (Fig. 28–30)

Drugs and Solutions

Normal saline (0.9% sodium chloride), 250 ml, is used with 5 ml of indigo carmine added, to check for tubal patency. Normal saline, 1000 ml, or lactated Ringer solution may also be used to irrigate the pelvis.

Physiological Monitoring

Because the procedure is performed endoscopically, blood loss is minimal. A Foley catheter is inserted into the patient's bladder and usually discontinued at the end of the procedure.

Specimens and Cultures

A D&C may be performed at the end of the procedure; therefore, curettage specimens are possible. All specimens are sent to the pathology laboratory routinely unless otherwise indicated.

Physician's Orders

Refer to the discussion of tuboplasty.

Laboratory and Diagnostic Studies

In addition to screening for recurrence of ovarian carcinoma, all patients require urinalysis and CBC. Results should be within normal limits. Patients with ovarian carcinoma require routine tests and additional ultrasound. Normal levels should be found in all test results.

Procedure

Incision and Exposure

No incision is made for the vaginal part of the procedure. Exposure of the cervix is obtained with a Sims retractor. The abdominal incision is made with a No. 11 blade, through the umbilicus.

Details

After the patient is placed in the lithotomy position, the legs are rotated downward to allow access to the

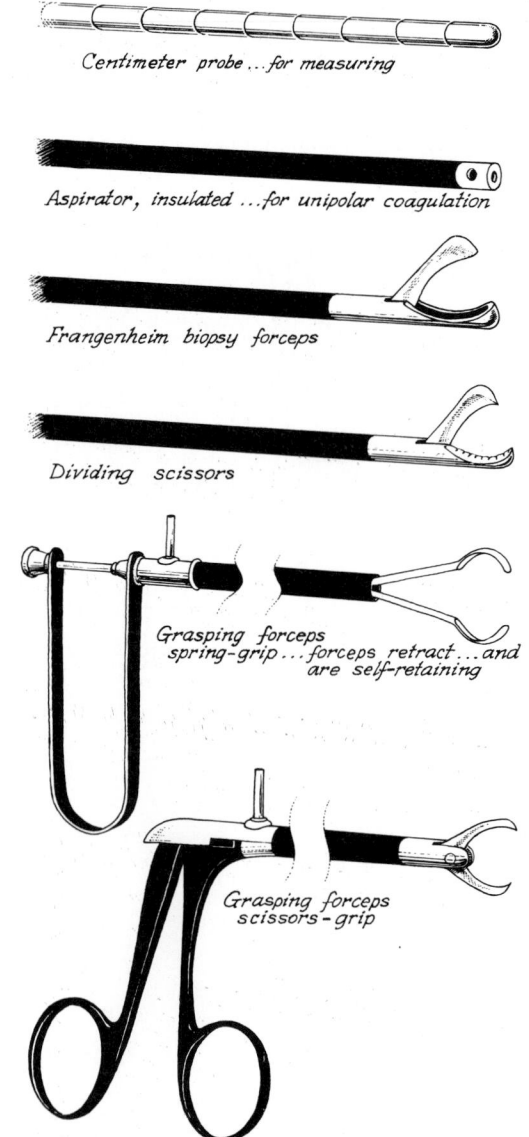

Centimeter probe . . . for measuring

Aspirator, insulated . . . for unipolar coagulation

Frangenheim biopsy forceps

Dividing scissors

Grasping forceps spring-grip . . . forceps retract . . . and are self-retaining

Grasping forceps scissors-grip

FIGURE 28–30. Manipulating instruments. (From Hulka, J. F. [1985]. *Textbook of laparoscopy*. Orlando, FL: Grune & Stratton.)

abdomen. A Foley catheter is inserted into the bladder and attached to a urinary drainage bag. Next, a Sims retractor is used to expose the cervix, after which a tenaculum is used to grasp the cervix. A Jarcho or Spackman cannula is inserted into the cervix and attached to the tenaculum.

Attention is focused on the abdomen. Towel clips are used to grasp the subumbilical area of the abdominal wall. A small incision is made with the No. 11 blade. The towel clips are elevated to allow easy advancement of the Verres needle. After the needle is in place, the carbon dioxide tubing is attached. One liter of carbon dioxide is allowed into the peritoneum, after which tympanic sound of percussion is tested at the suprapubic region, to indicate free diffusion of the gas in the peritoneal cavity. When 3 to 5 L of gas is in the abdomen, there is usually adequate distention. The Verres needle is removed at this time.

The incision is extended to allow for the 8-mm trocar and sleeve. After the sleeve is in the cavity, the trocar is removed. The laparoscope is inserted into the sleeve and the gas reconnected. The uterus is manipulated by holding the vaginal apparatus already in the vagina.

If a second puncture is needed, the lower abdominal wall is illuminated to select an avascular site for the incision. A small incision is made. A 3- or 5-mm trocar and sleeve are used. The surgeon may look through the laparoscope and use the second incision for operative instruments.

Indigo carmine may be injected through the Jarcho or Spackman cannula to check for tubal patency. Via the laparoscope, the dye may be seen flowing through the fallopian tubes, with any obstruction noted.

For tubal ligation, a 10-mm setup is used instead of the 8-mm trocar and sleeve. An operative laparoscope and electrocoagulation forceps are used. A cord is connected to the Kleppinger forceps, and each fallopian tube is thoroughly burned twice.

Closure

The laparoscope is removed from the sleeve. Carbon dioxide is suppressed from the abdomen. The sleeve is removed. If a second puncture apparatus was used, it is removed in the same fashion. All incisions are closed with 4–0 Vicryl suture. Antibiotic ointment and adhesive bandages are used for dressings.

The vaginal apparatus is gently removed, and the cervix is checked for any bleeding. Pressure is used to stop any bleeding that may occur.

Postoperative Care

The patient is taken to the postanesthesia care unit for a short time. Any bleeding is checked and noted. The patient is discharged the same day. The patient is instructed to take her temperature two times per day for 1 week and report if it is more than 100°F. Acetaminophen should be used for mild pain. Activity may be gradually increased. Referred pain may be experienced in the arm.

Potential Surgical Complications

Infection
Hemorrhage

PELVIC EXENTERATION

Definition

Pelvic exenteration is extensive surgery that involves the removal of fallopian tubes, ovaries, uterus, cervix, pelvic nodes, bladder, and distal ureters, rectum, and pelvic floor. In all instances, this procedure is an attempt to give a second chance for life, when nothing else is possible or recommended.

Indications

Pelvic exenteration is indicated in patients with carcinoma of the cervix who, after radiation therapy for stage IV disease, have tumor that recurs and erodes into the bladder and the rectum.

Related Surgical Procedures

Anterior exenteration
Posterior exenteration

Perioperative Nursing Implications

Anesthesia

These patients are premedicated before arriving in the OR suite. In many instances, an epidural catheter is inserted before anesthesia induction and is used for pain control postoperatively.

A general endotracheal anesthetic is used for the surgical procedure. Fentanyl is the most common narcotic used, with halothane, nitrous oxide, and enflurane used as inhalation drugs. Owing to the length of the procedure, arterial catheters are inserted.

Blood loss during the procedure can be excessive; blood samples are sent to the laboratory at regular intervals for arterial blood gas content analysis. Blood transfusions are always given. The circulating nurse should be available for retrieval and delivery of blood samples to the laboratory.

A nasogastric tube is requested by the surgeon after the procedure has begun.

Position

The patient is placed in the modified dorsal lithotomy position. To allow access by the anesthesiologist, both arms are extended on arm boards. The patient is also provided with an eggcrate mattress. Both legs should be wrapped with elastic (Ace) bandages or antiembolism stockings.

Creation and Maintenance of the Sterile Field

The skin should be shaved and prepared to include the total abdomen, the upper thighs, the perineum, and the internal vagina. The preparation is performed with povidone-iodine solution. The grounding pad is placed on the lower thigh.

The patient is draped with laparotomy as well as vaginal drapes. Two instrument tables are prepared for pelvic exenteration (upper or abdominal and lower or perineal). Both tables are set up at the beginning of the procedure. The scrub nurse may be positioned to the patient's right, with the instrument table close at hand. If a Mayo stand is used, it is positioned over the patient's right leg for the abdominal part of the procedure. The electrosurgical unit is placed to the right of the patient's head.

Equipment and Supplies

Upper table
    Major gynecology set (see above)
    Gastric and bowel set
    Hemoclips (medium and large)
    Pushers
    Magnetic pad
    Colostomy bags
    60-ml syringes (for washings)
    All other basic laparotomy instruments
    Skin staples
Available
    Autosuture
    Small Allis clamps
Lower table
    Dissecting set
    Plastic surgery set
    Surgical sponges
    Suction tubing
    Electrosurgical pencil
    Wound drains

Drugs and Solutions

Washings are obtained during the abdominal part of the procedure. A 1000-ml bag of Normosol-R is poured from a sterile spout into a solution basin with 5000 U of heparin added. Sixty-milliliter syringes are filled with the solution, and Pomeroy adaptors are attached. Each washing is then placed in sterile containers. No. 16 red rubber catheters may be used to obtain gutter washings. Warm irrigation solution is available for use.

Physiological Monitoring

The circulating nurse is available if requested to catheterize the patient. The catheter is removed after the ureters are severed from the bladder. Both the circulating and scrub nurses should be aware of blood loss and irrigating fluids used during the procedure. Blood loss is usually excessive.

Specimens and Cultures

For each washing taken, a separate cytology specimen form must be used. Samples may be pelvis, right and left subdiaphragm, and right and left gutters. Specimens include the uterus, the ovaries, the fallopian tubes, the bladder, the distal ureters, the rectum, and the lymph nodes.

The circulating nurse should have a large number of stamped pathology laboratory forms, printed patient labels, and specimen containers for routine and frozen sections.

Physician's Orders

The evening before surgery the patient must have a cleansing enema and shower. NPO orders are in effect after midnight, with a regular meal given for dinner. As ordered by the anesthesiologist, a sleeping pill is given.

Laboratory and Diagnostic Studies

The patient must have CBC, blood urea nitrogen, creatinine clearance, and liver function studies. Chest x-ray film and IV pyelogram are also ordered. In many instances, a barium enema is also included.

Procedure

Incision and Exposure

The abdomen is entered through a low midline incision. The retractor of choice is used. All bleeders are controlled with 3–0 Vicryl ties and suture ligatures, along with the electrocautery.

Details

The upper abdomen is explored. The right common iliac vein and artery are identified. Washings are taken at this time. Next, the aortic lymph nodes are palpated and any suspicious lymph nodes are removed, using scissors and forceps, and sent for frozen section examination. If the nodes are reported to be normal, the procedure continues.

The peritoneal incision is extended along the external

iliac vessels to the femoral canal. Again with the use of scissors and forceps, the lymphatic tissue is incised from the common veins.

The round ligaments (clamped with Heaney clamps) are ligated with heavy suture, cut, and tied, which opens the broad ligament. The lymphatic tissue is removed from the obturator fossa. The uterosacral ligaments are next clamped, cut, and tied at the pelvic brim.

The ureters are transected below the pelvic brim. The hypogastric artery and vein are clamped with Mixter clamps and tied at the bifurcation of the common iliac vessels. The lateral peritoneum of the mesentery of the rectosigmoid colon is opened. A Penrose drain is placed through an opening and used for retraction of the colon. The colon is clamped and transected with the GIA autosuture. The remaining mesentery to the colon is clamped and incised down to the sacrum.

The rectum is dissected from the sacrum and coccyx by blunt dissection. The stalks of rectum on both sides are clamped, incised, and tied down to the levator muscles.

The bladder is separated from the pubic symphysis. The lateral attachments of the bladder are clamped and incised on both sides. The anterior wall of the paravesical space and the posterior wall of the panrectal space are removed by dissecting the rectal stalks and bladder attachments.

The urethra is exposed and transected at the level of the levator, and the vagina is transected. The rectum is anastomosed to the descending colon. The intestinal loop urinary diversion is made from the sigmoid colon. The proximal sigmoid colon is transected with the GIA autosuture. The ureters are anastomosed to the sigmoid colon. The colon is anastomosed to the rectum. A wound drain is placed in the vagina. An omental flap is made and is moved into the pelvis. The omental flap holds the intestines out of the true pelvis.

Depending on the surgeon, it may not be necessary to do a perineal approach.

Closure

The abdomen is closed in the usual abdominal closure fashion.

Postoperative Care

The patient is admitted to the postanesthesia care unit or the surgical intensive care unit. Extensive postoperative care is required for these patients.

Nothing by mouth allowed until bowel sounds return
Intake and output measured
Daily weights obtained
Restricted bed rest

Dressing checks made
Antibiotic therapy given
Whole blood given as needed
Potassium administered as ordered by the surgeon
Heparin therapy given
Drains removed when no longer productive
Pain medications administered as needed

Discharge from the hospital is dependent on

ability to perform self-care
normal diet
adequate physical and mental ability
minimal drug requirements
stable weight
no fever for at least 5 days
understanding of possible complications

Potential Surgical Complications

Infection
Hemorrhage

ACKNOWLEDGMENT

This chapter is dedicated to my family, who always believed in me. But most of all this chapter is dedicated to my Grandmother "Annie," who always thought I was the greatest nurse who ever lived.

Bibliography

Cavanagh, D., Woods, R. E., O'Connor, T. C. F. (1978). *Obstetric emergencies* (2nd ed.). Hagerstown, MD: Harper & Row.

Cibils, L. A. (1975). *Gynecologic laparoscopy.* Philadelphia: Lea & Febiger.

Fuller, J. R. (1986). *Surgical technology: Principles and practice* (2nd ed.). Philadelphia: W. B. Saunders.

Golan, A., Barnan, S., Wexler, S., et al. (1989). Incompetence of the uterine cervix. *Obstretical and Gynecological Survey, 44,* 96–107.

Hacker, N. F., Moore, J. G. (Eds). (1986). *Essentials of obstetrics and gynecology.* Philadelphia: W. B. Saunders.

LeMaitre, G. D., Finnegan, J. A. (1980). *The patient in surgery: A guide for nurses* (4th ed.). Philadelphia: W. B. Saunders.

Newton, N., Newton, E. R. (Eds.). (1988). *Complications of gynecologic and obstetric management.* Philadelphia: W. B. Saunders.

Pivers, M. S. (Ed.). (1989). *Manual of gynecologic oncology and gynecology.* Boston: Little, Brown.

Rubin, S. C. (1988). Ovarian cancer: Diagnosis and surgical treatment. *AORN Journal, 47,* 1427–1437.

Sanz, L. E. (Ed.). (1988). *Gynecologic surgery.* Oradell, NJ: Medical Economics Books.

Siegler, A. M., Valle, R. F., Lindemann, H. J., Mencaglia, L. (1990). *Therapeutic hysteroscopy: Indications and techniques.* St. Louis: C. V. Mosby.

VanNagell, J. R., Barber, H. R. K. (Eds.). (1982). *Modern concepts of gynecologic oncology.* Boston, MA: John Wright.

Vontver, L. A., Gamette, K. R., Guzinski, G. M., et al. *Differential diagnosis: Gynecology.* New York: Arco Publishing.

Wells, M. P., Villano, K. (1985). Total abdominal hysterectomy: Perioperative patient care. *AORN Journal, 42* 368–373.

Wheeless, C. R., Jr. (1981). *Atlas of pelvic surgery.* Philadelphia: Lea & Febiger.

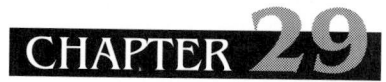
Otolaryngologic Surgery

Juan A. Bonilla and Gwendolyn Singleton

DEFINITION

The field of otolaryngologic surgery (i.e., ear, nose, throat, head, and neck surgery) has become extremely diversified during the past 50 years. The numerous different surgical procedures involving this part of the anatomy have led to subspecialty training in certain fields. The goals of most procedures in the ear, nose, and throat and the head and neck are

- the elimination of chronic infections
- the extirpation of tumors
- the preservation or improvement of hearing
- manipulation of the food and air passages when obstructed or injured

This chapter discusses the common procedures in the ear, within the nose and paranasal sinuses, and within the soft tissues of the oropharynx and head and neck.

ANATOMY

Ears

The *ears* are special sense organs located on both sides of the head and are involved in enabling hearing as well as maintaining balance. The ear is divided into the external, the middle, and the inner ear (Fig. 29–1). The external ear is made up of the visible auricle and the external auditory canal. The ear and canal act as a funnel for the transmission of air vibrations that are eventually transformed into understandable sound. The external auditory canal ends at the tympanic membrane, or eardrum. The eardrum is the division between the external ear and the middle ear.

On the other side of the tympanic membrane is the middle ear cavity, or tympanic cavity (see Fig. 29–1). Within the middle ear cavity are the three bones that are involved in the transmission and modification of sound energy. This energy is transported to the inner ear through the oval window. The first bone is called the malleus ("hammer"), the second is the incus ("anvil"), and the third bone is the stapes ("stirrup"). The footplate of the stapes sits within the oval window.

The inner ear is located deep within the temporal bone. It is composed of a bony portion as well as a membranous portion. The membranous portion contains a special fluid that is placed in motion when sound energy is transmitted from the tympanic membrane through the bones of hearing. Within the area called the bony labyrinth are the vestibule, the semicircular canals, and the cochlea. The vestibule and the semicir-

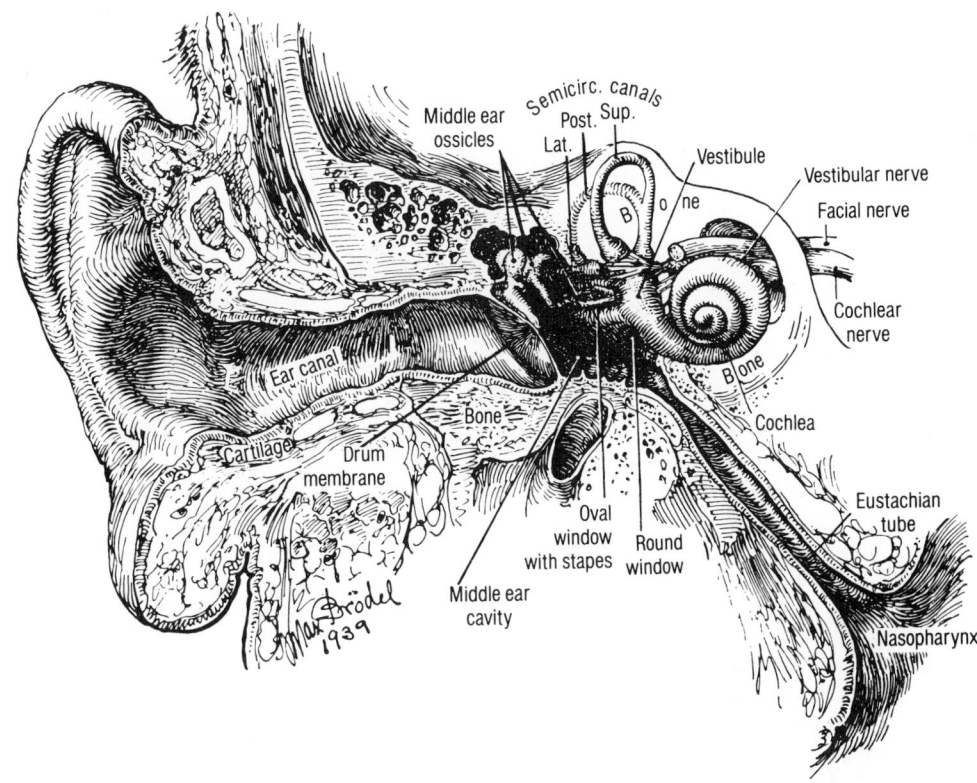

FIGURE 29–1. Ear anatomy. (From Adams, G., Boies, L., Hilger, P. [1989]. *Boies fundamentals of otolaryngology: A textbook of ear, nose, and throat diseases* [6th ed.] [p. 34]. Philadelphia: W. B. Saunders.)

cular canals are involved in balance mechanisms. The cochlea is the organ of hearing.

Nose and Paranasal Sinuses

The nose is made up of a combination of bone, cartilage, and mucous membrane (Fig. 29–2). The upper third of the external nose is composed of bone: the frontal, ethmoid, and maxillary bones. The lower two thirds of the nose is made up of cartilage. The internal nose contains openings on each side called the nares. The posterior openings into the nasopharynx are called choanae. The anterior skin-lined portion of the nasal cavity is called the vestibule.

The nasal septum divides the nose into two chambers

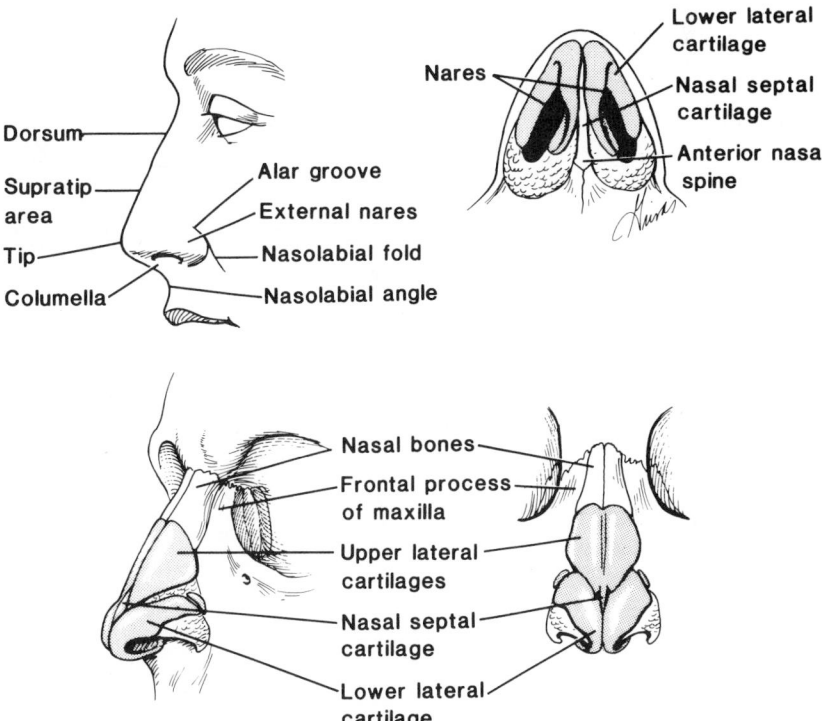

FIGURE 29–2. External portion of the nose. (From Adams, G., Boies, L., Hilger, P. [1989]. *Boies fundamentals of otolaryngology: A textbook of ear, nose, and throat diseases* [6th ed.] [p. 178]. Philadelphia: W. B. Saunders.)

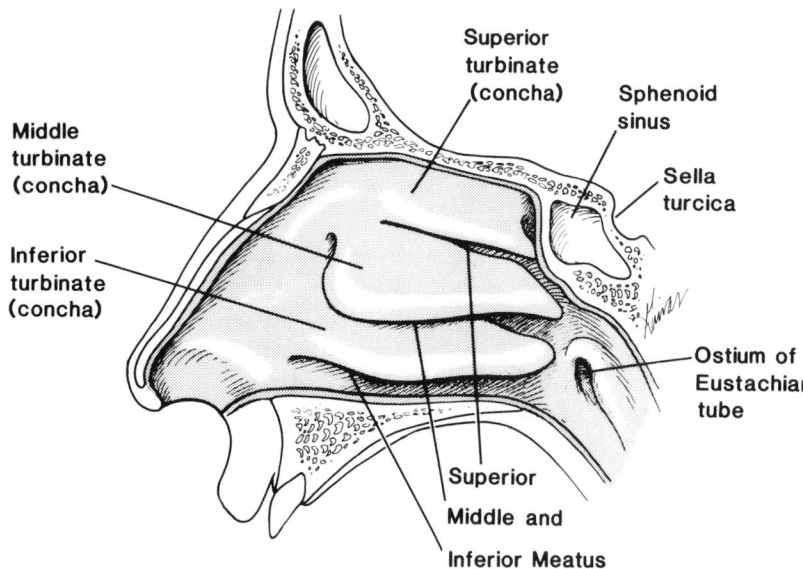

FIGURE 29–3. Anatomical structures of the lateral nasal wall. (From Adams, G., Boies, L., Hilger, P. [1989]. *Boies fundamentals of otolaryngology: A textbook of ear, nose, and throat diseases* [6th ed.] [p. 179]. Philadelphia: W. B. Saunders.)

lined by mucous membrane. The septum can become deviated and cause obstruction of the nasal airway. The nasal cavity communicates with the ear through the eustachian tube. The hard and soft palates divide the nasal cavity from the oral cavity. The lateral wall of the nasal cavity contains mucous membrane–lined bony projections called turbinates, or conchae (Fig. 29–3). Usually, there are bilateral inferior, middle, and superior turbinates. Rarely seen is a fourth turbinate called the supreme turbinate.

The grooves between the turbinates and the lateral nasal walls are called meati. The inferior meatus con-

tains the nasolacrimal duct opening. The lacrimal glands produce tears, which eventually flow into the nasal cavity. The middle meatus is the most important to know about. This is the one into which the maxillary, frontal, and anterior ethmoidal sinuses drain. The sphenoidal sinuses drain posteriorly and superiorly within the nasal cavity (Fig. 29–4).

The sinuses are air-filled pockets lined with mucous membranes. The maxillary sinuses are the largest and most accessible. The paranasal sinuses drain into the nasal cavity through openings called ostia. When these ostia become blocked, infections usually follow.

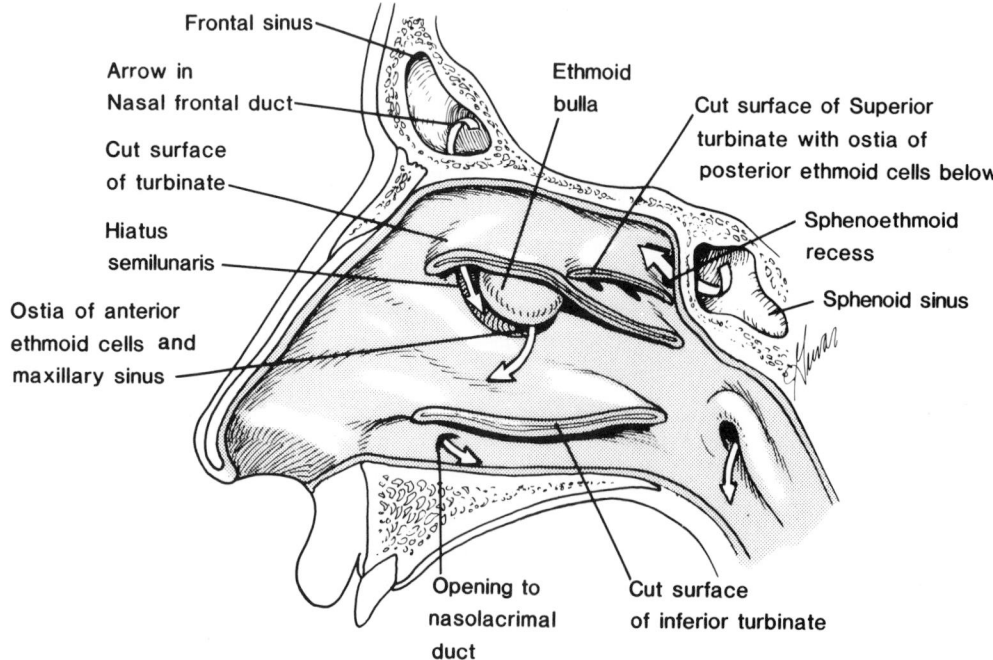

FIGURE 29–4. Lateral wall of the sinuses shown without the turbinates. *Arrows* indicate the flow of the drainage ducts. (From Adams, G., Boies, L., Hilger, P. [1989]. *Boies fundamentals of otolaryngology: A textbook of ear, nose, and throat diseases* [6th ed.] [p. 179]. Philadelphia: W. B. Saunders.)

The nasal cavity has a rich vascular supply from both the external and internal carotid arteries. The proximity to the brain and the orbit makes infections within the nasal cavity and sinuses potentially dangerous.

Tonsils and Adenoids

The *tonsils* are found within the oropharynx, which is posterior to the oral cavity (Fig. 29–5). The tonsils are part of the ring of Waldeyer of lymphoid tissue present in the throat. The tonsils are found between the folds of mucosa known as the anterior and posterior tonsillar pillars. They are usually seen on either side of the throat when the mouth is opened and the tongue is depressed. The ease of visualization depends on the size of the tonsils.

In contrast, the *adenoid* tissue, which is often called a pharyngeal tonsil, is not easily visualized. The adenoid tissue is found in the nasopharynx, which is the most superior portion of the throat. Although visualization of the adenoid is occluded by the soft palate and the uvula, the adenoid pad and the nasopharynx can be seen by using a mirror. In this indirect fashion, cooperative patients can be examined.

Parotid Gland

The *parotid gland* is the largest of the major salivary glands. The gland is found on either side of the face in

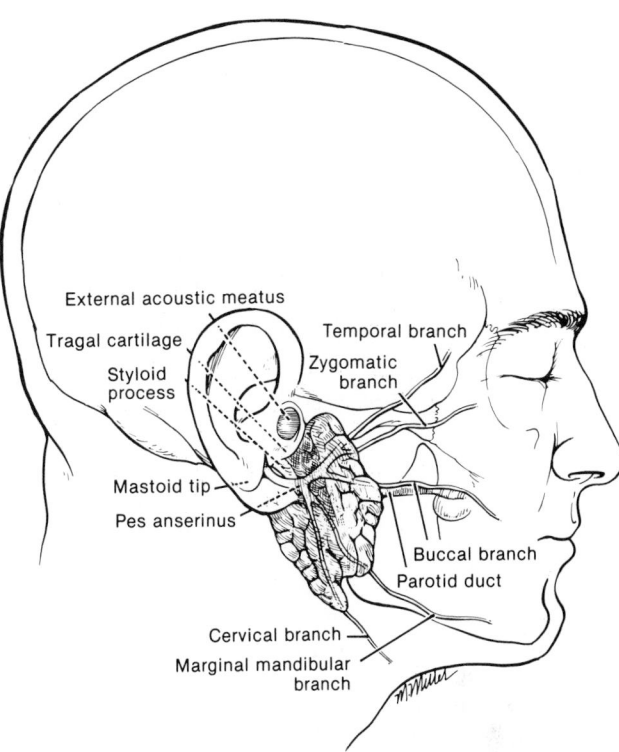

FIGURE 29–6. The parotid gland. (From Meyerhoff, W., Rice, D. [1992]. *Otolaryngology—Head and neck surgery* [p. 555]. Philadelphia: W. B. Saunders.)

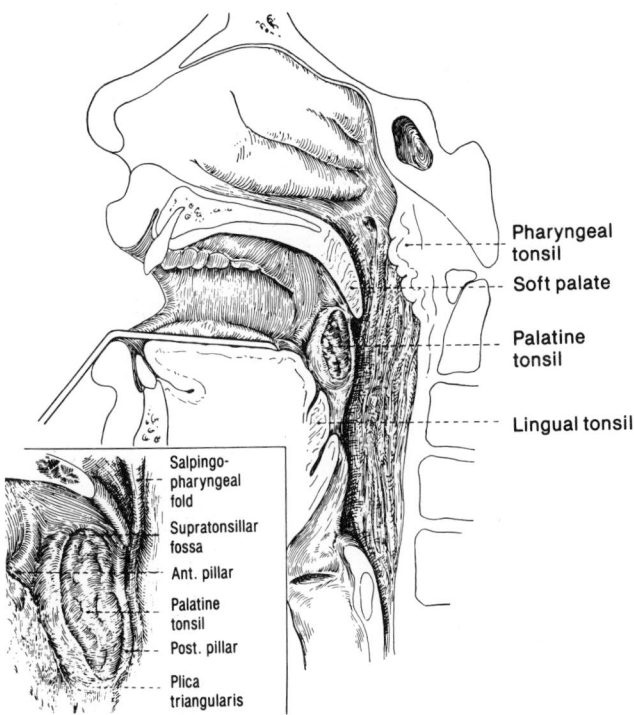

FIGURE 29–5. Tonsil and oropharynx. Inset shows the actual tonsil bed and surrounding tonsillar area. (From Adams, G., Boies, L., Hilger, P. [1989]. *Boies fundamentals of otolaryngology: A textbook of ear, nose, and throat diseases.* [6th ed.] [p. 276]. Philadelphia: W. B. Saunders.)

the area of the angle of the mandible (Fig. 29–6). The salivary glands deliver their secretory product, saliva, into the oral cavity and the oropharynx. Saliva functions as a lubricant and an acid buffer and also contributes to the digestion of food. Diseases affecting the salivary glands are seen as either alterations in the production of saliva or abnormalities of the gland itself.

The parotid gland consists of two portions. There is a superficial lobe, as well as a deep lobe that is in contact with the parapharyngeal space. The parotid gland empties its contents through the parotid duct (also known as Stensen duct). It enters the oral cavity opposite the second upper molar tooth.

The facial nerve is the most important structure associated intimately with the parotid gland. The most superficial portion of the facial nerve passes through the main substance of the parotid gland. It divides into five main branches: temporal, zygomatic, buccal, mandibular, and cervical. The mandibular branch is especially important because it lies deep under the platysma muscle in the neck.

Trachea

Examination of the neck involves identification of palpable structures (Fig. 29–7). In infants, the most easily palpable structures are different from those in the adult. In the adult, the most prominent structure in the neck is the thyroid cartilage, or the Adam's apple. This is usually found along the midline of the neck. Imme-

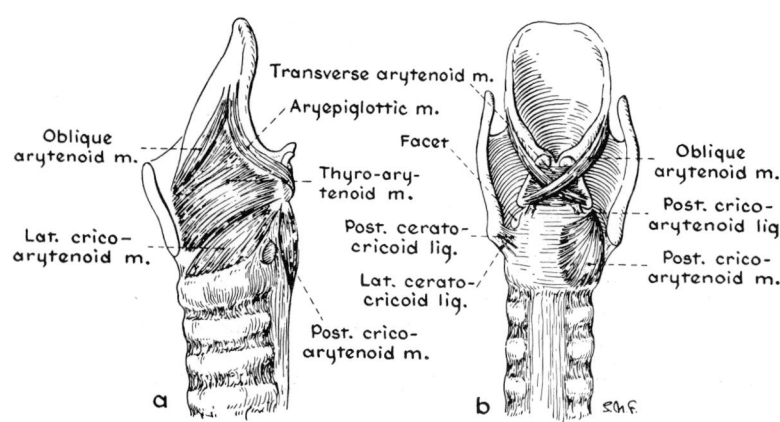

FIGURE 29–7. Trachea and thyroid cartilage. *a*, Side view. *b*, Posterior view. (From Adams, G., Boies, L., Hilger, P. [1989]. *Boies fundamentals of otolaryngology: A textbook of ear, nose, and throat diseases* [6th ed.] [p. 386]. Philadelphia: W. B. Saunders.)

diately below this prominent cartilage is another easily palpable structure—the cricoid cartilage. In adults, the cricothyroid membrane is easily palpable between the cricoid and the thyroid cartilage most of the time. The cricothyroid membrane can be entered in an emergency situation in most adults.

In infants up to 2 months of age, the most palpable structure is usually the hyoid bone. This horseshoe-shaped bone is found superior to the thyroid cartilage. Most infants and young children have short necks with a large amount of subcutaneous fat, which makes palpation difficult. In addition, the cartilages are much softer. Therefore, emergency access through the neck into a pediatric airway is much more difficult than in the adult.

Larynx

The *larynx* is found anteriorly between the lowermost portion of the pharynx superiorly and the trachea (windpipe) inferiorly (Fig. 29–8). It consists of three major cartilages supported by different ligaments and muscles. These cartilages are the thyroid cartilage, the cricoid cartilage directly beneath it, and the arytenoid cartilage, which is behind the thyroid gland and joined to the cricoid cartilage.

A function of the larynx is to modify the air being expelled from the lungs and allow this air column to be used by the tongue, cheeks, and lips to produce intelligible speech. Intelligible speech can still occur if the larynx is absent. The most important function of the

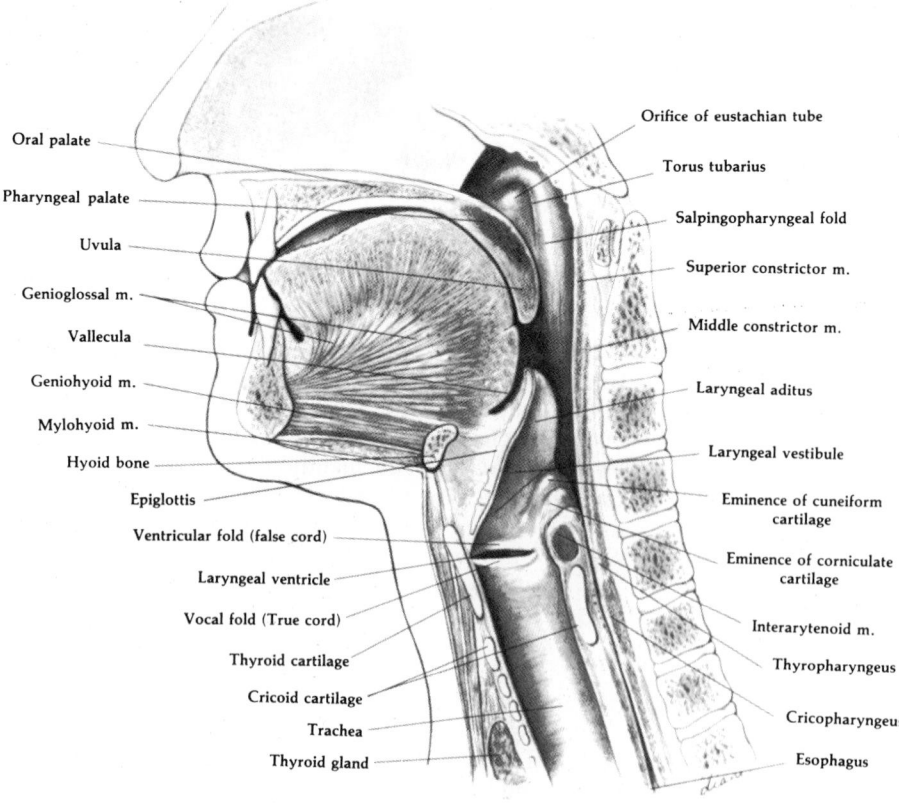

FIGURE 29–8. Larynx and neck. (From Bosma J. [1988]. Functional anatomy of the upper airway during development. In D. P. Matthew, G. Sant'Ambrogio [Eds.], *Respiratory function of the upper airway* [p. 51]. New York: Marcel Dekker, Inc.)

larynx, however, is not speech production but protection of the respiratory passages to prevent aspiration.

Within the larynx are found the vocal cords. There are false vocal cords, which are upper folds within the larynx, and true vocal cords. The vocal cords perform the vibratory function that aids in phonation. The vocal cords are innervated by the recurrent laryngeal nerve. This nerve originates from the vagus, or 10th cranial, nerve.

SURGICAL PROCEDURES OF THE EAR

The ear has been studied since ancient times. Hippocrates in 400 BC was the first to clearly describe acute otitis media. In the mid-17th century, Duverney, who is often called the father of otology, published the first monograph on otology. He was the first anatomist to describe the mastoid air cells communicating with the middle ear cavity. He also established that pus coming from the ear did not originate in the brain.

Infections of the ear and mastoid were deadly before the advent of antibiotics. The operations designed at the birth of otology revolved around the elimination of infection. It was not until the 19th century that operations to cure infection were successfully performed on a regular basis. In the early 1900s, the operating microscope added a new dimension to ear operations designed to cure infection and deafness. With the advent of antimicrobials, the necessity for operative intervention within the ear decreased dramatically. The most common surgical procedure performed in the ear today is the insertion of ventilation tubes.

Myringotomy

Definition and Indications

Myringotomy refers to the incision of the tympanic membrane (eardrum) to provide ventilation to the middle ear with a pressure-equalizing tube, to facilitate drainage of middle ear fluid, or to obtain cultures (Adams et al., 1989, p. 119).

Myringotomy is either diagnostic or therapeutic. It is usually performed on a pediatric patient who has had chronic middle ear effusions or recurrent acute otitis media. Other indications for this procedure include

- chronic serous otitis media that has not responded to conservative management
- chronic negative middle ear pressure and resultant atelectasis of the tympanic membrane
- the development of persistent negative middle ear pressure in patients undergoing hyperbaric oxygen treatment
- an accompaniment to reconstructive procedures in which the eustachian tube dysfunction is considered marginal (Adams et al., 1989, p. 120)

Related Surgical Procedures

None

Perioperative Nursing Implications

Anesthesia

Most myringotomies are performed under general inhalation anesthesia. The use of intravenous (IV) catheters is usually not necessary, but the decision is made by the anesthetist. The procedure can be performed under local anesthesia. This type of anesthetic, however, is typically reserved for older children and adults.

Position

The patient is placed in the supine position. After general anesthesia is induced and appropriate monitoring devices are placed, the procedure is initiated by turning the patient's head with the operative ear facing the surgeon.

Creation and Maintenance of the Sterile Field

Myringotomy is considered by some surgeons as a minor procedure. It does, however, deserve the same preparation as for any invasive surgical procedure. The ear is usually draped with sterile towels only. Before any sterile towels are placed, the microscope should be in position to be easily swung into the operative field. A sterile sheet may or may not be placed over the chest and body of the patient. The skin preparation is determined by the surgeon. Many surgeons use alcohol or iodophor solution. Some surgeons do not request skin preparation. If the ear is prepared, the circulating nurse should include the ear, the postauricular area, and the face. The scrub nurse may stand next to the surgeon or across from him or her and close to the Mayo stand.

Equipment and Supplies

A dedicated myringotomy tray should be available. Table 29–1 lists recommended instruments for a myringotomy set. The different types of ventilation tubes available can be confusing to the surgical staff. The ventilation tube is usually chosen by the surgeon before or at the time of the procedure. Therefore, it is wise to have the ventilation tubes located where they can be

TABLE 29–1. MYRINGOTOMY INSTRUMENTS

Wire loop or cerumen remover
Alligator forceps
Beaver handle and myringotomy blade (No. 7100 or 7120)
45-degree pick
90-degree pick
Rosen pick
Nos. 3, 5, and 7 Baron suction tubes

easily accessible to the operating room (OR) personnel. A microscope with either a 200- or a 250-mm focal length lens is most often used.

Drugs and Solutions

Normal saline
Iodophor solution
Otic antibiotic solution

Physiological Monitoring

Myringotomies are normally quick surgical procedures. The patient may or may not be intubated. The circulating nurse must be readily available to assist the anesthetist, especially during initial induction of and recovery from anesthesia.

Specimens and Cultures

A culture may be taken to determine the type of microorganism present.

Physician's Orders

The patient is given liquids when awake and is discharged when she or he is alert and stable.

Laboratory and Diagnostic Studies

Complete blood count (CBC) and urinalysis, if indicated, are obtained.

Procedure

Exposure and Incision

An ear speculum is inserted in the external auditory canal while the ear is viewed under the microscope. Cerumen is usually removed with cerumen spoons. After this is done, the ear can be irrigated with alcohol or the iodophor solution. Iodophor use is usually followed by copious irrigation with normal saline. After the tympanic membrane has been identified and described by the surgeon, a myringotomy scalpel is used to incise the tympanic membrane (Fig. 29–9). After the incision is made, it is imperative to have appropriate Baron suction tips that are used to aspirate any middle ear effusions. Because some of the effusions may be tenacious, duplicate suction catheters should be available.

Details

The various ventilation tubes are then inserted through the myringotomy incision using either alligator forceps or special introducers. Mounting of the ventilation tube is at the discretion of the surgeon. The scrub nurse should be aware of the preference of the surgeon. It is important at the time of mounting of the ventilation tube that a minimal amount of contact exists between the gloves of the scrub nurse or the surgeon and the ventilation tube. The ventilation tube should be primarily handled with the tip of the alligator forceps or the introducer. The alligator forceps or the introducer should be handed to the surgeon so that the surgeon does not have to look away from the microscope. A 45-degree pick or a curved Rosen pick may also be used for proper positioning of the tube.

Closure

After the tube is placed, an antibiotic solution may or may not be used by the surgeon. If it is used, it is introduced by placing the drops through the ear speculum or with a syringe. A cotton ball is usually placed in the ear canal after the instillation of antibiotic solutions. Occasionally, a small amount of bleeding occurs. Because blood can occlude the lumen of the ventilation tube, vasoconstricting solutions should be available for instillation into the ear before the patient's departure from the OR.

Postoperative Care

After the procedure is completed, the patient is awakened in the OR and is then transported to the recovery room. Because the procedure is short, the patient usually awakens quickly. If the patient is a child, the postanesthesia period can be traumatic. The child should be reunited with the parent as soon as it is feasible. There is no dressing. However, cotton may be placed in the ears.

Potential Surgical Complications

Otorrhea
Bleeding

Tympanoplasty

Definition and Indications

Tympanoplasty is a broad term that has been used to refer to any procedure performed to repair perforations within the eardrum or repair defects of middle ear structures for the purpose of restoring sound conduction pathways. Simple tympanoplasty can be done to protect middle ear structures from direct exposure owing to loss of the membrane cover. Tympanoplasties are classified as types 1 through 5.

Type 1 tympanoplasty is the simple closure of a perforation in the tympanic membrane. Usually, for this type, the ossicular chain is normal. The operation involves placing a graft on the tympanic membrane in the area of the perforation. The graft acts as a scaffold for epithelialization and closure of the perforation. This restores the continuity of the tympanic membrane to the ossicular chain. Different grafts can be used to include vein and perichondrium (the covering immedi-

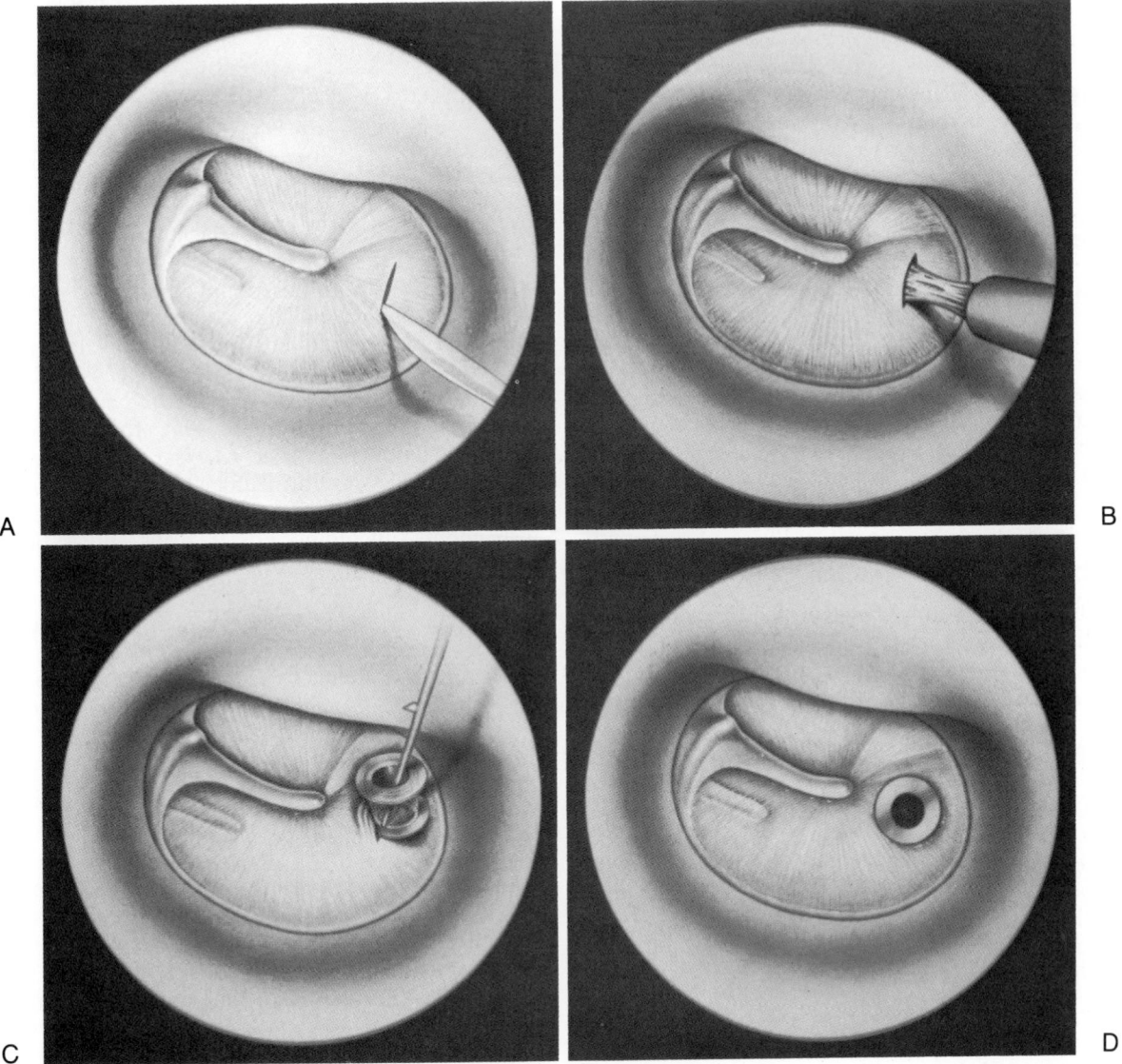

A

B

C

D

FIGURE 29–9. *A,* Myringotomy incision. *B,* Aspiration of fluid. *C,* Insertion of ventilation tube. *D,* Ventilation tube in place. (From Paparella M. M., Shumrick, D. A. [eds.], *Otolaryngology* [Vol. 2, p. 90]. Philadelphia: W. B. Saunders.)

ately next to cartilage). The most common material used, however, is the fascia covering the temporalis muscle. This muscle is found within the scalp in the area just above the ear.

Tympanoplasty types 2 through 4 also involve placing a graft on the ossicles. In these types of tympanoplasties, one or more of the ossicles has been destroyed owing to infection. In type 5 tympanoplasty, the graft is placed immediately next to a small opening in one of the semicircular canals. The graft seals the middle ear and provides preservation of sound conduction. This is performed when all of the ossicles are missing.

Related Surgical Procedures

None

Perioperative Nursing Implications

Anesthesia

Tympanoplasty can be performed under local anesthesia, but general anesthesia is usually preferred by most surgeons. One of the techniques used is hypotensive anesthesia, which helps create a bloodless field. If nitrous oxide is used, it is discontinued before the graft is placed. Nitrous oxide diffuses into the middle ear cavity and leads to disruption of the grafting procedure.

Position

Most likely, the surgeon performs this procedure while sitting. Before transferring the patient to the OR bed, turn the bed so that the patient's head rests on the foot of the bed and the feet are positioned at the head of the bed. This facilitates placement of the base of the microscope under the OR bed and enables the surgeon to position his or her feet under the bed. The patient is placed in the supine position, close to the edge of the bed, with the head turned and the operative ear up and stabilized. A doughnut-shaped stockinet or small headrest support device is used to stabilize the head and protect the nonoperative ear. The circulating nurse should ensure that the nonoperative ear is within the hole of the doughnut or headrest to avoid pressure on the ear.

Creation and Maintenance of the Sterile Field

The ear and the hair immediately around the ear may or may not be shaved. The operating microscope is usually placed at the head of the OR bed. It is draped in a sterile fashion, because it will be manipulated by the surgeon. At times, the surgeon may examine the ear before the circulating nurse scrubs and prepares the patient. Therefore, a simple myringotomy set should be available for this purpose. After the patient's head has been positioned, the ear can be prepared with a variety

of antibacterial solutions. The preparation should include the ear, the postauricular area, and the face just past the midline.

The eye on the operative side is taped closed with an eye occluder. After this is done, a plastic drape with a preformed hole can be pressed onto the skin with the ear protruding through the hole. Lint-free drapes are preferred. It is imperative that gloves used by the surgeon and the scrub assistant be free from powder and lint. Formation of granulomas within the middle and inner ear has been reported to cause irreversible hearing loss.

Equipment and Supplies

As for any otological procedure, a proper assortment of otological instruments is necessary. Most of these instruments are used in conjunction with the operating microscope. Because many of these instruments are unique for otological procedures, it is important for the scrub assistant to be fully familiar with the instruments. Different sets are available commercially and include a variety of fine instruments for the mobilization of tissue within a small space. A variety of fine ossicular instruments are also essential. Appropriate suction catheters are also found within these sets. In addition to the microinstruments, a basic surgical set should also be available. This should include fine scissors, such as iris and Metzenbaum scissors, to harvest a graft. Bone instruments, including power drills, must be readily available if drilling becomes necessary during a simple tympanoplasty.

Table 29–2 lists a sample tympanoplasty set. Other supplies include bone wax, oxidized cellulose, absorbable hemostatic sponges, and a nerve stimulator (in rare cases the facial nerve may be encountered). The surgeon may use .05 Silastic sheeting rather than the patient's temporalis fascia autograft.

Drugs and Solutions*

Lidocaine (Xylocaine) 1% with 1:100,000 epinephrine (Adrenalin)
1:1000 epinephrine
Neosporin ointment
Colistin sulfate (Coly-Mycin) otic suspension
Absorbable hemostatic sponges or oxidized cellulose
Tis-U-Sol solution

Physiological Monitoring

Tympanoplasty surgery can be a short procedure or it can take several hours, depending on the surgeon's findings. If the procedure is performed under local anesthesia, constant monitoring of the patient's electro-

---

*The drugs and solutions listed in this chapter are examples of the agents that the surgeon may choose to use during the procedure. The types of agents employed vary with the preferences of the surgeon.

TABLE 29–2. **TYMPANOPLASTY SET**
Sickle knife
Lancet knife
Round (weapon) knife
Flap knife
Rosen knife
Roller knife
Stapes knife
Tympanoplasty knife
Micro–cup forceps: right, left, and straight
Alligator forceps: fine plain or serrated
Bellucci scissors
45-degree pick
90-degree pick
Rosen pick
Drum elevator
Gimick elevator
Duckbill elevator (3 sizes)
Fisch excavators: left and right
Microcurets
Iris and tenotomy scissors
Iris forceps with and without teeth
Teflon block

cardiogram (ECG), blood pressure, and oxygen saturation by pulse oximetry is essential. The patient is asked to lie supine with the head turned in one position for a period of time; therefore, the patient's comfort level is monitored constantly. Comfort measures such as padding for elbows and heels are supplied after positioning the patient on the OR bed. A pillow under the knees is offered to reduce pressure on the back. The patient may even be placed in a flexed (lawn chair) position for comfort, with care not to compromise adequate operating position for the surgeon.

If the patient is placed under general anesthesia, the same comfort measures are applied. The circulating nurse must be readily available to assist the anesthetist during induction of and emergence from anesthesia. The suction must be in close reach of the anesthetist.

Specimens and Cultures

Specimens may include excess tissue used for the graft and/or remnants of the tympanic membrane. Cultures are taken as indicated by clinical findings.

Physician's Orders

The patient is given a regular diet. The IV catheter should be kept open until the patient is taking liquids successfully. Antiemetic and analgesic drugs are administered. The patient can ambulate depending on comfort level.

Laboratory and Diagnostic Studies

CBC, urinalysis, chest x-ray films, and ECG are obtained as indicated. The surgeon may also order

- audiogram with pure-tone air and bone conduction curves with adequate narrow-band masking as well as speech discrimination scores

- mastoid x-ray films
- computed tomographic (CT) scans (may help in determining ossicular defects and cholesteatoma size and extension)

Procedure

Incision and Exposure

The operation usually begins with an injection of a local anesthetic mixed with epinephrine. The injections are performed in a four-quadrant fashion within the external auditory canal. Incisions are then made within the canal skin at 6 and 12 o'clock positions. These incisions are connected with different canal microknives. This forms a flap. The flap is raised medially until the entire fibrous portion of the tympanic membrane is identified.

Before beginning the procedure or at the surgeon's discretion, the graft can be taken from the temporalis muscle fascia. The incision is made within the hairline using standard surgical scalpels. The incision is carried down through the subcutaneous tissue until the fascia of the muscle can be identified (Fig. 29–10). A portion of the fascial layer is removed that is slightly larger than the size of the perforation to be repaired. After the graft has been harvested, it is usually given to the surgical assistant or the scrub person for preparation. The graft is prepared by compressing it between a fascia press forceps. Then it is placed on a Teflon block for drying. A dry graft allows the surgeon better pliability during the grafting stage.

Details

After the perforation is identified, different micropicks are used to freshen the margin of the perforation. This can also be done with fine curets or cup-biting forceps. Next, the previously created tympanomeatal flap is raised superiorly (Fig. 29–11). Absorbable gelatin sponge is then placed within the middle ear cavity to act as a support for the graft. The graft is then taken and placed in the medial surface of the tympanic membrane. After the graft is placed in its proper position, the tympanomeatal flap is brought down to its normal position. The external auditory canal is then packed with absorbable gelatin. Antibiotic solution or ointment can also be used for this purpose.

Closure

A wide variety of techniques exist for packing the external auditory canal. The scrub person should inquire as to the surgeon's preference. If a simple tympanoplasty was performed without any external incisions, the ear can be dressed in a variety of ways. Dressings are not necessary, however, if the incisions were all within the external auditory canal. A mastoid dressing is described below. The area of grafting is closed in a standard fashion using absorbable suture for the subcutaneous tissue and nonabsorbable suture for the skin.

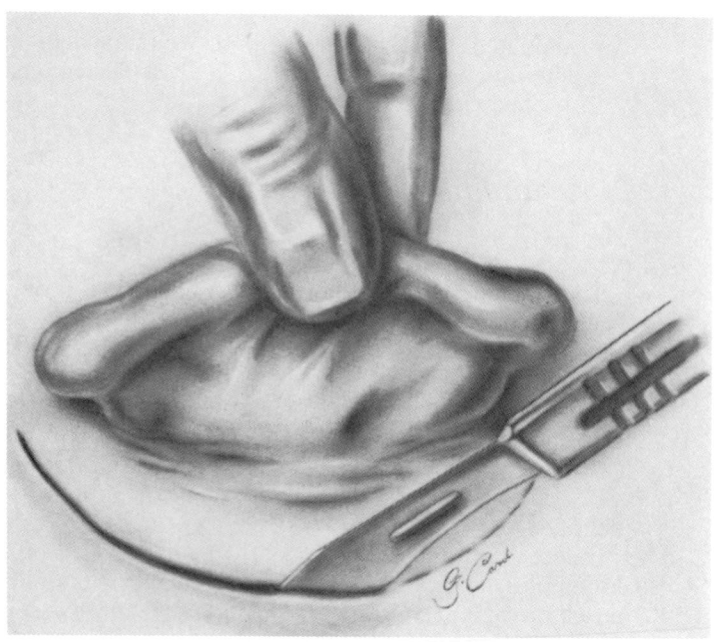

FIGURE 29–10. Incision for tympanoplasty. (From Glasscock, M. E., III, Miller, G. W. [1976]. Intact canal wall tympanoplasty in the management of cholesteatoma. *Laryngoscope, 86,* 1639.)

Postoperative Care

The patient is immediately transported to the recovery room. Typical postoperative orders include the administration of antinausea medication as well as pain medication. Most tympanoplasties of the simple type can be performed on an outpatient basis. The patients are instructed to keep water away from the operative ear until further advised. If the procedure was performed through the external canal only, the dressing may be an adhesive bandage (Band-Aid). If a postauricular incision was created, however, a pressure bandage of fluffs (Kerlix) and Kling bandage is used to wrap around the head and over the operative ear.

Potential Surgical Complications

As with any wound, there is always the potential for infection within the operated area. The graft site rarely becomes infected. However, hematomas forming in this area have been reported. Additional complications include the failure of the graft to take, with a persistence of the perforation.

Mastoidectomy

Definition and Indications

A *mastoidectomy* is performed for eradication of the mastoid air cells to relieve complications of acute or chronic mastoiditis. Mastoidectomy may or may not be done in conjunction with a tympanoplasty. In addition, a mastoidectomy may be performed along with an ossicular reconstruction.

A *simple* mastoidectomy involves a postauricular incision through which the air cells of the mastoid process are eradicated by drilling through the bone with burrs. The external canal and the middle ear are at times not involved (Fig. 29–12). A *modified radical* mastoidectomy involves a removal of the portion of the ear canal, allowing drainage from the mastoid into the canal. The tympanic membrane and middle ear ossicles are preserved. A *radical* mastoidectomy is performed for severe chronic mastoiditis. In this procedure, the middle ear cavity and the mastoid antrum are combined into a large

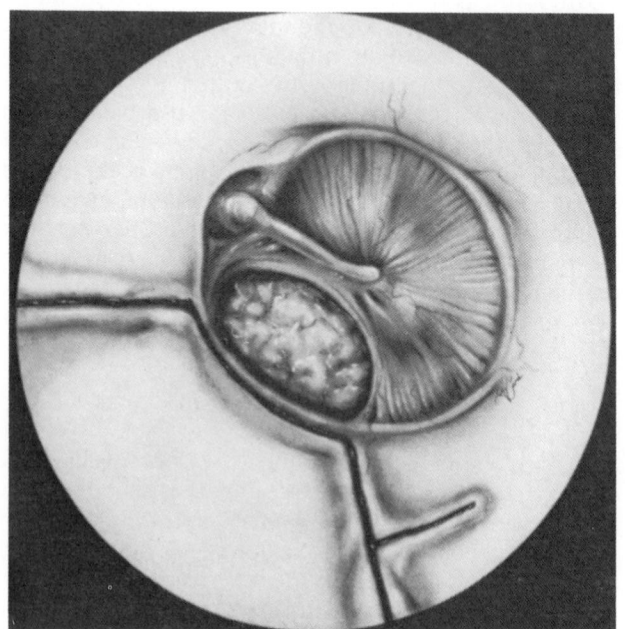

FIGURE 29–11. Perforation and flaps for tympanoplasty. (From Glasscock, M. E., III, Miller, G. W. [1976]. Intact canal wall tympanoplasty in the management of cholesteatoma. *Laryngoscope, 86,* 1639.)

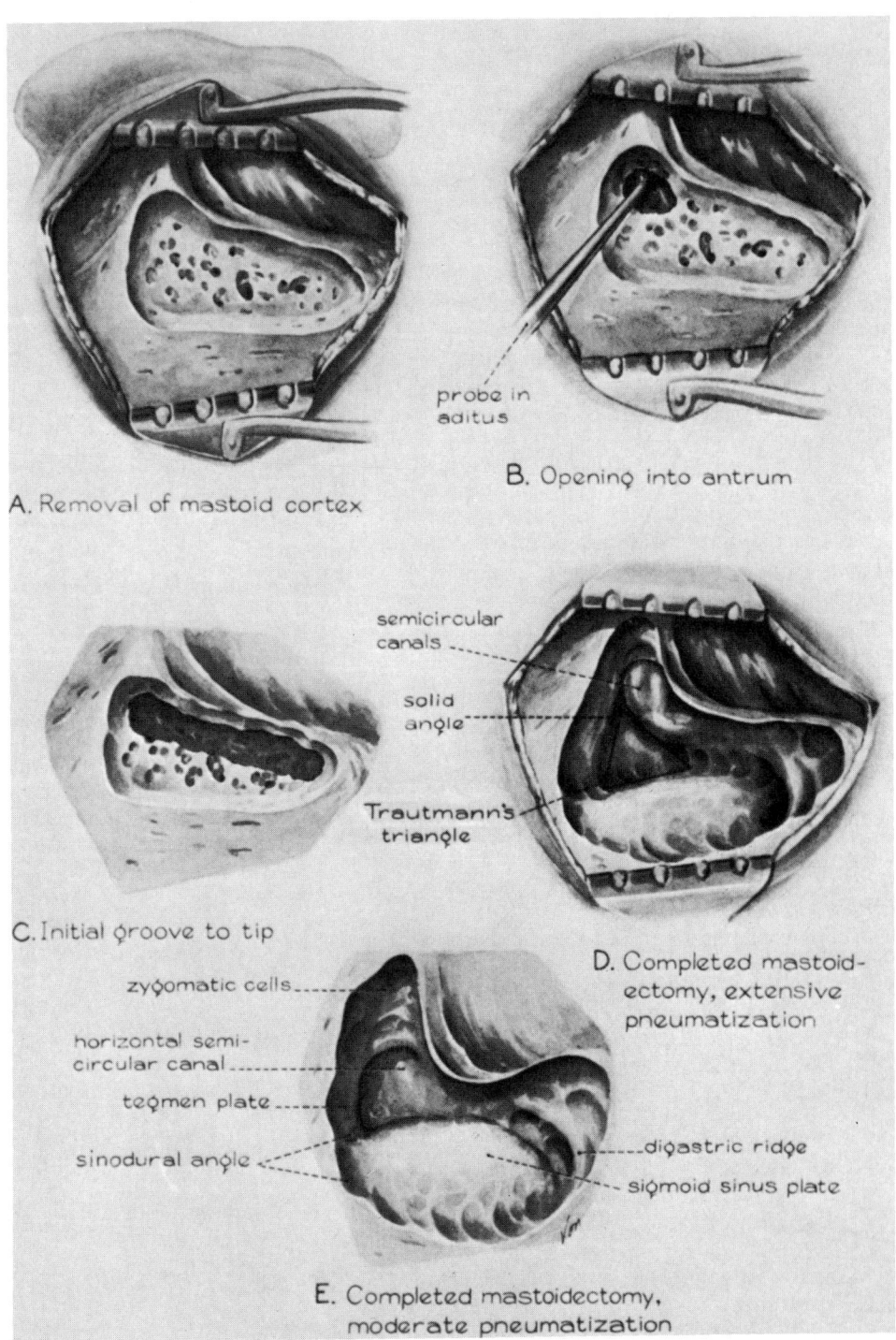

A. Removal of mastoid cortex

B. Opening into antrum

probe in aditus

C. Initial groove to tip

semicircular canals

solid angle

Trautmann's triangle

D. Completed mastoid-ectomy, extensive pneumatization

zygomatic cells

horizontal semi-circular canal

tegmen plate

sinodural angle

digastric ridge

sigmoid sinus plate

E. Completed mastoidectomy, moderate pneumatization

FIGURE 29–12. Simple mastoidectomy. (From Glasscock, M., Shambaugh, G. [1990]. *Surgery of the ear* [4th ed.] [p. 225]. Philadelphia: W. B. Saunders.)

single cavity. Periodically, this cavity is inspected and cleaned on an outpatient basis. Usually, the ossicles and the tympanic membrane are entirely removed. Throughout these procedures, an additional structure that becomes important to identify and protect is the facial nerve.

Related Surgical Procedures

None

Perioperative Nursing Implications

Anesthesia

As for other ear procedures, mastoidectomy is performed using general hypotensive anesthesia. Before the procedure is started, the surgeon often injects a combination of local anesthetic with epinephrine.

Position

The patient's head is turned with the operative side up and stabilized. As for tympanoplasty, the OR bed is reversed before positioning the patient. The basic principles described above are also used for mastoidectomy as well as other middle ear procedures.

Creation and Maintenance of the Sterile Field

The sterile field is created by shaving behind the ear and preparing the ear and the surrounding area with an antibiotic solution. The ear is covered with a plastic drape with a preformed hole. The operating microscope is also draped with a sterile plastic drape.

Equipment and Supplies

In addition to a tympanoplasty set, the following instruments should be included for a mastoidectomy:

- Elevators
- Incudostapedial joint knife
- Myringotomy knife
- Picks: 90 degree and 40 degree; curved, straight, and right angle
- Knives: Guilford, tympanoplastic sickle shaped
- Knives: Rosen, House
- Strut caliper
- Tabb knives: 45 degree and 90 degree
- Weitlaner retractors, Wullstein retractors
- Rongeurs
- Suction irrigation system
- Rosen suction tube, sizes 18 to 24
- House adapter
- Absorbable gelatin sponge (Gelfoam) press
- Shea ear specula (Mailhot and Slezak, 1992, pp. 8–9)

Micro ear instruments and an air-powered drill with a variety of burrs must be available. The burrs are of two types. These are designated as cutting burrs and diamond burrs. Cottonoids and cotton balls moistened with Tis-U-Sol are often used. They must always be counted. At times, solutions of diluted epinephrine are used to assist in hemostasis. Prosthetic devices for reconstruction of the ossicular chain must be readily available in a wide variety of types and sizes. Because the facial nerve is at risk during a mastoidectomy, nerve stimulators may be used to identify the facial nerve. Evoked potential audiometry can also be used to monitor the facial nerve.

Drugs and Solutions

Lidocaine 1% with 1:100,000 epinephrine
Gelfoam 100
1:1000 epinephrine
Cortisporin ointment
Cortisporin Otic suspension
Tis-U-Sol Solution

Physiological Monitoring

During mastoidectomy, the patient is placed under general anesthesia (see the discussion of tympanoplasty).

Specimens and Cultures

Mastoid bone, granulation tissue, and/or cholesteatoma

Physician's Orders

The patient is given IV fluids and antibiotics. A regular diet is ordered. Antiemetic and analgesic drugs are administered. The patient is advised not to use straws with liquids and to sneeze with the mouth open.

Laboratory and Diagnostic Studies

See the discussion of tympanoplasty.

Procedure

Incision and Exposure

Mastoidectomy can involve only a postauricular incision. Most often, however, the procedure is combined with a tympanoplasty. This is better known as a tympanomastoidectomy. The procedure is started by palpating the tip of the mastoid process. After external landmarks have been identified, a postauricular incision is made close to the postauricular sulcus. This incision is made with a surgical blade or cautery. The microscope is usually not used for this portion of the procedure.

A dissection is carried down to the temporalis fascia superiorly and down through the periosteum just below the temporalis muscle insertion. At this time, a portion of temporalis muscle fascia is obtained if a graft will be placed later during the procedure. If the procedure is going to be combined with a tympanoplasty, external auditory canal incisions are made as described above.

After the tympanomeatal flap is elevated, the operation proceeds through the postauricular incision and, if necessary, through the ear canal. The postauricular incision, however, exposes the ear canal also. After the periosteum is exposed, it is elevated anteriorly with an elevator, such as a 4-mm periosteal elevator. After the external auditory canal incision is visualized through the postauricular incision, different canal instruments can be used to expose the middle ear fully through the canal. A self-retaining retractor is placed and opened widely. At this point, the air-powered drill is used with the largest available cutting burr.

Details

After the dissection has proceeded beyond the superficial bony landmarks, a microscope is brought in for finer detail. Depending on the indications for the operation, the middle ear can be entered from the mastoid approach as well. It is important that the surgeon be as comfortably seated as possible. It is also important that the scrub nurse have a thorough knowledge of the anatomy and the procedure to anticipate the use of the appropriate instruments. Ideally, the surgeon should never have to look away from the microscope for instruments. A surgeon should be able to request an instrument by name and have it handed to him or her by the scrub assistant.

If reconstructive procedures are indicated, the surgeon selects from a wide variety of prosthetic devices. If a tympanic membrane perforation is to be repaired, the previously harvested graft is used in a manner similar to that described above.

Closure

The postauricular wound is copiously irrigated and the wound is closed by approximating the previously raised periosteum. Periosteum is usually closed with absorbable sutures of the surgeon's choice. The subcutaneous tissues are then reapproximated in the postauricular area. A drain may be placed and brought out through the most inferior portion of the postauricular incision. The skin is usually closed with a nylon or polypropylene (Prolene) stitch. A subcuticular suture may be used to alleviate the necessity for suture removal later.

Again, the preferences of the surgeon should be investigated before the procedure is started. After the postauricular incision is closed, the ear canal is examined in the usual fashion. A variety of ear specula are used to visualize the canal. The tympanomeatal flap is replaced and the external auditory canal is packed as previously described. Postoperatively, a mastoid dressing is used. A nonadhering bandage is placed behind the ear. The postauricular incision is then supported with gauze squares. Rolls of self-adhering gauze are used to surround the head from the occiput to the forehead. Gauze may be used to place pressure on the wound to prevent a hematoma.

Postoperative Care

The patient is transferred immediately to the recovery room. After operations of the mastoid and the middle ear, it is important to assess the hearing capability of the patient as well as the facial nerve function. As soon as the patient is conscious, different tuning fork tests may be used to assess hearing. A facial function evaluation is also routinely performed (e.g., smiling, wrinkling of the nose on the operative side, and closing of the eye).

Potential Surgical Complications

Hearing loss
Facial nerve injury
Vertigo
Taste changes
Bleeding and hematoma formation
Infection

Stapedectomy

Definition and Indications

Stapedectomy refers to the removal of the stapes. In some patients, a conductive hearing loss is identified. A common reason for this hearing loss is the formation of spongy bone within the capsule of the bony labyrinth of the inner ear. In such conditions, normal bone is replaced by vascular otosclerotic bone, which eventually involves the footplate of the stapes. The stapes thus becomes locked and unable to vibrate. This condition, commonly known as *otosclerosis,* is a hereditary defect. The procedure of stapedectomy with the insertion of a prosthesis has been developed to restore hearing to the ear.

The indications for a stapedectomy involve primarily the finding of a conductive hearing loss without any evidence of other middle ear disease.

Related Surgical Procedures

Stapedotomy

Perioperative Nursing Implications

Anesthesia

As for other ear procedures, stapedectomy is usually performed under general anesthesia. In cooperative adults, however, local anesthesia may be used so that the patient can assist the surgeon by informing her or him of an immediate improvement in hearing.

Position

The patient is positioned as described for tympanoplasty.

Creation and Maintenance of the Sterile Field

The sterile field is created and maintained as for other ear procedures. The position of the sterile field is identical to that for other ear procedures.

Equipment and Supplies

All microinstruments for ear procedures should be available, to include fine stapes dissectors and manipulators. A variety of prosthetic devices have been described for use in this procedure. A tympanoplasty set is used with the additions of the following:

- Hough hoe excavators: 45 degree and 90 degree
- Footplate picks: 1 mm and 2 mm
- Straight pick or 30-degree obtuse pick
- Perforator
- Crimper: House and/or McGee
- Strut caliper (measuring stick)
- Prostheses of different sizes and shapes
- House incudostapedial joint knife
- Guilford-Wright joint knife

Drugs and Solutions

See the discussion of mastoidectomy.

Physiological Monitoring

See the discussion of tympanoplasty.

Specimens and Cultures

Stapes superstructure

Physician's Orders

See the discussion of tympanoplasty.

Laboratory and Diagnostic Studies

See the discussion of tympanoplasty.

Procedure

Incision and Exposure

A tympanomeatal flap is raised as previously described for simple tympanoplasty. The fibrous annulus of the tympanic membrane is identified and lifted superiorly with a tympanomeatal flap (Fig. 29–13). Oftentimes, a small portion of bone from the edge of the bony ear canal is removed for better visualization of the joint between the incus and the stapes. The chorda tympani nerve is located in this area. Care is taken not to injure this nerve, which supplies taste to the lateral portion of the tongue on that side. Microinstruments are used to sever the connection between the incus and the stapes. The stapes bone is fractured and removed along with the remnant footplate.

A graft is also necessary during this procedure. This graft may be vein, perichondrium, fascia, fat, or absorbable hemostatic sponges. The graft is placed over the oval window of the inner ear.

Details

After the prosthesis has been selected, the previously obtained graft is placed over the oval window where the stapes footplate previously existed. A prosthesis is then inserted and connected from the incus to the graft. This restores sound conduction. If the operation is being performed under local anesthesia, the surgeon can reposition the tympanic membrane and talk to the patient while testing for a hearing improvement. As in other microsurgical procedures, the operating microscope must be used.

Closure

The tympanomeatal flap is replaced as previously described.

Postoperative Care

The postoperative care is the same as that for other ear procedures.

Potential Surgical Complications

Hearing loss
A change in taste
Injury to the facial nerve

SURGICAL PROCEDURES OF THE NOSE AND PARANASAL SINUSES

Operations inside the nose and sinuses are primarily performed to correct obstruction or alleviate infection. Other operations have been designed to control intractable nosebleeds. Tumors within the nasal cavity and sinuses are rare. When tumors are discovered, however, extensive resection of these structures is often necessary.

Special Instruments, Supplies, and Equipment

A dedicated nasal set should always be available for surgical procedures within the nasal cavity. This set usually includes a variety of elevators, dissectors, curved scissors, and curets, plus nasal specula of different lengths. Dedicated sinus endoscopy sets should be readily available in ORs that provide otolaryngologic services. The scrub nurse should be thoroughly familiar with the names of the various forceps that are often used in endoscopic sinus surgery. The use of different lasers within the nasal cavity has been undertaken.

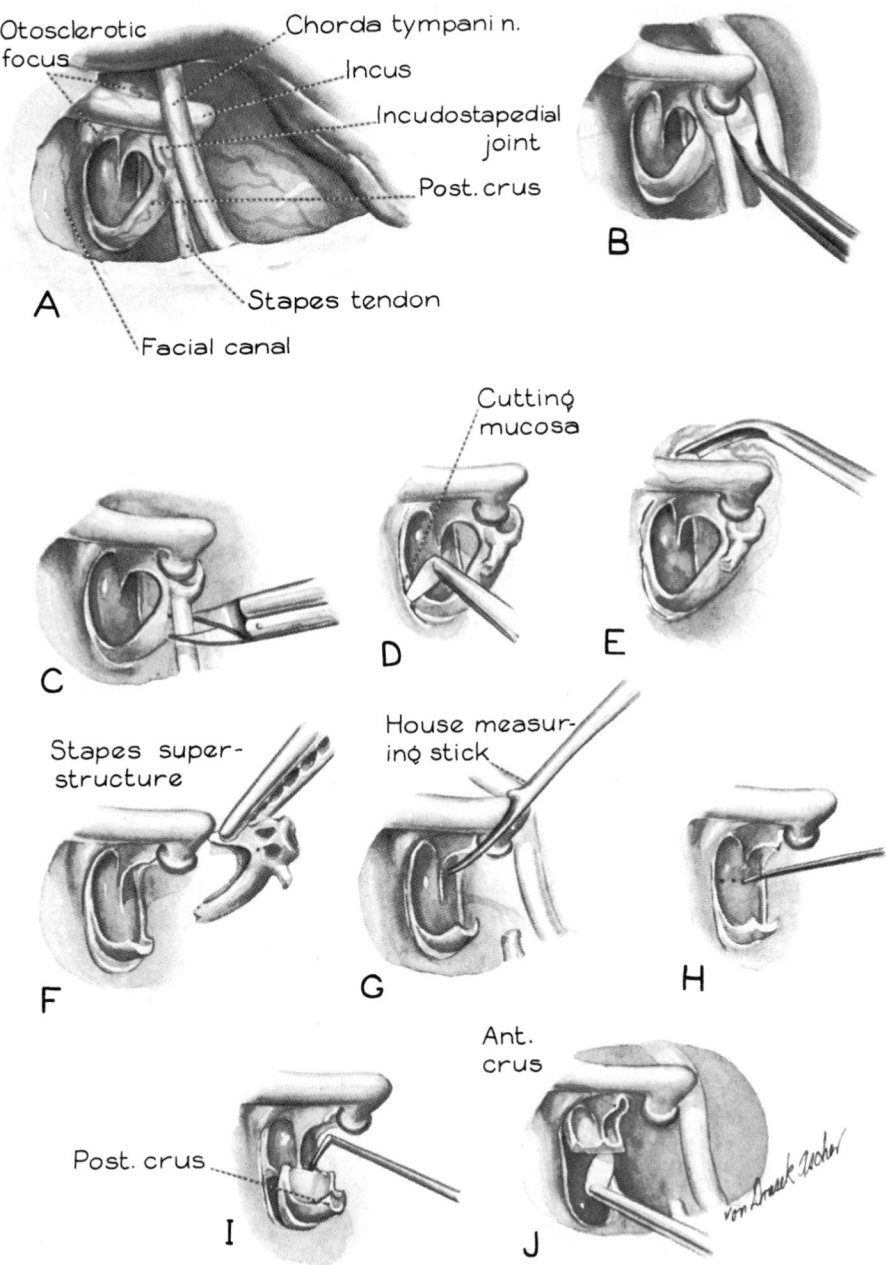

FIGURE 29–13. Stapedectomy procedure. (From Glasscock, M., Shambaugh, G. [1990]. *Surgery of the ear* [4th ed.] [p. 398]. Philadelphia: W. B. Saunders.)

Septoplasty (Septorhinoplasty)

Definition and Indications

Septoplasty, or septorhinoplasty, refers to the excision of the cartilaginous or bony portions of the nasal septum that lie between the flaps of the mucous membrane and the perichondrium (Fig. 29–14).

The primary indications for septoplasty or septorhinoplasty are relief of obstruction resulting from nasal deformity. The deformity might be only within the internal nasal cavity, but it is frequently seen in conjunction with the deviation of the external nose as well. Deviation of the septum often leads to other problems besides obstruction of the nasal airflow. Severe deviations are aggravating factors in recurrent sinusitis. When there are defects of the bony framework, the bones of the nose must be reshaped. Therefore, the preoperative evaluation of the entire external and internal nose is essential.

Related Surgical Procedures

Submucous resection

Perioperative Nursing Implications

Anesthesia

Septoplasty and septorhinoplasty are often performed under local anesthesia with conscious IV sedation. When this is done, cocaine solutions can be applied intranasally on cottonoids to provide vasoconstriction and anesthesia. Other agents often used include lidocaine hydrochloride in addition to oxymetazoline (Afrin). These drugs can cause adverse reactions in the patient. The

initial symptoms consist of central nervous system stimulation, which is eventually followed by cardiovascular depression. Usually mild symptoms, such as mild excitation, can be seen if the patient is awake. If the patient is under general anesthesia, an increase in heart rate is frequently the only finding. If general anesthesia is going to be used for the procedure, often a throat pack is placed in the back of the throat after the patient is intubated to decrease the chance of aspiration of blood.

Position

The patient is usually placed in the supine position. A headrest should be available to stabilize the head. The same comfort measures are used as for tympanoplasty patients.

Creation and Maintenance of the Sterile Field

Even though the nasal membranes are contaminated, the mucus within the sinuses should be considered sterile; therefore, a sterile field is created.

Equipment and Supplies

Because illumination is usually provided by the endoscope, or a surgical headlight, it must be in working order. On rare occasions, a microscope may be used. If endoscopes are used, appropriate light connectors for each type of endoscope must be available. The entire lighting mechanism must be thoroughly checked before initiation of the procedure. Verify with the surgeon his or her preference for nasal packing and/or splinting supplies and have these available for use at the end of the procedure.

Drugs and Solutions

Lidocaine 1% with 1:1000 epinephrine
Cocaine solution or crystals
Antibiotic ointment or cream
Gelfoam
Neosporin 1%
1:1000 epinephrine

Physiological Monitoring

The patient must be monitored at all times by vital signs measurement, ECG, and pulse oximeter. The circulating nurse must always record the amount of local anesthesia that is administered. All sponges and cottonoids must be counted. Because the cottonoids that are commonly used are small, they can present a hazard if miscounted, or not tagged. Throughout the procedure, cottonoids soaked in a vasoconstricting agent such as oxymetazoline are used. Suction must be available at all times, along with varying sizes of suction catheters.

Specimens and Cultures

Nasal cartilage and bone
Turbinates

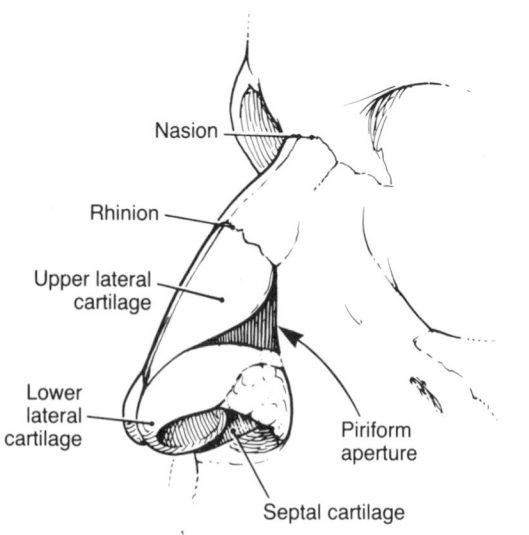

FIGURE 29–14. Anatomy of the nose. (From Meyerhoff, W., Rice, D. [1992]. *Otolaryngology—Head and neck surgery* [p. 464]. Philadelphia: W. B. Saunders.)

Labels on figure:
Nasion
Rhinion
Upper lateral cartilage
Lower lateral cartilage
Piriform aperture
Septal cartilage

Physician's Orders

Keep the IV catheter open until the patient is tolerating liquids. Administer analgesics for pain and antiemetics for nausea. Advise the patient not to drink with straws and to sneeze with the mouth open.

Laboratory and Diagnostic Studies

Routine CBC, urinalysis, prothrombin time (PT), and partial thromboplastin time (PTT) are obtained. Before procedures within the nose or the sinuses are started, x-ray films or CT scans are often obtained to evaluate the problem fully. It is essential that these be present in the OR.

Procedure

Incision and Exposure

Unless endoscopes are used along with a camera and monitor, procedures inside the nose can be difficult to follow by the scrub nurse. The initial portion of the procedure involves the placement of local anesthetic–soaked sponges or cottonoids, as well as the injection of a local anesthetic and epinephrine solution. After this is done, an appropriate time for vasoconstriction is allowed, and the nose is examined with a nasal speculum. The initial incision is made inside the nose along the tip of the nasal septum. The initial steps involve the separation of the soft tissues, which include the mucous membrane and underlying perichondrium, from the cartilaginous and bony septum. In a previously traumatized nose, this may be a difficult aspect of the operation. Different elevators, such as the Cottle elevator, are used to lift the perichondrium off the septum.

Details

After the deformed portion of the septum is identified, it may be removed, straightened, or replaced. A variety of instruments often found in nasal sets are used for this purpose. If the external nasal framework is also to be reshaped (rhinoplasty), this is accomplished using a variety of osteotomes as well as mallets.

Closure

After the nose is shaped in the desired way, and the internal septal deviation is corrected, it is imperative that attempts be made to stabilize the internal and external nasal framework. This can be done in a variety of ways. Tight nasal packing has been used in the past. More commonly, however, internal nasal splints such as Doyle splints may be used to stabilize the septum. Teflon sheeting has also been used for this purpose. The internal splints are stabilized with nonabsorbable sutures. Before placement of the splints, the previously made mucosal incisions are closed using small absorbable sutures. Different ways of stabilizing the external nasal framework have been proposed. Plaster is still used and is effective. Commercially available rigid shields can protect the external nose also. At the completion of the procedure, the throat pack must be removed.

Postoperative Care

After the operation, the patient is transferred to the recovery room. The head of the bed should be elevated to lessen edema. Analgesics are often prescribed to reduce the discomfort. At times, sedation is necessary in the postoperative period. A nasal drip pad is often in place under the nose. Because there might be packing inside the nose, the patient is breathing primarily through the mouth. This necessitates good oral care. If the nose is packed bilaterally, humidified oxygen is often given via face mask. However, intake of oral fluids must not be started until the effects of the local anesthetic are gone. If oral fluids are started too early, aspiration could occur. Most septoplastys and septorhinoplastys are performed on an outpatient basis. Therefore, discharge instructions should be discussed at length with the patient.

Potential Surgical Complications

Bleeding

Endoscopic Sinus Surgery

Definition and Indications

Endoscopic sinus surgery refers to procedures performed on the sinus cavities via endoscopic resection. With the advent of sinus endoscopes, the extent of visualization inside the nose as well as knowledge of its anatomy and physiology have dramatically improved. Endoscopes allow precise operations within the nasal cavity. Indications for endoscopic sinus procedures include the removal of diseased mucosa and resection of the necessary bony portions of the nasal cavity to establish natural drainage of the paranasal sinuses.

Patients come to the OR for endoscopic sinus surgery only after an extensive medical and allergic evaluation. When medical treatment has failed and the patients persist with sinusitis, the surgeon often recommends surgical intervention. A septoplasty may or may not be performed at the time of the endoscopic procedure. Occasionally, septoplasty becomes necessary to gain access to the nasal cavity with the endoscopes. The extent of the procedure depends on the location of the diseased mucosa and the extent of bony abnormalities within the nasal cavity and sinuses.

Related Surgical Procedures

Caldwell-Luc procedure
External ethmoidectomy

Perioperative Nursing Implications

Anesthesia

As for other nasal procedures, endoscopic sinus procedures can be performed under local anesthesia. However, general anesthesia is preferred because of the inability to anesthetize posterior portions of the nose. The principles previously discussed for septoplasty and septorhinoplasty must be followed.

Position

See the discussion of septoplasty.

Creation and Maintenance of the Sterile Field

See the discussion of septoplasty.

Equipment and Supplies

Of greatest importance is the availability and thorough knowledge of the appropriate equipment. Complications of the operation have occurred in the past because of lack of appropriate instrumentation. Commercially available endoscopic sinus surgery sets contain a wide variety of telescopes. The endoscopes are usually either 2.7 or 4 mm in diameter. These have 0-, 25-, 30-, 70-, and 120-degree viewing angles (Fig. 29–15). Endoscopes require an external light source; therefore, precaution should be taken in case of burnout of the bulb. Also needed is a camera with a color monitor and a video recorder. A designated endoscopy cart housing all video equipment is essential.

Lasers have been advocated for use intranasally. This, however, is somewhat controversial. If the laser is used, all appropriate precautions as established by the laser safety standards of the hospital must be followed.

Drugs and Solutions

See the discussion of septoplasty.

Physiological Monitoring

See the discussion of septoplasty.

Specimens and Cultures

Nasal cartilage and bone
Contents of different sinuses (e.g., ethmoidal and maxillary)

Physician's Orders

See the discussion of septoplasty.

Laboratory and Diagnostic Studies

Routine laboratory studies as described for septoplasty are performed. Of utmost importance, is the availability of previously obtained CT scans. Because the CT scan provides the "road map" for the surgeon, the patient should not come into the OR unless the CT scan is readily available.

Procedure

Incision and Exposure

The procedure is usually initiated as for a septoplasty. Local anesthetic or vasoconstricting solutions are used. These are placed intranasally on soaked cottonoids. They are placed in the area of the operation (i.e., the middle meatus) (Fig. 29–16). The area to be operated on is injected with local anesthetic and epinephrine solutions. If a septoplasty is going to be combined with the operation, this is performed first. After the cotto-

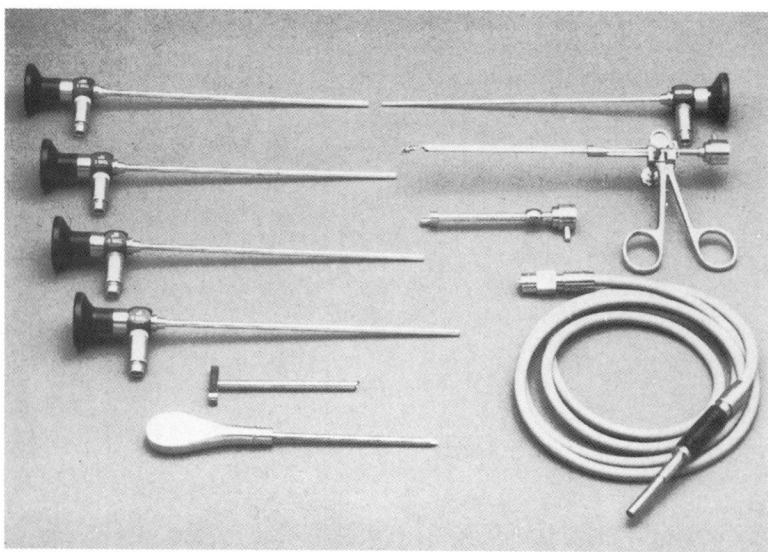

FIGURE 29–15. Endoscopic instruments. (From Adams, G., Boies, L., Hilger, P. [1989]. *Boies fundamentals of otolaryngology: A textbook of ear, nose, and throat diseases* [6th ed.] [p. 259]. Philadelphia: W. B. Saunders.)

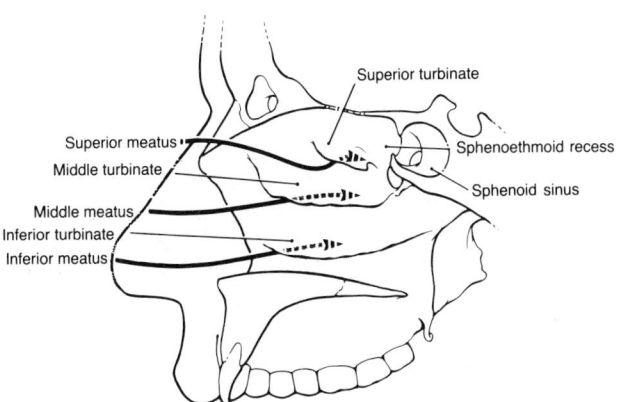

FIGURE 29–16. Location of turbinates and meati for endoscopic sinus surgery. (From Meyerhoff, W., Rice, D. [1992]. *Otolaryngology—Head and neck surgery* [p. 465]. Philadelphia: W. B. Saunders.)

noids have been left in place to allow for vasoconstriction, the operation is initiated.

Different sharp instruments, such as sickle-shaped knives and scissors, are used for the initial incisions within the middle meatus. A wide variety of straight and angled-biting forceps (usually available in the endoscopic sinus surgery sets) are used for removal of the diseased bony abnormality as well as mucosa. A wide variety of curved suction catheters are also used. The telescope is inserted intranasally and advanced into the ethmoidal sinus, and if necessary the sphenoidal sinus. The sinus endoscopes are used to visualize anteriorly within the nasal cavity and also into the frontal sinus.

Details

Because the operation proceeds in close proximity to the eye and the brain, care is taken to identify the walls of the orbit and the base of the skull. It is important not to have the eyes taped shut. If the orbit is accidentally entered, what might be perceived as nasal mucosa could be orbital contents. When pulling on these contents, movement of the eyeball is seen. This can be occluded if the eyes are taped shut.

After the diseased mucosa and bony abnormalities have been removed from within the nasal cavity, evaluation of the operative field reveals a common cavity between the anterior and posterior ethmoidal cells. However, if diseased mucosa is not encountered in the posterior portion of the ethmoidal cavity, it is not disturbed. Backward cutting antral punches are used to widen the maxillary sinus ostia.

Closure

As the procedure is concluded, hemostasis is obtained with either bipolar electrocoagulation or suction cautery. Because the operation is performed between the lateral nasal wall and the middle turbinate, stents are used that are later removed, to prevent the formation of scarring.

Different materials have been used; commercially available Merocel sponges have been designed for this purpose. Most commonly, however, rolled absorbable gelatin film (Gelfilm) dressing is used as a stent within the operated cavity. This is removed at a later date. Usually, no drains or packing is necessary. If extensive bleeding is encountered, however, an anterior nasal pack might be left in place temporarily.

Postoperative Care

The same nasal dressing as described for septoplasty is applied. Principles previously described are applicable in this situation as well. Of utmost importance, however, is the assessment of vision. Reports of complications stemming from swelling around the eye to blindness have been reported. It is critical that this be evaluated as early as possible. If difficulty with vision is encountered, the surgeon must be notified immediately. Further procedures might become necessary to prevent blindness. If the base of the skull has accidentally been entered, this might not be immediately known. However, profuse clear drainage from the nose may indicate cerebrospinal fluid. Again, the surgeon must be notified immediately.

Potential Surgical Complications

Blindness
Perforation of the base of skull with subsequent central nervous system infection
Injury to the lacrimal duct
Bleeding

Caldwell-Luc Procedure

Definition and Indications

The *Caldwell-Luc procedure,* also known as a radical antrostomy, refers to the incision into the canine fossa of the superior maxilla and "exposure of the antrum for excision of bony diseased portions of the antral wall and contents of the sinus, or establishment of drainage by means of a counteropening into the nose through the inferior meatus" (Meeker and Rothrock, 1991, p. 539).

The Caldwell-Luc operation has been a standard procedure for the sinus surgeon. Additional thought and improved knowledge of the physiology of the sinuses have decreased the use of this operation. However, there are still times when tremendous amount of diseased mucosa and polyps exist within the maxillary sinus. This operation is designed to gain access to the maxillary sinus through an incision underneath the upper lip in the area of the anterior wall of the maxillary sinus. Sinus endoscopes have often been used to visualize maxillary sinus contents also. A trocar can be used to penetrate the anterior wall of the maxillary sinus. After the trocar has entered the sinus, the scope can be placed through a sheath into the sinus. This helps in assessing the extent of the maxillary sinus operation.

Related Surgical Procedures

Creation of nasal antral windows (antrostomy)

Perioperative Nursing Implications

Anesthesia

Often, the Caldwell-Luc operation is performed in conjunction with other intranasal procedures. Therefore, previously discussed anesthesia regimens should be followed.

Position

See the discussion of septoplasty.

Creation and Maintenance of the Sterile Field

The patient is prepared and draped as previously described for nasal procedures.

Equipment and Supplies

A general nose set is used. Also used is a Caldwell-Luc set, which includes an antral punch and Coakley antrum curets.

Drugs and Solutions

See the discussion of septoplasty.

Physiological Monitoring

See the discussion of septoplasty.

Specimens and Cultures

- Polyps
- Diseased nasal mucosa

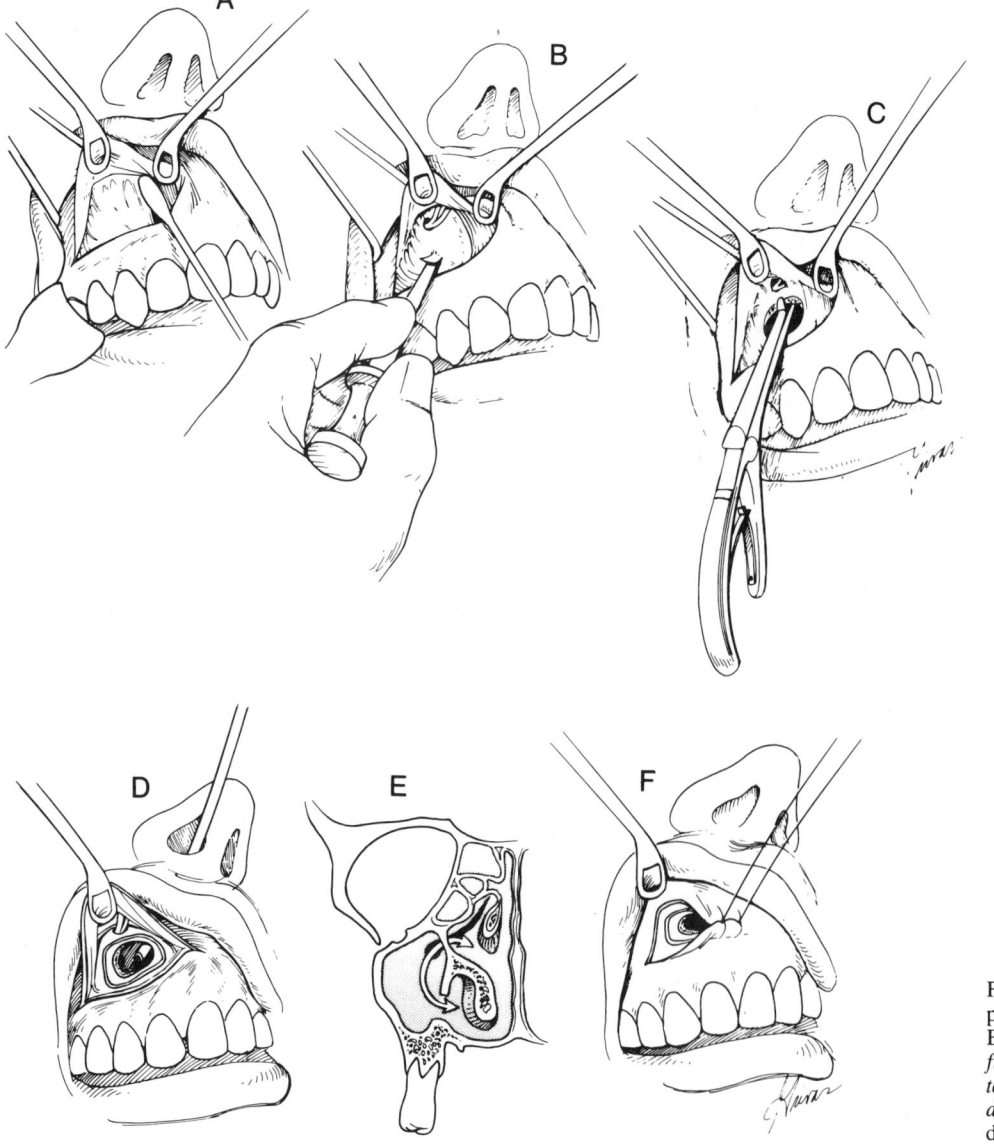

FIGURE 29–17. Caldwell-Luc procedure. (From Adams, G., Boies, L., Hilger, P. [1989]. *Boies fundamentals of otolaryngology: A textbook of ear, nose, and throat diseases* [6th ed.] [p. 258]. Philadelphia: W. B. Saunders.)

Physician's Orders

See the discussion of septoplasty.

Laboratory and Diagnostic Studies

Routine CBC, urinalysis, PT, PTT, CT scan, and sinus x-ray films are obtained.

Procedure

Incision and Exposure

The maxillary sinus to be operated is approached through an incision in the oral mucous membrane above the canine teeth. This mucosal flap is retracted until periosteum is incised (Fig. 29–17). A section of maxillary bone is cut out to gain access into the maxillary sinus.

Details

Through this opening, polyps or diseased mucosa is removed. Through the nasal cavity, a flap and opening is created into the maxillary sinus through the inferior meatus. After this connection has been created, the sinus is packed with gauze impregnated with antibiotic ointment. One end of the gauze is brought out through the opening made in the nasal cavity. This packing is eventually removed through the nose. After the gauze is in place, care must be taken not to lose the end of the gauze that is brought out through the nasal cavity.

Closure

The periosteum is reapproximated and the mucosal incision is closed with absorbable suture.

Postoperative Care

Postoperative care is similar to that for other intranasal procedures previously described.

Potential Surgical Complications

Injury to the roots of the teeth in children
Injury to the infraorbital nerve leading to anesthesia of the cheek
Injury to the orbital contents
Injury to the tooth sockets
Edema

Closed Repair of Nasal Fracture

Definition

Closed repair of nasal fracture refers to the manipulation of a nasal fracture without incision. This procedure is often performed after trauma to the face. Intranasal manipulation can be used immediately after the injury. Occasionally, elevation of depressed bone or cartilage can be performed and the nose reshaped to its normal position.

Indications

The indications for closed reduction primarily involve the finding of depressed nasal bones or cartilage. The reduction should be performed as soon as possible. A delay of just 3 to 4 days in children can lead to unsuccessful reduction. In adults, the delay can be as long as 7 days. Beyond this time, the bony structures are extremely difficult to manipulate.

Related Surgical Procedures

None

Perioperative Nursing Implications

Anesthesia

Most procedures to reduce the nasal cavity are most comfortably performed under general anesthesia. This is especially true in children. However, local anesthesia can be used and previously described principles followed.

Position

See the discussion of septoplasty.

Creation and Maintenance of the Sterile Field

See the discussion of septoplasty.

Equipment and Supplies

- General nose set or designated closed nasal fracture set
- Headlight

Drugs and Solutions

See the discussion of septoplasty.

Physiological Monitoring

See the discussion of septoplasty.

Specimens and Cultures

None

Physician's Orders

See the discussion of septoplasty.

Laboratory and Diagnostic Studies

CBC and urinalysis are obtained.

Procedure

Intranasal manipulation is performed with a variety of blunt instruments. A Boies elevator is often used intranasally to elevate nasal bony depression. Different types of forceps are also available for this purpose. It is important to know that clinical evaluation of the nose is far more important than x-ray evaluation. Therefore, x-ray films are not necessarily obtained. Even if the operation is performed under general anesthesia, topical anesthesia and vasoconstrictors are placed on soaked cottonoids intranasally. Previously described substances such as cocaine or oxymetazoline can be used.

After the desired reduction is obtained, it is important to stabilize the nose externally. The same principles should be used as for stabilization of the patient who has had a rhinoplasty.

Postoperative Care

See the discussion of septoplasty.

Potential Surgical Complications

The complications of closed reduction are few. However, an undesirable result can occur that would necessitate a formal rhinoplasty at a later date. Unmanageable bleeding is rarely encountered. Nasal packing might be used temporarily to control a nosebleed after the manipulation. Additional complications have been reported if nasal packing is used. Some of these complications are infectious, such as toxic shock syndrome.

SURGICAL PROCEDURES OF THE OROPHARYNX AND HEAD AND NECK

Tonsillectomy and Adenoidectomy

Definition and Indications

Tonsillectomy and adenoidectomy refers to the excision of the pharyngeal tonsils and adenoids. No operation has attracted as much attention and heated controversy. Tonsillectomy and adenoidectomy is the most common major head and neck operation performed in children.

Indications

The indications for tonsillectomy and adenoidectomy have varied throughout the years. The three most common indications, however, are chronic infections, obstruction of breathing (Fig. 29–18), and excisional biopsy in the evaluation of tonsillar tumors. Tonsillectomy and adenoidectomy are not always performed at the same time. Different indications exist for removal of the adenoid pad only. For example, the adenoid tissue affects the middle ear. Studies revealing the effects of adenoidectomy on chronic otitis media are well known. Therefore, the decision to perform an adenoidectomy does not always include a tonsillectomy. Sometimes, a tonsillectomy alone is performed. Most adenoidal tissue involutes with age. The decision to remove it depends on the symptoms associated with an enlarged adenoid pad.

Related Surgical Procedures

None

Perioperative Nursing Implications

Anesthesia

Most tonsillectomies and adenoidectomies are performed under general anesthesia. Local anesthesia has been used successfully in adults. The description below, however, is primarily for the patient under general anesthesia.

Position

The patient is usually in a supine position and is placed on the OR bed with his or her head at the foot. This facilitates the surgeon's comfortable access to the patient. If the patient has the procedure under local anesthesia, the semi-Fowler position may be preferable.

Creation and Maintenance of the Sterile Field

Tonsillectomy and adenoidectomy is not considered a sterile procedure. Hospital policy specifies whether the patient is or is not draped. The surgeon and scrub nurse, however, should don sterile gowns and gloves and wear appropriate head covering, eye protection, and a surgical mask according to universal precaution guidelines. The surgeon may sit at the head of the OR bed or stand at the side of the bed.

Lighting into the oral cavity is usually obtained with a headlight. Overhead lights, however, have been used. Lighting is superior, nevertheless, with a headlight. After the patient has been intubated, the table may be turned to suit the surgeon. The patient's head is draped to cover the eyes, which have been taped by the anesthetist.

If the surgeon sits at the head of the bed, a mouth gag is inserted to depress the tongue and expose the oropharynx. Most often, a Crowe-Davis or palate-type mouth gag is used for this purpose. These gags are designed to open the oral cavity while simultaneously depressing the tongue. After this is obtained, the gag is secured to a suspension apparatus. Different suspension apparatus designs are available. Most commonly, how-

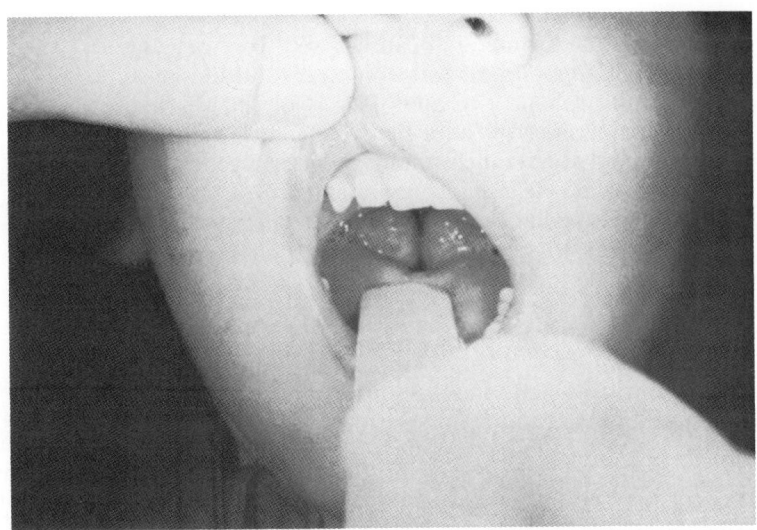

FIGURE 29–18. Tonsils obstructing the oropharynx. (From Meyerhoff, W., Rice, D. [1992]. *Otolaryngology—Head and neck surgery* [p. 650]. Philadelphia: W. B. Saunders.)

ever, suspension is obtained by placing the tongue blade on a Mayo stand. This is probably the most common way of suspending the mouth gag; however, independent suspension apparatuses are superior. Independent suspension apparatuses provide free movement of the table without having the worry of the Mayo stand height or location.

Because a tonsillectomy and adenoidectomy can be a bloody procedure, appropriate suctioning with Yankauer tips is required. The incision and dissection have been described in a number of ways. A cold knife, electrocautery, and laser have been used to perform the operation. There have been different advocates for the various techniques. To this day, no single technique is considered superior. There should be an effort, however, to decrease intraoperative bleeding. After the oropharynx is exposed, the decision is made to begin either the adenoidectomy first or the tonsillectomy. Sometimes removal of the adenoid tissue first allows more time for packing of the nasopharynx and easier hemostasis.

Equipment and Supplies

A tonsil and adenoid set is needed, as well as the surgeon-preferred mouth gag. These may range from the Jennings, to Crowe-Davis, to a palate-type mouth gag. The nurse may anticipate the use of a Crowe-Davis mouth gag if the surgeon sits or stands at the patient's head during the procedure. The Jennings mouth gag, however, is more routinely used if the surgeon stands at the patient's side during the procedure.

The suction coagulator electrocautery is necessary, and the possible use of a handswitch pencil cautery should be anticipated. Be aware that the foot pedal of the electrocautery is necessary for the use of the suction coagulator. As for the use of all electrical equipment, the nurse should ensure that these pieces of equipment are operating correctly before the beginning of the procedure. If the laser is used, all laser precautions should be in place before the procedure.

Drugs and Solutions

Normal saline
Lidocaine 1% with 1:100,000 epinephrine
Phenylephrine (Neo-Synephrine)
Tannic acid
Bismuth subgallate
1:1000 epinephrine
Defogging solution (Antifog, pHisoHex)

Physiological Monitoring

The patient is monitored at all times as for previously described procedures.

Specimens and Cultures

Right and left tonsils
Adenoid tissue

Physician's Orders

The IV catheter is maintained at a keep-open rate until the patient is taking fluids without nausea and vomiting. The patient is given a soft diet. The following are administered: an analgesic of the surgeon's preference for pain (most common is acetaminophen with codeine), promethazine suppository for nausea, and dexamethasone for swelling.

Laboratory and Diagnostic Studies

CBC, urinalysis, PT, and PTT are obtained.

Procedure

Incision and Exposure

The procedure is initiated by making a decision whether the tonsillectomy or the adenoidectomy will be performed first. The tonsillectomy is performed as follows: The tonsil is retracted with an Allis or similar tonsil clamp. Other material can be used to retract the tonsil as well. Sometimes, a 0-plain catgut suture is used on a curved urological needle. This is placed through the tonsillar tissue itself in a figure-of-eight knot. This provides good retraction without fragmenting the tonsillar tissue, which can happen with clamps. By retracting the tonsil medially, the anterior pillar is incised by whatever means the surgeon decides.

Details

As previously mentioned, a knife, electrocautery, or lasers can be used for this purpose. The incision is carried down until the capsule of the tonsil becomes visible. Using blunt and sharp dissection, the capsule of the tonsil is exposed from the tonsillar fossa. Having the availability of suction cautery helps in the hemostasis. As the dissection continues, the superior pole of the tonsil is exposed and retracted from the tonsillar fossa. As blood vessels are encountered, they may be either cauterized or tied with suture. Slip knots of 2–0 or 3–0 catgut are placed around these vessels. The tonsil dissection then continues until the most inferior portion of the tonsil is exposed. At this time, the tonsil is removed from the tonsillar fossa with a snare, or with sharp dissection using electrocautery, laser, or scissors. After this is performed, the fossa of the tonsil is carefully inspected and any bleeding vessel is either cauterized or clamped and tied. The opposite tonsil is then removed in a similar fashion. An adenoidectomy should be performed with indirect vision using a mirror. A "blind" adenoidectomy is discouraged because the eustachian orifice can be injured.

The easiest way to expose the nasopharynx is by placing soft rubber catheters through the nasal cavity and bringing them out through the oral cavity. Before the catheters are placed through the nose, the surgeon often inspects the soft palate. This is important to identify congenital defects of the palate that might be a contraindication to an adenoidectomy. These catheters can then be used to retract the soft palate. Using a dental mirror that has been defogged with defogging solution, the surgeon can visualize the nasopharynx. Only in this way can the eustachian tube orifices be identified and protected.

Different devices have been designed to remove the adenoid tissue. A variety of adenoid curets are available and are most commonly used to scrape the lymphoid tissue from the nasopharynx. Different basket punches also exist to remove any loose fragments of lymphoid tissue. The adenoidectomy is a somewhat more difficult procedure, because of the possibility of leaving fragments of lymphoid tissue in the nasopharynx. Hemostasis is usually obtained with packing as well as the suction cautery. It must be emphasized that, when suction cautery is used, the eustachian tube orifice must always be in full view to prevent debilitating scarring and intractable middle ear problems.

Closure

Before the procedure is terminated, a final inspection is performed to evaluate for any bleeding sites. The nasopharynx can be irrigated with ice or room temperature normal saline. The stomach contents should be suctioned out before the procedure is terminated to decrease the chance of postoperative nausea and vomiting.

Postoperative Care

Because bleeding from the operated area is the most dreaded complication, this must be watched for at all times in the immediate postoperative period. Any bleeding must be reported to the surgeon immediately. When the patient is transferred to the recovery room, he or she is often lying on the side. This decreases the chance of aspiration of blood or secretions. Analgesia is almost always required for the patients. The discomfort after a tonsillectomy and adenoidectomy is often underemphasized. A balance must be made between narcotic administration and depression of the central nervous system. Analgesia is attempted; however, too much sedation should be avoided to prevent aspiration.

A liquid diet is initiated only if the patient is awake enough to ask. Antiemetic medication is also often prescribed.

Potential Surgical Complications

Bleeding that can be life-threatening
Pain and inability to swallow, which can cause dehydration in young children
Injury to the eustachian tube orifices
Aspiration of blood, leading to pulmonary complications
Aspiration, leading to airway obstruction and respiratory arrest

Parotidectomy

Definition and Indications

Parotidectomy refers to the partial or complete excision of the parotid gland. The most common reason to excise the parotid gland is the presence of tumors within the gland itself. Most lesions growing within the parotid gland are benign. The minimal operation performed for these tumors is a superficial or lateral parotidectomy. Malignant lesions often necessitate the removal of the entire parotid gland, including the deep lobe. At times, a radical neck dissection or other more radical procedures are combined with a parotidectomy. However, for most parotid tumors, a lateral parotidectomy with preservation of the deep lobe and the facial nerve is all that is necessary.

Related Surgical Procedures

None

Perioperative Nursing Implications

Anesthesia

Operations performed on the parotid gland are always done under general anesthesia. It is critical that no neuromuscular blockade be used during the procedure. This is because identification of the facial nerve is often made not only with visualization but also by stimulation using a nerve stimulator. If blockade has been given, the nerve is not stimulated. This might lead to inadvertent severing of facial nerve branches.

Position

The position of the patient is supine with the affected side of the face up. A small roll underneath the shoulders, as well as a headrest, provides stabilization of the area.

Creation and Maintenance of the Sterile Field

This is a sterile procedure and therefore different from previously described techniques within the oral cavity or nasal cavity. Maintenance of a sterile field is critical and follows standard sterile field principles. Because parotidectomy can be a lengthy procedure, padding must be provided for pressure points. After the patient is asleep and intubated and appropriate positioning has been obtained, the patient's face is prepared with antimicrobial solutions. The face is draped from the level of the forehead down to the level of the clavicle on the operative side. It is often a good idea to place a cotton ball or other type of wick into the ear canal to prevent preparation solutions from entering the ear canal.

It is important that the face be visible at all times. Stimulation of the facial nerve leads to movement of the muscles of facial expression. Therefore, the ability to see movement in the face is of utmost importance. A self-adhering plastic drape can be used to cover the entire face and neck. Some surgeons prefer not to do this and just keep the face exposed. Towels are used to create a sterile field. Lint-free sterile drapes are then used to cover the patient inferiorly and superiorly.

Equipment and Supplies

A general plastic set, a nerve stimulator, special parotid retractors, and bipolar cautery should be available.

Drugs and Solutions

None

Physiological Monitoring

Because a parotidectomy can be a lengthy procedure, the patient's comfort and safety are important. All bony prominences are padded to decrease the risk of nerve damage and a pillow is offered for under the knees to decrease back strain. The routine ECG, blood pressure, and oxygen saturation are monitored by the anesthetist. The circulating nurse should be aware of monitoring and assist the anesthetist as necessary.

Specimens and Cultures

Parotid tissue

Physician's Orders

A regular diet is given. The IV catheter is kept open until the patient is tolerating fluids. Antiemetic and analgesic of physician's choice are administered. Check for facial function. The patient can be up ad lib.

Laboratory and Diagnostic Studies

CBC, urinalysis, and CT scan are obtained.

Procedure

Incision and Exposure

The incision is made immediately in front of the ear following natural skin creases. The incision extends below the earlobe and into the neck below the angle of the jaw. The incision is carried down into the neck to provide full visualization of the facial nerve. Anterior and posterior skin flaps are developed. This incision is carried down sharply using a blade until the fascia overlying the parotid gland is seen. Unipolar electrocautery should be used carefully because transmission to and subsequent injury of the facial nerve may occur. It is better to provide electrocautery using a bipolar mode.

Details

After the parotid fascia is identified, the next portion of the procedure involves careful dissection using curved clamps to separate the gland from the mastoid process and the cartilage of the external auditory canal. At times, there is troublesome bleeding, which can usually be controlled with bipolar cautery. The tail of the parotid gland is then separated from the anterior and superior portion of the sternocleidomastoid muscle.

The most important portion of the operation is the identification of the main trunk of the facial nerve. Using a small curved or delicate Crile clamp, the parotid fascia is carefully elevated. The fascia is then transected carefully and the main trunk is identified. At times, identification is difficult. The cartilage of the external auditory canal can be used as a guide to finding the main trunk. After the main trunk is identified, the dissection proceeds anteriorly and laterally. It is critical that the dissection follow the trunk of the facial nerve. The branches of the facial nerve are identified most easily in this fashion. At times, the main trunk is not found readily. Identification of a superficial branch can be made and followed posteriorly and deeply to the main trunk. However, the safest technique is to identify the main trunk and pursue the course of the branches in a posterior-to-anterior fashion. The nerve stimulator here becomes important to trace small branches of the facial nerve. As the branches of the facial nerve become visible, the substance of the parotid gland and the lesion within it can be dissected away safely. After the freed portion of the superficial lobe is dissected from the facial nerve branches, the parotid duct is transected and ligated at the anterior wound margin.

Closure

After the parotid gland and the lesion are removed from the operative field, the nerve fibers are again identified. Any areas of bleeding are either ligated with small silk ties or cauterized using bipolar cautery. The previously raised flaps are then reapproximated using 4–0 or 5–0 absorbable suture and the skin is closed using 5–0 or 6–0 nonabsorbable suture material. A small tissue drain, preferably a suction drain, may be placed in the most dependent portion of the wound.

Postoperative Care

A firm pressure dressing (similar to the previously described mastoid dressing) is used. However, the self-adherent gauze is used in a similar fashion to a modified Barton dressing. Care must be taken to support the external ear. After the wound is dressed, the patient is transferred to the recovery room. One of the most important aspects of transfer, especially if a suction drain is placed, is to prevent accidental dislodging of the suction drain.

After the patient is awake, the facial nerve can be examined by asking the patient to follow commands regarding facial expressions. Analgesics are usually ordered. The amount of discomfort is usually that of a pressure sensation from the pressure dressing. The dressing is left in place for at least 24 to 48 hours. After this, the dressing is changed and the wound evaluated. The suction drain is removed at the surgeon's discretion.

Potential Surgical Complications

Facial nerve injury, temporary or permanent (if a branch or main trunk is sectioned, immediate repair is indicated)
Bleeding with subsequent hematoma formation
Recurrence of the lesion
Abnormal sweating on the side of the face

Tracheotomy

Definition and Indications

Tracheotomies are performed to form an artificial opening into the trachea, or windpipe. Adult and pediatric tracheotomy procedures are different.

The indications for tracheotomy vary but they are all for a maintenance of an artificial airway:

- Prolonged intubation or need to undergo ventilation
- Upper airway obstruction in which orotracheal intubation is difficult or not possible
- Pulmonary toilet and cleaning of secretions

A permanent tracheotomy is always performed when there is a laryngectomy, or removal of the voice box.

Related Surgical Procedures

None

Perioperative Nursing Implications

Anesthesia

Tracheotomies are often performed under local anesthesia in adults. General anesthesia, however, is preferred in the pediatric patient. A small amount of local anesthetic with vasoconstricting agents may be used to infiltrate the skin in the area of the incision.

Position

Several important aspects of positioning exist when performing a tracheotomy. Unless it is contraindicated, the neck is hyperextended. A roll is placed under the shoulders. In young children, the chin is pulled superiorly as much as possible. Tape may be used to help further in hyperextending a child's neck. The tape can be secured from the chin to the head of the OR bed. The surface landmarks of the neck are identified.

Creation and Maintenance of the Sterile Field

Even though the respiratory system is entered, the procedure should be considered sterile. A marking pen can be used to mark the structures that have been palpated. The skin incision can be either horizontal or vertical. The neck is prepared with antimicrobial solution, and sterile drapes are applied in standard fashion.

Equipment and Supplies

In a young child, appropriate pediatric instruments are required. This may include smaller curved hemostats than in an adult tracheotomy set, as well as fine tissue forceps. In addition, a wide variety of sizes and types of tracheotomy tubes are essential. A discussion of the different types of tracheotomy tubes is beyond the scope of this chapter, but sizes ranging from those small enough to fit premature babies to those suitable for the largest adult must be readily available.

Drugs and Solutions

Lidocaine 1% with 1:100,000 epinephrine
Lubricant jelly
Lidocaine 4% transtracheal injection

Physiological Monitoring

If the procedure is performed under general anesthesia, routine care as discussed for previous procedures should be maintained. However, if the procedure is done under local anesthesia, it is vital that the circulating nurse explain the procedure and the sensations that the patient will experience before the procedure. The placement of a shoulder roll, the application of the electrocautery dispersive pad and possible wrist restraints, and the feeling of "loss of breath" are all critical to explain to the patient. During this procedure, the nurse plays a vital role in decreasing the patient's anxiety level by being close at hand. ECG, respirations, blood pressure, and pulse oximetry are monitored throughout the procedure.

Specimens and Cultures

None

Physician's Orders

The physician orders a chest x-ray film, tracheostomy care as necessary, continuation of IV fluid administration, pulmonary function studies if indicated, and respiratory therapy if necessary.

Laboratory and Diagnostic Studies

CBC, urinalysis, and a chest x-ray film are obtained.

Procedure

Incision and Exposure

A vertical incision technique is described. After the skin incision has been made, it is carried deep through the platysma muscle (Fig. 29–19A). It is carried down until the fascia in the midline between the small strap muscles of the neck is identified. The fascia is then incised in a sharp fashion using either a blade or an electrocautery unit. The strap muscles are then retracted laterally. This usually exposes the thyroid gland isthmus (i.e., the connection between both sides of the thyroid gland). A decision must be made at this time whether the isthmus of the thyroid gland will be transected or merely retracted (Fig. 29–19B). If a decision is made to transect the thyroid gland, curved hemostats are used to dissect the gland gently from the trachea below. The gland is transected between two curved hemostats and ligated using absorbable 3–0 suture material. This facilitates visualization of the structures below.

Details

The cricoid cartilage should be in full visibility. As the surgeon prepares to enter the windpipe, the surgical scrub assistant must have the tracheotomy tube prepared and available to be inserted. The anesthetist is notified that the airway will be entered. The technique of entering the airway varies in children and adults. In adults, a No. 11 blade knife can be used to cut a window of cartilage in the area of the second, third, or fourth tracheal arch (Fig. 29–19C). A flap of tracheal cartilage has also been advocated.

In young infants, however, before the airway is entered, it is important to place silk stay ties on the lateral portion of the trachea. These can be used to help bring the trachea out into the neck incision in case of accidental decannulation. Also in the pediatric population, a sharp blade that is short (a Beaver 6900 blade is ideal) can be used to incise the tracheal arches. In the pediatric population, a portion of the tracheal arch is not removed. Instead an incision is made along the third, fourth, and at times, fifth tracheal arch.

After elevating the tracheal ring (Fig. 29–19D), the surgeon places the tracheotomy tube, complete with obturator, through the opening. The tracheotomy ties and a syringe to inflate the cuff are attached to the tube. The obturator is removed and an inner cannula is inserted. Sterile anesthesia connectors are then used to connect a tracheotomy tube to the anesthesia machine if the tube selected is not designed with the appropriate connector.

Closure

After the airway has been established, the tracheotomy tube can be secured using the tracheotomy ties usually included in tracheotomy tube sets. In addition, for extra protection, the flanges of the tracheotomy tube may be sutured to the skin of the neck.

Postoperative Care

In the immediate postoperative period, a chest x-ray film should be obtained, especially for young infants. The possibility of pneumothorax exists in the younger patient. In addition, even small tracheotomy tubes are at times too long in the very young patient. This can cause the tracheotomy tube tip to ventilate only one side of the chest. Visualization of the tube tip on a chest x-ray film helps prevent this complication. The excessive incision can be approximated using a single skin nonabsorbable suture in the young patient. However, care must be taken not to create an airtight wound. This is

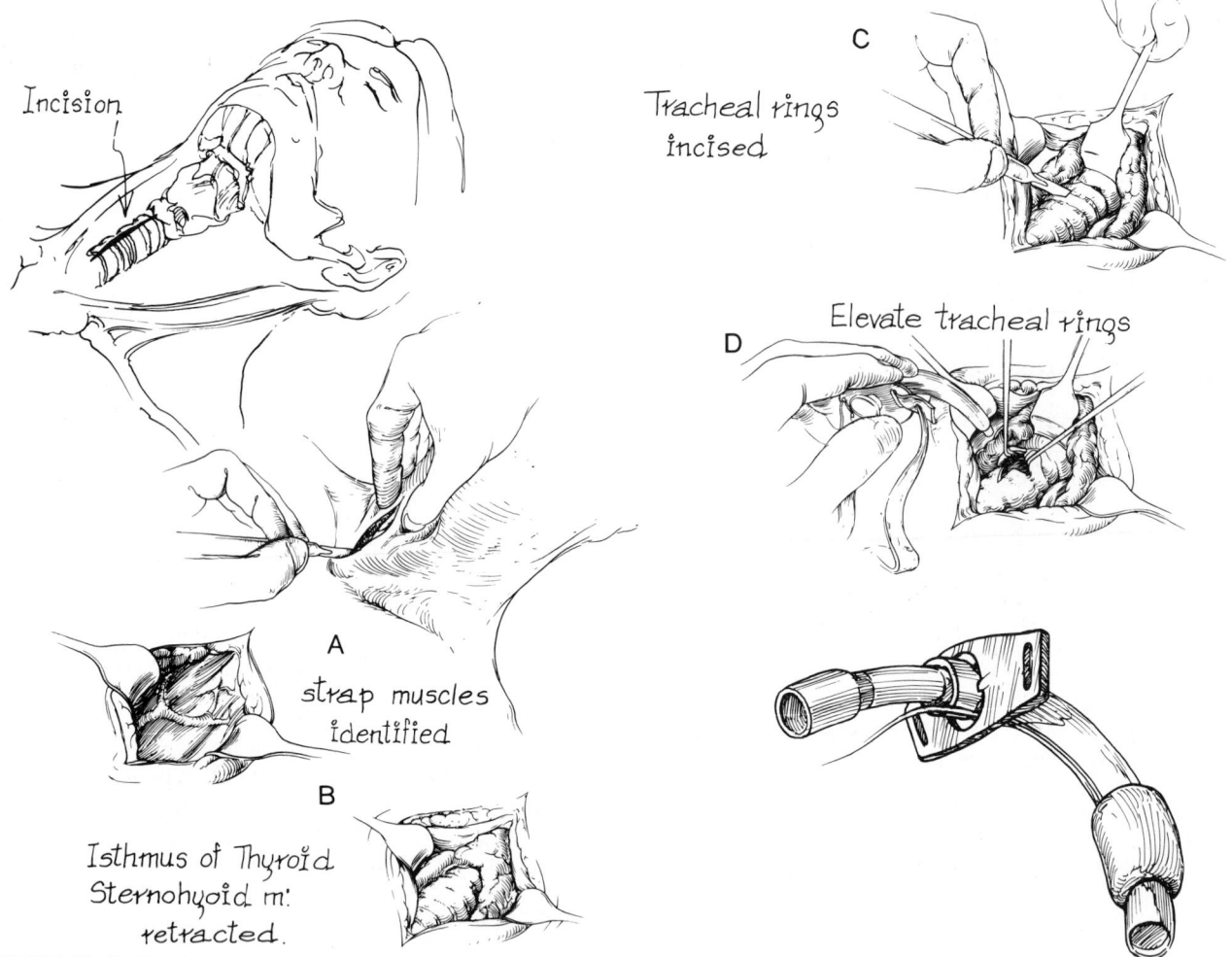

Incision

C

Tracheal rings
incised

D

Elevate tracheal rings

A

strap muscles
identified

B

Isthmus of Thyroid
Sternohyoid m.
retracted.

FIGURE 29–19. Tracheotomy procedure. (From Bailey, B., Biller, H. [1985]. *Surgery of the larynx* [pp. 404, 405]. Philadelphia: W. B. Saunders.)

because air escape from a tracheotomy tube almost always occurs. If the wound is closed tightly, there can be air dissection into the subcutaneous tissues.

As the patient is transported to either the recovery room or the intensive care unit, the most important portion of the transport is prevention of accidental dislodging of the tracheotomy tube. Elbow restraints should be used to prevent young children from pulling at the tracheotomy tube. If necessary, sedation is ordered by the surgeon. Performing pediatric tracheotomies should be discouraged in settings in which pediatric intensive care units are not readily available. The nursing staff is critical in preventing accidental decannulation and subsequent tragedies. Most patients require frequent suctioning of secretions in the first 24 hours. Additional tracheotomy tubes of the size used must always accompany the patient. The previously placed tracheal stay sutures should be marked right and left. In case of accidental decannulation, these sutures may be used to elevate the trachea and aid in replacement of the tracheotomy tube. The obturator is secured to the head of the patient's bed at all times to aid in replacement of the tube.

Potential Surgical Complications

Intraoperative complications, including injury to the nerves of the vocal cords and injury to large blood vessels abnormally located in the area of the incision

Pneumothorax

Accidental decannulation during the postoperative period, especially in children

Pneumonia

Infections in the area of the skin or within the trachea

Formation of a tracheoesophageal fistula

Tracheal stenosis

Erosion of blood vessels leading to fatal hemorrhage

Total Laryngectomy and Radical Neck Dissection

Definition and Indications

Total laryngectomy refers to the excision of the "cartilaginous larynx, hyoid bone, and the strap muscles connected to the larynx and possible removal of the preepiglottic space with the lesion" (Meeker and Rothrock, 1991, p. 567). *Radical neck dissection* refers to excision of a tumor, the surrounding anatomical structures, and lymph nodes on the affected side of the neck.

The indications for partial or total removal of the larynx and radical neck dissection are primarily the treatment of cancer. Because patients undergoing laryngectomy or neck dissection are usually heavy alcohol and tobacco users, their overall medical condition must be fully evaluated. At times, preoperative or adjuvant chemotherapy is also advocated.

Related Surgical Procedures

Hemilaryngectomy or partial laryngectomy
Supraglottic laryngectomy

Perioperative Nursing Implications

Anesthesia

The anesthesia implications are usually identical to those described above for a tracheotomy under general anesthesia. The anesthesiologist should be positioned to the side of the patient on the unaffected side of the neck. Usually, an arterial line is placed. Blood gas levels are often monitored.

Position

The positioning implications are usually identical to those described above for a tracheotomy. If an accompanying neck dissection is to be performed, the head might need to be turned to the appropriate side. The comfort and safety devices described above for the ear procedures are used.

Creation and Maintenance of the Sterile Field

The entire face, including the ears, the neck, and the chest to the nipple line should be prepared with povidone-iodine (Betadine) scrub and paint. If necessary, the chest should be shaved. If a tracheostomy stoma is present, include the stoma in the preparation. Avoid getting solutions, however, in the stoma. If the surgeon intends to obtain a graft, prepare the thigh. The initial tracheostomy site is painted with povidone-iodine. The sterile field is created using a head and neck drape pack. Care is taken in lifting the patient's head for application of the head drape, and the anesthetist is informed before this is done. The patient is then draped with appropriate sterile sheets.

Equipment and Supplies

A general plastic set, a tracheostomy set, a vascular set, biolar cautery, a headlight, a nerve stimulator, an eggcrate or gel pad for the OR bed, a hyperthermia blanket, a scale for weighing sponges, antiembolism stockings (these may be applied on the nursing unit before transfer to the OR), a nasogastric feeding tube, a closed suction drain, bone cutters and an oscillating saw (for partial laryngectomy), a Foley catheter, and tracheostomy and/or laryngectomy tubes are assembled.

Drugs and Solutions

Lidocaine 1% with 1:100,000 epinephrine
Oxidized regenerated cellulose (Surgicel)
Lidocaine 4%
Hetastarch (Hespan) for anesthesia
Demineralized water for the hyperthermia blanket
Antibiotic of surgeon's preference

Physiological Monitoring

Most neck cancer cases are lengthy, therefore, a Foley catheter is usually inserted. In addition, a nasal feeding tube is usually passed through one naris down to the level of the throat. At the end of the procedure, this feeding tube is advanced into the esophagus and into the stomach. This tube is used to feed the patient in the postoperative period.

The sponges are weighed throughout the procedure to obtain an estimate of blood loss during the procedure. The patient's temperature is also monitored with a rectal probe. An oral temperature probe is contraindicated to decrease the number of tubes in the surgical field. Blood gas and electrolyte values are monitored throughout the procedure.

Specimens and Cultures

Contents of the neck to include the jugular vein, the 11th cranial nerve, the sternocleidomastoid muscle and the submandibular salivary gland, the ipsilateral portion of the throid gland, and the larynx are the surgical specimens.

Physician's Orders

The physician orders an IV, antibiotics of choice, the use of drains to suction, nothing by mouth for 48 hours, admittance to the intensive care unit, and a chest x-ray film. Vital signs are obtained every hour for 4 hours and then every 4 hours. Mouth care and tracheotomy care are given as necessary. Oxygen is given per tracheotomy collar at 5 L/minute. Analgesics and antiemetics of choice are ordered. The patient is advanced to tube feeding every 4 hours and is up to a chair on the first postoperative day.

Laboratory and Diagnostic Studies

CBC, urinalysis, PT, PTT, SMA 15, electrolyte values, a chest x-ray film, and CT scan are obtained.

Procedure

Incision and Exposure

After the neck has been prepared and draped as described above, a decision is made about the skin incision. If a laryngectomy is going to be performed without a neck dissection, the head should stay in the midline and be hyperextended. If a partial laryngectomy (i.e., a vertical or supraglottic laryngectomy) is the operative procedure, appropriate horizontal incisions are planned. If the procedure is to be a total laryngectomy without neck dissection, the incision is usually a midline vertical incision.

Because the operation is most commonly performed in conjunction with a neck dissection, the incisions planned can vary at the discretion of the surgeon. The description below is for the most comprehensive of laryngectomy procedures (a total laryngectomy and radical neck dissection).

The goal of the neck dissection is to remove all lymph-bearing tissue from the midline anteriorly to the trapezius muscle posteriorly and also from the mandible superiorly to the clavicle inferiorly. All of this tissue between the deep cervical fascia and the platysma muscle externally is removed, except for the carotid artery system and the vagus, phrenic, and hypoglossal nerves. The brachial plexus is also preserved.

The contents of the neck that are removed include the jugular vein, the 11th cranial nerve, the sternocleidomastoid muscle, and the submandibular salivary gland. Sometimes, the spinal accessory (the 11th cranial) nerve can be preserved.

When the operation is combined with a total laryngectomy, the larynx, the midportion of the hyoid bone, and the epiglottis are also removed. Inferiorly, the laryngectomy also includes at least one or two tracheal arches. The patient requires a permanent tracheotomy.

Various skin incisions have been described. One of the most common incisions is made from the area just lateral to the chin, extending in a curvilinear fashion posteriorly to the mastoid process. Inferiorly low in the neck, the incision is made to include a circular portion of skin in the midline at the site of the tracheotomy. This incision extends approximately two fingerbreadths above the clavicle and curves back down posteriorly close to the edge of the anterior border of the trapezius muscle. The superior and inferior incisions are connected through an incision made in an S-type fashion. The skin flaps are then elevated, including the platysma muscle.

After the flaps have been raised, care must be exercised that the external jugular vein is not accidentally cut. The vein should instead be doubly ligated with tie and suture ligature and then transected. The inferior border of the sternocleidomastoid muscle is identified and a clamp is placed under the muscle. The muscle is then sectioned and retracted superiorly. The carotid sheath is then identified and the internal jugular vein is isolated. Care is taken to preserve the vagus nerve also present within the carotid sheath.

Details

A proximal suture ligature and a distal silk tie are placed above and below, respectively, the line of tran-

section of the internal jugular vein. The vein is then sectioned. The muscle with internal jugular vein and associated lymph nodes and fat is raised superiorly. The radical neck dissection specimen also includes transection of the strap muscles immediately superficial to the larynx and trachea. At this time, the ipsilateral portion of the thyroid gland is transected and also taken with the specimen. The trachea is now entered and endotracheal anesthesia is directed into the distal portion of the trachea. The upper portion of the specimen includes the tracheal arches and the entire larynx. The uppermost portion of the laryngeal complex includes the hyoid bone. The hyoid bone is transected from all the attachments to the muscles of the throat and tongue. As the dissection continues, the junction of the upper end of the esophagus with the lower end of the hypopharynx becomes visible. After this is done, the specimen, including the larynx and the upper portion of the trachea, is in connection with the radical neck specimen.

The pharyngeal defect is in the shape of a T. The remainder of the neck contents including the contents of the submandibular space, described above, are lifted superiorly. Throughout this submandibular space are large arteries and veins that necessitate suture ligatures. In addition, the duct of the submandibular gland must be ligated. After this is done, the entire specimen is attached in the posterior and superior portion. The dissection is now carried from the anterior to the posterior direction until the internal jugular vein limits the dissection. At this time, a double ligation of the internal jugular vein is performed. A suture ligature is placed as well. The vein is then transected. The remaining portion includes the tail of the parotid, which is transected along with the attachment of the sternocleidomastoid muscle. Many vessels are encountered in this area and need ligation.

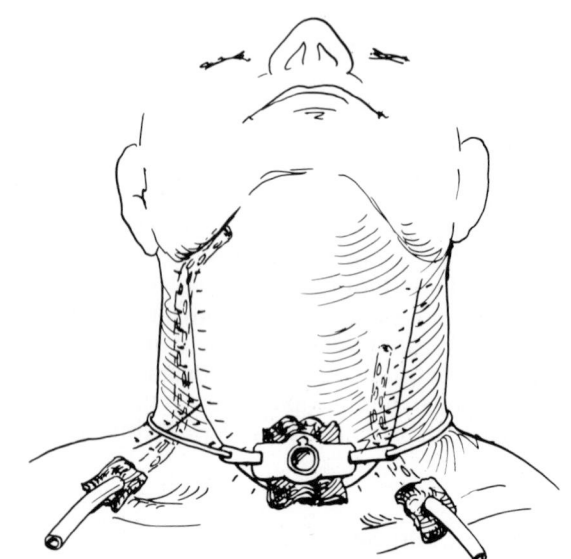

FIGURE 29–20. Total laryngectomy. (From Bailey, B., Biller, H. [1985]. *Surgery of the larynx* [p. 344]. Philadelphia: W. B. Saunders.)

These include a supraglottic laryngectomy in which the epiglottis, false vocal cords, and hyoid bone are removed, but the rest of the larynx is preserved. Also possible is a vertical or frontolateral hemilaryngectomy. With any conservation laryngectomies, a prophylactic tracheotomy is always performed.

Voice rehabilitation is a critical part of the short- and long-term follow-up of patients who have had any type of laryngectomy. Many surgeons advocate immediate insertion of a voice prosthesis after a total laryngectomy. Different types of prostheses exist. Other ways of communicating include esophageal speech, an electrolarynx, or simply, a writing tablet and pencil. Before a patient undergoes a laryngectomy, extensive preoperative counseling should be given on voice rehabilitation. The perioperatve nurse can make the transition to loss of the voice easier by being sensitive to the needs of this type of patient.

Postoperative Care

After the procedure is completed, a pressure dressing is applied, taking care not to occlude the laryngectomy opening. Many patients undergoing a lengthy oncological procedure stay in an intensive care unit setting overnight, or longer. Analgesics and antiemetics are given. Intense humidification to the airway is given as well. Care must be taken not to dislodge the suction drains.

Potential Surgical Complications

Injury to uninvolved nerves as well as laceration of large blood vessels of the neck
Injury to the lung pleura leading to a pneumothorax
Necrosis of the skin and exposure of the carotid artery, leading to exsanguinating hemorrhage
Fistula formation between the pharynx or esophagus and the skin after laryngectomy
Recurrence of tumor
Stenosis of the remaining pharynx and esophagus

Bibliography

Adams, G., Boies, L., Hilger, P. (1989). *Boies fundamentals of otolaryngology: A textbook of ear, nose, and throat diseases* (6th ed.). Philadelphia: W. B. Saunders.
Bailey, B., Biller, H. (1985). *Surgery of the larynx*. Philadelphia: W. B. Saunders.
Glasscock, M., Shambaugh, G. (1990). *Surgery of the ear* (4th ed.). Philadelphia: W. B. Saunders.
Mailhot, C., Slezak, L. (Eds.). (1992). *Advanced training for operative room clinical specialties. Module 12: Mastodectomy and tympanoplasty* (pp. 8–9). Stanford, CA: Medcom.
Meeker, M. Rothrock, J. (Eds.). (1991). *Alexander's care of the patient in surgery* (9th ed.). St. Louis. Mosby Year Book.
Meyerhoff, W., Rice, D. (1992). *Otolaryngology—Head and neck surgery*. Philadelphia: W. B. Saunders.

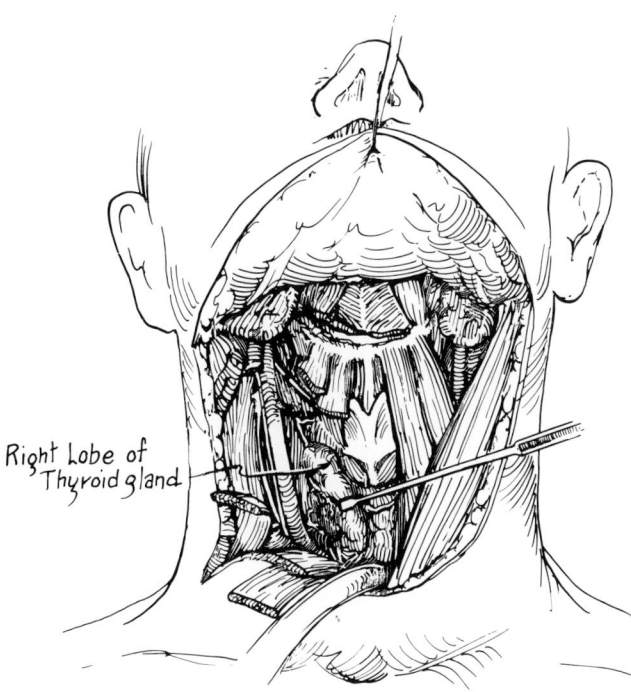

Right Lobe of Thyroid gland

FIGURE 29–21. Partial laryngectomy. (From Bailey, B., Biller, H. [1984]. *Surgery of the larynx* [p. 344]. Philadelphia: W. B. Saunders.)

Closure

The entire specimen, including the larynx, is now removed from the operative field. Through the T-shaped pharyngeal defect, the nasal feeding tube that was placed at the beginning of the procedure is advanced until it is visible within the operative field. It is then directed into the distal esophagus and the defect is closed over it. The defect is closed in a continuous inverting fashion using an absorbable suture of the surgeon's preference. The entire neck wound is then ready for closure.

The wound is copiously irrigated with either normal saline or an antibiotic solution. A two-layer closure using absorbable suture is employed for the approximation of the platysma muscle and subcutaneous tissue. To close the skin, nonabsorbable suture or skin staples are used. The distal trachea is sutured to the skin using interrupted, nonabsorbable sutures. Two suction drains are used, taking care not to place them directly over the carotid artery (Fig. 29–20).

Appropriately sized laryngectomy tubes should be available. Laryngectomy tubes are similar to tracheotomy tubes, except that they are usually shorter and of wider inner diameters. The preparation of the tubes before insertion is identical to that for tracheotomy tubes.

Partial Laryngectomy. There are times when a total laryngectomy is not necessary (Fig. 29–21). In malignancies of the larynx for which adequate margins can be obtained, preservation of a portion of larynx is preferred. In this way, a more functional voice can be obtained. Different procedures have been described.

SPECIAL POPULATIONS

CHAPTER 30

Pediatric Surgery

Robin Moushey, Candice Hawley, and Barbara Diomede

All children should be tirelessly noisy, playful, grubby-handed except at meal times, soiling and tearing such clothes as they need to wear, bringing not only the joy of childhood into the house but the dust and mud as well; in short, everything that makes the quiet and order of sickness and nursing impossible.

GEORGE BERNARD SHAW

Pediatric surgery is not surgery on small adults. Not only are the procedures often exclusive to pediatric surgery, but preoperative, intraoperative, and postoperative interventions differ markedly. Pediatric patients vary from neonates (Fig. 30–1) to adolescents and young adults; thus, the perioperative nurse must possess knowledge of the stages of growth and development. These are relatively simple statements with overwhelming implications for all hospital staff caring for children inside and outside the operating room (OR). The care of children is a unique and freestanding specialty. Instruments must be modified drastically for the variance in the size of pediatric patients. Appropriate suture and needles must also be available. Children do not act like adults in their physiological and psychological responses and so should not be treated as such.

The impetus to develop pediatric surgery as a separate entity began with a few pioneers more than 40 years ago. The first organization for pediatric surgeons in North America was founded in 1948. Entire hospitals dedicated solely to the care of children were built. Dr. Potts clearly saw the need to develop pediatric surgery as a unique and separate entity. He said, "I have often wondered what sort of scar, how deep and how serious, is left on the heart of a child who is torn from his parents and suddenly tossed into a hospital environment associated in his mind with insecurity and pain."

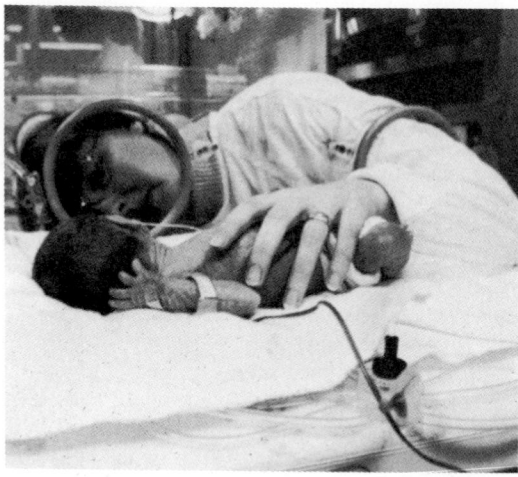

FIGURE 30–1. Mother in "en face" position with her premature infant. (From Klaus, M. H., Fanaroff, A. A. [1986]. *Care of the high-risk neonate* [3rd ed.]. Philadelphia, W. B. Saunders.)

DEVELOPMENT OF PEDIATRIC SURGERY

There have been many advances in pediatric surgery in the past decade. Although the perfection of surgical technique is all-encompassing, several factors have contributed to the successful outcomes of pediatric surgery patients.

Surgical developments were accompanied by advances in the training of pediatric anesthetists. The enhancement of knowledge of children's responses to anesthetic agents and the sheer increase in the number of anesthetists solely dedicated to children's health have greatly increased the safety when a young child is anesthetized. The location of children's operating and postanesthesia care units (PACUs), or recovery rooms, in close proximity to patient units and family waiting rooms is instrumental in fostering family-centered care. Equipment developed with children in mind is key to the surgeons' ability to operate in an effective and efficient manner. Environmental temperatures elevated to avoid hypothermia and cold stress in the infant can do just as much as proper fluid administration to avoid serious postoperative complications for the child.

Other far-reaching developments in pediatrics have occurred that affect the child, the family, the surgeon, and the nurse even before the surgery occurs. Many pediatric centers are focusing much time, money, and effort on becoming level I trauma centers. With the commitment to this program comes the development of transport teams. By air, land, or even sea, children are coming to hospitals after a traumatic birth or accident more quickly than in previous decades. The limited evaluative time spent by the surgeon in the emergency room is enhanced by preliminary care provided by colleagues in the field so that the need for OR time and rooms can be determined before the child reaches the medical center. Trauma and OR teams who had to be called in from home are now available in house 24 hours

a day to avoid any moments lost in stabilizing the child in readiness for possible surgery. Computed tomographic scanners are available to hasten diagnosis before surgery, but their use also protects the child from unnecessary surgical intervention. However, the final judgment as to whether a child goes to surgery is still based on the skillful examination of a pediatric surgeon.

Commensurate with the skill of the pediatric surgeon is the pediatric nursing care both inside and outside the OR. The child undergoing surgery needs skilled nursing care. The margin for error is small in the young child and almost nonexistent in the infant. Nurses well versed in the psychological and physiological responses of the child should be involved throughout the surgical experience. Thus, perioperative nursing becomes a process that encompasses care delivered before, during, and after the surgical intervention.

Postoperative developments that have hastened successful postoperative recovery in children are training of staff and advances in equipment, for both the PACU and the pediatric and neonatal intensive care units. Again, both units should be located with easy access to the surgeons and the surgical suite. Sophisticated monitoring abilities and quick retrieval of crucial laboratory values allow optimal postoperative assessment. Aggressive fluid and nutritional therapy early in the child's postoperative course enhances the child's ability to stabilize and recover. Careful management of intravenous (IV) catheters (both peripheral and central) enables delivery of needed fluids and medications without the setback of nosocomial infection. Postoperatively, the pediatric patient usually emerges from anesthesia much more rapidly than the adult patient and usually resumes normal activities more rapidly as well.

PHYSIOLOGICAL UNIQUENESS OF CHILDREN

Airway/Pulmonary Management

Children differ physiologically from adults in several variables that can affect surgical outcomes. Airway management is a priority because of the decreased diameter of the trachea in children. Cartilage development before muscle growth also makes the airway more prone to collapse than in the adult. If cold stress, hypoglycemia, hypovolemia, and sepsis occur, the young child is susceptible to respiratory arrest.

The lung buds develop within the mediastinum at 24 days of life, bronchial development is completed by 12 weeks, and the lobes of the lung are present at the 16th week (Krauss, 1976). Alveolar growth continues from 24 weeks of gestational life to birth. However, at the moment of birth, the number of saccules and primitive alveoli is 8% of the number in adults. The alveolar maturation continues until 8 to 10 years of age (Krishna et al., 1981).

To satisfy increased oxygen demands, alveolar ventilation in children is twice that of adults. The respiratory rate increases faster than the volume of air. This leads to decreased respiratory reserves related to functional and structural immaturity as well as increased anesthetic requirements in relationship to size. The uptake of anesthesia is faster in children because of increased alveolar ventilation and cardiac output (Krishna et al., 1981).

Temperature Regulation

Maintaining body temperature is difficult for all young children. The pediatric patient, especially the neonate, tends to become hypothermic during anesthesia and surgery. Thermoregulation is difficult because the young child suffers heat loss more than the adult in response to a variety of factors. Children have a larger surface area in relationship to size. They possess a thin layer of subcutaneous fat. They also have a decreased ability to produce heat because they do not have the ability to shiver nor have chemical thermogenesis in brown adipose tissue. Maintaining normal body temperature can be a challenge, especially in premature or critically ill patients. The room temperature is kept above 80°F and the patient is placed on a warming blanket. Radiant heat lights are directed at the child during induction of anesthesia, skin preparation, and emergence from anesthesia. Wrapping the patient's extremities and head in plastic wrap or bags helps to prevent heat loss. Only warm irrigation fluids are used. Care must be taken to prevent pooling of skin preparation solution. The skin of pediatric patients has increased sensitivity, which can result in burns, especially when the skin is brought into contact with a heating blanket. Pediatric electrocautery grounding pads are used on infants. Placement on the lower back and upper buttocks provides adequate contact and also helps prevent contact of preparation solution and the grounding pad.

A body temperature registering below 35° represents a cold injury that can be associated with respiratory depression, hypoglycemia, acidosis, and sepsis. The greatest risk of intraoperative hypothermia is usually manifested in the postanesthesia recovery period.

Energy Stores

Infants undergoing surgery may have an increased risk of hypoglycemia. Glycogen stores can be decreased in children small for gestational age and those with malnutrition and hypoxia. It is essential to replace glucose in the infant and young child during surgery (Krishna et al., 1981). Cold stress, sepsis, and hypoxia add extra metabolic and energy requirements for the young child. Anesthesia, surgical trauma, and sepsis also may increase energy requirements by 10 to 15% for as long as 3 weeks (Rowe, 1979). Often, these factors are interrelated. Hypoglycemia compounds cold stress, and oxygen and fluid requirements subject the child to septic risks. Desaturation occurs much more rapidly in infants than in adults. Owing to reduced circulating blood volume in small children, every effort must be made to prevent what may at first appear to be slight hemorrhage. Correspondingly, the administration of intravenous (IV) fluids must be monitored closely to prevent fluid overload. Increased demands for oxygen and fluid result in greater energy need, which contributes to energy losses and therefore contribute to cold stress and sepsis. Constant surveillance is needed to prevent these damaging occurrences.

Much energy is required for the child to keep warm, and the increased metabolic rate in young children often consumes their already meager energy stores. Glycogen storage usually occurs immediately before birth. The infant depends on glycolysis until glucose is supplied by an exogenous source. Although fat tissue is usually the largest energy supply, this may be limited in an infant who is not full term. By 3 hours after birth, all the hepatic glycogen may have been used, and muscle glycogen stores are completely utilized by 48 hours (Rowe, 1980).

Fluid Balance

Crucial to physiological needs is the child's need to maintain proper fluid balance. Again, their needs differ from those of adults because children have a larger percentage of their body weight in extracellular water than do adults. Infants can have 70 to 90% of their body weight in water. Children's increased metabolic rates also increase their need for fluids. Increased evaporative water losses come from increased surface area and a thinner epidermis. A crying child may double his or her fluid loss. Radiant heat warmers and phototherapy also increase water losses. Children who have fevers and are undergoing ventilation also require additional fluids.

To add to the difficulty of maintaining fluid balance, children have a limited renal function. Their glomerulofiltration rate is 25% of that of an adult. Their kidneys are immature and have a decreased ability to concentrate urine. All these factors contribute to the need for increased administration of maintenance fluids during surgery, but extra replacement fluids are necessary when there are major alterations in fluid shifts or balances when a child undergoes major surgery.

Third spacing can occur in children postoperatively as a result of peritoneal irritation caused by intestinal perforation, peritonitis, or enterocolitis. During the surgical procedure, capillary and lymphatic drainage can occur throughout the intestinal tract. This damage causes increased capillary permeability, which may lead to leakage of fluid, electrolytes, and proteins from the capillary space to the interstitial and intracellular spaces. The spillage of bowel contents causes a loss of gastrointestinal tone and decreased peristaltic activity. The inflammatory response causes bacteria, fecal material, and intestinal juices to pour into the peritoneal cavity, mimicking a "peritoneal burn" (Rowe, 1980). The loss of osmotic activity from the intravascular space to the interstitial and intracellular spaces causes more fluid to leave the capillaries. Children undergoing surgery have increased need for fluid replacement simply because of age, which is compounded when they lose fluids from the procedure and then have a large amount of needed reserve fluid sequestered in lost spaces. Children can require 1½ to 2 times maintenance fluids to sustain fluid volume and blood pressure postoperatively until the capillaries begin to heal and the lymphatics return to work. By 24 to 48 hours after surgery, the kidneys, if they have been well hydrated, begin the process of diuresis, and fluid administration can be decreased.

Cardiovascular System

Infants possess certain cardiovascular characteristics that can affect their postoperative course. The right and left ventricles are almost equal in muscular thickness at birth. The foramen ovale and ductus arteriosus, although functionally closed, are anatomically patent. The foramen ovale closes at 3 months to 1 year, whereas the ductus arteriosus, although functionally closed at 10 to 15 days, does not close anatomically until 2 months. The pulmonary arterioles in young children have increased muscularity and extreme vasoreactivity.

The primary deterrent to closure of the ductus arteriosus is believed to be increased arterial carbon dioxide tension, which has a direct constricting effect on smooth muscle. The neonate undergoing surgery can sustain many physiological insults. Hypoxia, acidosis, and increased pulmonary vascular volume can all produce intense pulmonary vasoconstriction (Krishna et al., 1981). Pulmonary arterial hypertension and increasing blood pressure occur, causing the ductus arteriosus to dilate. When the right-sided heart pressure exceeds the left-sided heart pressure, the right-to-left shunt develops across the foramen ovale and ductus arteriosus. A large volume of blood passes into the left side of the heart and descending aorta without first traversing the lungs (Rowe, 1980). This causes further increases in pulmonary vascular resistance and can develop into persistent fetal circulation. Although most commonly seen in the infant with diaphragmatic hernia, this is a risk for all neonates undergoing surgery.

Thus, there are unique physiological characteristics that make children different from adults. These differences are also observed in the normal ranges for laboratory studies. Table 30–1 presents normal findings in common preoperative blood tests for pediatric patients.

PSYCHOSOCIAL ALTERATION AND THE SURGICAL EXPERIENCE

Reactions to Hospitalization and Surgery

Children also differ in their psychological responses and reactions to surgery and the OR environment.

It never ceases to be interesting to watch the reaction of children entering a hospital for an operation. It varies all the way from childish bravado to sheer panic. A seven-year-old boy was brought in because of a question of hernia. Examination proved there was no hernia; and as the boy left the examining room he made a gesture of wiping sweat from his brow and exclaimed, "Boy, that was a close one." A younger child clarified his position after I had explained to him that he would have to have an operation. He said, "I hate you, you stinker." Another little boy said in response to what he considered bad news, "You know what? Lions eat people, and I hope they eat you." One will not have to worry that such children will have repressions.

POTTS (1956)

The optimal approach to the child facing surgery is an overall acceptance of their behaviors. They also need information to process so that they can gain some mastery and control over their OR experience. Appendix A presents an example of a preoperative teaching program for pediatric surgical outpatients.

Although children's responses to hospitalization and surgery are varied, there some fears that children commonly experience. The immediate fear is separation from loved ones and things. This includes feelings of abandonment, thoughts of punishment, and fears of rejection. The hospitalized child may respond to her or his parents in various ways because of the blame she or he places on them. The child may exhibit indifference or even reject the parent. At times, the children may cling to the nurse in the presence of the parent. If the child is old enough, his or her verbalizing this anger helps to restore the parent-child relationship.

Real and fantasy fears of pain and injury include all the apprehensions regarding procedures, injections, anesthesia, and surgery. Freud (1952) noted that the child reacts more to the fantasy aroused by the procedure than to the procedure itself. It is difficult for the child to differentiate between pain from within and pain imposed from without. A child often points to her or his parents or the nurse and says, "You hurt me!" (Erickson, 1967). Fear of death has been reported to be one aspect of pain that is difficult for the child to bear (Schultz, 1971).

Honesty is essential when dealing with children and pain. They need to know when something will or will not hurt. "But woe unto him who breaks faith in promising that nothing bad is going to happen and then hurts the child" (Potts, 1956). The nature of the illness or injury affects the thoughts of the child and can produce concerns regarding body image, feelings of guilt, and fears of death.

Children in the past experienced unnecessary pain because adults feared that children could not tolerate sufficient pain medication. Pain management in children has reached acceptance and success. Pain services have been developed in some children's hospitals to act as resources to all health care services and patients.

The child between the ages of 1 and 4 years seems to be most vulnerable to the effects of separation during hospitalization. Children of ages 2 to 4 years show the most severe reactions to hospitalization. Younger chil-

TABLE 30–1. NORMAL FINDINGS IN COMMON PREOPERATIVE BLOOD TESTS FOR PEDIATRIC PATIENTS

Test	Normal Range		Test	Normal Range	
Potassium (mmol/L)	Newborn:	3.9–5.9	Partial thromboplastin time	Premature (48 h):	7.35–7.5
	Infant:	4.1–5.3		Birth, full term:	7.11–7.36
	Child:	3.4–4.7		5–10 min:	7.09–7.3
	Thereafter:	3.5–5.1		30 min:	7.21–7.38
Sodium (mmol/L)	Newborn:	134–146		>1 h:	7.26–7.49
	Infant:	139–146		1 d:	7.29–7.45
	Child:	138–145		Thereafter:	7.35–7.45
	Thereafter:	136–146		Must be corrected for body	
Chloride (mmol/L)	Cord:	96–104		temperature	
	Newborn:	97–110	White blood cell count	Birth:	9–30
	Thereafter:	98–106	(1000 cells/mm³ [ul])	24 h:	9.4–34
Carbon dioxide (mmol/L)	Cord:	14–22		1 mo:	5–19.5
	Premature:	14–27		1–3 y:	6–17.5
	Newborn:	13–22		4–7 y:	5.5–15.5
	Infant:	20–28		8–13 y:	4.5–13.5
	Child:	20–28		Adult:	4.5–11
	Thereafter:	23–30	Hemoglobin (g/dl)	1–3 d (capillary):	14.5–22.5
				2 mo:	.9–14.
Glucose (fasting) (mg/dl)	Cord:	45–96		6–12 y:	11.5–15.5
	Premature:	20–60		12–18 y,	
	Neonate:	30–60		Male:	13–16
	Newborn,			Female:	12–16
	1 d:	40–60		18–49 y,	
	>1 d:	50–90		Male:	13.5–17.5
	Child:	60–100		Female:	12–16
	Adult:	70–105	Hematocrit (% of packed	1 d (capillary):	48–69
Creatinine (mg/dl)	Cord:	0.6–1.2	red blood cells)	2 d:	48–75
	Newborn:	0.3–1		3 d:	44–72
	Infant:	0.2–0.4		2 mo:	28–42
	Child:	0.3–0.7		6–12 y:	35–45
	Adolescent:	0.5–1.0		12–18 y,	
	Adult,			Male:	37–49
	Male:	0.6–1.2		Female:	36–46
	Female:	0.5–1.1		18–49 y,	
Blood urea nitrogen (mg/dl)	Cord:	21–40		Male:	41–53
	Premature (1 wk):	3–25		Female:	36–46
	Newborn:	3–12			
	Infant or child:	5–18			
	Thereafter:	7–18			
Prothrombin time	In general: 11–15 s (varies with type of thromboplastin)				
	Newborn:	prolonged by 2–3 s			

Adapted from Behrman, R. E., Vaughan, V. C. (Eds.). (1987). *Nelson textbook of pediatrics* (13th ed.) (pp. 1535–1558). Philadelphia: W. B. Saunders.

dren often view hospitalization as punishment for various misdeeds. Generally, before 4 years of age, separation anxiety is the greatest crisis for the child, whereas the child older than 4 years has more problems coping with the illness than the separation.

Body Image

A child younger than 2 years of age is keenly aware of body intactness and experiences fear of mutilation during medical procedures. For example, a child often is reassured if a Band-Aid is used to cover the spot of injection, thus addressing the fear of blood loss (Erickson, 1967). A child of 4 or 5 years wants to cooperate during procedures but she or he may need some time to prepare. The child's having some say in how prepa-

ration for the procedure is accomplished helps him or her to cooperate.

The preschool child has fears of body mutilation and reacts to any violation of body integrity. These children often misinterpret the meaning of procedures. Their intense imagination often distorts explanations that they may receive. These misinterpretations often evoke anxiety and regression.

The school-age child is often outnumbered and overshadowed by younger children in the hospital setting. His or her fantasy life at this time is still vivid. Although the younger child may blame parents and other relatives for an illness, the school-age child often blames herself or himself. The child needs his or her parent change when he or she is ill. Fears of death become more pronounced at this age. The responses to illness and hospitalization are usually anger and hurt. The school-age child's expression of anxiety is usually increased activity. The older child may also show regression and anxiety because of fear of genital inadequacy, muscular weakness, and loss of body control. The fear of body mutilation is more intense if the child's head or genitals are involved (Whaley and Wong, 1979).

The school-age and the preschool child have certain fears and reactions to surgery. They often wonder what will be done while they are under anesthesia, what will be removed, and whether or not they will die. All these fears may result in aggressive behavior if they are not resolved (Erickson, 1967).

An intact motor system helps create a good body image. A child learns about the world through muscular activity. When this activity is cut off, the child feels trapped. It is thought that immobilization may be the most difficult part of illness for the child (Erickson, 1965). The child may feel punished and threatened. The inability to move is a threat to self-preservation and promotes feelings of anxiety and aggression in the child. Immobility reactivates the dependence-independence struggle and the activity-passivity struggle. The normal reaction to restriction is preoccupation with activity.

Coping

The immobilized child gets upset from loneliness, sensory deprivation, and intolerable tension. To be inactive and prone connotes death to children and they have to fight it. Immobility often breeds fears and fantasies (Erickson, 1965). The child may defy the restrictions or become rigid and frozen. The child cannot vent anger on those responsible for the immobility so she or he may turn the anger inward and become depressed, withdrawn, quiet, and subdued. Some goals are to help these children feel understood and mobilize their resources to increase their control over aggression.

The child may react to hospitalization in various ways. These reactions may include regression, anger, aggression, depression, denial of illness, and withdrawal.

The child's reactions to procedures may be caused by the resentment of intrusion into his or her body or a fantasy of what is being done. These reasons may cause the child to fight to try to ward off the danger to his or her body. This fight-or-flight reaction to perceived danger is a universal response (Erickson, 1967). The child may attack procedures in place of expressing feelings about separation and punishment. This acting out behavior may also be exacerbated by the lack of knowledge the child may have about his or her body, lack of knowledge about what is wrong with it, and confusion over what is being done to diagnose or treat it.

Adult anger felt by the child as a result of these reactions often makes the child feel overpowered, ashamed, and angry. These feelings evoke more anxiety in the child, which in turn leads to more unacceptable behavior. The child has to learn quickly to trust the staff to establish a healthy adaptation to the hospital. If the child is unable to do this, she or he will keep feelings under rigid control or aggressively act them out.

Preparation for Hospitalization and Surgery

Preparation for the hospital needs to begin before admission. It is often necessary to prepare parents before one can prepare the child. Preparation needs to be accepted as part of the treatment received in the hospital. The value of good preparation often appears afterward in the speed of recuperation and freedom from neurotic symptoms. The goal is to provide the child with appropriate information so that he or she is able to master the situation or at least gain some control over the situation to cope with the impending danger that he or she may experience.

The nurse needs to understand the behavior of the family at home to really understand the child. Thereby, a family assessment has to be made, if possible, at the time of the child's admission to the hospital. To assess the family, one should consider the cultural background and economic level. The development, composition, and experiences of the family should also be considered.

Information on preparatory communications should be based on how the child will feel and what he or she can do. The timing of preparation is also important. Freud (1952) stated that, if the preparation is done too early, too much time is left to activate unconscious fantasies and fears. If not enough time is given, however, the ego has too little time to prepare defenses adequately (Fig. 30–2).

When asked to illustrate a concept or object, the child

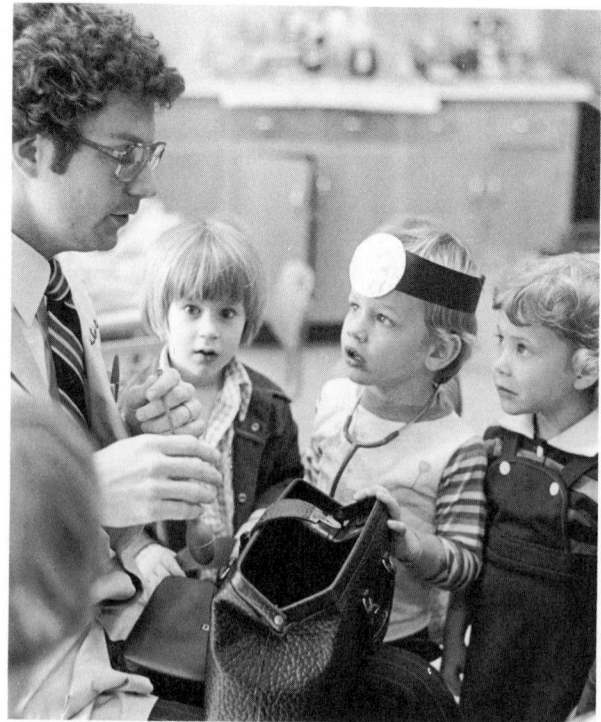

FIGURE 30–2. A nurse prepares a group of preschool children for hospitalization. (From Marlow, D. R., Redding, B. A. [1988]. *Textbook of pediatric nursing* [6th ed.]. Philadelphia: W. B. Saunders.)

draws what he or she knows rather than what he or she sees. If a child has an erroneous idea about an object, seeing the object may correct the false idea. Showing him or her another child, however, may not help with acceptance of the same treatment.

The young child learns on the concrete level. She or he gains knowledge through the use of the senses. Meanings are associated with objects through vision and touch. The child needs to manipulate the object himself or herself. He or she has problems connecting one idea with another and connecting an idea with an object. She or he cannot make generalizations or logical deductions.

The child younger than 4 years of age may not require an explanation of anatomy and physiology. One needs to stress the equipment and care used in treating the child. These young children do not comprehend the statement that taking medicine will make them better again. The child relates more easily to concrete ideas (e.g., he or she will be able to ride a tricycle again like the little boy in a picture).

The older child wants a reason for every procedure. Equipment is not as important as specific information about what is going to happen because the child becomes more interested in what is to be done and why it is to be done. Gellert's (1962) study of the body showed that children identified contents of the body in terms of what they observed being put into or coming out of it. All ages of children should understand what body parts will be involved in surgery and should be reassured that no other part of the body will be operated on. Establishing trust through all the information presented to the child is as important as the preparation. Ask the child about his or her ideas of what will happen.

Methodology

Various methods have been used to prepare the child for hospitalization. Play and puppet therapy can help explain procedures to the child. The child can passively observe the situation or join in with lively participation. Through this therapy, the nurse can observe the play and its effects concerning the child. Other methods that can be used to prepare the child before the actual admission are hospital tours, kindergarten visits by nurses, preadmission parties, home visits by a nurse from the hospital, programs presented by the school nurse concerning hospitalization, and various pamphlets or books written by hospital staff or lay people.

Preoperatively, young patients can be helped to adjust to unfamiliar surroundings by being allowed to bring a stuffed animal or other toy that can remain with them throughout their surgical experience. Allowing the patient to play with equipment (e.g., a stethoscope and a blood pressure cuff) before the physical examination as well as to use the equipment on the toy at the time of the examination effectively reduces the child's anxiety (Fig. 30–3).

The use of an induction room in the pediatric setting has proved invaluable. The child and a family member are escorted to a pleasant room, often decorated with cartoon characters, yet fully stocked with anesthetic supplies. The room is located adjacent to the OR suites. A family member holds the child on his or her lap, and mask anesthesia is induced. This begets a sense of security for both the child and the family member. After the child is anesthetized, the family member is directed to the waiting area while the child is transported to the OR. In the age range of 18 months to 4 years, the induction room works well to reduce separation anxiety.

During mask induction, children respond well to a story told in a soft tone of voice. A story featuring Oscar the Grouch from Sesame Street is especially effective—when an agent (e.g., halothane) is introduced, the child can be told to imagine that the "bad" smell is from Oscar's trash can. Transparent anesthesia masks are used to decrease claustrophobia. A few drops of flavoring (e.g., vanilla extract, cherry, and bubble

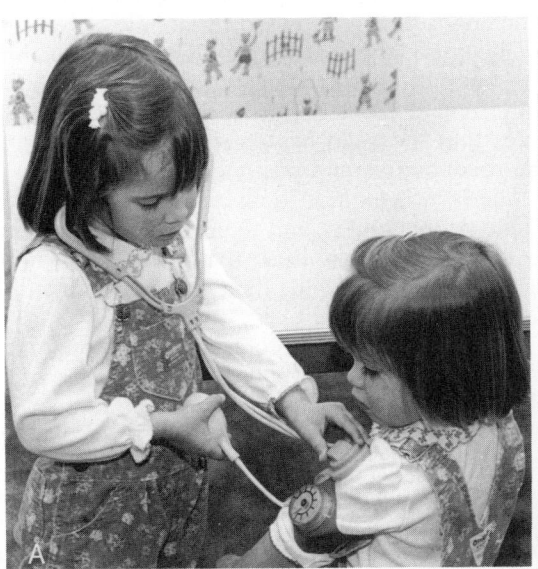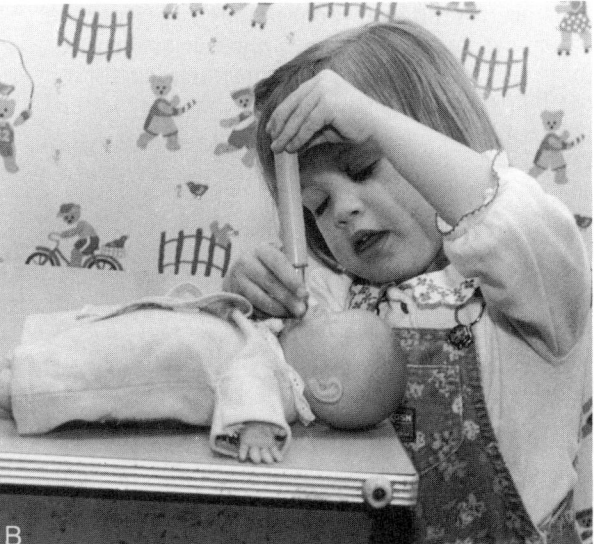

FIGURE 30–3. Preschool children "play out" their hospital experiences. *A,* Although their technique leaves something to be desired, the girls are engrossed in their play. *B,* This child was fed by gavage during her hospital stay and now carries out the procedure on her doll. (From Marlow, D. R., Redding, B. A. [1988]. *Textbook of pediatric nursing* [6th ed.]. Philadelphia: W. B. Saunders.)

gum) are applied to the inside of the mask to make the experience more pleasant. Again, if children are allowed to choose the flavor, they retain some sense of control.

Unlike the case for adults, children are allowed to come to the OR wearing their own clothing if they are reluctant to change into hospital garb. They are often upset when someone removes their shoes. Particularly in the emergent situation, allowing them to retain their clothing, thus salvaging part of their sense of control, considerably reduces their anxiety. The clothing is removed from the room immediately after anesthesia induction.

Some methods to improve preparation for the child in the future include

comprehensive community involvement emphasizing parental education and children's play regarding hospitalization and surgery

special careers for people involved in teaching and preparation children for surgery

tours of the hospital on weekends and evenings to provide exposure to the environment (see Appendix A)

PERIOPERATIVE NURSING: THE COLLABORATIVE PROCESS

Supporting children and their families throughout the surgical experience entails a collaborative nursing effort. The child is seen by a variety of caregivers, all with different roles and responsibilities, preoperatively, intraoperatively, and postoperatively. All these people contribute to the perioperative experience of the child and the family. Program development that meets the needs of children and their families has to be a collaborative effort.

Collaboration combines the power and energy of diversified roles. Clinical, managerial, and educational components are essential to program development, especially when caring for children in and out of the OR. Pooling of power creates an energy force that lets things happen. It helps make the system work for the betterment of patient outcomes (Moushey et al., 1988).

A Collaborative Project

A strong determination and desire to give clear, consistent information to children and their families is key to enhanced patient outcomes. This concern led to the development of a perioperative committee at St. Louis Children's Hospital spearheaded by management, clinicians, and educators working in collaboration. This brought together nursing resources that complemented one another and enhanced the completion of the committee's tasks. When nurses have varied roles, power can be utilized as a shared process if an open and trusting communication pattern exists.

Overall goals of the group were to

1. coordinate the varied resources involved in preparing children for hospitalization and surgery to promote efficient use of time and money
2. evaluate the effectiveness of preparation in the preadmission, preoperative, intraoperative, and postoperative period through quality assurance monitoring and research endeavors
3. coordinate resources to provide optimal outreach programs for the community
4. provide an avenue for collaboration and problem solving among professionals who prepare children for hospitalization procedures

Specific goals of the perioperative committee were manifested in the development of a coloring book describing significant preoperative and postoperative events; a slide show, program, and tour presented by the PACU staff; and a perioperative teaching tool that documents both the preparation and teaching of the child before surgery.

To coordinate both the individual and group teaching and to minimize an overload of information given by the various nurses involved in the perioperative teaching process, a tool was developed by the perioperative committee. The tool was designed as the front side of the basic surgical check list and has a threefold purpose (Fig. 30–4). First, it is an overall guide as to what could be reviewed in preoperative teaching. Second, it coordinates the various resource people involved in the teaching process, with the goal of decreasing actual nursing time while increasing the effectiveness of the information-giving process. Third, it serves as the complete documentation of the teaching and is a permanent part of the patient's record (Fig. 30–5).

Use of the Perioperative Tool

This tool is utilized for all children going to surgery. If the child is too young to receive the information, the teaching is directed toward the family.

Filling out the tool is relatively easy, but there are a few helpful hints to keep in mind. If the child attends the group session, the nurse just circles yes. This indicates that the child has received all the information in the preoperative and postoperative topics for teaching.

The section on individual teaching is the responsibility of the people on the unit to cover. Some notation needs to be made in this area. If all the information is not applicable to the child, then it is marked as not applicable.

If the child is unable to go to the preoperative group session, the nurse is responsible for all topics of teaching. She or he may call on resource people whenever needed if she or he is unable to complete the teaching. Other resources may be the preoperative teaching book and preoperative teaching pictures, which are the same as the slide shows in the group session. These resources are kept on the surgical unit and include a basket of preoperative teaching aids (e.g., anesthesia mask, gowns, surgical mask, gloves, OR hats, IV bottle and

St. Louis Children's Hospital
Surgical Check List

Pt. called for: Date _____ Time _____

Name of OR person calling _____

Time leaving unit _____ Sent to _____

Allergies _____

	PREOP			ON CALL
Initial or mark "NA" as items completed				Check or mark "NA"

Assigned Shift	Initial/NA		Check/NA
N	_____	1. NPO after _____ (Please write in actual time)	1. _____
E	_____	2. CBC (within 48 hrs) results in chart	2. _____
E	_____	3. UA (within 48 hrs) results in chart	3. _____
E	_____	4. Permit signed by parent or legal guardian	4. _____
E	_____	5. Consent form accurately specifies procedure	5. _____
E	_____	6. ID band on (legible, numbers accurate)	6. _____
E	_____	7. Allergy bands on (legible, complete)	7. _____
E	_____	8. Allergy sticker on front of chart	8. _____
N	_____	9. Extra, appropriate ID band(s) taped in chart	9. _____
E	_____	10. History and physical documented	10. _____
E	_____	11. Weight _____ on: Date: _____	11. _____
E	_____	12. B/P (within 24 hrs) _____ on: Date: _____	12. _____
N	_____	13. OR called and notified of isolation: Date _____	13. _____
E	_____	14. Prep done: Date _____ Type _____	14. _____
N	_____	15. Order sheets (all old orders and blank page) in chart	15. _____
E	_____	16. Nail polish removed from fingers and toes	16. _____
N	_____	17. Addressograph plate on front of chart	17. _____
N	_____	18. Med. Administration Guide in chart	18. _____
N	_____	19. Supplies/equipment ordered/obtained	19. _____
		20. Voided on call	20. _____
		21. Preop given and charted on Med. Guide and Order Sheet	21. _____
		22. Glasses/contacts/hair accessories/jewelry removed	22. _____
		23. Dental prosthesis removed	23. _____
		24. TPR documented on Bedside Record	24. _____
		25. Bedside Records (last 48 hrs. worth) in chart	25. _____
		26. Old chart, if ordered	26. _____
		27. Transport note in Progress Notes	27. _____

Ok'd for transport by _____ RN

Transported by _____

FIGURE 30–4. Perioperative nursing tool—basic surgical check list. (Courtesy of St. Louis Children's Hospital.)

St. Louis Children's Hospital
Perioperative Teaching Record

Date/Time of Surgery _____

	Yes	No	NA
Previous OR Experience			
Attended Preop Slide Show — Patient			
Attended Preop Slide Show — Parent			
Coloring Book Given			
Pictures/Equipment Shown			
Informed of Support/Resource Personnel			

Scheduled Procedure:

Topic for Teaching	Date	Teacher's Initials	Patient/Family Response
PREOP:			
NPO			
Vital signs/blood work			
Toys/pacifier to go to OR			
Who goes to OR with patient			
Mode of transportation			
Where parents can wait			
Holding area			
OR clothes			
Or environment (tile; lights; table; heart monitor; instrument trays)			
Anesthesia (mask/IV)			
POSTOP:			
Recovery Room (O_2 mask)			
Return to room			
Diet advancement			
IVs			
INDIVIDUAL TEACHING:			
Time NPO begins			
Time of surgery			
Preop medication			
Tubes (N/G; Foley; Drain)			
Dressings			
Activity			
Pain/discomfort			

COMMENTS: *(Specific patient and family needs)*

SIGNATURES:

Staff Nurse   OR Nurse   Other

FIGURE 30–5. Perioperative nursing tool—perioperative teaching record. (Courtesy of St. Louis Children's Hospital.)

tubing, blood pressure cuff, stethoscope, and more objects to help the children visualize and understand what will be happening to them).

Placing a bracket and initialing the large topics for teaching is appropriate in most cases.

If the nurse notes an unusual reaction or comments from the child and the family regarding the information given, this should be documented. The PACU nurse should call the nursing units and inform the nurses if the child and family exhibit unusual behavior during the preoperative slide show.

The preoperative teaching record is utilized for all patients going to surgery. There should be documentation that the nurse assessed the need for preoperative teaching.

If the child has had recent surgery experience, simply comment that the child has undergone surgery recently and note whether the child verbalizes an understanding of the OR and postoperative routine.

If emergency surgery is contemplated, often neither the child nor the family can comprehend teaching; pain or extreme anxiety may cloud their understanding. In this case, the nurse may comment, "the child needed relief from discomfort and timing was not appropriate to proceed with teaching," or "the family is experiencing much stress and is unable to process information concerning surgical routine; will answer questions and give added information after the child returns from PACU."

It is hoped that the perioperative tool provides the information that the nurse would like to have about children and their family before entering their room the morning of surgery.

This is a permanent part of the record and no further documentation is needed.

SUMMARY

In spite of careful preparation, children who are discharged often have fears that something was done to them that they do not know about. Often, they have not worked out all their fears and anger during hospitalization and they need time at home to continue to adapt to the situation. The parents need to realize this fact and must be supported in accepting some changes in their child's behavior.

Although surgery may be a fearful experience, it can also be beneficial to the development of the child. Some children leave the hospital with renewed courage and vigor.

Hospitalization may be seen as a growth experience. The child may learn identification with the nurse and the physician. He or she may have learned to achieve mastery over the environment and may have gained in self-awareness. There are also innumerable stimuli for development in the hospital.

Hospitalization and surgery interrupt the illness cycle and speed recovery. The family is mobilized around the needs of the child, attention is given to the child, and it is hoped that the child will realize that her or his worst fears and fantasies did not happen. The child's return to normal preoperative behavior is the ultimate goal.

Most surgeries in children occur because of congenital anomalies or conditions that are acquired soon after birth. Few major surgeries in children are elective, and therefore preparation time may be minimal. For this reason, the perioperative nurse has to be acutely aware of the specific needs of the child and OR procedures as well as the surgeon's preferences. Efficient and timely nursing interventions are crucial in all facets of the child's care.

Collaboration strengthens and interlocks all our nursing roles and functions. Nurses bring a part of themselves, a part of their values, and a part of their expertise to accomplish common goals. Every nurse involved in the care of a child undergoing surgery is a collaborator.

The nurse on the surgical unit needs updated information from the OR nurse to provide preoperative teaching of the child and the family in an optimal manner. The nurse in the OR depends on the skill of the unit nurse to assess the child preoperatively; the OR staff shares intraoperative information with the family and guides postoperative care on the surgical unit. The PACU nurse is another essential link in providing information to both families and nursing staffs on the units.

Each nurse has to value other health care team members as integral parts of the caring process or else the collaborative modality is lost. The ultimate outcome of collaboration is better patient care. However, there are other rewards. Job satisfaction is increased. The collaborative model fosters improved communication and understanding among health care professionals.

Professional and personal growth and development is a direct outcome of learning about varied nursing roles. Caring for the child and the family serves as the bond that draws the OR or PACU nurse and the unit nurse to cooperate. When responsibility and accountability are shared, work environments of mutual support rather than competitions are created.

POTENTIAL ALTERATIONS IN FUNCTIONAL HEALTH PATTERNS

The perioperative nurse sees many alterations in the young child facing surgery. These physiological and psychological alterations influence the role of the nurse in the preoperative, intraoperative, and postoperative periods. Although nursing diagnoses vary from child to child, depending on growth and development needs, there are some consistent diagnoses that affect all children.

Common nursing diagnoses and interventions are discussed. Some of these are

high risk for infection
high risk for impaired skin integrity
high risk for fluid volume deficit
high risk for intraoperative hypothermia
high risk for ineffective breathing patterns
alteration in comfort: pain
fear

Health Perception–Health Management Pattern

Diagnosis

High risk for infection

Definition

Presence of risk factors for the child to experience a postoperative wound infection

Risk Factors

- Immature immune response
- Poor nutritional state
- Thin epidermis
- Small surface area
- Immature ability to handle respiratory secretions
- Inability to control bowel and bladder functions
- Surgical incision
- Anesthesia
- Invasive monitoring
- Central catheters
- Total parenteral nutrition infusion
- Ostomies
- Open wounds
- Blood sampling
- Traumatic delivery
- Trauma or accident

Expected Outcome

The child does not experience a postoperative wound infection.

Perioperative Nursing Interventions

Utilize aseptic technique to prevent cross-contamination when working with wounds, ostomies, and central catheters, especially when they are in close proximity.
Protect the thin epidermis through meticulous wound care.
Keep wounds clean and protected.
Prepare central catheters with povidone-iodine (Betadine) and use discriminately
Perform a preoperative assessment of predisposing factors for infection.
Perform minimal shave preparation.
Follow the surgeon's preferences and aseptic technique for surgical skin preparation.
Instruct caregivers on wound care postoperatively.
Maintain correct wound drainage system.
Maintain sterile technique by monitoring self, surgical team, and sterile field.
Provide antibiotic irrigation as necessary.
Prevent foreign bodies from entering the surgical wound.
Assess and document the patient's condition preoperatively to determine preexisting infection and the potential for infection.

Be aware of suite airflow requirements to prevent dispersion of dust and airborne particles.
Control traffic in rooms.
Monitor all persons entering the OR for adherence to aseptic technique.
Spot clean areas contaminated with fluids from the surgical field.
Assist with dressing application using aseptic technique.
Provide antibiotics for irrigation and IV therapy.
Note wound classification.
Isolate potential contamination.

Nutritional-Metabolic Pattern

Diagnosis

High risk for impaired skin integrity

Definition

Presence of risk factors for the child to experience a disruption of the skin surface, destruction of skin layers, or invasion of body surfaces during the perioperative period (Gordon, 1987, p. 88)

Risk Factors

- Thin epidermis
- Decrease in normal skin lubricants
- Decrease in subcutaneous fat
- Surgical incision
- Infection
- Poor nutritional state
- Drainage in contact with the skin
- Open wounds
- Ostomies
- Invasive monitoring
- Application of extraneous objects such as electrosurgical dispersive electrode, pneumatic tourniquet, tape, casting material, adhesive drapes
- Application of chemical agents such as prepping solutions

Expected Outcome

The child's skin integrity is maintained.

Perioperative Nursing Interventions

Assess and document skin integrity.
Cover open wounds.
Remove excess prepping solution.
Prevent pooling of prepping solution.
Limit pressure on the skin by using padding when positioning (pad bony prominences and support devices).
Use nonirritating tape.
Confine drainage to avoid skin contact.
Place electrosurgery pad appropriately.
Use an appropriate preparation solution (avoid pooling of the solution in contact with the skin).

Limit shave preparation.
Use Montgomery tapes as appropriate.
Monitor the scrub team to avoid skin pressure.
Carefully remove adhesive drapes.
Monitor the use of the electrosurgical pencil.

Diagnosis

High risk for fluid volume deficit

Definition

Presence of risk factors for the child to experience a decrease in fluid volume during the perioperative period

Risk Factors

- Large body surface area in relation to size
- Immature kidney function
- Increased fluid needs due to increased percentage of body weight in water (infant's body weight 80% water compared with adult 50–60% of body weight in water)
- Inability to concentrate urine
- Increased volume of gastrointestinal secretions
- Surgery
- Anesthesia
- Exposed epidermis leading to increased evaporative water losses
- Poor IV access
- Narrow margin between adequate hydration and fluid overload
- Increased losses from the gastrointestinal tract due to nasogastric tubes and ostomies
- Increased fluid losses from seizures, fever, crying, time spent undergoing ventilation, suctioning, and nothing-by-mouth (NPO) status

Expected Outcome

Adequate fluid volume is maintained.
The kidneys remain perfused and output is 1 ml/kg/hour.
Blood pressure is maintained.
Vital signs remain stable.
Blood urea nitrogen and creatinine values are within normal limits.
The child maintains body temperature.

Perioperative Nursing Interventions

Assess the patient's condition preoperatively with laboratory results and determine the potential for problems (e.g., dehydration and electrolyte imbalances). Communicate with anesthesia personnel and the surgical team.

Be aware of the decreased circulating volume of infants and children and the importance of effective retraction and suctioning to increase visualization and to reduce potential blood loss. Also be aware of effective use of suture and the electrocautery pencil for achieving hemostasis and identification and clamping of a bleeding vessel.

Have instruments for clamping and suture readily available for ligating vessels.
Monitor electrocautery unit settings and keep the pencil tip clean for effective use.
Keep clean laparotomy pad available
Be prepared to use hemostatic agents (e.g., oxidized regenerated cellulose
Measure irrigation fluids and assist in blood loss calculations.
Assess and document the preoperative fluid volume status and the potential for fluid balance problems.
Maintain fluid therapy.
Have available
    IV solutions and blood products
    hemostatic agents
    a large volume of laparotomy sponges and sutures for hemostasis
    supplies for pressure dressing
Monitor electrocautery effectiveness and settings.
Monitor intake and output.
Keep a running total of fluid in suction containers and display blood laparotomy sponges for an estimation of bloody loss.
Document and report to the PACU problems with fluid volume and interventions.

Diagnosis

High risk for intraoperative hypothermia

Definition

Presence of risk factors for the child to experience a decrease in body temperature during surgery

Risk Factors

- Thin epidermis
- Large body surface in relation to size
- Thin layer of subcutaneous fat
- Chemical thermogenesis in brown adipose tissue
- Exposure of the epidermis to the outside environment
- Increased evaporative water loss
- Exposure of internal organs
- Exposure to cold IV fluids and skin preparation solutions
- Age (neonate)
- Low body weight

Expected Outcome

The child's body temperature is maintained within normal limits throughout the perioperative period.

Perioperative Nursing Interventions

Perform a preoperative assessment including laboratory data results, paying specific attention to the patient's age and the presence of anemia. All infants, but especially premature infants, have difficulty maintaining body temperature. Anemic patients are at risk for hypothermia.

Keep the patient covered during transport.

Increase the OR temperature to 85°F.

Position the patient on a heating blanket protected with sheets at 100°F.

Have warming lights available.

Place plastic around the extremities and head to reduce heat loss.

Monitor the patient's temperature and skin color.

Minimize the area of the surgical site preparation to limit the area of skin exposed to circulating air.

Cover as much skin area as possible during draping.

For abdominal surgery, reduce heat loss by placing plastic bags around the bowel.

Achieve good exposure through retraction and suctioning to allow abdominal contents to remain in the abdominal cavity when possible.

Arrange for a radiant heat warmer in the PACU.

Document and report to the PACU staff any problems with the patient's body temperature.

Activity-Exercise Pattern

Diagnosis

High risk for ineffective breathing patterns

Definition

Presence of risk factors for the child to experience respiration inadequate to maintain sufficient oxygen for cellular requirements during the perioperative period

Risk Factors

- Age (neonate or infant)
- Chest surgery
- Abdominal surgery
- Decreased ability to handle oral secretions
- Large size of infant head compared with the adult head (attaining a good "stiff" position for alignment of the airway axes is more difficult)
- Large tongue size of the infant compared with the adult tongue (laryngoscopy and visualization of the larynx are more difficult)
- Position of the vocal cords in the infant (makes the airway seem anterior, resulting in difficulty when trying to visualize the larynx with laryngoscopy)
- Difference in metabolic requirements and oxygen consumption in neonates and infants (a neonate may require 6 ml/kg/min of oxygen compared with 3 ml/kg/min in an adult)
- Presence of fetal hemoglobin during the first 6 months of life (fetal hemoglobin has more affinity for oxygen, thus allowing more oxygen to be carried to the tissues but less to be released at the tissue level)
- Nonshivering thermogenesis to produce body heat (can be detrimental because oxygen consumption and carbon dioxide production increase)
- Alveolar minute ventilation in the neonate, which is twice that of an adult (requires an increase in ventilatory rate to meet metabolic demands for oxygen consumption and carbon dioxide elimination)
- Smaller residual capacity in the neonate and infant (causes faster desaturation rate as compared with that in an adult) (Fontana, 1993, pp. 33–37)

Expected Outcome

The child's respirations are adequate to maintain sufficient oxygen to meet cellular requirements.

Perioperative Interventions

Assess preoperatively the respiratory status and communicate with anesthesia personnel and the surgical team.

Monitor the color of blood during surgery.

Position the patient for maximal lung expansion appropriate for the procedure.

Monitor the surgical team to prevent decreased ventilation due to pressure on the chest.

Assess the color of the patient's blood.

Preoperatively, assess the patient's respiratory status and NPO status and document.

Assist anesthesia personnel during anesthesia induction and intubation.

  Do not use a pillow under the head during intubation.

  Augment head extension by placing a rolled towel under the shoulders, if necessary.

  Listen for changes in the pulse oximeter.

  Assist with physical control of the patient during early induction.

  Assist with suctioning for visualization and with forceps for nasal intubation.

  Apply cricoid pressure to prevent laryngospasm, if needed.

  Assist with medication administration if laryngospasm occurs.

Document and report to the PACU problems with airway management.

Carefully monitor oxygen therapy.

Avoid cold stressors.

Decrease the energy requirements of child to decrease oxygen consumption.

Arrange for respiratory support equipment for the OR, PACU, or intensive care unit.

Cognitive-Perceptual Pattern

Diagnosis

Alteration in comfort: pain

Definition

Verbal report by the child and presence of emotional or physiological indicators of severe discomfort (pain) (Gordon, 1987, p. 172)

Defining Characteristics

- Verbal or nonverbal communication of pain
- Guarding or protective behavior
- Self-focusing
- Narrowed focus as evidenced by an altered perception of time, withdrawal from social contact, and impaired thought processes
- Moaning and crying
- Facial mask of pain as evidenced by a lack of luster in the eyes, a "beaten" appearance, fixed or scattered movement, and facial grimace
- Alteration in muscle tone, which may range from listless to rigid
- Autonomic response (diaphoresis, increased blood pressure and pulse, pupillary dilatation, and increased or decreased respiratory rate) (Gordon, 1987, p. 172)

Related Factors

- Surgery
- Intrusive procedures
- Lack of knowledge concerning pain management techniques (Gordon, 1987, p. 172)

Expected Outcome

The child comfort level is sufficient throughout the perioperative period.

Perioperative Nursing Interventions

Assess the patient's comfort level or level of pain.
Provide support for the parents.
Collaborate with anesthesia personnel to manage pain.
Reposition the patient, if necessary.
Provide local medication, as necessary.

Self-perception—Self-concept Pattern

Diagnosis

Fear

Definition

A feeling of dread experienced by the child, related to impending surgery, hospitalization, and intrusive procedures. The child perceives these events as a threat or danger to the self (Gordon, 1987, p. 198)

Defining Characteristics

- Describes or acts out the focus of perceived threat or danger
- Describes or acts out feelings of dread, nervousness, or concern about impending surgery, hospitalization, and intrusive procedures
- Verbalizes an expectation of danger to the self
- Increased questioning or information seeking
- Restless behavior
- Narrowed focus of attention that progresses to fixed attention on the impending event

- Diaphoresis
- Increased heart rate
- Increased respiratory rate
- Crying
- Clinging to a parent or other significant person
- Combative behavior to caregiver
- Decreased ability to express concerns and describe sensations (Gordon, 1987, p. 198)

Related Factors

- Lack of cognitive understanding concerning hospitalization, surgery, and intrusive procedures
- Fantasy thoughts
- Active imagination
- Sensed parental fear or anxiety
- Perceived inability to control event (Gordon, 1987, p. 198)

Expected Outcome

The child exhibits signs of control and expresses feelings (verbal or nonverbal) of security during the perioperative period.

Perioperative Nursing Interventions

Explain to the child procedures that he or she will experience in terms of sensations.
Allow the child to express concerns through the use of therapeutic play (have the child bring a favorite toy).
Show children the equipment they will see (preoperative teaching party).
Plan preparation according to the child's developmental level (see above).
Involve children in their own care.
Have parents present during anesthesia induction, if appropriate.
Provide information to parents and take action to reduce parental anxiety and fear.
Provide periodic reports to the parents during surgery.
Provide a quiet OR environment.

PROCEDURES

The perioperative nurse prepares for each of the following cases in a similar manner. The differences in each procedure are discussed.

Inguinal Herniorrhaphy

Definition

Inguinal herniorrhaphy is the most common surgical procedure performed by the pediatric surgeon. The majority of pediatric hernias are indirect and are due to congenital persistence of the processus vaginalis. The processus vaginalis, an extension of the peritoneal cavity through the internal inguinal ring (Rowe and Lloyd, 1986), closes spontaneously after the testis descends from the abdominal cavity to the scrotum. When it remains patent, the potential for herniation exists. In males (who account for 60% of inguinal hernia patients [Rowe and Lloyd, 1986]), the content of the hernia is usually bowel, with the fallopian tube and/or ovary being most common in females. In older children, omentum is often seen. Inguinal hernias are most frequently diagnosed in the first year of life, with premature infants having a significantly higher incidence than full-term infants (Marlow and Redding, 1988).

Indications

The patient has a history of an intermittent swelling in the groin. A thickening and silkiness of the spermatic cord as it crosses the pubic tubercle (silk glove sign) can be palpated (Rowe and Lloyd, 1986). If the hernia has been incarcerated, redness, swelling, and tenderness may be present. The possibility of incarceration with the potential strangulation and resultant necrosis of hernia sac contents results in the performance of this surgery soon after the diagnosis.

Pediatric inguinal herniorrhaphies are usually done on a same-day-surgery basis.

Perioperative Nursing Implications

General anesthesia is administered. In young children, endotracheal anesthesia is used, whereas mask anesthesia is often used in older children. After induction, a caudal anesthetic is administered to control intraoperative and postoperative pain. If a caudal anesthetic is not used, ilioinguinal block is performed by the surgeon during the procedure.

Procedure

The hernia is repaired by high ligation of the sac at the level of the internal ring. A transverse skin crease incision is made in the natural folds of skin in the inguinal region. The subcutaneous tissues are dissected along the spermatic cord through Scarpa fascia down to the external ring. In young patients, the internal ring lies just below the external ring, which makes it possible to achieve high ligation without incising the external oblique muscle, as is necessary for older patients. The hernia sac is visualized and, in males, the vessels and vas deferens are identified.

A clamp is placed on the sac, and the vessels and vas deferens are gently stripped from the hernia sac by grasping connective tissue, being careful never to grasp the vas deferens. In females, the hernia sac is identified with the round ligament. The fallopian tube is attached at the neck of the sac and must be avoided during ligation. Preperitoneal fat is identified, ensuring high ligation. The hernia is reduced and an instrument such as a slotted spoon may be used. The hernia sac is placed through the narrow slot, and the bowl of the spoon prevents structures from entering the sac. The sac is

ligated at the level of the internal ring with suture according to the surgeon's preference. A portion of the sac is usually removed and sent for routine pathological examination. Occasionally, the internal ring must be narrowed with a few sutures placed from the transversalis fascia to the inferior aspect of the ring (Rowe and Lloyd, 1986). The external oblique muscle, if opened, and Scarpa fascia are closed with interrupted suture. The skin is closed, usually with a running subcuticular suture, and dressings are applied—adhesive strips or collodion (a fast drying, occlusive liquid).

Postoperative Care

Discharge from same-day surgery takes place after the effects of general anesthesia have dissipated and the patient is able to retain oral fluids. Because of the caudal anesthesia or the ilioinguinal block, immediate postoperative pain is not usually a problem and later pain can be controlled with acetaminophen. Young pediatric patients usually have no activity restrictions, and older pediatric patients can usually resume strenuous activities in 2 to 3 weeks. The skin suture for pediatric patients is usually absorbable, thereby eliminating the need for suture removal. The dressings are kept dry for approximately 1 week. Special instructions for cleaning the area should be given to parents who have infants in diapers.

Potential Surgical Complications

Possible complications include recurrence, accidental ligation of sac contents, and damage to the spermatic cord during dissection from the sac.

Repair of Hydrocele or Undescended Testis

Definition and Indications

Hydroceles in the pediatric population are variants of inguinal hernias in which fluid accumulates owing to communication with the peritoneal cavity (Atwell, 1988). The procedure is similar, with the addition of opening the hydrocele, draining the fluid, and often removing a portion of the sac to prevent reaccumulation.

Undescended testis is another condition related to the inguinal hernia. The procedure is inguinal herniorrhaphy or ligation of the patent processus vaginalis, mobilization of the testis, and orchiopexy (fixation of the testis in the scrotum), usually by placing the testis in a pouch formed under dartos muscle.

Perioperative Nursing Implications

The scrub nurses select equipment and supplies and organize the room, using sterile technique. For this procedure, an electrocautery unit and, for infants, a warming blanket and possibly warming lights are used. Supplies consist of basic draping materials, gowns, gloves, x-ray detectable sponges, electrocautery handpiece, No. 15 scalpel blades, basins, dissecting sponges (e.g., peanuts or Kittner dissecting sponges), syringes and a needle for local anesthesia if ilioinguinal block is to be done, dressings (usually adhesive strips or collodion), and for larger patients, a Penrose drain to surround the spermatic cord. Suture is opened according to the surgeon's preference to include suture on taper needles for ligation of the sac and closing the external oblique muscle and fascia and usually fine absorbable suture on a cutting needle for a subcuticular skin closure.

Instruments, as always in pediatric surgery, are modified for patient size. Curved and straight mosquito clamps, dissecting scissors, smooth forceps (often vascular forceps) for manipulation of the hernia sac, forceps with teeth for opening and closing, small retractors, a Babcock or Allis clamp to place around the spermatic cord, and if desired, a hernia spoon are prepared.

Because most inguinal hernia patients are admitted for same-day surgery, the perioperative nurse meets the patient and the family in the holding area. The patient and the procedure are verified, the chart is reviewed, and the surgery permit and the history and physical examination results are noted, paying special attention to whether the procedure involves left, right, or both sides. The patient and family are questioned as to allergies and NPO status. As discussed above, the patient and the family are evaluated, and appropriate nursing interventions are used. They are escorted to the induction room or the patient is taken to the OR.

Procedure

General anesthesia is induced by mask for most children, with IV induction used primarily in adolescents. Constant assessment by the circulating nurse of the patient is required during induction. Endotracheal tubes are usually inserted in young patients, while in older patients anesthesia is usually maintained by mask. Standard anesthesia monitors are applied: electrocardiographic monitor, blood pressure monitor, and pulse oximeter. As for all infants and young children, maintenance of normal body temperature is important. Wrapping the extremities and head prevents heat loss.

The patient is placed in a supine position and the skin is prepared with povidone-iodine scrub and/or paint (or other solutions) from the umbilicus to the midthigh. Care is taken to prevent pooling of the povidone-iodine solution. Burns can occur when the skin is in contact with povidone-iodine and a warming blanket. Warm sterile saline is placed on the back table, along with any local anesthetic if an ilioinguinal block is to be administered.

The scrub nurse assists in draping and places the sterile Mayo stand over the foot of the table. The positions of the surgical team members must be monitored when the patient is an infant to prevent pressure on small extremities. As always, although hemorrhage is rare, the scrub nurse must be prepared with clamps, cautery, or suture. During sac manipulation, forceps without teeth (preferably vascular forceps) should be used to avoid tearing the sac, which may lead to recurrence. Owing to the use of small incisions in pediatric surgery, the scrub nurse may be required to assist in retracting. The portion of the hernia sac removed, which is often small, is sent for routine pathological examination.

Potential Surgical Complications

One complication of this surgery is recurrence. One possible cause is tearing of the sac beyond the internal ring. The registered nurse first assistant must provide adequate exposure, especially considering the size of the incision. Using only smooth forceps when handling the hernia sac is essential. Another complication is injury to the vas deferens. Adequate exposure and handling of only surrounding tissue, never the vas deferens, are critical.

Pyloromyotomy

Definition

Pyloromyotomy is the treatment of choice for congenital hypertrophic pyloric stenosis. Pyloric stenosis is a condition in which there is an obstruction at the pyloric sphincter due to hypertrophy of circular muscle (Fig. 30–6). It is most often seen in infants at 2 to 4 weeks of age. There is a strong familial association. Males are affected four times as often as females, with a high incidence of first-born males being affected (Benson, 1986).

Indications

The first symptom of pyloric stenosis is occasional vomiting, which increases in frequency and becomes projectile. The vomitus usually does not contain bile because the obstruction occurs proximal to the ampulla of Vater (Marlow and Redding, 1988). Occasionally, the vomitus is brown or blood streaked because of broken capillaries from the forceful vomiting. The hypertrophied muscle can usually be palpated as a firm, movable mass in the right upper quadrant, the olive. Other associated symptoms include dehydration, weight loss, and general failure to thrive. Peristalsis can often be identified as a wave from the left upper quadrant to the right. On barium swallow examination, diagnosis is made from evidence of active peristalsis with delayed or absent emptying (Marlow and Redding, 1988).

Although the condition is being recognized earlier with the resultant decrease in severity of symptoms, dehydration and acid-base imbalances are still a major concern.

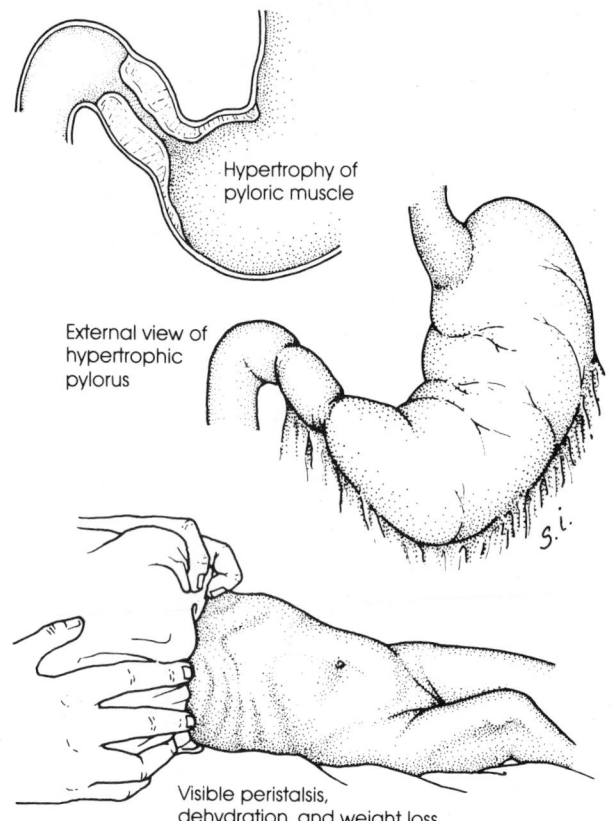

FIGURE 30–6. Pyloric stenosis. (From Marlow, D. R., Redding, B. A. [1988]. *Textbook of pediatric nursing* [6th ed.]. Philadelphia: W. B. Saunders.)

Perioperative Nursing Implications

Preoperatively, low serum potassium and sodium levels, decrease in serum chloride concentration with an increase in pH and carbon dioxide, and increased hematocrit and hemoglobin values can be expected (Marlow and Redding, 1988). Appropriate IV therapy is initiated, and the procedure is usually performed within 24 hours of hospitalization.

Procedure

General anesthesia is induced via endotracheal tube. The Ramstedt procedure consists of splitting the muscle of the hypertrophic pylorus leaving the mucosa intact. The Ramstedt technique does not reapproximate the muscle, although this was used in the past. A right transverse incision is made through subcutaneous tissue; external oblique, internal oblique, and transversus abdominis muscles; and the peritoneum (Spitz, 1988c). An incision is then made through the muscle of the anterior pylorus from the junction of the pylorus and duodenum to the antrum of the stomach (approximately 2–3 cm) (Spitz, 1988c). A blunt instrument is used to split the muscle fibers—often curved jaws of a hemostat or a pyloric spreader—with care to avoid perforation of the mucosa. Air can be placed in the stomach per nasogas-

tric tube to check for perforations. The pylorus is returned to the abdominal cavity and, after verification of hemostasis, the incision is closed according to the surgeon's preference. Adhesive strips and possibly a small dressing are applied.

Postoperative Care

Postoperatively, the nasogastric tube is removed when the patient has completely recovered from anesthesia, unless there has been a perforation, in which case it is usually left in place for 24 to 48 hours. The patient is begun on oral feedings approximately 6 to 8 hours after surgery. The surgeon's preferences result in a variety of feeding regimens, usually beginning with sugar water and progressing to weak formula and then to full-strength formula. Because vomiting continues to be of concern, the infant's head is elevated after feeding and the child is placed on his or her right side (Marlow and Redding, 1988).

Potential Surgical Complications

Complications of this procedure are rare. There is danger of peritonitis if a mucosal tear goes unrecognized and consequently unrepaired. Failure to split the muscle completely could result in unrelieved projectile vomiting.

Bowel Resection for Necrotizing Enterocolitis

Definition

Necrotizing enterocolitis is characterized by necrosis of the mucosa of the colon and/or small intestine, usually associated with prematurity. The condition is seen more often because of the increased viability of small neonates (Marlow and Redding, 1988). Stressful conditions resulting in decreased blood flow to the bowel are thought to be causative. The condition is usually diagnosed in the first 4 weeks of life.

Indications

Symptoms include abdominal distention, temperature instability, gastric retention, bile-stained vomitus, bloody feces, periods of apnea progressing to lethargy, and jaundice and metabolic acidosis. Radiography shows multiple areas of small-bowel dilation and, if perforation has occurred, free air in the abdomen.

Perioperative Nursing Implications

Preoperatively, the patient is kept NPO, IV therapy and antibiotic therapy are begun, and a nasogastric tube is inserted.

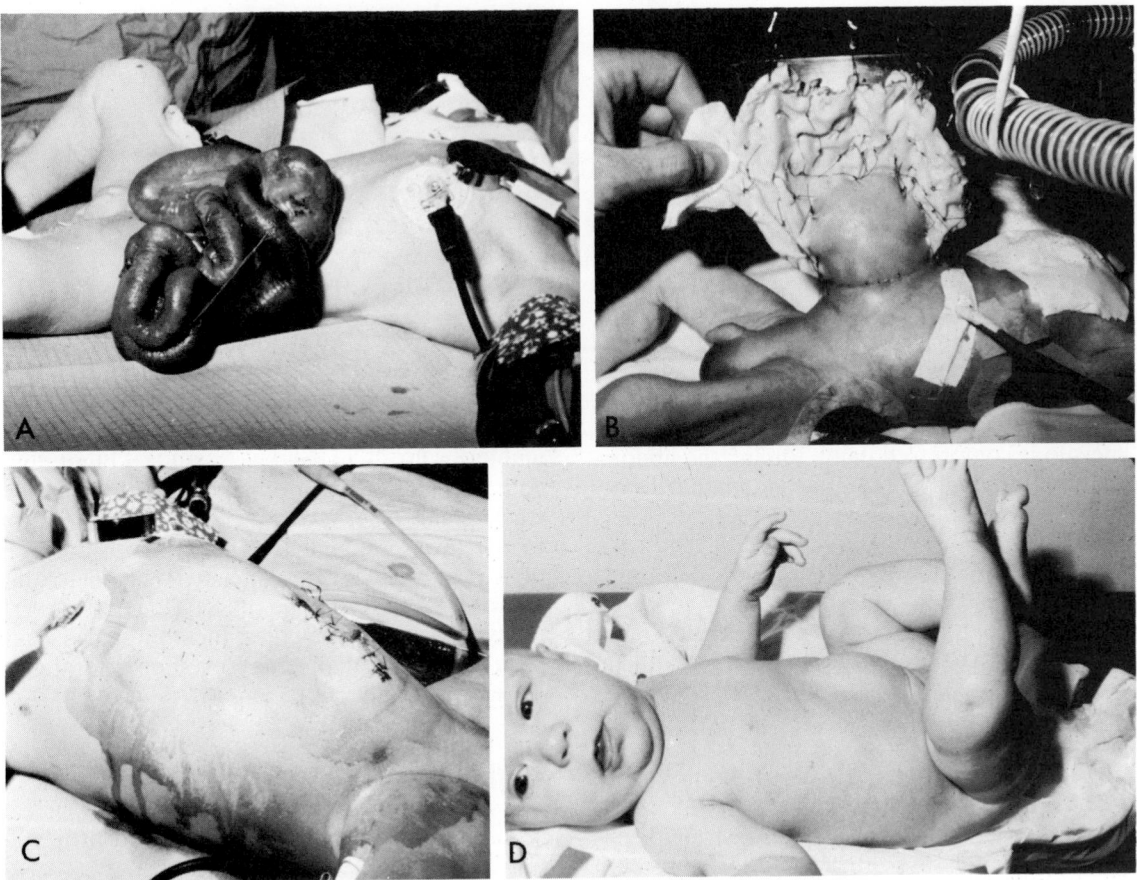

FIGURE 30–7. Omphalocele, a herniation of the abdominal viscera at the umbilicus. *A*, In this infant, the sac that usually surrounds the viscera is not present. Note the empty abdomen. *B*, A silo is being used. *C*, The abdominal wall defect is closed. *D*, This healthy infant has a slight bulge at the site of the defect. (Courtesy of Louise Schnaufer, M.D., Children's Hospital of Philadelphia.) (From Marlow, D. R., Redding, B. A. [1988]. *Textbook of pediatric nursing* [6th ed.]. Philadelphia: W. B. Saunders.)

Procedure

The condition is surgically treated by identifying areas of necrosis and resecting them. The patient is placed supine and a transverse supraumbilical incision is made (Dickson, 1988b). Necrosis is most often found in the terminal ileum and less frequently in the ascending colon and the splenic flexure (Dickson, 1988b). All bowel with definite necrosis should be resected and all bowel of questionable viability should be left. Multiple enterostomies are made at points of resection. Although somewhat controversial, when necrosis is localized and surrounding tissue is healthy, primary anastomosis may be performed (Rowe, 1986). A feeding gastrostomy tube may be inserted. The abdomen is closed with interrupted suture on taper needles and subcuticular skin closure is performed.

Postoperative Care

Postoperatively, IV and antibiotic therapy are continued. There may be a need for ventilatory assistance. The enterostomies are drained into closed containers—small ostomy bags are available. Takedown of the enterostomies is done when the infant is fully recovered.

Omphalocele and Gastroschisis Closure

Definition and Indications

An *omphalocele* is a defect in the anterior abdominal wall at the umbilicus; it consists of an avascular membranous sac with a wide base into which the liver has herniated (Fig. 30–7). *Gastroschisis* is an opening usually to the right of the umbilicus that has no sac and results in small intestine and possibly large intestine protruding from it. This bowel is abnormally thick and edematous and the opening in the abdominal wall is small.

Perioperative Nursing Implications

Preoperatively, care must be taken to avoid pressure or traction on the sac or herniated bowel. Sterile saline-soaked dressings are applied.

Procedure

Closure of both conditions is similar. In the omphalocele, the sac may be resected and the liver returned to the abdominal cavity, and the abdominal wall is repaired. The sac may also be left in place to prevent abdominal contents from adhering to the skin (Spitz, 1988b). Often, removal of the sac is necessary to stretch the abdominal wall to accommodate the abdominal contents. In gastroschisis, the defect is enlarged and the bowel is returned to the abdominal cavity and primary closure is attempted. In both cases, if the abdominal wall is too tight to allow primary closure, a "silo" of material such as Silastic sheeting may be constructed, which is sutured to the abdominal wall to cover the defect. The silo is compressed daily, forcing the abdominal contents to gradually enter the abdominal cavity until primary closure can be obtained.

Postoperative Care

Postoperatively, peripheral hyperalimentation and antibiotic therapy are used.

Potential Surgical Complications

Observation for edema of the lower extremities is necessary to detect pressure on the inferior vena cava that results when the abdominal cavity is closed under too much tension. Especially with gastroschisis (because the defect causes exposure of the bowel with no sac to protect it), infection is a concern.

Repair of Esophageal Atresia with Tracheoesophageal Fistula

Definition

Esophageal atresia is often associated with tracheoesophageal fistula. There are four different presentations: (1) a blind upper esophageal pouch with a lower esophageal pouch, which is connected to the stomach and has a fistula to the trachea; (2) a blind upper pouch with no fistula; (3) an upper pouch that connects to the trachea and may be blind or have a narrow connection to the lower esophagus; and (4) both the blind upper pouch and the lower pouch connected to the trachea (Marlow and Redding, 1988) (Fig. 30–8). There are many associated anomalies, including cardiac anomalies, gastrointestinal malformations, imperforate anus, and Vater syndrome.

Indications

The patient has initial symptoms of drooling, frothy saliva, choking, and cyanosis. Gastric secretions enter

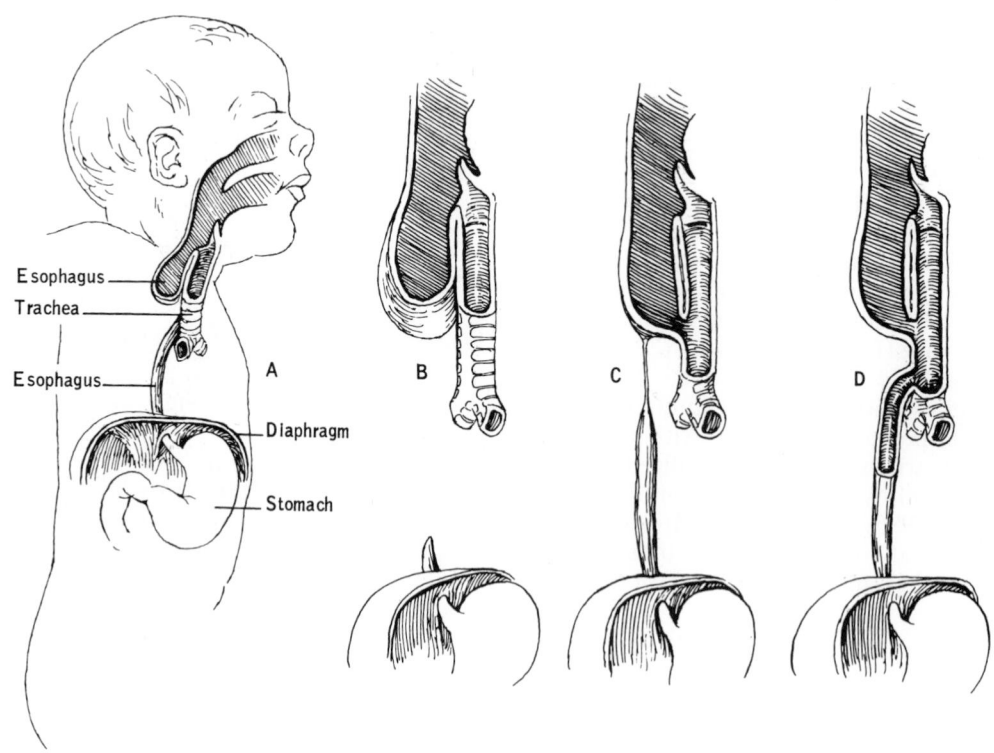

FIGURE 30–8. Atresia of the esophagus. *A,* Most common form. The lower esophagus communicates with the trachea. *B,* The upper esophagus ends in a blind pouch. The lower esophagus ends in a blind pouch. The lower segment does not communicate with the trachea. *C,* The upper esophagus ends in the trachea. A cordlike connection with the lower esophagus may or may not be present. *D,* Both upper and lower portions of the esophagus connect with the trachea. (From Marlow, D. R., Redding, B. A. [1988]. *Textbook of pediatric nursing* [6th ed.]. Philadelphia: W. B. Saunders.)

the lungs through the fistula and result in recurrent chemical pneumonitis. On radiographic examination, air is seen in the intestine if there is a fistula between the trachea and the lower pouch. Attempts to pass an esophageal tube are unsuccessful.

Perioperative Nursing Implications

Preoperatively, the patient may need ventilatory assistance. Antibiotics are initiated as well as IV therapy. The patient is kept NPO.

Procedure

The repair is accomplished by restoring continuity of the esophagus while ligating the fistula. The patient is placed on his or her left side with the right arm extended above the head. Thoracotomy is performed through an incision in the fourth intercostal space. Every attempt is made to avoid perforation of the thoracic cavity. A rib spreader is inserted and the azygos vein is identified, ligated, and divided (Wright, 1988). Care is taken to avoid the vagus nerve. The upper pouch can be identified by having anesthesia personnel put pressure on a bougie inserted into the esophagus. The lower esophagus and fistula are identified and the fistula is ligated proximal to the trachea and divided. The upper pouch is spatulated to facilitate anastomosis of the two pouches. The other varieties of this condition are repaired in similar fashion.

If the distance between the upper and lower pouches in the condition without fistula can be seen radiographically to be large, dilation with mercury-filled bougies is performed periodically according to the surgeon's preference with the hope that eventually primary anastomosis can be performed. If the distance is too great, colon interposition may be necessary.

A retropleural drain is usually placed, and closure is performed with suture on taper needles for muscle layers and subcutaneous tissues and a fine suture on a small cutting needle is used for subcuticular closure of the skin.

Postoperative Care

Postoperatively, IV therapy, administration of antibiotics, and chest tube connection to drainage are necessary treatments.

Potential Surgical Complications

Complications include a possible tracheal edema due to dissection of the trachea, leakage of the anastomosis, and tracheomalacia (softening of the tissue of the trachea with resultant collapse of a segment), resulting in a need for aortopexy.

Repair of Diaphragmatic Hernia

Definition

Diaphragmatic hernia is a condition in which a defect of the diaphragmatic muscle allows the abdominal contents to enter the thoracic cavity (Marlow and Redding, 1988) (Fig. 30–9). Emergency surgery is performed because of the severity of the symptoms. Acute respiratory distress and respiratory and metabolic acidosis make this condition life threatening. The hernia is usually on the left side, with the contents being the small intestine, the stomach, the left lobe of the liver, the spleen, and most of the colon. The right-sided hernia usually contains the liver and some small and large bowel.

Indications

Along with respiratory distress and acidosis, cyanosis, retractions, decreased breath sounds, displacement of the heart to the right side of the chest, auscultation of bowel sounds in the chest, and a scaphoid abdomen are seen. Fortunately, this condition can often be detected on prenatal ultrasound, resulting in preparation for resuscitation at birth and immediate surgery. As the infant cries and swallows air, the intestine that has herniated becomes filled with gas and increases mediastinal pressure, which, if severe, leads to shock and hypoxia (Marlow and Redding, 1988).

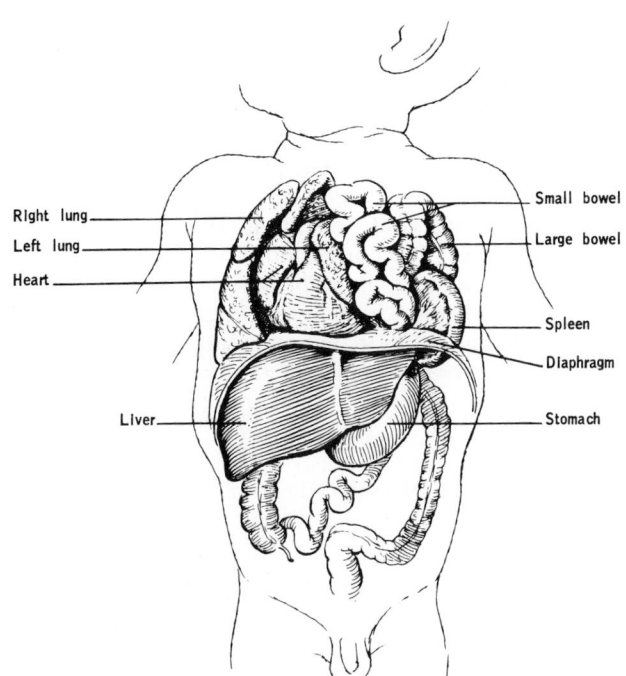

FIGURE 30–9. Diaphragmatic hernia. The abdominal viscera have herniated into the thorax. The thoracic viscera have been displaced and compressed. (From Marlow, D. R., Redding, B. A. [1988]. *Textbook of pediatric nursing* [6th ed.]. Philadelphia: W. B. Saunders.)

Perioperative Nursing Implications

Preoperatively, a nasogastric tube is placed, 100% oxygen is administered, and ventilator assistance is given if needed. An umbilical arterial catheter is inserted for drawing blood for blood gas determination. Vasodilators are given to decrease pulmonary arterial pressure (Anderson, 1986).

Procedure

Anesthesia is induced with awake intubation. The repair is accomplished by replacing the contents of the hernia in the abdominal cavity and closing the defect. If the hernia is on the right side, a transthoracic approach may be used. More commonly, the hernia is on the left side and an abdominal approach is used. A left subcostal incision is made. The hernia contents are reduced and the sac is resected if present. The posterior and anterior margins of the diaphragm are approximated with suture of the surgeon's preference. If the posterior margin is absent, suture may be placed around the ribs (Spitz, 1988a). A prosthetic material such as Dacron or Silastic may be used to close the defect. Chest tubes are placed. If the abdominal cavity is too small to accommodate the contents of the hernia without placing too much pressure on abdominal organs, the skin only may be closed to increase the space. A gastrostomy tube is usually placed.

Postoperative Care

Postoperatively, parenteral nutrition is given owing to prolonged ileus (Spitz, 1988a). If ventilation is being assisted, careful, gradual weaning is begun.

Potential Surgical Complications

A period that lasts several hours to several days (referred to as the honeymoon) is characterized by generalized improvement only to be followed by sudden worsening because of increased pulmonary pressure from persistent fetal circulation resulting in respiratory failure and increased right-to-left shunting. This condition can be treated with vasodilators (Anderson, 1986).

Nissen Fundoplication

Definition

Nissen fundoplication is a procedure to treat gastroesophageal reflux, which is usually a result of a central nervous system disorder (Marlow and Redding, 1988). Other conditions such as esophageal atresia and malrotation may be accompanied by gastroesophageal reflux. Reflux of stomach contents into the esophagus and vomiting may be caused by failure of the distal esophageal sphincter.

Indications

Patients with gastroesophageal reflux have vomiting, failure to thrive, and recurrent aspiration pneumonia. The esophagus may become ulcerated owing to contact with gastric juices, which, if allowed to progress, may develop into esophageal stricture.

Barium swallow examination is performed to identify esophageal stricture or ulceration and the degree of gastroesophageal reflux (Spitz, 1988b). The pH of the distal esophagus may be measured during a 24-hour period, with a pH of less than 4 identified as significant.

Perioperative Nursing Implications

Preoperatively, the patient should be positioned with his or her head elevated to prevent aspiration (Spitz, 1988b). Frequent small feedings are initiated after bowel functioning returns.

Procedure

Nissen fundoplication consists of wrapping a portion of the fundus of the stomach circumferentially around the distal esophagus. Endotracheal general anesthesia is induced. The patient is placed supine and a mercury-filled bougie or nasogastric tube is passed into the distal esophagus to ensure that the wrap is not too tight. A midline incision is made. The stomach is separated from the spleen at the proximal greater curvature (Spitz, 1988b). The short gastric vessels are ligated and divided with care to avoid the vagus nerve. The distal esophagus is mobilized, and a Penrose drain or umbilical tape can be placed around the esophagus, which can be used to provide traction to facilitate placement of sutures through the gastric and esophageal muscles at the site of the wrap. Prevention of movement of the fundoplication into the posterior mediastinum is accomplished by suturing the diaphragmatic hiatus to the fundoplication (Spitz, 1988b). A feeding gastrostomy may be formed, and closure with interrupted sutures and subcuticular closure of the skin is performed.

Postoperative Care

Postoperatively, the nasogastric tube is left in place and IV therapy continues until the ileus has resolved (Spitz, 1988b).

Potential Surgical Complications

A wrap that is too tight results in difficulty with swallowing; a wrap that is too loose results in continued gastroesophageal reflux and prolapse of the fundoplication into the posterior mediastinum, causing difficulty in swallowing.

Kasai Procedure

Definition

The Kasai procedure, or hepatic portoenterostomy, is performed for the treatment of biliary atresia. Biliary atresia is a condition in which there is absence or obstruction of bile ducts (Marlow and Redding, 1988). There are three basic types: (1) the extrahepatic ducts are patent proximally and obstructed distally; (2) there is patency of the gallbladder, cystic duct, and common duct with occlusion of the hepatic duct proximally; and (3) most frequently, the entire duct system is absent or obstructed (Lilly, 1986). Associated anomalies include intestinal malrotation, polysplenia, preduodenal portal vein, and absence of the inferior vena cava.

Indications

In the first 2 to 3 weeks of life, an olive-green jaundice becomes apparent. Dark urine, light and puttylike feces, hepatomegaly, abdominal distention, and failure to thrive, along with irritability and restlessness, are symptoms of biliary atresia.

Perioperative Nursing Implications

Percutaneous liver biopsy is performed. Radioisotope imaging shows decreased clearance of hepatocytes with concurrent increased excretion (Lilly, 1986). Ultrasound shows a reduction in size and contents of the gallbladder.

Procedure

The Kasai procedure consists of resection of the nonfunctional hepatic ducts and anastomosis of the jejunum to the transected duct at the liver hilum (Lilly, 1986). A right subcostal incision is made. The rectus muscle is incised to provide exposure of the right lobe of the liver. The gallbladder is mobilized and cholangiography is performed. If patency of the biliary tree cannot be visualized, the extrahepatic ducts are removed and a Roux-en-Y is performed by anastomosing a segment of jejunum to the liver hilus (Howard, 1988). An end-to-side anastomosis restores intestinal continuity. The porta hepatis is often the site of drain placement. The abdomen is closed with interrupted suture and a subcuticular skin closure is performed.

Postoperative Care

Postoperatively, a nasogastric tube is left in place until bowel sounds return. IV administration of antibiotics is continued for approximately 7 days. A diet high in protein and low in fats is needed because of the inability of these patients to absorb fat. Cholestyramine, which binds intraluminal biles, may be administered (Marlow and Redding, 1988).

Potential Surgical Complications

Complications of this medical therapy include intestinal obstruction and increased sebaceous gland secretion. Water-soluble vitamins are given. Drainage of bile is measured and replaced.

Cholangitis is a major complication. An elevated temperature, tenderness of the right upper quadrant, decreased bile drainage, and jaundice are indicative of cholangitis. Portal hypertension is another possible complication.

If jaundice and other associated symptoms persist after surgical intervention, liver transplantation may be the treatment of choice.

Bibliography

Abbott, N., Hanses, P., Lewis, K. (1970, November). Dress rehearsal for the hospital. *American Journal of Nursing*, pp. 2360–2362.

Ambler, M. (1967, March). Disciplining hospitalized toddlers. *American Journal of Nursing*, pp. 472–573.

Anderson, K. D. (1986). Congenital diaphragmatic hernia. In K. J. Welch, J. G. Randolph, M. M. Ravitch, et al. (Eds.), *Pediatric surgery* (4th ed.) (pp. 589–602). Chicago: Year Book Medical.

Atwell, J. D. (1988). Inguinal hernia and hydrocele. In H. Dudley, D. Carter, R. C. G. Russell (Eds.), *Operative surgery: Paediatric surgery* (4th ed.) (pp. 207–217). Stoneham, MA: Butterworth.

Barton, P. (1962, March). Play as a tool of nursing. *Nursing Outlook*, pp. 162–164.

Bates, T., Broome, M. (1986). Preparation of children for hospitalization and surgery: A review of the literature. *Journal of Pediatric Nursing*, *1*(4), 230–239.

Beal, J. (1983). Preparing children for hospital procedures. In J. Beal (Ed.), *Issues in advanced practice in pediatric nursing* (pp. 3–23). Reston, VA: Reston Publishing.

Benson, C. D. (1986). Infantile hypertrophic pyloric stenosis. In K. J. Welch, J. G. Randolph, M. M. Ravitch, et al. (Eds.), *Pediatric surgery* (4th ed.) (pp. 811–815). Chicago: Year Book Medical.

Berman, D. (1966, November). Pediatric nurses as mothers see them. *American Journal of Nursing*, pp. 2429–2431.

Billington, G. (1972, April). Play program reduces children's anxiety, speeds recovery. *Modern Hospital*, pp. 990–992.

Blake, F. (1969, November). Immobilized youth. *American Journal of Nursing*, *69*(11), 109–115.

Bowley, A. (1961). *The psychological care of the child in the hospital*. London: E. S. Livingstone.

Branstetter, E. (1969, January). The young child's response to hospitalization. *American Journal of Public Health*, pp. 92–97.

Conway, B., Mandelco, B., Trufant, J., Scoblic, M. (1970, May). The seventh right. *American Journal of Nursing*, pp. 1040–1043.

Dickson, J. A. S. (1988a). Exomphalos/omphalocele. In H. Dudley, D. Carter, R. C. G. Russell (Eds.), *Operative surgery: Paediatric surgery* (4th ed.) (pp. 229–239). Stoneham, MA: Butterworth.

Dickson, J. A. S. (1988b). Necrotizing enterocolitis. In H. Dudley, D. Carter, R. C. G. Russell (Eds.), *Operative surgery: Paediatric surgery* (4th ed.) (pp. 336–348). Stoneham, MA: Butterworth.

Dombro, R., Haas, B. (1970). His family in the hospital. *The chronically ill child and his family*. Springfield, IL: Charles C Thomas.

Englebardt, S. (1969, December). Care by parent relieves emotional strain on children, financial strain on parents. *Modern Hospital*, pp. 94–97.

Erickson, F. (1958, September). Reactions of children to hospital experience, *Nursing Outlook*, pp. 501–504.

Erickson, F. (1965). When 6–12 year olds are ill. *Nursing Outlook*, *13*, 48–50.

Erickson, F. (1967). Helping the child maintain behavioral control. *Nursing Clinics of North America*, *2*(4), 695–703.

Fontana, J. (1993). Anesthetic considerations for neonatal and infant patients. *Seminars in Perioperative Nursing 2(1)*, 33–37.

Freud, A. (1952). The role of bodily illness in the mental life of children. In A. Freud (Ed.), *The psychoanalytic study of the child* (Vol. 7, pp. 69–81).

Gellert, E. (1962). Children's conceptions of the content and function of the human body. *Genetic Psychology Monographs, 65,* 293.

Hales-Tooke, A. (1968, May-June). Improving hospital care for children. *Children,* pp. 116–118.

Hardgrove, G., Dawson, R. (1972). *Parents and children in the hospital.* Boston: Little, Brown.

Howard, E. R. (1988). Surgery for biliary atresia. In H. Dudley, D. Carter, R. C. G. Russell (Eds.), *Operative surgery: Paediatric surgery* (4th ed.) (pp. 443–453). Stoneham, MA: Butterworth.

Jolly, H. (1969, October). Clever chaos. *Hospitals,* pp. 51–55.

Kraus, A. N. (1976). Physiology. In S. F. Redo (Ed.), *Principles of surgery in the first six months of life* (pp. 1–16). New York: Harper & Row.

Krishna, G., Haselby, K., Rao, C. (1981). Current concepts in pediatric anesthesia with emphasis on the newborn infant. *Surgical Clinics of North America, 61,* 997–1011.

Langford, W. (1961, October). The child in the pediatric hospital: Adaptation to illness and hospitalizations. *American Journal of Orthopsychiatry,* pp. 667–683.

Lilly, J. R. (1986). Biliary atresia: The jaundiced infant. In K. J. Welch, J. G. Randolph, M. M. Ravitch, et al. (Eds.), *Pediatric surgery* (4th ed.) (pp. 1047–1056). Chicago: Year Book Medical.

Lindheim, R., Glaser, H., Coffin, C. (1972). *Changing hospital environments for children.* Cambridge, MA: Harvard University Press.

Luck, S. (1990). Preoperative evaluation and preparation. In J. Raffensperger (Ed.), *Swenson's pediatric surgery* (5th ed.) (pp. 8–12). Norwalk, CT: Appleton & Lange.

Marlow, D. R., Redding, B. A. (1988). *Textbook of pediatric nursing* (6th ed.). Philadelphia: W. B. Saunders.

Mason, E. (1965). The hospitalized child—his emotional needs. *New England Journal of Medicine, 272,* 406–414.

Mellish, R. (1969). Preparation of a child for hospitalization and surgery. *Pediatric Clinics of North America, 16,* 543–553.

Moushey, R., Sinacore, L., Diomede, B. (1988). A perioperative teaching program: A collaborative process. *Journal of Pediatric Nursing, 3*(1), 40–45.

Oremland, E., J. (1973). *The effects of hospitalization on children.* Springfield, IL: Charles C Thomas.

Petrillo, M. (1968, July). Preventing hospital trauma in pediatric patients. *American Journal of Nursing,* pp. 1468–1473.

Petrillo, M., Sanger, S. (1972). *Emotional care of hospitalized children.* Philadelphia: J. B. Lippincott.

Plank, E. (1962). *Working with children in hospitals.* Cleveland: Western Reserve University.

Polley, T. Z., Jr., Coran, A. G. (1986). Special problems in management of pediatric trauma. *Critical Care Clinics, 2*(4), 775–787.

Potts, W. (1956). The heart of a child. *JAMA, 161,* 487–490.

Rowe, M. I. (1979). Preoperative and postoperative management: The physiologic approach. In M. M. Ravitch, K. J. Welch, C. D. Benson, et al. (Eds.), *Pediatric surgery* (3rd ed.) (pp. 39–50). Chicago: Year Book Medical.

Rowe, M. (1980). Physiology of the pediatric surgery patient. In T. Holder, K. Ashcraft (Eds.), *Pediatric surgery* (pp. 1–26). Philadelphia: W. B. Saunders.

Rowe, M. I. (1986). Necrotizing enterocolitis. In K. J. Welch, J. G. Randolph, M. M. Ravitch, et al. (Eds.), *Pediatric surgery* (4th ed.) (pp. 944–958). Chicago: Year Book Medical.

Rowe, M. I., Lloyd, D. A. (1986). Inguinal hernia. In K. J. Welch, J. G. Randolph, M. M. Ravitch, et al. (Eds.), *Pediatric surgery* (4th ed.) (pp. 770–793). Chicago: Year Book Medical.

Scahill, M. (1969). Preparing children for procedures and operations. *Nursing Outlook, 17,* 205–211.

Schultz, N. (1971). How children perceive pain. *Nursing Outlook, 19*(10), 116–121.

Seleng, F., Luck, S. (1990). Care of the child in the operating room. In J. Raffeusperger (Ed.), *Swenson's pediatric surgery* (5th ed.) (pp. 17–25). Norwalk, CT: Appleton & Lange.

Spitz, L. (1988a). Congenital diaphragmatic hernia and eventration. In H. Dudley, D. Carter, R. C. G. Russell (Eds.), *Operative surgery: Paediatric surgery* (4th ed.) (pp. 146–154). Stoneham, MA: Butterworth.

Spitz, L. (1988b). Nissen fundoplication. In H. Dudley, D. Carter, R. C. G. Russell (Eds.), *Operative surgery: Paediatric surgery* (4th ed.) (pp. 240–247). Stoneham, MA: Butterworth.

Spitz, L. (1988c). Pyloromyotomy. In H. Dudley, D. Carter, R. C. G. Russell (Eds.), *Operative surgery: Paediatric surgery* (4th ed.) (pp. 267–273). Stoneham, MA: Butterworth.

Whaley, L., Wong, D. (1979). *Nursing care of infants and children.* St. Louis: C. V. Mosby.

Wright, V. (1988). Oesophageal atresia and tracheo-oesophageal fistula. In H. Dudley, D. Carter, R. C. G. Russell (Eds.), *Operative surgery: Paediatric surgery* (4th ed.) (pp. 116–126). Stoneham, MA: Butterworth.

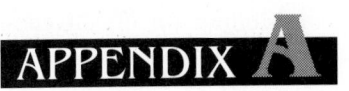

Reaching Different Learners with the Same Message: The Outpatient Presurgical Experience

Program Goals

- To decrease the uncertainty and anxiety of children and families regarding the patient's surgical experience by imparting information in a format specifically composed to provide
    sensory, sequence, and process information
    developmentally and cognitively relevant information
    language-appropriate information
- To establish trust between patients and their families and the hospital staff
- To promote emotional expression and personal coping with the surgical experience, as well as other related hospital experiences
- To enhance partnership between and among
    the patient
    the family
    physicians
    the hospital staff

Reaching Different Learners with the Same Message: The Preoperative Teaching Experience

Some key elements are used for implementing a presurgical education program designed to impart multivariant information to a multivariant group of learners.

- Determine the information to be shared.
    Solicit mutual agreement among key hospital staff regarding information specific to each area compiled to form a master teaching plan.

Courtesy of Child Life Services, Santa Rosa Children's Hospital, San Antonio, TX.

Explain the sequence of events in the complete hospital experience; include the ranges of time frames and sensory experiences.

Explain possible emotional responses and offer a variety of coping strategies for the different group participants to support their role in the surgical process.

- Translate and record information from the master teaching plan.
    Record the translation with good-quality audio equipment and tapes.
    Use individual battery-operated, portable cassette players with headphones for group members requesting the translation service.
    Provide a brief taped introduction and explanation before the tour process begins to include operating instructions for cassette players.
    Include transition information between tour modules to provide the listener with orientation information specific to the tour process itself.
    Translate with vocabulary from local dialect, *not* the formal language.
    Recommend use of the cassette player for children 5 to 6 years of age and older, with adult supervision for all under 12 years old.
- Involve knowledgeable staff.
    Include staff who are knowledgeable in child development and learning theories.
    Include staff who have knowledge of and are sensitive to the patient's and the family's hospital experiences.
    Train staff to implement a variety of teaching techniques.
    Include and/or train staff who are knowledgeable in the primary languages common in the community.
    Include and/or train staff to strengthen cultural sensitivities.

Train staff in the master teaching plan to facilitate their time management parallelling the taped translation.

● Monitor for effectiveness and implement changes, if necessary.

Implement a quality assurance plan indicating patient outcomes from the master teaching objectives.

Track and address questions that are frequently repeated.

Make changes in the master teaching plan and translation masters, as well as user copies.

Provide inservice training or update all instructor staff on all changes in the master teaching plan.

Tour

I. Children's Outpatient Surgery
   A. Indicate to parents that the children's outpatient surgery (COPS) waiting area will be where they report on the day of surgery at their designated time.
   B. Point out the playroom and mention its purposes:
      1. To provide diversion while waiting for pre-registration or tour class to begin.
      2. To provide diversion preoperatively.
      3. To increase activity postoperatively.
      4. To provide a place for parents to bring juice or a popsicle postoperatively to aid in drinking process.
   C. Lock the playroom door before taking the tour group unless Saturday surgery patients are waiting.
   D. Select a clean, unoccupied day surgery room. Point out the following items:
      1. Different bed types and side rails
      2. Control buttons
      3. Bedside table
      4. Television
      5. Telephone
      6. Bathroom with emergency pull chain
      7. Light switches
      8. Closets
         a. Plastic bags provided to keep belongings in.
         b. Storage space for other items such as strollers and baby carrier until the family returns from surgery.
      9. Different sizes of hospital gowns
      10. Blood pressure machine and cuff
      11. IVAC and disposable probe covers
   E. Note that patients may want to bring their own slippers, robe, and security items (e.g., blanket, pacifier, and stuffed animal).
   F. Explain that criteria for discharge are specified per the physician's orders.

```
Ask parents if there are any questions.
```

II. Surgical Floor Suite
   A. Single elevator or hallway to holding area
      1. Move to the surgical floor via the single elevator from the COPS floor.
      2. Point out the following:
         a. Patients may ride the gurney (bed with wheels), be carried by a family member, or walk up to the surgical holding area.
         b. If the patient rides on the gurney, safety belts must be worn.
   B. OR holding area
      1. The room for surgeons or physicians, nurses, and anesthesiologist to meet with the patient and parents is shown.
         a. The medical staff reviews patient history and laboratory work and checks the signatures on permit.
         b. Parents can bring questions written down for the physicians to answer at this time.
      2. The holding area is limited to parents only. Other family members need to wait across the hall in the family waiting area. Parents of the patient join them when the patient goes to surgery.
      3. When the patient is cleared for surgery, the patient rides on the gurney with physicians and/or nurses to the operating area. Parents are asked to wait in the waiting area. Point out the importance of having at least one parent available in the family waiting area at all times, if possible.
   C. Hallway or parent waiting area
      1. Point out the following features and locations:
         a. Restrooms
         b. Pay phone
         c. Refreshments
            1) Coffee available (suggest that parents restrict their intake because caffeine tends to agitate and makes coping harder)
            2) Cafeteria
         d. Use of elevators
      2. Explain that no eating is allowed in the family waiting area and suggest eating before coming to the hospital or later in the day during or after surgery is finished.
      3. No smoking is permitted in the building, smoking is permitted in the first floor patio, outside.
      4. Explain the sibling policy in the OR area and, if applicable, the sibling policy elsewhere on other units.
         a. No sibling is left unattended without a parent in the third floor playroom.
         b. Remind parents that their attention is focused on their child in surgery and it will be difficult for them to supervise and attend to the needs of their other children.

5. Point out that this is the area for saying your good-byes, giving kisses, and reassuring the child that you will wait for him or her.
6. If parents must leave the waiting area, they should tell the volunteer at the desk in the waiting area (a volunteer is present in the morning only) or tell the holding room staff.

Ask parents if there are any questions.

D. Main entry doors to surgical suites
   1. Open the electrical doors, look in to observe OR staff (dressed in scrubs ["pajamas"]), and wave to greet the friendly staff.
   2. Explain that patients will enter through the electrical doors on the "bed with wheels" with the physicians and nurses on the day of surgery. The tour enters OR area through adjacent electrical doors.
E. Parallel/hallway proceeding to designated OR
   1. Point out any staff in uniform
      a. Scrubs
      b. Caps
      c. Masks
      d. Shoe covers or booties
      e. Friendly people dressed up
   2. Note
      a. Long hallways
      b. Cool temperature
F. Designated and prepared OR (pulmonary or cystoscopy)
   1. Introduce and discuss the following:
      a. Table with safety belt
      b. Green sheet, blanket
      c. Blood pressure cuff ("arm hugs")
      d. Heart monitor with leads, "stickers"
      e. Anesthesia mask and other possible options for anesthesia are:
         1) Sometimes an IV catheter is placed on the nursing floor to begin antibiotic therapy; in this case, presedation may be given into the IV in the holding area.
         2) Sometimes presedation is given orally either on the nursing floor or in the holding area.
         3) Sometimes no presedation is given and an anesthetic ("air" or "gas") is given through a mask in the OR. (Different aromas may be available, such as a strawberry smell; ask the anesthesiologist.)
         4) Regardless of the anesthetic method used, an IV catheter is placed before the patient reaches the PACU (usually while the patient is asleep in the OR).

Ask parents if there are any questions.

Stress the importance of directing specific questions to the physician or the anesthesiologist about the type of anesthesia that their child will be receiving. Suggest that unique or individual questions be written for the physician.

G. PACU (wake-up room)
   1. Hallway outside the recovery room
      a. Patients usually stay approximately 1 hour; however, the time may vary.
      b. Mention to the parents that the recovery room is shared with adult patients after surgery and can get busy.
      c. One parent at a time may visit child at bedside briefly; parents can sometimes hold or rock their child depending on postoperative conditions.
      d. A staff member (nurse or volunteer) escorts the parent to the recovery area from the family waiting area.
      e. Explain to the parents that they may be asked to leave the recovery area if another patient is in distress. Advise them to leave quickly and follow the staff's instructions. At these times, recovery room staff split into teams—one to help the patient in distress and one to attend to the remaining patients.
      f. If staff have not come for the parents to see your child, advise them *please to be patient*. Staff are busy providing postoperative care sometimes to more than one patient.
   2. In the recovery area, introduce and discuss the use and purpose of the following items. Have patients touch, wear, smell, or demonstrate these items as appropriate.
      a. Heart monitor or leads ("stickers")
      b. IVAC and disposable probe covers
      c. Wrist or ankle restraints
      d. Pulse oximeter
      e. Oxygen nasal cannula, mask, or hose
      f. Staff
      g. Gurney
      h. Emesis basin
      i. Warm blankets

Ask parents if there are any questions.
Resuggest that questions be written and brought in on day of surgery.

III. Tour Conclusion
   A. Return to the elevators. Review and discuss the following:
      1. Refer to COPS child life specialist on the day and time of surgery for further questions.

2. Provide directions to exits, cars, and bus stops.
3. Disperse the tour group to appropriate place.
   a. Laboratory
   b. Radiology department
   c. Outpatient surgery area

> At the end of the translation, *collect the tape players.*

4. Two optional tour sites:
   a. Laboratory
      1) Guide those needing laboratory procedures.
      2) Offer any support, explanation, or coping tips needed.
   b. Radiology department
      1) Guide those needing an x-ray film to the appropriate place.
      2) Offer any support, explanation, or coping tips needed.
5. Return to the COPS to prepare for the next tour group.

Teaching Materials Used for Instructor Preparation

Children's Outpatient Surgery Patient Room Items for Display

1. Blood pressure machine or Dinamapp
2. Blood pressure cuffs in different sizes
3. IVAC pump or probe covers
4. Patient gowns in different sizes

Carried Items of Display on Tour

1. "Stickers" for leads
2. Arm or leg restraints
3. Ball-point pen
4. Two extra AA batteries

Operating Room Items for Display

1. Scrubs ("pajamas")
2. Caps
3. Masks
4. Shoe covers or booties
5. Table with safety belt
6. Blood pressure cuffs
7. Different types and sizes of masks
8. Heart monitor, leads, "stickers"
9. Sink with knee attachment and soap pump on the floor

Items in Patient Take-home Bags

1. Adhesive bandage (Band-Aid)
2. Tongue blade
3. Two cotton balls
4. Patient identification band with insert
5. Oral syringe
6. Two alcohol pads
7. Medicine cup
8. Mask
9. Cap
10. Sticker
11. *Child Life at Children's Hospital* brochure
12. "Parents Can Help" bookmark
13. "Suggestions to Parents Before Discharge from the Hospital" sheet

Geriatric Surgery

Nancy Girard

The wiser mind
Mourns less for what age takes away
Than what it leaves behind.

W. WORDSWORTH, THE FOUNTAIN, 1800

America's emergence as a graying society has had a profound impact on society and on health care needs. In 1987, the average life expectancy was 75 years, with men living 71.2 and women 78.2 years (National Center for Health Statistics, 1986). In 1987, 59% of the population was 65 to 74 years of age, and 41% was 75 years and older. If growth of the aging population continues at the present rate, it is projected that by 2080, the 65 to 74 age group will decrease to 47%, and the 75 and over group will increase to over 55% (U.S. Dept. of Commerce, 1989) (Table 31–1). The continued growth of the aging population (Fig. 31–1) will greatly impact those who will be paying the living and health care expenses of the elderly (Fig. 31–2). Thus, the acute health care crisis will continue unless the impact of aging is addressed.

The expansion of the elderly has contributed to further descriptive categories: over 65 (old), over 75 (old-old), and over 85 (oldest-old) (Rice, 1989).

Along with the high-priced, life-sustaining technology that is needed for patients of advanced age, nurses skilled in operating that technology are also needed. These advanced nursing skills are used in assisting with surgical interventions to extend or improve the quality of life or to provide palliation of untreatable conditions.

IMPACT ON HEALTH CARE DELIVERY SYSTEMS

The impact of societal aging on the health care delivery systems is seen in changes occurring today. These changes include financial and society trends and health care policies. More hospitals are becoming acute care facilities, with older adults occupying up to 70% of the beds (Rice, 1989). Many studies show that elderly patients generally have a two to three times greater risk of death for any given surgical procedure than do middle-aged adults. This greater risk is due to not only the physiological changes of aging, but also the greater incidence of pathological processes affecting the elderly (Johnson, 1988).

Delivery methods are changing to meet the needs of this older society. Hospitals are adding ambulatory surgery centers, in part because they are especially relevant to the needs of the elderly. Crawford (1985) identified five reasons that ambulatory surgery is especially beneficial to the older patient:

1. There is a decreased incidence of hospital-acquired complications, such as infection and pneumonia.
2. Patients are less traumatized emotionally and psychologically than if they are hospitalized.
3. The environment is not as foreign as that of the hospital, leading to less confusion and better coping ability.
4. It costs less for the patient. Many third-party

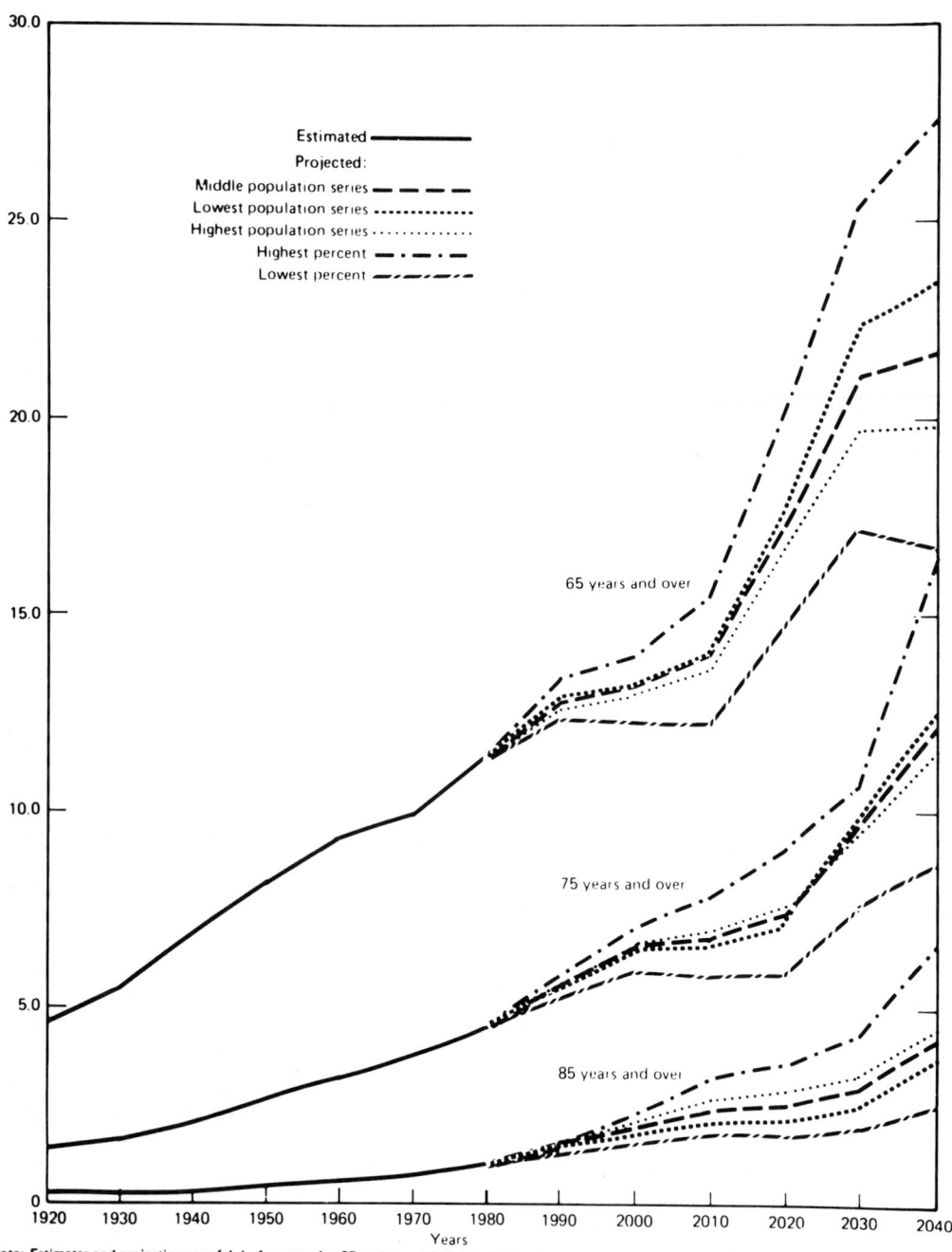

Note: Estimates and projections as of July 1, except for 85 and over, 1920-30, which relate to April 1; points are plotted for years ending in zero.

FIGURE 31–1. Percentage of the total population in the older ages: 1900–2040. (From U.S. Bureau of the Census: *Demographics and socioeconomic aspects of the aging in the United States*. Series P-23, No 138. Washington, D.C., 1984.)

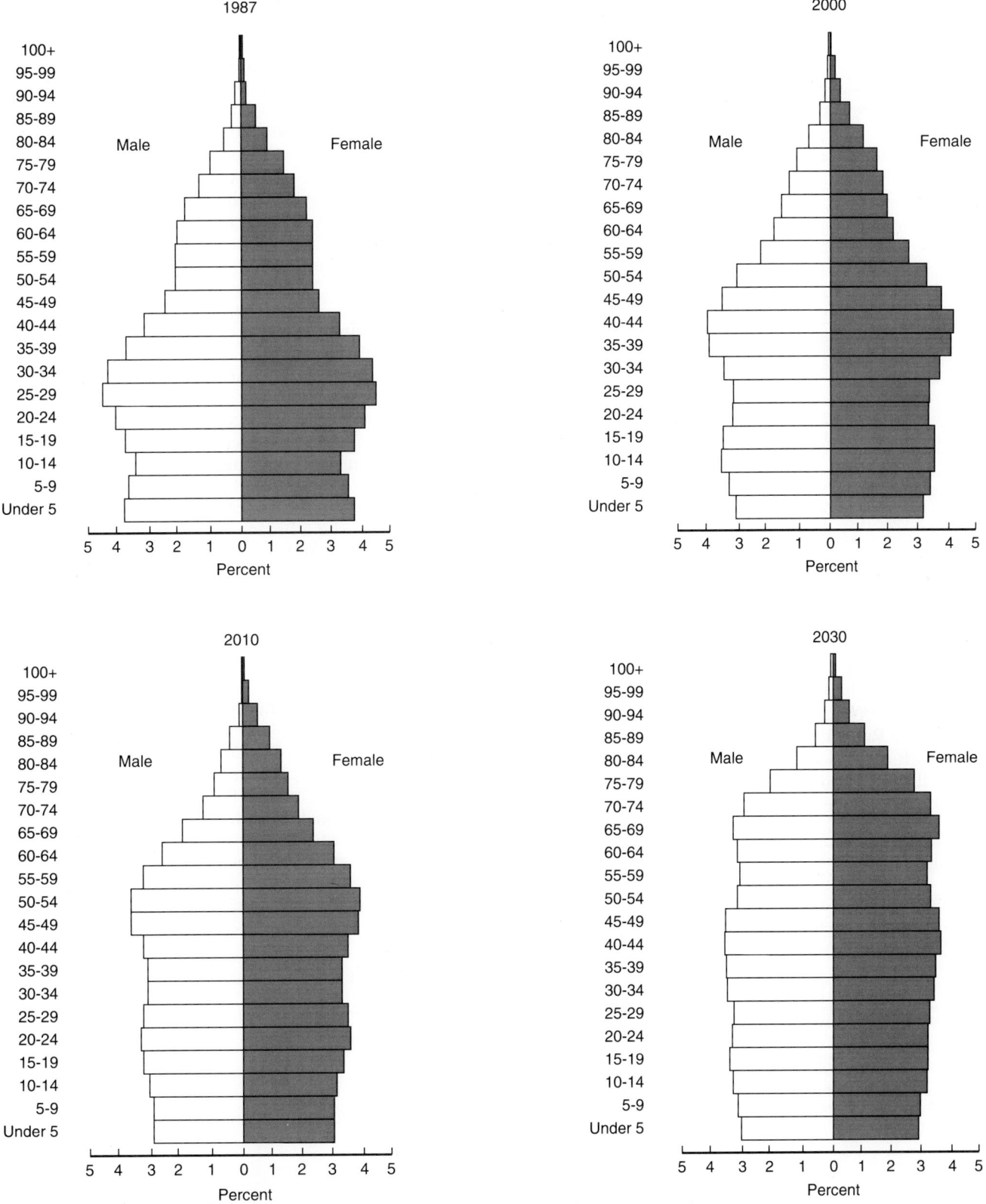

FIGURE 31–2. Age distribution of the U.S. population: 1987, 2000, 2010 and 2030. (From U.S. Dept. of Commerce, Bureau of the Census: *Projections of the population of the United States by age, sex, and race: 1988 to 2080.* Washington, D.C., 1989.)

Year	Age 65–74 Years (%)	Age 75–84 Years (%)	Age 85 Years and Over (%)	Median Age of 65-and-Over Population
TABLE 31–1. PERCENTAGE OF PERSONS AGE 65 AND OVER IN SELECTED AGE GROUPS: 1960–2080				
Estimates:				
1960	66.3	28.1	5.6	71.9
1965	64.4	29.7	5.9	72.3
1970	62.1	30.7	7.1	72.6
1975	61.3	30.7	8.0	72.5
1980	60.9	30.3	8.8	72.8
1985	59.6	31.0	9.4	73.0
1987	59.2	31.2	9.6	73.1
Projections:				
1990	58.2	31.5	10.3	73.3
1995	56.1	32.3	11.6	73.8
2000	52.3	34.4	13.3	74.5
2005	50.8	34.5	14.7	74.2
2010	53.4	31.0	15.5	74.2
2020	59.5	27.7	12.8	73.0
2030	54.9	32.8	12.4	74.0
2040	45.2	36.8	18.0	76.1
2050	46.1	31.6	22.3	76.1
2080	44.6	31.7	23.7	76.4

U.S. Dept. of Commerce, Bureau of the Census. (1989). *Projections of the population of the United States by age, sex, and race: 1988 to 2080.* Washington, D.C.

reimbursement agencies pay for only ambulatory surgery intervention.
5. Elderly patients can have more contact with their family and support network.

Medicare and Medicaid funds constitute nearly 10% of the federal budget, and many of the elderly utilize this method of payment for surgery. The institution of Diagnostic Related Grouping affects inpatient surgical interventions, and in the near future, ambulatory surgery will also be affected by similar developing federal regulations.

LEGAL IMPLICATIONS

When an older adult has surgery, an important legal consideration is that of informed consent. An informed consent recognizes the personal autonomy of the patient to make a decision about what happens to his or her body. In other words, a patient has the right to decide who will perform interventions or touch his or her body (Fig. 31–3). As a patient gets older, the right to determine treatment should become stronger, not weaker (Kapp and Bigot, 1985). Physicians' delegation of obtaining an informed consent to nurses or other health care personnel has been discussed widely in nursing literature. However, the general legal principle is that each health care professional must obtain consent for the intervention that he or she expects to perform (Kapp and Bigot, 1985). Nurses can certainly clarify and explain, but the physician should return to see the patient if there is uncertainty or questions about the surgical procedure.

Two theories about the elderly are applicable to failure to obtain informed consent: the negligence theory and the battery theory.

The negligence theory states that a health care professional has failed to give care to a particular patient, according to minimally acceptable standards. This includes obtaining surgical consent. The forms should contain certain important facts, such as major potential complications of anesthesia or the surgical procedure. Failure to mention these facts when obtaining a patient's signature could be a breach of duties and be considered negligence (Kapp and Bigot, 1985).

The battery theory is related to when someone does something physical to the patient that he or she does not want done. For example, a surgical procedure is other than that signed for (e.g., removing a left foot when the consent was for a right foot amputation) (Kapp and Bigot, 1985, p. 18).

In addition to negligence and battery, other legal areas are of special interest for the older population. These include giving voluntary valid consent and having competency to give consent. Voluntary consent means that a patient must be free to choose, and there cannot be any "force, fraud, deceit, duress, constraint or coercion to that patient" (Kapp and Bigot, 1985, p. 23). For example, a violation could occur when a patient is forced into undergoing a surgical intervention such as an amputation or when no alternative treatments are presented. This is not as common as coercion, in which the

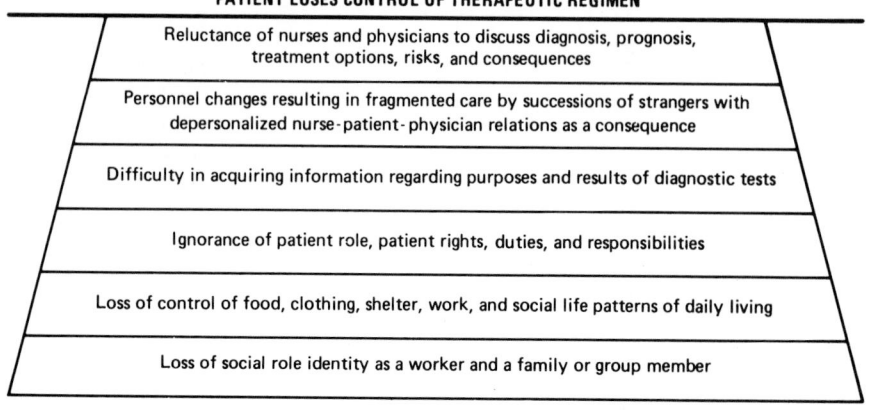

PATIENT LOSES CONTROL OF THERAPEUTIC REGIMEN

Reluctance of nurses and physicians to discuss diagnosis, prognosis, treatment options, risks, and consequences

Personnel changes resulting in fragmented care by successions of strangers with depersonalized nurse-patient-physician relations as a consequence

Difficulty in acquiring information regarding purposes and results of diagnostic tests

Ignorance of patient role, patient rights, duties, and responsibilities

Loss of control of food, clothing, shelter, work, and social life patterns of daily living

Loss of social role identity as a worker and a family or group member

FIGURE 31–3. Constraints on the patient's participation in health care decisions. (From Bandman, E. L., Bandman, B. [1985]. Ethical decision making in nursing: Values and guidelines. In E. L. Bandman, B. Bandman [Eds.], *Nursing ethics in the lifespan.* Norwalk, CT: Appleton-Century-Crofts.)

older adult may be consciously or unconsciously manipulated into having an unwanted surgical procedure. Kapp and Bigot (1985, p. 24) identified five questionable legal areas in which coercion may occur:

1. Patients are institutionalized or in the custody of another, often their children.
2. Patients are committed or involuntarily retained.
3. Patients have physical or mental impairments that make them more susceptible to coercion.
4. Patients want only to please others and do what others ask (their perception may be that they will not continue to get adequate care if they refuse).
5. Patients are unable to obtain or are financially incapable of obtaining independent advice and consultation.

A patient must also be mentally competent to sign a surgical consent. If a patient has been declared incompetent by a health care institution (de facto incompetence), she or he may not have been declared so in a court of law (de jure incompetence) (Kapp and Bigot, 1985). However, usually, an older adult's family members make compassionate and competent decisions when surgery is needed.

There are general exceptions to the informed consent requirements (Kapp and Bigot, 1985):

Legally required interventions: When treatment is required immediately to save a life or to prevent serious effects to the patient's health, but the patient is unable to give consent and it cannot be obtained from anyone else, intervention is appropriate. The patient probably would not refuse the treatment if he or she were able to give consent.

Emergency situations: The health care provider must show that it was not possible to obtain consent from the patient and that there was an immediate threat of death or permanent disability to the patient.

Waiver: The patient can waive, or relinquish, the right to be informed. Many older patients hold surgeons in great esteem—if the surgeon says they must have surgery, they do.

Therapeutic privilege: Kapp and Bigot (1985, p. 53) stated that therapeutic privilege occurs when a professional, such as a surgeon, withholds information about a patient's diagnosis or treatment. This is usually done because it is believed that telling patients information might cause them considerable psychological trauma and upset them so much that they would be unable to make a rational decision about their own treatment. Before making an independent decision to withhold information, the health care professional is advised to get a consultation about his or her decision.

Commonly known risks: When the risk of a treatment or procedure is known by the patient because of past experiences, or when the information is known to the average patient, the health care professional is not required to disclose the risk.

DEFINING THE TERM ELDERLY

There have been many attempts to define the term elderly. In the past, elderly was defined as the time of mandatory retirement—65 years. With modern health care and the expanded life span, some investigators have defined 70 to 75 years as young old, 75 to 90 years as middle old, and older than 90 years as old old (Jackson, 1988). Birren and Warner Schaie (1990) identified four types of age and aging:

1. Biological age: The person's biological status is compared with that of others of the same chronological age. It is measured by the functional abilities of the vital organs. A person with a young biological age has a longer life span than others of the same chronological age.
2. Psychological age: How well individuals can adapt to changing environmental demands is influenced by the functioning ability of systems such as the central nervous system and the cardiovascular system. It includes intelligence, memory, learning, skills, feeling, motivation, and emotions.
3. Functional age: One's capacity level for functioning in a given society, relative to others of the same age, is closely related to psychological age.
4. Social age: The individual is compared with societal expectations of roles and behavior. Does the person behave older or younger than expected for the chronological age?

In considering the various definitions of aging and elderly, it is more useful to the perioperative nurse to consider the individual. Assessment should consider more factors than simply the patient's chronological age in planning care. A 75-year-old person who is biologically, functionally, and psychologically much younger than her or his chronological age may withstand the surgery much better than a person of 50 years who is older in every category.

BIOLOGICAL AND PSYCHOSOCIAL ASPECTS OF AGING

Physiological Changes

Cardiovascular System

The incidence of death by ischemic heart disease increases sharply with advancing age for both men and women. It remains the major cause of death and disability of the elderly. There are three main areas of deterioration in the aging heart: the pumping ability, the conduction system, and the biochemical system.

The heart becomes a less effective pump for many reasons (Table 31–2). There is damage or change in the muscle fibers, reduced strength and efficiency of contractions, and decreased functioning due to valvular

TABLE 31–2. PHYSIOLOGICAL CARDIOVASCULAR CHANGES WITH AGING

Resting
Heart rate—unchanged
Left ventricular stroke volume—↑
Cardiac output—↓
Left ventricular end-diastolic pressure—unchanged
Ejection time—↑
Systolic blood pressure—↑
Systemic vascular resistance—↑
Exercise
Maximal heart rate—↓
Maximal oxygen consumption—↓
Arteriovenous oxygen difference—↓
Maximal cardiac output—↓
Left ventricular end-diastolic pressure—↑
Systolic blood pressure—↑
Systemic vascular resistance—↑

Modified from Schrier, R. (1982). *Clinical internal medicine in the aged.* Philadelphia: W. B. Saunders.

changes. Throughout the body, the arteries become clogged and less elastic (Harris, 1978).

The conduction system may have been damaged by past ischemic attacks, affecting the nodal areas in the heart. Tachycardia and arrhythmias become more prevalent and obvious. Johnson (1988) and Goldman (1983) found that a myocardial infarction 3 months before surgery is associated with a 39% chance of death due to other myocardial infarctions or cardiac complications. If the surgery can be postponed until 3 to 6 months after a myocardial infarction, the mortality in surgical patients drops to 15%, and after 6 months, it falls to a 5% risk.

The contractility and irritability of the myocardium slow in the aging heart. The heart functions well when there is adequate rest but has problems when tachycar-dia occurs (Harris, 1978). Patients may verbalize palpitations of the heart or say that it skips a beat occasionally. The biochemical system may be damaged from past acute and chronic systemic conditions such as myocardial infarction, diabetes mellitus, and obstructive respiratory disease. Furthermore, the aged heart has a decreased ability to utilize oxygen (Goldman, 1983).

Common conditions in the elderly are ischemic heart disease, hypertension, congestive heart failure, endocarditis, arrhythmias, and conductive disruptions (Birren and Warner Schaie, 1990). The most common vascular problems include chronic and acute arterial occlusions, aneurysms, phlebitis, cerebrovascular accidents, and varicosities. Surgeries most commonly performed for disorders of the elderly cardiovascular system include revascularization surgery, insertion of pacemakers, and surgery for degenerative calcific valvular disease (Fig. 31–4). All general anesthesic agents may affect the aging heart because of their impact on myocardial function, preload, and heart rate.

Respiratory System

Normal changes in the respiratory system also occur (Table 31–3). There is a decreased ability of the chest wall to expand during inspiration, which is due to the shortening of the vertebral column and loss of muscle mass in the shoulder and chest area. The lungs lose some of their elasticity. The alveolar walls thicken, and the alveoli are larger as well as decreased in numbers (Steffl, 1984). These changes lead to a decrease in the vital capacity and tidal volume, as well as generalized decreased tissue oxygenation. Between the ages of 20 and 80 years there is a loss of 40% in the amount of air a person can move through the lungs (Sheehy, 1982). Because respiratory changes, like other physiological

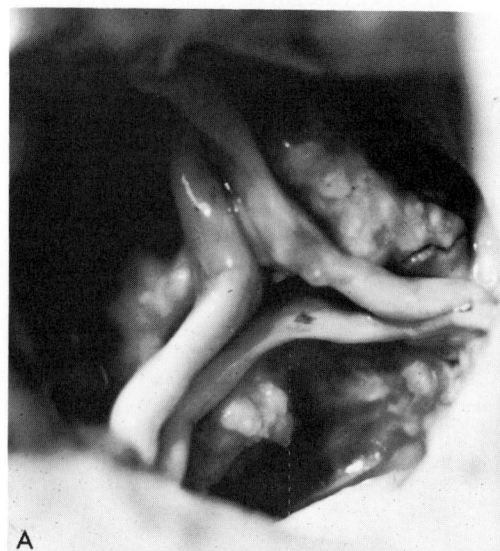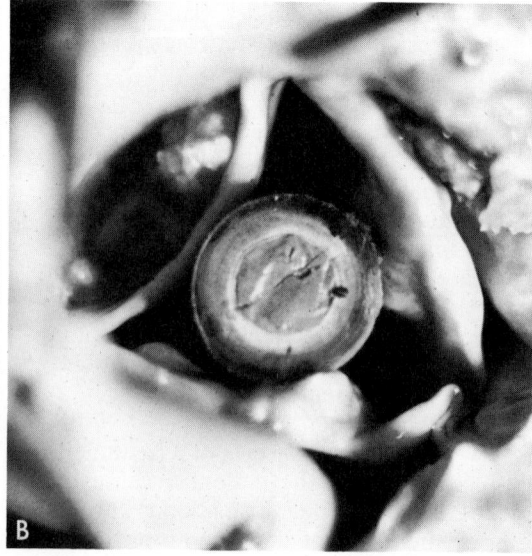

FIGURE 31–4. Degenerative calcific aortic stenosis. *A,* Heavily calcified tricuspid aortic valve from an 81-year-old woman with a 90 mm Hg aortic valve gradient. *B,* Wax pencil placed in the aortic valve orifice demonstrates that no commissural fusion was contributing to the obstruction in this degenerative process. (From Schrier, R. W. [1982]. *Clinical internal medicine in the aged.* Philadelphia: W. B. Saunders.)

TABLE 31–3. EFFECTS OF AGING ON THE RESPIRATORY SYSTEM

Respiratory Abnormality	Physiological Basis	Clinical Disorders
Decline in bellows function	Increased chest wall stiffness Loss of elastic recoil Decreased respiratory muscle strength Increased airway collapsibility	"Senile" emphysema
Abnormal gas exchange	Ventilation-perfusion mismatch Reduced diffusing for carbon monoxide Increased alveolar-arterial oxygen gradient	Arterial hypoxemia Decreased exercise tolerance
Abnormal breathing pattern	Diminished responsiveness to hypoxemia and hypercarbia Changing set point for ventilation due to fluctuating level of wakefulness	Cheyne-Stokes breathing Periodic breathing
Upper airway obstruction	Decreased airway muscle tone due to loss of wakefulness stimulus, decreased metabolic respiratory drive	Snoring, sleep apnea, hypopnea, oxygen desaturation
Altered lung host-defense	Decreased ciliary action Impaired cough mechanism Decreased IgA production ?Decreased phagocytic function of alveolar macrophages	Increased susceptibility to infection (pneumonia and chronic bronchitis)

From Schrier, R. W. (1982). *Clinical internal medicine in the aged.* Philadelphia: W. B. Saunders.

changes in the elderly, occur naturally with time, the well elderly patient adjusts to the decreased oxygenation and adapts well until trauma such as surgery intervenes and disrupts the balance.

The pathophysiological changes in the aging respiratory system are a major cause of mortality and morbidity in older adults after surgery. The aging patient has less physiological endurance to withstand surgery, as well as less energy to recover quickly, than younger patients. They have a decreased ability to cough productively, along with increased potential for pulmonary infections (Lewis and Collier, 1992). The most common surgeries performed in the elderly are for neoplasms of the lung (especially for patients with a long history of smoking) and endoscopic procedures. Because older people have a low tolerance for hypoxia, careful attention must be paid to these patients after surgery. The most frequent postoperative complications are pulmonary insufficiency, atelectasis, and pneumonia (Johnson, 1983).

Musculoskeletal System

There are changes with age in the muscle, bones, and joints of the musculoskeletal system. The changes in the muscle fibers are minimal in normal aging. There may be loss of type II muscle fibers, which are the fast twitch fibers that are involved in producing motor activity. There are few changes in muscle fiber function. It has been suggested that the decline in motor performance in the elderly is due more to a decline in tissue oxygenation and central nervous system functioning than to changes in the muscle fibers themselves (McCarter, 1985). With decreased activity, the muscle mass of an individual decreases, leading to flabby and weak muscles. Adipose cells increase in women and decrease in men (Girard, 1985). Strength also decreases if the person does not maintain an active exercise schedule.

Bones decrease in mass for several reasons. In women, demineralization and protein matrix loss occur after menopause (Lewis and Collier, 1992). Osteoporosis is twice as common in women as in men. There is more bone resorption than formation, leading to fragile, "Swiss cheese" bones.

There is an inability of the body to produce or use adequate calcium or phosphorus in making new bones, so bones fracture more easily and take longer to heal. Height decreases with age owing to the thinning of the vertebral disks and the general shortening of the vertebral column. There is an increase in joint rigidity because of chronic conditions such as arthritis. This reduces the general range-of-motion ability. The legs become more resistant to passive range of motion (Jessup, 1984). There is some shrinkage of tendons and atrophy of muscles, which further limit movement.

The aging joints may deteriorate with noninflammatory or inflammatory conditions. They may fuse or enlarge, leading to the bony joints common in the elderly.

The most common musculoskeletal surgeries are for degenerative joint disease, specifically total joint replacement. These surgeries often increase the quality of life for the elderly patient. Other frequent surgeries are those for repairs of fractures and dislocations and amputations. Postoperative complications include hemorrhage, emboli or thrombus formation, nonunion, nonhealing, and infection.

Gastrointestinal System

With age come many changes throughout the gastrointestinal tract. Oral and dental problems may prevent adequate intake of nourishment. The older adult may have pathophysiological problems such as dysphagia (difficulty swallowing), decreased esophageal peristalsis, and inefficiency of the esophageal sphincter. Liquids may be difficult to swallow, and some foods, such as tomatoes and oranges, may cause abnormal gastric motility (Bartol and Heitkemper, 1979). Gastric atrophy may cause the inability to metabolize iron. Malabsorption changes cause folic acid deficiencies. Lack of gastric intrinsic factors could lead to vitamin B_{12} deficiencies (Knudson, 1984). Hiatal hernias are common, occurring in 40 to 60% of people older than 60 years (Sklar, 1978). Medical conditions such as diverticulosis and cholelithiasis occur more frequently in the elderly (Bartol and Heitkemper, 1979; Goldman et al., 1978). Constipation can be a problem in older adults owing to decreased peristalsis and elasticity of the intestinal tract (Knudsen, 1984). Atrophy of mucus secretion glands, leading to decreased secretion products in the colon, adds to the problem. Lack of adequate fluid, bulk, and roughage in the diet and a decrease in exercise, along with the intake of constipating medications, add to the problem (Bowles et al., 1981; Hull et al., 1980).

Because of the above mentioned changes, elderly surgical patients are more prone to undernourishment (Table 31–4). They may have a deficiency in vitamins and minerals, which delays wound healing. They may be anemic, which further adds to their hypoxic condition and poor tissue perfusion. IV administration of electrolytes, particularly potassium, may be needed preoperatively to hydrate the elderly patient. The patient should have a nutritional assessment as far in advance of the proposed surgery as possible. A good nutritional status increases the chances of a smooth recovery and decreases potential complications.

Some of the more common surgeries of the gastrointestinal tract are gastric surgeries, ostomies, and surgeries for neoplasms. If enemas are ordered preoperatively, the perioperative nurse should be aware that there may be incomplete emptying owing to the sluggish peristalsis of the bowel and atrophy of abdominal muscle walls. This could result in contamination of the surgical field by involuntary expulsion of feces, or by leakage of feces into the abdominal cavity after the surgical incision. Elderly patients are slow healing, especially after abdominal surgery, even if fecal contamination has not occurred. The risk of wound infection may be higher than in young patients because of surgical contamination, poor tissue perfusion, malnutrition, or chronic diseases.

Genitourinary Tract

The genitourinary tract and renal system are affected by normal aging. In males, glanular and stomal tissues continue to develop, which may lead to benign prostatic hypertrophy, or hyperplasia of the prostate gland. Approximately 30% of white males older than 50 years have benign prostatic hypertrophy and the incidence increases with age (Jaffe, 1978; Knudson, 1984b). The urinary bladder walls become thickened, may lose muscle tone and function, and have a diminished capacity. There may also be loss of sphincter control (Lewis and Collier, 1992). The urine that cannot be excreted (residual urine) can lead to distention of the ureters. This may affect renal functioning by causing atrophy and insufficiency.

The older person is thus more prone to bladder and kidney infections during the invasive perioperative period. The aging kidney loses some of its ability to filter and clear substances from the blood. There is also an increase in tubular reabsorption, which may affect the patient's hydration status. Kidney function decreases 50% from age 20 to age 90 years (Lewis and Collier, 1992). This loss of renal function greatly affects the ability of older surgical patients to filter and clear medication and anesthesia from their systems. There is increased protein in the urine, an increased blood urea nitrogen level, and an increased potential for electrolyte imbalance.

Common genitourinary surgeries are transurethral resections of the prostate, cystoscopies, and surgeries for neoplasms throughout the genitourinary system. Postoperative complications in the elderly include urinary tract infections, urinary retention or incontinence, hemorrhage, electrolyte imbalances, and renal failure.

Skin

The most apparent changes of aging occur in the skin. Normally, there is a general thinning of the epidermis, or outer layer of the skin (Fig. 31–5). Epidermal cells are larger and more irregular and reproduce more slowly than in young skin. This is the reason older skin appears thinner and more translucent. The middle skin layer, or dermis, contains the blood vessels, nerves, subcutaneous glands, and hair follicles (Matteson and McConnell, 1988). There is a decrease in the amount of collagen in the dermis, which leads to decreased skin strength and elasticity. The small circulatory vessels become fragile, clogged, and fewer in number. This leads to poor peripheral perfusion and tissue anoxia. Any further pressure, such as from positioning in the operating room (OR), may quickly lead to pressure sores (Table 31–5).

These aging changes make the skin more fragile and friable. It is easier to produce shearing and skin tears when moving and positioning the patient. Dragging, instead of lifting, the patient across the OR bed may produce skin burns. Aging skin is also more prone to chemical, electrical, and tape injuries because of the decreased cell reproduction and increased sensitivity.

Common surgical procedures are done for skin cancers (Fig. 31–6) and skin grafts and free tissue transplants for pressure sores. Healing may be delayed in the elderly, and they are more likely to have postoperative infections.

Immune System

Aging adults have alterations in their immune systems, and hence their ability to resist infections. Throughout the life span, a person is continually ex-

TABLE 31–4. PHYSICAL SIGNS OF MALNUTRITION

Body Area	Normal Appearance	Signs Associated with Malnutrition
Hair	Shiny; firm; not easily plucked	Lack of natural shine; hair dull and dry; thin and sparse; hair fine, silky and straight, color changes (flag sign); can be easily plucked
Face	Skin color uniform; smooth, pink, healthy appearance; not swollen	Skin color loss (depigmentation); skin dark over cheeks and under eyes (malar and supraorbital pigmentation); lumpiness or flakiness of skin of nose and mouth; swollen face; enlarged parotid glands; scaling of skin around nostrils (nasolabial seborrhea)
Eyes	Bright, clear, shiny; no sores at corners of eyelids; membranes healthy pink and moist. No prominent blood vessels or mound of tissue on sclera	Eye membranes are pale (pale conjunctivae); redness of membranes (conjunctival injection); Bitot spots; redness and fissuring of eyelid corners (angular palpebritis); dryness of eye membranes (conjunctival xerosis); cornea has dull appearance (corneal xerosis); cornea is soft (keratomalacia); scar on cornea; ring of fine blood vessels around corner (circumcorneal injection)
Lips	Smooth, not chapped or swollen	Redness and swelling of mouth or lips (cheilosis), especially at corners of mouth (angular fissures and scars)
Tongue	Deep red in appearance; not swollen or smooth	Swelling; scarlet and raw tongue; magenta (purplish) color of tongue; smooth tongue; swollen sores; hyperemic and hypertrophic papillae; and atrophic papillae
Teeth	No cavities; no pain; bright	May be missing or erupting abnormally; gray or black spots (fluorosis); cavities (caries)
Gums	Healthy; red; do not bleed; not swollen	"Spongy" and bleed easily; recession of gums
Glands	Face not swollen	Thyroid enlargement (front and neck); parotid enlargement (cheeks become swollen)
Skin	No signs of rashes, swellings, dark or light spots	Dryness of skin (xerosis); sandpaper feel of skin (follicular hyperkeratosis); flakiness of skin; skin swollen and dark; red, swollen pigmentation of exposed areas (pellagrous dermatosis); excessive lightness or darkness of skin (dyspigmentation); black and blue marks due to skin bleeding (petechiae); lack of fat under skin
Nails	Firm, pink	Nails are spoon shaped (koilonychia); brittle, ridged nails
Muscular and skeletal systems	Good muscle tone; some fat under skin; can walk or run without pain	Muscles have "wasted" appearance; baby's skull bones are thin and soft (craniotabes); round swelling of front and side of head (frontal and parietal bossing); swelling of ends of bones (epiphyseal enlargement); small bumps on both sides of chest wall (on ribs)—beading of ribs; baby's soft spot on head does not harden at proper time (persistently open anterior fontanelle); knock-knees or bowlegs; bleeding into muscle (musculoskeletal hemorrhages); person cannot get up or walk properly
Internal systems:		
Cardiovascular	Normal heart rate and rhythm; no murmurs or abnormal rhythms; normal blood pressure for age	Rapid heart rate (above 100 beats/minute tachycardia); enlarged heart; abnormal rhythm; elevated blood pressure
Gastrointestinal	No palpable organs or masses (in children, however, liver edge may be palpable)	Liver enlargement; enlargement of spleen (usually indicates other associated diseases)
Nervous	Psychological stability; normal reflexes	Mental irritability and confusion; burning and tingling of hands and feet (paresthesia); loss of position and vibratory sense; weakness and tenderness of muscles (may result in inability to walk); decrease and loss of ankle and knee reflexes

From Nutrition assessment in health programs, part I—Methodology, clinical assessment of nutrition status. (1973). *American Journal of Public Health, 63*(Suppl.), 18. Copyright American Public Health Association.

YOUNG ADULT   OLD ADULT

Stratum corneum
Epidermis
Melanocytes
Basement membrane
Dermis
Capillary loops

FIGURE 31–5. Histological changes associated with aging in normal human skin. Note flattening of the dermoepidermal junction and shortening of capillary loops in older skin. Variability in the size and shape of epidermal cells, irregular stratum corneum, and loss of melanocytes are also apparent. Age-associated loss of dermal thickness and subcutaneous fat is not shown, because the diagram includes only the epidermis and superficial or papillary dermis. (From Gilchrest, B. A. [1982]. Skin. In J. W. Rowe, R. W. Besdine [Eds.], *Health and disease in old age*. Boston: Little, Brown.)

posed to all kinds of substances and microorganisms, which are called antigens. Immunity develops as the body produces antibodies to fight against the antigens of a specific substance or microorganism (Phair, 1983). This can result from deliberate vaccinations, or from unplanned, repeated exposure to the antigen. Studies of skin testing in older adults have shown that there is a decreased ability to respond to new antigens (Phair et al., 1978a). There appears to be a rise in serum immunoglobulin concentrations as people grow older (Phair, 1983); however, a study by Buckley and associates (1974) found that there is a decrease in immunoglobulin G (IgG) with age, which leads to a higher mortality. IgG cells migrate from bone marrow and are part of the humoral immune system. They are important in helping the patient resist disease and are responsible for "remembering" the antigens of most bacteria, viruses, and fungi. Other immunoglobulins are IgA, IgM, IgE, and IgD (Phair, 1983).

Besides the humoral immune system, the body also has a cellular immune system (Fig. 31–7). The most well known is the T-cell, which is mediated by the thymus. This T-cell (also called T-lymphocyte) immunity has been shown to be altered in the aging immune system (Gilles et al., 1981). The T-cell is also vital in the body's resistance to infection. Gardner (1980) suggested that alteration in the cellular immune response in the aged is related to the development of neoplastic diseases, autoimmune responses, and degenerative diseases, as well as increased suseptibility to infection. Changes in the membrane of the T-cell may cause functional changes in the lymphocyte response to antigens. The membrane viscosity in T-cells seems to be related to the ratio of cholesterol to phospholipids in serum.

Because of these alterations in the aging immune system, there is a decreased ability of the body to protect itself against invasion by both endogenous (normally present within the body) and exogenous (outside the body) microorganisms. The most common place for invasion of microorganisms in the hospital is in the OR. The combined factors of decreased immunity, increased stress, and invasive procedures threaten the older adult with infections, which hinder recovery. Therefore, the

TABLE 31–5. RISK FACTORS FOR ALTERED SKIN INTEGRITY IN THE ELDERLY

Factor	Implications
Dermal Ulcers	
Increased likelihood of immobility	Increased potential for injury and trauma
	Increased likelihood of pressure sores
Increased incidence of peripheral vascular disease	Increased potential for ischemic ulcers (e.g., arterial ulcers)
	Increased potential for venous insufficiency
Increased prevalence of nutritional deficiency	Prolonged wound healing
	Reduced immunocompetence
Increased prevalence of peripheral neuropathy	Increased potential for injury or trauma
Increased prevalence of cerebellar dysfunction	Same
Rashes	
Increased drug use	Increased potential for allergic or toxic drug reactions
Increased incidence of herpes zoster	Increased potential for skin infection
Decreased immunocompetence	Increased potential for superinfection of rash
Increased prevalence of dry skin	Decreased protection against chemical irritants
Increased incidence of incontinence	Increased exposure to chemical irritants (e.g., urine)

From Matteson, M. A., McConnell, E. S. (1988). *Gerontological nursing: Concepts and practice*. Philadelphia: W. B. Saunders.

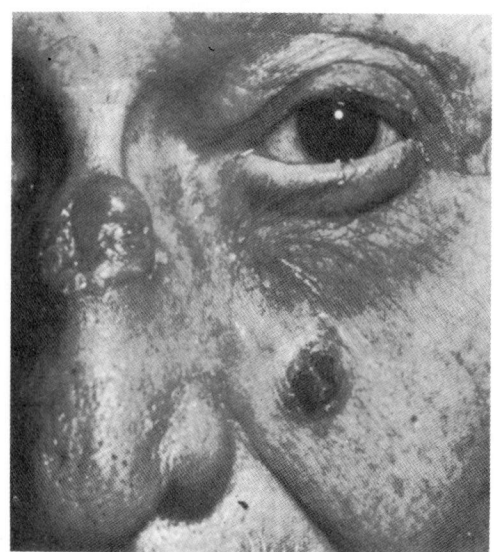

FIGURE 31–6. Basal cell carcinomas on the bridge of the nose and the left cheek of an 80-year-old woman. (From Domonkos, A. N., Arnold, H. L., Jr., Odom, R. B. [1982]. *Andrews' diseases of the skin*. Philadelphia: W. B. Saunders.)

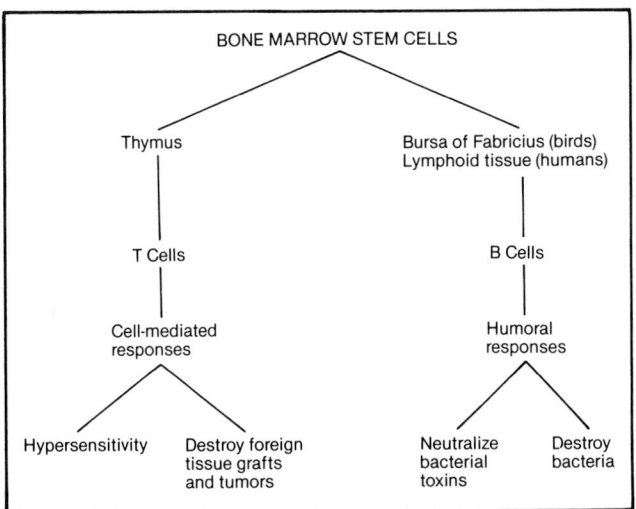

FIGURE 31–7. The immunologic process. (From Matteson, M. A., McConnell, E. S. [1988]. *Gerontological nursing: Concepts and Practice*. Philadelphia: W. B. Saunders.)

perioperative nurse must give attention to the total perioperative period when caring for an elderly patient. Strict and conscientious adherence to the principles of aseptic technique and the monitoring and controlling of the environment are essential.

Central Nervous System

The central nervous system, as with all the other systems in the body, is affected by aging. The effects may not be evident in the well elderly, and some experts say that the loss of cognitive abilities is a result of disease processes and not normal aging. *Secondary aging* is defined as the changes in the central nervous system caused by trauma, illness, and extreme stress (Ripple et al., 1982). There are, however, some definitive changes throughout the central nervous system. These changes are important for the perioperative nurse to assess to get a clear picture of the patient preoperatively. Baseline findings are vital to care of the elderly, so that postoperative confusion and delirium are not attributed to senility when they are due to the anesthesia and physiological insult of the surgical procedure (Tangorra, 1982) (Table 31–6).

Physiologically, both the brain and the autonomic nervous system have normal deterioration with age. The aging brain loses cells, which may lead to slight shrinkage of the brain and a slight decrease in extracellular space. Degenerative changes may also occur in the autonomic nervous system. The sympathetic and parasympathetic systems are impaired owing to ganglia degeneration, and the autonomic reflex response is slowed. (However, deep tendon reflexes remain unchanged in the healthy aging person.) These changes decrease the fine motor movement ability and may also affect gross motor movements. Therefore, the ability of a patient to perform psychomotor skills may be slowed. For example, if an ambulatory surgical patient must learn to

perform surgical wound dressing changes before discharge from the hospital, the perioperative nurse should allow extra time for hands-on practice. The patient may understand the concepts clearly but may have a problem with actually doing the skill.

Further changes in the central nervous system may be seen in the altered balance of an older patient. Balance is affected because of loss of control of random movements, which originate in the brain stem and cerebellum. Vertigo, or dizziness, can be present because of the cerebrovascular changes. Ambulation may be further affected by a less efficient kinesthetic sense, with the older person walking with a parkinsonlike gait (Sheehy, 1982). Knowledge of these changes is particularly significant for nurses working in outpatient surgery centers. Postoperatively, the normal aging changes affecting balance and motion, combined with anesthesia and drugs, make the patient at high risk for falls (Girard, 1985). When the patient walks, extra care must be taken to support and protect him or her.

Another important change the nurse should be aware of is that occurring in the thermoregulatory center of the hypothalamus and in skin receptors. Postsympathetic nerve endings become less sensitive, so tolerance decreases to heat and increases to cold. At the same time, the threshold for peripheral vasodilation and sweating increases. These changes cause decreased perceptions and sensitivity to cold (Matteson and McConnell, 1988). Thus, perioperative nurses should protect older patients from hypothermia, even if they state that they are not cold.

Because of the impaired heat-regulating mechanism, the patient is more likely to adapt to the temperature of the environment and develop hypothermia from the

TABLE 31–6. **COMMON CAUSES OF POSTOPERATIVE CONFUSION IN ELDERLY PERSONS**	
Environmental	Metabolic
Intensive care unit	Hypoxia
Intubation	Acid-base disturbance
Restraints	Hyponatremia
Isolation	Hyperosmolar coma
Traction devices	Acute renal failure
Sensory deprivation	Infection
Decreased auditory acuity	Sepsis
Marginal visual acuity	Pneumonia
Bandages and dressings	Urinary tract infection
Untoward drug reactions	Wound infection
Anesthetic agents	Meningitis
Narcotics	
Hypnotics	
Antiemetics	
Tranquilizers	
Vascular	
Myocardial infarction	
Stroke	
Pulmonary embolism	
Hemorrhage	
Shock	
Congestive heart failure	

From Koin, D. (1984). Surgical concerns. In C. K. Cassell, J. R. Walsh (Eds.), *Geriatric medicine* (Vol. 2). New York: Springer-Verlag.

cold OR. The older patient should be covered with a warm blanket during surgery unless it is contraindicated by the surgical procedure. There are also commercial blankets available to prevent hypothermia. Postoperatively, if the patient's temperature has decreased significantly, rewarming should take place gradually. Rewarming an older adult too rapidly can lead to many potential complications, including hypoxia, acid-base disturbances, pulmonary edema, pneumonia, dehydration, hyperglycemia, and acute tubular necrosis (Kolanosk and Gunter, 1983).

In addition to the above central nervous system changes, there are sensory changes in the older adult that the perioperative nurse should be aware of.

Vision

Changes of aging are especially prevalent in the eye. The size of the pupil diminishes with age, as does acuity and lens accommodation. These changes are called *presbyopia,* or old age vision. Other visual changes that develop with age include sensitivity to glare, altered color and depth perception, and peripheral vision changes (Sheehy, 1982). The ability to see color changes with age because the lens becomes yellow and transmits less violet light. The older adult is less able to distinguish blues and greens. This can be a definite problem if a patient is being given discharge instructions for taking medications that are blue and green. For example, telling patients to take the "blue pill twice a day and the green pill at bedtime" may cause incorrect self-medication. The lens may also be affected by disease and develop opacities, or cataract formations (Sheehy, 1982). This is so common that removal of cataracts is the most frequent eye surgery performed for the elderly.

Patients who are admitted to the hospital for surgeries other than eye surgery are aware of their decreased vision. They may have special glasses that they feel strongly about leaving on as long as possible. The nurse should allow this and make sure that the glasses, which are expensive, are safely confined for return to the patent after surgery.

The majority of eye surgeries for the elderly are performed in ambulatory surgery centers. Several things can be done in these environments to promote a more comfortable atmosphere for these patients. Yellow, orange, or red colors are easier on aging eyes. Lighting that is incandescent rather than fluorescent also makes a room more comfortable for the elderly patient. Glare

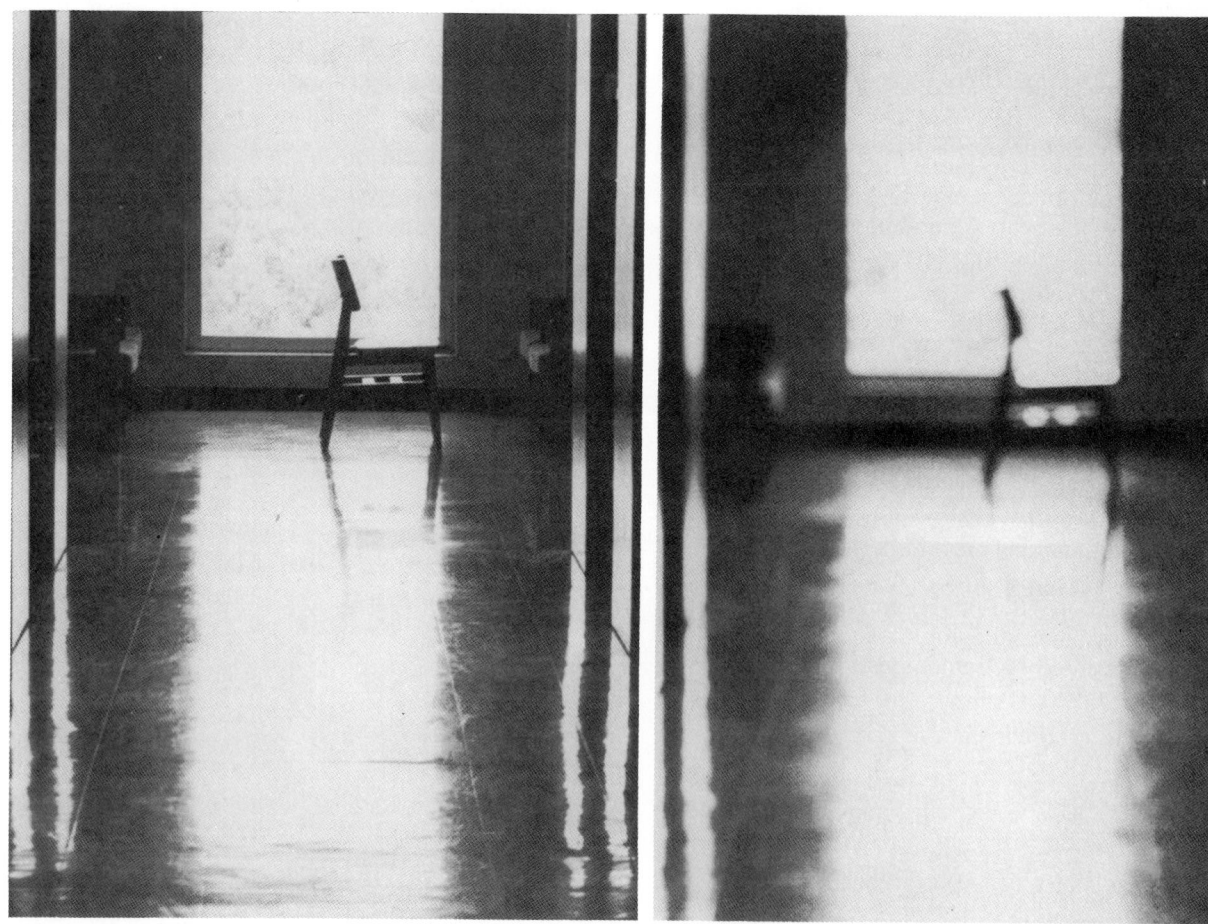

A   B

FIGURE 31–8. Age-related changes in visual acuity are demonstrated in *B,* which is a photographic simulation of the scene in *A* as a 70- to 80-year-old person might see it. Elderly people have an increased susceptibility to glare. (Photographs by Steve Matteson. From Matteson, M. A., McConnell, E. S. [1988]. *Gerontological nursing: Concepts and Practice.* Philadelphia: W. B. Saunders.)

is irritating to older adults. For example, bright sunlight or examining lights that shine on bright floors or surfaces can be distracting (Fig. 31–8). When doing admission procedures or taking histories, bright lights should be behind patients rather than facing them. Window glare can be minimized with carpeting and curtains or blinds. Because eye adaption to light takes longer with age, patients should not go from a dark to a light room, or vice versa. All rooms, such as change rooms and bathrooms, should be similarly lit. Consent forms and other written material should be in large, dark print to facilitate reading and comprehension. Using a teaching combination of visual and audio formats and demonstrations is also helpful.

By reducing the stress the elderly patient has because of his or her eye changes and inability to see clearly, the perioperative nurse can help make the surgical experience less traumatic.

Hearing

The aging hearing system has changes in both function and structure. The two primary functions are hearing and maintaining balance. There are three main types of functional hearing loss. Conductive loss occurs when there are changes with normal sound vibrations in the external and middle ear. Sensorineural loss occurs with damage to the cranial nerve VII (auditory nerve) in the inner ear. The third type is a mixed loss, which occurs to both the conductive and sensorineural functions.

Structural changes take place in the whole auditory system. The external ear becomes dry and wrinkled. The ceruminal glands decrease in function, leading to drier ear wax in the canal. This happens more frequently in older men and may lead to wax impactions, which further decrease hearing. In the middle ear, the eardrum thickens or may be scarred from past events. This decreases or distorts sounds waves passing through the eardrum to the inner ear. The inner ear changes include loss of nerve fibers, and atrophy of the organ of Corti and stria vascularis. The vestibular structures also degenerate, which may also affect the person's balance (Knox, 1977; Matteson and McConnell, 1988).

Ten percent of older adults who are 65 to 75 years of age, and more than 25% of those older than 75 years, have hearing loss (Fig. 31–9). This progressive hearing loss is called *presbycusis*. It is characterized by the inability to hear soft sounds and high-frequency tones. This causes poor discrimination in hearing consonants, especially s, t, f, and g (Knox, 1977). Men usually hear the low frequencies better and women hear the higher ones.

There is a problem of screening out background noises, which interfere with hearing. Loud background sounds may drown out the quiet speech of the perioperative nurse. It may also be difficult for the elderly patient to interpret and understand fast speech. These hearing changes may adversely affect the patient's perception of the surgical experiences. For example, if a patient is having cataract surgery under local anesthesia

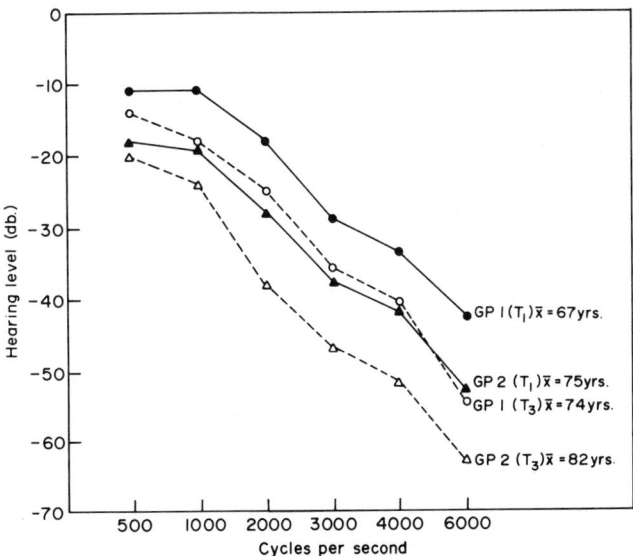

FIGURE 31–9. Average hearing threshold levels for group 1 (subjects initially examined at age 60 to 69 years) and for group 2 (subjects initially examined at age 70 to 79 years) at tests 1 and 3. (Figure from Carl Eisdorfer and Frances Wilkie, "Auditory Changes," in *Normal Aging II*, ed. Erdman Palmore. Copyright 1974 by Duke University Press. Reprinted by permission.)

and there is background noise, he or she may not be able to hear instructions and may become frightened.

The perioperative nurse should always be aware that the mechanical, sensory, and neural changes in hearing may cause fear, insecurity, or bewilderment in the elderly patient. Shouting may help an elderly patient with conductive hearing loss, but it does not help if there is neural damage. Patients with neural loss should have the nurse sit near enough so that they can read lips (if they can see them). Clear enunciations, lack of mumbling, and not dropping the voice level at the end of sentences also help the patient hear and understand perioperative teaching.

Touch

The sense of touch may diminish in the elderly. Diminished sensory receptors in the skin may prevent the patient from reacting to noxious stimuli, such as heat and pain. This may be further affected by the decrease of circulation to the sensory receptors. The perioperative nurse needs to be aware of the safety needs of these patients and prevent burns, pressure sores, or other skin problems due to lack of a pulling-away reaction by the patient. Elderly patients may have problems picking up and manipulating small articles because of the diminished sense of touch in the fingertips (Fig. 31–10). They may appear clumsy when doing skills such as drawing up and self-administering insulin. The nurse may have to be aware of the patients' frustrations and creatively help patients learn alternative ways to do necessary self-care skills before they are discharged.

While the elderly may have lost some touch sensations, they have not lost the need to be touched. The perioperative nurse should consider these psychological

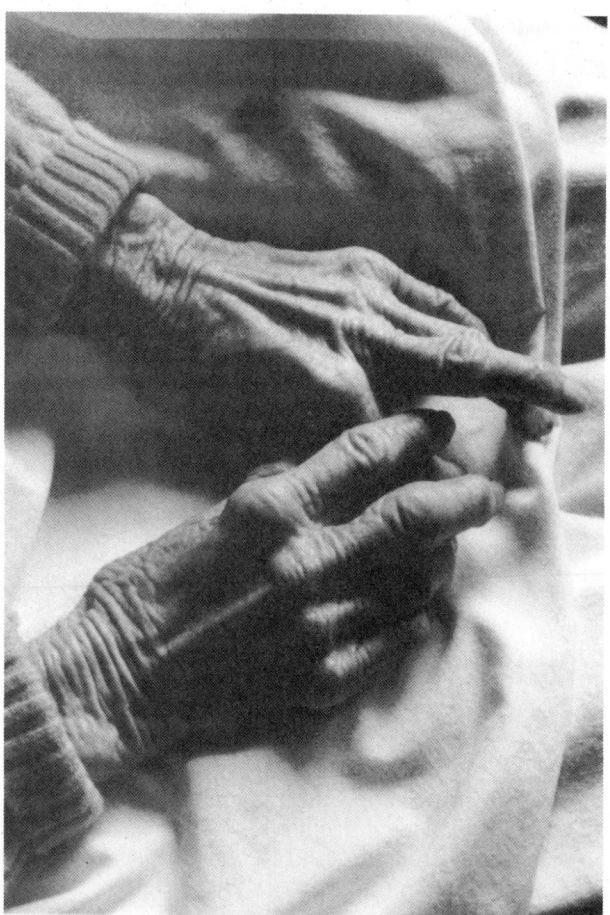

FIGURE 31–10. Elderly people have diminished sensory receptors and sense of touch in their fingertips. They may have problems picking up and manipulating small items and doing self-care skills. (From Matteson, M. A., McConnell, E. S. [1988]. *Gerontological nursing: Concepts and practice.* Philadelphia: W. B. Saunders.)

needs and offer to hold the patient's hand during induction of anesthesia or other stressful times during the surgical intervention.

Taste and Smell

Taste buds atrophy after the age of 50 years. The atrophy progresses from the front of the mouth to the back of the tongue. Older people have a sweetness threshold that is about three times less sensitive than that of a young adult (Knox, 1977). The sense of smell begins declining after the age of 40 years. The average 60-year-old person can detect smells only half as well as a 20-year-old person. There is fiber loss in the olfactory bulb and degeneration in the parietal lobe (Matteson and McConnell, 1988). The changes in taste and smell affect an elderly patient's interest in food. If an older adult has had ambulatory surgery, she or he may not want to eat the mandatory nourishment before discharge. The nurse may have to prepare special food or present it in a different way to encourage the patient to eat.

Cognitive Abilities

Memory

When older adults are hospitalized for surgery, or come in to have ambulatory surgery, the health care providers must ensure that they go home to be as autonomous and independent as possible. Therefore, teaching is a priority. The perioperative nurse should have a working knowledge about how older adults learn to be effective as a teacher. Learning theorists in the past believed that the ability of older adults to learn declines after the age of 40 years and is significantly affected by age 60 years (Cross, 1986). Many health care workers also mistakenly believe that every older adult is senile and cannot learn, instead of understanding the physiological effects on cognitive ability of anesthesia, drugs, and the stress of surgery. Further, extenuating factors such as past abilities, education, disease processes, and life style have been identified as affecting intelligence and learning (Ripple et al., 1982). If older adults have retained their intelligence, they should be able to learn, no matter what their age.

Physiologically, as discussed above, in normal aging, there are changes in the central nervous system that may affect the ability to learn. The brain of a human is a marvelous thing, with a tremendous ability to learn, store, and retrieve information. This is called memory. It is the function of the central nervous system to regulate and perform memory tasks. Specifically, glial cells and neurons act at the cellular level to support the brain function. Most neurons are long lived and do not die and redivide after early infancy. Thus, neurons persist for a lifetime. This stability and consistency allow the accumulation of memory and learning (Birren, 1986). Because neurons do not regenerate, their destruction may adversely affect learning. Any factor that damages these cells may affect the ability to learn. The damage may be from trauma, such as injury directly to the brain, or from degenerative illnesses, which affect the blood flow and oxygenation.

Brain tissue is extremely sensitive to lack of oxygen and begins deteriorating immediately without it. For example, a decrease of 20% in oxygen supply to the brain causes confusion, anxiety, or delirium. Lack of oxygen for 1 minute can lead to irreparable damage, and lack of oxygen for 3 to 5 minutes leads to brain death.

In examining age-related intellectual changes in the older adult, memory has been a major focus of gerontological research. A three-stage model of memory was defined by Murdock (1967):

The stages are

1. Sensory memory: The fleeting perceptions of the visual, auditory, olfactory, and tactile senses are information received by the senses for an extremely brief moment. "Visual memory lasts about ½ second to 1 second, auditory memory about 2 seconds" (Ciocon and Potter, 1988). It does not pass into primary memory.

2. Primary memory: Primary memory includes what is passed on by the sensory information if it has not been deleted by decay or other subsequent stimuli. It is also brief storage and is usually just "what you have in mind" (Ciocon and Potter, 1988).

3. Secondary memory: Long-term memory includes all that is known.

The elderly have sensory changes in seeing and hearing, but there seems to be no change in the sensory memory with age. Primary memory, although brief, appears to play an important part in learning. In one study designed to test primary memory, the researchers gave a series of letters verbally to subjects. Young subjects could recall about 7 or 9 letters, whereas older subjects could remember about 5 to 6 letters (Botwinick and Storandt, 1974). However, even though retrieval and speed of recall are less in older adults, there is general agreement that there is no great loss in primary memory with age. Research with secondary memory, on the other hand, reported substantial changes with age (Poon, 1985). The ability to acquire new information or retrieve it is affected. It is thought that both acquisition and retrieval defects develop with age. Memory failure seems to occur most frequently in older adults when there are physical or emotional needs that interfere.

The implications of this research for perioperative nurses are that older adults can learn. However, they may need to have smaller amounts of information given to them frequently before it is retained. In addition, because of retrieval problems, all postoperative discharge instructions should be written and given to the patient to take home.

Decision Making

The decision to have surgery is just one of many that older patients may have to make when they are admitted to the hospital. Although many patients are independent enough to make wise decisions, others become confused in a strange environment and from learned helplessness (Matteson and McConnell, 1988). The health care team must communicate closely with both the patient and the family to make the best decision possible (Fig. 31–11). As discussed above, informed consent is the most important decision the elderly surgical patient must make.

Learning and Teaching Implications

How do older adults function as learners? Adults usually function in crystallized intelligence, which considers the person's experience, education, and learning. Ripple and associates (1982, p. 564) stated that crystallized intelligence "consists of mental abilities such as information content, verbal comprehension, social intelligence and number facility."

Learning cannot proceed if the elderly patient has certain unmet needs. These needs should be considered

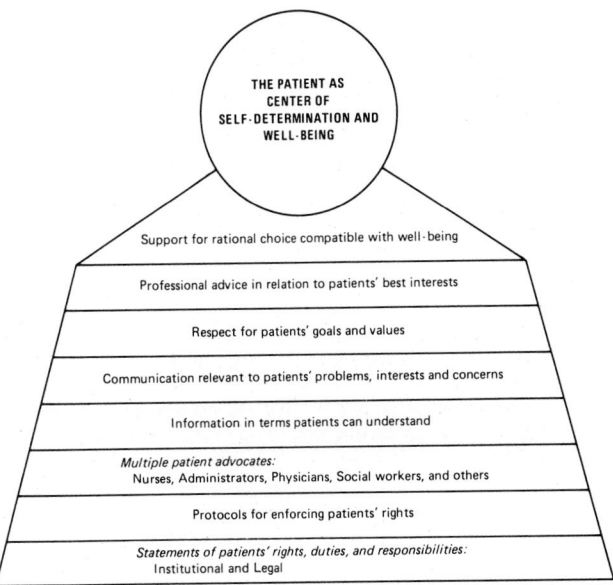

FIGURE 31–11. Factors that foster patient participation in health care decisions. (From Bandman, E. L., Bandman, B. [1985]. Ethical decision making in nursing: Values and guidelines. In E. L. Bandman, B. Bandman [Eds.], *Nursing ethics in the lifespan.* Norwalk, CT: Appleton-Century-Crofts.)

a priority by the perioperative nurse when planning education for older adults, particularly when teaching patients in the presurgical or postsurgical periods. The alignment of two need concepts (emotional reaction to the trauma of surgery and Maslow's hierarchy of human needs) should be considered in the elderly patient undergoing surgery (Fox, 1986). If older adults have strong anxieties, fears, or worries, memory deficits become more pronounced and it is harder for them to comprehend and retrieve information that may be vital to their welfare (Eysenck, 1979).

Research has given guidelines to use in helping elderly patients accomplish their most effective learning. After the needs that may be barriers to learning are met, the older adult should be emotionally capable of learning. Relaxation techniques, with progressive muscle relaxation, increase the ability of the elderly to learn. Any pain the patient has should be dealt with before beginning a teaching session. After the patient is prepared and the environment is conducive to learning, some strategies for effective teaching can be used.

Internal memory strategies employed to counter secondary memory deficits can include rehearsal, imagery, categorization, the use of mnemonics, and practice (Ciocon and Potter, 1988). External memory aids include lists, notes, calendars, reminders from other people, and articles or items that trigger memory. Visual aids are extremely important because of the elderly patient's hearing degeneration, which adversely affects communication and understanding.

There are also strategies to counteract the physiological sensory changes that hinder communication, therefore decreasing learning. Teaching should be done in a quiet environment. Environmental distractions and

TABLE 31–7. TEACHING STRATEGIES FOR THE ELDERLY PATIENT

1. Sit facing the learner so that he or she can watch lip movements and facial expressions.
2. Speak slowly.
3. Keep the voice pitch low because low sounds are easier to hear than high sounds.
4. Present one idea at a time; give one topic at a time.
5. Emphasize concrete rather than abstract ideas.
6. Compare new information with the person's past experiences.
7. Allow for a longer time for the patient to think and react.
8. Keep sessions short because of physical fatigue.
9. Use audio, visual, and tactile teaching aids.
10. Ask for frequent feedback to move information to secondary storage.
11. All patients to set their own goals and learning when possible.
12. Remember that older adults learn what is important to them and what positively affects their lives.
13. Preoperatively, older adults prefer sensory information: what they will see, hear, feel, and smell.

background noise greatly interfere with hearing when presbycusis is present.

In teaching one on one (e.g., a nurse teaching an older adult patient specific preoperative information), there are strategies that are recommended to improve learning (Fielo and Rizzolo, 1988; Girard, 1985) (Table 31–7). (Refer to Chapter 5 for in-depth general information on patient and family teaching.)

Psychological and Emotional Aspects

Developmental Theories

Many theorists have considered human development as occurring during the entire life span. A brief summary of the most well-known theories, and their significance to aging, are presented. For further study, the reader is referred to psychological and developmental textbooks.

One of the most well-known developmental theories applicable to nursing is that of Erikson. Erikson (1959) presented a psychosocial theory of development across the age span. He believed that people go through seven stages of development during a normal life span, with ego integrity being the last stage. If the individual resolves the psychological conflicts encountered in each stage, he or she successfully progresses to the next stage. Erikson did not explore the last stages of life as well as he did the early stages. Basically, he seemed to believe that anticipating and accepting one's death is the final stage. He suggested that there is a shift in values at this time and that a person has intrinsic worth. The main desire of the elderly person is the need for recognition of his or her dignity (Erikson, 1963).

This has profound implications for the perioperative nurse, because the patient encounters multiple compromising situations during the perioperative period, which have the potential for robbing him or her of dignity. Some ways that the nurse can protect the elderly pa-

tient's dignity include calling patients by their formal name (e.g., Mrs. rather than Grandma or her first name), being careful not to invade their body space without asking permission (May I listen to your stomach with this stethoscope?), and not overly exposing them when preparing or transferring them.

Another developmental theorist is Havighurst, who wrote his theory in 1953. He defined later maturity as being 60 years and older. He defined the aging person's necessary activities as

1. *adjusting to decreasing physical strength and health*
2. *adjustment to retirement and reduced income*
3. *adjusting to death of spouse*
4. *establishing an explicit affiliation with one's own group*
5. *adopting and adapting social roles in a flexible way*
6. *establishing satisfactory physical living arrangements*

A period of crisis occurs at retirement. The aging person must adapt successfully to his or her new role by developing new patterns of leisure to replace what was previously society-valued work (Table 31–8).

Levinson (1978) divided life into four cycles of 25 years each, the last being late adulthood. He referred to these cycles as the "seasons" of a person's life. In the last season, the person finalizes activities and promotes the establishment of a new generation.

The staff perioperative nurse does not have contact for a sufficient length of time to assist the patient in accomplishing the goals of life's stages and adjusting to these stages. By being aware of them, however, the nurse may help by arranging contact of the patient with the appropriate human resources to facilitate health and wellness across the developmental continuum. Some of these resources may be the family, the perioperative clinical nurse specialist, a pastoral service, a social service, and home health care services.

Needs Theory

Maslow (1970) defined a heirarchy of human needs. These needs are physiological needs (requirements), safety and security, love and belonging, and self-esteem and self-actualization. During surgery, the basic physiological needs of oxygen and hydration are a priority. Only after those are met can other needs be addressed. Because the needs are hierarchical in Maslow's scheme, a lower need must always be met before a higher need is recognized by the person. Maslow's theory explains much about human motivation and learning. A need must be satisfied before anything else can happen. Age is not as important, according to Maslow, as the needs of an individual. However, the elderly patient may have different needs than the young because of normal physiological changes of aging.

When the perioperative nurse plans teaching for a patient related to surgical intervention, he or she must evaluate the needs of the patient and attend to the immediate needs first. The nurse should also be aware

TABLE 31–8. HAVIGHURST'S TAXONOMY OF LEISURE BEHAVIOR

Pattern I	Challenging new experiences: focus is on meeting new people, having fun
Pattern II	Instrumental service: accomplishing useful things such as service to family or church
Pattern III	Expressive pleasure: the opposite of pattern II, activities such as game playing, but not novel activities
Pattern IV	Mildly active time filling: watching television, visiting with relatives
Pattern V	Ordinary routines expanded to fill the week
Pattern VI	Apathetic
Pattern VII	No free time

From Matteson, M. A., McConnell, G. S. (1988). *Gerontological nursing: Concepts and practice*. Philadelphia: W. B. Saunders.

that obtaining information about the surgery may or may not be an overwhelming need of the elderly.

POTENTIAL ALTERATIONS IN FUNCTIONAL HEALTH PATTERNS

Health Perception–Health Management Pattern

Diagnosis

High risk for infection

Definition

Presence of risk factors for the patient to experience a nosocomial infection following surgery

Risk Factors

- Decreased immunocompetence system
- Presence of compromising chronic diseases
- Decline in respiratory system defenses
- Decreased protective ability of the skin
- Declining protective ability of the gastrointestinal system
- Aging alterations in the genitourinary system
- Surgery
- Anesthesia
- Invasive monitoring and replacement techniques
- Breaks in aseptic technique

Expected Outcome

The patient is free from a nosocomial infection following surgery.

The wound heals without infection.
There is no urinary tract infection.
The respiratory status remains within the patient's norm.
Venous or arterial insertion sites remain free from infection.

Perioperative Nursing Interventions

Carefully prepare and decontaminate the skin and the surgical site.
Monitor the white blood cell count and differential count.
Maintain optimal surgical conscience.
Use impeccable aseptic technique.
Monitor the aseptic technique of other team members carefully.
Utilize careful aseptic techniques in inserting invasive devices, especially indwelling catheters.
Monitor team members' use of aseptic technique.
Document nursing care plans and their implementation.
Confer with infection control personnel to obtain information on postoperative infections in surgical patients.

Nutritional-Metabolic Pattern

Diagnosis

High risk for fluid volume deficit

Definition

Presence of risk factors for the patient to experience a decrease in circulating fluid volume during the perioperative period

Risk Factors

- Decreased ability of the kidney to concentrate urine
- Decreased renal functioning related to aging
- Decreased oral fluid volume intake
- Vomiting or diarrhea
- Decreased circulating blood volume

Expected Outcome

The patient maintains adequate fluid volume intake and hydration.

Perioperative Nursing Interventions

Monitor fluid volume replacement.
Have an indwelling catheter and insertion kit available.
Preoperatively, assess skin turgor, edema, urine output, and oral or IV fluid intake.
If there is significant bleeding, weigh sponges during surgery to determine the need for fluid or blood replacement.
Be prepared to obtain IV fluids and blood products for replacement.
Measure urine output during surgical procedure.

Diagnosis

High risk for impaired skin integrity

Definition

Presence of risk factors for the patient to experience a disruption or destruction of the skin surface during the perioperative period

Risk Factors

- Thinning or decreased epidermis and adipose tissue
- Decreased peripheral vascular circulation
- Increased peripheral neuropathy
- Improper transferring, moving, positioning, and padding
- Use of strong chemical antimicrobials
- Use of adhesive tape

Expected Outcome

The patient maintains intact skin during the surgical intervention, with the exception of the surgical site.

Perioperative Nursing Interventions

Assess skin integrity before surgery and document any rashes, sores, or skin disruptions.

Prepare the surgical site gently and carefully preoperatively. Remove hair only when absolutely necessary. If the patient has no allergies, consider using depilatory creams rather than shaving with a razor.

Apply the safety belt firmly, but avoid pressure. Pad if necessary.

Use nontoxic chemicals when doing the skin preparation. Carefully decontaminate the skin to decrease postoperative infections.

Select a nonirritating, broad-spectrum, antimicrobial agent for the skin preparation.

If using a liquid agent, allow the skin to dry before draping.

Wipe the surgical area with normal saline after the procedure to remove irritating chemicals such as povidone-iodine.

Position the patient carefully, padding all pressure points and areas where circulation may be restricted.

Be careful not to perforate the skin with towel clamps.

Have extra sterile pads available for padding if needed. (Do not have the circulator open these until requested.)

Pad retraction sites with sponges or pads and maintain gentle retraction at the surgical site.

Have paper tape or Montgomery straps available for dressing the surgical incision.

Use paper tape to prevent skin tape tears.

Transfer the patient from the gurney to the OR bed by lifting rather than dragging to prevent shearing skin tears. Use a lift sheet when possible.

Evaluate all skin areas immediately postoperatively and document any changes from the preoperative status.

Diagnosis

High risk for altered body temperature; hypothermia

Definition

Presence of risk factors for the patient to experience a decreased body temperature during the intraoperative period

Risk Factors

- Impaired thermoregulation
- Diminished peripheral vascular circulation
- Administration of drugs and anesthesia
- Surgical procedure requirements (e.g., renal or cardiac surgery)
- Exposure to a cold environment
- Lack of adequate covering
- Preoperative drug administration

Expected Outcome

The patient is free from complications associated with hypothermia during the perioperative period (hypoxia, acid-base disturbances, pulmonary edema, pneumonia, dehydration, hyperglycemia, and acute tubular necrosis).

Perioperative Nursing Interventions

Assess the potential for hypothermia preoperatively
  Determine the normal and present body temperature range.
  Assess skin color (pallor?).
  Check the color of the hands and feet (bluish? cyanotic?).
  Note the patient's age (the older, the more prone to hypothermia).
  Note the presence of systemic diseases, such as Raynaud disease, peripheral vascular disease, and diabetes mellitus.

Do not unnecessarily expose the patient to the external environment during preoperative or operative skin preparation.

Cover the patient with a warm blanket or a hypothermia blanket during surgery

Cover the patient's head with a cap or towel intraoperatively.

Observe vital sign monitors for evidence of hypothermia complications.

Be aware that shivering and ventricular fibrillation may occur and bleeding is decreased owing to vasoconstriction if the patient's body temperature is 35°C or lower.

Monitor for signs of hypothermia more closely if a surgical procedure calls for cooling with drugs, solutions, or slush.

Monitor the patient's temperature throughout surgery.

Report hypothermia potential and nursing actions taken intraoperatively to the postanesthesia care unit nurses.

If actual hypothermia results from surgical intervention, communicate with the postanesthesia care unit nurses before the end of surgery. Effective warming procedures can then be available immediately after surgery.

Document and evaluate all interventions.

Diagnosis

Altered nutrition: less than body requirements

Definition

Insufficient intake of nutrients to meet metabolic needs (Gordon, 1987, p. 68)

Defining Characteristics

- Emaciation
- Weight 20% or more below ideal body weight
- Capillary fragility
- Inadequate food intake
- Pale conjunctiva/mucous membranes
- Tiredness
- Excessive hair loss
- Poor muscle tone
- Abdominal manifestations (hyperactive bowel, cramping, pain)
- Diarrhea or steatorrhea

Related Factors

- Gastrointestinal changes of aging
- Presence of chronic diseases
- Administration of drugs
- Use of alcohol
- Presence of mechanical problems
- Lack of ability to care for self
- Dysphagia or oral problems
- Knowledge deficit

Expected Outcome

The patient is in the best possible nutritional state before surgery.

Perioperative Nursing Interventions

Obtain the patient's weight and height. Note any recent change.

Assess the status of nutrition preoperatively.

Inspect the skin for signs of nutritional deficiencies:

Note signs of vitamin deficiencies: eczema; dry, rough skin; "sheet hemorrhages" on thighs and calves, cracking of the lips; and inflammation of the gums.

Note signs of protein, zinc, or vitamin deficiencies: chronic, nonhealing skin ulcers and edema of the hands and feet.

Monitor laboratory values (Matteson and McConnell, 1988, p. 639).

	Acceptable	Deficient
Hemoglobin (gm/100 ml)		
Males	12–14	<12
Females	10–12	<10
Hematocrit (packed cell volume in %)		
Males	37–44	<37
Females	31–38	<31
Serum albumin (gm/100 ml)	2.8–3.5	<2.8
Serum protein (gm/100 ml)	6–6.5	<6

Practice careful use of aseptic technique.

Be aware that pressure sores may develop within 2 hours if there is a nutritional lack of serum protein and vitamins, along with other deficiencies.

Pad bony prominences well.

Be prepared for complications during surgery that may arise because of undernourishment:

Bleeding problems

Arrhythmias

Activity-Exercise Pattern

Diagnosis

Impaired physical mobility

Definition

Limited ability for independent movement

Defining Characteristics

- Inability to move
- Limited range of motion
- Decreased muscle strength, control, or mass
- Impaired coordination (Gordon, 1987, p. 128)

Related Factors

- Aging musculoskeletal system
- Chronic disease conditions
- Falls
- Trauma to nonoperative joints
- Nerve damage from unrelieved pressure

Expected Outcome

Safety is maintained and trauma to the musculoskeletal system is minimized.

Perioperative Nursing Interventions

Assess the patient.

Inspect joints for range of motion and pain.

Test the patient's muscle strength and grip strength.

Assess the patient's balance when the patient is sitting and standing.

Assess the patient's transfer ability.

Assess the patient's walking ability.

Assess the ability of the patient to flex the spine if regional anesthesia is planned.

Evaluate any neurovascular deficits, such as bradykinesia and diabetic neuropathies.

Transfer the patient to the OR bed gently.

Monitor the patient's shoulder range of motion and do not overextend.

Avoid hyperextension of the patient's elbows, knees, and neck.

Assist the patient to flex the spine for regional anesthesia. Allow time for stiff vertebrae and muscles to conform to their optimal level of stretch.

If marked osteoporosis is present, log roll the patient for lateral position. When positioning for lithotomy, flex and raise both the patient's knees at the same time. Extreme caution prevents fracture of the head of the femoral head.

Ensure that the patient's fingers, hands, toes, and feet are not cramped or resting against metal before applying sterile drapes.

Monitor team members to avoid their leaning or resting on the patient during surgery.

Evaluate the patient's neuromuscular status postoperatively.

Diagnosis

High risk for altered peripheral tissue perfusion

Definition

Presence of risk factors for the patient to experience impaired peripheral circulation

Risk Factors

- Decreases in cardiac output and respiration at a cellular level
- Disruption of microcirculation by mechanical pressure, positioning, and immobility

Expected Outcome

The patient maintains adequate peripheral circulation, and the formation of emboli and/or thrombus is minimized.

Perioperative Nursing Interventions

Assess the patient's cardiac status by taking vital signs, reviewing the electrocardiogram, prothrombin time and partial thromboplastin time, and other studies as ordered.

Note a past history of clotting problems or emboli formation.

Take the patient's smoking history.

Assess the past history of recurrent leg ulcers.

Assess the presence of chronic diseases such as diabetes mellitus, chronic obstructive pulmonary disease, malnutrition, and circulatory diseases.

Preoperatively, teach the patient to flex and extend the knees and hips and to dorsiflex and extend the ankles. Demonstrate and practice. Stress that the patient needs to do this or the nurses do this for her or him immediately after surgery.

Position the patient carefully, making sure that the ankles are not crossed and there is no pressure on the feet.

Observe the patient's position before sterile draping.

Apply antiembolism devices or stockings during surgery.

Cognitive-Perceptual Pattern

Diagnosis

Decisional conflict

Definition

A state of uncertainty the patient experiences about the appropriate action to take when the choice among competing actions involves risk, actual or potential loss, or a challenge to personal values (Gordon, 1987, p. 194)

Defining Characteristics

- Delayed decision making
- Vacillation in decision making
- Verbal expressions of distress or anxiety
- Physiological manifestations such as increased heart rate, respiration, blood pressure, and diaphoresis (Gordon, 1987, p. 194)

Related Factors

- Incomplete or confusing information regarding the surgery
- Informational overload
- Ineffective communication techniques
- Inadequate time to consider surgical implications
- Fear of surgical outcomes

Expected Outcome

The decision-making ability of the patient and significant others is supported.

Perioperative Nursing Interventions

Recognize and compensate for normal aging changes that may affect the communication of preoperative surgical information (e.g., hearing, seeing, and memory deficits).

Clarify and repeat the surgeon's explanations as needed for comprehension and understanding.

Assess the patient's decision-making ability.

Consider the cultural implications of making decisions. Include appropriate family members in the decision. (The patient may not be the one who makes the final decision.)

Provide emotional and psychological support if the patient exhibits anxiety and fears.

Respect and accept the patient's final decision.

Allow adequate time to ensure that all forms for consent are correctly completed.

Diagnosis

Altered thought processes

Definition

Discrepancy between the patient's actual cognitive operation (thought processes) and expected cognitive operations for chronological age (Gordon, 1987, p. 192)

Defining Characteristics

- Disorientation or confusion during the preoperative period
- Failure to remember information about the surgery given preoperatively
- Impaired attention span
- Inappropriate behavior
- Impaired perception
- Impaired judgment
- Impaired decision making
- Egocentricity (Gordon, 1987, p. 192)

Related Factors

- Sensory overload
- Disorders of memory
- Inappropriate response to commands or directions
- Inaccurate interpretation of the environment

Expected Outcome

Perioperatively, the patient is protected from physical injury that may result from altered thought processes and experiences optimal postoperative recovery.

Perioperative Nursing Interventions

Preoperatively, assess and monitor the physiological factors that may affect the patient's thought processes:

Hypoxia

Imbalance in glucose levels

Altered metabolism that could affect the central nervous system

Drug interactions or adverse reactions

Central nervous system abnormalities, such as tumors and infarcts

Note that the patient may misinterpret commands or directions intraoperatively.

Assess the patient's ability to think and reason.

Assess the patient's orientation to time, place, and event.

Assess the patient's cognitive abilities.

Assess the patient's short-term memory.

Verbally list a series of items and have patient repeat them back. He or she should normally be able to remember three to seven items.

Do preoperative teaching on one thing, and ask the patient to repeat it 15 minutes later.

Assign one nurse to coordinate care and to communicate with the family.

Supply written reminders that may help remembering (e.g., place a note on the wall to practice deep breathing every hour if the patient can read and see).

Provide frequent verbal reminders during the perioperative period (e.g., ask patients not to move and to keep their hands away from their faces).

Use pictures to increase recognition memory.

Document the patient's preoperative mental status.

Adjust preoperative and discharge teaching needs to accommodate patient and family needs.

Communicate decreased cognitive ability to other members of the health care team.

Diagnosis

Knowledge deficit

Definition

Inability to explain information or demonstrate required skills (e.g., self-care skills or skills necessary for rehabilitation) related to the surgical experience

Defining Characteristics

- Patient's verbal responses or questions indicate inadequate understanding, misinterpretation, and misconception of information concerning the perioperative period or the reason for surgery
- Noncompliance with previous instructions or prescribed therapeutic regimen
- Inability to perform or inadequate performance of a critical self-care or rehabilitative skill
- Hysterical, hostile, agitated, or apathetic behaviors (Gordon, 1987, p. 186)

Related Factors

- Altered thought processes
- Uncompensated memory loss
- Impaired hearing
- Inability to use teaching materials (cultural-language differences)
- Impaired vision
- Fear, anxiety (Gordon, 1987, p. 186)

Expected Outcome

The patient's knowledge about surgical intervention is adequate for the patient's needs.

Perioperative Nursing Interventions

Assess the patient for sensory impairments (vision, hearing) and, if present, implement appropriate interventions.

Be aware of the elderly person's potential inability to hear or understand directions given to him or her intraoperatively. Pay particular attention to the patient's communication needs if regional or local anesthesia is used.

Allow the patient to use communication aids as long as possible. Secure glasses or hearing aids in a safe place or give to a family member during surgery.

Sit next to the patient and speak distinctly.

Face the patient so that he or she can read lips.

Use large, dark print for reading matter.

Draw or use illustrations for clarification.

Assess the patient's knowledge level and need to know. Older patients tend to want sensory information about intraoperative events (e.g., what they will hear, see, and feel), rather than procedural information.

Provide preoperative teaching. Demonstrations and patient practice of turning, coughing, deep breathing, and ambulating are vital. Older patients should be told about the postoperative environment (e.g., the intensive care unit) and the presence of tubes, drains, or machines. They often worry about pain, so should be reassured that they will be watched and can have medication when they need it.

Provide discharge instructions. For ambulatory surgery, elderly patients especially need written discharge instructions. The family or caregiver must also be aware of the instructions.

Diagnosis

Sensory perceptual alteration: sensory overload

Definition

Information or environmental stimuli greater than the usual amount of information or stimuli a patient is used to receiving

Defining Characteristics

- Irritability
- Anxiety
- Disorientation
- Sleeplessness
- Decisional-conflict manifestations
- Complaints of tiredness
- Complaints of muscle tension (Gordon, 1987, p. 182)

Related Factors

- Extensive information regarding surgical intervention
- Environmental complexity (Gordon, 1987, p. 182)

Expected Outcome

An environment and informational system that the elderly surgical patient can control is maintained.

Perioperative Nursing Interventions

Recognize sensory overload by the patient's verbal or nonverbal communications.

Minimize the number of people from the surgical team who visit the patient preoperatively.

Have one contact person coordinate the total perioperative experience.

Give information only at a need-to-know level.

Teach only vital, life-sustaining self-practices, such as taking medication and performing dressing changes postoperatively.

Provide anticipatory sensory information about the surgical procedure.

Develop with the patient a mutually agreed on method for the patient to signal a need for help during the perioperative period.

Teach the family about the impact of sensory perceptual alterations, with recommendations for care.

Self-perception—Self-concept Pattern

Diagnosis

Fear: death, mutilation, loss of body part or function, loss of independence

Definition

The patient has feelings of dread related to an identifiable source that he or she believes is a threat or danger (Gordon, 1987, p. 198)

Defining Characteristics

- Describes the threat
- Verbalizes feelings of dread, nervousness, or concern about surgery
- Verbalizes expected danger to self related to surgery
- Restlessness
- Voice tremor
- Excessive talking
- Hand tremor and increased muscle tension
- Narrowed focus to fixed focus on impending surgery
- Diaphoresis
- Increased heart and respiratory rates (Gordon, 1987, p. 198)

Related Factors

- Knowledge deficit
- Perceived inability to control the event (Gordon, 1987, p. 198)

Expected Outcome

The patient and the family are assisted in coping with fear.

Perioperative Nursing Interventions

(Also see the discussion of anxiety below.)

Alert the anesthesiologist and the surgeon preoperatively, if fear is moderate to extreme.

Recognize that overwhelming, realistic fear may interfere with other nursing and medical goals.

Establish a relationship preoperatively, so that the patient believes that there is an ally intraoperatively.

Allow the patient an opportunity preoperatively to share fears.

Use active listening techniques.

Recognize that some patients may feel more free to discuss fears with someone chronologically or culturally their peer.

Offer to arrange contact with other health care team members if the patient desires, such as a chaplain, a social services worker, or a hospice nurse.

Diagnosis

Anxiety

Definition

Vague or uneasy feelings expressed by the patient concerning impending activities or events associated with the perioperative period

Defining Characteristics

- Verbal expressions of apprehension, uncertainty, fear, distress, worry concerning the perioperative period or expected surgical outcome
- Verbal expressions of helplessness concerning impending surgery
- Overexcited, rattled, jittery behavior
- Restlessness
- Focus on self
- Insomnia
- Physiological manifestations such as diaphoresis and increased heart rate, pulse, and respirations
- Increased tension
- Foot shuffling, hand and arm movements, trembling, hand tremor, shakiness
- Facial tension, poor eye contact, voice quivering (Gordon, 1987, p. 202)

Related Factors

- Impending surgery that may result in a potential, uncertain change in health, role status, or environment

Expected Outcome

The patient's preoperative anxiety level is decreased.

Perioperative Nursing Interventions

Assess the patient's anxiety level preoperatively.

Consider the physiological effects of surgical stress on the elderly patient and anticipate needs during the intraoperative period. Consider the effects of
    increased immunosuppression
    decreased blood flow to the kidneys, with decreased urine output
    increased gluconeogenesis
    increased vasoconstriction
    increased respiratory and heart rate

Suggest preoperative antianxiety medication if needed.

Strengthen the patient's support systems by including the family and significant others in preoperative teaching.

Assess the patient's past coping skills (how did he or she react to stress in the past?).

Use a quiet, confident demeanor around the patient.

Answer or clarify questions in a positive way to instill hope.

Teach relaxation and breathing techniques.

Provide a therapeutic environment.

    Assist in maintaining a quiet and supportive atmosphere during the intraoperative period. Ask for supplies in a quiet voice, do not talk during anesthesia induction, and maintain minimal conversation if the patient has a local anesthetic. Take precautions to protect the patient from noxious sounds if the patient has received a local anesthetic.

Diagnosis

Hopelessness

Definition

A state in which the patient sees limited or no alternatives or personal choices available and is unable to mobilize energy on his or her behalf (Gordon, 1987, p. 212)

Defining Characteristics

- Passive behaviors
- Decreased talking
- Decreased affect
- Lack of initiative to actively participate during perioperative period or rehabilitation
- Decreased response to stimuli
- Behaviors that attempt to shut out others (closing eyes, turning head away)
- Decreased appetite
- Increased sleep (Gordon, 1987, p. 212)

Related Factors

- Nonelective or life-sustaining surgery
- Differing opinion between the patient and the health care team as to the need for surgery
- Family pressure for surgery
- Deteriorating physiological or psychological condition

Expected Outcome

The patient maintains realistic hope throughout the perioperative period.

Perioperative Nursing Interventions

Assess the presence of hope by seeing if the patient can
discuss the future
actively question all treatments
mobilize resources in her or his own defense
Maintain the patient's hope.
Reassure the patient and the family that the patient will be given the best care during the intraoperative period.
Reassure the patient that the surgeon and the surgical team are the best available.
After surgery, tell the patient what he or she will be able to do after discharge from the hospital.
Do not become overly hopeful or cheerful. Aging patients may feel that their despair and sorrow are considered unimportant.

Coping–Stress Tolerance Pattern

Diagnosis

Ineffective individual coping

Definition

Impairment of adaptive behaviors and abilities for meeting the demands and rules related to daily living (Gordon, 1987, p. 284)

Defining Characteristics

- Verbally expresses inability to cope
- Does not ask for help
- Does not effectively solve problems
- Manifests anxiety and fear
- Describes personal life stress
- Does not meet role expectations
- Does not meet basic needs
- Altered social interaction
- Manifests destructive behavior toward self or others
- Digestive, bowel, appetite disturbances
- Chronic fatigue or sleep pattern disturbance
- Attempts verbal manipulation (Gordon, 1987, p. 284)

Related Factors

- Inability of the patient to adapt to the basic demands of the surgical intervention
- Knowledge deficit
- Problem-solving skills deficit (Gordon, 1987, p. 284)

Expected Outcome

The patient is assisted in coping with the impending surgery.

Perioperative Nursing Interventions

Assess the autonomic stress response of the patient: measure pulse, respiration, and blood pressure.
Observe for signs of self-neglect.
Assess the patient's mental status.
Be supportive to the patient.
Assess the patient's coping skills and communicate with other members of the health care team regarding the patient's status.
Identify ineffective coping with surgical crises. Be aware that different cultures may have different ideas and behaviors regarding the appropriateness of a particular coping response.
Report potential problems to all members of the surgical team.
Identify the patient's stress level (see the discussion of anxiety).
Define behavior characteristics.
Note verbalizations of an inability to cope.
Note an inability to meet the health care personnel's expectations regarding surgery.
Intervene if the patient exhibits destructive behavior, such as deliberately pulling out IV or indwelling catheters.
Enlist the aid of family, volunteers, or other potential network for patient so that surgery may proceed without incident.

Bibliography

Abbey, J. (1976). Digestive disorders in the aged. In I. Burnside (Ed.), *Nursing and the aged* (p. 346). New York: McGraw-Hill.

Bandman, E., Bandman, B. (1985). *Nursing ethics through the life span* (2nd ed.). Norwalk, CT: Appleton-Century-Crofts.

Bartol, M. A., Heitkemper, M. (1979). Gastrointestinal problems. In D. L. Carnevali, M. Patrick (Eds.), *Nursing management for the elderly*. Philadelphia: J. B. Lippincott.

Birren, J. (1986). The process of aging: Growing up and growing old. In A. Pifer, L. Bronte (Eds.), *Our aging society*. New York: W. W. Norton.

Birren, J. E., Warner Schaie, K. (1990). *Handbook of the psychology of aging* (3rd ed.). San Diego: Academic Press.

Botwinick, J., Arenberg, D. (1976). Disparate time spans in sequential studies of aging. *Experimental Aging Research, 2,* 55–61.

Bowles, L. T., Portnoi, V., Kenney, R. (1981). Wear and tear: Common biological changes of aging. *Geriatrics, 36*(4), 77–86.

Buckley, C. E., Buckley, E. G., Dorsey, F. C. (1974). Longitudinal changes in serum immunoglobulin levels in older humans. *Federation Proceedings 33,* 2036.

Ciocon, J., Potter, J. (1988). Age-related changes in human memory: Normal and abnormal. *Geriatrics, 43*(10), 43–48.

Crawford, F. J. (1985). Ambulatory surgery. *AORN Journal, 41,* 356–359.

Crosby, D., Rees, G. (1985). Anesthesia and surgery in the elderly. In M. S. J. Pathy (Ed.), *Principles and practice of geriatric medicine* (pp. 1167–1192). New York: Wiley.

Cross, K. P. (1982). *Adults as learners*. San Francisco: Jossey Bass Publishers.

Dean, A. F. (1987). The aging surgical patient: Historical overview, implications and nursing care. *Perioperative Nursing Quarterly, 3*(1), 1–7.

DelGuercio, L. R. M., Cohn, J. D. (1980). Monitoring operative risks in the elderly. *JAMA, 243,* 1350–1355.

Dobb, R. B. (1983). Anesthesia. In F. U. Steinberg (Ed.), *Care of the geriatric patient*. St. Louis: C. V. Mosby.

Domonkos, A. N., Arnold, H. L., Odom, R. B. (1982). *Andrew's diseases of the skin*. Philadelphia: W. B. Saunders.

Duncalf, D., Kepes, E. R. (1986). Geriatric anesthesia. In I. Rossman (Ed.), *Clinical geriatrics* (3rd ed.) (pp. 494–510). Philadelphia: J. B. Lippincott.

Eisendorfer, C., Wilkie, E. (1974). Auditory changes. In E. Palmore (Ed.), *Normal aging II*. Durham, NC: Duke University Press.

Erikson, E. H. (1959). Identity and the life cycle. *Psychological Issues, 1,* 50–100.

Eysenck, M. W. (1979). Anxiety, learning and memory: A reconceptualization. *Journal of Research in Personality, 13,* 363–385.

Fielo, S., Rizzolo, M. A. (1988, April). Handle with caring: Meeting elderly clients' special learning needs. *Nursing and Health Care,* pp. 189–195.

Fox, V. (1986). Patient teaching. Understanding the needs of the adult learner. *AORN Journal, 44,* 234–242.

Frishman, W. H. (1983, January). The aging heart. *Transition,* pp. 39–53.

Gardner, I. (1980). The effect of aging on susceptibility to infection. *Reviews of Infectious Diseases, 2,* 801.

Gilles, S., Kozak, R., Durante, M., Weksler, M. (1981). Immunological studies of aging: Decreased production of and response to T-cell growth factor by lymphocytes from aged humans. *Journal of Clinical Investigation, 67,* 937.

Girard, N. J. (1985). *The elderly surgical patient* [Film]. Danbury, CT: An AORN/Davis + Geck Film. Davis + Geck Surgical Film Library.

Goldman, L. (1983). Cardiac risks and complications of noncardiac surgery. *Annals of Surgery, 198,* 780.

Goldman, L., Caldera, D. L., Southwick, F. S., et al. (1978). Cardiac risk factors and complications in non-cardiac surgery. *Medicine, 57,* 357.

Gordon, M. (1987). *Manual of nursing diagnosis 1986–1987.* New York: McGraw-Hill.

Harris, R. (1978). Special problems of geriatric patients with heart disease. In W. Reichel (Ed.), *Clinical aspects of aging.* Baltimore: Williams & Wilkins.

Hogstel, M. O., Taylor-Martof, M. (1988). Perioperative care. In M. O. Hogstel (Ed.), *Nursing care of the older adult* (pp. 335–353). New York: Wiley.

Howe, R. B. (1983). Anemia in the elderly. *Postgraduate Medicine, 73*(4), 153–160.

Hull, C., Greco, R. S., Brooks, D. L. (1980). Alleviation of constipation in the elderly by dietary fiber supplementation. *Journal of American Geriatrics Society, 28,* 410–414.

Jackson, M. F. (1988). High risk surgical patients. *Journal of Gerontological Nursing, 14*(1), 8–15.

Jaffe, J. W. (1978). Common lower urinary tract problems in older persons. In W. Reichel (Ed.), *Clinical aspects of aging.* Baltimore: Williams & Wilkins.

Jessup, L. (1984). The integument. In B. Steffl (Ed.), *Handbook of gerontological nursing* (p. 173). New York: Van Nostrand Reinhold.

Jessup, L. (1984). The musculoskeletal and nervous system. In B. Steffl (Ed.), *Handbook of gerontological nursing* (p. 207). New York: Van Nostrand Reinhold.

Johnson, J. C. (1983). The medical evaluation and management of the elderly surgical patient. *Journal of American Geriatrics Society, 31,* 621.

Johnson, J. C. (1988). Surgical assessment in the elderly. *Geriatrics, 43*(Suppl.), 83–90.

Kapp, M. B., Bigot, A. (1985). *Geriatrics and the law. Patient rights and professional responsibilities* (pp. 15–42). New York: Springer.

Knox, A. (1977). Physical condition. In *Adult development and learning* (pp. 245–316). San Francisco, CA: Jossey-Bass.

Knudson, F. S. (1984a). Cardiovascular conditions in older adults. In B. Steffl (Ed.), *Handbook of gerontological nursing* (p. 221). New York: Van Nostrand Reinhold.

Knudson, F. (1984b). Gastrointestinal and metabolic problems in older adults. In B. Steffl (Ed.), *Handbook of gerontological nursing* (p. 234). New York: Van Nostrand Reinhold.

Knudson, F. (1984c). Genitourinary and gynecological problems in older adults. In B. Steffl (Ed.), *Handbook of gerontological nursing* (p. 259). New York: Van Nostrand Reinhold.

Knudson, F. (1984d). Respiratory conditions in older adults. In B. Steffl (Ed.), *Handbook of gerontological nursing* (p. 251). New York: Van Nostrand Reinhold.

Koin, D. (1984). Surgical concerns. In C. K. Cassel, J. R. Walsh (Eds.), *Geriatric medicine* (Vol. 2, pp. 275–288). New York: Springer-Verlag.

Kolanosk, A. M., Gunter, L. M. (1989). Thermal stress in the aged. *Journal of Gerontological Nursing, 9*(1), 13–15.

Levinson, D. J. (1978). *The seasons of a man's life.* New York: Alfred A. Knopf.

Lewis, S., Collier, I. C. (1992). *Medical-surgical nursing: Assessment and management of clinical problems.* St. Louis: Mosby/Year Book.

Linn, B. S., Linn, M. W., Jensen, J. (1983). Surgical stress in the healthy elderly. *Journal of American Geriatric Nursing, 31,* 544–548.

Linn, B. S. (1983). Surgery and the elderly patient. In R. Cape, R. M. Coe, I. Rossman (Eds.), *Fundamentals of geriatric medicine* (pp. 309–319). New York: Raven Press.

Maslow, A. H. (1970). *Motivation and personality* (2nd ed.). New York: Alfred A. Knopf.

Matteson, M. A., McConnell, E. S. (1988). Care of the older surgical patient. In M. A. Matteson, E. S. McConnell, *Gerontological nursing: Concepts and practice* (pp. 735–741). Philadelphia: W. B. Saunders.

McCarter, R. (1985). *Age and the neuromuscular system* [Lecture]. San Antonio TX: University of Texas Health Science Center.

Morrissey, K., Schein, C. J. (1986). Surgical problems in the aged. In I. Rossman (Ed.), *Clinical geriatrics* (3rd ed.) (pp. 472–493). Philadelphia: J. B. Lippincott.

Murdock, B. B. (1967). Recent developments in short term memory. *British Journal of Psychology, 58,* 421–433.

National Center for Health Statistics (1986). *Health, United States, 1985.* DHHS Pub No (PHS) 87-1232. Washington, DC: U.S. Government Printing Office.

Phair, J. P. (1983). Host defense in the aged. In R. A. Gleckman, N. M. Gantz (Eds.), *Infection in the elderly* (pp. 1–11). Boston: Little, Brown.

Phair, J. P., Kauffman, C. A., Bjornson, A., et al. (1978a). Failure to respond to influenza vaccine in the aged: Correlation with B-cell number and function. *Journal of Laboratory Clinical Medicine, 92,* 822.

Phair, J. P., Kauffman, C. A., Bjornson, A., et al. (1978b). Host defenses in the aged: Evaluation of components of the inflammatory and immune response. *Journal of Infectious Diseases, 138,* 67.

Pomorski, M. E. (1983). Surgical care for the aged patient: The decision-making process. *Nursing Clinics of North America, 18,* 365–372.

Poon, L. W. (1985). Differences in human memory with aging: Nature, causes, and clinical implications. In J. E. Birren, K. W. Schaie (Eds.), *Handbook of the psychology of aging.* New York: Van Nostrand Reinhold.

Rice, D. (1989). The characteristics and health of the elderly. In C. Eisdorfer, D. Kessler, A. Spector (Eds.), *Caring for the elderly: Reshaping health policy.* Baltimore: Johns Hopkins University Press.

Ripple, R., Biehler, R. F., Jaquish, G. A. (1982). *Human development.* Boston: Houghton Mifflin.

Rivnay, B., Bergman, S., Skinitzky, M., Globersen, A. (1980). Correlations between membrane viscosity, serum cholesterol, lymphocyte activation and ageing in man. *Mechanisms of Ageing and Development, 12,* 119.

Roberts, S. (1976). Cardiopulmonary abnormalities in aging. In I. Burnside (Ed.), *Nursing and the aged* (p. 286). New York: McGraw-Hill.

Roberts, S. (1976). Renal abnormalities in aging. In I. Burnside (Ed.), *Nursing and the aged* (p. 317). New York: McGraw-Hill.

Santos, A. L., Galperin, A. (1979). Surgical mortality in the elderly. *Journal of American Geriatrics Society, 923,* 42–46.

Schrier, R. W. (1982). *Clinical medicine in the aged.* Philadelphia: W. B. Saunders.

Schrier, R. W. (1990). *Geriatric medicine.* Philadelphia: W. B. Saunders.

Seymour, D. G., Pringle, R. (1982). A new method of auditing surgical mortality rates: Application to a group of elderly general surgical patients. *British Journal of Medicine, 284,* 1539–1542.

Shanck, A. H. (1976). Musculoskeletal problems in aging. In I. Burnside (Ed.), *Nursing and the aged* (p. 365). New York: McGraw-Hill.

Sheehy, T. W. (1982). An overview of geriatric medicine. *Resident and Staff Physician,* June, 29–40.

Sklar, M. (1978). Gastrointestinal disease in the aged. In W. Reichel (Ed.), *Clinical aspects of aging.* Baltimore: Williams & Wilkins.

Steen, P. A., Tinker, J. H., Tarhan, S. (1978). Myocardial reinfarction after anesthesia and surgery. *JAMA, 239,* 2566.

Steffl, B. (1984). *Handbook of gerontological nursing.* New York: Van Nostrand Reinhold.

Tangorra, K. H. (1982, September-October). Your attitude toward the elderly—and how they affect your nursing care. *Nursing Life,* pp. 57–63.

United States Bureau of the Census (1984). Projections of the population of the United States, 1983 to 2080. *Current Population Reports,* Series P-25, No 952. Washington, DC: U.S. Government Printing Office.

U.S. Department of Commerce, Bureau of the Census (1989). *Projections of the population of the United States by age, sex, and race: 1988 to 2080.* Washington, DC.: U.S. Government Printing Office.

Van Buren, C. T. (1984). Surgery in the older patient. In A. J. Levenson D. M. Porter (Eds.), *An introduction to gerontology and geriatrics: A multidisciplinary approach* (pp. 341–355). Springfield, IL: Charles C Thomas.

Walker, M. L. (1986). Growing old. *AORN Journal, 43,* 887–890.

Watchel, T. J. (1981). How to limit the risks of elective surgery. *Geriatrics, 36*(11), 95–99.

White, N. E. (1984). Surgical conditions in the elderly. In B. Steffl (Ed.), *Handbook of gerontological nursing* (p. 286). New York: Van Nostrand Reinhold.

Wolanin, M. O., Steffl, B. (1984). Neurological disorders of the elderly. In B. Steffl (Ed.), *Handbook of gerontological nursing* (p. 303). New York: Van Nostrand Reinhold.

PERIOPERATIVE ISSUES: MANAGEMENT AND EDUCATION

CHAPTER 32

Perioperative Nursing Staff Development

Linda Brazen

Each of us is either a stumbling block or a stepping stone.

LEE NOEL

As health care institutions, agencies, and organizations redefine their missions, educators "who can bring the greatest efficiency to diagnosing the learning need[s] and applying the appropriate resources to meet [these needs for all personnel] will be in greatest demand" (Huntsman, 1987).

The role of the clinical education nurse in educating, training, and developing staff varies from institution to institution. Perioperative nurses direct perioperative quality assessment programs; write policies and procedures; and serve as liaisons to schools of nursing, preceptors to nursing students as they rotate through the operating room, and mentors to graduate students. Most importantly, however, these nurses conduct orientation programs for new perioperative nursing staff members and direct the staff education program.

CONDUCTING AN ORIENTATION PROGRAM

Orientation is a method of providing professional education, as well as professional socialization. Orientation as a method is how a person acquires the necessary knowledge and skill (abilities) to fulfill expected work services. As such, orientation places a person in a state of information dependency.

The value system of the orientation setting fosters attitudes about roles and responsibilities expected in the work place. The socialization process inherent in orientation is how a person internalizes the value system of the service setting. The socialization dimension of orientation places a person in a state of information discovery.

Both the method and process involve a teaching role, a learning role, and content to be taught and learned.

This section presents these elements of nursing orientation in the operating room setting.

Orientation Frameworks

Characteristics of a health care organization that influence an orientation program are its philosophy, type (i.e., government, private, teaching, specialty, general), size, and geographic location. These characteristics drive the human, economic, and physical resources for planning and, most importantly, for implementing one of three approaches to orientation: centralized, decentralized, or coordinated. Although each has its strengths, each strength has a weakness or limitation, especially with regard to the operating room (OR) care setting.

A *centralized approach* may facilitate institutional information, but it also contains aspects that are nonspecific to unit needs. During a centralized orientation program, a newly employed staff nurse who, for example, has chosen to practice in the OR may spend the greater part of one orientation day "needing to know" how to document a medical nursing admission. This information will probably not be utilized in the OR setting. On the other hand, in a *decentralized approach,* specialty units such as the OR may be busy, and institutional information that does affect newly employed nurses may not be presented (e.g., fire safety). The *coordinated organizational approach* to orientation avoids duplication of efforts and responsibility and allows for options in program design. Nonetheless, its limitations are directly related to the degree to which the centralized or decentralized approach predominates.

It is not unusual for a new employee to participate in an institutional orientation and then undergo orientation in his or her chosen clinical specialty department. Currently some organizations are designing OR orientation programs further by delimiting the new employees' orientation to subspecialty service tracks (Fig. 32–1) and/or perioperative services.

Creating Learning Experiences

Philosophically, no one can be *taught* anything. However, it is possible to create an environment that will make it possible for someone to learn.

Learning is not a matter of filling a void with information. Instead, it is a process of internally reorganizing thought patterns, perceptions, assumptions, attitudes, feelings, and skills and successfully testing this reorganization in relation to and in the work setting. Learning can take place effectively only when the atmosphere in the teaching-learning interaction reduces threats and defensiveness and provides support during the process of changing patterns of thought and behavior.

It is obvious that learning is affected by this important intangible known as *climate*. In general, people learn most readily in a warm and friendly atmosphere. They tend to produce more and feel more secure when this environment is also business-like and work centered.

Powerful learning environments acknowledge, encourage, and legitimatize the learner's uncertainty of knowledge (Colucciello, 1988). The outcome of a powerful learning experience is growth and change in a learner, in his or her behavior, and in his or her interpersonal self-actualization.

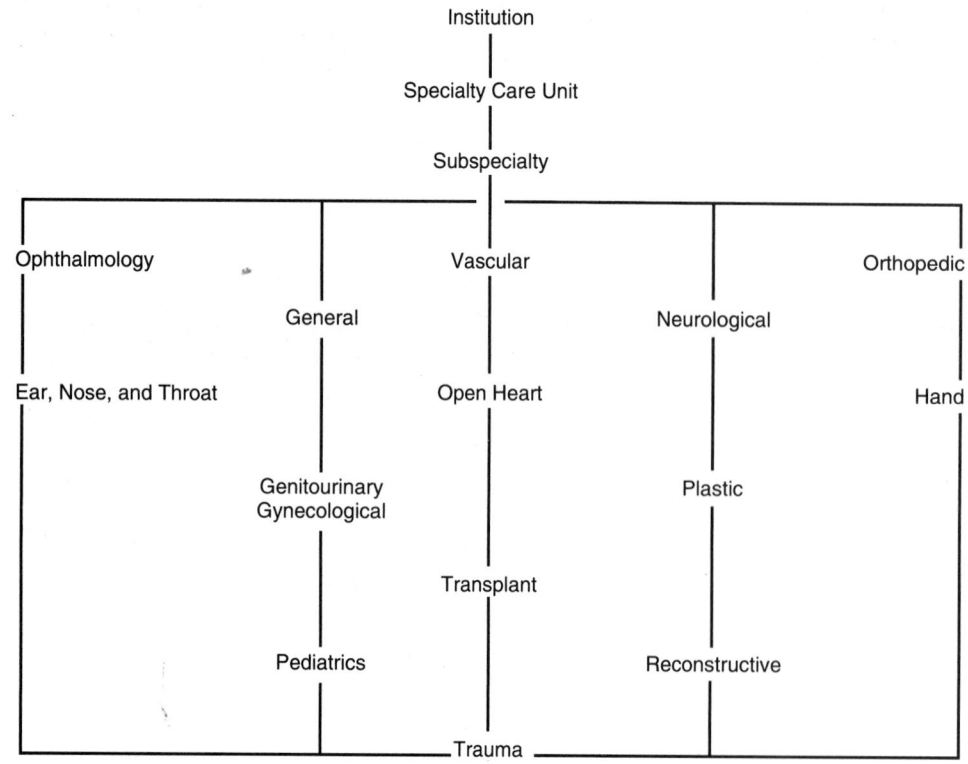

FIGURE 32–1. Mapping of subspecialty orientations.

THE ORIENTATION TEACHER

Nurses responsible for orientation activities are usually expert clinicians with a desire to share their expertise. Successful teaching enhances successful learning, and vice versa. A coordinated interdepartmental approach is necessary to identify the extent of involvement of staff in the orientation program.

Orientation teachers in the OR guide and facilitate the process of teaching-learning. At a minimum, a teacher is a registered nurse with knowledge of and skill in OR nursing practice. In addition to these two qualifications, an ideal teacher is certified in perioperative nursing practice and has knowledge of and skill in nursing education and adult education.

As registered nurses, orientation teachers provide the learner with a broad knowledge base. The clinical teacher should be aware of current developments in nursing and in the general area of health and should be familiar with the environment of the employing institution and the OR.

Certification in perioperative nursing practice (CNOR) status is a considerable asset for a clinical teacher and places his or her achievement level on a continuum between competency and excellence in perioperative nursing. Such achievement affirms that the perioperative nurse models consistent application of the nursing process and adheres to identified standards of perioperative nursing practice.

The orientation teacher must also have knowledge and skill with regard to curriculum, program design, and teaching. To be an educator, a philosophy about teaching and educational activities that has evolved from academic background and clinical experience is essential.

The teacher must understand the needs of the adult learner and the principles of adult education.

Teacher-Centered Learning

Teacher-centered learning is a traditional approach to learning—that is, the teacher decides what should be learned. The teacher-centered approach to learning is not inappropriate for teaching OR skills; its success as an efficient method of instruction is due to the fact that the learner does not know what skill is necessary for the role and therefore cannot identify learning needs.

This educational approach only considers teaching the "how-to's" and thus is inappropriate as a sole or long-term means of education in the OR. Teaching strategies that compel learners to discover more complex ways of making meaning and using knowledge in the OR care setting are needed to augment teacher-centered learning.

Learner-Centered Learning

The ability to provide learners with educational experiences to service their learning needs presumes that the learner can identify his or her needs; subsequently, the teacher can identify an appropriate learning experience. Like teacher-centered learning, learner-centered learning is not an independent approach to learning. Learner-centered learning should take place alongside teacher-centered learning in an OR orientation program.

Learner-centered learning is predicated on adult learning theory. Briefly, adult education is a process based on an individual's maturity and motivation gained from past experiences; it is not based on a learner's chronological age. This is an important, albeit abstract, construct for the teacher in a learner-centered experience to grasp, as the core of the process is an interactive one.

Experiences in learner-centered learning require creativity on the part of the teacher. Learner-centered learning, within the problem-solving framework, is "thinking" learning. The learner relates and/or combines two or more acquired principles to produce a new or higher level of practice. The nursing literature is beginning to address learner-centered learning as part of the interaction of adult education and the process of problem solving (Bratton, 1987).

THE LEARNER

Students entering nursing education are a diverse group. Their instructors have been challenged by the electronic media to make learning fun. After graduation, the student comes to the traditional health care setting with assertive learning expectations.

Learners with OR or nursing experience who are new to an institution are predictably true adult learners. Adult learners may need to unlearn in order to learn. Therefore, they may not respond to traditional teaching methods and may thrive when nontraditional methods are utilized. Nontraditional teaching methods that challenge the adult learner are capable of providing multiple learning experiences simultaneously.

CONTENT OF AN ORIENTATION PROGRAM

In this era of accountability, it is important to base any educational programming, especially orientation, on validated teaching and learning principles. Clinical educators must include flexible experiences that facilitate an individual's identified learning needs. Developing a learner's basic abilities into critical thinking, problem-solving, and decision-making capacities is the "heart and soul" of clinical education.

The best planned learning provides for a steady cumulative sequence of successful behaviors. A new learner in the OR may, on the first clinical day, express a desire to "scrub on a total hip." The behavior expected at that level of practice, as well as the knowledge and skill building required to achieve that competency, need to be discussed. However, if the situation allows, an observational double scrub experience early in the orientation would probably facilitate the learner's motivation.

In orientation, a learner is dependent on information to clarify work responsibilities and discover his or her role in the workplace. Core content elements commonly found in orientation programs include philosophy, goals, needs assessment, objectives, topics, methods, and evaluation.

A *philosophy* provides a written foundation that gives meaning to and clarifies the programs that an institution supports. The departmental philosophy must be consistent with the institutional philosophy. Knowledge of institutional and department philosophies and commitment to the beliefs stated are vital for all orientation teachers. Awareness of the professional organization's philosophy of perioperative nursing practice can also enhance appreciation of OR nursing. Orientation teachers need to promote institutional, departmental, and professional organizational philosophies and standards. Learners should be encouraged to draft their own philosophy of nursing, as well as their own philosophy of OR nursing. These philosophies can be utilized as baseline measurements of the socialization dimension of orientation.

Goals for institutional and departmental orientation programs give broad, general, decentralized direction to the teacher and learner regarding implementation of the philosophy. Goals are not directives. They describe how the roles and responsibilities of individuals in the institution contribute as a collective to the philosophy.

Needs Assessment

Achieving established goals and progressing from one level to the next requires the goals to have sets of educational experiences. A needs assessment defines these experiences.

A *needs assessment* is the element of orientation that identifies what a learner knows versus what the learner needs to know in order to meet the expectations of the role.

Needs are assessed by soliciting input about the learning behaviors expected of employees from OR managers and clinical experts. The orientation teacher then has the responsibility to formalize the input within the philosophy of the institution and the philosophy of the department.

Assessing what an orientee knows can be as simple as having the orientee complete a check list or as complex as having the orientee complete a learning style index. The orientation teacher uses this information as a baseline to (1) identify educational needs (needs that can be satisfied by a learning experience) and (2) establish learning objectives.

Learning Objectives

Learning objectives describe how assessed educational needs will be met within the practice setting. These can be program or learner related. Program-related objectives describe a broad behavior change that will occur as a result of participating in an orientation program.

Learner-related objectives describe changes that the learner will achieve in order to address the role and responsibilities inherent in the new work setting. Learner-related objectives also describe how the individual's behavior will change as a result of participating in the orientation program. Specific behaviors that can be measured by performance are developed to identify how the learner will progress from basic competency toward excellence. As necessary in an OR setting, the program and learner objectives may be individualized and/or may be further defined by objectives for subspecialty rotations.

Activity Content

Overall, objectives organize the instructional activities of the orientation program that a learner will be involved in and enable the learner to "see" the proposed learning plan. Learners can internalize and assess the congruency of their own learning styles within the proposed activities. Discussion and any alterations can then be negotiated with the various people involved in the orientation program.

Alterations should be supported and encouraged, especially for the adult learner. The means of achieving program and individual objectives, however, should not compromise patient safety, should be within the scope of nurse practice acts, should enhance the learning experience, and should meld the new employee's socialization with his or her new service-related responsibilities.

The *topics* that can be included in an orientation's curriculum are endless. Frameworks of curriculum can be conceptualized within the phases of perioperative practice (pre-, intra-, postoperative), within competency behaviors that use the nursing process, and/or within the knowledge and skill content areas of certified perioperative nursing practice.

Remember: the learning plan reflects the philosophy of the OR and the goals of the orientation program. The framework for identifying topics flows from the concepts identified in the philosophy and goals. For example, if research is a major institutional goal, it would not be unusual for patients to be participating in drug studies. An OR orientation program topic would need to include research, guidelines, and ethics of patient participation.

Teaching-Learning Methods

Operationalizing orientation topics is directly related to *teaching-learning methods*; these are the "how" of assisting the learner to learn identified topics. Traditional teaching-learning methods include, but are not limited to, lecture, assigned readings, discussion, and observation. These traditional methods are appropriate if either the program or individual objectives relate to some knowledge or skill the learner needs to know. If the objectives relate to some knowledge or skill the learner needs to apply, then participative teaching-learning methods such as demonstrations with return or group work are more appropriate.

Institutional orientation programs utilize both traditional and participative teaching-learning methods. For example, one program objective may be to know the responsibilities of the job; an appropriate teaching-learning method would be to read and discuss job descriptions. However, a program objective that requires health care personnel to be trained in basic life support essentially requires a demonstration that these skills can be applied.

OR orientation program objectives and the individual's learning objectives also combine both traditional and participative teaching-learning methods. Job descriptions and policies can be read, reviewed, and discussed. The learner can observe the expert clinician. In an OR orientation program, traditional teaching-learning methods such as these comprise teacher-centered learning. The reader will recall that teacher-centered learning is inappropriate as a sole means of OR orientation.

The variety and diversity of subspecialties in an OR department mandate that the majority of any orientation program consist of participative teaching-learning methods. Preceptorships are a common participative teaching-learning method utilized to implement orientation content as a method and a process.

Preceptorship Program

A *preceptorship program* is a participative teaching-learning method that can be used successfully for all types of nurse learners (i.e., students, adult learners, or new graduates). Preceptorships are a transitional model of orientation education. They bridge the discrepancy, or gap, between learning needs and proficiency, education, and service. Licensure as a registered nurse assumes a safe practitioner level, and initial competence is attained in relation to defined objectives. However, continuing competence and intellectual curiosity in a learner's clinical expertise can be enhanced with a preceptor. Caty and Scott (1988, p. 21) state that, in addition to clinical knowledge and skill, preceptors help nurses learn, ". . . the realities of daily nursing practice with all its joys and frustrations" (p. 21). In other words, preceptors as a method of orientation facilitate the process of orientation.

Current literature, as well as AORN's *Preceptor Guide for Perioperative Nursing Practice* (1993), describes a preceptor as a registered nurse, experienced in perioperative nursing practice, who has a specific responsibility to provide and direct learning experiences for the learner. The preceptor acts to facilitate learning within the perioperative setting. Thus, the learner is able to satisfactorily meet the goals and objectives of the orientation program. The RN preceptor takes on the role of teacher, role model, and mentor. Reference

to preceptors as subject matter experts reflects the roles collectively (Allanach, 1988).

In addition to assisting with learning experiences and facilitating a learner's individualized knowledge and skill building, a preceptor has a responsibility as a clinical professional to focus the novice's role expectations. A study by McCloskey and McCain (1987, p. 20) found the following:

Over their first year of work all nurses employed . . . reported decreased job satisfaction, decreased organizational commitment, and decreased professionalism. This happened with both new graduates and experienced nurses alike; only Master's prepared nurses did not report this decline. . . . Results suggest that employers need to assess the initial expectations of new nurses and either meet more of those expectations or help new nurses form more realistic expectations about their jobs.

Preceptorship is a role wherein expert clinical professionals volunteer to be responsible for a learner's learning, not a learner's practice. A preceptor commits to life-long learning and sharing information. As a voluntary role, compensation is not expected, yet the time involved in planning, implementing, and evaluating a learning experience is demanding.

Supporting a preceptor program must be an organizational commitment. Economic as well as human resources (i.e., the quantity and quality of available nursing staff) must be critically assessed.

The organization considering establishing a preceptor program to orient students or new employees to the OR should realize that such an action will involve an outlay in terms of time, money, and personnel. Financially, the cost provides a significant savings compared with the expense of recruiting and orienting new nurses to replace those who have left (McLean, 1987). Preceptorships, however, may not be appropriate or cost effective if the program is a one-time effort. Alternately, a large number of individuals needing this program at once may overwhelm the system. Developing the program is time consuming, especially the process of precepting the preceptor to precept. When considering a preceptor program, it should be remembered that the program may be less effective as a whole if there are only novice preceptors to pair with learners who are themselves novices.

Overall, precepting provides opportunities to apply interpersonal skills, develop and demonstrate leadership potential, and receive recognition for expertise in a specialty area. It also provides numerous opportunities to enhance teaching skills while promoting and encouraging advanced practice. The sponsoring facility will usually find that the program enhances patient care, improves staff morale, and often increases the motivation of the entire staff to pursue learning. A preceptor program can attract nurses desiring challenge and growth. Thus, such a program has the potential to serve as a vehicle for employee retention, as well as to enhance recruitment.

On-The-Job Training

On-the-job (OTJ) training is a concept whose implications for a departmental orientation program stem from business and education fields. OTJ training is focused on the acquisition and competent performance of requisite skills. The most common business example of OTJ training is the assembly line worker.

A newly employed assembly line worker without assembly line experience needs to acquire essential manual (and possibly verbal and mental) skills to accomplish the tasks of the job. A competent level of behavior is achieved when pre-established criteria are met (e.g., *x* amount of items assembled in *x* amount of time). Achieving the criteria provides observable and measurable evidence that requisite skills have been mastered.

OTJ training is not so simply applied in clinically intensive OR education activities, especially in the novice level skill period of orientation. Overall, the nursing roles and responsibilities have numerous diverse inherent tasks that can be simple or complex. A newly employed OR nurse and a nurse without OR experience both need OTJ training, but using a conceptual teaching-learning method.

As a conceptual teaching-learning method, OTJ training combines specific skill acquisition with general knowledge bases. Knowledge (i.e., knowing what to do and how to do it) is enhanced with experience. Skill (i.e., verbally, mentally, or manually manipulating people, things, or information) is enhanced with practice. Having knowledge does not mean that the skill can be performed. Performing a skill competently does not mean there is an appropriate knowledge base.

In the OR, nursing care skill without knowledge or knowledge without skill precipitates an unsafe level of practice. Conceptually, then, OTJ training relative to OR orientation programs requires interactive teaching-learning experiences. The application of knowledge and skill appropriate to a patient care situation is simultaneously demonstrated and explained in real care situations by an expert clinician. The learner concurrently sees the skill performed and hears the knowledge base associated with the skill.

Knowledge building and skill building parallel each other along the continuum of professional excellence. A patient care situation in perioperative nursing practice requires an orientation teacher to use general nursing knowledge bases, such as the nursing process, with specific nursing skill bases (e.g., the length of instruments compared with the depth of the surgical anatomy). Problem solving according to general knowledge and specific skills carries a novice's learning through the numerous, diverse, complex and simple tasks inherent in perioperative nursing care. Striving to consistently develop knowledge and skill using OTJ training as a conceptual teaching-learning method also de-emphasizes the OTJ business training philosophy of "we've always done it this way."

Table 32–1 describes general nursing knowledge bases applicable to perioperative nursing practice. Table

TABLE 32–1. GENERAL PERIOPERATIVE NURSING KNOWLEDGE* BASES

The Nursing Process:	A systemic approach to nursing practice utilizing problem-solving techniques.
Perioperative Nursing Practice:	Providing care to surgical patients, with primary emphasis on the intraoperative period and responsibility for preoperative assessment and postoperative evaluation.
Preoperative period:	Begins when the decision for surgical intervention is made and ends with transfer of the patient to the operating room bed.
Intraoperative period:	Begins when the patient is transferred to the operating room bed and ends with admission to the recovery area.
Postoperative period:	Begins with admission of the patient to the recovery area and ends with the resolution of surgical sequelae.
A Safe Environment:	The physical and psychological aspects of the surgical environment.
The Surgical Procedure:	Technical aspects and anatomical approach used during surgical intervention.
Scrubbing:	The functions of the nurse who is scrubbed, wears sterile gown and gloves, and who indirectly participates in patient care by handing instruments, preparing and handing suture, and caring for sterile supplies and equipment during the surgical procedure.
Circulating:	The functions of the nurse who is not scrubbed, does not wear sterile gown and gloves, and is free to move about and assist other personnel. This nurse coordinates the activities of the room, prepares an environment conducive to patient safety, and carries out nursing care that involves direct interaction with the patient.

*Knowledge is knowing what to do.

32–2 demonstrates how the nursing process as a knowledge base can be integrated with specific perioperative nursing skills.

Evaluation

Evaluation is an ongoing activity, although it is more commonly associated in education as the final formal step of an OR orientation program. Throughout the program, the learner's progress, the teacher's performance, the teaching-learning interaction, and the learning

TABLE 32–2. GENERAL PERIOPERATIVE NURSING SKILL* BASES

Perioperative role	Implementation
Assessment	Aseptic technique
Professional role	Apparel
Definition	Scrubs
Scope of care	Gowning/gloving
responsibility	Skin preparation
Functions	Traffic
Patient record	Draping
Consents	Electrosurgical grounding
Medical and nursing data	Devices
Patient/family/significant	Elements
other	Positioning principles
Interviewing	Surgical implications
Physical assessment	Nursing roles and
Psychological assessment	responsibilities
Teaching-learning process	Counts
Collaboration	Types
Communication	Rationale
Group dynamics	Methods
Professional ethics	Patient care management
Team roles/relationships	Time
Nursing diagnosis	Resources
Recording/reporting	Patients
Documentation	Psychological monitoring
Planning	Emotional status
Goal development	Support
Priorities	Communication
Patient outcomes	Records/reports
Measurable criteria	Documentation
Factors affecting goal	Evaluation
attainment	Goals/criteria
Infection control	Nursing activities/responses
Environmental control	Methods
Sterilization	Goals/criteria
Preparation, storage, and	Documentation
maintenance of supplies	Quality assurance
Skin integrity	Documentation
Wound healing	Reassessment
Skin preparation	
Safety	
Electrical	
Equipment	
Anesthesia	
Radiation	
Disaster	
Immune system responses	
Fluids and electrolytes	
Physiological responses	
Monitoring	
Effects of imbalances	
Nursing activities	
Patient responses	
Sociocultural and ethnic	
factors	
Patients' rights	
Rehabilitation	
Participation	
Nursing care plans	
Nursing care planning	
Standards of perioperative	
nursing practice	
Communication	
Recommended practices	

*Skill is defined as the proficient manual, verbal, or mental manipulation of information, people, or things. Skill embodies observable, quantifiable, and measurable performance variables.

environment are monitored for learning quality, growth in learning, and professional development. Lunn and Humphries (1986) have delineated the following five purposes of evaluation:

1. Acquiring and processing the evidence needed to improve the teaching-learning process.
2. Validating data obtained through a variety of methods and from several sources.
3. Determining whether goals and objectives are being attained. Data may indicate goals and objectives are unrealistic and need to be revised.
4. Controlling quality, as each step in the teaching-learning process can be assessed for effectiveness and determination made about needed program revisions.
5. Ascertaining whether alternative procedures are equally effective in achieving program goals and objectives.

An OR orientation program should have a number of methods for evaluation. This variety of methods allows learning to be validated according to an individual learner. Learning outcomes should not vary, and judgment about competent patient care giving should be consistent across the evaluation methods. A variety is suggested, because the type of nurse learner varies. Pencil-and-paper tests may demotivate an adult learner. Alternately, skills checklists may provide a feeling of accomplishment and consequently motivate a new employee. The orientation teacher should provide the learner with guidance in the evaluation method most appropriate to his or her learning style. Whatever the methods available or the method utilized, evaluation of the evaluation methods is continuous. The resources allocated to nurse teachers and nurse learners in orientation programs create and maintain powerful professional nursing care settings. The needs of the individual, as well as the needs of the department, are well balanced within the needs of the organization and the organization's mission to the people it serves.

DIRECTING A PERIOPERATIVE STAFF EDUCATION PROGRAM

The nature of programming educational activities for a perioperative nursing staff is more complex than the centralized/decentralized concept described in the section on conducting an orientation program. Presently, programming inservices and continuing education (CE) for perioperative nursing staffs are related primarily to the programming pattern of the employing health care setting. There is no standard. In some settings, for example, inservice and CE activities are within the critical care budget; in others, the OR is considered a separate unit, but the presurgical and postanesthesia care unit nursing staffs receive inservice and CE monies from a medical-surgical nursing fund.

There is a paucity of literature describing the advantages, disadvantages, challenges, and changes nonstandardized educational programming presents to the individual administrator, director, staff educator, and nursing staff in perioperative practice. However, as an economic issue, education is always acknowledged as an investment, not an expense. It is vital, therefore, to establish who sets priorities and coordinates education functions (Waterstrade, 1988). Other issues to be addressed in standardization are the acquisition and allocation of educational staff within time, as well as financial, parameters (Borden and Noll, 1986).

The process, purpose, and function of staff education as a specialty area of perioperative practice—including appropriate service delivery mechanisms, the role of the peer educator, and the development and presentation of educational programs—seems to be an evolving discipline. This section is a blueprint for a perioperative staff education program. It is a curriculum of topics for the perioperative nurse with clinical credibility and a philosophical commitment to the educational development of peers, but without the resources to obtain a formal academic education.

Definition of Perioperative Staff Education

Perioperative nursing staff education is a unit contained within the interrelated parts of orientation, inservice, and continuing education. The interrelationship is such that there is a small amount of overlap between orientation and the other activities, but a considerable amount of overlap between inservice and CE programs (Tiessen, 1987).

The role of the staff educator focuses on the incorporation of adult learning principles and the belief that the educational process fosters growth and development of individuals and enables them to achieve goals and potentials. The focus on the involvement of learners in the total learning process and the incorporation of teaching strategies that promote action and involvement are foremost (Tobin and Beeler, 1988).

Staff Development

The ANA defines staff development as

. . . a process consisting of orientation, inservice education, and continuing education for the purpose of promoting the development of personnel within any employment setting consistent with the goals and responsibilities of the employer.

(ANA, STANDARDS FOR CONTINUING EDUCATION IN NURSING, 1984, p. 5.)

Inservice Education

Inservice education consists of activities intended to assist the professional nurse to acquire, maintain, and/or increase competence in fulfilling the assigned responsibilities specific to the expectations of the employer.

Critical Characteristics
Content: Reflects employer's goals and service commitments; includes, but is not limited to, review of

previously learned skills.
Application: Knowledge and skills are specific to a given employment setting and are immediately applicable by the learner.

(ANA, STANDARDS FOR CONTINUING EDUCATION IN NURSING, 1984, p. 5.)

Inservice education must be differentiated from orientation activities. Orientation requirements are clearly defined. Staff educators, as orientation teachers, are responsible for facilitating a learner's movement from a generic, safe level of nursing to that of initial competence in relation to defined objectives. Staff educators responsible for inservice education, however, focus on peer learning activities that are "specific to the expectations of the employer." Inservices may develop specialty nursing knowledge and skill or attitudes. Most common to perioperative nursing staff are presentations by service/product representatives. However, the ANA key to presentations being classified as inservice is an emphasis on patient care aspects and nursing practice implications, not on products. The ANA standards specifically state that nursing practice must be addressed by a registered nurse.

Continuing Education

Continuing education in nursing consists of those planned educational activities intended to build upon the educational and experiential bases of the professional nurse for the enhancement of practice, education, administration, research, or theory development to the end of improving the health of the public.

Critical Characteristics
Content: Current and emerging concepts, principles, practices, theories, and/or research in or related to nursing.
Application: Immediate or futuristic application in meeting nursing practice needs or goals of the learner. Knowledge and skills may be utilized in a variety of nursing practice and education settings.

(ANA, STANDARDS FOR CONTINUING EDUCATION IN NURSING, 1984, p. 5.)

Continuing education may take place in the work setting or be offered through a variety of external sources. Contact hours for activities are granted by nursing organizations that have received accreditation. The criteria that must be met before contact hours are awarded need to be developed within a perioperative nursing focus. Perioperative staff education activities wherein a registered nurse facilitates the learning process by discussing nursing implications of patient care services and/or products may be considered CE, and therefore, participants may be eligible to receive contact hours.

The Perioperative Staff Educator

Geber (1988) believes that education activities evolved within health care settings for three primary reasons:

1. Management perceived a recurring problem that to date had been resolved only by outside consultants. An in-house program was proposed as more cost effective.
2. The apparent success at another facility or as documented in the health care literature instigated management to establish an educator position in hopes of capturing a market.
3. A legal mandate, such as a set of safety regulations or Federal rules, prompted establishment of an education program.

Deciding on an appropriate person to coordinate perioperative education, training and development is usually a matter of deciding whether educational experience or company experience is more critical. Candidates for the position are screened accordingly. A person without company experience needs time to learn the nuances and jargon; a person without educational experience needs to commit to adult learning and instructional media study. It is important to remember that a deficit of either will require time and resources for development.

In the perioperative setting, it is not astute to hire a person with adult education experience but no perioperative clinical experience. However, it is rare to find a perioperative nurse with both formal academic preparation in adult education and clinical expertise. Therefore, developing the inexperienced nurse educator is a mutually negotiated action between the director/manager and the person hired.

Conedera and Schoessler (1987, p. 175) described five qualifications the director of an acute care setting should consider when hiring an inexperienced nurse educator:

1. Affective skills (self-motivation, positive attitude toward learning, tolerance of ambiguity, flexibility, and innovation)
2. Presentation skills
3. Program development skills
4. Knowledge of adult learning theory
5. Ability to function in the department and the institution

The candidate should also explore and commit to the set of questions posed by Tobin and Beeler (1987, p. 93):

● Have I internalized the concept of life-long learning? Am I goal oriented? If not, why not?
● Do I have knowledge and skill in adult learning, group dynamics, curriculum development, teaching strategies, communication, evaluation, research, marketing, health care economics, and nursing information systems?
● If not, do I seek learning opportunities that will continually upgrade my knowledge and skills in these areas?

Finally, a mutually negotiated action plan for the inexperienced educator mandates time lines. Time lines may vary according to the reasons the perioperative education program was initiated, but one year is a recurrent indicator in the literature. A year allows the educator to establish goals, develop communication relationships with clinical leaders, and become aware of internal and external resources. The director/manager needs to support these experiences financially, verbally, and with documentation.

Principles of Adult Learning

Traditional learning, also known as the pedagogical model, is the one all of us have had the most experience with. Teaching in institutions is largely pedagogically oriented. Even in educators, the pedagogical model comes quickly to mind and often takes control of activities. Pedagogy has dominated education practices since the seventh century.

Five assumptions about the activity's participant are inherent in the pedagogical model:

1. The participant is a dependent personality. The teacher is expected to take full responsibility for making decisions about what is to be learned, how and when it should be learned, and whether it has been learned. The role of the participant is to carry out the teacher's directions passively.
2. The participant enters into an activity with little experience that can be used in the learning process. The experience of the teacher/trainer is what is important.
3. The participant needs to be told what he or she must learn in order to advance to or achieve the next level.
4. The participant in the activity has a subject-centered orientation. Learning means acquiring subject matter.
5. People are motivated to participate by external pressures from parents, teachers, employers, the consequences of failure, grades, certificates, etc.

Table 32–3 highlights the teaching implications of the pedagogical model.

Andragogy, a philosophical orientation for educating adults, forms the organizing framework for nursing's educational activities. Malcolm Knowles is credited with the promotion of adult education as a practice model. However, andragogy is an evolved educational process that is influenced by behavioral, gestalt, cognitive, and humanistic theories of education. The following five assumptions underlie the andragogical model of learning:

1. The learner is self-directing. Adult learners want to take responsibility for their own lives, including the planning, implementing, and evaluating of their learning activities.
2. The learner enters an educational activity with a great deal of experience. This experience is a resource for the learner as well as for others.
3. Adults are ready to learn when they perceive a need to know or do something in order to perform more effectively in some aspect of their lives. Their

TABLE 32–3. IMPLICATIONS OF THE PEDAGOGICAL MODEL

The basic concern of people with a pedagogical orientation is *content*:
- What needs to be covered
- How to organize
- Logical sequence
- Efficient transmission

readiness to learn may be stimulated by helping them to assess the gaps between where they are now and where they want and need to be.

4. Adults are motivated to learn after they experience a need in their life situation. For that reason, learning needs to be problem focused.
5. Adults are motivated to learn because of internal factors such as self-esteem, recognition, better quality of life, greater self-confidence, or the opportunity for self-actualization.

Table 32–4 highlights the implications of the educator within the andragogical model.

In the academic world, andragogy attracted attention because of "turf wars" between those who delivered training and those who designed it. The adult education camp often faulted the instructional design contingent for being so concerned with the methodology and outcomes of instruction as to lose sight of the learner in the process. Adult educators saw Knowles' theory about the unique characteristics of adult learners and the adult learning process as a great source of power in the battle over which factor really makes more difference in education: the learner or the program design.

In the business world, trainers also welcomed an alternative to the traditionally mechanistic model of workplace education in which workers had little, if any, input into the design and content of their learning. Knowles' theory was considered a door through which employees could increasingly direct and control their own on the job training.

The theoretical debate regarding pedagogy and adult education relative to its application to perioperative nursing as practiced in a clinically intensive care setting deserves comment. In 1984, in a teaching methodology course, a pedagogical theory of education was integrated with andragogy and quasitested in the OR clinical environment (Brazen, unpublished research, 1984). Although deemed appropriate and successful to student and participants, it was not acceptable to the graduate program faculty. It is ironic that the same year Knowles himself altered his concept.

I now regard the pedagogical and andragogical models as parallel, not antithetical. For centuries, educators had only one model, the pedagogical model, to go on. In some situations, such as when learners of whatever age are entering a totally strange territory of content or are confronting a machine they have never seen before, they may be truly dependent on didactic instruction before they can take much initiative in their own

learning; in such situations, the pedagogical strategies would be appreciated.

(KNOWLES AND COWORKERS, 1984, p. 13)

To date, the challenges to Knowles' assumptions leave only the quality and quantity of experience brought to an activity as a universal characteristic of an adult learner (Feuer and Geber, 1988). Andragogy and pedagogy are increasingly accepted as dichotomous models of human learning. In the current concept of education, learning is considered a problem-solving process rather than a set of rules used to answer a question.

Regardless of these recent changes, the principles of adult learning, inclusive of adult education theory, are a necessary knowledge and skill base for perioperative staff educators. The components of perioperative staff education programs parallel those of educational activities in other nursing units. Although educational activities are not routinely submitted for contact hours, a proactive educator can improve the learning product, process, and function of the perioperative staff by developing the topic according to adult education concepts. Standard 4 of the ANA CE Standards can be used as a framework for development.

Standard 4.   Educational Design

The continuing education design for each activity consists of planned, organized, and evaluated learning experiences based on the principles of adult learning.

Rationale
Assumptions about adults as learners have implications for educational design.

Structure Criterion
An educational design based on adult learning principles is employed.

Process Criteria
Through the educational design the provider:
1. *assesses learning needs of the target audience.*
2. *plans continuing activities which reflect identified needs of the target population.*
3. *states behavioral objectives for each continuing education activity.*
4. *selects content for each continuing education activity in relation to objectives.*

TABLE 32–4. IMPLICATIONS OF THE ANDRAGOGICAL MODEL

The basic concern of people with an andragogical orientation is *process*:

- Physical and psychological climate setting
- Involving learners in:
  - Planning for their learning
  - Diagnosing their own needs for learning
  - Formulating their own learning objectives
  - Designing learning plans
  - Evaluating their own learning outcomes
- Helping learners carry out their learning plans

5. relates content to nursing knowledge or nursing practice.
6. selects teaching methods for each continuing education activity in relation to objectives, content, and principles of adult learning.
7. ensures availability of adequate resources, including qualified faculty, to implement each continuing education activity.
8. develops evaluation strategies for each continuing education activity in relation to objectives and to principles of adult learning.

Outcome Criteria
1. The educational design operationalizes principles of adult learning:
   a. the learner is represented in identifying learning needs
   b. content is relevant to an identified need
   c. teaching strategies experientially involve the learner
   d. the learner participates in the evaluation process
2. The design for each continuing education program includes a needs assessment, behavioral objectives, content outline, teaching methods, learning activities, resources, and evaluation strategies.

DESIGNING AN EDUCATIONAL ACTIVITY FOR PERIOPERATIVE STAFF

An educational design is the essence of a perioperative staff educator's practice. Educational designs for inservice and CE activities are developed, processed, and retained according to established criteria. The criteria that determine the implementation of an inservice are usually set forth by regulatory agencies.

It is critical for staff educators to understand the ANA definitions of inservice and continuing education and to develop either or both accordingly. The key to this understanding and development is the fact that the educational design criteria for contact hours are determined by the accreditation body that approves contact hours for the activity. For this, the educator has a number of resources. State nurse associations and specialty nursing organizations offer publications to guide the process of obtaining contact hours for CE activities.

Seminars and courses to enable the novice staff educator to develop and process core components of an educational design tool are also available. These core components are a common bond between inservices and CE for registered nurses. They are also the least understood by perioperative staff nurses who have accepted or been delegated a perioperative staff educator role.

Components

Needs Assessment

The process of needs assessment is identifying discrepancies (gaps) between what is known and/or practiced and what should be known and/or practiced as

defined by the learner, professional or employee, and society. These gaps are referred to as *learning needs.*

Identifying learning needs is the first step in planning the activity and ensures that the program design is relevant to its purpose. The staff educator considers the methods of assessing needs and chooses the method most conducive to the setting. As much information as possible is gathered from the people involved. The staff educator reviews the completed needs assessment tool and, through a qualitative analysis, categorizes the information according to the definitions of need types. Real educational type learning needs are most commonly the ones that are developed into CE or inservice activities.

Commonly used methods for assessing the learning needs of the adult learner include the following:

- The Questionnaire or Survey Method—learners chose from a list of topics.
- The Interview Method—sample learners representative of the target group are asked to express opinions and feelings on topics.
- Observation—especially useful in clinical practice settings.
- Review of Literature—for nursing issues and trends related to a specific group of learners.

Learning Objectives

Learning objectives describe behavioral changes expected in the participant as a result of attending the program. Learning objectives are occasionally simply termed "objectives," but this is incorrect. Participants are led to believe that objectives are what the teacher would do, not what they would be able to do as a result of attending the activity. Learning objectives direct the selection of content and describe the behavioral outcomes the participant is expected to achieve. Learning objectives describe what the learner will be able to *do*. They should flow naturally from the needs assessment and demonstrate the worth of a program in such a way that potential learners can determine the benefit of attending. Ultimately, they also provide a means for determining the learning that occurred (evaluation).

Learning objectives may be developed according to the category of behavior the educational activity is geared to influence. These categories of behavior change are called *domains.* There are three domains: psychomotor, cognitive, and affective. Each domain addresses learning (i.e., behavior change) in different areas. Table 32–5 identifies these behavior changes.

Domain	Behavior Change
TABLE 32–5. CATEGORIES OF BEHAVIOR CHANGE	
Psychomotor	Skills, responses, motor activities
Cognitive	Intellectual abilities and understanding
Affective	Attitudes, appreciations, values, interests, beliefs

In addition, each of the three domains has different levels the learning objectives may target. The levels for each domain are described and sample learning objectives given in Appendices A through C.

Most CE and inservice learning needs are cognitive. Participants desire more information on a topic in order to advance their knowledge base. To be behavioral, a learning objective must refer to the behavior of the student rather than that of the teacher and describe measurable behavior. Examples of verbs used for each level of the cognitive domain are listed in Appendix D. This list should be used to write CE and inservice learning objectives.

Activity Content

Each learning objective must have related content that reflects the andragogical model. *Content* refers to facts or concepts to be presented to achieve the objectives. As a general rule, the staff educator should design the CE or inservice activity in such a way that one learning objective is addressed for every hour of content. A perioperative example is included as Appendix E.

Teaching Methods

Teaching methods enhance or facilitate the learning process of adults. Most adults prefer to be actively involved in the learning process, and teaching methods should therefore encourage discovery, complement the delivery of content, stimulate interest, and involve as many human senses as possible.

The effectiveness of teaching methods is influenced by the level or the domain of the learning objective. For example, if the objective relates to the cognitive domain, teaching methods might consist of lectures, independent study, or readings. If the objective relates to the application level, methods might consist of role playing, clinical practice, or small group activities. Learner material is concerned with facilitating mastery of knowledge, reinforcing the ability to learn, and stimulating a desire for further learning; although it should reflect adult attitudes, it should also accommodate individual learners.

Evaluation

The rationale for evaluation is growth of the learner and quality of the teacher-learner method. An evaluation tool asks learners to rate or comment on their attainment of each learning objective and is completed at the end of each CE and/or inservice activity.

Compilation and analysis of the data collected from the evaluations can be used to structure future needs assessments. In light of performance, problem areas are identified and plans made to correct them. In this way, evaluation is an ongoing process providing the bridge or beginning point for future activities.

TRENDS IN PERIOPERATIVE NURSING EDUCATION

Inservice and CE activities need to be responsive to an extremely sophisticated consumer group: perioperative registered nurses. The nursing process framework can be used by staff educators as a model to consider perspectives of the trends this challenge presents.

Assessment

The discussion of entry into practice has been and is ongoing and will not be continued here except for an untested trend the issue seems to have spawned. That trend is certification.

Currently, more than 40 certifications are offered through a number of nursing associations and specialty nursing organizations. Nurses may choose to test at a generalist level or at a specialist level. Candidate status for the generalist examination requires RN licensure, and 1 year of nursing practice is suggested. Candidacy for a specialist examination also requires RN licensure, although the suggested practice requirement is more detailed.

It is interesting to consider whether the increase in the number of nurses who are voluntarily and successfully testing for certification is directly, if at all, related to the currently inaccessible option of baccalaureate completion programs. Nonetheless, the number of certified nurses and the areas of certification certainly influence the need for contact hours.

Planning

The title of clinical nurse specialist no longer requires an academic degree or advanced practice certificate. More likely, a clinical specialist is a nurse who has deliberately chosen to provide day-to-day direct patient care in a specific clinical area.

The increase in specialty nursing practice, but most importantly its acceptance by health care employers, has increased the planning demands on providers of continuing education. Not only are more activities needed, these activities must focus on more specific agenda items to meet the learning needs of the specialist. The traditional subspecialties of perioperative nursing practice present a staff educator with another planning challenge—i.e., an increase in the numerous and diverse learning needs of clinical nurse subspecialists.

In the current health care environment, planning must also address outside influences. This is a challenge to staff educators and individual specialists. Provision of learning opportunities through activities and the individual's responsibility and accountability to participate in lifelong learning are separate but interrelated items. The outcome is as follows:

Nurses are becoming more selective and are demanding more input into continuing education opportunities. This has prompted educators to provide more cost effective, non-traditional methods of continuing education as economic constraints have increased creative approaches.

(BRUNT, 1988, p. 175)

Implementation

Hierarchy support for the service is central to accurately servicing the consumer (i.e., the nurse). A staff education position or delegation of the role and responsibility without supporting the time, growth, and development that inservice and CE programs require demonstrates "lip service" to the concept. If education is a one-time activity or the facilitator is perceived as "staff," it is unlikely that participants will internalize the knowledge presented or its nursing practice implications.

Evaluation

Addressing real educational needs, presenting too much or not enough relevant information, and continually focusing on a popular or safe topic are issues included in evaluation. To date, the long-term ways CE fosters excellence in practice are purely speculative. A nurse may receive financial support to attend an activity, be inspired by a dynamic presentation, and yet not apply the learning to practice. Establishing the nursing practice effect and the nursing care affect of CE is the "$64,000 research question" for staff educators.

CONCLUSION

To date, few articles have reported on the functions, tasks, characteristics, and development of hospital-based education as a specialty area of nursing. Preliminary research regarding the learning needs and satisfaction with the teaching methods used to meet those needs have been shared in the nursing staff development circle (Brazen, 1991). Competencies of OR as well as of organizational nursing educators is ongoing (Brazen, 1993). Clearly, as health care is evolving, so are the role and position of education in the health care setting.

There is more to be learned about the scholarly discipline and the clinical practice of nursing than we can impart and absorb in formal education programs. Thus, programs must not be concerned with consciousness raising or assertiveness training, but with nursing in all of its rich and existing dimensions. Continuing education offerings in nursing must increase the intellectual capacities of the learners.

As the number of continuing education workshops, conferences, and seminars steadily increases, many nurses will find it more and more difficult to decide which of these educational programs to attend. Continuing education is a professional responsibility. Nurses already are aware of their responsibility to practice

competently. Continuing education is one way to help peers maintain and/or increase professional nursing competence. Knowledge of programming a perioperative staff educational activity will keep nurses on the cutting edge.

Bibliography

Allanach, B. C. (1988). Interviewing to evaluate preceptorship relationships. *Journal of Nursing Staff Development, 4*(4), pp. 152–157.

Association of Operating Room Nurses (1993). *Preceptor guide for perioperative nursing practice.* Denver.

Barber, E. (1987). Developing and maintaining a climate of support for staff development. *Journal of Nursing Staff Development, 3*(4), p. 150.

Borden, M., Noll, A. (1986). Increasing education staff without exceeding budget. *Journal of Healthcare Education and Training, 1*(1), p. 30.

Bowman, B., Wolkenheim, B. (1987). Learning needs are dynamic: The value of repeated assessment. *The Journal of Continuing Education in Nursing, 18*(4), p. 116.

Bratton, B. D. (1987). Systematic planning for teaching and learning. In H. L. Van Hoozer, B. D. Bratton, P. M. Ostmoe, et al. (Eds.). *The teaching process: Theory and practice in nursing.* East Norwalk, CT: Appleton-Century-Crofts.

Brazen, L. (1984). Pedagogy in perioperative clinical nursing examination. Unpublished research, p. 854.

Brazen, L. (1991). Meeting the learning needs of O.R. educators. Presentation at the First National Nursing Staff Developmental Conference. San Francisco, CA, p. 857.

Brazen, L. (1993). Roles, responsibilities and competency in staff development. Research in progress, p. 857.

Brunt, B. (1988). Continuing education and megatrends. *Journal of Nursing Staff Development, 4*(4), p. 174.

Buchanan, B., Glanville, C. (1988). The clinical nurse specialist as educator: Process and method. *Clinical Nurse Specialist, 2*(2), p. 82.

Byre, M. (1986). Skill acquisition. *AORN Journal, 43*(6), pp. 1312–1317.

Caty, S., Scott, B. (1988). Preceptors for pregraduates. *The Canadian Nurse, 84*(10), pp. 20–23.

Colucciello, M. L. (1988). Creating powerful learning environments. *Nursing Connections, 1*(2), pp. 23–33.

Conedera, F., Schoessler, M. (1987). Focus. *Journal of Nursing Staff Development, 3*(4), p. 175.

Davis, A. R. (1988). Developing teaching strategies based on new knowledge. *Journal of Nursing Education, 27*(4), pp. 156–160.

Feuer, D., Geber, B. (1988). Uh-oh . . . second thoughts about adult learning theory. *Training, 25*(12), p. 31.

Geber, B. (1988). Building a training department from scratch. *Training, 25*(9), p. 28.

Huntsman, A. (1987). The future role of the health care educator. *Journal of Healthcare Education and Training, 2*(2), p. 4.

Kelly, K., Carty, R., Haskell, C. (1988). Preparing nurses for staff development practice: An educational opportunity. *Journal of Nursing Staff Development, 4*(20), p. 50.

Klassens, E. L. (1988). Improving teaching for thinking. *Nurse Educator, 13*(6), pp. 15–19.

Knowles, M. (1980). *The modern practice of adult education from pedagogy to andragogy.* Chicago: Follett Publishing Company.

Knowles, M. (1984). *Andragogy in action.* San Francisco: Josey Bass.

Lunn, S., Humphries, S. (1986). *MILS—The staff development series II: Orientation—OR.* Denver, CO: Association of Operating Room Nurses, Inc.

Malek, C. J. (1986). A model for teaching critical thinking. *Nurse Educator, 11*(6), pp. 20–23.

McCloskey, J. C., McCain, B.E. (1987). Satisfaction, commitment and professionalism of newly employed nurses. *Image: Journal of Nursing Scholarship, 19*(1), pp. 20–24.

McLean, P. H. (1987). Reducing staff turnover: The preceptor connection. *Journal of Nursing Staff Development, 3*(4), pp. 20–23.

Nielsen, B. (1989). Applying andragogy in nursing continuing education. *The Journal of Continuing Education in Nursing, 20*(2), p. 86.

Standards for Continuing Education in Nursing. (1984). Kansas City, MO: American Nurses Association.

Standards for Nursing Staff Development. (1990). Kansas City, MO: American Nurses Association.

Tarcinale, M. (1988). The role of evaluation in instruction. *Journal of Nursing Staff Development, 4*(3), pp. 97–103.

Tiessen, J. (1987). Comprehensive staff development evaluation. *Journal of Nursing Staff Development, 3*(4), p. 9.

Tobin, H., Beeler, J. (1988). Roles and relationships of staff development educators. *Journal of Nursing Staff Development, 4*(3), p. 91.

Tribulski, J. (1987). Staff development: Practice ethics. *The Journal of Continuing Education in Nursing, 18*(1), p. 15.

Urden, L. D. (1989). Knowledge development in clinical practice. *The Journal of Continuing Education in Nursing, 20*(1), pp. 18–22.

Waterstrade, C. (1988). Developing a hospital wide education program. *Journal of Healthcare Education and Training,* p. 6.

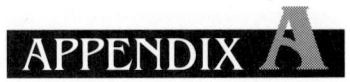

Psychomotor Domain

DESCRIPTION OF THE MAJOR CATEGORIES IN PSYCHOMOTOR DOMAIN

1. *Imitation.* The learner is exposed to an observable action and begins to make covert imitation of that action. This is then followed by overt performance of an act and capacity to repeat it.
2. *Manipulation.* Developing skill in following directions, performing selected actions, and fixing performance through necessary practice are emphasized. At this level, the learner is capable of performing an act according to instruction rather than only by observation, as in the case at the level of imitation.
3. *Precision.* Performance efficiency of a given act reaches a level of refinement. The learner performs the skill independently of a model or set of directions.
4. *Articulation.* Coordination of a series of acts emphasized by establishing an appropriate sequence or internal consistency among different acts (i.e., performance involves accuracy and control plus elements of speed and time).
5. *Naturalization.* A high level of proficiency is required to perform a single act skillfully to the extent that it becomes automatic and spontaneous.

PSYCHOMOTOR OR SKILL LEARNING: SAMPLE OBJECTIVES

1. Prepare within 15 minutes a sterile back table and Mayo stand with commonly used laparotomy instruments and equipment.
2. Draw a floor plan for a four-room operating suite that illustrates four principles of traffic control.
3. Withdraw 1.2 ml of sterile solution from a multiple-dose vial with a 5-ml syringe.
4. Unwrap a sterile article using principles of asepsis.

From Reilly, M. (Ed.). (1974). Play as exploratory learning. Troy, NY: Sage Publishing Company.

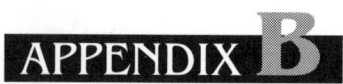

Cognitive Domain

DESCRIPTION OF THE MAJOR CATEGORIES IN THE COGNITIVE DOMAIN

1. *Knowledge.* Knowledge is defined as the remembering of previously learned material. This may involve the recall of a wide range of materials from specific facts to complete theories, but all that is required is the bringing to mind of the appropriate information. Knowledge represents the lowest level of learning outcomes in the cognitive domain.
2. *Comprehension.* Comprehension is defined as the ability to grasp the meaning of material. This may be shown by translating material from one form to another (words to numbers), by interpreting material (explaining or summarizing), and by estimating future trends (predicting consequences or effects). These learning outcomes go one step beyond the simple remembering of material and represent the lowest level of understanding.
3. *Application.* Application refers to the ability to use learned materials in new and concrete situations. This may include the application of such things as rules, methods, concepts, principles, laws, and theories. Learning outcomes in this area require a higher level of understanding than those under comprehension.
4. *Analysis.* Analysis refers to the ability to break down material into its component parts so that its organizational structure may be understood. This may include identification of the parts, analysis of the relationships between parts, and recognition of the organizational principles involved. Learning outcomes here represent a higher intellectual level than comprehension and application because they require an understanding of both the content and the structural form of the material.

5. *Synthesis.* Synthesis refers to the ability to put parts together to form a new whole. This may involve the production of a communication (theme or speech), a research proposal, or a set of abstract relations (scheme for classifying information). Learning outcomes in this area stress creative behaviors, with major emphasis on the formulation of new patterns or structures.
6. *Evaluation.* Evaluation is concerned with the ability to judge the value of material for a given purpose. The judgments are to be based on definite criteria. These may be internal criteria (organization) or external criteria (relevance to the purpose), and the student may determine the criteria or be given them. Learning outcomes in this area are highest in the cognitive hierarchy, because they contain elements of all of the other categories along with conscious value judgments based on clearly defined criteria.

COGNITIVE OR KNOWLEDGE LEARNING: SAMPLE OBJECTIVES

1. Given a list of six communicable diseases, underline three that produce a fever in the prodromal stage.
2. Given a list of functions of the professional OR nurse, identify at least five that are within your current job description.
3. Prepare a sample job description for the professional nurse in the OR using the criteria outlined.
4. Evaluate current practice for OR sanitation by comparing them with AORN Standards for OR Sanitation.

From Bloom, B. (1956). *Taxonomy of educational objectives; the classification of educational goals.* White Plains, NY: D. McKay Co.

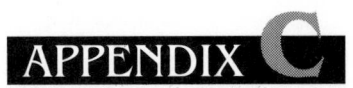

Affective Domain

DESCRIPTION OF THE MAJOR CATEGORIES IN THE AFFECTIVE DOMAIN

1. *Receiving.* Awareness or conscious recognition of the existence of a given condition.
2. *Responding.* Reacting overtly and voluntarily to a stimulus or phenomenon, and doing something with or about them. Emotional significance is attached to the stimulus.
3. *Valuing.* A step in the internalization process signified by the attachment of worth or belief. Behavior is sufficiently consistent and stable to be characteristic of a belief or attitude.
4. *Organization.* Development of values into organized systems after considering their interrelationships and establishing value priorities.

From Krathmohl, D. and Associates. (1964). *Taxonomy of education objectives.* White Plains, NY: D. McKay Co.

5. *Characterization by a Value or Value Complex.* Acting consistently in accordance with a value system. Beliefs, ideas, and attitudes are integrated into the person's total philosophy.

AFFECTIVE OR ATTITUDE LEARNING: SAMPLE OBJECTIVES

1. Write your own values with regard to change in professional nursing roles.
2. Express an opinion in relation to the guidelines for mandatory continuing education.
3. Determine a course of action that demonstrates effective resolution of a problem involving sexual behavior in the OR.

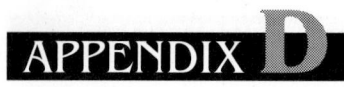

Verbs Used for Each Level of the Cognitive Domain

Knowledge

arrange	memorize
acquire	name
define	order
describe	recall
distinguish	recognize
duplicate	relate
identify	repeat
label	reproduce
list	state
match	

Application

apply	operate
choose	organize
classify	practice
demonstrate	relate
develop	restructure
employ	schedule
generalize	solve
illustrate	transfer
interpret	use

Synthesis

arrange	manage
assemble	modify
classify	organize
collect	originate
combine	plan
compose	prepare
construct	produce
create	propose
derive	set up
design	specify
develop	synthesize
document	transmit
formulate	write

Comprehension

classify	recognize
demonstrate	rephrase
describe	report
determine	restate
discuss	review
explain	rewrite
express	select
identify	summarize
indicate	tell
interpret	translate
locate	

Analysis

analyze	diagram
appraise	differentiate
calculate	discriminate
categorize	distinguish
classify	examine
compare	experiment
contrast	identify
criticize	inventory
deduce	question
detect	test

Evaluation

accuracy	estimate
appraise	evaluate
argue	judge
assess	predict
attach	rate
choose	score
compare	select
consider	standardize
contrast	support
decide	validate
defend	value

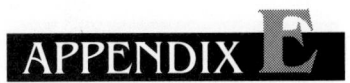

Example of Perioperative Activity Content

TITLE OF OFFERING: NURSING CARE OF A PATIENT RECEIVING A REGIONAL ANESTHETIC

Objectives	Content	Time Frame	Faculty	Teaching Method
By the end of this session, the participant will be able to:	List each topic to be covered and provide a description or outline of the content to be presented.	State the time frame for the topic.	List the presenter for each topic.	Describe the teaching method used for each.

Discuss pre-op preparation of the regional anesthesia patient.	Physical assessment
	Psychological assessment
	  Understanding of procedure
	  Preop teaching needs
	Paper preparation
	  Consent
	  Blood work
	  Radiographs
		8:00–8:30	Jane Smith, RN	Group discussion
				Lecture

List three measures used to alleviate anxiety in the regional anesthetized patient.	Physical measures
	  Position
	  Physical environment
	Communication
	  Explain procedure
	  Answer questions
	Medication
	  Effects
	  Precautions
		8:30–9:00	Jane Smith, RN	Lecture

	Questions and Answers	9:00–9:10	Jane Smith, RN	Evaluation/group discussion

CHAPTER 33

Developing Perioperative Nursing Department Policies and Procedures

Frances A. Koch

POLICIES
PROCEDURES
FORMAT OF THE POLICY AND
   PROCEDURE MANUAL
BASIC RULES OF WRITING POLICIES AND
   PROCEDURES

REVIEWING AND REVISING POLICIES AND
   PROCEDURES
ENFORCING POLICIES AND PROCEDURES
RETENTION OF POLICIES AND
   PROCEDURES

Policies and procedures are an important segment of the organizational framework of a perioperative nursing department. According to the Joint Commission on Accreditation of Healthcare Organizations (JCAHO), they are to be developed by the nursing executive, registered nurses, and designated nursing staff members and are to be defined in writing (JCAHO, 1992).

POLICIES

Policies are guidelines promulgated to assist in decision making and to ensure practice that is in compliance with standards. Policies identify responsibilities and describe actions. An effective manual serves the following functions:

1. *Promotes teamwork.* Having everyone do things the same way helps unite individuals into a team. Without effective policies and procedures, individuals are expected to learn a "new" way to do things each time they change operating rooms or specialty services.
2. *Provides clarity, consistency, and uniformity.* Written policies and procedures identify what is expected in a specific manner. The reader can envision clearly how to perform the task or can determine the parameters for decision making.

When action results from this clarity of purpose and/or function, staff performance will be the same from one time to the next and from one individual to another.
3. *Defines limits of authority and responsibility.* How do you know what to do, how far to go, and when to stop? Effective policies can identify limits.
4. *Aids in delegation.* Policies provide advance sanctioning of subordinates' decisions when they remain within policy guidelines (Haimann, 1973).
5. *Serves as a resource for accreditation and regulating agencies.* JCAHO assesses practice based on written policies and procedures. Institutions are held to the standard of practice defined in their policies and procedures. If an organization defines more stringent requirements than are stipulated in the *Accreditation Manual for Hospitals,* it will be required to meet its defined standard; otherwise, it will be judged by the standard prescribed by the accrediting body.
6. *Provides a basis for change.* Unless the current policy is known, it is impossible to know what needs to be altered. Without written policies, problems cannot be identified, and it is impossible to implement change.
7. *Ensures uniformity of action.* Through knowledge of policies, individuals are expected to perform according to the same standard and in the same manner.

8. *Establishes an avenue for consistent treatment of staff.* While patient care policies have the greatest impact on nursing care outcomes, personnel policies have the greatest impact on staff morale. Few things are more demoralizing to an operating room staff than inconsistent treatment of personnel, leading to remarks such as, "It isn't fair, I have already worked one holiday this year" or "Why doesn't Sally ever have to take call?" Staffing policies provide the framework for staff assignments. Documentation of staff assignments provides support for adherence to the policies.

9. *Provides a safeguard for nursing personnel when legal action ensues* (McKenzie, 1979). Nurses are held accountable for practice consistent with policies in place at the time of action. Adherence to policies provides a defense for action taken.

10. *Establishes a consistent level of expectation of personnel* (McKenzie, 1979). The remark "I didn't know I was supposed to do that" should never be heard. Orientation to the operating room must clearly identify each individual's responsibility to know and adhere to policies at all times.

11. *Forces management to think through the needs of the department and its employees* (Hestwood, 1988). Management is a fluid process requiring the ability to amalgamate sensory input with objective data to produce an effective outcome. Managers must continually seek input on policies/procedures from the staff, who know how tasks can be accomplished more easily. If the staff's suggestion is consistent with the standard of practice and scientific principles, the policy/procedure should be revised. Managers should not be afraid to make revisions based on staff input, as many times staff have a better understanding of the best way to accomplish a goal in the practice setting. Accepting staff recommendations affirms the manager's respect for staff members. *Always* give recognition to the staff members making the suggestion!

Policies are determined by managers; however, when staff members are included in the process, an increase in the use of the manual, as well as increased job satisfaction, can be anticipated (Douglass and Bevis, 1983).

PROCEDURES

Procedures are instructions that detail the steps to complete a task. Well-written and well-maintained procedures:

- Serve as reminders for infrequent tasks.
- Provide a resource for orienting new personnel.
- Facilitate cost containment by identifying necessary supplies and reducing waste.

- Increase productivity by decreasing time lost seeking answers.

FORMAT OF THE POLICY AND PROCEDURE MANUAL

Policy and procedure manuals should be developed according to prescribed guidelines that are determined before initiation of work.

A loose-leaf configuration works best, as it allows for additions and deletions. Ringed binders are readily available and relatively inexpensive. Pressboard report covers are also effective. They are less expensive but somewhat more difficult to disassemble for changes.

The organization of the contents must be decided. Divisions by subject facilitate location of a particular policy. Common divisions include Administration, Infection Control, and Safety and Quality Assurance (or Personnel and Patient Care).

The policies and procedures covered in the manual are listed in a Table of Contents. A numbering system that is simple and allows for changes must be established. For example:

Administration
1. Time off
  1.1 Vacation
  1.2 Personal Days
  1.3 Education Days

An appropriate page layout must be determined. Basic information should always appear in the same location. The following information should always be included (Fig. 33–1):

- Logo
- Title
- Number
- Authorizing signature/approving body
- Review date
- Revision date

The layout original should be maintained on file.

The format for the body of the document must be decided. The information to be included will vary with individual documents.

It is possible to have a policy without a procedure or a procedure without a policy. Procedures also have different components. The purpose may be included in a document if that information is unclear in the policy statement but not if the information is redundant.

Procedures may require the inclusion of equipment or supply lists. References should always be listed. The documentation should be specific, including page number.

Basic guidelines for development of a policy and procedure manual include the following:

1. Use short, concise sentences.
2. Use consistent sentence structure and phraseology.

INSTITUTIONAL LOGO

☐ POLICY NO. _____

PAGE 1 OF_____

OPERATING ROOM SERVICES

TITLE

APPROVED BY

DATE

FIGURE 33–1. Basic information for all policies. (Courtesy of Henry Ford Hospital, Grosse Point, MI.)

3. Use correct and consistent punctuation.
4. Use action verbs, when possible.
5. Always use the same tense. Present tense is preferable.
6. Use second person ("you") if possible. The same person should be used consistently.
7. Use acceptable abbreviations and format.
8. Remember the rules for using an outline format: "Every A should have its B, at least; and every 1 its 2" (Baker, 1973).
9. Avoid specific information that may change frequently (e.g., use titles instead of individual names). Avoid telephone numbers unless they are definitely assigned to a function (e.g., the Fire Department number).

BASIC RULES OF WRITING POLICIES AND PROCEDURES

Departmental policies and procedures must be consistent with institutional policies and procedures and should not conflict with other departmental policies and procedures. Exceptions should be identified.

Procedures require careful research into standards of care and performance standards for equipment. They require careful attention to detail and should provide sufficient depth for those unfamiliar with the procedure to either complete it effectively or identify the need to seek assistance (Figs. 33–2 through 33–4).

Certain policies/procedures cross departmental lines and require collaboration to ensure compliance with standards of another discipline. The degree of sophistication of the policy will dictate the direction for development. If a cooperative effort is needed to accomplish a task, the policy/procedure should be drafted and submitted to the other department for approval.

If the policy/procedure involves standards established by another discipline (e.g., blood banking), ask for assistance. Probably there are written policies that can be modified for use in the operation room.

All interdepartmental policies should be approved by all departments concerned.

Operating room policies/procedures are usually approved by the nursing director of the operating room; however, there may be policies or procedures that require approval from other individuals. Policies/procedures that involve sanctioning physicians should be signed by the appropriate physician administrator (e.g., Chief of Surgery).

A sample policy and procedure list is shown in Table 33–1.

REVIEWING AND REVISING POLICIES AND PROCEDURES

There must always be a system for policy and procedure review and revision. Each policy and procedure should be reviewed at a predetermined interval, as established by policy, and also any time there has been a change or there is a question of current appropriateness. The JCAHO stipulates a three-year review cycle for policies and procedures except for infection control policies and procedures. "All policies and procedures related to infection surveillance, prevention and control activities in all departmental services are to be reviewed and approved at least every two years" (JCAHO, 1992).

A simple way to implement a review is to divide the policy and procedure manual into 12 equal sections. A review document listing each policy and/or procedure should be completed to identify the review month for each document (Fig. 33–5).

The month preceding the review date, the list of policies and procedures to be reviewed is distributed. The goal of the review process is two-fold:

1. To ensure compliance with current standards.
2. To verify accuracy.

Staff input is essential, not only to provide assurance that the procedure is correctly documented, but also to ensure staff involvement and increase compliance.

This input is evaluated by the manager and shared, as appropriate, with the management team. Valid recommendations are incorporated in the draft revision, and the revision is reviewed by the management team. Approved revisions are then shared with the staff, posted, and placed in the manual. There must be a system for maintenance of policy and procedure manuals, and the responsibility for actually placing new documents in the manual must be assigned. However, very few things are "etched in stone." Most policies/procedures change with time and circumstances; changes should be made whenever the need for change

Text continued on page 871

Safety

☒ POLICY NO. ___322___

PAGE 1 OF _1_____

OPERATING ROOM SERVICES

TITLE

Safe Use of
Glutaraldehyde

APPROVED BY   DATE

POLICY: Glutaraldehyde is a known chemical hazard that can be irritating
            to skin, mucous membranes, and the respiratory tract. To ensure
            employee safety, personnel are required to:

            A. Wear disposable face masks to decrease inhalation.
            B. Keep the solution covered when soaking instruments.
            C. Wear goggles or a face shield to decrease the chance of
                splatter to eyes.
            D. Remove clothing wet with liquid glutaraldehyde immediately.
            E. Place solution containers in a well-ventilated area.

FIGURE 33–2. Example of a policy statement. (Courtesy of Henry Ford Hospital, Grosse Point, MI.)

Administration

☒ POLICY NO. ___204___

PAGE 1 OF _1_____

OPERATING ROOM SERVICES

TITLE

Licensure

APPROVED BY   DATE

POLICY: Registered nurses must have a current license to practice nursing.

PROCEDURE: 1. All licensed personnel must present their license to the Department of OR Services
                  Administration upon employment. A copy is made and kept on file in the department of
                  OR Services as required by the Board of Nursing.

              2. The current license must be presented before the March 31 deadline of the year
                  the license is due to expire.

              3. Failure to present licenses by the March 31 deadline of the year of expiration may
                  result in suspension without pay until proof of licensure is provided.

              4. If a graduate nurse fails the state board examination, he or she may transfer to
                  Operating Room Technician status until the examinations are successfully completed.

FIGURE 33–3. Example of a policy and procedure statement. (Courtesy of Henry Ford Hospital, Grosse Point, MI.)

<u>Patient Care</u>

☒ POLICY NO. ___104___

PAGE 1 OF __4__

OPERATING ROOM SERVICES

TITLE

Cardiopulmonary
Resuscitation (Blue Alert)

APPROVED BY

DATE

POLICY:

1. Cardiopulmonary resuscitation may be instituted by any member of the operating team who has successfully completed Basic Life Support (BLS) training.

2. The anesthesiologist and the staff physician shall be notified when a cardiac emergency occurs.

3. Call a Blue Alert by depressing the Blue Alert Button available in each OR.

4. The anesthesiologist and/or the surgeon will direct the code.

PROCEDURE:

1. When a cardiac or respiratory arrest occurs, the patient is assessed by anesthesia personnel or the surgeon, who declares the arrest and announces the time for the patient's record.

2. The circulating nurse activates the Blue Alert Red Button.

3. CPR is initiated by a qualified team member, as requested by the physician directing the code, until help arrives. The time is noted by the circulating nurse.

4. The crash cart is brought to the room, opened, and plugged in, and the defibrillator is readied for use.

5. Anesthesia personnel will prepare and give medications as needed, noting the time and dosage. The circulating nurse will assist when needed, making notes on the medication list* reflecting medications administered, dosage, and time administered.

6. If a consultation is needed, dial 61234 and ask the operator to page whatever specific service you need "STAT FOR THE OR."

7. The scrub nurse should maintain the sterile field, if appropriate.

8. The circulating nurse will share the medication notes with anesthesia personnel to verify medication administration, dosages, and times. The medication notes are then discarded.

A

FIGURE 33–4. *A,* Example of a policy and procedure statement for cardiopulmonary resuscitation. (Courtesy of Henry Ford Hospital, Grosse Point, MI.)

Medication Notes

ITEM	DOSE	TIME	DOSE	TIME	DOSE	TIME	DOSE	TIME
Edrophonium chloride (Tensilon), 10 mg/ml								
Dobutamine								
Bretylium, 50 mg/ml								
Phenylephrine hydrochloride (Neo-Synephrine)								
Verapamil								
Propranolol hydrochloride (Inderal)								
Epinephrine								
Dexamethasone (Hexadrol)								
Digoxin (Lanoxin)								
Deslanoside (Cedilanid-D)								
Atropine								
Isoproterenol hydrochloride (Isuprel)								
Norepinephrine bitartrate (Levophed)								
Retinene								
Metaraminol bitartrate (Aramine)								
Sodium chloride for injection								
Procainamide hydrochloride (Pronestyl)								
Methylprednisolone sodium succinate (Solu-Medrol)								
Water for injection								
Furosemide (Lasix)								
Lidocaine (Xylocaine)								
Heparin sodium (Liquaemin Sodium)								
Dopamine (Intropin)								
Potassium chloride for injection								
Sodium bicarbonate								
Aminophylline								
Calcium chloride								

B

FIGURE 33–4 *Continued B*, Example of medication notes that are attached to a cardiopulmonary resuscitation policy and procedure statement. (Courtesy of Henry Ford Hospital, Grosse Point, MI.)

POLICIES–1989	REVISED	IN BOOK
JULY		
Medical services representatives #114		
Students, visitors, and guests #126		
ID and care of surgical specimens #112		
Presurgical skin preparation #119		
AUGUST		
Emergency CABG following coronary angioplasty #108		
Cardiopulmonary resuscitation #104		
Patient safety in transit #118		
SEPTEMBER		
Scheduling of OR personnel #206		
OR dress code #117		
Safety during laser surgery #314		
OCTOBER		
Credentialing doctor for laser surgery #106		
Scheduling of laser surgery #122		
Staff surgeon presence in OR #124		
Scheduling surgical procedure #123		

FIGURE 33–5. Example of schedule for review of policies and procedures. (Courtesy of Henry Ford Hospital, Grosse Point, MI.)

TABLE 33–1. POLICY AND PROCEDURE LIST

Administration
  Management—responsibility and accountability
  Preoperative nursing assessment
  Staffing pattern
  Emergency access for level I and level II emergency services
  Pharmacy inspection
  Scheduling policies and procedures
  Preoperative instructions for patients
  Record retention
  Credentialing, physician
  Credentialing, laser surgery
  Credentialing, nonphysician
  Cardiopulmonary resuscitation certification requirements
  Licensure
  Informed consent
  Handling of legal evidence
  Vacation scheduling
  Observation in the operating room
  Loan of equipment, supplies, and instrumentation
  Supplies—restocking and rotation
  Staff surgeon presence in operating room
  On-call
  Attendance
  Education meeting days
Infection control
  Principles of asepsis
  Sterilization and disinfection
  Maintenance and surveillance of sterilization equipment
  Sanitation of rooms and equipment
  Selection of draping and gowning materials
  Preoperative skin or body cavity preparation of patients
  Wearing apparel for surgery and anesthesia personnel
  Traffic control
  Receiving, decontamination, cleaning, preparing, disinfecting, and sterilizing reusable items
  Shelf life of sterile items
  Recall of products—internal and external
  Management of patients with communicable diseases
  Handling of materials
  Assembly, wrapping, storage, distribution, and quality control of sterile equipment and medical supplies
  Use of sterilization process monitors
  Selection, storage, handling, use, and disposition of disposable items
  Reuse of disposable items
  Reprocessing of disposable items to be reused
Safety protection of personnel
  Hazardous waste identification, handling, use, storage, and disposition
  Monitoring of radiation exposure
  Safe use of radioactive materials and imaging equipment
  Handling of specimens
  Storage and handling of blood and blood components
  Identification and disposal of outdated or unusable drugs
  Distribution and administration of controlled drugs
  Equipment testing—prior to use and annually
  Orientation and continuing education of users
  Counts—sponges, sharps, instruments
  Patient transportation
  Traffic pattern
  Patient identification
  Incident reporting
  Laser safety
  Fire safety

This list of policies and procedures is provided to identify specific policies and procedures that may be useful, but it is not intended to be inclusive or in any way a "recipe" for what is needed in any particular institution.

is identified. Advise staff on changes promptly and monitor compliance.

ENFORCING POLICIES AND PROCEDURES

Policies and procedures must be enforced. Compliance with policies/procedures requires continual monitoring. Each member of the perioperative team is responsible for being alert to infractions. Just as a "sterile" conscience must be developed, so must a "policy/procedure" conscience be developed. Policy/procedure enforcement should not be punitive unless there is no alternative. If policies/procedures are current, practical, effective, efficient, and result in a positive outcome, punitive enforcement should not be necessary. Compliance can be achieved by identifying how the policy/procedure helps the patient or employee. Policies/procedures written with staff input tend to have staff support. If an individual refuses to adhere to a policy/procedure, the disciplinary process must be initiated, beginning with documentation of expectations, time of expected compliance, and the result of noncompliance.

If noncompliant behavior is demonstrated by a physician member of the team, staff nurses are empowered to enforce the policy/procedure. The process should begin by having the nurse share the policy/procedure with the physician in an assertive manner. If the physician refuses to comply, the behavior must be reported to a manager. The appropriate action is dependent on the nature of the infraction. If the action is pending and may affect patient outcome, a manager must be summoned immediately. If the infraction has been completed or will not affect patient outcome, the behavior should be shared, in writing, with a manager, so that she or he can discuss the reason for the policy/procedure with the physician in a positive conference.

It is every staff member's responsibility to monitor compliance and correct violations. Adherence to policies and procedures should be a criterion for performance-based appraisal. An important part of managers' performance appraisal is the support of policies and procedures and compliance of staff.

During orientation, it should be documented in the newly employed nurse's record that all policies and procedures were reviewed. When a new policy or procedure is adopted, it should be presented at an inservice session, and it may be worthwhile to have nurses sign a notation for their file stating that they have reviewed the new policy or procedure (Creighton, 1987).

RETENTION OF POLICIES AND PROCEDURES

Copies of all previous policies and procedures must be maintained on file, as any legal decisions will be based on the policy or procedure in force at the time the alleged problem arose.

Compliance with policies and procedures demonstrates that the nurse meets the institution's standard of care (Creighton, 1987).

Bibliography

Baker, S. (1973). *The practical stylist* (3rd ed.). New York: Thomas Y. Crowell.

Barras, A. (1985). Developing an effective policy and procedure manual. *Medical Laboratory Observer, 17*(6), 28–33.

Campbell, J. M. (1983). The personnel policy manual. *Pediatric Nursing, May/June,* 209, 229.

Creighton, H. (1987). Legal implications of policy and procedure manual—part I. *Nursing Management, 18*(4), 22–28.

Creighton, H. (1987). Legal implications of policy and procedure manual—part II. *Nursing Management, 18*(5), 16–18.

Douglass, L. M., Bevis, E. A. (1983). *Nursing management and leadership in action* (4th ed.). St. Louis: C. V. Mosby.

Gross, R. C. (1985). The development of a format for a policy and procedure manual for allied health administration. *Journal of Allied Health, 14,* 395–402.

Haimann, T. (1973). *Supervisory management for health care institutions.* St. Louis: The Catholic Hospital Association.

Hestwood, T. M. (1988). Make policy manuals useful and relevant. *Personal Journal, April,* 43–46.

Holle, M. L., Blatchely, M. E. (1982). *Introduction to Leadership and Management in Nursing.* Monterey, CA: Wadsworth Health Sciences Division.

Joint Commission on Accreditation of Healthcare Organizations. (1992). *Accreditation Manual for Hospitals.* Chicago: JCAHO.

McKenzie, R. (1979). Structural standards developing a service philosophy and a policy manual. *The Lamp, December,* 5–6.

Morton, P. G. (1985). A hospital nursing education manual. *Journal of Nursing Staff Development, Summer,* 61–67.

Nardecchia, M. A., Myers, M. F. (1980). The policy manual: a basis for legal protection. *Nursing Administration Quarterly, 5*(1), 57–62.

Price, C. (1984). *The Management Guide For Developing Group Practice Personnel Policies, Procedures and Employee Handbooks.* Denver, CO: Medical Group Management Association.

Rawland, H. S., Rawland, B. L. (eds.). (1985). *Nursing Administration Handbook* (2nd ed.). Rockville, D: Aspen.

Smith, J. M. (1988). *Operating Room Update.* Palas Verdes Estates, CA: Academy Medical Systems, Inc.

Smith-Marker, C. (1988). *The Marker Model for Nursing Standards OR Applications.* Boulder, CO: OR Manager.

Stevens, B. J. (1985). *The Nurse As Executive* (3rd ed.). Rockville, MD: Aspen.

Thomas, D. O. (1987). How to survive an accreditation review. *RN, April,* 17–20.

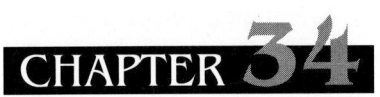
Financial Management for the Perioperative Nursing Manager

Jeannie Botsford

FINANCIAL MANAGEMENT IN THE CURRENT HEALTH CARE ENVIRONMENT

Perioperative nurse managers must understand financial management and have astute business skills to function effectively in the ever-changing economic environment of health care. Deregulation and the rationing of health care services have significantly changed the role and responsibilities of the perioperative nurse manager. Financial management of the operating room has expanded beyond the concept of an isolated unit to a much broader perspective; the chief financial officer no longer simply tells the perioperative nurse manager how much money is allocated for the surgery department for the coming fiscal year. The operating room must be run like a business; it must be financially responsible and profit oriented. Administrators look for fiscal accountability as part of management effectiveness. Changing roles and increased responsibilities have expanded the perspective and potential for financial leadership.

The health care industry will continue to change as we approach the turn of the century. Managing in the midst of these changes mandates the use of all learned and acquired skills. Understanding financial management and keeping abreast of changes are key factors in developing a financial management strategy for the perioperative nurse manager.

Federal Regulations

Federal regulations, fixed reimbursement, and competitive contracting all affect the financial picture and, ultimately, the institution's profit or loss (Grimaldi, 1983) The perioperative nurse manager must be knowledgeable about regulations governing the health care delivery system and aware of how they impact the management of the operating room. As the resident expert, the perioperative nurse manager can best determine how surgical care can be delivered economically. The key to success is keeping the cost of service down while maintaining a high level of operational performance. The manager must draw on knowledge of strategy, courage, innovation, and tenacity to be an effective financial manager and achieve a leadership position in the institution's financial arena.

Economic Implications

Understanding the economic implications of the changing reimbursement system is paramount for the

873

nurse participating in financial management. Managers must be knowledgeable about regulations in the health care delivery system and be aware of how they affect the operation of surgical services.

DRGs and Fixed Reimbursement

The diagnosis-related group (DRG) prospective reimbursement system has significantly affected the revenue-generating potential of the operating room. Fixed-rate reimbursement is an important concept for the manager to understand in light of surgical charges that might appear profitable but in fact are not when only a percentage of the charges is actually reimbursed.

Understanding how much money is generated for a specific surgical procedure can help the operating room manager determine how much to spend on labor and supplies to ensure profitability for the department.

Coping with fixed reimbursement has made competition between hospitals fierce. Hospitals have to re-evaluate how to attract physicians and patients to the hospital to ensure solvency. Negotiating and contracting with preferred-provider organizations and health care maintenance organizations have become crucial elements for the management in health care institutions (Bernam and Weeks, 1982).

Perioperative nurse managers must identify outside resources and seek individuals within their institution who can assist them in understanding the economic constraints and how they affect the surgical department. A DRG coordinator or contract coordinator who can assist in giving information and advice to the perioperative nurse manager is usually available in the hospital's finance department.

Challenges and Opportunities

Many nurse managers experience apprehension and anxiety when faced with participating in budget preparation and being accountable for the financial functioning of their department. Perioperative managers practicing in the current complex financial environment must be challenged and motivated to expand their knowledge base to include such components as the budget process, cost accounting, break-even analysis, and the ability to read and understand the financial statements (Weston and Brigham, 1986). These tools will better equip the manager to defend expenditures, justify equipment purchases, and participate effectively in hospital-wide financial operations.

The more knowledge and understanding the nurse manager has about the financial operation of the specialty unit and the institution in general, the greater will be his or her ability to control decisions and effect change. Financial accountability will enable the manager to negotiate from a position of strength and influence decision making.

Strategy

Understanding change and its effects is a crucial aspect of the perioperative manager's strategy. It is important to train oneself to respond to change rather than to react, and to be able to adapt one's own action plan. Programming oneself to analyze situations and develop a plan to handle change on one's own terms helps managers to feel they are in control.

Financial management challenges the participant to use knowledge, strategy, and savvy to gain desired results. How that knowledge is acquired and used, not just knowledge itself, can determine success or failure as a manager. The ability to use political savvy to sway opinion is a key aspect of the successful manager's job. Reframing a question or repositioning oneself in a situation allows the manager to present ideas from a different perspective or set of circumstances. This is important when the manager feels that a favorite project may not be approved. Often, by reframing the question or changing the perspective from which the approach was made, one can alter the outcome in a positive way.

Two important strategies must be kept in mind when dealing in financial management. First, the manager must persevere and identify any adjustments, adaptations, or flexible elements that can be applied to the situation. Managers must know their negotiating position and predetermine what they are willing to trade off in order to attain something else. Second, it is essential not to get discouraged during tough times so that the long-term rewards of sound fiscal management can be realized.

The operating room manager must be prepared to fight for budgeted dollars, identified programs, and projects that are crucial to the success of the department.

MANAGEMENT INFORMATION SYSTEMS

Establishing a systematic and orderly system to capture and retain information is essential for managing economically and understanding the dynamics of financial management. Modern information systems supply in-depth data necessary for accurate cost accounting and up-to-date analysis of the current financial status of the department (Austin, 1983). Computer software systems store and expand information and provide statistics to assist the operating room manager in establishing accurate data and recognizing trends.

Computer systems may not be available in all institutions, and if one is not available, a manual system can be implemented. The better organized the manual system, the easier it will be to enter the information into a computer system later.

Surgical statistics must be readily available to the manager who seeks to affect decision making and support projects that are being pursued. The ability to relate current data, case mix, cost per unit of service, physician activity, trends, and the percentage of growth will place the manager in a position of perceived command and authority. The credibility of the perioperative manager will be destroyed by the inability to retrieve and relate current data. The ability to sway opinions and affect decision making can be the difference between success or failure.

Computerized information systems in the operating room can be an asset to the functioning of the department and can assist in financial management. A well-developed and integrated system must have the capacity for on-line scheduling, maintenance of preference cards, printing of the daily schedule, billing, and accumulation of statistics. This will enhance the functioning and capability of the surgery manager (Widhalm, 1988). Careful planning and assessment of department and institutional needs will ensure that an appropriate computerized system is selected.

A computerized case cart system can save time and energy by identifying supplies needed for surgical procedures. A printout of the next day's schedule, including the physician's preference file (PPF) for each specific surgeon and procedure, will expedite early and accurate selection of items and supplies for each procedure.

Budgeting, statistical reporting, quality assurance (QA) analysis, staff credentialing, and the staff scheduling are all capabilities of a modern computerized system. These functions should be available to the perioperative manager through a well-programmed information system.

Computer technology is instrumental in assisting the manager to meet the challenges of cost-effective management. Future innovations for surgical services will include hand-held computers used by the circulating nurse in each operating room suite; these will assist in timely inputing of data and charging of supplies. Interdepartmental communications will be improved when blood banks, pathology, and radiology reports are expedited by computer systems installed in each operating room suite.

The surgery department is a vital part of the institution's overall revenues and expenses and therefore is a prime area in which computerized systems can help track the DRG cost reimbursement factor. Cost analysis of patient care according to surgical procedure becomes an accurate measurement tool for the nurse manager to identify and justify costs for effective financial management.

portant role in product evaluation and purchasing decisions for equipment and supplies used in the surgery department. Product standardization is essential for cost effectiveness and efficiency in procurement of supplies. Factors that must be considered are availability, delivery, reliability of service, packaging, and storage.

Maintaining appropriate volume in the surgery department can be a challenge because of the unpredictable nature of the case mix and emergency procedures. Patient care may be compromised when understocking occurs, whereas overstocking results in poor utilization of storage space and financial resources. Computerized inventory systems can provide up-to-date analysis of product availability and product usage and identify the need for reordering by reducing inventory when the item is used and billed.

Control of inventory can cause conflict when a surgeon is emphatic about a particular type and brand of product and the operating room manager has been mandated to cut costs. One approach to resolve this dilemma is to establish an internal inventory product standardization committee within the surgery department. Participants should include the surgery director, the chief of surgery, the assistant director assigned to oversee inventory management, and a representative from the material management department. Cooperation can be gained by identifying less frequently used items that can be removed from the inventory and having the chief of surgery make the recommendation at the Department of Surgery monthly meeting. The chances of the recommendation being accepted are increased because of the participation and presentation by surgeon to his or her fellow colleagues. Significant reduction of inventory can be achieved by this method without undesired turmoil and stress.

Inventory management is directly related to control of supplies, which is carried out by purchasing policies, an internal control mechanism within the surgery department, and accounts payable management. To achieve inventory control, the cooperative efforts of central services, materials management, and surgery personnel must be realized. Monthly task force meetings or a quality circle committee comprised of representatives from identified departments will enhance the cooperative effort and result in effective problem solving and financial savings. Time and money can be saved through these combined efforts when cost-consciousness is increased and a cost-effective action implemented.

INVENTORY MANAGEMENT

Inventory control is one of the most vital components in keeping overhead costs and cost per unit of service down. When inventory management is inadequate, large amounts of department capital may be tied up in inventory and thus are unavailable for other expenditures. A financially astute manager knows that inventory items and supplies translate into dollars.

The perioperative nurse manager must play an im-

BUDGETING: A MANAGEMENT TOOL

Budgeting is the heart of financial management, and the effective nurse manager knows that strong managers must learn to master the budget process. Basic fundamental skills are needed by managers to successfully meet the demands in health care. More than ever before, good fiscal management is needed to maximize limited reimbursement and the scarce resources that are available. Budgeting can improve efficiency and provide essential documentation to demonstrate compliance within institutional guidelines (Stechert, 1987). The budgeting process is a tool by which management plans are translated into financial terms and then evaluated in relation to financial and statistical criteria.

Goals and Objectives

For the budget to function as a tool, managers must establish goals and objectives to determine what activity will occur and what services will be provided and to identify the necessary equipment and supplies necessary to accomplish these activities. The perioperative nurse manager should know the institutional goals and establish department goals and objectives that will facilitate these institutional goals (Fig. 34–1).

Planning is the cornerstone to developing budgetary strategy and identifying the framework for monitoring and control. The Mission Statement and Strategic Plan of the institution will assist the manager in understanding and providing guidelines for participation.

Goals and objectives are necessary to identify needed changes to the existing programs and also to give direction and guidance for future programs or systems. These terms are often used interchangeably, but each has a specific meaning:

Goal: An end toward which effort is to be directed.
Objective: A milestone on the road to achieving a goal.

When goals and objectives are integrated as part of the budget process, they provide a means of recording the desired progress and identifying the difference between actual progress achieved and that that was targeted.

The hospital goals should include providing quality patient services to fulfill the needs of the community and delivering services in an efficient manner through good management of facilities and resources.

STATEMENT OF OBJECTIVE

ORIGINATOR:

DEPARTMENT: Surgery

PERFORMANCE PLANNING YEAR: FY _____

OBJECTIVE: WEIGHTED % _____

ACTION PLAN: (Steps to complete Objective and proposed completion date.)

REVIEW DATE:

RESOURCES REQUIRED:

HUMAN (FTES) _____ FINANCIAL ($) _____ PHYSICAL _____

RESULTS EXPECTED/BENEFIT TO ORGANIZATION:

    Cost reduction/financial savings.

METHOD OF EVALUATING RESULTS:

STATEMENT OF SHARED COMMITMENT:

SUBMITTED   DATE
SHARED COMMITMENT   DATE

APPROVED:

_____ DATE _____

_____ DATE _____

FIGURE 34–1. Statement of objective. (Courtesy of Henry Mayo Newhall Memorial Hospital, Valencia, CA.)

Department goals may focus on patient care programs, training and development, quality control, and intra- or interdepartmental functioning. Identified programs can be presented with other departments as shared goals, with commitment indicated by all affected directors approving the goal.

The criteria for effective goals and objectives are as follows:

- Goals and objectives must be *measurable*—stated in such a way that the degree to which they are attained can be measured.
- Goals and objectives must be *understandable*—fully understood by those who are responsible for their attainment.
- Goals and objectives must be *achievable*—attainment should be feasible within given constraints.

Financial planning contributes significantly to accomplishment of the stated goals and objectives. It provides the nurse manager with the ability to make critical decisions and provide direction for the department. When the strategic planning process is on line, the possibility of attaining the goals and objectives is greatly enhanced.

Whatever goals and objectives are formulated, they must be consistent and in harmony with the overall objectives and philosophy of the nursing department and institution (Koontz and O'Donnell, 1978).

Units of Service

Forecasting units of service (UOS) (e.g., surgery hours, procedures, cases, or patients) is a key component of the budget, affecting projected staffing needs and identifying expenses and revenues for the budget year.

Collecting accurate historical data is essential to successful budgeting and financial planning. This preliminary function should be given careful attention and analysis by the perioperative nurse manager (Appendices A, A1, and A2).

Forecasting is based on the assumption that trends and patterns have been established in the past. Internal and external factors must be considered carefully before any prediction of increase or decrease of activity is made. Key physicians must be consulted to accurately determine changes in surgical specialties, projected case mix, new procedures, or anticipated high and low seasonal activity. External factors might include unusual growth or decline in the hospital's service, economic fluctuation, or a shift to alternative methods of health care delivery (e.g., a free-standing ambulatory facility).

The manager must have input into and trust the UOS projection, as total support and accountability will be expected.

Position Control and Staffing Cost

The *position control* is a list of approved labor positions necessary to meet the staffing requirement for the surgery department. The position control displays the approved positions by category of personnel (e.g., registered nurses, certified operating room technicians, aides), as well as by the number of part-time equivalents (PTEs) or full-time equivalents (FTEs). An FTE is a unit of time that is equivalent to 40 hours of work per week, 80 hours per pay period, and 2080 hours per year.

Salary costs are divided into fixed and variable costs. Fixed labor costs are paid no matter what the volume of surgical procedures per fiscal year. Examples include salaries for the unit secretary, nursing manager, on-site staff for trauma response, and any other position that does not vary with the number of surgeries.

The *position control plan* is a projection of staffing requirements that determines how many FTEs will be required to assist with the forecasted number of surgical procedures in the budgeted year. The manager must identify how many PTEs and FTEs will be necessary to adequately cover the projected work load. This will depend on the number of surgical suites that will be open and the number of hours designated for elective and emergency surgeries as determined by surgery department policy.

Historical statistics must be carefully evaluated and implemented to determine correct projections for department coverage. Paid hours include worked time, also called productive time, and nonproductive time (i.e., sick time, vacation time, education, and on-call time) (Fig. 34–2 and Appendix B). Relief coverage for sick days, holidays, and vacations and weekend coverage must be calculated. On-call hours will also need to be identified and funds allocated accordingly for stand-by and call-back hours at the designated rate of pay.

Cost Accounting (Appendices C through G1)

Cost accounting is the process of identifying total costs and assigning them to specific items, procedures, or services provided within the surgery department. The principles and application of cost accounting are important concepts for the nurse manager to grasp. There is an ever-increasing expectation in the health care environment to reduce costs to coincide with the decline in fixed reimbursement. Outpatient reimbursement is becoming more regulated, and pressure to reduce costs will continue as the outpatient volume increases.

Line-item analysis and a breakdown of costs per procedure are essential management tools for surgical services. It enables the manager to make intelligent decisions regarding reduction of services, case mix, productivity assessment, and volume expansion.

The perioperative manager must know the components of costs, including supplies, overhead, direct and indirect costs, and fixed and variable labor costs. The ability to analyze profit or loss per procedure can then be made through a comparison of the total costs and the actual reimbursement received per procedure (Appendices D through G1).

NONPRODUCTIVE SALARY BUDGET

DEPARTMENT NAME, NUMBER

SPREAD OF NONPRODUCTIVE
SALARIES

DESCRIPTION	OCT	NOV	DEC	JAN	FEB	MAR	APR	MAY	JUNE	JULY	AUG	SEPT	TOTAL
A. Total holidays (from Exhibit A)	0	8	8	16	0	0	0	8	0	16	0	8	64
1. Bud. FTEs (flows from salary wksts)	0.00	0.00	0.00	0.00	0.00	0.00	0.00	0.00	0.00	0.00	0.00	0.00	0.00
2. Days in the month	31	30	31	31	28	31	30	31	30	31	31	30	365
3. Reg. accrual (handouts)	0.00	0.00	0.00	0.00	0.00	0.00	0.00	0.00	0.00	0.00	0.00	0.00	0.00
4. Vacation hours (2 + 3)	0	0	0	0	0	0	0	0	0	0	0	0	0
5. Holiday hours (A + 1)	0	0	0	0	0	0	0	0	0	0	0	0	0
6. Educ. other hours (best estimate)	0	0	0	0	0	0	0	0	0	0	0	0	0
7. Sick hours to be used (best estimate)	0	0	0	0	0	0	0	0	0	0	0	0	0
8. Total nonprod. hours	0	0	0	0	0	0	0	0	0	0	0	0	0
9. Dept. hourly rate (FROM SALARY WORKSHEETS)	0.00	0.00	0.00	0.00	0.00	0.00	0.00	0.00	0.00	0.00	0.00	0.00	0.00
10. Subtotal nonprod. to FXSTAFF	$0	$0	$0	$0	$0	$0	$0	$0	$0	$0	$0	$0	$0
11. Call, bonus, sick payoff, and other	$0	$0	$0	$0	$0	$0	$0	$0	$0	$0	$0	$0	$0
12. Nonprod. salary (To B-3)	$0	$0	$0	$0	$0	$0	$0	$0	$0	$0	$0	$0	$0

FIGURE 34–2. Nonproductive salary budget. (Courtesy of Henry Mayo Newhall Memorial Hospital, Valencia, CA.)

Fixed and Flexible Budgeting

A *fixed budget* (Appendix H) is based on a fixed level of annual activity or volume divided by 12 months to arrive at a monthly average. The fixed budget does not allow for monthly variations and thus is not the most desirable type of budget for the surgery department, as it cannot be easily adjusted to reflect actual activity levels in comparison with costs.

Flexible budgeting (Fig. 34–3 and Appendix I) requires more time and resources to develop but provides a more accurate evaluation of financial performance, regardless of activity level. It takes variations in volume into account, and the range of activity is estimated based on a projected range of volume from low to high. Flexible budgeting varies as the UOS changes. As the number of surgical procedures increases or decreases, expenses are adjusted up or down in a predetermined manner to reflect this variation. Fixed costs are not flexible, and consequently budget flexibility is directly related to variable costs resulting from an increase or decrease in surgical procedures.

Nonsalary Expenses

The cost of supplies are allocated as nonsalary expenses and should closely follow the UOS for the department. In budgeting, the manager should attempt to determine the relationship between actual nonsalary expense and department activity. The projected UOS or number of surgical procedures are used as a basis for identifying supply requirements, and these requirements are then translated into dollars.

Prices of supplies usually rise a certain amount each year depending on the rate of inflation. This rate must be identified and incorporated into the budget projections. The rate of inflation to use is established by the institution and is usually provided in the budget preparation packet.

Determining future needs is a vital part in calculating the supply budget. The manager must be informed as to any changes, new specialties, procedures, or services that might affect the use and need of supplies.

Supplies are categorized as medical or nonmedical, and it is important for the manager to ensure that correct subaccount numbers are assigned at the time of budgeting and costs appropriated as requisitions are made and supplies used throughout the fiscal year.

Capital Budget

The capital budget component of the budget includes supplies and equipment that cost more than a predetermined fixed amount (often $500) and has a life span of a designated number of years (usually three) (Fig. 34–4 and Appendix J). Equipment specified in the capital budget is nonexpendable and can be depreciated over a period of years.

Capital budget requests must include justification for purchase and as much documentation as possible (e.g., product and cost analysis, vendor information, number of years required to obtain return of the original investment [payback period], and the average rate of return on an investment [ROI]) (Hoffman, 1986).

Information should be provided about whether the requested item is a new piece of equipment or a replacement and which quarter of the fiscal year the requested item is to be purchased.

The more support and justification the nurse manager can provide for the capital budget requests, the more likely it is that these requests will be granted. Integration of capital equipment requests into a marketing plan will verify the need for specialized equipment for new procedures or services. This can be presented along with appropriate input and a documented request from the

VARIABLE STAFF ANNUAL SALARY BUDGET FORM

DEPARTMENT NAME

TRENDS DATA	MONTH NAME	
YTD productive salaries (trends)		0
YTD nonproductive salaries (trends)		0
YTD employee benefits (trends)		0
Variable avg. hourly rate (p/r rpts)		0.00
Merit increase % for balance of current fiscal year (see instructions)		0.00%
Merit increase for fiscal year 199☐		0.00%
Budgeted units of service		
Productive hours per unit of service		0.00
Fixed staff hours per week		0
Fixed staff hourly rate		0.00
Variable productive salaries		0
FY 199☐ fixed salary amount (computed)		0
Total productive salaries		0
Total productive hours		0
Total productive full-time equivalents		0.00

FIGURE 34–3. Variable staff annual salary budget. (Courtesy of Henry Mayo Newhall Memorial Hospital, Valencia, CA.)

surgeons involved (e.g., an orthopedic specialist requesting arthroscopy equipment expansion).

A cost-benefit analysis will demonstrate the cost of purchasing the piece of capital equipment and a comparison of that cost with the benefits that will be derived from use of that equipment. The perioperative manager must also be prepared to project the break-even point (i.e., the point at which the revenue generated covers the cost of equipment, based on the number of proce-dures done or the number of times the equipment is used).

Depreciation of expenses for items purchased in the capital budget should be calculated and included in the expense summary spreadsheet (Fig. 34–5).

Monitoring and Control

The budget proposal is only one segment of the overall budget process and financial management of the surgery department. Monitoring and control are essential functions that must follow budget approval to ensure adherence and successful implementation of the budget throughout the fiscal year.

A *variance* is the difference between the planned budgeted costs and the actual costs. Variances must be easily identifiable and will assist the manager in pinpointing trouble spots. The *variance report* is a method of using the budget as a comparison and evaluation tool. Budgeted figures are compared with actual figures to identify compliances with or deviations from the budget. An acceptable percentage of variance above or below the budget is usually established by the administration, and the manager must be able to justify variations from those standards and present solutions to correct the situation.

Monthly and year-to-date data must be used to identify and implement adjustments that must be made to manage the budget. Departmental reports should be made as soon as possible after the end of the month, addressing any problems and explaining corrective action taken. In this way, progress toward goals and objectives can be demonstrated, enabling the manager and administration to evaluate operational effectiveness.

Page 1   **SANTA CLARITA HEALTHCARE ASSOCIATION**
DEPARTMENTAL CAPITAL BUDGET SUMMARY
DEPARTMENT NAME

CO.	Dept. No.	Description	Qty.	Prty. Code	First Quarter	Second Quarter	Third Quarter	Fourth Quarter	199☐ Summary	199☐	199☐	Summary
			0						0			0
			0						0			0
			0						0			0
			0						0			0
			0						0			0
			0						0			0
			0						0			0
			0						0			0
			0						0			0
			0						0			0
			0						0			0
			0						0			0
			0						0			0
			0						0			0
			0						0			0
			0						0			0
			0						0			0
			0						0			0
			0			0	0	0	0	0	0	0	0

FIGURE 34–4. Departmental capital budget summary. (Courtesy of Santa Clarita Healthcare Association, Valencia, CA.)

SANTA CLARITA HEALTHCARE ASSOCIATION
CAPITAL EXPENDITURE JUSTIFICATION

Dept: _____ Replacement _____ New item _____ Remodel project _____

Item Description _____

_____

_____

_____

_____

Priority:
Cost (Incl. sales tax and freight)—Each $ _____ Qty. _____ = Total _____

Estimated life in years _____ Date needed: _____

Reasons and justification

_____

_____

_____

_____

_____

_____

_____

_____

_____

_____

_____

Approvals

Department Director _____ Date: _____

Contract Physician _____ Date: _____

Administrative Director _____ Date: _____

FIGURE 34–5. Capital expenditure justification. (Courtesy of Santa Clarita Healthcare Association, Valencia, CA.)

MARKETING

The principles of marketing management have direct application in the operating room and are so vital to its function that they cannot be left to a marketing administrator in a distant office. Each member of the surgical staff is part of the marketing team and is vital to selling operating services.

The perioperative nurse manager must develop a marketing strategy and communicate to the surgeons that the hospital wants their business. The surgery department and staff must be available to provide services in a convenient, cost-effective manner for both patient and physician. The surgeons are the primary target, because they direct the patient to the facility where a procedure will be done. Patients need to know the benefits of the services provided and will be attracted to a facility that has cultivated individualized patient care.

Hassle-free surgery scheduling and convenience in patient admission are vital components of a successful marketing plan to attract physicians and patients. Hospitals can expedite the process by computerized scheduling that links surgery with admitting; one phone call from the physician's office will initiate the scheduling and admitting process. Preadmission forms can be supplied to the physician's office to simplify and personalize admission of the surgery patient.

Scheduling meetings with key surgeons is a good marketing strategy and enables the perioperative nurse manager to obtain feedback as to how services are being received and information on how services can be improved from the surgeon's perspective.

The shift to ambulatory or short-stay surgery has opened up new areas of marketing possibilities for the perioperative nurse manager. By using the "four Ps" of marketing—Product, Promotion, Place, and Price—the nurse manager can attract future patients and physicians to the hospital and contribute to the success of the surgery department's expansion and growth.

The marketing strategy for the surgery department is based on organizational goals and objectives and defines a course of action by identifying the targeted market and allocating specific resources to achieve these goals.

Glossary of Budgetary Terms

Assets: Economic resources that can be expressed in monetary terms such as cash, accounts receivable, inventories, and equipment.

Balance sheet: A financial statement that reports the assets and liabilities of a company at one point in time.

Break-even point: The level of business volume at which total revenue equals total costs.

Budget: Projected financial statements used for comparison with actual performance to stimulate improvements in the use of an institution's resources in a planning and control process.

Capital equipment: A major purchase, usually defined as above a baseline cost with an expected life span.

Cost accounting: The process of identifying total costs and assigning them to the service that the company provides.

Cost center: A functional unit for which cost control and accountability can be assigned.

Cost per case: The expense to a department to provide specific intervention for a patient from admission to the time of discharge.

Depreciation: The process of recognizing a portion of the cost of an asset as an expense during each year of its estimated service life.

Expenditure: A liability arising from the acquisition of an asset.

Expense: A decrease in owner's equity resulting from operations.

Fixed cost: Costs that do not vary with the level of activity.

Income statement: A statement of revenues and expenses for a given period; a flow report.

Inflation: The erosion of real income by price increases.

Indirect cost: Those costs that are not readily identified with a particular department and are often allocated among departments.

Inventory: An asset record in which is recorded the purchase price of supply items held for patient use.

Liabilities: Present obligations resulting from past transactions that require an institution to pay money, provide goods, or perform services in the future.

Marketing: A human activity directed at satisfying needs and wants through the exchange process.

Marketing strategy: Set of objectives, policies, and rules that determine the institution's marketing efforts over time.

Net income: The amount by which total revenues exceed total expenses for a given period.

Net loss: The amount by which total expenses exceed total revenues for a given period.

Nonsalary budget: Supplies, linen, uniforms, services, repairs, maintenance, education, and depreciation.

Operating budget: Revenue and expense budget.

Overhead: Any cost of doing business other than a direct cost of a service.

Prospective reimbursement: Reimbursement-of-payment schedules that are set or determined before the services are delivered.

Purchase order: A document completed by the department setting forth quantities, description, price, and vendor for merchandise to be purchased.

Retrospective reimbursement: Reimbursement or payment for services after they are delivered or received.

Revenues: Actual or expected cash inflow as a result of departmental ongoing operations.

Return on investment: Return of income received from services of purchased capital equipment calculated by the cost of initial purchase minus depreciation.

Strategic plan: The managerial process of developing and maintaining a viable relationship between the organization and its environment by developing a mission, goals, strategies, and operational plans.

Variable budget: A budget designed to vary with volume of activity.

Bibliography

Austin, CJ. (1983). *Information systems for hospital administrators* (2nd ed.). Ann Arbor, MI: Health Administration Press.

Babtist, A. (1987). A general approach to costing procedures in ancillary departments. *Topics in Health Care Financing, 13* (4), 32–47.

Bernam, H., Weeks, L. (1982). *The financial management of hospitals* (5th ed.). Ann Arbor, MI: Health Administration Press.

Cleverly, W. (1986). *Essentials of healthcare finance* (2nd ed.). Rockville, MD: Aspen.

Coile, R. (1986). *The new hospital: Future strategies for a changing industry.* Rockville, MD: Aspen.

Cooper, PD. (1982). *Health care marketing management.* Rockville, MD: Aspen.

Finkler, S. (1984). *Budgeting concepts for nurse managers.* Orlando: Grune & Stratton.

Grimaldi, P.L. (1983). Public law 97–24B: The implications of prospective payment schedules. *Nurse Manager, 14*(2).

Groah, L.K. (1985). Preparing the O.R. budget: The nurse managers responsibility. *AORN Journal, 41*(3), 547–553.

Hoffman, F.M. (1986). The capital budget: Developing a capital expenditure proposal. *AORN Journal, 44*(4), 604–610.

Kerschner, M., Rooney, J. (1987). Utility cost accounting information for budgeting. *Topics in Health Care Financing, 13*(4), 56–66.

Kirk, R. (1981). *Nursing management tools.* Boston: Little, Brown.

Koontz, H., O'Donnell C. (1978). *Essentials of management.* New York: McGraw-Hill.

Krueger, D., Davidson, T. (1987). Alternative approaches to cost accounting. *Topics in Health Care Financing, 13*(4), 1–9.

Mark, B., Smith, H. (1987). *Essentials of finance in nursing.* Rockville, MD: Aspen.

Porter-O'grady, T. (1987). *Nursing finance, budgeting strategies for a new age.* Rockville, MD: Aspen.

Quayle, SN. (1978). Efficient costing and budgeting in the operating room theater. *National News, 15*(2), 11–14.

Schimmel, V., Cassandra, H. (1987). Measuring costs productive accounting versus ratio of costs to changes. *Topics in Health Care Financing, 13*(4), 78–86.

Slezak, L.G. (1986). A computerized operating room scheduling and utilization system. *Perioperative Nursing Quarterly, December,* pp 22–28.

Spitzer, R., Davivier, M. (1987). Nursing in the 1990's: Expanding opportunities. *Nursing Administration Quarterly, 11*(2), 55–61.

Stechert, K. (1987). Strategic budgeting in good times and bad. *Working Woman, June,* 87–91.

Strasen, L. (1987). *Key business skills for nurse managers.* Philadelphia: J.B. Lippincott.

Weston, J. F., Brigham, E. F. (1986). *Essentials of managerial finance* (7th ed.). Chicago, IL: Dryden Press.

Widhalm, S. (1988). Challenge and opportunity: Preparing for automation in the operating room. *Health Care, March,* 36–37.

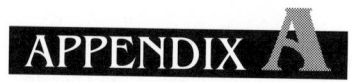

APPENDIX A

Instructions for Completing the Units of Service Forecast (FA Form) and Staffing Position Worksheet

PURPOSE

Projected units of service are the foundation for the budget process. Projected activity serves to guide revenue and salary and supply expenses, which comprise the bulk of your budget.

PROCEDURE

1. You will receive this form (Appendix A1) from the finance department already filled out except for the last two columns. The column entitled "Preliminary Projection" is the column you should complete.
2. Several procedures have been executed by the time you receive this form. First, Administration will have approved Primary Units of Service such as patient days, surgeries, and emergency room visits. Second, the Financial Analysis Department will have made a preliminary projection for your department using appropriate statistical methods and available subjective information.
3. Before entering your projections, it is strongly recommended that you compare the historical data shown on the form with your own records of activity.

4. The staffing position worksheet (Appendix A2) will aid you in making your projections. When completing the staffing worksheet, consider the relationship of your departmental activity to the primary units of service, historical trends, changes in service, departmental goals and objectives, anticipated physician utilization, and other observed activity patterns.

You should include shift differential in the monthly salary value for appropriate positions.

For the column "Classification No." on Appendix A1, enter the personnel classification code for that position. The classification number for each level of staffing must be supplied by the institution's Human Resources department.

The section entitled "Existing of Per Diem/Casual Positions" should be used to list the current and planned *annual* usage of per diem and casual employees. The planned FY 199☐ usage hours are converted into equivalent FTEs by dividing the total hours by 2080 (two decimal places).

The space labeled "Monthly Salary" is optional if you use Appendix E1. To complete this information, use your best estimate of your average monthly per diem/casual salary costs.

Complete the bottom two lines on the form to obtain total current monthly salaries and total FY 199☐ budgeted FTEs.

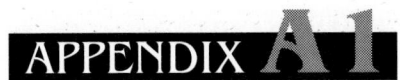

Units of Service Forecast— FY 199☐ (FA Form)

_____

| PREPARED BY | DATE | UNIT OF SERVICE | DEPARTMENT |

| APPROVED BY | DATE | | DEPARTMENT |

MONTH	ACTUAL	ACTUAL	ACTUAL	FY 199☐ CURRENT YEAR BUDGET	FY 199☐ CURRENT YEAR ACTUAL	FY 199☐ PRELIMINARY PROJECTION	APPROVED BUDGET
OCT.							
NOV.							
DEC.							
JAN.							
FEB.							
MAR.							
APR.							
MAY							
JUN.							
JUL.							
AUG.							
SEPT.							
TOTAL							

% Change From Prior Year

Annualized Actuals based on actual versus budget performance extended for remainder of the year. For Nursing Units:

Available Beds _____ Projected Census _____ Occupancy _____

Additional Comments: _____
_____
_____

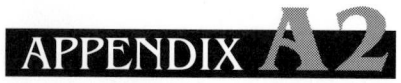

Staffing Position Worksheet

DEPARTMENT _____

Prepared by _____

Classification No.	POSITION CLASSIFICATIONS	APPROVED FTEs	CURRENT FTEs	BUDGETED FTEs	CURRENT MONTHLY SALARY
0		0.0	0.0	0.0	0
0		0.0	0.0	0.0	0
0		0.0	0.0	0.0	0
0		0.0	0.0	0.0	0
0		0.0	0.0	0.0	0
0		0.0	0.0	0.0	0
0		0.0	0.0	0.0	0
0		0.0	0.0	0.0	0
0		0.0	0.0	0.0	0
0		0.0	0.0	0.0	0
0		0.0	0.0	0.0	0
TOTAL FTEs AND SALARIES		0.0	0.0	0.0	0

EXISTING PER DIEM/CASUAL POSITIONS	CURRENT AVAIL HRS	PLANNED 1993 HRS	MONTHLY SALARY
	0	0	0
	0	0	0
	0	0	0
		P/D FTEs	
TOTAL PER DIEM HOURS	0	0.00	0
TOTAL SALARIES (PER DIEM PLUS REGU) TOTAL MONTHLY SALARY			0

Courtesy of Henry Mayo Newhall Memorial Hospital, Valencia, CA.

Instructions for Completing the Budgeted Nonproductive Salaries Form

The Budgeted Nonproductive Salaries Form (see Fig. 34–2) was developed to help compute nonproductive salary budgets. It is designed to provide a more accurate delineation of nonproductive salary expenses by budgeting expenses in the month that they occur. Several items can affect the spread of nonproductive salaries:

- *Holidays:* Both floating holidays and observed holidays are expensed to the departments when earned by the employee. This means that December, January, June, July, and September will have higher nonproductive costs, because they contain pay periods in which holidays are earned. The worksheet allows you to adjust for this by recording eight hours per employee per holiday.
- *Education and Orientation Hours:* Hours coded to these categories are recorded as nonproductive salary expense. The number of education hours should be recorded in the month in which the educational program is anticipated.
- *Sick Leave:* Sick time is charged to the department when it is used. Consequently, employees who take sick leave cause additional expense to be charged to the department. If there are times in which you

anticipate having employees out sick (e.g., during pregnancy or flu season), you should include the anticipated use of time in the appropriate time period.
- *Sick Leave Payouts:* These should be budgeted in each month based on the anticipated hours to be paid out in December as the hours are earned (one half of the eligible hours over 220 or a full hour for each hour over 320 hours). The system expenses over-220 and over-320 amounts each month as the hours are earned. Refer to your nonproductive salary reports to determine the monthly accrual.
- *Vacation and On-Call Time:* Each department accrues vacation time based on the seniority of personnel. You can determine your department's accrual rate by reviewing your paid time off reports. The accrual rate will increase on employees' anniversary dates when the amount of vacation time for which the employee is eligible increases. The department may also experience an increase in nonproductive salary expenses with each pay increase as the value of an employee's accrued hours increases. On-call time is also coded to nonproductive time and is included in the worksheet.

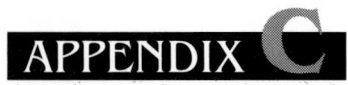

APPENDIX C

Instructions to Complete Supply Costs and Purchased Services Summary

PURPOSE

Annual supply costs will be developed for the yearly budget using this form. Additionally, both purchased medical services and other purchased services for the new budget year will result.

PROCEDURE

1. Complete the informational section at the top of the form (department name, etc.).

2. The section entitled "Supply Costs" should be self-explanatory. You will need the inflation multiplier for each supply category from Administration to complete the form.
   - _____ Inflation multiplier for medical supplies
   - _____ Inflation multiplier for nonmedical supplies
   - _____ Inflation multiplier for pharmaceuticals
   - _____ Inflation multiplier for food

3. Departments without specific units of service should use the number of months to calculate the year-to-date monthly expense.

4. Be prepared to discuss supply costs in detail at your budget hearing. Please list the major categories of supply usage in the departmental budget being presented and include explanations of why these supplies are needed. Include suggestions for cost reductions in your presentation.

5. List purchased medical services and other purchased services currently being used by your department. The column entitled "Natural Classification" should be determined by using the Trends Report and accounts payable distribution. Under each month, enter projected values for contract renewal dates. Expected increases and other changes to existing arrangements should be considered.
   a. After obtaining totals for the FY 199☐ budget, you should spread the total throughout the 12 months in Appendix G1 using an appropriate method.
   b. Be prepared to explain the need for the budgeted purchased services in detail and to demonstrate what actions you have taken to control costs in this area.

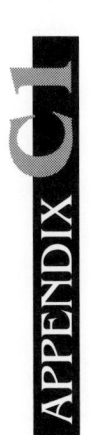

Monthly Budgeted Expense Data Entry Form

DEPARTMENT NAME, NUMBER

Prepared By _____

For Those Expenses Budgeted by Month Enter in the Appropriate Month Below _____

Natural Classification	Sub Acct		October	November	December	January	February	March	April	May	June	July	August	September	Total Direct Mths.	Enter UOS Amts Below / Spread by UOS
Productive salaries	2	00	0	0	0	0	0	0	0	0	0	0	0	0	0	0
Paid time off salaries	1	12	0	0	0	0	0	0	0	0	0	0	0	0	0	0
Subtotal salaries			0	0	0	0	0	0	0	0	0	0	0	0	0	0
Benefit (%)	0		0	0	0	0	0	0	0	0	0	0	0	0	0	0
Registry	1	19	0	0	0	0	0	0	0	0	0	0	0	0	0	0
Medical fees	1	21	0	0	0	0	0	0	0	0	0	0	0	0	0	0
Supplies—medical	1	20	0	0	0	0	0	0	0	0	0	0	0	0	0	0
Supplies—nonmedical	1	41	0	0	0	0	0	0	0	0	0	0	0	0	0	0
Supplies—food	1	46	0	0	0	0	0	0	0	0	0	0	0	0	0	0
Supplies—minor equip	1	43	0	0	0	0	0	0	0	0	0	0	0	0	0	0
Purch svcs—medical	1	49	0	0	0	0	0	0	0	0	0	0	0	0	0	0
Purch svcs—nonmed	1	61	0	0	0	0	0	0	0	0	0	0	0	0	0	0
Maintenance	1	66	0	0	0	0	0	0	0	0	0	0	0	0	0	0
Utilities	1	62	0	0	0	0	0	0	0	0	0	0	0	0	0	0
Equipment rental	1	85	0	0	0	0	0	0	0	0	0	0	0	0	0	0
Insurance	1	76	0	0	0	0	0	0	0	0	0	0	0	0	0	0
Depreciation	1	81	0	0	0	0	0	0	0	0	0	0	0	0	0	0
Interest (financing)	1	74	0	0	0	0	0	0	0	0	0	0	0	0	0	0
Legal and audit fees	1	68	0	0	0	0	0	0	0	0	0	0	0	0	0	0
Advertising	1	22	0	0	0	0	0	0	0	0	0	0	0	0	0	0
Employee-related exp	1	90	0	0	0	0	0	0	0	0	0	0	0	0	0	0
Transfer in costs	1	88	0	0	0	0	0	0	0	0	0	0	0	0	0	0
Transfer out costs	1	94	0	0	0	0	0	0	0	0	0	0	0	0	0	0
Other expenses	1	92	0	0	0	0	0	0	0	0	0	0	0	0	0	0
Subtotal expense		89	0	0	0	0	0	0	0	0	0	0	0	0	0	0
Units of svc	S.66		1	2	3	4	5	6	7	8	9	10	11	12	78.0	78.0
Productive hours	S.00		0.0	0.0	0.0	0.0	0.0	0.0	0.0	0.0	0.0	0.0	0.0	0.0	0.0	0.0
Pd time off hours	S.12		0	0	0	0	0	0	0	0	0	0	0	0	0	0
Full-time equivalents prod.			0.0	0.0	0.0	0.0	0.0	0.0	0.0	0.0	0.0	0.0	0.0	0.0	0.00	0.00
Revenue per unit			0.00	0.00	0.00	0.00	0.00	0.00	0.00	0.00	0.00	0.00	0.00	0.00	0.00	14.00

Courtesy of Henry Mayo Memorial Hospital, Valencia, CA.

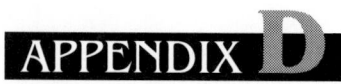
APPENDIX D

Form for Determining Natural Class for Intercompany Billings

DEPARTMENTS IN THE HOSPITAL

Actual	Budget	Description	Supplies or Services From
.38	330	Medical supplies	Drugs
.94	920	Transfers—other	Drugs
.61	410	Med. purchased svcs.	Extracorporeal
.62	415	Maintenance	Bio-Med
.62	415	Maintenance	Engineering
.66	420	Purchased svcs., other	Housekeeping
.66	420	Purchased svcs., other	Dietary (catering svcs.)
.43	345	Food (pantry supplies)	Dietary/purchasing
.87	560	Employee related	Education
.87	560	Physicals	Management group
.90	230	Advertising	Association/other
.66	420	Purchased svcs., other	Public relations

DEPARTMENTS IN THE ASSOCIATION

Actual	Budget	Description	Supplies or Services From
.38	330	Medical supplies	Drugs
.94	920	Medical supplies	Drugs
.62	415	Maintenance	Bio-Med
.62	415	Maintenance	Engineering
.66	420	Purchased svcs., other	Housekeeping
.66	420	Purchased svcs., other	Dietary (catering svcs.)
.43	345	Food (pantry supplies)	Dietary/purchasing
.87	560	Employee related	Education
.87	560	Physicals	Management group
.94	920	Purchased svcs., other	Public relations

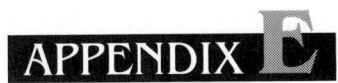

Instructions for Completing the Revenue and Expense Comparison Form

PURPOSE

This form provides a convenient tool for analyzing your FY 199☐ budget as compared with the current year's actual performance.

PROCEDURE

1. Complete the informational section at the top of the page.

2. Information from Adjusted Annualized Expense Worksheet (Appendix E1), column 5, should be entered in the first column of Appendix E2.

3. Enter the revenue, expenses, and units of service budgeted for this year in the second column.

4. Enter in the "FY 199☐ Budget" column the projected expenses and units of service (expenses from Appendix G1 and units of service from Appendix A1).

5. The first comparison column compares current year actual results with the current year budget. Carry the division to two decimal places.

6. The second comparison column compares the proposed budget with current year actual results. The division should be carried to two decimal places.

7. If the results in the last colum for any item are greater than 1.10 or less than 0.90, an explanation should be made as to the reason for the increase or decrease.

INSTRUCTIONS FOR THE REVENUE AND EXPENSE PER UNIT COMPARISON

1. Each category of expenses—actual annualized, budget 199☐ and budget 199☐—from the budget revenue and expense analysis completed earlier is to be divided by the appropriate units of service, and the result entered here. Please enter result to two decimal places. The comparison columns should be completed, and any variances of plus or minus 10% must be explained.

2. Those departments without specific departmental units of service should use total patient days in this calculation.

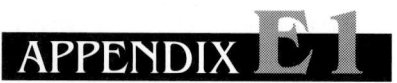
Budget Revenue and Expense Per Unit

DEPARTMENT NAME, NUMBER

DESCRIPTION	(1) ANNUALIZED FY 199☐ ACTUAL	(2) FY 199☐ BUDGET	(3) COMPARISON (2)/(1)	(4) FY 199☐ BUDGET	(5) COMPARISON (4)/(1)
UNITS OF SERVICE	1	1	100.00%	1	100.00%
REVENUE PER UNIT	0.00	0.00	0.00%	0.00	0.00%
(NAT. CLASS) EXPENSES:					
(00.) Productive salaries	0.00	0.00	0.00%	0.00	0.00%
(.12) Nonproductive salaries	0.00	0.00	0.00%	0.00	0.00%
Total Salaries	0.00	0.00	0.00%	0.00	0.00%
(.19) Benefits	0.00	0.00	0.00%	0.00	0.00%
(.21) Registry	0.00	0.00	0.00%	0.00	0.00%
(.20) Med. fees	0.00	0.00	0.00%	0.00	0.00%
(.41) Med. supplies	0.00	0.00	0.00%	0.00	0.00%
(.46) Nonmed supplies	0.00	0.00	0.00%	0.00	0.00%
(.43) Food	0.00	0.00	0.00%	0.00	0.00%
(.49) Minor equipment	0.00	0.00	0.00%	0.00	0.00%
(.61) Med. purch. svs.	0.00	0.00	0.00%	0.00	0.00%
(.66) Nonmed purch. svs.	0.00	0.00	0.00%	0.00	0.00%
(.62) Maintenance	0.00	0.00	0.00%	0.00	0.00%
(.85) Utilities	0.00	0.00	0.00%	0.00	0.00%
(.76) Equip. rental	0.00	0.00	0.00%	0.00	0.00%
(.81) Insurance	0.00	0.00	0.00%	0.00	0.00%
(.74) Depreciation	0.00	0.00	0.00%	0.00	0.00%
(.68) Interest	0.00	0.00	0.00%	0.00	0.00%
(.23) Legal and audit	0.00	0.00	0.00%	0.00	0.00%
(.90) Advertising	0.00	0.00	0.00%	0.00	0.00%
(.87) Employee-related	0.00	0.00	0.00%	0.00	0.00%
(.94) Transfer in	0.00	0.00	0.00%	0.00	0.00%
(.92) Transfer out	0.00	0.00	0.00%	0.00	0.00%
(.89) Other expenses	0.00	0.00	0.00%	0.00	0.00%
Total expense	0.00	0.00	0.00%	0.00	0.00%
Contribution margin	0.00	0.00	0.00%	0.00	0.00%

Explanation of significant variances %

Courtesy of Henry Mayo Memorial Hospital, Valencia, CA.

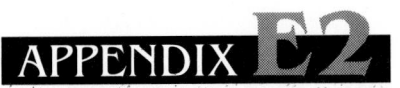

Budget Revenue and Expense Analysis

DEPARTMENT NAME, NUMBER
INFORMATION FROM NONSALARY WORKSHEET FOR 1 AND 4

DESCRIPTION	(1) ANNUALIZED FY 199☐ ACTUAL	(2) FY 199☐ BUDGET	(3) COMPARISON (2)/(1)	(4) FY 199☐ BUDGET	(5) COMPARISON (4)/(1)
UNITS OF SERVICE	1	1	100.00%	1	100.00%
REVENUE PER UNIT	0.00	0.00	0.00%	0.00	0.00%
REVENUE	0	0	0.00%	0	0.00%
(NAT. CLASS) EXPENSES:					
(00.) Productive salaries	0	0	0.00%	0	0.00%
(.12) Nonproductive salaries	0	0	0.00%	0	0.00%
Total Salaries	0	0	0.00%	0	0.00%
(.19) Benefits	0	0	0.00%	0	0.00%
(.21) Registry	0	0	0.00%	0	0.00%
(.20) Med. fees	0	0	0.00%	0	0.00%
(.41) Med. supplies	0	0	0.00%	0	0.00%
(.46) Nonmed. supplies	0	0	0.00%	0	0.00%
(.43) Food	0	0	0.00%	0	0.00%
(.49) Minor equipment	0	0	0.00%	0	0.00%
(.61) Med. purch. svs.	0	0	0.00%	0	0.00%
(.66) Nonmed. purch. svs.	0	0	0.00%	0	0.00%
(.62) Maintenance	0	0	0.00%	0	0.00%
(.85) Utilities	0	0	0.00%	0	0.00%
(.76) Equip. rental	0	0	0.00%	0	0.00%
(.81) Insurance	0	0	0.00%	0	0.00%
(.74) Depreciation	0	0	0.00%	0	0.00%
(.68) Interest	0	0	0.00%	0	0.00%
(.23) Legal and audit	0	0	0.00%	0	0.00%
(.90) Advertising	0	0	0.00%	0	0.00%
(.87) Employee-related	0	0	0.00%	0	0.00%
(.94) Transfer in	0	0	0.00%	0	0.00%
(.92) Transfer out	0	0	0.00%	0	0.00%
(.89) Other expenses	0	0	0.00%	0	0.00%
Total expense	0	0	0.00%	0	0.00%
Contribution margin	0	0	0.00%	0	0.00%

Explanation of significant variance %

_____

_____

_____

_____

Courtesy of Henry Mayo Memorial Hospital, Valencia, CA.

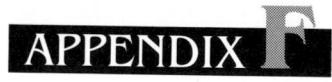
Instructions for Completing the Departmental Adjusted Annualized Expense Worksheet

PURPOSE

This form will help you in comparing your annualized expenditures with your current-year budget.

PROCEDURE

1. Fill in the actual departmental expenses from your most recent Trends Report. Enter the annualizing factor for the date of the Trends Report in column 2 and multiply column 2 times column 1.

2. In column 4 you should enter on the appropriate line:
   a. Additional expenditures that you anticipate will begin to occur on a regular basis before the end of the current fiscal year but are not yet reflected on your current trends.
   b. Reclassifications of expenses between natural classifications if reflected incorrectly in current year-to-date trends.
   c. Deletion of one-time nonrecurring expenses reflected on your current trends that should not be budgeted in the following year.
   On a separate page, a brief explanation should be made for all items entered onto column 4.

3. You arrive at column 5 by taking column 3 plus or minus the amounts listed in column 4.

4. The estimates in column 5 are then carried forward to the Revenue and Expense Analysis (see Appendix E1).

Date Of Trends Report	Column 2 Annualizing Factor
October	12.000
November	6.000
December	4.000
January	3.000
February	2.400
March	2.000
April	1.714
May	1.500
June	1.333
July	1.200
August	1.091
September	1.000

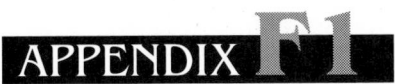
Detail of Subaccounts: Natural Class (Budget Code) Groups for Expenses

PRODUCTION SALARY (110)
.00 Management and supervision
.01 Technician and specialist
.02 Registered nurses
.03 Licensed vocational nurses
.04 Aides and orderlies
.05 Clerical and other administrative
.06 Environmental and food service
.07 Physicians
.08 Non-physician medical practitioners
.09 Other salaries and wages

PAID LEAVE, HOLIDAY AND SALARY
   CONT. (120)
.12 Vacation, holiday, and sick leave

REGISTRY PERSONNEL (130)
.21 Registry personnel

EMPLOYEE BENEFITS (140)
.10 FICA
.11 Unemployment and disability insurance
.13 Group health insurance
.14 Group life insurance
.15 Pension and retirement
.16 Workers' compensation insurance
.17 Deferred equity investment contract
.18 Group life benefit
.19 Miscellaneous

MEDICAL FEES AND COMMISSIONS
   (210)
.20 Medical fees—physicians
.26 Medical—non-patient care

LEGAL, AUDIT, AND CONSULTING
   FEES (220)
.22 Consulting and management
.23 Legal
.24 Audit
.25 Other

ADVERTISING (230)
.90 Advertising

MEDICAL SUPPLIES (330)
.27–.30 Reserved for future use
.31 Prosthesis
.32 Sutures and surgical needles
.33 Surgical packs and sheets
.34 Surgical supplies—general
.35 Anesthetic materials
.36 Oxygen and other medical gases
.37 IV solutions
.38 Pharmaceuticals
.39 Radioactive materials
.40 Radiology films
.41 Other medical care materials and
   supplies

NONMEDICAL SUPPLIES (340)
.44 Linen and bedding
.45 Cleaning supplies
.46 Office and administrative supplies
.47 Employee wearing apparel
.50 Other nonmedical supplies
.51 Printing and duplicating
.52 Inventory obsolescence
.53–.59 Reserved for future use

FOOD (345)
.42 Food—meats, fish, and poultry
.43 Food—other

MINOR EQUIPMENT (350)
.48 Instruments and minor medical
   equipment
.49 Other minor equipment

PURCHASED MEDICAL SERVICES
   (410)
.60 Reserved for future use
.61 Medical

MAINTENANCE (415)
.62 Repairs and maintenance

OTHER PURCHASED SERVICES (420)
.63 Medical school contracts
.65 Collection agencies
.66 Other—purchased services

HOSPITAL SERVICES (430)
.64 Management services

DEPRECIATION AND AMORTIZATION
   (510)
.72 Depreciation and amortization—land
   improvements
.72 Depreciation and amortization—building
   improvements
.73 Depreciation and amortization—leasehold
   improvements
.74 Depreciation and amortization—
   equipment

RENTAL/LEASE COST (520)
.75 Rental/lease cost—buildings/land
.76 Rental/lease cost—equipment

FINANCING COSTS (530)
.67 Reserved for future use
.68 Other financing costs
.69 Bond interest
.70 Financing amortization

UTILITIES (540)
.77 Utilities—electricity
.78 Utilities—gas
.79 Utilities—water
.80 Utilities—other
.85 Telephone/Telegraph

INSURANCE (550)
.81 Insurance—professional liability
.82 Insurance—other

EMPLOYEE RELATED EXPENSE (560)
.86 Dues and subscriptions
.87 Outside training
.88 Travel

OTHER EXPENSES (590)
.83 Licenses and taxes (other than on income)
.84 Other unassigned costs
.89 Other expenses
.96–.99 Reserved for future use

INTERDEPT. TRANSFERS TO OTHER
   DEPTS. (910)
.91 Transfers to other hospital depts.—labor
.92 Transfers to other hospital depts.—suppl.
   and other exp.

INTERDEPT. TRANSFERS FROM OTHER
   DEPTS. (920)
.93 Transfers from other hospital depts.—
   labor
.94 Transfers from other hospital depts.—
   suppl.

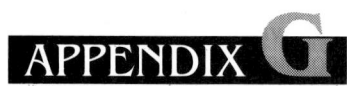

APPENDIX G

Instructions for Completing the Department Expense Budget Summary

PURPOSE

This form (Appendix G1) has been revised for input into the computer. It shows all departmental expenses on a single page and is the document used to keypunch data into the computer system. The original documents will be given to the financial analyst, and photocopies will be retained by the hospital.

PROCEDURE

1. First complete the informational section at the top of the form (department name, etc.). If Appendix G1 pertains to more than one cost center, make sure you use the "key" department number that controls your Trends Report.

2. Productive and nonproductive annual salaries have already been calculated on the salary worksheet (Appendix E1), and the results are transferred to

Appendix G1. Similarly, supply costs and purchased services can be transferred from the Supplies and Purchased Services Worksheet to Appendix G1.

3. Employee benefits are to be calculated by multiplying the appropriate percentage for each month times the total productive salary for each month. The employee benefits percentage is included on your key information handout from Administration. Multiply each month by the appropriate percentage for that month and enter the result on the benefits line in Appendix G1. Those departments using a variable staffing format must enter their monthly productive salaries from Appendix E1 in order to complete the benefits calculation.

4. Units of service, FTEs, and revenue per unit must be entered on the Appendix G1.

5. Total the annual column to determine your total departmental expense. Then double-check this total for accuracy.

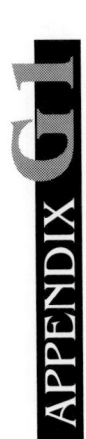
Budget Summary

Department Approval   Date

DEPARTMENT NAME, NUMBER   Dept.

Prepared By:

Approved By: Approval Date

Natural Classification	Sub Acct	Oct	Nov	Dec	Jan	Feb	March	April	May	June	July	Aug	Sept	Total
Productive salaries	2 00	0	0	0	0	0	0	0	0	0	0	0	0	0
Paid time off salaries	1 12	0	0	0	0	0	0	0	0	0	0	0	0	0
Subtotal salaries		0.00	0.00	0.00	0.00	0.00	0.00	0.00	0.00	0.00	0.00	0.00	0.00	0.00
Benefit (%) 0.00%	1 19	0	0	0	0	0	0	0	0	0	0	0	0	0
Registry	1 21	0	0	0	0	0	0	0	0	0	0	0	0	0
Medical fees	1 20	0	0	0	0	0	0	0	0	0	0	0	0	0
Supplies—medical	1 41	0	0	0	0	0	0	0	0	0	0	0	0	0
Supplies—nonmedical	1 46	0	0	0	0	0	0	0	0	0	0	0	0	0
Supplies—food	1 43	0	0	0	0	0	0	0	0	0	0	0	0	0
Supplies—minor equip	1 49	0	0	0	0	0	0	0	0	0	0	0	0	0
Purch svcs—medical	1 61	0	0	0	0	0	0	0	0	0	0	0	0	0
Purch svcs—nonmed	1 66	0	0	0	0	0	0	0	0	0	0	0	0	0
Maintenance	1 62	0	0	0	0	0	0	0	0	0	0	0	0	0
Utilities	1 85	0	0	0	0	0	0	0	0	0	0	0	0	0
Equipment rental	1 76	0	0	0	0	0	0	0	0	0	0	0	0	0
Insurance	1 81	0	0	0	0	0	0	0	0	0	0	0	0	0
Depreciation	1 74	0	0	0	0	0	0	0	0	0	0	0	0	0
Interest (financing)	1 68	0	0	0	0	0	0	0	0	0	0	0	0	0
Legal and audit fees	1 22	0	0	0	0	0	0	0	0	0	0	0	0	0
Advertising	1 90	0	0	0	0	0	0	0	0	0	0	0	0	0
Employee-related exp	1 88	0	0	0	0	0	0	0	0	0	0	0	0	0
Transfer in costs	1 94	0	0	0	0	0	0	0	0	0	0	0	0	0
Transfer out costs	1 92	0	0	0	0	0	0	0	0	0	0	0	0	0
Other expenses	1 89	0	0	0	0	0	0	0	0	0	0	0	0	0
Subtotal expense		0	0	0	0	0	0	0	0	0	0	0	0	0
Units of svc	S.66	1	2	3	4	5	6	7	8	9	10	11	12	78
Product hours	S.00	0	0	0	0	0	0	0	0	0	0	0	0	0
Pd time off hours	S.12	0	0	0	0	0	0	0	0	0	0	0	0	0
Full-time equivalents		0.00	0.00	0.00	0.00	0.00	0.00	0.00	0.00	0.00	0.00	0.00	0.00	0.00
Revenue per unit		0.00	0.00	0.00	0.00	0.00	0.00	0.00	0.00	0.00	0.00	0.00	0.00	0.00
Gross revenue		0	0	0	0	0	0	0	0	0	0	0	0	0
Contractual allowances		0	0	0	0	0	0	0	0	0	0	0	0	0
Contribution margin		0	0	0	0	0	0	0	0	0	0	0	0	0

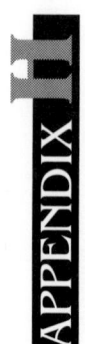

APPENDIX H

Fixed Staff Annual Salary Budget

DEPARTMENT NAME, NUMBER

AUTHORIZED POSITION	REVIEW DATE	Month the Year Code (?1)	OCTOBER MONTHLY SALARY	YEARLY MERIT INCR	NO. OF FTEs	1 OCT	2 NOV	3 DEC	4 JAN	5 FEB	6 MAR	7 APR	8 MAY	9 JUN	10 JUL	11 AUG	12 SEP	TOTAL
7-DAY STAFFING	Revw. Dte	0	0	0.0%	0.0	0	0	0	0	0	0	0	0	0	0	0	0	0
7-DAY STAFFING	Revw. Dte	0	0	0.0%	0.0	0	0	0	0	0	0	0	0	0	0	0	0	0
7-DAY STAFFING	Revw. Dte	0	0	0.0%	0.0	0	0	0	0	0	0	0	0	0	0	0	0	0
7-DAY STAFFING	Revw. Dte	0	0	0.0%	0.0	0	0	0	0	0	0	0	0	0	0	0	0	0
7-DAY STAFFING	Revw. Dte	0	0	0.0%	0.0	0	0	0	0	0	0	0	0	0	0	0	0	0
7-DAY STAFFING	Revw. Dte	0	0	0.0%	0.0	0	0	0	0	0	0	0	0	0	0	0	0	0
7-DAY STAFFING	Revw. Dte	0	0	0.0%	0.0	0	0	0	0	0	0	0	0	0	0	0	0	0
7-DAY STAFFING	Revw. Dte	0	0	0.0%	0.0	0	0	0	0	0	0	0	0	0	0	0	0	0
7-DAY STAFFING	Revw. Dte	0	0	0.0%	0.0	0	0	0	0	0	0	0	0	0	0	0	0	0
7-DAY STAFFING	Revw. Dte	0	0	0.0%	0.0	0	0	0	0	0	0	0	0	0	0	0	0	0
7-DAY STAFFING	Revw. Dte	0	0	0.0%	0.0	0	0	0	0	0	0	0	0	0	0	0	0	0
7-DAY STAFFING	Revw. Dte	0	0	0.0%	0.0	0	0	0	0	0	0	0	0	0	0	0	0	0
7-DAY STAFFING	Revw. Dte	0	0	0.0%	0.0	0	0	0	0	0	0	0	0	0	0	0	0	0
7-DAY STAFFING	Revw. Dte	0	0	0.0%	0.0	0	0	0	0	0	0	0	0	0	0	0	0	0
7-DAY STAFFING	Revw. Dte	0	0	0.0%	0.0	0	0	0	0	0	0	0	0	0	0	0	0	0
7-DAY STAFFING	Revw. Dte	0	0	0.0%	0.0	0	0	0	0	0	0	0	0	0	0	0	0	0
7-DAY STAFFING	Revw. Dte	0	0	0.0%	0.0	0	0	0	0	0	0	0	0	0	0	0	0	0
5-DAY STAFFING	Revw. Dte	0	0	0.0%	0.0	0	0	0	0	0	0	0	0	0	0	0	0	0
5-DAY STAFFING	Revw. Dte	0	0	0.0%	0.0	0	0	0	0	0	0	0	0	0	0	0	0	0
5-DAY STAFFING	Revw. Dte	0	0	0.0%	0.0	0	0	0	0	0	0	0	0	0	0	0	0	0
5-DAY STAFFING	Revw. Dte	0	0	0.0%	0.0	0	0	0	0	0	0	0	0	0	0	0	0	0
5-DAY STAFFING	Revw. Dte	0	0	0.0%	0.0	0	0	0	0	0	0	0	0	0	0	0	0	0
5-DAY STAFFING	Revw. Dte	0	0	0.0%	0.0	0	0	0	0	0	0	0	0	0	0	0	0	0
5-DAY STAFFING	Revw. Dte	0	0	0.0%	0.0	0	0	0	0	0	0	0	0	0	0	0	0	0
TOTAL SALARIES			0															
TOTAL FTEs					0.0	0.0	0.0	0.0	0.0	0.0	0.0	0.0	0.0	0.0	0.0	0.0	0.0	0.0

NONPRODUCTIVE REDUCTION FACTOR FROM NONPRODUCTIVE WORKSHEET 0 0 0 0 0 0 0 0 0 0 0 0 0

PRODUCTIVE $ (TO LINE 019, FORM B-3)
(TOTAL SALARIES MINUS NONPRODUCTIVE $) 0 0 0 0 0 0 0 0 0 0 0 0 0

WORKING DAYS 5-DAY

Courtesy of Henry Mayo Memorial Hospital, Valencia, CA.

898

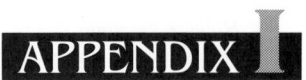

Variable Staff Annual Salary Budget Form

COMPANY _____

VARIABLE STAFF ANNUAL SALARY BUDGET FORM (S-2V)

Trends As Of _____

_____
Fiscal Year

Month

Prepared by: _____   Department: _____

Date: _____   Department #: _____

Total budgeted FTEs: _____   Budgeted UOS (annual total): _____

COMPUTATIONS:

1. Average productive hourly rate: _____ Period from: _____ to _____
   (From Trends)

2. Inflation percentage for current average hourly rate to bring to level in effect at beginning of fiscal year.

   _____ × _____ = _____ × _____ = _____
   (Current avg., from line 1)　(Previous year inflation %)　(Avg. hourly rate for　(Previous year inflation %)　Avg. previous rate
   　　　　　　　　　　　　　　　　　　　　　　　　beginning of budget year)

3. Fixed and flexible staffing
   a. *Flexible Staffing*

   _____ × _____ × _____ = _____ ÷ _____ = _____
   　(Hrs/UOS)　　　(Budgeted UOS)　　(Hourly rate, from　　(Flex. salary amt.)　　UOS　　Flex. salary per
   　　　　　　　　　　　　　　　　　　line 2)　　　　　　　　　　　　　　　　　　　　　UOS

   b. *Fixed Staffing*
   Avg. hourly rate for fixed employees: _____ (if different from line 1)

   _____ × _____ = _____ ÷ 12 = _____
   (Total hrs. fixed staffing　(Avg. hourly rate from　(Fixed salary amount)　Monthly fixed salary
   × hrs/wk × 52 weeks)　above, or line 1)

   c. *Salary Totals*

   _____ + _____ = _____
   (Flexible salary amt., from line a above)　(Fixed salary amt., from line b)　Salary subtotal for flexible and fixed
   　　　　　　　　　　　　　　　　　　　　　　　　　　staffing

   d. *FTEs Productive*

   _____ ÷ 2080 = _____ _____ _____
   Prod. hours flex.　　　Flex. FTEs　　Total FTEs　　FTE UOS Budget
   UOS × UOS

   _____ ÷ 2080 = _____ _____ _____
   Fixed hours　　　Fixed FTEs　　YTD FTEs from Trends　　FTE per UOS Trends

899

4. Other items
   a. *New Employee Orientation*

   _____ × _____ × _____ = _____
   (No. of hrs per orientation)   (No. of employees for   (Avg. hourly rate, from line 6)   Total cost for orientation
                                        orientation)

   b. *Holiday Premium Pay*
   8-hour employees and 12-hour employees (first 8 hours):

   _____ × _____ × _____ = _____
   (No. FTEs × 8 hrs)   (½ avg. hourly rate, from   (No. of holidays of premium   Total premium pay, 8-hour
                                        line 6)   pay)   and 12-hour employees (first 8
                                                                                                                 hrs)

   12-hour employees (last 4 hours):

   _____ × _____ × _____ = _____
   (No. FTEs × 4 hrs)   (3 × avg. hourly rate, from   (No. of holidays of premium   Total premium pay, 12-hour
                                        line 6)   pay)   employees (last 4 hrs)

   _____ + _____ = _____
   Total premium pay (8-hr —   Total premium pay (12-hr,   Total premium pay
   12-hr)   last 4 hrs)

   c. *Sick Leave Payoff*
   Total number of employees receiving sick leave payoff _____ = _____
                                                                         Total sick leave payoff

   d. *Mandatory Classes*

   _____ × _____ 8 hrs/class _____ × _____ = _____
   (No. of employees)   (Avg. hourly rate, from line 6)   Total for mandatory classes

   e. *CPR*

   _____ × _____ 8 hrs/class _____ × _____ = _____
   (No. of employees)   (Avg. hourly rate, from line 6)   Total for CPR

5. Spread of Salaries

	(1) UOS	(2) Fixed Salary	(3) Flexible Cost/UOS	(4) Monthly Productive Salaries		UOS	Fixed Salary	Flexible Cost/UOS	Monthly Productive Salaries
Oct.					Apr.				
Nov.					May				
Dec.					June				
Jan.					July				
Feb.					Aug.				
Mar.					Sept.				
Total:	____		____	____		____			____
Grand Total:	====		====	====		====			====

(1) Approved UOS from form FA.
(2) Monthly fixed salary, from 3(b).
(3) Flex. salary per unit of service, from 3(a).
(4) Multiply column 1 (UOS) × column 3 (Flexible Cost per UOS) and add the result to column 2 (Fixed Salary) to obtain the monthly productive salary figure.

Capital Budget

Any expenditure in excess of certain dollar values (including sales tax and shipping charges) specified by the Administration for remodeling, furnishings, or equipment having a usable life of more than three years is classified as a capital expenditure.

Values specified by Administration are as follows:

$ _____ for equipment or furnishings
$ _____ for remodeling projects

Example: Assuming that a specified value of $500 for equipment purchases has been set by Administration, an order for six chairs costing $150.00 each would not be capitalized, even though the total cost for the order would be $900.00. It is the individual cost of items that should be measured against the specified limit. In this example, the chairs should be included as a departmental expense on the B-3 form in the minor equipment category.

Figures 34–4 and 34–5 show the capital budget worksheets to be completed for anticipated expenditures during FY 199☐. Figure 34–4 is a summary of the capital items requested. Figure 34–5 is to be used to justify the purchase of each requested item. Instructions for the completion of these forms follow.

CAPITAL BUDGET SUMMARY (Fig. 34–4)

On completion of the informational section at the top of the form, each item requested should be listed in order of importance (priority). For example, the capital item that is most important and necessary for the department to meet its goals and objectives for the new fiscal year would be assigned priority number 1. The next most important item would be assigned as second priority, etc. Each item listed must have a different priority number.

A checkmark should be placed in the appropriate box to indicate which quarter you expect the expenditure to occur. Any item purchased during October, November, or December of 199☐ will fall within the first quarter of the fiscal year. Any item expected to be purchased in July, August, or September of 199☐ will fall within the fourth quarter.

The "Functional Code" column indicates why the expenditure is considered necessary. The three codes to be used are as follows:

1. *Replacement Item.* Items needed to replace worn-out or obsolete equipment or furnishings that are required to maintain current programs relative to the department's approved 199☐ objectives.

2. *New Item.* Items considered desirable for economic or other reasons or items that are necessary to improve or expand current programs included in the 1988 goals and objectives.

3. *Remodeling Project.* Items included in a conversion or remodeling project that involves changes to the physical structure surrounding the department. Each item listed should be given a functional code.

CAPITAL EXPENDITURE JUSTIFICATION (Fig. 34–5)

This form should be completed for each item listed on Figure 34–4. The reasons why the acquisition is necessary, as well as the projected economic benefits (if any), should be clearly stated.

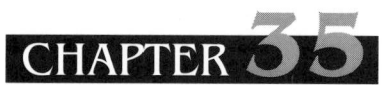

CHAPTER 35

Staffing and Scheduling

Inez E. Tenzer

Staffing and scheduling appropriately qualified personnel is a creative challenge confronting all managers. Every facility is unique, and its needs require individual consideration when applying management formulas or suggestions. Staffing must be predicated on the known, with flexibility to accommodate unpredictable events. As budgetary constraints continue to affect daily practices, departments are expected to provide service, maintain quality, be adaptable to change, and remain fiscally intact. There are a number of steps to take before determining the classification and number of staff required in a particular operating room (OR) suite. It is important to be aware of OR demand and utilization and the goals of the organization in relation to the surgical services provided. Developing operational definitions permits a common frame of reference for all who will be involved in the staffing and scheduling aspects between and within departments. As with any generic element that is customized to fit a specific situation, definitions vary among institutions and individuals.

This chapter will include six sections: surgery scheduling, data collection and forecasting, staffing, ambulatory care, regulatory standards, the budgeting process, and scheduling of staff. The sections are not intended to be sequential, reflecting the process you would use when assessing or planning staffing/scheduling patterns. Hopefully, the individual sections will serve as a resource for your unique needs. Which comes first: the schedule, the staff, or the budget? Each factor is dependent on the others, but development of a specific area will depend on the need at the particular time. If an OR department is in its infancy and undergoing the preliminary stages of development, historical information may be nonexistent, and the approach may require looking at the type of services to be provided, the number of surgeons expected to use the facility, and the number of ORs to open. Staffing guidelines and budget may then follow.

SURGERY SCHEDULING

Surgery scheduling is critical to the efficiency of and effective provision of service by the OR, regardless of the type of setting (i.e., acute care or ambulatory). There are two major scheduling methods—open and block scheduling—with offshoots developed to adapt to different circumstances.

Open Scheduling

Open scheduling provides OR time on a first-come basis and is most frequently used in community or private practice facilities.

Block Scheduling

Traditional Block Scheduling

Traditional block scheduling is the allocation of available scheduled hours divided into AM and PM time

902

periods, Monday through Friday. Weekend and evening blocks are incorporated into the traditional block schedule if necessary. Customarily, blocks range 3½ to 4 hours in length. This form of scheduling is commonly used in departments where surgeons are salaried and considered to be part of the institution's staff (Appendix A).

Creative Block Scheduling

Creative block scheduling is similar to traditional scheduling, with the exception of the time periods assigned. A creative block schedule develops block time by actual or projected surgeon need according to the type of surgeries performed and the average time required by the surgeon. For example, Surgeon A generally requires a minimum of 6 hours to complete a surgery because of the complexity of the procedure. Surgeon B most frequently schedules less complex surgeries of shorter duration. The creative block schedule can accommodate these needs by creating a total block of 10 hours, subdivided into 6-hour and 4-hour segments. There are several advantages of creative block scheduling: a realistic amount of time is provided, runover into someone else's block is minimized, and the schedule is better controlled. Disadvantages include the impact a unique time frame has on the surgeon's nonoperative responsibilities and the coordination required for both surgical and nonsurgical demands. Staffing becomes an issue because the block time is elective and requires dedicated coverage exclusive of emergencies and urgencies (Fig. 35–1). Provision of staff for such situations must be considered.

Mixed Scheduling

Mixed scheduling combines block and open scheduling, thereby providing surgeons who desire specific OR time with a more predictable surgical calendar while accommodating surgeons who want or need more flexible time arrangements (Fig. 35–2). However, it is advisable to obtain approval from OR committee members when instituting or changing a scheduling system. In a mixed scheduling system, certain hours will most likely be designated for block use. However, any type of scheduling method requires a definition of the routine hours of service, the days of the week, and the policy and procedure to cope with emergency and urgent surgeries. Temporary or permanent adjustments in the block or expansion of allocated or open time may be necessary due to increased volume, special requests, or practice changes (Appendix B). It is not uncommon for weekend and evening elective hours to be offered to absorb volume fluctuations or accommodate special situations. Periodic evaluation of the scheduling mechanism is recommended to identify problems, establish trends, track efficiency, and revise the plan or procedure, if necessary.

In the block scheduling approach, productivity is determined by block utilization, or the percentage of allocated time used by the service or surgeon (Table 35–1). If block time is released, there is no adjustment. Usually there are guidelines for releasing block time (e.g., release must be made a certain number of days in advance to allow for scheduling another surgeon or service; the Perioperative Director or designee must be notified so that the computations can be adjusted, if necessary) (Appendix C). With block scheduling, utilization by one service of another service's time will be reflected in out-of-block hours, resulting in a report that reflects an overall lower block utilization. This information may be misinterpreted as an inefficient use of OR time. To prevent this misinterpretation, the room utilization rate, which indicates the amount of time used in the specified OR during available hours of service, should be reviewed. If automated reporting is available, information should be requested according to the elective hours of operation against which ORs are usually measured. The room utilization rate is also the tool to use when evaluating efficiency with the open scheduling system.

The target utilization rate for elective hours varies with each department. A number of factors must be considered, and even these may not be the deciding elements. The amount of time required during elective hours to schedule the more unpredictable surgeries (i.e.,

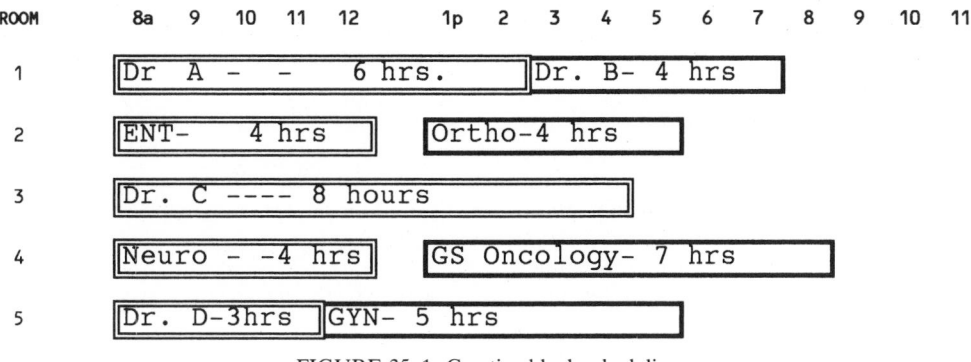

FIGURE 35–1. Creative block scheduling.

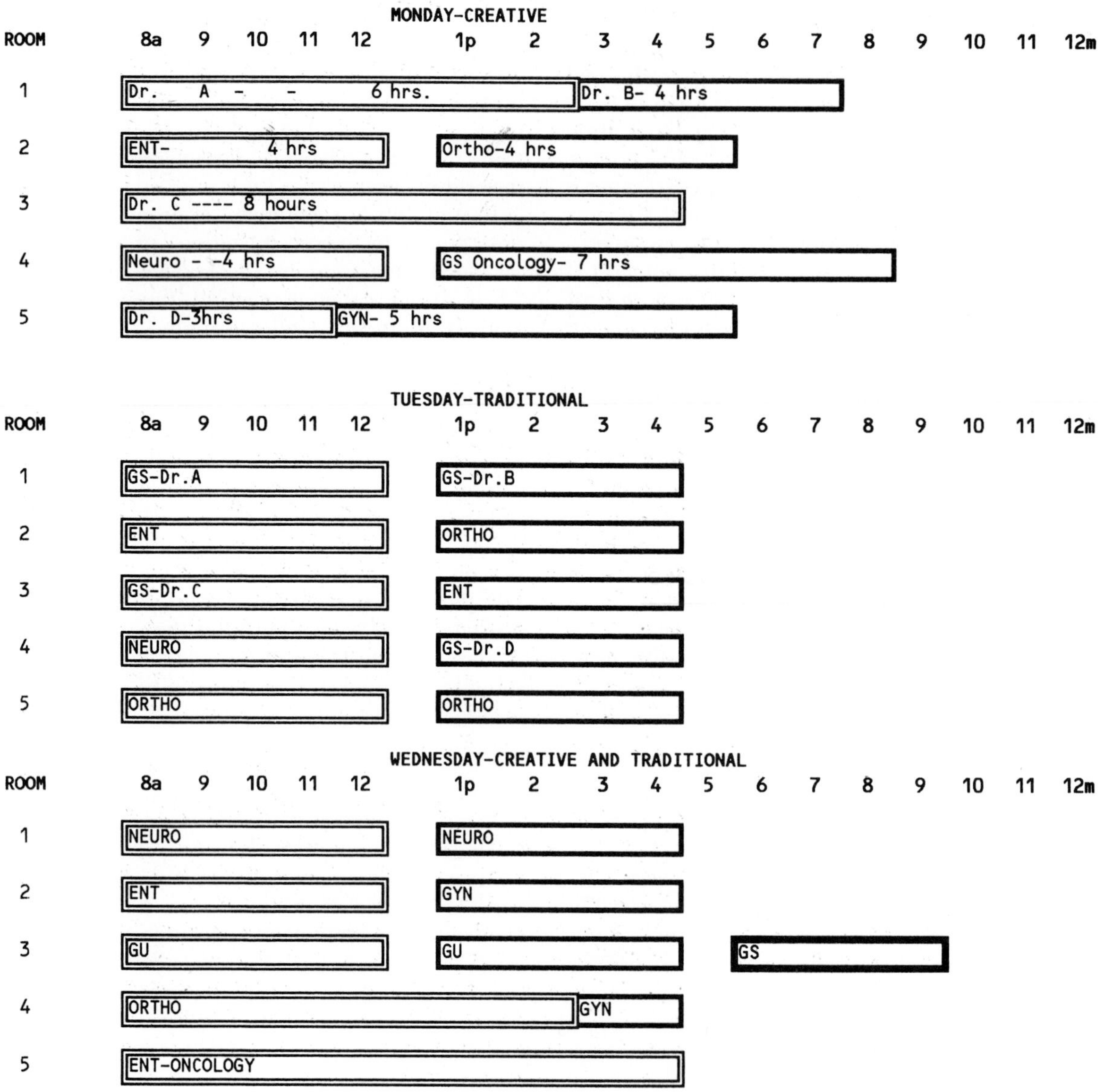

MONDAY-CREATIVE

ROOM	8a	9	10	11	12		1p	2	3	4	5	6	7	8	9	10	11	12m

Room	Schedule
1	Dr. A - - 6 hrs. / Dr. B- 4 hrs
2	ENT- 4 hrs / Ortho-4 hrs
3	Dr. C ---- 8 hours
4	Neuro - -4 hrs / GS Oncology- 7 hrs
5	Dr. D-3hrs / GYN- 5 hrs

TUESDAY-TRADITIONAL

ROOM	8a	9	10	11	12		1p	2	3	4	5	6	7	8	9	10	11	12m

Room	Morning	Afternoon
1	GS-Dr.A	GS-Dr.B
2	ENT	ORTHO
3	GS-Dr.C	ENT
4	NEURO	GS-Dr.D
5	ORTHO	ORTHO

WEDNESDAY-CREATIVE AND TRADITIONAL

ROOM	8a	9	10	11	12		1p	2	3	4	5	6	7	8	9	10	11	12m

Room	Schedule
1	NEURO / NEURO
2	ENT / GYN
3	GU / GU / GS
4	ORTHO / GYN
5	ENT-ONCOLOGY

FIGURE 35–2. Mixed block scheduling.

TABLE 35–1. BLOCK UTILIZATION BY SERVICE

MONTH_____

SERVICE	ALLOCATED HOURS	IN BLOCK HOURS	% OF BLOCK UTILIZATION	OUT OF BLOCK HRS.
GENERAL SURGERY	493.00	435.93	88.42	369.90
CARDIOVASCULAR	517.50	424.41	82.01	203.36
GYN	168.50	132.40	80.00	125.71
OPHTHALMOLOGY	0.00	0.00	0.00	12.05
ORTHOPEDICS	338.50	287.72	85.00	85.80
NEUROSURGERY	192.50	148.96	77.38	63.58
PLASTIC	40.00	32.00	80.00	11.96
UROLOGY	237.50	194.75	82.00	65.13
CYSTOSCOPY	345.00	258.75	75.00	15.31
ORAL/MAXILLO	63.50	45.91	72.29	36.03
ENT	320.00	241.71	75.53	74.83
TOTAL	2716.00	2202.54	81.09	1063.66

USAGE IS BASED UPON PATIENT ROOM IN TO ROOM OUT TIMES WITH PRE-DETERMINED SET-UP AND CLEAN-UP TIMES INCLUDED.

Courtesy of Kaiser Medical Center, Los Angeles, CA.

emergencies and urgencies) determines the target rate. For example, if short-notice situations equal 15% of the elective hours, a block or elective hours utilization rate of 75 to 80% would be reasonable. At the same time, add-on procedures may constitute a significant portion of the schedule because of the type of surgeon's office or clinic practice and would need to be considered. Any other facility-specific characteristics that affect efficiency and utilization rates must be included in the analysis. The most important step is the acceptance of the target utilization rate for the particular OR by the Administration, surgeons, and other key staff. It is extremely helpful to have a concrete method to determine productivity that can be understood by all. Once again, defining terms is essential to establishing a common frame of reference; this prevents conflicts in interpretation of the data and provides consistent application of the terms. A sample of definitions for scheduling purposes may include the following:

Scheduled surgery: Scheduled at least 48 hours in advance.

Add-on surgery: Scheduled after the preliminary schedule is printed.

Urgent surgery: Scheduled 24 hours before the surgery date.

Emergency surgery: Scheduled on the day the surgery is required to be performed.

With an automated scheduling system, definitions may be incorporated into the data base and identified when the surgery is scheduled. The type of surgery scheduled has no relationship to the condition of the patient as defined for scheduling criteria.

DATA COLLECTION AND FORECASTING

Data Collection

With the technological advances available for collecting data and generating reports in a multitude of formats, most facilities probably have more information than can be evaluated. However, the advantages of automated systems justify their cost when such systems are used appropriately. The data must be critically reviewed for accuracy and promptly corrected when necessary before results are published. Establishment of credible documents is essential for future use and current proposals. When computerization is available, depending on focus and need, reports may be routinely printed on a monthly, weekly, or daily basis; occasionally data may be required many times throughout the day. Quarterly and yearly analyses may consist of cumulative statistics from frequently generated reports or information required only on an intermittent basis. Popular data reports include but are not limited to the following:

1. OR Utilization: Percentage of OR time used based on time available; can be formatted to reflect specific hours (e.g., elective time frames).
2. Surgeon Profile: Length of operative time per procedure, from beginning to end.
3. Room Turnover: Time from patient out to next patient in within the same OR (Appendix D).
4. Patient Turnover: Time from the operation stop of one patient to the operation start of the next patient in the same OR.
5. Admission Type: Inpatient, outpatient, same-day admit (Appendix E).
6. Scheduling Type: Scheduled, add-on, urgent, emergency; this can be expanded to include specific time frames (Appendix F).
7. Staff Profile: Staff participation in surgeries by type, assignment, number, and frequency.
8. Surgeon Productivity: Number of surgeries by type and by the amount of time needed per procedure.
9. Runover Report: Number of surgeries started during designated hours and running over into the next time frame (Appendix G).
10. Delay Study: Describes the delay factors by service, surgeon, and frequency (Appendix H)
11. Cancellations: Surgeries cancelled on the day of surgery.
12. Equipment Usage—type and frequency.
13. Implant Log—type and frequency of implants inserted; can include patient, day, or time.
14. OR Usage Time Spread: Describes the number of rooms in use at specific intervals during requested time frames (Appendix I).
15. OR Usage: Graphic display of the OR Usage Time Spread (Appendix J).

Once the data are entered into the system, the information can be manipulated according to individual preference and can be called for when needed. Computerization can potentially provide a dynamic mechanism for assessing the changing environment. Usually, the ability to respond to the need is slow because of extraneous factors required to implement changes (e.g., developing the plan, obtaining approval if necessary, allocating resources, communicating with the appropriate people, and determining and coping with the impact of the change on other departments' systems). Some statistics may be considered "sensitive" (e.g., those reflecting surgeon productivity and length of surgical time per procedure). This information needs to be shared on a selective basis and used in a discriminating manner for scheduling purposes. One statistic that is difficult to obtain by automation is the number of surgeries pending during a specific time frame. When identifying volume during selected hours, the data do not reflect those surgeries placed on hold or queuing for the first available

time and staff on the day of surgery. If this information is desirable, manual collection may be required (Fig. 35–3).

EXAMPLE: APPLYING STATISTICAL INFORMATION TO DETERMINE EVENING STAFFING

For the purposes of correlation, consider the information in Appendices I and J to represent 3 months of data. (Three to 6 months of statistics should be collected, using normal months in which there were no unusual occurrences to skew the customary experience [e.g., volume reduction as a result of blood shortage, or temporary volume increase to accommodate special scheduling demands].) Without actually using the numbers, the following analysis may be employed:

1. Determine the average number of rooms in use each day at various time frames.
2. Evaluate the pending surgeries, including the wait time for emergencies or elective cases that are delayed (see Fig. 35–3). This information is important when justifying a change in staffing. Every facility formally or informally establishes an acceptable time factor for OR access. If room availability consistently exceeds this factor, it is necessary to assess the accuracy of the factor or find solutions to reduce the wait time.
3. Identify factors influencing case volume and distribution into evenings.
4. Compare the number of staff currently scheduled and their distribution of hours.
5. Identify the number of staff required to cover the hours of OR demand.
6. Develop a staffing strategy to accommodate OR volume and distribution.
7. Review budgetary impact and prepare a proposal, if necessary.
8. Obtain approval from and/or inform appropriate sources (Administration, Personnel Department, Bargaining Units, staff, surgeons, Anesthesiology, other departments) that may be affected by the change.

When computerization is not available, manual compilation of data may be required. Under these circumstances, prioritizing the information desired is critical to providing essential data without taxing resources. Statistics are valuable tools for maintaining an awareness of department activity on many levels and need to be provided to surgeons, staff, Anesthesiology and Administration. Each group may have a particular focus of interest, and superfluous information may result in a waste of time and paper. If possible, it may be prudent to distribute a summary sheet that synopsizes generically relevant data and to provide specific reports on request (Table 35–2).

Forecasting

Forecasting is the projection of the number of patients and defined services anticipated to be required during a

P.M. CASES PENDING AT 1530

DAY OF WEEK_____   # CASES ON HOLD AT 1515_____

DATE_____   # CASES ON HOLD AT 1550_____

STAFFING (EXCLUDING MGR.)

# STAFF AVAILABLE	SCHEDULED	ACTUAL	#STAFF OVERTIME	O.T. HOURS
1530-1730	_____	_____	_____	_____
1730-1800	_____	_____	_____	_____
1800-2000	_____	_____	_____	_____
2000-2350	_____	_____	_____	_____

MANAGER AT DESK_____   MANAGER IN ROOM_____(AMT. OF TIME)

CASES PLACED ON HOLD

SURGERY	TIME SCHED.	TIME DESIRED	TIME PT. READY	O.R. AVAIL.	ELECTIVE HOLD	ADD-ON	EMERG.

FIGURE 35–3. Data collection sheet to supplement automated systems. (Courtesy of Kaiser Medical Center, Los Angeles, CA.)

TABLE 35–2. SUMMARY OF PERIOPERATIVE STATISTICS

PERIOPERATIVE STAT SUMMARY

MONTH	CASES	%BLK UTIL.	OP	SDA	HOUSE PT.	# DELAYS	% TOTAL	REMARKS
				ADMIT STATUS		DELAYS		
JAN								
FEB								
MARCH								
APRIL								
MAY								
JUNE								
JULY								
AUGUST								
SEPT.								
OCT.								
NOV.								
DEC.								
TOTAL								

Courtesy of Kaiser Medical Center, Los Angeles, CA.

specified time frame, usually a period of 1 to 5 years. Changes in health care require yearly, if not more frequent, reviews to reassess projections and adjust them as indicated. Budget preparations are based on forecast projections and obviously affect staffing and scheduling in the OR. Historical information, current data, and potential changes in practice, surgeon staff, and organizational mission are considered when determining the direction of the facility. Forecasting is a fundamental component of the budget process and will be discussed in the section entitled "Budgeting Process."

STAFFING

Policy

"The hospital provides nursing services to meet the nursing care needs of patients who receive care throughout the hospital" (JCAHO, 1989). The structural standards for Perioperative Services require a description of the unit, the types of services provided, and the staffing provisions for every contingency occurring within the department. Appendices K through M are examples of policies relating to staffing in the OR. An acuity factor has been used in nursing services for many years but has not been applied to the OR until recently. Addi-

tional personnel were assigned to a room when indicated, but the criteria for the change were not usually documented. In 1988, JCAHO surveyors began emphasizing an OR-related acuity system; however, published material was based on a charging structure for revenue purposes, not based on staffing patterns. The Association of Operating Room Nurses (AORN) appointed a committee to develop a patient classification system for the OR. Appendix N shows a revised policy originally developed by Massino and Spies from Kaiser Medical Center, Woodland Hills, CA.

Staffing Plan

When determining staffing requirements, it is important to define terms to provide a common frame of reference and consistency in application of methodology. Staffing "is a process to determine the appropriate number, by category, of nursing personnel to provide care of a predetermined quality to a specific number of patients. A Staffing Plan or Pattern is the number of staff by category required by shift and day of the week for a designated census or workload" (Lawrenz, 1987). Once created, the staffing plan can be translated into a budgetary format.

Ordinarily, development of a staffing plan is unit based according to specified criteria and guidelines. The system of preparing and maintaining the staffing plan may be centralized or decentralized. A centralized system consists of a focal source such as a Staffing Office that performs the staffing/scheduling function for a group of services. A decentralized system places the responsibility for the staffing plan with the unit or service.

In the OR, a basic staffing assumption is that at least one registered nurse (RN) will be in each OR serving as the circulating nurse. A worksheet to identify the coverage required is a dynamic tool that may be updated and revised as necessary. A simplified worksheet is depicted in Table 35–3 and includes a sample staffing plan, explained in the text. Although volume is a critical factor, the number of rooms available for scheduling are a primary influence on the number of personnel scheduled on a given day during specific hours.

Staffing Issues

In an early study conducted by the Cleveland Clinic, results from a questionnaire indicated that many nurses left the profession because of the rigidity of scheduling, rotating shifts, and weekend and night assignments. (Newby, 1980). In 1987, nursing turnover was estimated to be at 20% and increasing (*HRA*, 1987). In the 1990s, with the dramatic economic pressures on the majority

TABLE 35–3. STAFFING WORKSHEET

7:30A–4P	MONDAY	TUESDAY	WEDNES.	THURS.	FRIDAY	SAT.	SUNDAY
FIXED							
Mgr.	3.0	3.0	3.0	3.0	3.0	0.0	0.0
Clerk	1.0	1.0	1.0	1.0	1.0	0.0	0.0
Orderly	2.0	2.0	2.0	2.0	2.0	1.0	1.0
SUBTOTAL	6.0	6.0	6.0	6.0	6.0	1.0	1.0
ROOMS SCHED.	10+	10+	10+	10+	10+	1	1
	2 CYSTO	2 CYSTO	2 CYSTO	2 CYSTO	2 CYSTO		
VARIABLE							
#Staff Required–*	22.0	22.0	22.0	22.0	22.0	2.0	2.0
Special Procedure (laser,cell saver)	0.0	1.0	0.0	1.0	0.0	0.0	0.0
TOTAL	28.0	29.0	28.0	29.0	28.0	3.0	3.0
3P–11:00P							
FIXED							
Mgr.	1.0	1.0	1.0	1.0	1.0	0.0	0.0
Clerk	1.0	1.0	1.0	1.0	1.0	0.0	0.0
Orderly	1.0	1.0	1.0	1.0	1.0	1.0	1.0
SUBTOTAL	3.0	3.0	3.0	3.0	3.0	1.0	1.0
ROOMS SCHED.	1	1	1	1	1	1	1
VARIABLE							
#Staff Required–*	2.0	2.0	2.0	2.0	2.0	2.0	2.0
SUBTOTAL	5.0	5.0	5.0	5.0	5.0	3.0	3.0
11:00P–7:30A							
FIXED							
Orderly	1.0	1.0	1.0	1.0	1.0	1.0	1.0
ROOMS SCHED.	1	1	1	1	1	1	1
VARIABLE							
#Staff Required–*	2.0	2.0	2.0	2.0	2.0	2.0	2.0
SUBTOTAL	3.0	3.0	3.0	3.0	3.0	3.0	3.0
TOTAL	36.0	37.0	36.0	37.0	36.0	9.0	9.0

*2 STAFF/ROOM; CYSTO = 1 PERSON/ROOM

of households, resulting in the return of the other spouse to the workforce, those figures are likely to change, albeit temporarily. Statistics for the OR are unavailable. Replacing RNs in the Nursing Department takes approximately 90 days (AHA, 1987); filling perioperative positions usually takes longer because of the specialized education and experience required. Nationwide, 78.7% of the total RN population is employed (Morse, 1987). Based on the statistics, unemployed nurses are probably not an appropriate target for recruitment. Part-time staff, constituting 27% of the total pool of RNs, are a more likely source of increasing staffing potential (Westfall, 1988). As permanent employees of the institution, part-time personnel are considered members of the staff; their schedules are based on mutual need of the individual and employer, and their lighter schedules provide the option for expansion of hours or days as need dictates.

Many years ago the nursing profession accepted the necessity of rotating shifts to provide coverage for off hours. However, it has become widely accepted that individuals cannot effectively violate their circadian rhythm and cope well with schedules that require them to work on opposing shifts. According to the literature, rotating shifts on a permanent basis is not a satisfactory solution to staffing vacant positions. Studies indicate that workers who rotate shifts (other than day shift) suffer from increased fatigue, nervousness, and insufficient sleep and have an increased number of accidents at work. In addition, leisure time is reduced, and home life is disrupted (Rose, 1984). When staff members volunteer because the rotation temporarily meets their needs or solves an immediate problem, rotation may serve to address a staffing issue. When possible, it is more functional for the employee and the department to hire permanently into off-shift positions.

Staffing Options

Fixed and Variable Personnel. Two categories—fixed or constant and variable or flex—are frequently used to describe staffing hours. Fixed/constant personnel are required regardless of volume, rooms, or cases and do not perform direct patient care activities; these include managers, clerks, and often nursing attendants or orderlies. Variable/flex personnel are required to perform direct patient care; the number is adjusted according to projected volume. Staffing is initially predicated on the number of people required to be present to meet the criteria of the staffing guidelines. A replacement factor must be identified to allow for coverage during vacation, sick leave, compassionate leave, jury duty, or education time. Usually the fixed positions are not replaced except for orderlies; variable positions are replaced 75 to 100% of the time, depending on the shift and responsibilities of the particular positions. Nonworked hours are nonproductive hours that are paid but not worked. The worksheet visually informs the manager of the minimum number of staff required to be present during the specified hours of the days of the week. Coverage for breaks and lunch may be included in the basic staffing plan to formulate an inclusive pattern. The budget process will then convert personnel into hours and respective full-time equivalents (FTEs), which are "the number of employees needed to cover the number of hours or shifts required during a period of time (by week, pay period, year) and are calculated using 2080 hours a year or 80 hours a pay period" (Lawrenz, 1987).

Planning coverage to ensure compliance with the staffing plan offers the opportunity for a variety of creative approaches. The traditional 8-hour shift is preferred by many and is a mainstay of the OR. However, a number of alternative methods complement the unpredictability of the department's activity and may be desirable to staff. Variable shifts are those hours assigned outside the routinely scheduled shifts (e.g., 9:00–5:30 PM, 10:00–6:30 PM). Variable shifts have many advantages for both the department and personnel. The hours are usually designed to provide relief for breaks and meals and coverage for surgical procedures that run over into the later shift. In the event of a reduced number of staff at the beginning of the day shift, variable shift personnel may be available for preshifting, with the understanding that they will work to the end of their usual shift, if necessary.

Flexible Staffing. *Flexible staffing* is the development of alternative shifts of defined time frames differing from the customary 8-hour shift (e.g., 12-hour, 10-hour, 6-hour, 5-hour, or 4-hour shifts). Alternative or flexible shifts are popular with people who are able to cope with expanded hours in order to have additional days off. Similarly, shortened shifts are appealing to those who prefer having additional time off during the day. Flexible shifts in the OR provide an effective mechanism for using personnel in relation to department activity and controlling the payroll budget. Of course, overtime provisions for expanded shifts need to be considered in relation to the financial impact compared with the FTEs. Overtime may be less costly at times in comparison to employing additional FTE personnel with salary and benefits. Before implementing flexible staffing, it is important to identify the goals to be achieved by this method. In the OR, overtime is frequently necessary but usually is not scheduled 6 weeks in advance. Knowing that a lengthened day awaits them 3 or 4 days a week can be fatiguing for personnel and counterproductive. If expanded shifts are to be initiated, it is necessary to determine the hours to be covered, the number of positions required, the days of the week most frequently in need of the coverage, the impact of the reduced coverage on specific days, and the mechanism used to ensure adequate staffing every shift of every day. Staff also need to consider the impact of reduced hours on their retirement benefits. Adjustable hours are appealing to those who enjoy variety and have the ability to change their schedules on short notice. Staff may be hired for a total number of hours per pay period with the shifts varied to suit the activity of the department.

Job Sharing. Job sharing provides an opportunity for one position to be shared by two or more employees.

Usually the responsibilities of the position are assumed by the individuals to promote continuity of care. In the OR, depending on the staffing assignment, continuity of positional responsibilities may or may not be an issue. It is possible to hire part-time employees into one position and give them different assignments on their scheduled days. The difference between part-time classification and job sharing seems to rest with the accountability of the employees to the requirements of the position.

Per Diem Staff. Per diem staff, who are employed by the facility and scheduled on an as-needed basis, contribute significantly to ensuring adequate staffing in a more controlled manner. Usually, a higher hourly rate is paid in lieu of benefits; the individual is considered a member of the staff and may be prescheduled for specific time frames.

Stand-by Hours. Stand-by hours are those hours a staff person is scheduled to be available to work, with financial compensation provided for this availability and additional compensation earned when the person is called in to work. Stand-by requirements vary with location and type of facility. In some situations personnel are expected to be able to respond within 20 minutes; others may be required to remain on the premises. Stand-by hours can be used to provide supplemental staffing capability or to serve as the primary coverage for a particular shift.

Perioperative Courses. Perioperative courses are an intermediate approach to meeting a staffing deficit. The advantages and disadvantages must be carefully weighed before implementation, and adequate educational support must be provided throughout the program and orientation. Many courses are 4 to 6 months in duration; may require a fee or, conversely, may pay a stipend or salary to the learner; incorporate orientation into the total time frame; or add a specific transition time at the completion of the program. With budgetary factors an ever-present force, the length of nonproductive time for the learner must be considered when developing the curriculum, and creative teaching approaches must be integrated into the program design. After completion of a program, there is a period of adjustment when the learner gradually makes the transition from student to orientee/new hire to accepted member of the staff. From a personal perspective, it frequently takes 18 months (6 months for the program, 2 months for orientation, and 10 months for the adaptation period) before the learner begins to feel comfortable in his or her new role and is productively contributing to the department.

Internal Staffing Pool. An internal staffing pool is similar to a registry but is based in house. Full-time employees who are oriented to the department agree to work on a supplemental basis. Considerations for maintaining the pool include flexibility of scheduling staff, demonstrated competency of skills, and good attendance.

Travel Nurses. Travel nurses are employed by some facilities and have been a successful adjunct to staffing (DeLaney, 1988). The contractual agreement ensures commitment of an individual who is well prepared for the assignment to serve as a reliable staff member for a specified period of time (OR Focus, 1988). Although the cost of a travel nurse is usually higher than that for traditional registry personnel, the investment may be worth the expenditure if such nurses fulfill a needed staffing gap.

Registry Personnel. Registry personnel are employed by outside agencies contracted to provide staff to the facility on an as-needed basis. Within appropriate time frames, registry personnel may be cancelled if the OR schedule or staffing no longer warrants their assistance. The advantages and disadvantages to using a registry must be considered on an individual basis.

Regardless of the staffing patterns developed, personnel must have sufficient knowledge and skill to perform their responsibilities. Their performance requires periodic evaluation, and their skills should be assessed on an ongoing basis with a systematic plan for review and updating.

AMBULATORY CARE

The standards and requirements for ambulatory surgery centers generally are the same as for inpatient facilities, especially if such centers are to receive government reimbursement. If it is a free-standing center, the primary difficulty in developing a staffing plan revolves around the erratic surgery schedule. It is impossible to predict volume, and yet staffing must be rigidly monitored to prevent over- or understaffing. Although achieving an equitable balance is challenging, a few strategies appear to be successful. Employing an all-RN staff permits flexibility and cross-training with the post-anesthesia care unit; using a core of full-time RNs supplemented by a large pool of part-time and some per diem employees allows for the surgery fluctuations. However, a staff of RNs might not be cost effective. A more practical plan might use surgical technologists in the scrub nurse role. As with any staffing plan, recruiting qualified staff is not always easy. Free-standing centers have some advantages that may attract nurses. Work schedules are designed for weekdays during daytime hours; weekend and stand-by hours are not required, and the environment is less intense than in inpatient or acute care settings (*OR Manager*, 1987). Ambulatory surgery ORs attached to a hospital may develop a separate staff roster or routinely rotate staff from the inpatient OR. Internal staff pools are not as critical in this model, because the "inpatient" OR may be able to provide the back-up personnel. If supplemental staff are required, they may be assigned to the "inpatient" OR, where their hours and costs are more easily absorbed, and used in either the inpatient or the outpatient area, as needed.

REGULATORY STANDARDS

A number of licensing and regulatory standards dictate staffing and scheduling practices. The Joint Commission on Accreditation of Healthcare Organizations (JCAHO), the federal government, and the Department of Health Services all set standards via legislation and regulations. Each state describes its relationship to the federal government in its state constitution. For example, in California, state regulations supersede federal regulations, which means that the requirements contained in the California Administrative Code (CAC), administered by the Department of Health, are California's primary guidelines. However, federal regulations that are not in contradiction to the CAC must be followed. Often the state requirements are more stringent than the federal. Because regulatory standards are subject to change, references for such standards are best obtained from the hospital administration or respective agency. Although not directly describing staffing, the Board of Nursing and the nurse practice act in each individual state will reflect the way nursing is to be practiced, which will affect staffing patterns.

BUDGETING PROCESS

The budgeting process is determined by the financial department of the organization. Payroll budgets are usually prepared concurrently with nonpayroll budgets but will be the sole focus of this section. Preparing the payroll budget, including documents, data, and methodology, is a process that is specific to each facility and/or organization. Figure 35–4 is an example of a form used by an organization. As the budget process evolves, more information is provided on the form, requiring the department manager to verify the figures and make adjustments for projected changes and to justify the adjustments. Most preliminary budgets for the following year are developed 4 to 6 months in advance, with occasional opportunity provided to reassess volume indicators closer to the target date. In a prepaid system where membership fees must be determined with ample time for notifying contracting groups, an initial forecast for rate-determining purposes may be implemented. Because dues are predicated on these rate calculations, the final operational budget is expected to be very similar to the rate forecast. Therefore, forecasted figures must be developed with the same detail and attention used for the final budget.

Components. There are two components of the budget: productive time (the actual hours worked, regular and overtime) and nonproductive time (hours paid but not worked [vacation, sick leave, holidays, education]). These are separated on the budget worksheets (Lawrenz, 1987). Converting the required number of personnel into hours and relative FTEs must also take into account the benefit replacement factor (paid to work ratio, or Pd/Wk) hours. If an employee is to be replaced 100% of the time while on nonproductive time off, the replacement factor will be equal to the nonproductive portion of the budget. For example, if nonproductive time equals 19% of paid hours and if 100% replacement is required, then the 19% will be included for FTE replacement. If replacement will be for only 75% of the time, then 75% of the 19% nonproductive time, or 14.25%, will be included for replacement FTE. Volume for the OR is described in minutes, hours, or occasionally the number of surgeries. If surgeries are the volume indicator, an average length of time per surgery must be calculated. Hours worked per workload unit (HWkd/WLU) is the unit of measure of the cost of staff hours for each unit of the volume of service. The department history determines hours worked per workload unit, and the manager must determine if that will change based on new practices or trends. Often, the hours worked per workload unit and the paid to work ratio may not be negotiable, and staffing is expected to remain the same for the next year despite extraneous influences. The challenge becomes to devise creative methods to comply with the directive, such as evaluating the staffing mix, reducing overtime, and changing staffing patterns. Hours worked per workload unit may not be a significant measurement if the accepted practice is to staff all ORs on weekdays during daytime hours and to staff a specific number of rooms during other times, regardless of volume. An assortment of methods—historical, zero-based, and flexible budgeting—are used to prepare the payroll budget.

For the purpose of this chapter, the model OR will be a 10-room suite, with integrated inpatient and outpatient services, in which all subspecialties are performed except cardiac surgery and containing two cystoscopy rooms; it is staffed 24 hours each day, 7 days a week.

Historical Approach. Figure 35–5 illustrates volume projection using historical data and demonstrates a 1-year projection in preparation for the following budget year. The history reveals an erratic volume over the previous 3 years; the current year-to-date volume, when annualized, is less than the lowest year. With consideration for expected changes, the projected volume appears reasonable in relation to the historical experience and future needs. An example of the historical approach follows:

EXAMPLE: HISTORICAL APPROACH TO BUDGETING

Volume = 17,000 hours (annualized hours based on YTD activity)
HWkd/WLU = 6.75 (given)
Pd/Wk Ratio = 1.171 = 17.1% hours not worked
    17,000 hours × 6.75 HWkd/WLU = 114,750 hours worked
    114,750 hours worked × 17.1% hours not worked = 19,622 hours not worked
    114,750 + 19,622 hours = 134,372 paid hours
    134,372 paid hours ÷ 2,080 hours = 64.6 FTEs

PAYROLL OPERATING BUDGET

DEPARTMENT_____

| Prepared by | Date | Approved by | Date |

STAFFING AT PAY PERIOD I

Job Code	Job Description	FTES PAID				HOURS PAID				
		PP I Day	PP I Eve	PP I Nite	Total	PP I Day	PP I Eve	PP I Nite	Total	Annual Hrs
	SUBTOTAL									

STAFF ADDITIONS AND DELETIONS AFTER PAY PERIOD I (EFFECTIVE WITH PAY PERIOD NO. INDICATED)

Job Code	Job Description	FTES PAID				HOURS PAID				
		Day	Eve	Nite	Total	Day	Eve	Nite	Total	Annual Hrs
	SUBTOTAL									
	TOTAL									(1)

HOURS PAID AND NOT WORKED

Prev. Yr.___ Hrs.Wkd	CATEGORY	Yr.___Proj. Hours
	SICK LEAVE	
	VACATION	
	HOLIDAY	
	EDUCATION	
	TRAINING	
	MISCELLANEOUS	
	TOTAL	

WORK LOAD UNIT DESCRIPTION

WORK LOAD VOLUME	
	(2)

BUDGET SUMMARY

Est.% of Hrs.Wk	Hours Worked	
	Regular	
	O/T-1.5	
	O/T-2.0	
	O/T-2.5	
	HOL.2.5	
100.0%	TOTAL --------->	(3)
	RATIO OF PAID TO WORKED HOURS-(1) ÷ (3)	
HOURS WORKED PER WORK LOAD UNIT (3)÷(2)------>		

FIGURE 35–4. Payroll operating budget. (Courtesy of Kaiser Medical Center, Los Angeles, CA.)

VOLUME PROJECTION

Ten (10) room suite, integrated In-patient and Out-patient surgeries; all subspecialties except Cardiac are performed; two (2) cysto rooms are staffed M-F, 8 hours/day. The unit is staffed 24 hours, 7 days per week for a minimum of room after hours and week-ends.

Historical Data:

Year	Actual Volume
19____	21,000 hours
19____	19,300 hours
19____	20,000 hours

CURRENT YEAR	ACTUAL VOLUME YTD JAN.-JUNE	FACTORS
19____	9600 HOURS	*INCLUDES CHRISTMAS, N.Y. HOLIDAY WEEKS- REDUCED ELECTIVE SCHEDULE 4 DAYS ONE(1) ROOM OPEN FOR EMERGENCIES:
	9600-6 MOS.=1600 HRS/MOS 1600 HRSx12 MOS.=19200/YR. ANNUALIZED VOLUME	9 RMSx8 HRS.=72 HRS./DAY 72 HRSx4 DAYS=288 HRS. 288 HRSx80% UTILIZATION= **PROJECTED REDUCTION OF 230 HOURS.**
		*EXPANSION OF SCHEDULING HRS.: SAT. 1 ROOM=6 HRS. 6 HRS.x50 SATURDAYS= **PROJECTED INCREASE OF 350 HOURS.**
		INCREASE = 350 HOURS <u>REDUCTION= 230 HOURS</u> FACTORS = 120 HOURS INC.

19200 HOURS ANNUALIZED VOLUME
<u> 120 HOURS FACTOR TOTAL</u>
19320 HOURS PROJECTED 19__ VOLUME

FIGURE 35–5. Volume projection using historical data and showing a 1-year projection for the coming budget year.

64.6 FTEs are then divided into the appropriate categories of personnel required to assume all the responsibilities of the department (Fig. 35–6). Adjustments may be included for anticipated variations in any of the historical data. New programs or technology may require additional staffing considerations; an unusual occurrence slanting the figures higher or lower will require evaluation and a decision on whether to adjust the FTE allotment.

Zero-based Budgeting. Zero-based budgeting is the development of staffing complement based on need rather than on historical data. An example of a zero-based approach follows.

EXAMPLE: ZERO-BASED APPROACH TO BUDGETING

- Determine the number of rooms to staff and time frame.

  10 rooms + 2 cysto. 7:30 AM–4:00 PM (2 staff/room; 1 staff/cysto)
  1 room .... 4:00 PM–7:30 AM

- Provide for a replacement factor.

  100% replacement for variable staff with exception of two variable shift RNs.
  No replacement for fixed staff (managers, etc.)

- Identify special considerations such as new programs, new technology, and access demands.

  Laser usage increased to approximately 16 hours/week on weekdays.
     16 hours ÷ 40 hours/week = 0.4 FTE
  Weekend staffing: 2 staff at 8 hours each.
     16 hours/shift ÷ 40 hours/week
       = 0.4 FTE/shift
       = 1 orderly at 8 hours/day
     8 hours ÷ 40 hours/week = 0.2 FTE/day

- Develop personnel hours.

  Orderlies—need to be replaced
  One orderly scheduled 5 days/week, day shift, and one scheduled 7 days/week. One orderly scheduled 7 days/week, all other shifts.
     Day Shift: 8 hours × 5 days = 40 hours ÷ 40 hours = 1.0 FTE
     Day Shift: 8 hours × 7 days = 56 hours ÷ 40 hours = 1.4 FTE
     Evenings: 8 hours × 7 days = 56 hours ÷ 40 hours = 1.4 FTE
     Nights: 8 hours × 7 days = 56 hours ÷ 40 hours = 1.4 FTE
  Clerk scheduled 8 hours, 5 days weekdays and evenings and not replaced.
  There are four exempt staff—not replaced.

The FTEs described for replacement will then be distributed to the appropriate categories of personnel requiring replacement.

Note the variance of FTEs and hours worked per workload unit between historical and zero-based approaches. The hours worked per workload unit was given in the historical approach, and it was calculated in the zero-based after the personnel hours were determined.

Flexible Budgeting. Flexible budgeting provides for FTEs to be earned based on fluctuations in volume. Table 35–4 shows an example of this type of process. The following table extracts the YTD information in Table 35–4 to demonstrate the method used to arrive at the Earned figure.

	FTEs Worked/Pay Period				Volume	
Budgeted HWkd/WLU	Budget	Actual	Earned		Budgeted/Pay Period	Actual
6.15	58.05	60.21	58.92		743 hours	766 hours

Method: Actual volume = 766 hours × 6.15 budgeted HWkd/WLU
        = 4710.9 FTE hours
4710.9 ÷ 80 hours pay period = 58.88 earned FTEs

The flexible budget is a retrospective assessment of what has already occurred and provides a dynamic tool for monitoring productivity and budgetary compliance.

Other Budgeting Methods. There is one method that is quick and simple and does not require complicated calculations. Calculate the number of staff required for each OR to be scheduled and add 0.5 to each room for the replacement factor. The number of the other classification of personnel must still be added for a total FTE projection. For example:

10 rooms = 20 staff on days
2 cysto = 2 staff
Add the .5 per room (cysto = total of .5) to achieve a total of 5.5 replacement factor.
Total FTE required for running 10 rooms + 2 cysto = 27.5.

Other shifts and classification of personnel and fixed positions must then be added to that figure. Compare this approach to one used previously to determine the variance and realistic reflection of your staffing needs.

Budgetary Reports. Budgetary reports are another component of automated systems and are usually collected and distributed by the Financial Department. Aside from reports that describe payroll variances, which compare worked and nonworked budgeted hours to actual hours and dollars by personnel classification, a labor and volume report may be issued; this is useful when reviewing staffing patterns and guidelines in relation to productivity. Using Table 35–4 as a visual guide, consider the following analysis:

- Productivity (budget index) is reported in columns (10) and (11). 1.00 is equivalent to 100% utilization of staff in relation to volume. A budget index of 1.00 or greater is interpreted as a more productive output. The budget index is derived by dividing budgeted HWkd/WLU (D) by the actual HWkd/WLU (7) (using pay period 01: 6.15 ÷ 6.96

PROJECTING PERSONNEL HOURS

FULL TIME EQUIVALENTS (FTE'S)

REQUIREMENTS	DAYS	VARIABLE	EVENINGS	NIGHTS	TOTAL
ROOMS 1-10	20.0		2.0	2.0	24.0
CYSTO X 2	2.0(1/RM)				2.0
SATURDAY	.4		.4	.4	1.2
SUNDAY	.4		.4	.4	1.2
RUNOVERS		2.0(NOT REPLACED)			2.0
LASER NURSE					
(2days/wk=16 hrs.=.4)	.4				.4
ORDERLY	2.4		1.4	1.4	5.2
CLERK	1.0		1.0		2.0
TOTAL	26.6	2.0	5.2	4.2	38.0 FTE'S

TOTAL 36 FTE'S WILL REQUIRE REPLACEMENT; IF 1.171 = PAID TO WORK RATIO, 17.1% IS USED AS THE REPLACEMENT FACTOR FOR DETERMINING HOW MANY FTE'S ARE NEEDED TO COVER FOR NON-PRODUCTIVE (NON-WORKED) HOURS SUCH AS SICK TIME, VACATION, EDUCATION.

      *36 FTE'S X 17.1% = 6.15 FTE'S OR 6.0 REPLACEMENT FTE'S.

      *2.0 FTE'S WILL NOT BE REPLACED (RUNOVER TEAM)

      *4.0 FTE'S EXEMPT STAFF WHO ARE NOT REPLACED(SUPERVISOR,HEAD NURSE, EDUCATOR LEADER, UNIT MANAGER)

              FTE'S = 38.0 FOR SCHEDULED COVERAGE
                     6.0 FOR REPLACEMENT
                     4.0 FIXED EXEMPT STAFF
    TOTAL FTE'S = 48.0

CONVERSION OF FTE'S TO HOURS

TOTAL FTE'S = 48.0 X 2080 HOURS = 99840 HOURS

        99840 HOURS X 17.1% (NON-WORKED) = 17072 NON-WORKED HOURS

        99840 HOURS − 17072 HOURS = 82768 WORKED HOURS

PROJECTED VOLUME = 17,000 HOURS

        82768 WORKED HOURS ÷ 17,000 HOURS = 4.86 HWD/WLU

FIGURE 35–6. Projecting personnel hours.

TABLE 35–4. COST CENTER LABOR AND VOLUME REPORT

YEAR _____

DEPARTMENT _____

(A) WORKLOAD UNIT: OR Hrs
(B) PROJECTED VOL./YEAR: 19320 Hrs
(C) AVERAGE VOL./PAY PERIOD: 743 Hrs
(D) BUDGETED HWkd/WLU: 6.15

Pay Period (1)		FTEs Worked					HWkd/ WLU (7)	Workload Volume		Budget Index	
Ending	Nos.	Budget (2)	Actual (3)	Earned (4)	Budget Variance (5) (2)-(3)	Earned Variance (6) (4)-(3)		Current (8)	YTD (9)	Current (10)	YTD (11)
01/02/_____	01	51.28	40.75	36.05	10.52	−4.70	6.96	469	469	0.88	0.88
01/16/_____	02	57.04	62.88	61.87	−5.84	−1.00	6.25	805	1274	0.98	0.94
01/30/_____	03	59.55	65.08	67.71	−5.53	2.63	5.91	881	2155	1.04	0.98
02/13/_____	04	60.13	64.16	63.95	−4.04	0.22	6.17	832	2987	1.00	0.99
02/27/_____	05	59.67	59.72	58.57	−0.05	−1.16	6.27	762	3729	0.98	0.98
03/13/_____	06	60.64	68.70	65.41	−8.06	−3.29	6.46	851	4600	0.95	0.98
YTD AVERAGE		58.05	60.21	58.92	−2.16	−1.29	6.28	766		0.97	
ADJ. YTD AVERAGE		59.44	64.10	63.50	−4.66	−0.60	6.21	826	4131	0.99	

Courtesy of Kaiser Medical Center, Los Angeles, CA.

= 0.88). YTD average, based on 6 pay periods (1), = 0.97 budget index (10). In pay periods 03 and 04, exceeding 100% productivity may reflect the use of overtime or premium paid hours but requires further exploration to identify the underlying factors.

- Volume is slightly increased (8) compared to budgeted volume indicated in (C).
- HWkd/WLU (7) is higher than budgeted (D), indicating increased staffing hours for the volume experienced.
- Actual FTEs are higher than budgeted (3, 2, 5).
- Earned FTEs (4) (which provide flexible budgeting aspects) are lower than actual FTEs (3), which indicates that staffing hours exceed the actual volume.

If you consider pay period 01, the extreme results reflect the holiday working hours, which traditionally are reduced. Overtime may be increased if stand-by teams are called in more frequently and if holidays worked are paid at premium rates. To evaluate labor and volume, it may be beneficial to adjust the YTD average by deleting the outer pay period 01 and recalculating on 5 pay periods, rather than 6. Reviewing the adjusted YTD average presents a different picture:

- Budget index = 0.99 (increase of 0.1)
- Volume is significantly higher compared to budget.
- HWkd/WLU is still higher but is less than the unadjusted figure.
- Actual FTEs are significantly higher than budgeted but are less surprising in relation to the higher volume.
- Earned FTEs are minimally lower than actual FTEs, which indicates the impact of increased volume on staffing needs.

More detailed analysis is required to consider the factors contributing to the increased HWkd/WLU compared to budget, such as additional staff provided for surgical procedures, changes in fixed staffing positions, premium pay for worked hours (8 hours worked at 1.5 times is calculated at 12 hours). If staffing hours are increased to provide for specific patient care needs, departmental operations, or contractual obligations without an increase in volume, the hours worked per unit will be increased and productivity will appear to be less (budget index <1). It is not unrealistic to expect to use overtime to cope with fluctuations in volume. However, relying on extended staff hours or people working on scheduled days off is not a preferred practice. A consistent trend of over 100% productivity justifies increasing or redistributing staff. The hours cost more when premium pay is provided for overtime. It is important to establish an acceptable level of overtime as a baseline indicator and to closely monitor deviations.

SCHEDULING STAFF

A department's ability to function effectively depends a great deal on the scheduling of the people required to perform the work. Compatibility of the schedule with individual and service needs will enhance efficiency and increase work performance (Dunham et al., 1987). *Scheduling* is the assignment of appropriately skilled, knowledgeable personnel to a service area for specific hours and days of the week to meet the needs of the department.

A number of scheduling methods have evolved over the years and are applicable to the OR. *Master scheduling* "assigns an equitable number of desirable and undesirable shifts and days off to employees to meet the requirements of the staffing plan" (Lawrenz, 1987) (Appendices O and P).

Cyclical scheduling occurs when each employee is placed in a group, and each group repeats the same schedule over a period of time. Ordinarily, cyclical scheduling involves a greater number of staff during days but may include all staff members if different shifts are covered by the entire group. In the OR, cyclical scheduling provides a predetermined weekend pattern that allows staff to know their weekend commitment for as long as the groups remain intact. Some changes will occur if vacancies disrupt the group composition or vacations require coverage not available from other sources (Appendix Q).

Self-scheduling places the primary responsibility of developing a staff schedule on the employee, using specific guidelines. Flexible hours and self-scheduling became popular in the early 1980s as the nursing shortage began affecting the availability of RNs. Implementing a self-scheduling system requires thorough preplanning that incorporates staff nurses and managers into the preliminary stages. The method must be accepted by staff if it is to be successful. Creating a staffing schedule requires manipulation, negotiation, patience, and flexibility to cope with changes. Frequently, employees feel it is easier to let someone else do the work, even if the end result is undesirable. The OR is suitable for self-scheduling because it is self-contained. Staff do not usually float to other areas and often identify their preferred work schedules and stand-by schedules. In such a situation, the manager may be recording requests on the schedule and ensuring an adequate number of appropriate personnel, but the staff members are basically creating their own schedules. As part of the initial phase, a scheduling proctor or coordinator should be selected to review the schedule, coordinate adjustments, and facilitate the overall process. Conflicts may be handled by the proctor or, if unresolved, by the manager. Establishing guidelines for staff is a key element in the process. Guidelines provide the boundaries for flexible staff scheduling. Unit-specific information should include the number or ratio of staff per shift, acuity factors, special considerations, how to resolve a scheduling conflict, time frames, approval mechanism, special requests, and how to change schedules. As with any change in practice, the self-scheduling system needs to be reassessed and revised as necessary.

Tracking and revising schedules is a laborious task, and the schedule may be difficult to maintain without errors. A manual tracking system is a common method whether the function is centralized, decentralized, or self-scheduled. Once a master scheduling tool is completed, individual unit schedules are posted in the specific service area. All adjustments are made on the master schedule, which is usually divided into weekly components for ease of handling and access.

Automated staff scheduling systems have the potential to reduce the labor intensity involved in producing unit-specific schedules, prevent rewriting information, avoid deletion of information when numerous changes are made, and provide updated copies of the schedule whenever requested. Most frequently, the OR retains control of the schedule when a centralized system is in place. Some automated system models have the ability to track educational attendance, licensing, and certification expirations. Of course, the effectiveness of the automated system depends on timely, accurate input of data.

When staff are represented by a collective bargaining agreement, contract practices will prevail unless otherwise negotiated. Before instituting alternative staffing arrangements, the Fair Labor policies, bargaining unit contracts, and state laws should be reviewed. The Fair Labor Standards Act of 1938 regulates the number of hours an employee may work and establishes the overtime provisions for hours worked in excess of the maximum.

The following description of scheduling restraints and limitations is extracted from the scheduling workbook by Lawrenz (1987). Overtime pay in hospitals may be based on one 40-hour work week or the pay period.

In the 40-hour option, employees must have two days off in every work week. In the second option, employees may work as many as seven 8-hour shifts in one week, as long as they do not exceed ten 8-hour shifts within a two-week period. In the 40-hour option, overtime is not paid if an employee works more than 8 hours in a 24-hour period. However, hours in excess of 40 within one work week are paid at overtime.
The institution is allowed to choose the starting day of the work week. With a policy of every other weekend off, this choice of work week becomes important in providing the flexibility desired by both hospitals and employees.

In the OR, the issue of Specialist versus Generalist is crucial when considering staff composition and scheduling guidelines. The versatility of the Generalist provides flexibility and maximum utilization of personnel. However, as surgical procedures progress in complexity and technological requirements, the expectation that employees can increase their knowledge and skill in all subspecialties is unrealistic. In smaller suites the Generalist is a necessity for efficient, cost-effective management of the department. The volume of some procedures is usually unevenly distributed throughout the services, and focusing on a particular service would not be practical.

Larger departments lend themselves well to the Specialist approach, especially when the volume and types of surgeries are able to support the concept. Various systems are designed to accommodate the Specialist option. A selected number of staff either volunteer or are assigned to a primary subspecialty with the expectation that they will maintain their skills in other areas, which is especially important when employees are scheduled for weekends and stand-by. In many facilities, one individual is identified as a service coordinator or team leader and serves as the resource for the subspecialty, checking inventory, teaching in the area, and ensuring the availability of well-functioning equipment. If a "clinical ladder" is in place, the Specialist may be integrated into the plan on the clinical tract. If a Specialist concept is initiated, scheduling decisions will need to consider how the limited scope of primary practice will affect off-hours scheduling such as weekends and holidays. How does the Specialist concentrate on a specific service area during the week and be prepared to perform safely and knowledgeably in other high-tech areas on the weekends? Ensuring updating of skills and demonstration of competency then becomes a triad challenge involving the employee, the department's educator, and the manager.

CONCLUSION

Appropriate staffing and effective scheduling are a challenge. They offer an opportunity to be creative while performing routinized, logically sequenced tasks. Regardless of the method or the process used, it is important to identify the desired outcome and then develop the guidelines or objectives that will provide the means to accomplish them. Formulas, patterns, recommendations, and experiences are tools with which to work. Every OR is unique and, as such, is deserving of a customized plan that best reflects the activity and trends of the department. Organizational and departmental culture, geographic location, surgical diversity, available resources (both human and financial), and the physical plant are only a few factors that will influence the staffing and scheduling process. The following key points should be remembered:

1. Identify desirable outcomes.
2. Remember that patient safety is the primary responsibility.
3. Provide knowledgeable, skilled staff that can perform safely and efficiently.
4. Attempt to match staff needs with department needs to promote an effective, harmonious environment.

5. Develop guidelines and plans that reflect the department's unique needs.
6. Use staff in decision-making whenever feasible.
7. Periodically monitor and evaluate staffing schedules and revise them as necessary.
8. Be prepared to let go of some traditions and "get creative."
9. Try not to get discouraged when the volume of surgeries exceeds staffing capability.
10. Keep Administration informed of potential and actual staffing/scheduling issues.
11. If staffing resources are limited despite creative attempts, assess the scheduling of surgical procedures. It may be necessary to propose a reduction in the number of rooms scheduled or to consider a different approach in scheduling procedures.
12. Ensure compliance with regulatory requirements and accrediting standards.

Bibliography

Accreditation manual for hospitals (1989, p. 273). Chicago: The Joint Commission on Accreditation of Healthcare Organizations.

The nursing shortage: facts, figures and feelings. (1987, p. viii). Chicago: American Hospital Association.

Dunham, R. B., Pierce, J. L., Castaneda, M. B. (1987). Alternative work schedules: two field quasi-experiments. *Personnel Psychology, 40,* 215–241.

Human Resources Administrator (1987, August). *Nursing shortage near crisis.* Chicago, IL.

Lawrenz, E. (1987). *Staffing and scheduling workbook.* Montclair, NJ: Lawrenz-Madden-Sofio, Inc..

Morse, L. E. (1987). Hospital personnel supply v demand. *California Association Hospital & Health Systems Insight, II,* 9.

Newby, J. M., Jr. (1980, September). Study supports hiring more part-time RNs. *Hospitals,* 71–73.

OR Focus. (1988). Filling the staffing gap. *OR Focus, 5.* Baxter Healthcare Corporation, McGaw Park, IL.

Staffing in freestanding surgery centers (1987). *OR Manager, 3,* 10.

Rose, M. (1984, April). Shiftwork, how does it affect you? *American Journal of Nursing,* 442–447.

Westfall, P. G. (1988, September/October). Legal staffing issues and the nursing shortage. *California Nursing Review, 16,* 19–20, 28–32.

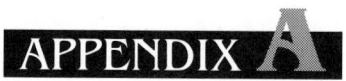

Traditional Block Scheduling

BLOCK SCHEDULE – YEAR_____

A.M.

ROOM	MONDAY	TUESDAY	WEDNESDAY	THURSDAY	FRIDAY
1	ENT	ENT	ENT	ENT	ENT
2	GS	ORTHO	GS	EYE	GS
3	ENT	ENT	ENT	GYN	ENT
4	ORTHO	EYE	GS	GS	GS-PLASTIC
5	NEURO	NEURO	NEURO	NEURO	NEURO
6	GYN-ONCOLOGY	GYN-RADIUM	NEURO	GYN-ONCOLOGY	ORTHO
7	GU	GU	GU	GS	GS-PEDS
8	GU-ONCOLOGY	GU	GU	GU	GU-ONCOLOGY
9	EYE	ORTHO	ENT	ORTHO	ORTHO
10	CARDIAC	CARDIAC	CARDIAC	CARDIAC	CARDIAC
11	ORTHO	ORTHO	GS	GS	ORTHO
12	CARDIAC	CARDIAC	CARDIAC	CARDIAC	CARDIAC
14	CARDIAC	CARDIAC	CARDIAC	CARDIAC	CARDIAC
CYSTO	CYSTO	CYSTO	CYSTO	CYSTO	CYSTO
CYSTO	CYSTO	CYSTO	CYSTO	CYSTO	CYSTO

P.M.

ROOM	MONDAY	TUESDAY	WEDNESDAY	THURSDAY	FRIDAY
1	GS	ENT	ENT	ENT	ENT
2	GS	ORTHO	ORTHO	GS-THORACIC	GS-PV
3	ENT	ORTHO	ENT	GS	EYE
4	EYE	GS	GS-ONCOLGY	GU	GS-ONCOLOGY
5	NEURO	NEURO	ORTHO	ENT	NEURO
6	GYN-ONCOLOGY	GS	NEURO	GYN-ONCOLOGY	ORTHO
7	GU	ENT	GS	ENT	GU-ONCOLOGY
8	GU-ONCOLOGY	GU	GYN	ORTHO	ENT
9	ORTHO	ORTHO	NEURO	ORTHO	ORTHO
10	CARDIAC	CARDIAC	CARDIAC	CARDIAC	CARDIAC
11	GS	GS	ORTHO	GS-PV	GS-PV
12	CARDIAC	CARDIAC	CARDIAC	CARDIAC	CARDIAC
14	CARDIAC	CARDIAC	CARDIAC	CARDIAC	CARDIAC
CYSTO	CYSTO	CYSTO	CYSTO	CYSTO	CYSTO
CYSTO	CYSTO	CYSTO	CYSTO	CYSTO	CYSTO

Courtesy of Kaiser Medical Center, Los Angeles, CA.

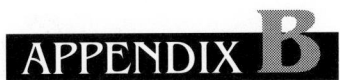

Block Schedule Revision Form

TO: DATE:
                                                       FROM:

SUBJECT: Block Schedule Revisions   EXTENSION:
                                                       CC:

_____

DELETE	**ADD**	**CHANGE**

Dept:_____ Surgeon:_____

Original Schedule:_____

New Schedule:_____

Effective Date:_____

Remarks:_____
_____
_____

Courtesy of Kaiser Medical Center, Los Angeles, CA.

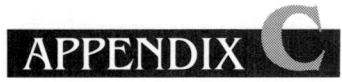

Monthly OR Block Time Release Notification Form

Department_____Date Submitted_____

Surgeon:_____

Effective Dates of Releases	**AM or PM**	**Reason**		
		Vac	**S/L**	**Ed**	**Other**
_____/_____/_____	_____/_____	_____/_____/_____/_____
_____/_____/_____	_____/_____	_____/_____/_____/_____
_____/_____/_____	_____/_____	_____/_____/_____/_____
_____/_____/_____	_____/_____	_____/_____/_____/_____
_____/_____/_____	_____/_____	_____/_____/_____/_____

To be completed by O.R. Scheduling Department

Date Received: _____ Date Posted: _____

Date Submitted to O.R._____

To be completed by O.R. Department:

Date Received:_____ Date Reassigned:_____

Date Submitted to Scheduling:_____

Reassigned to: Department: _____

        Surgeon: _____

White: Scheduling Dept. Pink: O.R. Yellow: Scheduling Goldenrod: Surgical Department

Courtesy of Kaiser Medical Center, Los Angeles, CA.

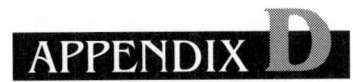

Room Turnover Between Cases

HOSPITAL X OPERATING ROOM DEPARTMENT
Turnaround Time Between Cases (Clean-up/Set-up)

SERVICE	INPATIENT/SDA			OUTPATIENT			TOTAL	TOTAL
	TIME	CASES		TIME	CASES		TIME	CASES
Cardiovascular	28.43	7		0.00	0		28.43	7
Cystoscopy	22,05	37		20,56	9		21.76	46
ENT	24.31	26		15.70	73		17.96	99
Ophthalmology	13.25	12		12.84	76		12.90	88
General/Thoracic/PV	21.63	92		18.86	57		20.57	149
	(average)			(average)			(average)	
TOTAL	21.93	174		13.59	215		20.32	389

Courtesy of Kaiser Medical Center, Los Angeles, CA.

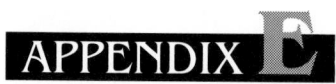

Type of Surgical Admission by Service

TYPE OF SURGICAL ADMIT

MONTH OF _____

SERVICES	OUTPATIENT		INPATIENT		SAME DAY		TOTAL
	COUNT	% OF TOTAL	COUNT	% OF TOTAL	COUNT	% OF TOTAL	
GENERAL SURGERY	63	30.29	88	42.31	57	27.40	208
PERIPHERAL VASCULAR	2	6.45	26	83.87	3	9.68	31
THORACIC	3	15.00	14	70.00	3	15.00	20
CARDIOVASCULAR	1	0.80	123	98.40	1	0.80	125
GYN	37	34.26	35	32.41	36	33.33	108
OPHTHALMOLOGY	0	0.00	4	100.00	0	0.00	4
ORTHOPEDICS	37	43.02	28	32.56	21	24.62	86
NEURO	6	12.77	20	42.55	21	44.68	47
TOTAL	149	23.68	338	53.73	142	22.57	629

Courtesy of Kaiser Medical Center, Los Angeles, CA.

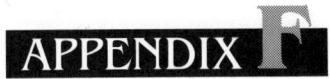

Number of Cases by Service and Scheduling Priority

CASES BY SERVICE AND SCHEDULING
MONTH OF _____

SERVICES	SCHEDULED		ADD-ON		URGENT		EMERGENCY		TOTAL
	COUNT	% OF TOTAL	COUNT	% OF TOTAL	COUNT	% OF TOTAL	COUNT	% OF TOTAL	
GENERAL SURGERY	121	58.17	29	13.94	9	4.33	49	23.56	208
PERIPHERAL VASCULAR	11	35.48	7	22.58	7	22.58	6	19.35	31
THORACIC	14	70.00	4	20.00	1	5.00	1	5.00	20
CARDIOVASCULAR	83	66.40	20	16.00	11	8.80	11	8.80	125
GYN	52	48.15	2	1.85	10	9.26	44	40.74	108
OPHTHALMOLOGY	0	0.00	0	0.00	4	100.00	0	0.00	4
ORTHOPEDICS	59	68.690	17	19.77	5	5.81	5	5.81	86
NEURO	35	74.47	6	12.77	1	2.13	5	10.64	47
TOTAL	375	60.00	85	13.60	44	7.00	121	19.36	625

Courtesy of Kaiser Medical Center, Los Angeles, CA.

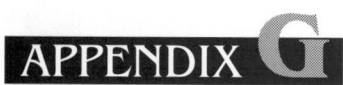

Runover Report

RUNOVER REPORT

(CASES WHICH RAN BEYOND 5:00 P.M.)

DAY OF WEEK_____

OVERTIME AFTER 5p(HRS)	GENERAL	NEURO	GYN	ORTHO	TOTAL
0–1	2.61	0.42	0.40	1.39	4.82
1–2	1.46	0.33	0.33	0.31	2.43
2–3	0.73	0.07	0.07	0.14	1.01
4–5	0.38	0.09	0.00	0.02	0.49
TOTAL	5.18	0.91	0.8	1.86	8.75

TYPE OF SCHEDULE	GENERAL	NEURO	GYN	ORTHO	TOTAL
SCHEDULED	2.92	0.54	1.25	0.96	5.67
ADD-ON	1.65	0.31	0.12	0.45	2.53
URGENT	0.38	0.09	0	0.05	0.52
EMERGENCY	0.31	0.12	0.14	0.14	0.71
TOTAL	5.26	1.06	1.51	1.6	9.43

Courtesy of Kaiser Medical Center, Los Angeles, CA.

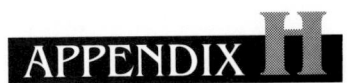

Delay Statistics by Service

DELAY FIRST CASE IN THE MORNING-(DELAY= PT NOT IN ROOM BY 7:15)
MONTH____

SERVICE	INPATIENT/SDA		OUTPATIENTS		TOTAL	
	TIME-MIN.	CASES	TIME-MIN.	CASES	TIME-MIN.	CASES
CARDIOVASCULAR	8.69	61	0.00	0	9.84	61
CYSTOSCOPY	21.91	53	16.67	9	21.15	62
ENT	26.50	20	18.96	53	21.03	73
OPHTHALMOLOGY	18.33	12	22.98	48	21.33	60
GENERAL SURGERY	26.15	89	20.00	36	24.38	125
NEUROSURGERY	24.80	50	20.91	11	24.10	61
TOTAL	126.38	285.00	99.52	157.00	121.83	442.00

Courtesy of Kaiser Medical Center, Los Angeles, CA.

927

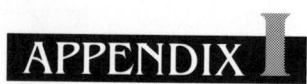

OR Usage Time Spread

OPERATING ROOM USAGE TIMESPREAD
OPERATING ROOMS 1 - 10
FOR THE MONTH OF _____

DATE: _____

TIME SPREAD	OPERATIONS IN PROGRESS
0700-0714	2
0715-0729	3
0730-0744	3
0745-0759	10
0800-0814	10
0815-0829	10
0830-0844	10
0845-0859	10
0900-0914	10
0915-0929	9
0930-0944	9
0945-0959	9
1000-1014	9
1015-1029	10
1030-1044	8
1045-1059	8
1100-1114	9
1115-1129	10

Time Spread covers the entire 24 hours or any segment indicated by the requestor.

Courtesy of Kaiser Medical Center, Los Angeles, CA.

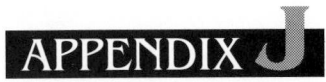
Graph of OR Usage Time Spread

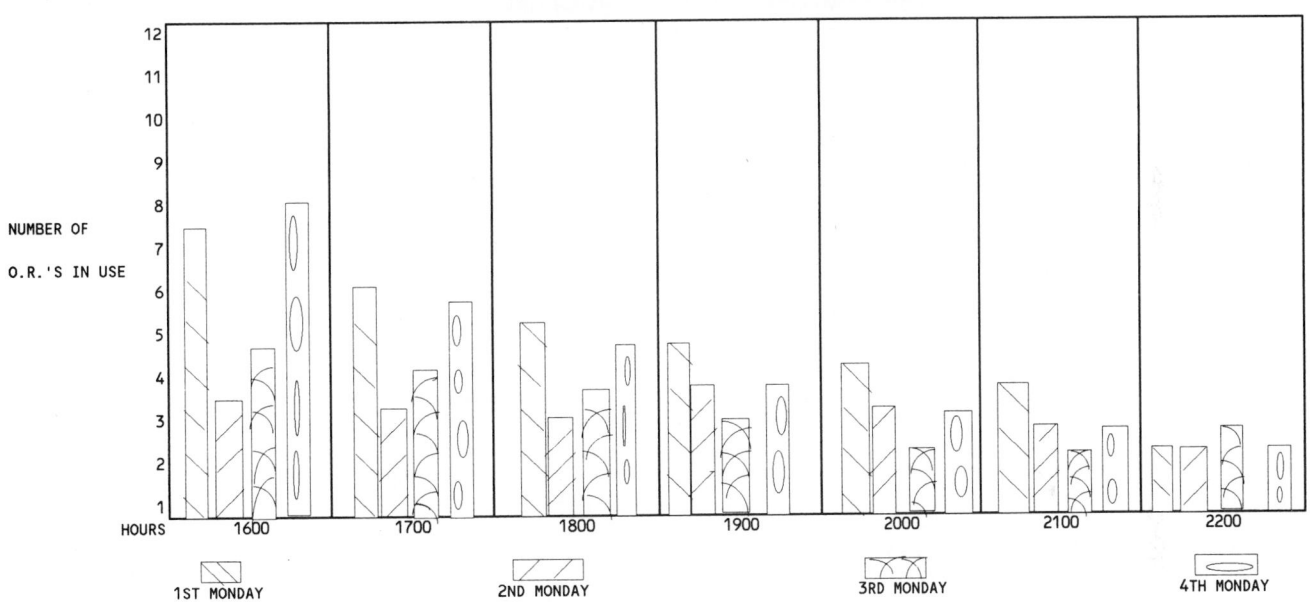

OPERATING ROOM USAGE (PER HOUR)
DAY OF WEEK OF ___MONTH ____YEAR

Courtesy of Kaiser Medical Center, Los Angeles, CA.

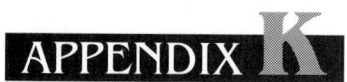

Policy and Procedure: Staffing the OR

POLICY AND PROCEDURE

SECTION:	PERIOPERATIVE NURSING STRUCTURE	NUMBER: _____
TITLE:	STAFFING THE OPERATING ROOM	EFFECTIVE DATE:
		REVISION DATE:

REVIEW DATES: PAGE NUMBER

References: Standardized Procedure - NO   Procedure - NO

MAIN OR

Educated, trained, skilled staff are provided on a 24 hour, 7 day/week basis. Staff assignments are made according to each patient's health status and surgical procedure. A minimum of one (1) scrub assistant (**RN** or **CST**), and one (1) **RN** circulator are provided per patient, with the exception of **Cystoscopies**. One(1) **RN** circulator is provided per patient in the **Cystoscopy** area.

P.M.'s- A minimum of two operating rooms will be staffed for emergency surgeries. In the event of insufficient staffing, personnel may be obtained by the following alternatives: overtime, stand-by, per diem, registry.
Nights-One (1) team is on duty, 11:30 P.M. - 7:30 A.M., 7 days per week. In addition, one (1) team on stand-by.
Week-ends- Two (2) teams are on duty from 7:30 A.M. to 4:00 P.M. Saturday for coverage of elective and emergency surgeries. Two (2) teams are on stand-by for the same hours. One (1) team is on duty, and one team is on stand-by for each 8 hour shift from 3:15 P.M. Saturday to 11:45 P.M. Sunday.

SATELLITE SURGERY:

Hours of operation are from 8:00 A.M. - 4:00 P.M., Monday through Friday. Trained, skilled staff are provided from 7:30 A.M. to 5:30 P.M. Patients requiring surgery other than during these hours are transferred to the main O.R. according to health status and requirements for care.

APPROVALS

Courtesy of Kaiser Medical Center, Los Angeles, CA.

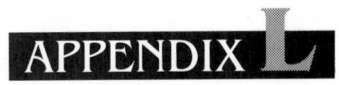

Policy and Procedure: Staffing the OR—Additional Staff

POLICY AND PROCEDURE

SECTION: **PERIOPERATIVE NURSING STRUCTURE**   NUMBER: _____

TITLE: **STAFFING THE OPERATING ROOM**   EFFECTIVE
                                                    DATE:
                                                REVISION
                                                  DATE:

REVIEW DATES: **PAGE NUMBER**

References: Standardized Procedure - NO   Procedure - NO

ADDITIONAL STAFF

In the event staffing needs exceed the minimum number of personnel scheduled, additional staff are usually available from our internal labor poole, comprised of unassigned staff and variable shift personnel. If the department's internal labor poole cannot provide sufficient staffing, per diem and registry staff will be utilized; overtime will be employed, as necessary. Perioperative Nursing Managers and the Clinical Nurse Specialist will assist with patient care activities, as necessary. In the event alternative staffing options are unsuccessful or inefficient, operating rooms will be delayed until staff is available.

DELAY OF CASES- will be decided upon according to the following criteria:
- a. health status of the patient
- b. urgency of the procedure
- c. psycho-social impact to the patient
- d. M.D. availability
- e. impact on the schedule

After hours, stand-by personnel are available to provide assistance. If necessary, additional personnel may be obtained by the Perioperative Manager on-call.

APPROVALS

Courtesy of Kaiser Medical Center, Los Angeles, CA.

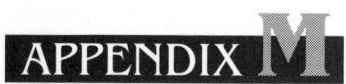

Policy and Procedure: Scope of Practice for Perioperative Nursing

POLICY AND PROCEDURE

SECTION:	**PERIOPERATIVE NURSING STRUCTURE**	NUMBER: _____
TITLE:	**SCOPE OF PRACTICE FOR**	EFFECTIVE
	PERIOPERATIVE NURSING	DATE:
		REVISION
		DATE:

REVIEW DATES: _____ PAGE NUMBER

References: Standardized Procedure - NO   Procedure - NO

1. On an annual basis, to coincide with the performance evaluation, each member will complete the assessment tool. Learner R.N. will be required to perform a minimum of one (1) double circulate and solo circulate on each procedure identified.

2. Learner Certified Surgical Technologist will perform a minimum of two (2) double scrub and solo scrub on each procedure identified under the supervision of a R.N.

3. The Clinical Supervisor of the Operating Room will assume responsibility for updating and maintaining trained, skilled staff on a 24 hour, 7 day/week basis by collaborating with the Assistant Supervisor of each O.R. wing.

APPROVALS

Courtesy of Kaiser Medical Center, Los Angeles, CA.

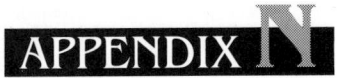

Policy and Procedure: Acuity Based Staffing for the OR

POLICY AND PROCEDURE

SECTION:	**PERIOPERATIVE NURSING STRUCTURE**
TITLE:	**ACUITY BASED STAFFING FOR**
	THE OPERATING ROOM

NUMBER: _____
EFFECTIVE
DATE:
REVISION
     DATE:

REVIEW DATES: **PAGE NUMBER**

Purpose: To establish guidelines for staff assignment related to the level of care required, as determined by the acuity of the patient, surgical procedure and/or technology.

Policy:

I. Basic Staffing, for each operative procedure, with the exception of Cysto, is comprised of a ratio of two (2) qualified Perioperative Staff, at least one of whom is a Registered Nurse (RN) per patient. The RN will assume the role of the circulating RN and CST or second RN will assume the role of the scrub person. The CST is under the direct supervision of the Circulating RN. The Cystoscopy O.R. is a 1:1 ratio and requires 1 RN at all times.

Additional staff will be provided (refer to Staffing Policy) at any time during the procedure when acuity is greater than 2:1 ratio and 1:1 ratio respectively. In the event the acuity of the patient requires additional staff, personnel may be provided by Certified Nurse Anesthetists (CRNA's).

II. In the O.R., there are three categories of acuity on which staffing ratios will be determined, for all or part of the surgery: patient, surgical procedure and technological needs.

A. Patient factors which may require a ratio of 3:1 (2:1-Cysto)
 1. Physical condition of the patient such as hemodynamic imbalance, severe blood loss, severe active bleeding, unstable vital signs, malignant hyperthermia.
 2. Emotional distress of the patient.

B. Surgical procedure factors which may require a ratio of 3:1 (2:1-Cysto):
 1. Multiple procedures occurring simultaneously.
 2. Multiple trauma procedures occurring simultaneously.
 3. Cysto reverts to Open Procedure
 4. Life threatening conditions including but not limited to:
     4.1 Ruptured aortic aneurysm
     4.2 Stab wounds to the heart
     4.3 Ruptured ectopic pregnancy
     4.4 Cardiac Arrest

C. Technological factors which may require a ratio of 3:1 (2:-Cysto):
 1. Cell Saver- one RN will operate and be accountable for the use of the Cell Saver.
 2. Laser- an appropriately trained staff person is responsible for the safe operation of the Laser.
 3. Use of an unusual amount of specialty equipment.

D. In addition, 3:1 (2;1-Cysto) staffing will be provided in cases, as judged on an individual basis, where an extra qualified RN or CST is necessary due to an unusual or urgent factor and when care of the patient presents physical danger to self and/or others.

APPROVALS

Courtesy of Phyllis Massino and Margaret Spres, Kaiser Medical Center, Woodland Hills, CA.

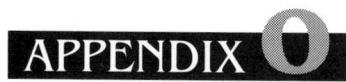

Sample Master Schedule

VARIABLE POSITIONS

DAYS	NAME	WK I S	M	T	W	TH	F	S	WK II S	M	T	W	TH	F	S	WK III S	M	T	W	TH	F	S	WK IV S	M	T	W	TH	F	S
RN		7A	R	X	X	X	X	R	R	X	X	X	X	X	R	R	X	X	X	X	X	R	R	X	X	X	X	X	R
RN		R	X	X	X	R	X	7A	7A	R	X	X	X	X	R	R	X	X	X	X	X	R	R	X	X	X	X	X	R
RN		R	X	X	X	X	X	R	R	X	X	R	X	X	7A	7A	X	R	X	X	X	R	R	X	X	X	X	X	R
RN		R	X	X	X	X	X	R	R	X	X	X	X	X	R	R	X	X	R	X	X	7A	7A	X	R	X	X	X	R
RN		R	X	X	X	X	X	R	R	X	X	ED	X	X	R	R	X	X	X	X	X	R	R	X	X	X	R	X	7A
RN		R	X	X	X	X	X	R	R	X	X	X	X	X	R	R	X	X	X	X	X	R	7A	R	X	X	X	X	R
TECH		R	X	X	X	X	R	7A	7A	X	R	X	X	X	R	R	X	X	X	X	X	R	R	X	X	X	X	X	R
TECH		7A	X	R	X	X	X	R	R	X	X	X	X	X	R	R	V	V	V	V	V	R	R	X	X	X	X	X	R
TECH		R	X	X	X	X	X	R	R	X	X	X	X	R	7A	7A	R	X	X	X	X	R	R	X	X	X	X	X	R
PT-RN		R	7A				7A	R	R		7A	7A			R	R	7A	7A	7A	7A	7A	R	R		7A		7A	R	7A
PT-RN		R		7A		7A		R	R	7A				7A	R	R			7A		7A	R	R	7A				7A	R
PD-RN											7A					7A	7A												

EVENINGS

DAYS	NAME	WK I S	M	T	W	TH	F	S	WK II S	M	T	W	TH	F	S	WK III S	M	T	W	TH	F	S	WK IV S	M	T	W	TH	F	S
RN		3P	R	X	X	X	X	R	R	X	X	X	X	X	R	R	X	X	X	X	X	R	R	X	X	X	X	X	R
RN		R	X	X	X	X	R	3P	3P	X	R	X	X	X	R	R	X	X	X	X	X	R	R	X	X	X	X	X	R
RN		R	X	X	X	X	X	R	R	X	X	R	X	X	3P	3P	R	X	X	X	X	R	R	X	X	X	X	X	R
RN		R	X	X	X	X	X	R	R	X	X	X	X	X	R	R	X	X	X	X	ED	R	R	X	X	X	X	X	R
TECH		3P	X	R	X	X	X	R	R	X	X	X	X	X	R	R	X	X	X	X	X	R	R	X	X	X	R	X	3P
TECH		R	X	X	X	X	X	R	R	X	X	X	X	X	R	R	X	X	X	X	R	3P	3P	X	R	SL	SL	SL	R
PT-RN		V						3P	3P						3P	3P						3P	3P			3P	3P	3P	3P

NIGHTS

DAYS	NAME	WK I S	M	T	W	TH	F	S	WK II S	M	T	W	TH	F	S	WK III S	M	T	W	TH	F	S	WK IV S	M	T	W	TH	F	S
RN		11P	R					R	R					R	11P	11P			R			R	R				R		11P
TECH		R			R		11P		11P	R					R	R				R	11P		11P	R					R
PT-RN		11P					11P		11P												11P		11P						
PT-RN		R	TR																	11P	11P							R	11P

R-DAY OFF
V-VACATION
SL-SICK LEAVE
ED-EDUCATION
TR-TRAINING

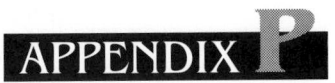
Sample Master Schedule: Ambulatory Surgery

WEEK   I   II   III   IV

POSITION	NAME	S	M	T	W	TH	F	S	S	M	T	W	TH	F	S	S	M	T	W	TH	F	S	S	M	T	W	TH	F	S
FT-RN		R	X	X	X	X	X	R	R	X	X	X	X	X	R	R	X	X	X	X	X	R	R	X	X	X	X	X	R
FT-TECH		R	V	V	V	V	V	R	R	X	X	X	X	X	R	R	X	X	X	X	X	R	R	X	X	X	X	X	R
PT-RN		R	X	X	X				R	R	X	X	X				R	R	X	X	X				R	R	X	X	X			R
PT-RN		R			X	X	X	R	R			X	X	X	R	R			X	X	X	R	R			X	X	X	R
PT-TECH		R	X	X				R	R	X	X				R	R	X	X				R	R	X	X				R
PT-TECH		R				X	X	R	R				X	X	R	R				X	X	R	R				X	X	R
PD-RN			X	X	X	X	X																						
PD-RN																													
PACU-FLOAT		R	X	X	X	X	X	R	R	X	X	X	X	X	R	R	X	X	X	X	X	R	R	X	X	X	X	X	R
PACU-FLOAT		R	X	X	X	X	X	R	R	X	X	X	X	X	R	R	X	X	X	X	X	R	R	X	X	X	X	X	R

R-Day Off
V-Vacation

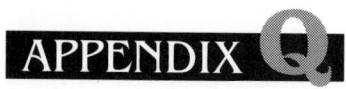

Cyclical Weekend Schedule

CYCLICAL SCHEDULE
(FOR 6 WEEK SCHEDULE)

GROUP I EMPLOYEE	WEEKEND	GROUP II EMPLOYEE	WEEKEND	GROUP III EMPLOYEE	WEEKEND
1	1ST	9	3RD	17	5TH
2	1ST	10	3RD	18	5TH
3	1ST	11	3RD	19	5TH
4	1ST	12	3RD	20	5TH
5	2ND	13	4TH	21	6TH
6	2ND	14	4TH	22	6TH
7	2ND	15	4TH	23	6TH
8	2ND	16	4TH	24	6TH

EMPLOYEE 25, 26, ETC. ARE USED TO FILL IN FOR VACATION, SICK TIME, SPECIAL REQUESTS.

CHAPTER 36

Perioperative Nursing Job Descriptions and Performance Appraisals

Noreen E. McHugh, Mary Bradley, and Mark L. Phippen

A *job description* lists the duties, responsibilities, and requirements of a particular job and serves as a standard by which an employee may be rated during the annual performance evaluation. Well-written job descriptions and performance appraisals are essential for quality perioperative nursing care.

This chapter describes the elements of an effective job description, provides guidelines for writing job descriptions, discusses problems frequently encountered when completing an evaluation tool, and suggests strategies for minimizing the effects of rating errors. Examples of job descriptions and criteria-based performance appraisals for perioperative nurses engaged in clinical practice and assistive personnel working in the perioperative area are provided.

STANDARDS

Well-written job descriptions and performance appraisals are based on standards of clinical practice, which in turn flow from standards of patient care. Figure 36–1 illustrates how job descriptions and performance appraisals flow from standards of patient care.

A *standard of patient care* describes a basic level of care a patient can expect to receive during his or her hospitalization. Appendix A provides an example of standards of patient care for a perioperative nursing services department. Note that the standard is categorized into five major headings: patient care process, teaching, discharge planning, safety, infection control, and respect. These headings correspond to quality assessment and improvement aspects of care frequently used by health care institutions.

The standards for clinical practice shown in Appendix B were derived from the standards of patient care. They focus on the process of providing perioperative nursing care and the performance of professional role activities, rather than on what the patient can expect to receive during the perioperative period. The professional and assistive personnel job descriptions presented in Appendices C through M and the examples of performance appraisals presented in Appendices N and O were developed using the standards for clinical practice shown in Appendix B. Appendix P presents performance appraisal scoring guidelines.

JOB DESCRIPTIONS

The Joint Commission for Accreditation of Healthcare Organizations (JCAHO) requires job descriptions for each position classification of registered nurses and assistive personnel (JCAHO, 1992). Job descriptions

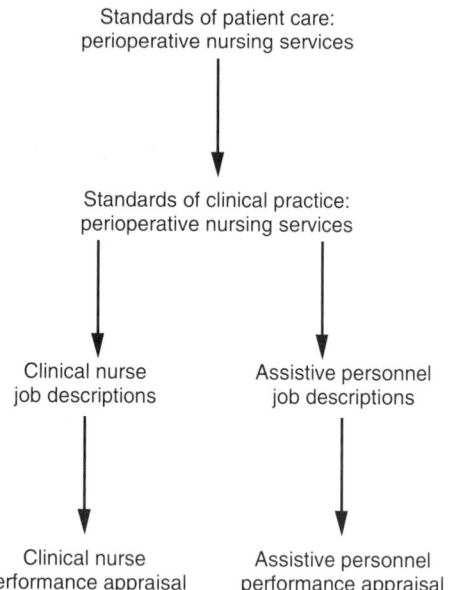

FIGURE 36–1. Flow chart showing how job descriptions and performance appraisals develop from standards of patient care.

should specify standards of performance and delineate the functions, responsibilities, and specific qualifications of each classification. Other requirements include a periodic review of job descriptions and revision as needed to reflect current job requirements. Job descriptions should be on file and accessible to employees when hired or on request.

An effective job description has four basic subdivisions: heading, job summary, duties performed, and personal requirements (Metzger, 1981).

Heading

The importance of selecting an appropriate job title is essential and should not be underestimated. "Social behaviorists have pointed out repeatedly the important roles that status and recognition play in the motivation of employees. Not only should the selected title distinguish a job from every other job in the organization, it should also be fully acceptable to the incumbents" (Metzger, 1981). When writing the job description, the heading should include the following:

- Job title
- Alternate job title (if appropriate)
- Department in which job is assigned
- Title of supervisor responsible for the job
- Position code number
- Date of approval

Job Summary

The job summary briefly describes the objective and purpose of the job and delineates how the job differs from other jobs. When writing the job summary, words

should be carefully used to achieve the maximum amount of meaning (Otis and Leukart, 1948). The hours of work, shift information, and overtime requirements should be included.

Duties Performed

A complete description of the duties of a job is given in the duties performed section. When writing and organizing this section (Patton et al., 1964)

- arrange duties in logical order, either in order of importance or chronologically within the work cycle;
- state the duties clearly and concisely;
- begin each statement with an active, functional verb in the present tense;
- avoid vague, ambiguous generalizations by using specific words; and
- indicate whether duties are regular or occasional by estimating the percentage of time spent on each activity.

In addition, the description of duties performed should state the minimum requirements expected.

Personal Requirements

The personal requirements section, also referred to as the job specifications section, describes the skills needed to perform the job and the physical demands of the job. The most common factors found in a job specification are as follows:

- *Education and training.* Formal education or courses required to provide minimum knowledge and background for the job, including specialized training and licensing, if applicable.
- *Experience.* Minimum experience necessary to perform the job requirement effectively.
- *Physical demands.* Specific physical tasks required and the percentage of time spent on the tasks, stating in measurable terms the amount of strength, endurance, or physical strain required to perform the job. For example, the amount of time spent sitting, climbing, lifting, walking, pulling, bending, and stretching should be delineated.
- *Mental, visual, and hearing demands.* The amount and nature of mental, visual, and aural alertness required to perform the job.
- *Initiative, judgment, and creative ability.* The extent and range of independent action, exercise of judgment, decision making, and planning required in the job.
- *Working conditions.* The positive and negative aspects of the working conditions (e.g., extremes of hot, cold, wet, glaring light, noise, odors).
- *Health hazards.* Health hazards that may exist even though recognized safety procedures and devices are in place (e.g., exposure to chemical fumes or to infectious materials).

- *Machines, tools, and equipment operated.* Equipment routinely used (e.g., lasers, microscopes, sharps, electrosurgical devices).
- *Financial responsibility.* Financial responsibilities in terms of accounting, budgeting, record keeping, equipment and supplies, and other duties related to hospital income or expense.
- *Reports and records.* The responsibility for the development and maintenance of records and reports.
- *Contacts.* External as well as internal contacts for meeting, working, instructing, guiding, or influencing other persons (e.g., hospital staff, patients, visitors, vendors).
- *Supervision.* The extent of responsibility for supervising the work of others including level of authority, the decision to hire, fire, and discipline, and the distribution of work to employees.

In addition, a section should be provided to describe any special comments about the position not covered in other sections of the job description. Finally, the signature of the department representative authorized to approve the job description must be included.

WRITING JOB DESCRIPTIONS

The following are some guidelines for writing job descriptions:

- Be clear and concise. Use nontechnical language whenever possible. A job description should explain the objectives, duties, and responsibilities of a job so precisely that they are understandable to a layperson.
- Start each sentence with an active, present-tense verb in describing the duties of a job.
- Avoid the narrative form.
- Refer to job titles rather than names. For example, use "Reports to Head Nurse" rather than "Reports to Mary Jones."
- Describe what a job incumbent does instead of attempting to explain a procedure that must be used.
- Be precise in defining responsibility.
- Focus the job description on the duties of the job rather than the person performing the duties.

UPDATING JOB DESCRIPTIONS

After a job description has been written, evaluated, analyzed, and approved, it should be reviewed periodically to ensure that it adequately describes the work currently being performed. Whenever significant changes are introduced into the job requirements, it is necessary to change the job description. The following are examples of changes that require revision of the job description:

- Restructuring of the department that results in the realignment of several jobs into new positions that involve a change of difficulty or responsibility.
- A change in technology resulting in either the need for special knowledge or elimination of a job function.
- A change in the physical facilities resulting in an alteration in the way in which functions of the job are performed.

USES OF JOB DESCRIPTIONS

A thorough knowledge of all hospital jobs is necessary to carry out many personnel and human resource activities both internally and externally.

Internal Uses

- *Recruitment and placement.* Staffing activities require that job requirements be known and specified. The job description provides an effective guide for recruiting and hiring qualified individuals.
- *Transfers and promotions.* The job description aids employees in making educated transfer decisions and in considering a promotion.
- *Job evaluation.* The job description is a vital component of the process to determine the relative value of one job to other jobs within the hospital. The job description is directly related to each position's salary range and the salary potential designated for the position.
- *Wage and salary surveys.* The job description provides a method of comparing rates of pay for similar jobs in other institutions.
- *Performance appraisal.* The job description defines the minimum requirements for a job and the tasks to be performed. It is a tool used in appraising employee performance and can provide the information necessary to develop performance standards.
- *Health and safety.* The job description provides data on health factors and safety hazards.

External Uses

- *Fair Labor Standards Act.* The job description provides a basis for determining whether a job is exempt from the provisions of the Fair Labor Standards Act.
- *Equal Employment Opportunity.* The job description provides the basis for determining whether personnel and human resource activities are discriminatory because they are not job related. When something other than the job and its requirements serves as the basis for a particular decision or type of treatment, the employer must be able to demonstrate the job relatedness of the activity in question through the job description.

- *Occupational Safety and Health Act (OSHA).* Regulations under OSHA describe the obligations for safety standards for both employers and employees. Statements in the job description regarding health and safety factors clarify such obligations.
- *Equal Pay Act.* Discrepancies in wages must be justified by actual differences in job functions and not mere dissimilarities in job titles. The job description can assist in justifying the discrepancies in pay.

PERFORMANCE APPRAISALS

Well-written job descriptions provide the foundation for building an effective job evaluation program. With an effective program in place, managers are able to assess the performance of their subordinates. This enables them to observe and scrutinize the work of subordinates from the standpoint of how well the employee is performing and provides data on how the employee can improve performance. An effective program forces the manager to act when he or she "is unwilling or unable to deal with a problem employee because of a desire to avoid conflict" (Rakich et al., 1985).

A formal appraisal system serves another important purpose. Employees have a right to know how well they are doing and what can be done to improve job performance. Most employees want to know what supervisors think of their work. This desire to know stems from psychological issues dealing with self-worth and a need for reassurance.

USES OF PERFORMANCE APPRAISALS

Performance evaluations yield important information for both employee and manager. This information can be used to

- compare an individual's actual performance to expected standards by collecting information and assessing whether an employee is performing satisfactorily or unsatisfactorily;
- identify different levels of competence and determine appropriate interventions such as inservice education, reassignment, or promotion;
- identify individuals who may require additional counseling or assistance for purposes of providing direction toward an appropriate support program;
- assess the quality of the manager's supervision and effectiveness of leadership style; and
- determine compensation or reward based on performance.

Performance appraisal systems provide feedback to both employee and manager. The information generated can be useful in identifying individuals whose performance is exemplary and worthy of recognition.

Likewise, unsatisfactory performance can be identified, appropriate interventions formulated, and objectives established.

PROBLEMS

Appraisal systems are based on the development and measurement of standards of performance. The evaluator faces a number of problems when completing an evaluation tool. Some of these problems include the following (Levitz, 1981; Rakich et al., 1985):

- Performance standards are often not operational or have no bearing on the performance of the job.
- All evaluators may not agree on the definition of evaluation standards. Terms such as "outstanding," "satisfactory," or "unsatisfactory" may mean different things to different evaluators.
- Some evaluators do not give low ratings for fear of alienating the employee, while others are more critical and take the stand that no one is "outstanding." These evaluators are likely to rate all employees within a narrow range (i.e., rating toward the mean).
- Halo effect. The manager may tend to rate an employee high on each factor being rated based on only one outstanding characteristic, such as quantity of work. Values may be assigned without the benefit of a critical analysis of each performance standard.
- Isolated events. Rather than evaluate an employee's overall performance, a manager may focus attention on isolated or recent events. This can have positive or negative consequences.
- Subjectivity. The evaluator's own biases toward the individual being evaluated can influence the overall interpretation of a performance appraisal.
- Inadequate preparation of the evaluator. A manager may be influenced by favoritism when making judgments regarding performance. In this situation, individuals may be judged on popularity rather than actual performance.

Levitz (1981) suggests some possible ways to minimize the effects of rating errors:

- Focus criteria on a single job activity.
- Observe performance regularly.
- Define terms clearly or eliminate if no clear definition is possible.
- Provide training for managers in techniques or methods of evaluation.
- Ensure that raters do not have to evaluate large groups of subordinates.
- Ensure that evaluation criteria are clearly stated and are meaningful to the task being performed.

In summary, well-written job descriptions and performance appraisals based on standards of patient care and clinical practice are essential for quality patient care in the perioperative setting. In fact, they are the blueprint for excellence in patient care.

Standards of Patient Care: Perioperative Nursing Services

PATIENT CARE PROCESS

The patient will receive care that reflects an ongoing process of management of his or her health status.

Assessment

The patient will receive a physiological assessment on admission to the operating room and ongoing assessments of his or her physiological health status during the perioperative period. The patient can expect to have his or her

- identity, operative procedure, and operative permit verified;
- skin checked for rashes, bruises, lesions, and previous incisions;
- range of motion assessed;
- diagnostic studies reviewed (laboratory values and radiograph results) and abnormal results reported to the physician;
- blood pressure, temperature, pulse, and respirations assessed;
- abnormalities, injuries, previous surgery, and reactions to previous anesthetics noted;
- internal and external prostheses/implants identified;
- sensory impairments noted;
- nutritional status identified (NPO status and weight);
- allergies verified;
- physiological health status communicated to appropriate health team members; and
- physiological health status documented in the health record.

The patient will receive a psychosocial assessment on admission to the operating room. The patient can expect to have his or her

- perception of surgery and expectation of care assessed,
- coping mechanisms assessed,
- ability to understand assessed,
- knowledge level determined,
- religious preference identified, and
- psychosocial health status communicated to appropriate health team members and documented in the health record.

The patient will have nursing diagnoses appropriate to the perioperative period identified. The patient can expect the registered nurse to identify his or her

- risk for intraoperative injury related to positioning, extraneous objects, or chemical, physical, and electrical hazards;
- risk for nosocomial infection;
- risk for alteration in body temperature during the procedure;
- risk for fluid deficit during the procedure;
- risk for ineffective airway clearance during the procedure;
- risk for alterations in breathing patterns during the procedure;
- risk for alterations in cardiac output during the procedure;
- risk for self-care deficit following the procedure; and
- knowledge deficit related to the physiological and psychological responses to the surgical or invasive procedure.

Plan

The patient's care will be planned based on problems/needs identified in the assessment. The patient can expect a perioperative plan of care that ensures he or she will

- be free from injury related to positioning, extraneous objects, or chemical, physical, and electrical hazards;

Adapted with permission from Association of Operating Room Nurses. (1992). *Standards and recommended practices for perioperative nursing.* Competency statements in perioperative nursing; Standards of perioperative clinical practice; Patient outcomes: Standards of perioperative care. Denver.

941

- be free from nosocomial infection;
- have body temperature maintained;
- have fluid and electrolyte balance maintained;
- have effective airway clearance;
- have breathing patterns maintained;
- have cardiac output maintained;
- have potential self-care deficits identified; and
- have knowledge concerning the expected physiological and psychological responses to the planned procedure.

Intervention

The patient will receive perioperative nursing care according to an established plan of care. The patient can expect to

- be safely transported to and from the surgical suite;
- receive care in an aseptic environment;
- have equipment and supplies provided based on identified needs;
- have equipment and supplies provided in a timely and efficient manner;
- have scrub and circulating personnel perform their duties in a competent manner;
- have sponge, sharps, and instrument counts performed according to operating room policy;
- have drugs, blood, and solutions administered according to hospital and operating room policy;
- be physiologically monitored during surgery; and
- have the surgical environment monitored and controlled.

Evaluation

The patient will receive ongoing evaluations of the effectiveness of the care provided. The patient can expect to be evaluated for

- injury related to positioning, extraneous objects, or chemical, physical, and electrical hazards;
- nosocomial infection;
- maintenance of body temperature;
- fluid deficit;
- ineffective airway clearance;
- alterations in breathing patterns;
- alterations in cardiac output;
- potential self-care deficits; and
- knowledge of the physiological and psychological responses to surgical intervention.

TEACHING

The patient and/or family will be knowledgeable about what to expect during the perioperative period. The patient and/or family can expect to have

- teaching needs identified,
- readiness to learn assessed,

- instruction designed based on identified needs, and
- the effectiveness of teaching evaluated.

DISCHARGE PLANNING

The patient will be prepared for discharge from the operating room to the postanesthesia care unit or nursing unit through coordination of resources and communication of pertinent clinical information. The patient can expect to have

- his or her physiological and psychosocial status communicated to the postanesthesia care unit or nursing unit personnel, and
- intraoperative complications that may affect postoperative course or hospital discharge communicated to appropriate personnel.

SAFETY

The patient can expect to receive care in a safe environment according to the Association of Operating Room Nurses (AORN) *Recommended Practices and Operating Room Policies and Procedures*. The patient can expect the perioperative nursing team to

- adhere to Operating Room safety policies and procedures;
- incorporate into practice the principles delineated in *Recommended Practices for Electrosurgery, Laser Safety in the Practice Setting, Positioning the Surgical Patient, Radiological Safety in the Practice Setting, Safe Care Through Identification of Potential Hazards in the Surgical Environment, Use of the Pneumatic Tourniquet,* and *Sponge, Sharps, and Instrument Counts;* and
- maintain awareness and take appropriate actions relative to known allergies and/or previous anesthetic incidents.

INFECTION CONTROL

The patient can expect to receive care in an aseptic environment according to *Recommended Practices and Operating Room Policies and Procedures*. The patient can expect the perioperative nursing team to

- adhere to Operating Room infection control policies and procedures;
- incorporate into practice the principles delineated in *Recommended Practices for Basic Aseptic Technique, Care of Instruments, Scopes, and Powered Surgical Instruments, Cleaning and Processing Anesthesia Equipment, Operating Room Sanitation, Preoperative Skin Preparation of Patients, Sterilization and Disinfection, Surgical Attire, Surgical Hand*

Scrub, and *Traffic Patterns in the Surgical Suite;* and

- implement universal precautions and good hand-washing techniques.

RESPECT

The patient will retain personal identify, self-worth, and human rights during the intraoperative period. The patient can expect to have the perioperative nursing care team to

- demonstrate awareness of his or her rights as a patient,
- provide for privacy through maintaining confidentiality,
- provide for privacy through physical protection,
- identify and respect ethnic and spiritual beliefs,
- provide status reports to family members, and
- demonstrate awareness of the right to communicate in his or her native tongue.

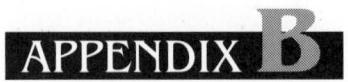

Standards of Clinical Practice: Perioperative Nursing Services

---

PATIENT CARE PROCESS

The nurse provides nursing care that reflects an ongoing process of management of the patient's health status.

Assessment

On patient admission to the operating room, the nurse collects physiological assessment data. Assessment of the patient's physiological health status is ongoing during the intraoperative period. The nurse

- identifies the patient and operative procedure;
- verifies the operative permit;
- checks the patient's skin for rashes, bruises, lesions, and previous incisions;
- assesses the patient's range of motion;
- reviews the patient's diagnostic studies (laboratory values and radiographic results) and reports abnormal results to the physician;
- assesses the patient's blood pressure, temperature, pulse, and respirations;
- notes patient abnormalities, injuries, previous surgery, and reactions to previous anesthetics;
- identifies the patient's internal and external prostheses/implants;
- notes the patient's sensory impairments;
- identifies the patient's nutritional status (NPO status and weight);
- verifies patient allergies;
- communicates the patient's physiological health status to appropriate health team members; and
- documents the patient's physiological health status in the health record.

On patient admission to the operating room, the nurse collects psychosocial assessment data. The nurse

- assesses the patient's perception of surgery and expectation of care,
- assesses the patient's coping mechanisms,
- assesses the patient's ability to understand,
- determines the patient's knowledge level,
- identifies the patient's religious preference,
- communicates the patient's psychosocial health status to appropriate health team members, and
- documents that status in the health record.

The nurse identifies nursing diagnoses appropriate to the perioperative period. The nurse will identify the patient's

- risk for intraoperative injury related to positioning, extraneous objects, or chemical, physical, and electrical hazards;
- risk for nosocomial infection;
- risk for alteration in body temperature during the procedure;
- risk for fluid deficit during the procedure;
- risk for ineffective airway clearance during the procedure;
- risk for alterations in breathing patterns during the procedure;
- risk for alterations in cardiac output during the procedure;
- risk for self-care deficit following the procedure; and
- knowledge deficit related to the physiological and psychological responses to the surgical or invasive procedure.

Plan

The nurse plans nursing care based on problems/needs identified in the assessment. The nurse will develop a plan of care that ensures that the patient

- is free from injury related to positioning, extra-

Adapted with permission from Association of Operating Room Nurses. (1992). *Standards and recommended practices for perioperative nursing.* Competency statements in perioperative nursing; Standards of perioperative clinical practice; Patient outcomes: Standards of perioperative care. Denver.

neous objects, or chemical, physical, and electrical hazards;

- is free from nosocomial infection;
- has body temperature maintained;
- has fluid and electrolyte balance maintained;
- has an effective airway clearance;
- has breathing patterns maintained;
- has cardiac output maintained;
- has potential self-care deficits identified; and
- has knowledge concerning the expected physiological and psychological responses to the planned procedure.

Intervention

The nurse provides nursing care according to an established plan of care. The nurse will

- ensure that the patient is safely transported to and from the surgical suite;
- provide care in an aseptic environment;
- provide equipment and supplies based on identified needs;
- provide equipment and supplies in a timely and efficient manner;
- ensure that scrub and circulating personnel perform their duties in a competent manner;
- perform sponge, sharps, and instrument counts according to operating room policy;
- administer drugs, blood, and solutions according to hospital and operating room policy;
- physiologically monitor the patient during surgery; and
- monitor and control the surgical environment.

Evaluation

The nurse performs ongoing evaluations of the effectiveness of the care provided. The nurse will evaluate the patient for

- injury related to positioning, extraneous objects, or chemical, physical, and electrical hazards;
- nosocomial infection;
- maintenance of body temperature;
- fluid deficit;
- ineffective airway clearance;
- alterations in breathing patterns;
- alterations in cardiac output;
- potential self-care deficits; and
- knowledge of the physiological and psychological responses to surgical intervention.

TEACHING

The nurse ensures that the patient and/or family are knowledgeable about what to expect during the perioperative periods. The nurse will

- identify teaching needs,
- assess readiness to learn,
- design strategies instruction based on identified needs, and
- evaluate the effectiveness of teaching.

DISCHARGE PLANNING

The nurse prepares the patient for discharge from the operating room to the postanesthesia care unit or nursing unit through coordination of resources and communication of pertinent clinical information. The nurse will

- communicate the patient's physiological and psychosocial status to postanesthesia care unit or nursing unit personnel, and
- communicate critical intraoperative events that may impact postoperative course or hospital discharge to appropriate personnel.

SAFETY

The nurse provides care in a safe environment according to *Recommended Practices and Operating Room Policies and Procedures*. The nurse will

- adhere to Operating Room safety policies and procedures;
- incorporate into practice the principles delineated in *Recommended Practices for Electrosurgery, Laser Safety in the Practice Setting, Positioning the Surgical Patient, Radiological Safety in the Practice Setting, Safe Care Through Identification of Potential Hazards in the Surgical Environment, Use of the Pneumatic Tourniquet,* and *Sponge, Sharps, and Instrument Counts;* and
- maintain awareness and take appropriate actions relative to known allergies and/or previous anesthetic incidents.

INFECTION CONTROL

The nurse creates and maintains an aseptic environment according to *Recommended Practices and Operating Room Policies and Procedures*. The nurse will

- adhere to Operating Room infection control policies and procedures;
- incorporate into practice the principles delineated in *Recommended Practices for Basic Aseptic Technique, Care of Instruments, Scopes, and Powered Surgical Instruments, Cleaning and Processing Anesthesia Equipment, Operating Room Sanitation, Preoperative Skin Preparation of Patients, Sterilization and Disinfection, Surgical Attire, Surgical Hand*

Scrub, and *Traffic Patterns in the Surgical Suite;* and

● implement universal precautions and good hand-washing techniques.

RESPECT

The nurse ensures that the patient's personal identity, self-worth, and human rights are protected during the perioperative period. The nurse will ensure that the nursing care team

● demonstrates awareness of the patient's rights as a patient,
● provides for privacy through maintaining confidentiality,
● provides for privacy through physical protection,
● identifies and respects ethnic and spiritual beliefs,
● provides status reports to family members, and
● demonstrates awareness of the patient's right to communicate in his or her native tongue.

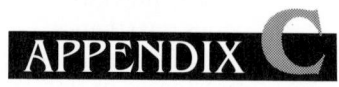

Perioperative Nurse I

POSITION IDENTIFICATION

1. Job Title: Perioperative Nurse I
2. Alternative Title: Operating Room Nurse I; Clinical Nurse I
3. Department: Perioperative Nursing Services
4. Supervisor: Department Head, Perioperative Nursing Services
5. Position Number:
6. Approved by: _____ Date: _____

POSITION SUMMARY

1. Under the general supervision of the Department Head, the Perioperative Nurse I is responsible for the perioperative nursing care of pediatric and adult surgical and endoscopy patients. The Perioperative Nurse I delivers care through the use of the nursing process as reflected in *Standards of Clinical Practice: Perioperative Nursing Services* and the *Standards of Perioperative Clinical Practice* in a manner that is cost effective without compromising quality of care. Expected practice behaviors include assessment, planning, implementation of perioperative nursing interventions, and evaluation.
2. The Perioperative Nurse I demonstrates competency to scrub and circulate for simple surgical and endoscopy procedures, scrub for complex surgical procedures in at least one surgical service, and circulate for complex surgical procedures in at least two surgical services.
3. Under the supervision of a qualified surgeon, the Perioperative Nurse I performs second assisting duties during the surgical procedure.
4. The Perioperative Nurse I participates in departmental quality assessment and improvement activities, meets hospital continuing education and cer-

tification requirements, participates in student teaching activities, upholds Nursing Services philosophy and objectives, contributes to organizational effectiveness, participates in professional nursing organizations, demonstrates knowledge of *Standards and Recommended Practices for Perioperative Nursing,* keeps abreast of professional literature, and demonstrates professional growth and development.
5. The Perioperative Nurse I works 8-hour rotating shifts as assigned by the Department Head; Weekend shifts and call are assigned on a rotating basis.

POSITION DUTIES*

1. Assesses the physiological health status of the patient on admission to the operating room and performs an ongoing assessment of the patient's physiological health status during the intraoperative period. The Perioperative Nurse I
   - verifies the patient's identity and planned operative procedure;
   - ensures that the operative permit is prepared, signed, and witnessed according to hospital policy and procedure;
   - inspects the patient's skin for rashes, bruises, lesions, and previous incisions;
   - determines the patient's range of motion;
   - reviews diagnostic studies (laboratory values and radiographic results) and reports abnormal results to the physician;

---

*Nursing process objectives adapted from Association of Operating Room Nurses (1992). Competency statements in perioperative nursing. In *Standards and recommended practices for perioperative nursing,* I:2-4–I:2-12, Denver.

Second assisting objectives from American College of Surgeons, American Hospital Association, Association of Surgical Technologists, American Medical Association. (1990). Proposed essentials and guidelines for an accredited educational program in surgical technology (draft document). Chicago, IL: American Medical Association, 1–17.

- checks the patient's blood pressure, temperature, pulse, and respirations;
- questions the patient about abnormalities, injuries, previous surgery, and reactions to previous anesthetics;
- identifies the presence of internal and external prostheses or implants;
- determines sensory impairments;
- assesses nutritional status, including NPO status and weight; and
- checks the patient for allergies.

2. Assesses psychological, sociocultural, and spiritual status on admission to the operating room. The Perioperative Nurse I
   - elicits the patient's perception of surgery and expectation of care,
   - identifies the patient's coping mechanisms,
   - determines the patient's ability to understand,
   - identifies the patient's knowledge level,
   - determines the patient's ethnic/cultural background, and
   - identifies religious preference.

3. Identifies nursing diagnoses appropriate to the intraoperative period. At a minimum, the Perioperative Nurse I identifies the patient's
   - risk for intraoperative injury related to positioning, extraneous objects, or chemical, physical, and electrical hazards;
   - risk for nosocomial infection;
   - risk for alteration in body temperature during the procedure;
   - risk for fluid deficit during the procedure;
   - risk for ineffective airway clearance during the procedure;
   - risk for alterations in breathing patterns during the procedure; and
   - knowledge deficit related to the physiological and psychological responses to the surgical or invasive procedure.

4. Plans care based on the patient's problems/needs identified in the assessment. The Perioperative Nurse I plans intraoperative care to ensure that the patient will
   - be free from injury related to positioning, extraneous objects, or chemical, physical, and electrical hazards;
   - be free from nosocomial infection;
   - have body temperature maintained;
   - have fluid and electrolyte balance maintained;
   - have effective airway clearance;
   - have breathing patterns maintained; and
   - have knowledge concerning the expected physiological and psychological responses to the planned procedure.

5. Implements perioperative nursing care according to an established plan of care and operating room policies and procedures. The Perioperative Nurse I
   - ensures that the patient is safely transported to and from the surgical suite;

- teaches the patient based on needs identified during the assessment;
- creates and maintains an aseptic surgical environment;
- counts sponges, sharps, and instruments according to operating room policy and procedure;
- provides equipment and supplies based on identified needs and in a timely, efficient, and safe manner;
- administers drugs, blood, and solutions according to hospital and operating room policy and procedure;
- physiologically monitors the patient during surgery;
- monitors and controls the surgical environment;
- positions the patient according to operating room policy and procedure;
- prepares and handles specimens and cultures according to operating room policy and procedure;
- supervises perioperative nursing associates and assistants assigned to perform the actions necessary to accomplish the identified goals;
- scrubs and circulates for simple surgical and endoscopy procedures;
- scrubs for complex surgical procedures in at least one surgical service; and
- circulates for complex surgical procedures in at least two surgical services.

6. Evaluates the effectiveness of the care provided. The Perioperative Nurse I evaluates the patient for
   - injury related to positioning, extraneous objects, or chemical, physical, and electrical hazards;
   - postoperative nosocomial infection;
   - maintenance of intraoperative body temperature;
   - intraoperative fluid deficit,
   - the presence of ineffective airway clearance during the intraoperative period,
   - alterations in breathing patterns during the intraoperative period, and
   - knowledge of the physiological and psychological responses to surgical intervention.

7. Communicates and documents perioperative nursing care. The Perioperative Nurse I
   - communicates the assessment, planning, implementation, and evaluation activities to appropriate health team members; and
   - documents the assessment, planning, implementation, and evaluation in the health record.

8. Serves as a second surgical assistant. The Perioperative Nurse I
   - holds retractors or instruments as directed by the surgeon,
   - sponges and suctions operative site,
   - applies electrocautery to clamps on bleeders,
   - cuts suture material as directed by the surgeon,

- connects drains to suction apparatus, and
- applies dressing to the closed wound.

ORGANIZATION AND PROFESSIONAL DEVELOPMENT RESPONSIBILITIES

1. The Perioperative Nurse I contributes to organization effectiveness and efficiency by
   - participating in quality assessment and improvement activities;
   - meeting hospital continuing education and certification requirements;
   - participating in student teaching activities, serving as a role model for professional nursing students rotating through the surgical suite, participating in the clinical instruction of professional nursing students and assistive personnel students, and assisting with the orientation of professional and paraprofessional employees;
   - upholding Nursing Services philosophy and objectives;
   - contributing to organizational effectiveness by demonstrating punctuality when reporting for duty, adhering to hospital policy concerning rest and lunch breaks, and completing assigned duties in an effective, efficient, and timely manner; and
   - demonstrating stewardship for hospital resources by adhering to established surgical charge protocols.
2. The Perioperative Nurse I demonstrates professional growth and development by
   - participating in professional nursing organizations,
   - demonstrating knowledge of *Standards and Recommended Practices for Perioperative Nursing,* and
   - keeping abreast of professional literature.

POSITION SPECIFICATIONS

1. Education and Training
   - Registered nurse
   - Graduate of a formal perioperative nursing course or documented on-the-job training
2. Experience
   - Entry-level position
3. Physical Demands
   - Constant walking, standing, bending, and stooping.
   - Pushing and pulling heavy objects such as gurneys, patient beds, and OR beds.
   - Must be able to lift patients, heavy boxes weighing up to 40 pounds, instrument sets weighing up to 20 pounds; must be able to lift surgical supplies above the head.

4. Mental, Visual, and Hearing Demands
   - Must be able to read, write, and understand English. Must be able to read supply labels, the surgical schedule, patient identification bracelets, and policies and procedures.
   - Must be able to read fine print.
   - Must be able to hear and follow verbal instructions.
5. Working Conditions
   - Must work in air-conditioned environment with a temperature of 65°–72°F and humidity of 45–55%. When assigned to assist with pediatric cases, temperature may be up to 85°–90°F.
   - Must wear hospital-provided scrub attire while on duty.
6. Hazards
   - Potential for cuts, bruises, muscle strains, and exposure to contagious diseases via blood and body fluids.
   - Potential for exposure to anesthetic waste gases, ethylene oxide, harsh disinfectants, sterilizing agents, exposure to high steam pressure and radiological environment.
   - Potential noise hazard from ultrasonic equipment when assigned to decontamination area.
7. Machines, Tools, and Equipment Operated
   - OR beds, fracture tables, recovery beds
   - Steam sterilizer, ultrasonic cleaner and dryer, and heat package sealing devices
   - Compressed gas gauges
   - Lasers, microscopes, sharps, electrosurgical devices, power instruments
8. Financial Responsibility
   - Must demonstrate stewardship behavior by conserving hospital resources (i.e., supplies).
9. Reports and Records
   - Completion of nursing documentation, charge records, incident reports, and other paperwork associated with position.
   - Communicates health status data to other team members as described in position duties.
10. Contacts
    - Must demonstrate hospital core values when interacting with visitors, patients, physicians, and nursing staff.
11. Supervisory Responsibilities
    - Perioperative nursing assistants; perioperative nursing associates; operating room materiels services technicians assigned to surgical procedures.
12. Worker Characteristics
    - Must maintain a neat, clean, professional appearance.
    - Willingness to work with employees at various levels of skill, knowledge, and abilities.
    - Must have understanding, patience, and tact in dealing with physicians and fellow workers.
    - Must pay attention to details.
    - Must be free of prejudice.
    - Must be self-motivated and work in an efficient and effective manner.

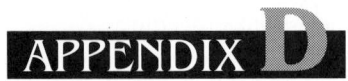

Perioperative Nurse II

POSITION IDENTIFICATION

1. Job Title: Perioperative Nurse II
2. Alternative Title: Operating Room Nurse II; Clinical Nurse II
3. Department: Perioperative Nursing Services
4. Supervisor: Department Head, Perioperative Nursing Services
5. Position Number:
6. Approved by: _____ Date: _____

POSITION SUMMARY

1. Under the general supervision of the Department Head, the Perioperative Nurse II is responsible for the perioperative nursing care of pediatric and adult surgical patients. The Perioperative Nurse II delivers care through the use of the nursing process as reflected in *Standards of Clinical Practice: Perioperative Nursing Services* and the *Standards of Perioperative Clinical Practice* in a manner that is cost effective without compromising quality of care. Expected practice behaviors include assessment, planning, implementation of perioperative nursing interventions, and evaluation.
2. The Perioperative Nurse II demonstrates competency to scrub and circulate for simple surgical and endoscopy procedures, scrub for complex surgical procedures in at least two surgical services, and circulate for complex surgical procedures in at least three surgical services.
3. Under the supervision of a qualified surgeon, the Perioperative Nurse II performs second assisting duties during the surgical procedure.
4. The Perioperative Nurse II serves as a professional and technical subject matter expert for at least one surgical service.
5. The Perioperative Nurse II serves as charge nurse for an identified shift.

6. The Perioperative Nurse II participates in departmental quality assessment and improvement activities, meets hospital continuing education and certification requirements, participates in student teaching activities, upholds Nursing Services philosophy and objectives, contributes to organizational effectiveness, participates in professional nursing organizations, demonstrates knowledge of *Standards and Recommended Practices for Perioperative Nursing,* keeps abreast of professional literature, and demonstrates professional growth and development.
7. The Perioperative Nurse II works 8-hour rotating shifts as assigned by the Department Head. Weekend shifts and call are assigned on a rotating basis.

POSITION DUTIES*

1. Assesses the physiological health status of the patient on admission to the operating room and performs an ongoing assessment of the patient's physiological health status during the intraoperative period. The Perioperative Nurse II
   - verifies the patient's identity and planned operative procedure;
   - ensures that the operative permit is prepared, signed, and witnessed according to hospital policy and procedure;
   - inspects the patient's skin for rashes, bruises, lesions, and previous incisions;
   - determines the patient's range of motion;

---

*Nursing process objectives adapted from Association of Operating Room Nurses (1992). Competency statements in perioperative nursing. In *Standards and recommended practices for perioperative nursing,* I:2-4–I:2-12, Denver.

Second assisting objectives from American College of Surgeons, American Hospital Association, Association of Surgical Technologists, American Medical Association. (1990). Proposed essentials and guidelines for an accredited educational program in surgical technology (draft document). Chicago, IL: American Medical Association, 1–17.

- reviews diagnostic studies (laboratory values and radiographic results) and reports abnormal results to the physician;
- checks the patient's blood pressure, temperature, pulse, and respirations;
- questions the patient about abnormalities, injuries, previous surgery, and reactions to previous anesthetics;
- identifies the presence of internal and external prostheses or implants;
- determines sensory impairments;
- assesses nutritional status, including NPO status and weight; and
- determines patient for allergies.

2. Assesses psychological, sociocultural, and spiritual status on admission to the operating room. The Perioperative Nurse II
   - elicits the patient's perception of surgery and expectation of care,
   - identifies the patient's coping mechanisms,
   - determines the patient's ability to understand,
   - identifies the patient's knowledge level,
   - determines the patient's ethnic/cultural background, and
   - identifies religious preference.

3. Identifies nursing diagnoses appropriate to the intraoperative and postoperative periods. At a minimum, the Perioperative Nurse II identifies the patient's
   - risk for intraoperative injury related to positioning, extraneous objects, or chemical, physical, and electrical hazards;
   - risk for nosocomial infection;
   - risk for alteration in body temperature during the procedure;
   - risk for fluid deficit during the procedure;
   - risk for ineffective airway clearance during the procedure;
   - risk for alterations in breathing patterns during the procedure;
   - risk for noncompliance to prescribed therapeutic regimens during the postoperative/rehabilitation period;
   - risk for self-care deficit during the postoperative/rehabilitation period; and
   - knowledge deficit related to the physiological and psychological responses to the surgical or invasive procedure.

4. Plans care based on the patient's problems/needs identified in the assessment. The Perioperative Nurse II plans intraoperative care to ensure that the patient will
   - be free from injury related to positioning, extraneous objects, or chemical, physical, and electrical hazards;
   - be free from nosocomial infection;
   - have body temperature maintained;
   - have fluid and electrolyte balance maintained;
   - have effective airway clearance;
   - have breathing patterns maintained;

- provide self-care during the postoperative/rehabilitation period;
- comply with prescribed therapeutic regimens during the postoperative/rehabilitation period; and
- have knowledge concerning the expected physiological and psychological responses to the planned procedure.

5. Implements perioperative nursing care according to an established plan of care and operating room policies and procedures. The Perioperative Nurse II
   - ensures that the patient is safely transported to and from the surgical suite;
   - teaches the patient-based needs identified during the assessment;
   - creates and maintains an aseptic surgical environment;
   - counts sponges, sharps, and instruments according to operating room policy and procedure;
   - provides equipment and supplies based on identified needs and in a timely, efficient, and safe manner;
   - administers drugs, blood, and solutions according to hospital and operating room policy and procedure;
   - physiologically monitors the patient during surgery;
   - monitors and controls the surgical environment;
   - positions the patient according to operating room policy and procedure;
   - prepares and handles specimens and cultures according to operating room policy and procedure;
   - supervises perioperative nursing associates and assistants assigned to perform the actions necessary to accomplish the identified goals;
   - scrubs and circulates for simple surgical and endoscopy procedures;
   - scrubs for complex surgical procedures in at least two surgical services; and
   - circulates for complex surgical procedures in at least three surgical services.

6. Evaluates the effectiveness of the care provided. The Perioperative Nurse II evaluates the patient for
   - injury related to positioning, extraneous objects, or chemical, physical, and electrical hazards;
   - postoperative nosocomial infection;
   - maintenance of intraoperative body temperature;
   - intraoperative fluid deficit;
   - the presence of ineffective airway clearance during the intraoperative period;
   - alterations in breathing patterns during the intraoperative period;
   - potential self-care deficits; and
   - knowledge of the physiological and psychological responses to surgical intervention.

7. Communicates and documents perioperative nursing care. The Perioperative Nurse II
   - communicates the assessment, planning, implementation, and evaluation activities to appropriate health team members; and
   - documents the assessment, planning, implementation, and evaluation in the health record.
8. Serves as a second surgical assistant. The Perioperative Nurse II
   - holds retractors or instruments as directed by the surgeon,
   - sponges and suctions operative site,
   - applies electrocautery to clamps on bleeders,
   - cuts suture material as directed by the surgeon,
   - connects drains to suction apparatus, and
   - applies dressing to the closed wound.
9. Serves as professional and technical subject matter expert for at least one surgical service. In this role, the Perioperative Nurse II
   - develops, implements, evaluates, and updates perioperative nursing practice guidelines, physician preference cards, and policies and procedures specific to surgical service;
   - collaborates with the Manager, Perioperative Nursing Services Business Operations personnel, and perioperative nursing associate assigned to surgical service to identify budget needs of a surgical specialty required to support the established nursing practice guidelines; to implement new procedures, procure specialty supplies, identify costs for the annual supply budget, develop the annual specialty equipment budget, and evaluate the quality and the effectiveness of equipment used by the surgical specialty;
   - collaborates with the perioperative nursing associate to inventory and orders specialty instruments, supplies, and equipment unique to surgical service;
   - demonstrates competency to operate all specialty instruments, supplies, and equipment unique to surgical service;
   - prepares and conducts professional and technical performance-oriented training programs related to specialty services for perioperative nursing personnel; and
   - serves as preceptor to perioperative nursing personnel rotating through specialty service.
10. Functions as the charge nurse on an identified shift. In this role, the Perioperative Nurse II
    - ensures that operating room policies and procedures are implemented,
    - makes patient care assignments based on identified patient needs and physician requirements,
    - ensures staffing patterns are adjusted according to policy and procedure, and
    - collaborates with physicians to ensure quality surgical patient care.

ORGANIZATION AND PROFESSIONAL DEVELOPMENT OBJECTIVES

1. The Perioperative Nurse II contributes to organization effectiveness and efficiency by
   - participating in quality assessment and improvement activities;
   - meeting hospital continuing education and certification requirements;
   - participating in student teaching activities, serving as a role model for professional nursing students rotating through surgical suite; participating in the clinical instruction of professional nursing students and assistive personnel students; and assisting with the orientation of professional and paraprofessional employees;
   - upholding Nursing Services philosophy and objectives;
   - contributing to organizational effectiveness by demonstrating punctuality when reporting for duty, adhering to hospital policy concerning rest and lunch breaks, and completing assigned duties in an effective, efficient, and timely manner; and
   - demonstrating stewardship for hospital resources by adhering to established surgical charge protocols.
2. The Perioperative Nurse II demonstrates professional growth and development by
   - participating in professional nursing organizations,
   - demonstrating knowledge of *Standards and Recommended Practices for Perioperative Nursing,* and
   - keeping abreast of professional literature.

POSITION SPECIFICATIONS

1. Education and Training
   - Registered nurse
   - Graduate of a formal perioperative nursing course or documented on-the-job training
   - Certification as a perioperative nurse (CNOR) highly desirable
2. Experience
   - 2½ years experience as a perioperative nurse
3. Physical Demands
   - Constant walking, standing, bending, and stooping.
   - Pushing and pulling heavy objects such as gurneys, patient beds, and OR tables.
   - Must be able to lift patients, heavy boxes weighing up to 40 pounds, instrument sets weighing up to 20 pounds; must be able to lift surgical supplies above the head.
4. Mental, Visual, and Hearing Demands

- Must be able to read, write, and understand English; must be able to read supply labels, the surgical schedule, patient identification bracelets, and policies and procedures.
- Must be able to read fine print.
- Must be able to hear and follow verbal instructions.

5. Working Conditions
  - Must work in air-conditioned environment with a temperature of 65°–72°F and humidity of 45–55%. When assigned to assist with pediatric cases, temperature may be up to 85°–90°F.
  - Must wear hospital-provided scrub attire while on duty.

6. Hazards
  - Potential for cuts, bruises, muscle strains, and exposure to contagious diseases via blood and body fluids
  - Potential for exposure to anesthetic waste gases, ethylene oxide, harsh disinfectants, sterilizing agents; exposure to high steam pressure and radiological environment
  - Potential noise hazard from ultrasonic equipment when assigned to decontamination area

7. Machines, Tools, and Equipment Operated
  - OR beds, fracture tables, recovery beds
  - Steam sterilizer, ultrasonic cleaner and dryer, and heat package sealing devices
  - Compressed gas gauges
  - Lasers, microscopes, sharps, electrosurgical devices, power instruments

8. Financial Responsibility
  - Must demonstrate stewardship behavior by conserving hospital resources (e.g., supplies, charging).

9. Reports and Records
  - Completes nursing documentation, charge records, incident reports, and other paperwork associated with position.
  - Communicates health status data to other team members as described in position duties.

10. Contacts
  - Must demonstrate hospital core values when interacting with visitors, patients, physicians, and nursing staff.

11. Supervisory Responsibilities
  - Perioperative nursing assistants; perioperative nursing associates; perioperative nurse I; operating room materiels services technicians assigned to surgical procedures.

12. Worker Characteristics
  - Must maintain a neat, clean, professional appearance.
  - Willingness to work with employees at various levels of skill, knowledge, and abilities.
  - Must have understanding, patience, and tact in dealing with physicians and fellow workers.
  - Must pay attention to details.
  - Must be free of prejudice.
  - Must be self-motivated and work in an efficient and effective manner.

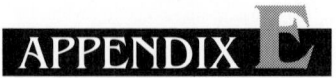

Perioperative Nurse III

POSITION IDENTIFICATION

1. Job Title: Perioperative Nurse III
2. Alternative Title: Operating Room Nurse III; Clinical Nurse III
3. Department: Perioperative Nursing Services
4. Supervisor: Department Head, Perioperative Nursing Services
5. Position Number:
6. Approved by: _____ Date: _____

POSITION SUMMARY

1. Under the general supervision of the Department Head, the Perioperative Nurse III is responsible for the perioperative nursing care of pediatric and adult surgical patients. The Perioperative Nurse III delivers care through the use of the nursing process as reflected in *Standards of Clinical Practice: Perioperative Nursing Services* and the *Standards of Perioperative Clinical Practice* in a manner that is cost effective without compromising quality of care. Expected practice behaviors include assessment, planning, implementation of perioperative nursing interventions, and evaluation.
2. The Perioperative Nurse III demonstrates competency to scrub and circulate for simple surgical and endoscopy procedures, scrub for complex surgical procedures in at least two surgical services, and circulate for complex surgical procedures in at least four surgical services.
3. Under the supervision of a qualified surgeon, the Perioperative Nurse III performs second assisting duties during the surgical procedure.
4. The Perioperative Nurse III serves as a professional and technical subject matter expert for at least two surgical services.

5. The Perioperative Nurse III serves as charge nurse for an identified shift.
6. The Perioperative Nurse III designs, implements, and evaluates systems to improve the quality of perioperative nursing patient care.
7. The Perioperative Nurse III assists the Department Head in the clinical evaluation of professional and paraprofessional perioperative nursing staff.
8. The Perioperative Nurse III participates in departmental quality assessment and improvement activities, meets hospital continuing education and certification requirements, participates in student teaching activities, upholds Nursing Services philosophy and objectives, contributes to organizational effectiveness, participates in professional nursing organizations, demonstrates knowledge of *Standards and Recommended Practices for Perioperative Nursing,* keeps abreast of professional literature, and demonstrates professional growth and development.
9. The Perioperative Nurse III works 8-hour rotating shifts as assigned by the Department Head. Weekend shifts and call are assigned on a rotating basis.

POSITION DUTIES*

1. Assesses the physiological health status of the patient on admission to the operating room and performs an ongoing assessment of the patient's

---

*Nursing process objectives adapted from Association of Operating Room Nurses (1992). Competency statements in perioperative nursing. In *Standards and recommended practices for perioperative nursing,* I:2-4–I:2-12, Denver.

Second assisting objectives from American College of Surgeons, American Hospital Association, Association of Surgical Technologists, American Medical Association. (1990). Proposed essentials and guidelines for an accredited educational program in surgical technology (draft document). Chicago, IL: American Medical Association, 1–17.

physiological health status during the intraoperative period. The Perioperative Nurse III

- verifies the patient's identity and planned operative procedure;
- ensures that the operative permit is prepared, signed, and witnessed according to hospital policy and procedure;
- inspects the patient's skin for rashes, bruises, lesions, and previous incisions;
- determines the patient's range of motion;
- reviews diagnostic studies (laboratory values and radiographic results) and reports abnormal results to the physician;
- checks the patient's blood pressure, temperature, pulse, and respirations;
- questions the patient about abnormalities, injuries, previous surgery, and reactions to previous anesthetics;
- identifies the presence of internal and external prostheses or implants;
- determines sensory impairments;
- assesses nutritional status, including NPO status and weight; and
- checks the patient for allergies.

2. Assesses patient's psychological, sociocultural, and spiritual status on admission to the operating room. The Perioperative Nurse III

- elicits the patient's perception of surgery and expectation of care,
- identifies the patient's coping mechanisms,
- determines the patient's ability to understand,
- identifies the patient's knowledge level,
- determines the patient's ethnic/cultural background, and
- identifies religious preference.

3. Identifies nursing diagnoses appropriate to the intraoperative and postoperative periods. At a minimum, the Perioperative Nurse III identifies the patient's

- risk for intraoperative injury related to positioning, extraneous objects, or chemical, physical, and electrical hazards;
- risk for nosocomial infection;
- risk for alteration in body temperature during the procedure;
- risk for fluid deficit during the procedure;
- risk for ineffective airway clearance during the procedure;
- risk for alterations in breathing patterns during the procedure;
- risk for noncompliance to prescribed therapeutic regimens during the postoperative/rehabilitation periods;
- risk for self-care deficit during the postoperative/rehabilitation period; and
- knowledge deficit related to the physiological and psychological responses to the surgical or invasive procedure.

4. Plans care based on the patient's problems/needs identified in the assessment. The Perioperative

Nurse III plans intraoperative and postoperative care to ensure that the patient will

- be free from injury related to positioning, extraneous objects, or chemical, physical, and electrical hazards;
- be free from nosocomial infection;
- have body temperature maintained;
- have fluid and electrolyte balance maintained;
- have effective airway clearance;
- have breathing patterns maintained;
- comply with prescribed therapeutic regimens during the postoperative/rehabilitation period;
- provide self-care during the postoperative/rehabilitation period; and
- have knowledge concerning the expected physiological and psychological responses to the planned procedure.

5. Implements perioperative nursing care according to an established plan of care and operating room policies and procedures. The Perioperative Nurse III

- ensures that the patient is safely transported to and from the surgical suite;
- teaches the patient-based needs identified during the assessment;
- creates and maintains an aseptic surgical environment;
- counts sponges, sharps, and instruments according to operating room policy and procedure;
- provides equipment and supplies based on identified needs and in a timely, efficient, and safe manner;
- administers drugs, blood, and solutions according to hospital and operating room policy and procedure;
- physiologically monitors the patient during surgery;
- monitors and controls the surgical environment;
- positions the patient according to operating policy and procedure;
- prepares and handles specimens and cultures according to operating room policy and procedure;
- supervises perioperative nursing associates and assistants assigned to perform the actions necessary to accomplish the identified goals;
- scrubs and circulates for simple surgical and endoscopy procedures;
- scrubs for complex surgical procedures in at least two surgical services; and
- circulates for complex surgical procedures in at least four surgical services;

6. Evaluates the effectiveness of the care provided. The Perioperative Nurse III evaluates the patient for

- injury related to positioning, extraneous objects, or chemical, physical, and electrical hazards;
- postoperative nosocomial infection;

- maintenance of intraoperative body temperature;
- intraoperative fluid deficit;
- the presence of ineffective airway clearance during the intraoperative period;
- alterations in breathing patterns during the intraoperative period;
- compliance with prescribed therapeutic regimens;
- provision of self-care; and
- knowledge of the physiological and psychological responses to surgical intervention.

7. Communicates and documents perioperative nursing care.
   - Communicates the assessment, planning, implementation, and evaluation activities to appropriate health team members.
   - Documents the assessment, planning, implementation, and evaluation in the health record.

8. Serves as a second surgical assistant. The Perioperative Nurse III
   - holds retractors or instruments as directed by the surgeon,
   - sponges and suctions operative site,
   - applies electrocautery to clamps on bleeders,
   - cuts suture material as directed by the surgeon,
   - connects drains to suction apparatus, and
   - applies dressing to the closed wound.

9. Serves as professional and technical subject matter expert for at least two surgical services. In this role, the Perioperative Nurse III
   - develops, implements, evaluates, and updates perioperative nursing practice guidelines, physician preference cards, and policies and procedures specific to surgical service;
   - collaborates with the Manager, Perioperative Nursing Services Business Operations personnel, and perioperative nursing associate assigned to surgical service to identify budget needs of a surgical specialty required to support the established nursing practice guidelines, implement new procedures, procure specialty supplies, identify costs for the annual supply budget, develop the annual specialty equipment budget, and evaluate the quality and the effectiveness of equipment used by the surgical specialty;
   - collaborates with the perioperative nursing associate to inventory and orders specialty instruments, supplies, and equipment unique to surgical service;
   - demonstrates competency to operate all specialty instruments, supplies, and equipment unique to surgical service;
   - prepares and conducts professional and technical performance-oriented training programs related to specialty services for perioperative nursing personnel; and
   - serves as preceptor to perioperative nursing personnel rotating through specialty service.

10. Functions as the charge nurse on an identified shift. In this role, the Perioperative Nurse III
    - ensures that operating room policies and procedures are implemented,
    - makes patient care assignments based on identified patient needs and physician requirements,
    - ensures staffing patterns are adjusted according to policy and procedure, and
    - collaborates with physicians to ensure quality surgical patient care.

11. Designs, implements, and evaluates systems to improve the quality of perioperative nursing patient care. In this role, the Perioperative Nurse III
    - designs, implements, and evaluates quality assessment and improvement tools;
    - collaborates with the Clinical Educator in the orientation of all new employees; and
    - collaborates with the Clinical Educator to plan appropriate learning experiences for all levels of staff.

12. Assists the Department Head in the clinical evaluation of professional and paraprofessional perioperative nursing staff. In this role the Perioperative Nurse III
    - participates in clinical evaluation of all levels of clinical personnel, and
    - completes written clinical performance appraisals at specified intervals for nursing personnel as assigned.

ORGANIZATION AND PROFESSIONAL DEVELOPMENT OBJECTIVES

1. The Perioperative Nurse III contributes to organization effectiveness and efficiency by
   - participating in quality assessment and improvement activities;
   - meeting hospital continuing education and certification requirements;
   - participating in student teaching activities, serving as a role model for professional nursing students rotating through the surgical suite, participating in the clinical instruction of professional nursing students and assistive personnel students, and assisting with the orientation of professional and paraprofessional employees;
   - upholding Nursing Services philosophy and objectives;
   - contributing to organizational effectiveness by demonstrating punctuality when reporting for duty, adhering to hospital policy concerning rest and lunch breaks, and completing assigned duties in an effective, efficient, and timely manner; and
   - demonstrating stewardship for hospital resources by adhering to established surgical charge protocols.

2. The Perioperative Nurse III demonstrates professional growth and development by
   - participating in professional nursing organizations,

- demonstrating knowledge of *Standards and Recommended Practices for Perioperative Nursing,* and
- keeping abreast of professional literature.

POSITION SPECIFICATIONS

1. Education and Training
   - Registered nurse
   - Graduate of a formal perioperative nursing course or documented on-the-job training
   - Certification as a perioperative nurse (CNOR) required
2. Experience
   - 4½ years experience as a Perioperative Nurse II
3. Physical Demands
   - Constant walking, standing, bending, and stooping.
   - Pushing and pulling heavy objects such as gurneys, patient beds, and OR beds.
   - Must be able to lift patients, heavy boxes weighing up to 40 pounds, and instrument sets weighing up to 20 pounds; must be able to lift surgical supplies above the head.
4. Mental, Visual, and Hearing Demands
   - Must be able to read, write, and understand English. Must be able to read supply labels, the surgical schedule, patient identification bracelets, and policies and procedures.
   - Must be able to read fine print.
   - Must be able to hear and follow verbal instructions.
5. Working Conditions
   - Must work in air-conditioned environment with a temperature of 65°–72°F and humidity of 45–55%. When assigned to assist with pediatric cases, temperature may be up to 85°–90°F.
   - Must wear hospital-provided scrub attire while on duty.
6. Hazards
   - Potential for cuts, bruises, muscle strains, and exposure to contagious diseases via blood and body fluids.
   - Potential for exposure to anesthetic waste gases, ethylene oxide, harsh disinfectants, sterilizing agents; exposure to high steam pressure and radiological environment.
   - Potential noise hazard from ultrasonic equipment when assigned to decontamination area.
7. Machines, Tools, and Equipment Operated
   - OR beds, fracture tables, recovery beds
   - Steam sterilizer, ultrasonic cleaner and dryer, and heat package sealing devices
   - Compressed gas gauges
   - Lasers, microscopes, sharps, electrosurgical devices, power instruments
8. Financial Responsibility
   - Must demonstrate stewardship behavior by conserving hospital resources (e.g., supplies, charging).
9. Reports and Records
   - Completion of nursing documentation, charge records, incident reports, and other paperwork associate with position.
   - Communicates health status data to other team members as described in position duties.
   - Completes performance evaluations and quality assessment and improvement documents, and writes policies and procedures.
10. Contacts
    - Must demonstrate hospital core values when interacting with visitors, patients, physicians, and nursing staff.
11. Supervisory Responsibilities
    - Perioperative nursing assistants; perioperative nursing associates; perioperative nurse I; operating room materiels services technicians assigned to surgical procedures.
12. Worker Characteristics
    - Must maintain a neat, clean, professional appearance.
    - Willingness to work with employees at various levels of skill, knowledge, and abilities.
    - Must have understanding, patience, and tact in dealing with physicians and fellow workers.
    - Must pay attention to details.
    - Must be free of prejudice.
    - Must be self-motivated and work in an efficient and effective manner.

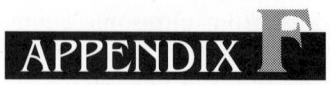

Perioperative Nursing Assistant I

POSITION IDENTIFICATION

1. Job Title: Perioperative Nursing Assistant I
2. Alternative Title: Orderly
3. Department: Perioperative Nursing Services
4. Supervisor: Department Head, Perioperative Nursing Services
5. Position Number:
6. Approved by: _____ Date: _____

POSITION SUMMARY

1. Under the supervision of a registered professional nurse or, as appropriate, a perioperative nursing associate, the Perioperative Nursing Assistant I participates as a member of the perioperative nursing team. The Perioperative Nursing Assistant I performs direct and indirect perioperative nursing tasks for patients having pediatric and adult surgical and endoscopy procedures. The primary focus of this position is patient transportation, application of casts and splints, preoperative skin preparation, maintenance of OR supply levels, and OR sanitation.
2. The Perioperative Nursing Assistant I performs all tasks in a manner that is cost effective without compromising quality of care, meets hospital continuing education and certification requirements, upholds Nursing Services philosophy and objectives, contributes to organizational effectiveness, and demonstrates career growth and development.
3. Under the supervision of an operating room materiels services technician, the Perioperative Nursing Assistant I performs basic operating room materiels services tasks.
4. The Perioperative Nursing Assistant I works 8-hour rotating shifts as assigned by the Department Head. Weekend shifts and call are assigned on a rotating basis.

POSITION DUTIES*

1. Preoperative Duties
   - Identifies the patient.
   - Ensures that extraneous objects such as jewelry and prostheses have been removed from the patient.
   - Transports patients to the surgical suite.
   - Performs shave preps.
   - Assists in selecting supplies and equipment for surgical procedures.
   - Assists in preparing the OR for surgical procedures.
   - Assists in preparing the operating room bed and sets up the fracture table.
   - Checks supplies and equipment needed for the surgical procedure.
   - Opens sterile packages using sterile technique.
2. Intraoperative Duties
   - Assists in placing and positioning the patient on the operating room bed for all surgical procedures.
   - Ties and secures sterile gowns.
   - Dons sterile gloves using the open-glove method.
   - Holds extremities during the operative prep.
   - Assists the surgeon in applying casts and splints.
3. Postoperative Duties
   - After local procedures, transports postoperative patients to the patient care unit.

*American College of Surgeons, American Hospital Association, Association of Surgical Technologists, American Medical Association. (1990). Proposed essentials and guidelines for an accredited educational program in surgical technology (draft document). Chicago, IL: American Medical Association, 1–17.

- Assists the registered nurse and anesthetist in transporting postoperative patients to the post-anesthesia recovery unit.
- Transports patient specimens, cultures, blood, and body fluids to pathology and the laboratory.
- Performs operating room sanitation tasks.
- Stocks operating rooms with supplies.
- Changes compressed air tanks.

4. Operating Room Materiels Services Duties
   - Receives, sorts, decontaminates, cleans, and sterilizes surgical items.
   - Loads and operates washer-sterilizers, dryers, ultrasonic cleaners, and sterilizers.
   - Wraps assembled instrument trays.
   - Stamps, dates, stores, and rotates items and issues sterile and nonsterile items and inspects for outdated items.
   - Cleans sterilizers and ultrasonic cleaners.
   - Uses and evaluates sterilizer test indicators.
   - Reports defective materiel or equipment to supervisor.

ORGANIZATIONAL RESPONSIBILITIES

1. Meets hospital continuing education requirements.
2. Upholds Nursing Services philosophy and objectives.
3. Contributes to organizational effectiveness by reporting for duty on time, adhering to hospital policy concerning rest and lunch breaks, and completing assigned duties in an effective, efficient, and timely manner.

POSITION SPECIFICATIONS

1. Education and Training
   - High school diploma or GED
2. Experience
   - Entry-level position
3. Physical Demands
   - Constant walking, standing, bending, and stooping.
   - Pushing and pulling heavy objects such as gurneys, patient beds, and OR beds.
   - Must be able to lift patients, heavy boxes weighing up to 40 pounds, and instrument sets weighing up to 20 pounds; must be able to lift surgical supplies above the head.

4. Mental, Visual, and Hearing Demands
   - Must be able to read, write, and understand English. Must be able to read supply labels, the surgical schedule, patient identification bracelets, and policies and procedures.
   - Must be able to read fine print.
   - Must be able to hear and follow verbal instructions.
5. Working Conditions
   - Must work in air-conditioned environment with a temperature of 65°–72°F and humidity of 45–55%. When assigned to assist with pediatric cases, temperature may be up to 85°–90°F.
   - Must wear hospital-provided scrub attire while on duty.
6. Hazards
   - Potential for cuts, bruises, muscle strains, and exposure to contagious diseases via blood and body fluids.
   - Potential for exposure to anesthetic waste gases, ethylene oxide, harsh disinfectants, sterilizing agents; exposure to high steam pressure and radiological environment.
   - Potential noise hazard from ultrasonic equipment when assigned to decontamination area.
7. Machines, Tools, and Equipment Operated
   - OR beds, fracture tables, recovery beds
   - Steam sterilizer, ultrasonic cleaner and dryer, and heat package sealing devices
   - Compressed gas gauges
8. Financial Responsibility
   - Must demonstrate stewardship behavior by conserving hospital resources (e.g., supplies).
9. Reports and Records
   - Verbal reports to registered nurse concerning the condition of the patient following transport to the operating room.
10. Contacts
    - Must demonstrate hospital core values when interacting with visitors, patients, physicians, and nursing staff.
11. Supervisory Responsibilities
    - None
12. Worker Characteristics
    - Must maintain a neat, clean, professional appearance.
    - Willingness to work with employees at various levels of skill, knowledge, and abilities.
    - Must have understanding, patience, and tact in dealing with physicians and fellow workers.
    - Must pay attention to details.
    - Must be free of prejudice.
    - Must be self-motivated and work in an efficient and effective manner.

Perioperative Nursing Assistant II

POSITION IDENTIFICATION

1. Job Title: Perioperative Nursing Assistant II
2. Alternative Title: Operating Room Technician; Surgical Technologist
3. Department: Perioperative Nursing Services
4. Supervisor: Department Head, Perioperative Nursing Services
5. Position Number:
6. Approved by: _____ Date: _____

POSITION SUMMARY

1. Under the supervision of a registered professional nurse or, as appropriate, a perioperative nursing associate, the Perioperative Nursing Assistant II participates as a member of the perioperative nursing team. The Perioperative Nursing Assistant II performs direct and indirect perioperative nursing tasks for patients having minor pediatric and adult surgical and endoscopy procedures and assists anesthesia personnel. The primary focus of this position is the scrub person role.
2. Under the supervision of an operating room materiels services technician, the Perioperative Nursing Assistant II performs basic operating room materiels services tasks.
3. Under the supervision of a qualified surgeon, the Perioperative Nursing Assistant II performs second assisting duties during the surgical procedure.
4. The Perioperative Nursing Assistant II performs all tasks in a manner that is cost effective without compromising quality of care, meets hospital continuing education and certification requirements, upholds Nursing Services philosophy and objectives, contributes to organizational effectiveness, and demonstrates career growth and development.

5. The Perioperative Nursing Assistant II works 8-hour rotating shifts as assigned by the Department Head. Weekend shifts and call are assigned on a rotating basis.

POSITION DUTIES*

1. Preoperative Duties
   - Identifies the patient.
   - Ensures that extraneous objects such as jewelry and prostheses have been removed from the patient.
   - Transports patients to the surgical suite.
   - Performs shave preps.
   - Assists in selecting supplies and equipment for surgical procedures.
   - Assists in preparing the OR for surgical procedures.
   - Assists in preparing the operating room bed and sets up the fracture table.
   - Checks supplies and equipment needed for the surgical procedure.
   - Opens sterile packages using sterile technique.
   - Sets up and prepares anesthesia equipment, monitors, and supplies for surgery.
   - Sets up intravenous fluids for administration.
2. Intraoperative Duties
   - Assists in placing and positioning the patient on the operating room bed for all surgical procedures.

---

*American College of Surgeons, American Hospital Association, Association of Surgical Technologists, American Medical Association (1990). Proposed essentials and guidelines for an accredited educational program in surgical technology (draft document). Chicago, IL: American Medical Association, 1–17.

- Ties and secures sterile gowns.
- Dons sterile gloves using the open-glove method.
- Holds extremities during the operative prep.
- Assists the surgeon in applying casts and splints.
- Applies monitor leads, pulse oximeters, and blood pressure cuffs.
- Assists anesthesia personnel with the administration of general, spinal, and regional anesthesia.
- Provides scrub services for minor surgical procedures.
- Provides scrub services for endoscopy procedures.
- Assists the surgeon in applying casts and splints.

3. Postoperative Duties
   - After local procedures, transports postoperative patients to the patient care unit.
   - Assists the registered nurse and anesthetist in transporting postoperative patients to the postanesthesia recovery unit.
   - Transports patient specimens, cultures, blood, and body fluids to pathology and the laboratory.
   - Performs operating room sanitation tasks.
   - Cleans anesthesia machines after use and changes breathing circuits.
   - Stocks operating rooms and anesthesia carts with supplies.
   - Changes compressed air tanks.

4. Operating Room Materiels Services Duties
   - Receives, sorts, decontaminates, cleans, and sterilizes surgical items.
   - Loads and operates washer-sterilizers, dryers, ultrasonic cleaners, and sterilizers.
   - Wraps assembled instrument trays.
   - Stamps, dates, stores, and rotates items and issues sterile and nonsterile items and inspects for outdated items.
   - Cleans sterilizers and ultrasonic cleaners.
   - Uses and evaluates sterilizer test indicators.
   - Reports defective materiel or equipment to supervisor.

5. Second Assisting Duties
   - Holds retractors or instruments as directed by the surgeon.
   - Sponges or suctions operative site.
   - Applies electrocautery to clamps on bleeders.
   - Cuts suture material as directed by the surgeon.
   - Connects drains to suction apparatus.
   - Applies dressing to the closed wound.

ORGANIZATIONAL RESPONSIBILITIES

1. Meets hospital continuing education requirements.
2. Upholds Nursing Services philosophy and objectives.
3. Contributes to organizational effectiveness by re-

porting for duty on time, adhering to hospital policy concerning rest and lunch breaks, and completing assigned duties in an effective, efficient, and timely manner.

POSITION SPECIFICATIONS

1. Education and Training
   - High school diploma or GED
   - Diploma from an accredited surgical technology program or documented on-the-job training program
2. Experience
   - Entry-level position
3. Physical Demands
   - Constant walking, standing, bending, and stooping.
   - Pushing and pulling heavy objects such as gurneys, patient beds, and OR beds.
   - Must be able to lift patients, heavy boxes weighing up to 40 pounds, and instrument sets weighing up to 20 pounds; must be able to lift surgical supplies above the head.
4. Mental, Visual, and Hearing Demands
   - Must be able to read, write, and understand English. Must be able to read supply labels, the surgical schedule, patient identification bracelets, and policies and procedures.
   - Must be able to read fine print.
   - Must be able to hear and follow verbal instructions.
5. Working Conditions
   - Must work in air-conditioned environment with a temperature of 65°–72°F and humidity of 45–55%. When assigned to assist with pediatric cases, temperature may be up to 85°–90°F.
   - Must wear hospital-provided scrub attire while on duty.
6. Hazards
   - Potential for cuts, bruises, muscle strains, and exposure to contagious diseases via blood and body fluids.
   - Potential for exposure to anesthetic waste gases, ethylene oxide, harsh disinfectants, sterilizing agents; exposure to high steam pressure and radiological environment.
   - Potential noise hazard from ultrasonic equipment when assigned to decontamination area.
7. Machines, Tools, and Equipment Operated
   - OR beds, fracture tables, recovery beds
   - Steam sterilizer, ultrasonic cleaner and dryer, and heat package sealing devices
   - Compressed gas gauges
   - Lasers, microscopes, sharps, electrosurgical devices, power instruments
8. Financial Responsibility
   - Must demonstrate stewardship behavior by conserving hospital resources (e.g., supplies).

9. Reports and Records
   - Verbal reports to registered nurse concerning the condition of the patient following transport to the operating room.
10. Contacts
   - Must demonstrate hospital core values when interacting with visitors, patients, physicians, and nursing staff.
11. Supervisory Responsibilities
   - None

12. Worker Characteristics
   - Must maintain a neat, clean, professional appearance.
   - Willingness to work with employees at various levels of skill, knowledge, and abilities.
   - Must have understanding, patience, and tact in dealing with physicians and fellow workers.
   - Must pay attention to details.
   - Must be free of prejudice.
   - Must be self-motivated and work in an efficient and effective manner.

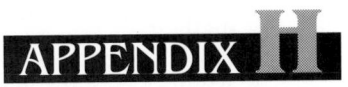

Perioperative Nursing Associate I

POSITION IDENTIFICATION

1. Job Title: Perioperative Nursing Associate I
2. Alternative Title: Operating Room Technician; Surgical Technologist
3. Department: Perioperative Nursing Services
4. Supervisor: Department Head, Perioperative Nursing Services
5. Position Number:
6. Approved by: _____ Date: _____

POSITION SUMMARY

1. Under the supervision of a registered nurse or, as appropriate, a senior perioperative nursing associate, the Perioperative Nursing Associate I participates as a member of the perioperative nursing team. The Perioperative Nursing Associate I performs direct and indirect perioperative nursing tasks for patients having pediatric and adult surgical and endoscopy procedures and assists anesthesia personnel. The primary focus of this position is the scrub person role.
2. The Perioperative Nursing Associate I performs basic operating room materiels services tasks.
3. Under the supervision of a qualified surgeon, the Perioperative Nursing Associate I performs second assisting duties during the surgical procedure.
4. The Perioperative Nursing Associate I performs all tasks in a manner that is cost effective without compromising quality of care, participates in the departmental quality assessment and improvement activities, meets hospital continuing education and certification requirements, participates in student teaching activities, upholds Nursing Services philosophy and objectives, contributes to organiza-

tional effectiveness, and demonstrates career growth and development.
5. The Perioperative Nursing Associate I works 8-hour rotating shifts as assigned by the Department Head. Weekend shifts and call are assigned on a rotating basis.

POSITION DUTIES*

1. Preoperative Duties
   - Identifies the patient.
   - Ensures that extraneous objects such as jewelry and prostheses have been removed from the patient.
   - Transports patients to the surgical suite.
   - Performs shave preps.
   - Assists in selecting supplies and equipment for surgical procedures.
   - Assists in preparing the OR for surgical procedures.
   - Assists in preparing the operating room bed and sets up the fracture table.
   - Checks supplies and equipment needed for the surgical procedure.
   - Opens sterile packages using sterile technique.
   - Sets up and prepares anesthesia equipment, monitors, and supplies for surgery.
   - Sets up intravenous fluids for administration.
2. Intraoperative Duties
   - Assists in placing and positioning the patient

---

*American College of Surgeons, American Hospital Association, Association of Surgical Technologists, American Medical Association (1990). Proposed essentials and guidelines for an accredited educational program in surgical technology (draft document). Chicago, IL: American Medical Association, 1–17.

on the operating room bed for all surgical procedures.
- Ties and secures sterile gowns.
- Dons sterile gloves using the open-glove method.
- Holds extremities during the operative prep.
- Applies monitor leads, pulse oximeters, and blood pressure cuffs.
- Assists anesthesia personnel with the administration of general, spinal, and regional anesthesia.
- Provides scrub services for minor surgical procedures.
- Provides scrub services for endoscopy procedures.
- Provides scrub services for major procedures in at least two surgical services.
- Assists the surgeon in applying casts and splints.

3. Postoperative Duties
- Transports postoperative patients to the patient care unit after local procedures.
- Assists the registered nurse and anesthetist in transporting postoperative patients to the post-anesthesia recovery unit.
- Transports patient specimens, cultures, blood, and body fluids to pathology and the laboratory.
- Performs operating room sanitation tasks.
- Cleans anesthesia machines after use and changes breathing circuits.
- Stocks operating rooms and anesthesia carts with supplies.
- Changes compressed air tanks.

4. Operating Room Materiels Services Duties
- Receives, sorts, decontaminates, cleans, and sterilizes surgical items.
- Loads and operates washer-sterilizers, dryers, ultrasonic cleaners, and sterilizers.
- Wraps assembled instrument trays.
- Stamps, dates, stores, and rotates items; issues sterile and nonsterile items; and inspects for outdated items.
- Cleans sterilizers and ultrasonic cleaners.
- Uses and evaluates sterilizer test indicators.
- Reports defective materiel or equipment to supervisor.

5. Second Assisting Duties
- Holds retractors or instruments as directed by the surgeon.
- Sponges or suctions operative site.
- Applies electrocautery to clamps on bleeders.
- Cuts suture material as directed by the surgeon.
- Connects drains to suction apparatus.
- Applies dressing to the closed wound.

ORGANIZATIONAL RESPONSIBILITIES

1. Meets hospital continuing education requirements.
2. Upholds nursing services philosophy and objectives.

3. Contributes to organizational effectiveness by reporting for duty on time, adhering to hospital policy concerning rest and lunch breaks, and completing assigned duties in an effective, efficient, and timely manner.

POSITION SPECIFICATIONS

1. Education and Training
- High school diploma or GED
- Diploma from an accredited surgical technology program or documented on-the-job training program

2. Experience
- One year experience as a perioperative nursing assistant II or operating room technician

3. Physical Demands
- Constant walking, standing, bending, and stooping.
- Pushing and pulling heavy objects such as gurneys, patient beds, and OR beds.
- Must be able to lift patients, heavy boxes weighing up to 40 pounds, and instrument sets weighing up to 20 pounds; must be able to lift surgical supplies above the head.

4. Mental, Visual, and Hearing Demands
- Must be able to read, write, and understand English. Must be able to read supply labels, the surgical schedule, patient identification bracelets, and policies and procedures.
- Must be able to read fine print.
- Must be able to hear and follow verbal instructions.

5. Working Conditions
- Must work in air-conditioned environment with a temperature of 65°–72°F and humidity of 45–55%. When assigned to assist with pediatric cases, temperature may be up to 85°–90°F.
- Must wear hospital-provided scrub attire while on duty.

6. Hazards
- Potential for cuts, bruises, muscle strains, and exposure to contagious diseases via blood and body fluids.
- Potential for exposure to anesthetic waste gases, ethylene oxide, harsh disinfectants, sterilizing agents; exposure to high steam pressure and radiological environment.
- Potential noise hazard from ultrasonic equipment when assigned to decontamination area.

7. Machines, Tools, and Equipment Operated
- OR beds, fracture tables, recovery beds
- Steam sterilizer, ultrasonic cleaner and dryer, and heat package sealing devices
- Compressed gas gauges
- Lasers, microscopes, sharps, electrosurgical devices, power instruments

8. Financial Responsibility
- Must demonstrate stewardship behavior by conserving hospital resources (e.g., supplies).

9. Reports and Records
   - Verbal reports to registered nurse concerning the condition of the patient following transport to the operating room.
10. Contacts
    - Must demonstrate hospital core values when interacting with visitors, patients, physicians, and nursing staff.
11. Supervisory Responsibilities
    - None
12. Worker Characteristics
    - Must maintain a neat, clean, professional appearance.
    - Willingness to work with employees at various levels of skill, knowledge, and abilities.
    - Must have understanding, patience, and tact in dealing with physicians and fellow workers.
    - Must pay attention to details.
    - Must be free of prejudice.
    - Must be self-motivated and work in an efficient and effective manner.

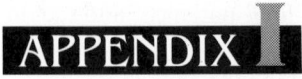

Perioperative Nursing Associate II

POSITION IDENTIFICATION

1. Job Title: Perioperative Nursing Associate II
2. Alternative Title: Operating Room Technician; Surgical Technologist
3. Department: Perioperative Nursing Services
4. Supervisor: Department Head, Perioperative Nursing Services
5. Position Number:
6. Approved by: _____ Date: _____

POSITION SUMMARY

1. Under the supervision of a registered nurse or, as appropriate, a senior perioperative nursing associate, the Perioperative Nursing Associate II participates as a member of the perioperative nursing team. Performs direct and indirect perioperative nursing tasks for patients having pediatric and adult surgical and endoscopy procedures, assists the registered nurse in the preoperative holding area, and assists anesthesia personnel. The primary focus of this position is the scrub person and assistant circulator roles.
2. The Perioperative Nursing Associate II performs basic operating room materiels services tasks.
3. Under the supervision of a qualified surgeon, the Perioperative Nursing Associate II performs second assisting duties during the surgical procedure.
4. In collaboration with a registered nurse, the Perioperative Nursing Associate II serves as a technical subject matter expert for at least one surgical service.
5. The Perioperative Nursing Associate II performs all tasks in a manner that is cost effective without compromising quality of care, participates in de-

partmental quality assessment and improvement activities, meets hospital continuing education and certification requirements, participates in student teaching activities, upholds Nursing Services philosophy and objectives, contributes to organizational effectiveness, and demonstrates career growth and development.
6. The Perioperative Nursing Associate II works 8-hour rotating shifts as assigned by the Department Head. Weekend shifts and call are assigned on a rotating basis.

POSITION DUTIES*

1. Preoperative Duties
   - Identifies the patient.
   - Ensures that extraneous objects such as jewelry and prostheses have been removed from the patient.
   - Transports patients to the surgical suite.
   - Performs shave preps.
   - Reviews the preoperative checklist in accordance with operating room policy and procedure.
   - Takes and records vital signs and reports deviations to physician or registered nurse.
   - Checks consent form to ensure that it conforms to hospital policy and procedure.
   - Checks physician's orders to ensure that all preoperative orders are completed.
   - Reviews laboratory data and reports deviations to physician or registered nurse.
   - Performs phlebotomy tasks.
   - Monitors intravenous infusions in accordance with operating room policy and procedure.

---

*American College of Surgeons, American Hospital Association, Association of Surgical Technologists, American Medical Association (1990). Proposed essentials and guidelines for an accredited educational program in surgical technology (draft document). Chicago, IL: American Medical Association, 1–17.

- Selects supplies and equipment for surgical procedures.
- Prepares the OR for surgical procedures.
- Prepares the operating room bed and sets up the fracture table.
- Checks supplies and equipment needed for the surgical procedure.
- Opens sterile packages using sterile technique.
- Sets up and prepares anesthesia equipment, monitors, and supplies for surgery.
- Sets up intravenous fluids for administration.

2. Intraoperative Duties
- Assists in placing and positioning the patient on the operating room bed for all surgical procedures.
- Ties and secures sterile gowns.
- Dons sterile gloves using the open-glove method.
- Holds extremities during the operative prep.
- Applies monitor leads, pulse oximeters, and blood pressure cuffs.
- Assists anesthesia personnel with the administration of general, spinal, and regional anesthesia.
- Assists the circulating perioperative nurse during major surgical procedures.
- Catheterizes the urinary bladder.
- Measures urinary output.
- Performs the operative scrub prep.
- Applies tourniquets and sets up the electrosurgical unit and other specialized surgical equipment.
- Weighs sponges and records blood loss.
- Collects and prepares surgical specimens and cultures.
- Prepares and operates Cavitron ultrasonic aspirator (CUSA), surgical lasers, laparoscopy insufflation equipment, and autotransfusion equipment.
- Completes the operative record and charge forms.
- Provides scrub services for minor surgical procedures.
- Provides scrub and circulating services for endoscopy procedures.
- Provides scrub services for major procedures in at least four surgical services.
- Assists the surgeon in applying casts and splints.

3. Postoperative Duties
- Transports postoperative patients to the patient care unit after local procedures.
- Assists the registered nurse and anesthetist in transporting postoperative patients to the postanesthesia recovery unit.
- Transports patient specimens, cultures, blood, and body fluids to pathology and the laboratory.
- Performs operating room sanitation tasks.
- Cleans anesthesia machines after use and changes breathing circuits.

- Stocks operating rooms and anesthesia carts with supplies.
- Changes compressed air tanks.

4. Operating Room Materiels Services Duties
- Receives, sorts, decontaminates, cleans, and sterilizes surgical items.
- Loads and operates washer-sterilizers, dryers, ultrasonic cleaners, and sterilizers.
- Wraps assembled instrument trays.
- Stamps, dates, stores, and rotates items; issues sterile and nonsterile items; and inspects for outdated items.
- Cleans sterilizers and ultrasonic cleaners.
- Uses and evaluates sterilizer test indicators.
- Reports defective materiel or equipment to supervisor.

5. Second Assisting Duties
- Holds retractors or instruments as directed by the surgeon.
- Sponges or suctions operative site.
- Applies electrocautery to clamps on bleeders.
- Cuts suture material as directed by the surgeon.
- Connects drains to suction apparatus.
- Applies dressing to the closed wound.

6. Technical Subject Matter Expert Duties
- In collaboration with a registered nurse, the Perioperative Nursing Associate II serves as a technical subject matter expert for at least one surgical service.
- Updates surgeon preference cards.
- Inventories and orders specialty instruments, supplies, and equipment unique to surgical service.
- Demonstrates competency to operate all specialty instruments, supplies, and equipment unique to surgical service.
- Prepares and conducts technical performance-oriented training programs related to specialty service for perioperative nursing personnel.
- Serves as preceptor to perioperative nursing associate personnel rotating through specialty service.

ORGANIZATIONAL REQUIREMENTS

1. Commensurate with skill level and experience, participates in departmental quality assessment and improvement activities.
2. Meets hospital continuing education and certification requirements.
3. Commensurate with skill level and experience, participates in student teaching activities by participating in the clinical instruction of operating room technician students, serving as a role model for OR technician students rotating through the surgical suite, and assisting with the orientation of employees.
4. Serves as clinical preceptor for new perioperative nursing assistant and associate services employees.

5. Teaches scrubbing skills to perioperative nursing students and perioperative nursing associate students.
6. Prepares and conducts technical performance-oriented training programs for perioperative nursing personnel.
7. Upholds nursing services philosophy and objectives.
8. Contributes to organizational effectiveness by reporting for duty on time, adhering to hospital policy concerning rest and lunch breaks, and completing assigned duties in an effective, efficient, and timely manner.

POSITION SPECIFICATIONS

1. Education and Training
   - High school diploma or GED
   - Diploma from an accredited surgical technology program or documented on-the-job training program
   - Certification as a surgical technologist preferred
2. Experience
   - Four years as a perioperative nursing associate I or operating room technician
3. Physical Demands
   - Constant walking, standing, bending, and stooping.
   - Pushing and pulling heavy objects such as gurneys, patient beds, and OR beds.
   - Must be able to lift patients, heavy boxes weighing up to 40 pounds, and instrument sets weighing up to 20 pounds; must be able to lift surgical supplies above the head.
4. Mental, Visual, and Hearing Demands
   - Must be able to read, write, and understand English. Must be able to read supply labels, the surgical schedule, patient identification bracelets, and policies and procedures.
   - Must be able to read fine print.
   - Must be able to hear and follow verbal instructions.
5. Working Conditions (specifies both the positive and negative aspects of the working conditions—extremes of hot, cold, wet, glaring light, noise, odors, etc.)
   - Must work in air-conditioned environment with a temperature of 65°–72°F and humidity of 45–55%. When assigned to assist with pediatric cases, temperature may be up to 85°–90°F.
   - Must wear hospital-provided scrub attire while on duty.
6. Hazards
   - Potential for cuts, bruises, muscle strains, and exposure to contagious diseases via blood and body fluids.
   - Potential for exposure to anesthetic waste gases, ethylene oxide, harsh disinfectants, sterilizing agents; exposure to high steam pressure and radiological environment.
   - Potential noise hazard from ultrasonic equipment when assigned to decontamination area.
7. Machines, Tools, and Equipment Operated
   - OR beds, fracture tables, recovery beds
   - Steam sterilizer, ultrasonic cleaner and dryer, and heat package sealing devices
   - Compressed gas gauges
   - Lasers, microscopes, sharps, electrosurgical devices, power instruments
8. Financial Responsibility
   - Responsible for exercising stewardship when using surgical supplies and equipment.
   - Responsible for inventory of equipment and supplies of an assigned surgical service.
   - Charges for supplies and equipment.
   - Collaborates with a perioperative nurse in identifying capital equipment needs for an assigned specialty service.
9. Reports and Records
   - Verbal report to registered nurse concerning the condition of the patient following transport to the operating room.
   - Completes the operative record as appropriate.
   - When assigned to assist the registered nurse in the holding area, records and reports assessment data.
10. Contacts
   - Must demonstrate hospital core values when interacting with visitors, patients, physicians, and nursing staff.
11. Supervisory Responsibilities
   - Junior perioperative nursing associates and perioperative nursing assistants.
12. Worker Characteristics
   - Must maintain a neat, clean, professional appearance.
   - Willingness to work with employees at various levels of skill, knowledge, and abilities.
   - Must have understanding, patience, and tact in dealing with physicians and fellow workers.
   - Must pay attention to details.
   - Must be free of prejudice.
   - Must be self-motivated and work in an efficient and effective manner.

Perioperative Nursing Associate III

POSITION IDENTIFICATION

1. Job Title: Perioperative Nursing Associate III
2. Alternative Title: Operating Room Technician; Surgical Technologist
3. Department: Perioperative Nursing Services
4. Supervisor: Department Head, Perioperative Nursing Services
5. Position Number:
6. Approved by: _____ Date: _____

POSITION SUMMARY

1. Under the supervision of a registered professional nurse who is immediately available, the Perioperative Nursing Associate III participates as a member of the perioperative nursing team. Performs preoperative holding area duties, performs direct and indirect perioperative nursing tasks for pediatric and adult patients having surgical and endoscopy procedures, assists the registered nurse in the preoperative holding area, and assists anesthesia personnel. The primary focus of this position is the scrub person, assistant circulator, and workflow coordinator roles.
2. The Perioperative Nursing Associate III demonstrates competency as an Operating Room Materiels Services Technician I.
3. Under the supervision of a qualified surgeon, the Perioperative Nursing Associate III performs second assisting duties during the surgical procedure.
4. The Perioperative Nursing Associate III serves as a technical subject matter expert for at least two surgical services.
5. In collaboration with the patient care coordinator and/or Department Head, assists in managing subordinates.
6. The Perioperative Nursing Associate III performs all tasks in a manner that is cost effective without compromising quality of care, participates in departmental quality assessment and improvement activities, meets hospital continuing education and certification requirements, participates in student teaching activities, upholds Nursing Services philosophy and objectives, contributes to organizational effectiveness, and demonstrates career growth and development.
7. The Perioperative Nursing Associate III works 8-hour rotating shifts as assigned by the Department Head. Weekend shifts and call are assigned on a rotating basis.

POSITION DUTIES*

1. Preoperative Duties
   - Identifies the patient.
   - Ensures that extraneous objects such as jewelry and prostheses have been removed from the patient.
   - Transports patients to the surgical suite.
   - Performs shave preps.
   - Reviews the preoperative checklist in accordance with operating room policy and procedure.
   - Takes and records vital signs and reports deviations to physician or registered nurse.
   - Checks consent form to ensure that it conforms to hospital policy and procedure.

---

*American College of Surgeons, American Hospital Association, Association of Surgical Technologists, American Medical Association (1990). Proposed essentials and guidelines for an accredited educational program in surgical technology (draft document). Chicago, IL: American Medical Association, 1–17.

969

- Checks physician's orders to ensure that all preoperative orders are completed.
- Reviews laboratory data and reports deviations to physician or registered nurse.
- Performs phlebotomy tasks.
- Monitors intravenous infusions in accordance with operating room policy and procedure.
- Selects supplies and equipment for surgical procedures.
- Prepares the OR for surgical procedures.
- Prepares the operating room bed and sets up the fracture table.
- Checks supplies and equipment needed for the surgical procedure.
- Opens sterile packages using sterile technique.
- Sets up and prepares anesthesia equipment, monitors, and supplies for surgery.
- Sets up intravenous fluids for administration.

2. Intraoperative Duties
- Assists in placing and positioning the patient on the operating room bed for all surgical procedures.
- Ties and secures sterile gowns.
- Dons sterile gloves using the open-glove method.
- Holds extremities during the operative prep.
- Applies monitor leads, pulse oximeters, and blood pressure cuffs.
- Assists anesthesia personnel with the administration of general, spinal, and regional anesthesia.
- Assists the circulating perioperative nurse during major surgical procedures.
- Under the supervision of a registered nurse who is immediately available, serves as the primary circulator for low-risk surgical procedures.
- Catheterizes the urinary bladder.
- Measures urinary output.
- Performs the operative scrub prep.
- Applies tourniquets and sets up the electrosurgical unit and other specialized surgical equipment.
- Weighs sponges and records blood loss.
- Collects and prepares surgical specimens and cultures.
- Prepares and operates CUSA, surgical lasers, laparoscopy insufflation equipment, and autotransfusion equipment.
- Completes the operative record and charge forms.
- Provides scrub services for minor surgical procedures.
- Provides scrub and circulating services for endoscopy procedures.
- Provides scrub services for major procedures in at least four surgical services.
- Assists the surgeon in applying casts and splints.

3. Postoperative Duties
- Transports postoperative patients to the patient care unit after local procedures.
- Assists the registered nurse and anesthetist in transporting postoperative patients to the post-anesthesia recovery unit.
- Reports the condition of the patient to post-anesthesia personnel.
- Transports patient specimens, cultures, blood, and body fluids to pathology and the laboratory.
- Performs operating room sanitation tasks.
- Cleans anesthesia machines after use and changes breathing circuits.
- Stocks operating rooms and anesthesia carts with supplies.
- Changes compressed air tanks.

4. Operating Room Materiels Services Duties
- Receives, sorts, inventories, decontaminates, cleans, examines, and sterilizes surgical items.
- Inspects and prepares surgical items for sterilization.
- Loads and operates washer-sterilizers, dryers, ultrasonic cleaners, and sterilizers.
- Stamps, dates, stores, and rotates items; issues sterile and nonsterile items; and inspects for outdated items.
- Uses and evaluates sterilizer test indicators.
- Inventories and maintains prescribed levels of sterile and nonsterile supplies for the operating room.
- Reports defective materiel or equipment and takes appropriate action to repair or replace items.
- Processes sterilizer test control registers.
- Implements procedures to ensure adherence to sterilization requirements, standards of conduct, cleanliness, technical accuracy, and safety regulations.
- Implements preventive maintenance programs in the OR.
- Maintains stock level of supplies and equipment.
- Requisitions, stores, and issues supplies.
- Teaches operating room materiels services skills to perioperative nurse students and perioperative nursing associate students.
- Prepares and conducts operating room materiels services performance-oriented training programs for perioperative nursing personnel.

5. Second Assisting Duties
- Holds retractors or instruments as directed by the surgeon.
- Sponges or suctions operative site.
- Applies electrocautery to clamps on bleeders.
- Cuts suture material as directed by the surgeon.
- Connects drains to suction apparatus.
- Applies dressing to the closed wound.

6. Technical Subject Matter Expert Duties
- In collaboration with a registered nurse, the Perioperative Nursing Associate III serves as a technical subject matter expert for at least two surgical services.
- Updates surgeon preference cards.
- Inventories and orders specialty instruments,

supplies, and equipment unique to surgical service.

- Demonstrates competency to operate all specialty instruments, supplies, and equipment unique to surgical service.
- Prepares and conducts technical performance-oriented training programs related to specialty service for perioperative nursing personnel.
- Serves as preceptor to perioperative nursing associate personnel rotating through specialty service.

7. Workflow Coordinator Duties
- In collaboration with patient care coordinator and/or Department Head, establishes work priorities, organizes work schedules, assigns duties, and instructs subordinate perioperative nursing associates and assistants in work techniques and procedures.
- Assists patient care coordinator with the operational management of a surgical suite.
- Evaluates subordinate personnel performance, counsels subordinate personnel, and prepares evaluation reports.
- Establishes, reviews, and revises technical operating room policies and procedures.

ORGANIZATIONAL REQUIREMENTS

1. Commensurate with skill level and experience, participates in departmental quality assessment and improvement activities.
2. Meets hospital continuing education and certification requirements.
3. Commensurate with skill level and experience, participates in student teaching activities by participating in the clinical instruction of operating room technician students, serving as a role model for OR technician students rotating through the surgical suite, and assisting with the orientation of employees.
4. Serves as clinical preceptor for new perioperative nursing assistant and associate services employees.
5. Teaches scrubbing skills to perioperative nursing students and perioperative nursing associate students.
6. Prepares and conducts technical performance-oriented training programs for perioperative nursing personnel.
7. Upholds nursing services philosophy and objectives.
8. Contributes to organizational effectiveness by reporting for duty on time, adhering to hospital policy concerning rest and lunch breaks, and completing assigned duties in an effective, efficient, and timely manner.

POSITION SPECIFICATIONS

1. Education and Training
- High school diploma or GED
- Diploma from an accredited surgical technology program or documented on-the-job training program
- Certification as a surgical technologist
2. Experience
- Seven years as a perioperative nursing associate II or operating room technician.
3. Physical Demands
- Constant walking, standing, bending, and stooping.
- Pushing and pulling heavy objects such as gurneys, patient beds, and OR beds.
- Must be able to lift patients, heavy boxes weighing up to 40 pounds, and instrument sets weighing up to 20 pounds; must be able to lift surgical supplies above the head.
4. Mental, Visual, and Hearing Demands
- Must be able to read, write, and understand English. Must be able to read supply labels, the surgical schedule, patient identification bracelets, and policies and procedures.
- Must be able to read fine print.
- Must be able to hear and follow verbal instructions.
5. Working Conditions.
- Must work in air-conditioned environment with a temperature of 65°–72°F and humidity of 45–55%. When assigned to assist with pediatric cases, temperature may be up to 85°–90°F.
- Must wear hospital-provided scrub attire while on duty.
6. Hazards
- Potential for cuts, bruises, muscle strains, and exposure to contagious diseases via blood and body fluids.
- Potential for exposure to anesthetic waste gases, ethylene oxide, harsh disinfectants, sterilizing agents; exposure to high steam pressure and radiological environment.
- Potential noise hazard from ultrasonic equipment when assigned to decontamination area.
7. Machines, Tools, and Equipment Operated
- OR beds, fracture tables, recovery beds
- Steam sterilizer, ultrasonic cleaner and dryer, and heat package sealing devices
- Compressed gas gauges
- Lasers, microscopes, sharps, electrosurgical devices, power instruments
8. Financial Responsibility
- Responsible for exercising stewardship when using surgical supplies and equipment.
- Responsible for inventory of equipment and supplies of an assigned surgical service.
- Responsible for charges for supplies and equipment.
- Collaborates with a perioperative nurse in identifying capital equipment needs for an assigned specialty service.
9. Reports and Records
- Verbally reports to registered nurse concerning the condition of the patient following transport to the operating room.
- Completes the operative record as appropriate.

- When assigned to assist the registered nurse in the holding area, records and reports assessment data.
10. Contacts
    - Must demonstrate hospital core values when interacting with visitors, patients, physicians, and nursing staff.
11. Supervisory Responsibilities
    - Junior perioperative nursing associates and perioperative nursing assistants.
12. Worker Characteristics

- Must maintain a neat, clean, professional appearance.
- Willingness to work with employees at various levels of skill, knowledge, and abilities.
- Must have understanding, patience, and tact in dealing with physicians and fellow workers.
- Must pay attention to details.
- Must be free of prejudice.
- Must be self-motivated and work in an efficient and effective manner.

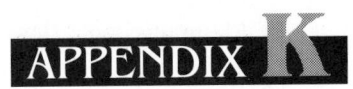

OR Materiels Services Technician I

POSITION IDENTIFICATION

1. Job Title: Operating Room Materiels Services Technician I
2. Alternative Title: Workroom Technician; Instrument Technician
3. Department: Perioperative Nursing Services
4. Supervisor: Department Head, Perioperative Nursing Services
5. Position Number:
6. Approved by: _____ Date: _____

POSITION SUMMARY

1. Under the supervision of a senior operating room materiels services technician, the Operating Room Materiels Services Technician I performs technical tasks that support clinical operations. The primary focus of this position is the performance of operating room materiels services tasks.
2. Under the supervision of a registered professional nurse or, as appropriate, a perioperative nursing associate, the Operating Room Materiels Services Technician I participates as a member of the perioperative nursing team. The Operating Room Materiels Services Technician I performs direct and indirect perioperative nursing tasks for pediatric and adult patients having minor surgical and endoscopy procedures and assists anesthesia personnel.
3. Under the supervision of a qualified surgeon, the Operating Room Materiels Services Technician I performs second assisting duties during the surgical procedure.
4. The Operating Room Materiels Services Technician I performs all tasks in a manner that is cost effective without compromising quality of care,

meets hospital continuing education and certification requirements, upholds Nursing Services philosophy and objectives, contributes to organizational effectiveness, and demonstrates career growth and development.
5. The Operating Room Materiels Services Technician I works 8-hour rotating shifts as assigned by the Department Head. Weekend shifts and call are assigned on a rotating basis.

POSITION DUTIES*

1. Operating Room Materiels Services Duties
   - Receives, sorts, inventories, decontaminates, cleans, examines, and sterilizes surgical items.
   - Inspects and prepares surgical items for sterilization.
   - Loads and operates washer-sterilizers, dryers, ultrasonic cleaners, and sterilizers.
   - Stamps, dates, stores, and rotates items; issues sterile and nonsterile items; and inspects for outdated items.
   - Uses and evaluates sterilizer test indicators.
   - Inventories and maintains prescribed levels of sterile and nonsterile supplies for the operating room.
   - Reports defective materiel or equipment and takes appropriate action to repair or replace items.
   - Processes sterilizer test control registers.
   - Implements procedures to ensure adherence to sterilization requirements, standards of con-

---

*The Field Manual, 8-38. Centralized Material Service/Section. Headquarters, Department of the Army, U.S. Army Publications Center, Baltimore, MD.

duct, cleanliness, technical accuracy, and safety regulations.

- Implements preventive maintenance programs in the OR.
- Maintains stock level of supplies and equipment.
- Requisitions, stores, and issues supplies.
- Teaches operating room materiels services skills to perioperative nurse students and perioperative nursing associate students.
- Prepares and conducts operating room materiels services performance-oriented training programs for perioperative nursing personnel.

2. Preoperative Duties
   - Identifies the patient.
   - Ensures that extraneous objects such as jewelry and prostheses have been removed from the patient.
   - Transports patients to the surgical suite.
   - Performs shave preps.
   - Assists in selecting supplies and equipment for surgical procedures.
   - Assists in preparing the OR for surgical procedures.
   - Assists in preparing the operating room bed and sets up the fracture table.
   - Checks supplies and equipment needed for the surgical procedure.
   - Opens sterile packages using sterile technique.
   - Sets up and prepares anesthesia equipment, monitors, and supplies for surgery.
   - Sets up intravenous fluids for administration.

3. Intraoperative Duties
   - Assists in placing and positioning the patient on the operating room bed for all surgical procedures.
   - Ties and secures sterile gowns.
   - Dons sterile gloves using the open-glove method.
   - Holds extremities during the operative prep.
   - Assists the surgeon in applying casts and splints.
   - Applies monitor leads, pulse oximeters, and blood pressure cuffs.
   - Assists anesthesia personnel with the administration of general, spinal, and regional anesthesia.
   - Provides scrub services for minor surgical procedures.
   - Provides scrub services for endoscopy procedures.
   - Assists the surgeon in applying casts and splints.

4. Postoperative Duties
   - Transports postoperative patients to the patient care unit after local procedures.
   - Assists the registered nurse and anesthetist in transporting postoperative patients to the post-anesthesia recovery unit.
   - Transports patient specimens, cultures, blood, and body fluids to pathology and the laboratory.
   - Performs operating room sanitation tasks.

- Cleans anesthesia machines after use and changes breathing circuits.
- Stocks operating rooms and anesthesia carts with supplies.
- Changes compressed air tanks.

5. Second Assisting Duties
   - Holds retractors or instruments as directed by the surgeon.
   - Sponges or suctions operative site.
   - Applies electrocautery to clamps on bleeders.
   - Cuts suture material as directed by the surgeon.
   - Connects drains to suction apparatus.
   - Applies dressing to the closed wound.

ORGANIZATIONAL RESPONSIBILITIES

1. Meets hospital continuing education requirements.
2. Upholds nursing services philosophy and objectives.
3. Contributes to organizational effectiveness by reporting for duty on time, adhering to hospital policy concerning rest and lunch breaks, and completing assigned duties in an effective, efficient, and timely manner.

POSITION SPECIFICATIONS

1. Education and Training
   - High school diploma or GED
   - Diploma from an accredited surgical technology program or documented on-the-job training program

2. Experience
   - One year as a perioperative nursing assistant II

3. Physical Demands
   - Constant walking, standing, bending, and stooping.
   - Pushing and pulling heavy objects such as gurneys, patient beds, and OR beds.
   - Must be able to lift patients, heavy boxes weighing up to 40 pounds, and instrument sets weighing up to 20 pounds; must be able to lift surgical supplies above the head.

4. Mental, Visual, and Hearing Demands
   - Must be able to read, write, and understand English. Must be able to read supply labels, the surgical schedule, patient identification bracelets, and policies and procedures.
   - Must be able to read fine print.
   - Must be able to hear and follow verbal instructions.

5. Working Conditions
   - Must work in air-conditioned environment with a temperature of 65°–72°F and humidity of 45–55%. When assigned to assist with pediatric cases, temperature may be up to 85°–90°F.
   - Must wear hospital-provided scrub attire while on duty.

6. Hazards
   - Potential for cuts, bruises, muscle strains, and exposure to contagious diseases via blood and body fluids.
   - Potential for exposure to anesthetic waste gases, ethylene oxide, harsh disinfectants, sterilizing agents; exposure to high steam pressure and radiological environment.
   - Potential noise hazard from ultrasonic equipment when assigned to decontamination area.
7. Machines, Tools, and Equipment Operated
   - OR beds, fracture tables, recovery beds
   - Steam sterilizer, ultrasonic cleaner and dryer, and heat package sealing devices
   - Compressed gas gauges
   - Lasers, microscopes, sharps, electrosurgical devices, power instruments
8. Financial Responsibility
   - Must demonstrate stewardship behavior by conserving hospital resources (e.g., supplies).
9. Reports and Records
   - Verbally reports to registered nurse concerning the condition of the patient following transport to the operating room.
   - Reports verbally and in writing to superiors concerning status of instruments and equipment.
10. Contacts
    - Must demonstrate hospital core values when interacting with visitors, patients, physicians, and nursing staff.
11. Supervisory Responsibilities
    - None
12. Worker Characteristics
    - Must maintain a neat, clean, professional appearance.
    - Willingness to work with employees at various levels of skill, knowledge, and abilities.
    - Must have understanding, patience, and tact in dealing with physicians and fellow workers.
    - Must pay attention to details.
    - Must be free of prejudice.
    - Must be self-motivated and work in an efficient and effective manner.

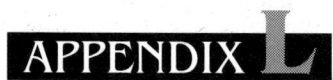

OR Materiels Services Technician II

POSITION IDENTIFICATION

1. Job Title: Operating Room Materiels Services Technician II
2. Alternative Title: Workroom Technician; Instrument Technician
3. Department: Perioperative Nursing Services
4. Supervisor: Department Head, Perioperative Nursing Services
5. Position Number:
6. Approved by: _____ Date: _____

POSITION SUMMARY

1. Under the supervision of a senior operating room materiels services technician, the Operating Room Materiels Services Technician II performs technician tasks that support clinical operations. The primary focus of this position is the performance of operating room materiels services tasks.
2. Under the supervision of a registered professional nurse or, as appropriate, a perioperative nursing associate, the Operating Room Materiels Services Technician II participates as a member of the perioperative nursing team. The Operating Room Materiels Services Technician II performs direct and indirect perioperative nursing tasks for pediatric and adult patients having minor surgical and endoscopy procedures and assists anesthesia personnel.
3. Under the supervision of a qualified surgeon, the Operating Room Materiels Services Technician II performs second assisting duties during the surgical procedure.
4. The Operating Room Materiels Services Technician II performs all tasks in a manner that is cost effective without compromising quality of care,

participates in departmental quality assessment and improvement activities, meets hospital continuing education and certification requirements, upholds Nursing Services philosophy and objectives, contributes to organizational effectiveness, and demonstrates career growth and development.

5. The Operating Room Materiels Services Technician II works 8-hour rotating shifts as assigned by the Department Head. Weekend shifts and call are assigned on a rotating basis.

POSITION DUTIES*

1. Operating Room Materiels Services Duties
   - Receives, sorts, inventories, decontaminates, cleans, examines, and sterilizes surgical items.
   - Inspects and prepares surgical items for sterilization.
   - Loads and operates washer-sterilizers, dryers, ultrasonic cleaners, and sterilizers.
   - Stamps, dates, stores, and rotates items; issues sterile and nonsterile items; and inspects for outdated items.
   - Uses and evaluates sterilizer test indicators.
   - Inventories and maintains prescribed levels of sterile and nonsterile supplies for the operating room.
   - Reports defective materiel or equipment and takes appropriate action to repair or replace items.
   - Processes sterilizer test control registers.
   - Implements procedures to ensure adherence to

---

*The Field Manual, 8-38. Centralized Material Service/Section. Headquarters, Department of the Army, U.S. Army Publications Center, Baltimore, MD.

sterilization requirements, standards of conduct, cleanliness, technical accuracy, and safety regulations.
- Implements preventive maintenance programs in the OR.
- Maintains stock level of supplies and equipment.
- Requisitions, stores, and issues supplies.
- Operates and troubleshoots all surgical instruments and equipment processed by operating room materiels services technicians.
- Implements systems to ensure that operating room charges for supplies, instruments, orthopedic hardware, prostheses, and equipment are recorded.
- Teaches operating room materiels services skills to perioperative nurse students and perioperative nursing associate students.
- Prepares and conducts operating room materiels services performance-oriented training programs for perioperative nursing personnel.

2. Preoperative Duties
- Identifies the patient.
- Ensures that extraneous objects such as jewelry and prostheses have been removed from the patient.
- Transports patients to the surgical suite.
- Performs shave preps.
- Assists in selecting supplies and equipment for surgical procedures.
- Assists in preparing the OR for surgical procedures.
- Assists in preparing the operating room bed and sets up the fracture table.
- Checks supplies and equipment needed for the surgical procedure.
- Opens sterile packages using sterile technique.
- Sets up and prepares anesthesia equipment, monitors, and supplies for surgery.
- Sets up intravenous fluids for administration.

3. Intraoperative Duties
- Assists in placing and positioning the patient on the operating room bed for all surgical procedures.
- Ties and secures sterile gowns.
- Dons sterile gloves using the open-glove method.
- Holds extremities during the operative prep.
- Assists the surgeon in applying casts and splints.
- Applies monitor leads, pulse oximeters, and blood pressure cuffs.
- Assists anesthesia personnel with the administration of general, spinal, and regional anesthesia.
- Provides scrub services for minor surgical procedures.
- Provides scrub services for endoscopy procedures.
- Assists the surgeon in applying casts and splints.

4. Postoperative Duties
- Transports postoperative patients to the patient care unit after local procedures.
- Assists the registered nurse and anesthetist in transporting postoperative patients to the post-anesthesia recovery unit.
- Transports patient specimens, cultures, blood, and body fluids to pathology and the laboratory.
- Performs operating room sanitation tasks.
- Cleans anesthesia machines after use and changes breathing circuits.
- Stocks operating rooms and anesthesia carts with supplies.
- Changes compressed air tanks.

5. Second Assisting Duties
- Holds retractors or instruments as directed by the surgeon.
- Sponges or suctions operative site.
- Applies electrocautery to clamps on bleeders.
- Cuts suture material as directed by the surgeon.
- Connects drains to suction apparatus.
- Applies dressing to the closed wound.

ORGANIZATIONAL RESPONSIBILITIES

1. Commensurate with skill level and experience, participates in departmental quality assessment and improvement activities.
2. Meets hospital continuing education and certification requirements.
3. Commensurate with skill level and experience, participates in student teaching activities by participating in the clinical instruction of operating room technician students, serving as a role model for OR technician students rotating through surgical suite, and assisting with the orientation of employees.
4. Serves as preceptor for new operating room materiels services technician employees.
5. Teaches operating room materiels services skills to perioperative nurse and operating room technician students.
6. Prepares and conducts technical performance-oriented training programs for perioperative nursing personnel.
7. Upholds nursing services philosophy and objectives.
8. Contributes to organizational effectiveness by reporting for duty on time, adhering to hospital policy concerning rest and lunch breaks, and completing assigned duties in an effective, efficient, and timely manner.

POSITION SPECIFICATIONS

1. Education and Training
- High school diploma or GED
- Diploma from an accredited surgical technology program or documented on-the-job training program

2. Experience
   - Four years; one as a perioperative nursing assistant II, and three as an operating room materiels services technician I
3. Physical Demands
   - Constant walking, standing, bending, and stooping.
   - Pushing and pulling heavy objects such as gurneys, patient beds, and OR beds.
   - Must be able to lift patients, heavy boxes weighing up to 40 pounds, and instrument sets weighing up to 20 pounds. Must be able to lift surgical supplies above the head.
4. Mental, Visual, and Hearing Demands
   - Must be able to read, write, and understand English. Must be able to read supply labels, the surgical schedule, patient identification bracelets, and policies and procedures.
   - Must be able to read fine print.
   - Must be able to hear and follow verbal instructions.
5. Working Conditions
   - Must work in air-conditioned environment with a temperature of 65°–72°F and humidity of 45–55%. When assigned to assist with pediatric cases, temperature may be up to 85°–90°F.
   - Must wear hospital-provided scrub attire while on duty.
6. Hazards
   - Potential for cuts, bruises, muscle strains, and exposure to contagious diseases via blood and body fluids.
   - Potential for exposure to anesthetic waste gases, ethylene oxide, harsh disinfectants, sterilizing agents; exposure to high steam pressure and radiological environment.
   - Potential noise hazard from ultrasonic equipment when assigned to decontamination area.
7. Machines, Tools, and Equipment Operated
   - OR beds, fracture tables, recovery beds
   - Steam sterilizer, ultrasonic cleaner and dryer, and heat package sealing devices
   - Compressed gas gauges
   - Lasers, microscopes, sharps, electrosurgical devices, power instruments
8. Financial Responsibility
   - Must demonstrate stewardship behavior by conserving hospital resources (e.g., supplies).
9. Reports and Records
   - Verbally reports to registered nurse concerning the condition of the patient following transport to the operating room.
   - Reports verbally and in writing to superiors concerning status of instruments and equipment.
10. Contacts
    - Must demonstrate hospital core values when interacting with visitors, patients, physicians, and nursing staff.
11. Supervisory Responsibilities
    - None
12. Worker Characteristics
    - Must maintain a neat, clean, professional appearance.
    - Willingness to work with employees at various levels of skill, knowledge, and abilities.
    - Must have understanding, patience, and tact in dealing with physicians and fellow workers.
    - Must pay attention to details.
    - Must be free of prejudice.
    - Must be self-motivated and work in an efficient and effective manner.

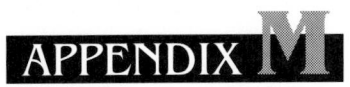

OR Materiels Services Technician III

1. Job Title: Operating Room Materiels Services Technician III
2. Alternative Title: Workroom Technician; Instrument Technician
3. Department: Perioperative Nursing Services
4. Supervisor: Department Head, Perioperative Nursing Services
5. Position Number:
6. Approved by: _____ Date: _____

POSITION SUMMARY

1. Under the supervision of the Department Head, the Operating Room Materiels Services Technician III manages operating room materiels services technicians and designs and implements systems that support clinical operations.
2. The Operating Room Materiels Services Technician III demonstrates competency as a Perioperative Nursing Associate I.
3. Under the supervision of a qualified surgeon, the Operating Room Materiels Services Technician III performs second assisting duties during the surgical procedure.
4. The Operating Room Materiels Services Technician III performs all tasks in a manner that is cost effective without compromising quality of care, participates in departmental quality assessment and improvement activities, meets hospital continuing education and certification requirements, upholds Nursing Services philosophy and objectives, contributes to organizational effectiveness, and demonstrates career growth and development.
5. The Operating Room Materiels Services Techni-

cian III works 8-hour rotating shifts as assigned by the Department Head. Weekend shifts and call are assigned on a rotating basis.

POSITION DUTIES*

1. Management Objectives
   - Establishes work priorities, organizes work schedules, assigns duties, and instructs subordinate operating room materiels services technicians in work techniques and procedures.
   - Establishes work priorities, assigns duties, and instructs perioperative nursing associate and assistant personnel assigned to the operating room materiels services section.
   - Assists the Department Head in managing the business operations of the surgical suite.
   - Evaluates subordinate personnel performance, counsels subordinate personnel, and prepares evaluation reports.
   - Establishes, reviews, and revises operating room materiels services policies and procedures.
   - Assists the Department Head with the coordination of operating room activities with support elements of the hospital.
   - Assists in implementing departmental quality improvement programs that monitor activities performed by operating room materiels services technicians.
   - Serves as surgery safety officer.

*The Field Manual, 8-38. Centralized Material Service/Section. Headquarters, Department of the Army, U.S. Army Publications Center, Baltimore, MD.

2. Operating Room Materiels Services Objectives
   - Designs and implements systems to receive, sort, inventory, decontaminate, clean, examine, and sterilize surgical items.
   - Designs and implements systems to inspect and prepare surgical items for sterilization.
   - Designs and implements systems for the utilization of washer-sterilizers, dryers, ultrasonic cleaners, and sterilizers.
   - Designs and implements systems that ensure quality control of sterile and nonsterile surgical items.
   - Ensures that inventories are conducted and prescribed levels of sterile and nonsterile supplies and equipment for the operating room are maintained.
   - Takes appropriate action to repair or replace defective materiel or equipment.
   - Ensures that sterilizer test control registers are processed.
   - Designs and implements procedures to ensure adherence to sterilization requirements, OR sanitation practices, and safety regulations.
   - Designs, supervises, and implements preventive maintenance programs in OR.
   - Establishes and maintains office files, technical publications library, and supply bulletins.
   - Establishes technical reports control system.
   - Prepares correspondence to industry vendors and other technical administrative reports.
   - Operates and troubleshoots all surgical instruments and equipment processed by operating room materiels services technicians.
   - Designs and implements systems to ensure that operating room charges for supplies, instruments, orthopedic hardware, prostheses, and equipment are recorded.
   - Teaches operating room materiels services skills to perioperative nursing students and perioperative nursing associate students.
   - Prepares and conducts operating room materiels services performance-oriented training programs for perioperative nursing personnel.
3. Preoperative Duties
   - Identifies the patient.
   - Ensures that extraneous objects such as jewelry and prostheses have been removed from the patient.
   - Transport patients to the surgical suite.
   - Performs shave preps.
   - Assists in selecting supplies and equipment for surgical procedures.
   - Assists in preparing the OR for surgical procedures.
   - Assists in preparing the operating room bed and sets up the fracture table.
   - Checks supplies and equipment needed for the surgical procedure.
   - Opens sterile packages using sterile technique.
   - Sets up and prepares anesthesia equipment, monitors, and supplies for surgery.
   - Sets up intravenous fluids for administration.
4. Intraoperative Duties
   - Assists in placing and positioning the patient on the operating room bed for all surgical procedures.
   - Ties and secures sterile gowns.
   - Dons sterile gloves using the open-glove method.
   - Holds extremities during the operative prep.
   - Applies monitor leads, pulse oximeters, and blood pressure cuffs.
   - Assists anesthesia personnel with the administration of general, spinal, and regional anesthesia.
   - Provides scrub services for minor surgical procedures.
   - Provides scrub services for endoscopy procedures.
   - Provides scrub services for major procedures in at least two surgical services.
   - Assists the surgeon in applying casts and splints.
5. Postoperative Duties
   - Transports postoperative patients to the patient care unit after local procedures.
   - Assists the registered nurse and anesthetist in transporting postoperative patients to the post-anesthesia recovery unit.
   - Transports patient specimens, cultures, blood, and body fluids to pathology and the laboratory.
   - Performs operating room sanitation tasks.
   - Cleans anesthesia machines after use and changes breathing circuits.
   - Stocks operating rooms and anesthesia carts with supplies.
   - Changes compressed air tanks.
6. Second Assisting Duties
   - Holds retractors or instruments as directed by the surgeon.
   - Sponges or suctions operative site.
   - Applies electrocautery to clamps on bleeders.
   - Cuts suture material as directed by the surgeon.
   - Connects drains to suction apparatus.
   - Applies dressing to the closed wound.

ORGANIZATIONAL REQUIREMENTS

1. Commensurate with skill level and experience, participates in departmental quality assessment and improvement activities.
2. Meets hospital continuing education and certification requirements.
3. Commensurate with skill level and experience, participates in student teaching activities by participating in the instruction of operating room technician students, serving as a role model for OR technician students rotating through surgical suite, and assisting with the orientation of employees.
4. Serves as preceptor for new operating room materiels services technician employees.
5. Teaches operating room materiels services skills to

perioperative nurse and operating room technician students.

6. Prepares and conducts technical performance-oriented training programs for perioperative nursing personnel.

7. Contributes to organizational effectiveness by reporting for duty on time, adhering to hospital policy concerning rest and lunch breaks, and completing assigned duties in an effective, efficient, and timely manner.

POSITION SPECIFICATIONS

1. Education and Training
   - High school diploma or GED
   - Diploma from an accredited surgical technology program or documented on-the-job training program
   - Certification as a surgical technologist required

2. Experience
   - Seven years (one as a perioperative nursing assistant II, three as an operating room materiels services technician I, and three as an operating room materiels services technician II) or equivalent experience

3. Physical Demands
   - Constant walking, standing, bending, and stooping.
   - Pushing and pulling heavy objects such as gurneys, patient beds, and OR beds.
   - Must be able to lift patients, heavy boxes weighing up to 40 pounds, and instrument sets weighing up to 20 pounds; must be able to lift surgical supplies above the head.

4. Mental, Visual, and Hearing Demands
   - Must be able to read, write, and understand English. Must be able to read supply labels, the surgical schedule, patient identification bracelets, and policies and procedures.
   - Must be able to read fine print.
   - Must be able to hear and follow verbal instructions.

5. Working Conditions
   - Must work in air-conditioned environment with a temperature of 65°–72°F and humidity of 45–55%. When assigned to assist with pediatric cases temperature may be up to 85°–90°F.
   - Must wear hospital-provided scrub attire while on duty.

6. Hazards
   - Potential for cuts, bruises, muscle strains, and exposure to contagious diseases via blood and body fluids.
   - Potential for exposure to anesthetic waste gases, ethylene oxide, harsh disinfectants, sterilizing agents; exposure to high steam pressure and radiological environment.
   - Potential noise hazard from ultrasonic equipment when assigned to decontamination area.

7. Machines, Tools, and Equipment Operated
   - OR beds, fracture tables, recovery beds.
   - Steam sterilizer, ultrasonic cleaner and dryer, and heat package sealing devices.
   - Compressed gas gauges.
   - Lasers, microscopes, sharps, electrosurgical devices, power instruments.

8. Financial Responsibility
   - Must demonstrate stewardship behavior by conserving hospital resources (e.g., supplies).

9. Reports and Records
   - Written and verbal reports to supervisor concerning status of instruments and equipment.
   - Maintenance of sterilization records.
   - Writing of policies and procedures.

10. Contacts
   - Must demonstrate hospital core values when interacting with visitors, patients, physicians, and nursing staff.

11. Supervisory Responsibilities
   - Junior operating room materiels services technicians and perioperative nursing assistants and associates assigned to the OR Materiels Section.

12. Worker Characteristics
   - Must maintain a neat, clean, professional appearance.
   - Willingness to work with employees at various levels of skill, knowledge, and abilities.
   - Must have understanding, patience, and tact in dealing with physicians and fellow workers.
   - Must pay attention to details.
   - Must be free of prejudice.
   - Must be self-motivated and work in an efficient and effective manner.

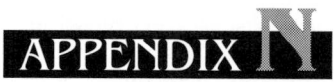

Perioperative Nurse III Performance Appraisal

EMPLOYEE NAME _____ **EVALUATION DATE** _____

Critical Performance Objectives	100	200	300	400	500	Weight	Score
Assesses the physiological health status of the patient on admission to the operating room and performs an ongoing assessment of the patient's physiological health status during the intraoperative period.						5%	
Assesses psychological, sociocultural, and spiritual status on admission to the operating room.						5%	
Identifies nursing diagnoses appropriate to the intraoperative and postoperative periods.						5%	
Plans care based on the patient's problems/needs identified in the assessment.						5%	
Implements perioperative nursing care according to an established plan of care and operating room policies and procedures.						5%	
Supervises perioperative nursing associates and assistants assigned to perform the actions necessary to accomplish the identified goals.						10%	
Scrubs and circulates for all simple surgical and endoscopy procedures.						10%	
Scrubs for complex surgical procedures in at least two surgical services.						10%	
Circulates for complex surgical procedures in at least four surgical services.						10%	
Serves as a second surgical assistant.						5%	
Evaluates the effectiveness of the care provided.						5%	
Communicates and documents perioperative nursing care.						5%	
Serves as professional and technical subject matter expert for at least two surgical services.						5%	
Functions as the charge nurse on an identified shift.						5%	
Designs, implements, and evaluates systems to improve the quality of perioperative nursing patient care.						5%	
Assists the Department Head in the clinical evaluation of professional and paraprofessional perioperative nursing staff.						5%	
						100%	
						TOTAL	

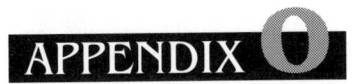
Perioperative Nursing Associate III Performance Appraisal

EMPLOYEE NAME _____ **EVALUATION DATE** _____

Critical Performance Objectives	100	200	300	400	500	Weight	Score
Preoperative duties						10%	
Intraoperative duties						15%	
Postoperative duties						5%	
Operating room materiels services duties						5%	
Second assisting duties						5%	
Technical subject matter expert duties						30%	
Workflow coordinator duties						30%	
						100%	
						TOTAL	

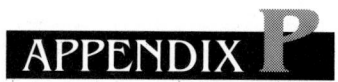

Performance Appraisal Scoring Guidelines

The scoring guidelines are identical for each performance appraisal.

Scoring Guideline

Actual score × weight = evaluation score for critical objective
Example: 300 × 5% = 15

Total Score for Performance Appraisal

100 =	Unacceptable performance
200 =	Needs improvement
300 =	Competent
400 =	Exceeds competency
500 =	Far exceeds competency

EVALUATOR SIGNATURE _____

EMPLOYEE SIGNATURE _____

Bibliography

Association of Operating Room Nurses, Inc. (1974). *What every OR supervisor should know.* Denver, CO: AORN.

Joint Commission for Accreditation of Healthcare Organizations. (1992). *Accreditation Manual for Hospitals—1992.* Chicago, IL: JCAHO.

Levitz G. (1981). Performance appraisal in health organizations. In N. Metzger (Ed.): *Handbook of health care human resource management.* Rockville, MD: Aspen, pp. 225–232.

Metzger, N. (1981). Job analysis and job description. In N. Metzger (Ed.): *Handbook of health care human resource management.* Rockville, MD: Aspen, pp. 157–172.

Otis, J. L., & Leukart, R. (1948). *Job evaluation.* Englewood Cliffs, NJ: Prentice Hall, p. 266.

Patton, J., Littlefield, C. L., Self, S. A. (1964). *Job evaluation: Text and cases.* Homewood, IL: Richard Irwin, Inc., pp. 93–94.

Rakichm, J. S., Longest, B., Darr, K. (1985). *Managing health services organizations.* Philadelphia, PA: W.B. Saunders, pp. 403–432.

CHAPTER 37

Quality Assessment and Improvement

Mark L. Phippen and Elaine Thomson Keith

DEFINITION OF QUALITY ASSESSMENT
   AND IMPROVEMENT
JCAHO Requirements
COLLECTING DATA
ORGANIZING DATA

EVALUATING CARE
TAKING ACTION TO IMPROVE CARE
DOCUMENTATION
AN EXAMPLE OF QUALITY IMPROVEMENT

Quality assessment and improvement provides the perioperative nurse with an opportunity for making a significant impact on the efficiency and effectiveness of perioperative nursing services, thereby reducing surgical costs and advancing the practice of perioperative nursing. This chapter presents a straightforward approach to quality assessment and improvement in the perioperative nursing arena.

DEFINITION OF QUALITY ASSESSMENT AND IMPROVEMENT

The Joint Commission on Accreditation of Healthcare Organizations (JCAHO) defines quality assessment and improvement as the "ongoing activities designed to objectively and systematically evaluate the quality of patient care and services, pursue opportunities to improve patient care and services, and resolve identified problems" (JCAHO, 1992, p. 234) It defines quality of patient care as "the degree to which patient care services increase the probability of desired patient outcomes and reduce the probability of undesired outcomes, given the current state of knowledge. Potential components of quality include the following: accessibility of care, appropriateness of care, continuity of care, effectiveness of care, efficacy of care, patient perspective issues, safety of the care environment, and timeliness of care" (JCAHO, 1992, p. 234).

JCAHO Requirements

JCAHO requires that the quality of care, including that provided to specific age groups, be monitored and evaluated in all patient care service areas. Specifically, directors for patient care service areas must ensure that their department or service identifies important aspects of care relevant to the department or service, identifies indicators for monitoring the quality of the important aspects of care, and evaluates the quality of care (JCAHO, 1992, p. 141).

Aspects of Care

The perioperative nursing services quality assessment and improvement team identifies those aspects of care that are most important to the health and safety of the patients receiving perioperative nursing care and services. The team examines those perioperative care activities and processes that

- occur frequently or affect large numbers of patients,
- place patients at risk of serious consequences if not provided correctly, or
- tend to produce problems for patients or staff (JCAHO, 1992, p. 142).

AORN's *Patient Outcomes: Standards of Perioperative Care* provides a framework for identifying pertinent aspects of care for the perioperative setting. Table 37–1 shows five aspects of care that are identified using the

TABLE 37–1. DEFINING ASPECTS OF CARE

Aspect of Care	AORN Outcome Standard
Patient and family teaching	The patient demonstrates knowledge of the physiological and psychological responses to surgical intervention.
Infection control	The patient is free from infection.
Skin integrity	The patient's skin integrity is maintained.
Patient safety	The patient is free from injury related to positioning, extraneous objects, or chemical, physical, and electrical hazards.
Discharge planning	The patient participates in the rehabilitation process.

Data from Association of Operating Room Nurses. (1992). *Standards and recommended practices for perioperative nursing* (pp. 7-1–7-2). Denver.

AORN outcome standards. Table 37–2 shows how each standard can be further subdivided to focus on specific patient care problems. The subdivided standards shown in Table 37–2 are derived from perioperative nursing diagnoses (Table 37–3).

Indicators

After important aspects of care are identified, the perioperative nursing services quality assessment and improvement team identifies indicators to monitor the quality of these important aspects of care. Such indicators may include clinical criteria, which are also called clinical standards, practice guidelines, or practice parameters. Reliable and valid indicators are stated in objective terms, are measurable, and are based on current knowledge and clinical experience (JCAHO, 1992, p. 143).

Indicators are classified as outcome, process, or structure. Outcome indicators focus on the results of the performance, or nonperformance, of a function or process. Process indicators focus on the actions taken by the perioperative nursing team to achieve the conditions or behaviors specified in the standard. Structure indicators focus on the resources required to perform the processes necessary to achieve the specified outcome standard.

Standards

Outcome standards (see Table 37–2), or other identified standards, should be used when identifying indicators for an important aspect of care. Measurable standards have identified clinical criteria that can be used to develop quality assessment and improvement indicators. Table 37–4 shows outcome, process, and structure indicators for skin integrity, an important aspect of care previously identified in Table 37–1. The

TABLE 37–2. SUBDIVIDED STANDARDS

Aspect of Care	AORN Outcome Standard	Subdivided Standards
Patient and family teaching	The patient demonstrates knowledge of the physiological and psychological responses to surgical intervention.	The patient demonstrates knowledge of the physiological responses to surgical intervention. The patient demonstrates knowledge of the psychological responses to surgical intervention.
Infection control	The patient is free from infection.	The patient is free from infection related to improper preparation of the surgical site. The patient is free from infection related to breaks in aseptic technique. The patient is free from infection related to improper sterilization techniques. The patient is free from infection related to improper high-level disinfection techniques.
Skin integrity	The patient's skin integrity is maintained.	The patient is free from impaired skin integrity related to use of the electrosurgical unit. The patient is free from impaired skin integrity related to positioning. The patient is free from impaired skin integrity related to pneumatic tourniquet use. The patient is free from impaired skin integrity related to the use of skin preparation or draping materials.
Patient safety	The patient is free from injury related to positioning, extraneous objects, or chemical, physical, and electrical hazards.	The patient is free from injury related to transportation to the surgical suite. The patient is free from injury related to positioning. The patient is free from injury related to pneumatic tourniquet use. The patient is free from injury related to retained foreign objects. The patient is free from injury related to electrosurgery. The patient is free from injury related to prepping solutions and other chemicals.
Discharge planning	The patient participates in the rehabilitation process.	The patient demonstrates self-care skills before discharge. The patient complies with therapeutic treatment regimens after discharge.

Data from Association of Operating Room Nurses. (1992). *Standards and recommended practices for perioperative nursing* (pp. 7-1–7-2). Denver.

TABLE 37–3. **NURSING DIAGNOSES RELATED TO OUTCOME STANDARDS**

Aspect of Care	Nursing Diagnosis	Standards
Patient and family teaching	Knowledge deficit	The patient demonstrates knowledge of the physiological responses to surgical intervention. The patient demonstrates knowledge of the psychological responses to surgical intervention.
Infection control	High risk for wound infection	The patient is free from infection related to improper preparation of the surgical site. The patient is free from infection related to breaks in aseptic technique. The patient is free from infection related to improper sterilization techniques. The patient is free from infection related to improper high-level disinfection techniques.
Skin integrity	High risk for impaired skin integrity	The patient is free from impaired skin integrity related to use of the electrosurgical unit. The patient is free from impaired skin integrity related to positioning. The patient is free from impaired skin integrity related to pneumatic tourniquet use. The patient is free from impaired skin integrity related to the use of skin preparation or draping materials.
Patient safety	High risk for injury	The patient is free from injury related to transportation to the surgical suite. The patient is free from injury related to positioning. The patient is free from injury related to pneumatic tourniquet use. The patient is free from injury related to retained foreign objects. The patient is free from injury related to electrosurgery. The patient is free from injury related to prepping solutions and other chemicals.
Discharge planning	High risk for self-care deficit after discharge	The patient demonstrates self-care skills before discharge.
	High risk for noncompliance to therapeutic treatment regimen after discharge.	The patient complies with therapeutic treatment regimens after discharge.

TABLE 37–4. INDICATORS

Aspect of care
  Skin integrity
Standard
  The patient's skin integrity is maintained.
Indicators
  Outcome: The patient is free from skin disruption and skin
    abrasion over bony prominences (name high-risk areas) after
    prone positioning.
  Process: Positioning devices are used when placing the patient in
    prone positioning. Egg crate padding is placed under the
    patient's knees, and a pillow is placed under the patient's feet.
  Structure: Positioning equipment is available when placing the
    patient in the prone position.
  • Gel positioning pads
  • Egg crate padding
  • Pillows
  • Chest rolls

example shown in Table 37–4 can serve as a model for developing indicators for all aspects of care.

Thresholds for Evaluation

After identifying indicators relevant to the important aspect of care being monitored and evaluated, the quality assessment and improvement team establishes thresholds for evaluation. Also know as trigger points, thresholds are levels or points at which an intensive evaluation of care or practice is initiated (AORN, 1993, p. 86). Thresholds are expressed in terms of percentages from 0% to 100% and are phrased in terms of compliance (e.g., 98% of the time, "x" will occur).

Determination of the thresholds depends on the specific indicator under evaluation. The higher the risk, the higher the required level of compliance. As an example, retained foreign bodies after surgery is considered a sentinel event. "A sentinel event requires individual case review for each occurrence" (AORN, 1993). When sentinel events occur, the quality assessment and improvement team, the manager, or another designated individual analyzes the event and draws conclusions concerning why the event happened. Recommendations are made, appropriate action is taken, and follow-up is planned. An appropriate outcome indicator concerning retained foreign bodies would state, "The patient is free from injury related to retained foreign bodies." Although the actual number of patients with retained foreign bodies may be low with respect to the total operative population, the risk of complications associated with retained foreign bodies is so great that 100% compliance with this indicator is required.

COLLECTING DATA

Data collection has several components: numerator and denominator identification, determination of the sources of data, and frequency of data collection.

Identifying Numerators and Denominators. The *numerator* is the number of times the behaviors or conditions specified in the indicator are met. The *denominator* represents the total number of patients, cases, records, or other variables surveyed or studied. The compliance rate for an indicator is calculated by dividing the numerator by the denominator. Figure 37–1 provides an example of numerator and denominator identification and calculation of an indicator compliance rate.

Data Sources. Data sources include the following:

- Patient records
- Observation of staff or patients
- Patient satisfaction questionnaires/interviews
- Department/service reports
- Medical staff quality improvement referrals
- Patient incident reports
- Interviews with patients/staff/physicians
- Infection control reports

Frequency of Data Collection. The frequency of data collection is "related to the frequency of the event or activity monitored; the significance of the event or activity monitored; and the extent to which the important aspect of care monitored by the indicator has been demonstrated to be problem-free" (JCAHO, 1992, p. 143).

Data collection should be spread throughout the week to assist in identifying whether problems exist on particular shifts or at certain times of the week. Data are collected at pre-established intervals, and data collection is coordinated between units. For example, if all the units within the perioperative department are going to monitor skin integrity at some point during the year, they should coordinate their quality assessment and improvement calendars so that it is monitored over the same time period. In addition to providing a large sample size, such coordination may help to identify areas where an opportunity for assessment and improvement exists and foster sharing of problem resolution strategies among units. Figure 37–2 provides an example of a data collection tool.

ORGANIZING DATA

After data are collected, they are organized by the quality assessment and improvement team to identify those situations in which an evaluation of the quality of

Numerator	95 (The total number of patients who are free from impaired skin integrity after prone positioning)
Denominator	100 (The total number of patients placed in the prone position)
	= 95% compliance

FIGURE 37–1. Calculating compliance.

Aspect of Care:		Numerator:																
Standard:		Denominator:																
Data Collector:	Date:	Method:	☐ Retrospective chart review ☐ Concurrent chart review ☐ Observation ☐ Other															

	Identification Data																	
Indicators	Y	N	Y	N	Y	N	Y	N	Y	N	Y	N	Y	N	Y	N	Y	N
1.																		
2.																		
3.																		
4.																		

FIGURE 37–2. Quality improvement data collection tool.

care is indicated. Evaluations are triggered by sentinel events, by levels or patterns/trends in the process or outcomes of care that are at significant variance with pre-established thresholds, and by patterns/trends in the process or outcomes of care (JCAHO, 1992, p. 143).

EVALUATING CARE

If data organization leads to an in-depth evaluation of an important aspect of care, the quality assessment and improvement team initiates a detailed analysis of the identified patterns/trends. The team looks for evidence of specific shift or unit involvement, unique patient population characteristics (e.g., age, diagnosis, and the type of admission), individuals that may represent a common trend, staff behavior problems, evidence of

staff knowledge deficit, and evidence of a systems deficit. The team identifies opportunities for improvement, or problems, in the quality of care. If the care of a perioperative nurse is analyzed, peers of the nurse review and participate in the analysis (JCAHO, 1992, p. 143). Figure 37–3 provides an example of a data compilation tool.

TAKING ACTION TO IMPROVE CARE

When the quality assessment and improvement team identifies a significant opportunity for improvement, or a problem, in the quality of care, the team determines the specific action that should be taken to improve the care or to correct the problem. The action designated by the team may include limited or full implementation of an improvement strategy. Action strategies should

Aspect of Care:		Numerator:		
Standard:		Denominator:		
Indicators	Threshold	Score	Analysis	
1.				
2.				
3.				
4.				

FIGURE 37–3. Quality improvement data compilation tool.

Aspect of Care:		Sentinel Event? ☐ Yes ☐ No	
Standard:		Numerator:	
Indicators:		Denominator:	
Threshold:	Score:	Monitoring Period:	

Conclusions	Recommendations	Action Taken	Follow Up

FIGURE 37–4. Quality improvement report.

specify who or what is expected to change and identify the person or group of people responsible for implementing the designated actions, what type of actions are appropriate, and when the change is expected to occur. Once implemented, the strategy for improvement is assessed through imitating or ongoing monitoring of care (JCAHO, 1992, p. 144).

DOCUMENTATION

The conclusions, recommendations, actions taken, and results of the actions taken are documented and reported through established channels. Figure 37–4 shows a form that can be used for documenting conclusions, recommendations, and actions taken. The quality assessment and improvement team summarizes the analysis documented on the compilation tool in the "Conclusions" column. Recommendations that require higher authority for implementation are listed in the "Recommendations" column. The actions taken to improve care and results of the actions are listed in the "Action Taken" column. In the "Follow-up" column the team lists plans for future monitoring to evaluate the results of the actions taken. Future plans should be specific and should clearly indicate when subsequent monitoring should occur. Follow-up plans may include a notation that monitoring will be initiated if a sentinel event occurs.

AN EXAMPLE OF QUALITY IMPROVEMENT

The following sentinel event occurred in a 22-room operating room suite in a major teaching medical center. This event triggered a quality assessment and improvement review.

The Event. During a 2-week period, three separate incidents of retained foreign bodies occurred. These events initiated an in-depth management review and subsequent referral to the perioperative nursing services quality assessment and improvement team for analysis, recommendations, and development of strategies for action. The event was recorded on the Quality Improvement Report of Problem Identification and Analysis shown in Figure 37–5.

Identifying the Aspect of Care, Standard, and Indicator. The quality assessment and improvement team determined that the aspect of care related to this event was patient safety. The standard that was not met was "The patient is free from injury related to retained foreign bodies." The indicator was identified as "Absence of retained sponge, sharps, instruments, and other surgical items after closure of the surgical wound." The aspect of care, standard, and indicator were identified on the Quality Improvement Report of Problem Identification and Analysis.

Analysis. The quality assessment and improvement team's analysis of this event revealed that a new policy

Problem	Aspect of Care	Standard	Indicators	Analysis
Sentinel Event? ☐ Yes ☐ No				

FIGURE 37–5. Quality improvement report of problem identification and analysis.

and procedure for sponge, sharps, and instruments had been implemented 2 weeks before the incidents. Furthermore, the old policy and procedure did not require extensive instrument counts. Staff members interviewed as part of the analysis reported that the procedure for counting instruments was difficult to implement and that confusion existed concerning what should be counted during a surgical procedure. They noted that traffic patterns in three operating rooms impeded work flow because of the placement of the count board. The count boards were placed in inconvenient areas and thus interfered with the circulating nurses' ability to immediately record the addition of items to the sterile field. Staff members also noted that an excessive number of personnel were frequently present during surgical procedures, which tended to distract the nurses, particularly during critical times such as when counting surgical items. The quality assessment and improvement team also noted that all staff involved with the incidents had fewer than 2 years of clinical experience. The analysis was recorded on the Quality Improvement Report of Problem Identification and Analysis.

Conclusions. The quality assessment and improvement team concluded that the incidents occurred because of

- a knowledge deficit concerning correct implementation of the new policy and procedure for counts and which surgical items (other than sponges, sharps, and instruments) should be counted during surgical procedures;
- staff inexperience;
- inappropriate traffic patterns related to positioning of the count board; and
- an excessive number of personnel assigned to or viewing surgical procedures

These conclusions were documented on the Quality Improvement Report.

Recommendations. The quality assessment and improvement team recommended the following to the operating room management team:

- mandatory inservice education concerning the new count policy and procedure for all registered nurses and surgical technologists,
- delineation in policy and procedure for items other than sponges, sharps, and instruments that should be counted;
- relocation of count boards to facilitate the immediate documentation of items added to the sterile field;
- assignment of tenured staff with novice staff;
- reduction in the number of personnel assigned to a room and viewing surgery; and
- a field visit by staff nurses and surgical technologists to another facility in which instrument counts had been successfully implemented.

These recommendations were documented on the Quality Improvement Report.

Action Taken. The operating room management team implemented the following actions:

- The clinical educator conducted a mandatory inservice education program concerning the new count policy and procedure for all registered nurses and surgical technologists.
- Count boards were relocated.
- The policy and procedure committee revised the new count policy and procedure to include a description of items that should be counted in addition to sponges, sharps, and instruments.
- Staffing patterns were reviewed by the operating room management team, and assignments were made to ensure that tenured staff were paired with novice staff.
- A field visit to another facility was arranged for five staff nurses and two surgical technologists.

The operating room management team recognized the impact of excessive personnel present during a surgical procedure but decided that limiting the number of personnel assigned to a room and viewing surgery would be difficult to achieve because of clinical affiliations with two nursing schools and one medical school. Actions taken were documented on the Quality Improvement Report.

Follow-up. The quality assessment and improvement team decided that additional monitoring would be necessary to determine whether staff were correctly implementing the count protocols delineated in the count policy and procedure. Using the same aspect of care (patient safety) and standard ("The patient is free from injury related to retained foreign bodies"), the following process indicators were identified by the team to measure compliance with count protocols:

1. The circulating nurse and scrub nurse count sponges, sharps, instruments, and other items listed in the policy and procedure in unison and aloud.
2. Counted items are recorded on the count board immediately after being added to the sterile field.
3. All items listed on the instrument count sheet are counted.
4. Protocols for incorrect counts are implemented according to policy and procedure.

The threshold for each indicator was set at 100%.

Next the quality assessment and improvement team defined the numerator and denominator. The numerator was defined as "the number of open-cavity abdominal and thoracic surgical cases in which the behavior described in the indicator was performed." The denominator was defined as "all open-cavity abdominal and thoracic surgical cases." The target sample was 30 cases.

Observers were selected, briefed on the intent of the monitoring, and instructed on how to collect the data.

The data collection tool was used to collect the data, and data were collected for 6 weeks. A total of 45 cases were observed. The results of monitoring and analysis were documented on the Quality Improvement Data Compilation Tool.

Indicators 1, 2, and 3 achieved a compliance rate of 100%. Indicator 4, however, had a compliance rate of 96%. Two perioperative nursing teams did not implement the appropriate protocols for incorrect counts. In the analysis, the quality assessment and improvement team reviewed the policy and procedure and determined that the protocols delineated the actions that should be taken for incorrect counts did not seem clear and possibly led to confusion among the staff involved with the incorrect counts. Because of this conclusion by the quality and improvement team, a randomly selected panel of five nurses also reviewed the protocols for incorrect counts. The panel concluded that the protocols lacked clarity. The quality assessment and improvement team concluded that the incidents of noncompliance were related to staff knowledge deficit owing to an ambiguous procedure statement. Recommendations were made to rewrite the new policy and procedure,

conduct another inservice program, and resurvey by observation. Using the same numerator and denominator previously defined, 40 cases were observed. Of these, there were four incidents of incorrect needle counts. Compliance with the behavior delineated in the indicator was 100%.

Because staff behaviors had changed and no additional incidents of retained foreign bodies occurred after the initial sentinel event, the quality assessment and improvement team decided that additional monitoring would not be necessary. The process of conducting counts, however, was placed on the quality improvement calendar for the upcoming year.

References

Association of Operating Room Nurses. (1992). *Standards and recommended practices for perioperative nursing*, Denver.
Joint Commission on Accreditation of Healthcare Organizations. (1992). *Accreditation Manual for Hospitals, 1993*. Chicago.

CHAPTER 38

Dealing with Regulatory Bodies

Linda Dickey White

Planning for an upcoming visit from a regulatory agency can test even the most experienced nurse managers. It does not seem to matter how well a department or unit functions, how up to date the policy and procedure manual is, or how current job descriptions and performance appraisals are; one cannot be sufficiently prepared for the visit. Dealing with regulatory agencies can cause bureaucratic nightmares for nurse managers who must decipher complex terminology that appears in small print and deal with the confusion that often occurs when implementing specific regulations. How is it that health care has come to be so stringently regulated? This chapter will describe the various agencies that currently regulate the health care environment and how they affect professional practice.

BEFORE REGULATION

The need for health care services has existed since the beginning of human's time on earth. These services were begun, embellished, and restructured over hundreds and thousands of years before regulation ever became an issue.

The earliest descriptions of surgery appear in the Edwin Smith Surgical Papyrus that dates back to 3000 B.C. The document identifies 48 surgical procedures ranging from the repair of flesh wounds to the repair of nasal and mandibular fractures and fractures of the long bones. In addition, anatomy, physiology, and pathology are accurately described.

As health care services became more sophisticated, the sick were brought to the marketplace where healers would discuss the patients' ailments, determine a treatment plan, and send them home to be cared for by families or friends.

The creation of hospitals was a result of the need to care for large numbers of sick people who could not be cared for in their homes. The word *hospital* comes from the Latin *hospitalis*, meaning house or institution for guests. Most of the early hospitals were operated by religious orders for the purpose of treating the poor or those too sick to be cared for at home. In the early 1700s, European cities and towns began building hospitals. These facilities were primarily established to serve the poor or victims of contagious diseases while the wealthy continued to be treated at home.

Surgery was sometimes performed in the home; newspapers were spread so that rugs would not be soiled, windows were covered so that neighbors could not look in, and straight-back chairs were tilted to achieve proper positioning for the patients.

It was not until the late 19th century that medical science made a significant improvement in the quality of health care. Before this time, surgical technique, as currently practiced, was nonexistent. Surgeons dressed in white coats that, in addition to protecting their clothing, contained their armamentarium. Sutures were conveniently wrapped around coat buttons, and pockets held blood-encrusted sponges that were readily available for reuse with each patient. An ordinary pin cushion, used to hold suture needles, was also kept in a pocket. Surgeons worked quickly, particularly when performing amputations, as their reputations were based on their speed. If this poor technique did not kill the patient, infection and/or shock usually did.

Perhaps the two most dramatic breakthroughs in the 19th century were the discovery of anesthesia and a beginning understanding of the principles of antisepsis. These contributions made it possible to perform painless surgery in an antiseptic environment.

INTRODUCTION OF REGULATION

In 1847 the American Medical Association was founded with the primary purpose of raising the standards for medical care in the United States and organizing licensure for physicians.

One of the first major pieces of national legislation affecting health care in the United States was the Pure Food and Drug Act of 1906, which brought about an end to the exciting and innovative era of patent medicines. Legislation on this issue was long in coming because of widespread opposition from the purveyors of patent medicines and rectifiers of whiskey. Support, however, came from drug manufacturers whose products already appeared in the National Formulary and the U.S. Pharmacopoeia. These manufacturers viewed legislation as an effective means of reducing competition from those who made their living enticing unsuspecting customers to purchase a variety of homemade concoctions. The actual passage of the law, however, was spawned by Sinclair Lewis, whose vivid description of the meat packing industry in *The Jungle* moved President Theodore Roosevelt into action with the legislature.

In 1917, the American College of Surgeons (ACS), founded in 1913, became the first professional organization to look at establishing standards of practice by developing a procedure for determining qualifications for those seeking application for fellowship in the college. The initial requirement was that a certain number of surgeries were to have been performed by each individual seeking admission. It also became apparent that standards were necessary for health care institutions, a need that led to the Hospital Standardization Program, which called for the creation of a uniform medical record format in which the physician could record activities. Thus, in addition to setting standards for physician practice, the ACS also introduced standardization for hospital care. The Catholic Hospital Association was the first hospital group to approve these standards, followed by the American Hospital Association.

Health care activity increased during the early years of this century until 1951, at which time the American College of Physicians, the American Hospital Association, and the American Medical Association joined forces with the ACS to form the Joint Commission for the Accreditation of Hospitals (JCAH). The JCAH was established as an extension of the evaluation process that was first outlined by the American College of Surgeons. During the years 1952 to 1961, physicians from the member organizations of JCAH performed surveys of hospitals seeking accreditation. By 1961 the Joint Commission had hired its own staff, and in 1964 it implemented a fee to hospitals seeking surveys for accreditation. In 1987, it was renamed the Joint Commission for Accreditation of Healthcare Organizations (JCAHO).

ERA OF REGULATION

In 1965 the Medicare Act (Title XVIII and Title XIX of the Social Security Act) was signed into law and regulations were instituted for hospitals seeking reimbursement for services provided to Medicare and Medicaid recipients. The act stipulated that hospitals already accredited by the JCAH were automatically eligible for reimbursement. Before 1965 the JCAH survey and accreditation process were voluntary, and hospitals were not obligated to participate, as the JCAH was a private, not-for-profit, voluntary, nongovernmental organization.

In 1972, the Social Security Act was again amended, and government involvement in the validating of commission survey results began. This marked the first official government involvement in establishing standards of care in the health care industry. The amendments of 1972 created the Professional Standard Review Organizations (PSROs). Although the Social Security Act stipulated that Medicare and Medicaid would pay for care that was medically necessary and of appropriate quality, these particular amendments stated that the determination of quality as well as medical necessity would be defined by these groups of local physicians.

In 1974 Congress passed Public Law 93-641, the National Health Planning and Resource Development Act, which mandated the creation of local Health Systems Agencies (HSAs). This law introduced federal controls over local jurisdictions by mandating the certificate of need (CON) requirement. The CON concept was designed to contain the growth of hospital facilities by focusing on availability, accessibility, cost, continuity, quality, and acceptability of services.

REGULATORY AGENCIES

Centers for Disease Control

The Centers for Disease Control (CDC) located in Atlanta, Georgia, is an agency of the U.S. Public Health Service. Its role is to protect the health of the public by way of national programs for the control and prevention of disease. The CDC was established in 1949 to provide health information and participate in research to locate the sources of epidemics.

Environmental Protection Agency

The Environmental Protection Agency (EPA) is charged with regulating pollution. An executive order signed by President Nixon in 1970 led to the creation of the EPA as an independent agency of the U.S. government. Its purpose is to collect data regarding sources of environmental damage and threats to human life. In addition to collecting such information, the EPA creates regulations to halt existing problems, investigates those who do not comply with its regulations, and enforces it decisions. Among other things, the EPA is concerned with air and water pollution, chemical and solid waste management and disposal, pesticides, toxic substances, radiation, noise, and heat.

Joint Commission for Accreditation of Healthcare Organizations

The JCAHO establishes standards and surveys institutions for compliance with these standards. These surveys are required if an institution is seeking accreditation from the JCAHO. Standards and surveys are currently in place for acute care hospitals, nonhospital-based psychiatric and substance abuse programs, long-term care facilities, home-care organizations, hospice programs, managed care providers, and ambulatory health care settings. The survey itself is designed to measure the degree to which an organization meets the standards established by the JCAHO and outlined in the accreditation manual for hospitals. It is the responsibility of the organization being surveyed to provide documentation demonstrating its compliance with the standards. If found to be in compliance, accreditation is provided for three years, even if the institution receives recommendations for improvement. A health care organization can seek accreditation after meeting certain eligibility requirements that include but are not limited to:

- Located in the United States or U.S. territories or possessions or serves as a military hospital;
- Maintains continuous service;
- Provides treatment such that patients would not be transferred for more intensive care;
- Maintains a governing body and organized medical and nursing services;
- Grants professional privileges appropriately;
- Provides registered nurse supervision

Another component of the 1972 amendments to the Social Security Act required that PSROs be established. The purpose of PSROs was to involve physicians in a continuing review of the quality as well as the cost of care received by recipients of Medicare, Medicaid, and other publicly funded programs. All facilities receiving funds via this mechanism were required to have both state as well as local PSROs in place by 1978. The reasons for this move were (1) health care professionals are the most appropriate individuals to evaluate the quality of health care, and (2) local peer review is the best way to ensure appropriate utilization of existing resources. One year after the amendments, in 1973, the JCAH included nursing and medical audits as a requirement for accreditation to verify that institutions were involved in continuous and ongoing evaluations of the quality of services provided. The nursing and medical professionals were then required to formulate criteria and implement means of evaluating care to assure the public that they were receiving optimal quality when they received services.

Food and Drug Administration

The Food and Drug Administration (FDA) is an agency of the U.S. Department of Health and Human Services. It oversees laws designed to guarantee pure food, safe cosmetics, and safe and effective biological products, drugs, and therapeutic devices. The FDA also monitors truthful labeling and safe packaging of products.

In 1971 the FDA assumed responsibility for enforcing the Radiation Control for Health and Safety Act of 1968, which called for the prevention of unnecessary exposure to radiation from electronic devices.

In 1976 the Medical Device Amendments were made to the Food, Drug and Cosmetic Act, giving broader powers to the FDA, including the authority to regulate medical devices. Other responsibilities of the FDA include developing new means of analyzing products and research on the effects of substances in animals as well as humans.

National Fire Protection Agency

The National Fire Protection Agency (NFPA), which gets its membership from the scientific and education community, is an organization concerned with the causes, prevention, and control of destructive fire. This agency was first organized in 1896 and incorporated in 1930 as a private, voluntary, charitable, and tax-exempt association.

The NFPA is involved with the development of fire safety and technical standards, information exchange, technical advisory services, public education research, and service to public protection agencies through the provision of information and advice.

Occupational Safety and Health Administration

By a nearly unanimous vote of Congress, the Occupational Safety and Health Act was passed into law in 1970. The purpose of the act was to assure a safe and healthy workplace with jobs that would not subject the work force to recognized hazards that could result in physical harm or even death.

Paving the way for this act were the politics of the 1960s, during which time there was renewed interest in the environment and concern about pollution and personal safety. Currently the Occupational Safety and Health Administration (OSHA) is considered to be quite a controversial organization. Workers speak of dissatisfaction with the slow response of the agency in establishing new standards and with the inadequate number of inspectors actually inspecting work sites. Likewise, employers are unhappy with OSHA largely because of its seeming unconcern regarding the cost of meeting standards and the excessive paperwork required by the agency.

PROFESSIONAL ORGANIZATIONS AND REGULATION

As previously mentioned, the American Medical Association was formally founded in 1847, and in 1912, the ACS was formally organized. The organization of registered nurses has its roots in England. A physician, Sir Henry Acland, proposed that nurses be centrally registered, follow a prescribed curriculum for education, and meet minimum standards of proficiency. Although this statement was first made in 1860, it was not until 1898 that the first public statement to license nurses was made in the United States. By 1903, four states—North Carolina, New Jersey, New York, and Virginia—required that nurses be licensed.

The American Nurses Association (ANA) was officially formed in 1911 as an extension of the Nurses Associated Alumnae of the United States and Canada and was a national organization with participation through membership in state nursing associations or individual memberships. By the following year (1912), 39 state nurses associations had been organized. Four years later, it was decided that membership would be through the states, and by 1923, all 48 states had licensure requirements following examination for registered nurses.

The ANA was restructured in 1952, and its functions were divided between two organizations: the ANA and the National League for Nursing (NLN). The ANA continued in its mission on behalf of individual nurses by maintaining progress through economic and general welfare issues, certification, and the development of standards to regulate professional practices. The NLN comprises individuals and agencies with an interest in the planning, coordinating, and implementation of educational programs for nurses. In 1984, the ANA took a stand that state nursing associations were the core of the ANA, and that membership in the national organization would be through membership in the state associations. Currently, the goal of the ANA is to strengthen the ANA and to maintain flexibility and autonomy for individual state professional organizations.

The Association of Operating Room Nurses (AORN) was officially founded on January 28, 1949, in New York City following an organizational meeting of 17 operating room supervisors. Founders of AORN battled both the NLN and the ANA until it was granted special status as a committee by the ANA. AORN's mission was to stimulate other operating room nurses into forming groups, to share knowledge among practitioners, to provide optimum patient care through educational programs, to make available for all nurses in the operating room a common body of knowledge, to motivate operating room nurses to share their experience with colleagues, and to establish an association that would benefit all professional registered nurses. Thirty chapters were in existence by the end of 1950, just one year after AORN began.

WHY REGULATE?

The 1970's has been described as the decade of regulation within the health care industry in the United States. It is clear that regulatory agencies, as well as regulations, have proliferated. Many speculate that in recent years regulation has increased because of concerns regarding the high cost of health care.

By the end of the 1980s, the United States was spending in excess of $0.5 trillion on health care. In future years, another $100 billion may be added to this annual total. Despite this large and ever-increasing amount of money, the number of people who are without health insurance continues to increase. Uncompensated care in the United States has increased from 4% in 1984 to approximately 8% in 1988. While government and private sector interests each are willing to control its own share of the health care market, neither sector is interested in footing the bill for the entire health care system. As a result, our present financing system is a combination of several different funding mechanisms. Although there is resistance on the part of the public to eliminate or decrease entitlement programs, there is not the same desire to create new groups or services within the existing health care structure.

Because the private insurance system is employer-based, the availability and the extent of benefits depend on the employer. On the one hand, our economy is shifting from one based on large manufacturing enterprises to one based on smaller, more service-oriented industries. At the same time, health insurance premiums are continuing to rise, in some cases by as much as 30%. Small employers are far less able to offer insurance to their employees at these high rates. Many small employers who do provide insurance coverage can only afford it on a limited basis, which means employees must pay a high percentage of their own health care costs. Those over the age of 65 or who are disabled have Medicare as their primary source of coverage, and although nearly all of the elderly participate in this program, it, too, has limits.

The other major public source of funding is Medicaid, which is actually a variety of programs that have been grouped together. First is the traditional welfare population, composed primarily of single parents and dependent children who meet some established state income eligibility criteria. This accounts for approximately 60% of all Medicaid recipients but only 40% of total Medicaid expenditures. Other groups that represent the majority of expenses include the aged and disabled; for many of these individuals, Medicaid is their only source of insurance for acute or chronic care needs. A major problem with the current Medicaid program is that there is variation in benefits from state to state. Because states have the ability to determine income and assets criteria for eligibility, scope of benefits, and level of payments to providers, there is widespread variation.

In addition to the increasing costs of health care, many feel that the health care industry is simply too large to be unregulated. Furthermore, because many believe that health care is a right, regulation must be imposed to secure that right for all citizens. Finally, many economists see the health care industry as a failure in the current marketplace, because health care must be provided to all, even those who cannot afford to pay for it. In the past, consumers were uninformed and often were unable to make choices about health care. This meant that demand was largely determined by the supplier of health care rather than by the consumer, and reimbursement for health care was based on charges, which meant that there was little or no incentive for health care providers to control costs.

In reviewing the economic changes that have faced health care in this century, an important event was the passage of the Social Security Act in 1965, which instituted regulations for hospitals seeking reimbursement for services provided to Medicare recipients. The act stipulated that hospitals already accredited by the JCAH were automatically eligible for reimbursement. Before 1965, the JCAH survey and accreditation process were voluntary and hospitals were not obligated to participate. The initial mission of the JCAH was to determine how health care would be provided in a way that would assure quality to the consumer. Although it remains voluntary, accreditation is essential to health care institutions seeking reimbursement from the government and other third-party payors. In addition, accreditation also signifies to the general public that a particular facility adheres to certain quality parameters.

Amendments to the Social Security Act, made in 1972, involved the government in validating commission survey results. Presently, the commission is composed of 24 commissioners from each of the following organizations: American College of Physicians, American College of Surgeons, American Dental Association, American Hospital Association, American Medical Association, and consumers. Although the ANA is not represented as a member of the commission, nursing is represented via the American Hospital Association.

One of the primary missions of the JCAHO is to stress quality assurance via requirements that health care facilities document problems and implement solutions to eliminate the problems identified. Quality assurance relies on a certain format for identifying problems. This documentation begins when an institution establishes certain quality assurance guidelines or standards that are based on structural, process, and outcome factors. Structural standards relate to policies and procedures (i.e., admission procedures, preoperative test requirements, or aseptic technique). Process standards focus on the actual delivery of care—that is to say, what is done and what is recorded by the nurse in the patient care record. The third category of standards is referred to as that of outcome standards which are used to document the outcome of nursing care. The collection of data via discharge surveys is another way that we can monitor the quality and effectiveness of care that is delivered and received by a patient.

Another economic change involves reimbursement mechanisms. Before 1984, Medicare paid hospitals and physicians after patients had been treated. However, in 1984 Congress passed a law that set cost guidelines and created 470 disease categories (diagnosis-related groups [DRGs]). Under this new system of prospective payment, providers received a predetermined payment for patients in a particular DRG. Providers could keep their surplus if treatment fees fell below the guidelines but must likewise absorb the loss if treatment costs exceeded the limit of payment. Many hospitals responded to this change in reimbursement by raising charges to people who had private insurance. This form of cost shifting provided a cushion for bad debts and charity expenses. In response, however, insurance companies began to bargain for discounts in an effort to decrease their expenses for health care. Alternative funding programs such as health maintenance organizations (HMOs) and preferred provider organizations (PPOs) began to appear in the health care funding scene. HMOs are organizations in which clients pay a fixed fee each month and may pay a minimum fee at the time care is actually given. PPOs developed as a result of insurance companies negotiating with health care providers to receive a discount from the provider in exchange for a guaranteed patient population.

REGULATION: THE FUTURE

This chapter has described the various regulatory agencies involved with the provision of health care services in the United States. The impact of these agencies and their regulations has had a noticeable effect on professional practice. Although the JCAHO may be the first regulatory agency that comes to mind when thinking about regulation in health care, it is only one of many agencies exerting influence on our practice. Because of the scope and complexity of the current health care industry, it is necessary to assure the public that they are receiving quality care. It is also necessary to demonstrate to third-party payors and to the government that the money providers receive in exchange for services is warranted. In a recent survey of more than 600 senior level executives from U.S. Fortune 500 companies, respondents were asked to identify issues that they considered to be of primary importance to the environment in which their companies operate. Those completing the surveys were from industrial companies as well as those involved in providing services. Regulatory factors were identified by the majority of respondents, which clearly indicates that regulation is seen as a crucial influence on the future.

External regulation has come from any of the aforementioned agencies, as well as from third-party payors. External regulation also comes from a society that looks to health care providers to make available and grant access to health care service for everyone regardless of their ability to pay. Internal regulation comes as a response of health care providers to external regulations. Internal regulations also come from organizations that proactively establish standards and measure their performance against those standards. Internal regulations are also created by individuals, by departments, and by those who are concerned with providing optimum service to the best of their abilities.

In recent years, Americans have seen the deregulation of several industries. Arguments can be made for and against such deregulation. It is not the purpose of this chapter to discuss the issue of deregulation in health care, but professionals must be mindful of this potential factor influencing the future delivery of health care services. Many providers feel strangled by regulations, overwhelmed by needless paperwork, and encumbered by requirements that seem meaningless.

The 1990s may well be remembered as the decade of quality. Many organizations are currently emphasizing quality in their services and in their dealing with customers. Mission statements and visions are being designed to attain and maintain higher levels of quality.

In pursuing quality, perioperative nurses must continue to be mindful of regulatory requirements and their impact on our practice. We must rely on regulations to guide us in the establishment of services, the monitoring of these services, and the evaluation of the outcomes of our efforts. It is also imperative that we use them as guidelines for improving the overall quality of the services that we offer to our patients. Quality is no longer identified by the professional but rather by our customers. The future of perioperative nursing will be shaped by our ability to use regulations to create new and innovative means of meeting the needs of our customers.

Bibliography

Driscoll, J. (1976). AORN in retrospect. *AORN Journal, 24*(1), 140.

Groah, L. K. (1983). *Operating room nursing: The perioperative role.* Reston, VA: Reston Publishing Co.

Joint Commission on Accreditation of Healthcare Organizations. (1990). *Accreditation manual for hospitals.* Chicago: JCAHO.

Schulz, R., and Johnson, A. C. (1983). *Management of hospitals* (2nd ed). New York: McGraw-Hill.

Thomson-Keith, E. (1989). Joint Commission standards: How AORN provides input. *AORN Journal, 50*(6), 1260–1262.

CHAPTER 39

Legislative Trends in Nursing: Implications for the Perioperative Nurse

Carla Willis and Alexia Green

The challenges faced by the nursing profession in the 1980s have led to a new decade of increasingly complex health care dilemmas. Each will leave its mark on the profession. What or who will determine nursing's future is in the hands of nurses. The choices are clear: become active and aggressive by influencing issues that will ultimately shape the health care system and the ability to control its contributions, or remain passive and apathetic, allowing others who are less knowledgeable and capable to direct the decision making governing the system in which nurses work. In either case, nurses will influence the outcome. They can either use influencing power to sculpt the outcomes they want or relinquish that power to others, giving them freedom to make decisions about health care that nursing will be responsible for implementing. Which alternative makes more sense?

Why then do many nurses resist becoming involved? Answers to this question range from feelings of powerlessness to perceptions of politics as "dirty or crooked." In either case, lack of knowledge of the political system and how it works fuels these feelings and reinforces the perception that individual nurses lack the power to effect positive changes in health care policies. Politics can be defined as influencing decisions and shaping outcomes. Again, passivity and inactivity in this process allow others to make those decisions. Few nurses would hesitate to speak out or become involved if they anticipated that a policy or procedure being written could result in questionable nursing practice in their workplace. The political or legislative arena is nothing more than a policy and procedure committee on a much broader scale, with an impact that is much more resounding. Because nurses are closest to the recipients of health care—patients or clients—they are suitably positioned to offer suggestions related to legislation affecting the delivery of that care. Legislators are beginning to recognize the value of input from the nursing sector (McQuide, 1989), and this recognition provides nurses with power to influence change.

UNDERSTANDING THE SYSTEM

The nurse must understand the institutional system and how to influence the system in a way that will produce the desired outcome to effect a policy or procedure change in the workplace. Health care policy changes are accomplished in a similar manner; however, the legislative process becomes the system in which the change is made.

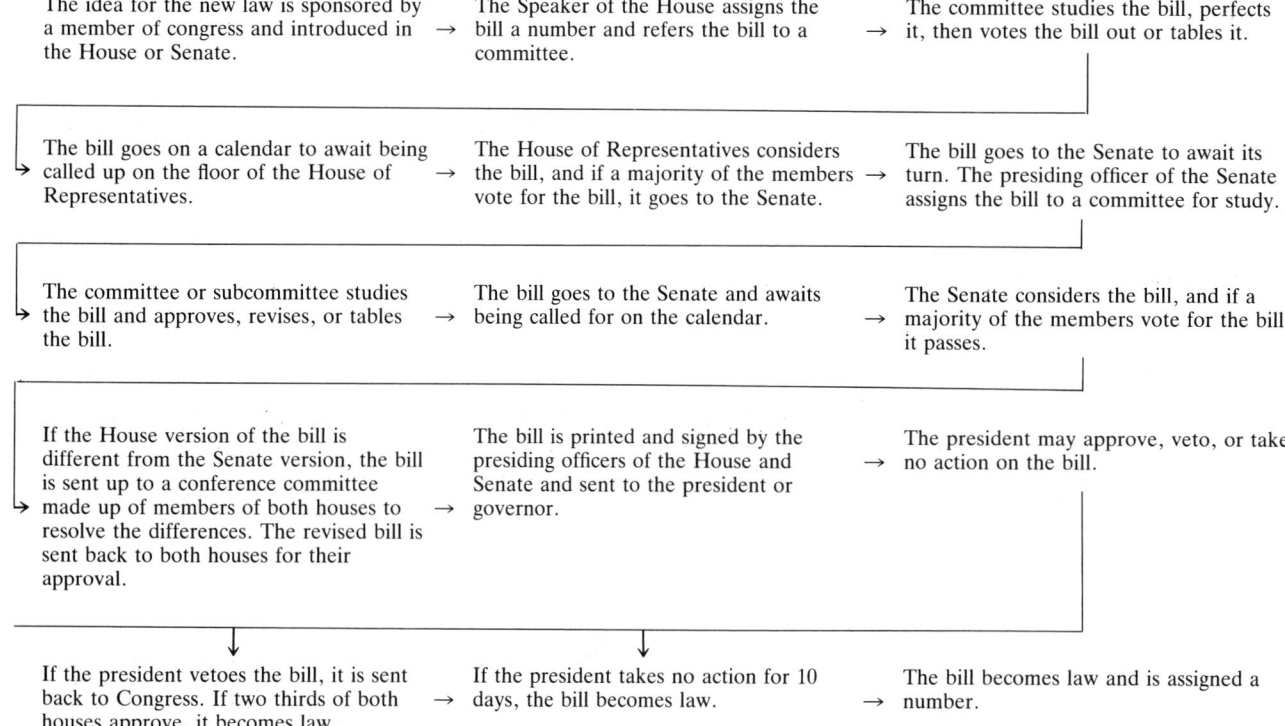

The idea for the new law is sponsored by a member of congress and introduced in the House or Senate. →	The Speaker of the House assigns the bill a number and refers the bill to a committee. →	The committee studies the bill, perfects it, then votes the bill out or tables it.
The bill goes on a calendar to await being called up on the floor of the House of Representatives. →	The House of Representatives considers the bill, and if a majority of the members vote for the bill, it goes to the Senate. →	The bill goes to the Senate to await its turn. The presiding officer of the Senate assigns the bill to a committee for study.
The committee or subcommittee studies the bill and approves, revises, or tables the bill. →	The bill goes to the Senate and awaits being called for on the calendar. →	The Senate considers the bill, and if a majority of the members vote for the bill, it passes.
If the House version of the bill is different from the Senate version, the bill is sent up to a conference committee made up of members of both houses to resolve the differences. The revised bill is sent back to both houses for their approval. →	The bill is printed and signed by the presiding officers of the House and Senate and sent to the president or governor. →	The president may approve, veto, or take no action on the bill.
If the president vetoes the bill, it is sent back to Congress. If two thirds of both houses approve, it becomes law. →	If the president takes no action for 10 days, the bill becomes law. →	The bill becomes law and is assigned a number.

FIGURE 39–1. Basic steps in the legislative process. (From Stevens, K. [1983]. *Power and influence: A source book for nurses*. New York, NY: Reprinted by permission of John Wiley & Sons, Inc., copyright © 1983.)

The government controls and administers policy, and the legislative system defines the parameters of this control and the methods of administration. The legislative system at the federal or state level consists of the constitution, statutes, regulations, and judicial opinion. The constitution outlines the powers of the governmental body and the functions of the branches. The three branches of the government are composed of the legislative branch, which makes laws; the executive branch, which enforces laws; and the judicial branch, which interprets laws. *Statutes* are the laws enacted by the legislature. *Regulations* are the rules established by an administrative body, considered part of the executive branch, that allow that body to carry out the laws or statutes that have been enacted. Judicial opinion is the rendering of an interpretation of laws by the judicial branch of the government.

Federal and state governments play somewhat different roles in health care. Generally speaking, the federal government determines health care policy on a broad scale by determining how resources will be allocated (e.g., who gets what kind of funding and which programs will be affected). "State and local governments monitor and regulate health care through legislation and regulations" (Mason, 1988). Federal and state governments perform these roles by enacting and carrying out legislation. How this legislation is developed is fundamental to understanding the process and its influence on the delivery of health care.

The legislative branch of government at the federal level, and in most cases at the state level, is bicameral—i.e., composed of two elected legislative bodies or chambers: the Senate and the House of Representatives. The names of these two bodies may vary from state to state, but their function is similar. At the federal level, the Senate is composed of two senators from each state. The number of members elected to the House of Representatives from each state is determined by the population of that state.

"Ideas for laws can come from a number of sources: citizens, nurses, governmental staff, elected officials, and special interest groups" (Jordan, 1983). However, to be introduced into one or both bodies of the legislature, a law must be sponsored by a member of that body. When initially introduced in a session of the legislature, an act or a statute is called a *bill*. This process is similar at both the state and federal level of government.

Bills introduced into the legislature are labeled with a number and a letter prefix. For example, the legislation introduced into the 101st Congress that would provide indirect Medicare payment for a registered nurse (RN) First Assistant was labeled S 125 when introduced into the Senate and HR 143 when introduced into the House of Representatives. Each bill was sponsored by a member of the respective body.

Once a bill is introduced into either the House or Senate, it enters a complicated process with many "political hoops" through which it must pass. A bill is vulnerable and may be killed at numerous points in the process. Part of this process includes scrutiny by various committees and subcommittees to which the bill is assigned for study. Figure 39–1 shows the basic steps through which a bill must pass. Once a bill has successfully passed through the various committees and subcommittees to which it was assigned, it proceeds to the entire assembly of that chamber. At this point it is debated, amended, passed, or defeated. Bills that are passed by one chamber go to the other chamber for consideration, where they undergo a similar process. The version of a bill passed by the House may be very different from that passed by the Senate. After being passed by both chambers, the bill is sent to a conference committee composed of members of both the House and the Senate. Members of this conference committee are responsible for working through differences in the two bills and reaching a compromise. The compromised version is then sent back to both chambers for final approval. If this final approval is obtained by both the House of Representatives and the Senate, the bill is sent to the President (or, in the case of states, the governor). This chief executive officer has the option of signing the bill, vetoing the bill, or sending it back to the legislature for reconsideration. The bill becomes law or statute only after it has been signed by the president or governor. Both the federal and state levels of government have provisions for overriding a veto so that a bill can still be passed.

A bill is frequently passed to an administrative agency for implementation after becoming a law. Administrative agencies then formulate rules or regulations determining how the law will be carried out. These rules and regulations carry the same weight as laws, for they must be followed for compliance to the law to be achieved. An example at the federal level is the Department of Health and Human Services (DHHS). This administrative body, among other duties, outlines regulations to which health care institutions must adhere to receive Medicare or Medicaid funding. The ability of this body's power to affect perioperative nursing was demonstrated in 1986 when the regulations determining the level at which personnel could perform circulating responsibilities in the operating room (OR) were changed. Before 1986, the regulations mandated that the OR circulator be a registered nurse:

> Only qualified registered nurses may perform circulating duties in the operating room, except that LPNs and surgical technologists may assist in circulatory duties under the direct supervision of a qualified registered nurse (Combs, 1986a).

When these regulations were again considered in 1986 by Dr. Otis Bowen, who was DHHS Secretary at that time, they were changed, allowing a less restrictive interpretation by institutions. The altered regulations stated:

> Qualified registered nurses may perform circulating duties in the operating room except that LPNs and surgical technologists in accordance with applicable state laws and approved medical staff policies and procedures may assist in circulating duties under the supervision of a qualified registered nurse who is immediately available to respond to emergencies (Combs, 1986b).

Federal administrative rules and regulations are often broad so as to apply to a variety of circumstances in many areas of the country. State administrative agencies promulgate rules or regulations that are narrowed in scope to meet needs in that particular state. An example of an administrative agency at the state level is the agency charged with governing nursing practice in that state. In Texas, the Board of Nurse Examiners enacts rules that govern the practice of nursing in that state. This particular board's impact on nursing is illustrated by Delegation Rules. These rules outline those tasks and responsibilities that a registered nurse in the state of Texas can and cannot delegate to an unlicensed person. Rule 218.7 identifies tasks that ". . . are not within the scope of sound professional nursing judgement to delegate . . ." (Nurse Practice Act, 1989). Outlined in this rule were nursing responsibilities that required physical, psychological, and social assessment; formulation of a plan of nursing care; implementation of the plan of care requiring professional nursing judgment; and evaluation of the patient's response to the care rendered. Therefore, the intent of these rules was to reinforce the need in Texas for the circulator in the OR to be a registered nurse. Thus, this action offset the loose interpretation of the DHHS regulations of 1986.

State legislation is the primary source of governmental power, as the federal government must operate within the powers enumerated by the Constitution. State government, however, has much broader powers not limited by the state or federal constitutions. States are given the authority to prescribe laws aimed at preserving public order, health safety, welfare, and morals (Wing, 1985). In this capacity, state legislation becomes more critical to nursing practice than federal legislation. The previous examples of federal and state intervention with regard to the RN circulator in the OR serve as illustrations of the impact that state level legislation can have on federal legislation in dictating parameters of nursing practice.

BASIC CONCEPTS OF POLITICAL POWER

Once nurses understand the political or legislative process, they can influence the process that will directly or indirectly support quality health care and sound nursing practice. Power is the ability to influence desired results (Stevens, 1983). Within the context of the political process, power then becomes the ability to influence desired laws. Power is the means of influencing members of the legislative or governmental arena.

Power can be exerted as an individual nurse, as a member of a nursing specialty group, or as a member of the nursing profession as a whole. First, nurses need to become knowledgeable about current legislation, rules, and regulations that affect nursing and health care. Also, nurses should be aware of a legislator's positions and voting records on legislation critical to nursing. As individuals, nurses can then use the power they have through their knowledge and expertise to influence their legislators regarding health care legislation. They can also share their expertise by testifying at public hearings concerning health care issues. Contributing to the campaigns of legislators is another important power that nurses have. Contributions can take the form of funds or time spent in working to help elect a particular candidate either because he or she is "friendly to nursing" (i.e., supports legislation critical to quality nursing and health care) or because he or she is opposing a candidate who is not favorably supportive of critical issues or legislation affecting nursing. As a member of a group, the nurse can enjoy a greater degree of power because of the "power in numbers" concept. Approximately 1 in 44 voters in this country is a registered nurse, and legislators are becoming aware of this fact. Nurses are a powerful political force that has been more or less dormant in this country until relatively recently. Nurses have the ability to transform that dormancy into a powerful driving force to bring about changes in the health care system. When a nursing group such as the Association of Operating Room Nurses (AORN) with more than 45,000 members aligns itself with the American Nurses Association and all its members communicate their position on a particular issue, legislators will listen. As nurses become more involved politically, other avenues of political power are open to them. Nurses can become lobbyists, political officers, or members of administrative and advisory councils or fulfill many other influential roles. To take advantage of these opportunities, nurses will have to recognize the power they already possess as individuals and work collectively to cultivate relationships with legislators who hold positions that can influence health policy and nursing practice.

NURSING'S ROLE IN THE POLITICAL PROCESS

Most nurses vote, but that is the extent of their political activity. Voting is simply not enough. If nurses care about their profession and the health care system, then they must do more. Nurses need to respond with creative strategies and with energy. It is time to be smart and strong, not dull and overwhelmed. Currently many nurses are becoming politically active. Important aspects of nursing's political activity include the professional associations' role, the consumer organizations' role, the role of other health care organizations, and the role of individual nurses.

Professional Associations

Nurses must continue to strive for increased political power, facing the fact that decisions and their outcomes revolve around those who have the power to exert influence. This can be accomplished most effectively through a collective organized effort with clear objectives. A professional nursing association provides one mechanism through which a nurse can become politically active. The professional association will have the most impact on health care legislation and nursing practice.

Factors that influence a professional association's potential political strength include size of membership, extent of formalization of the group, level of external and internal communication, economic resources, ability to compile and distribute information in a group effort, timing of effort, extent of personal resources and alliances, and degree of group cohesiveness (Dunn, 1983).

The power to promote change is inherent in a cohesive professional association such as the American Nurses Association (ANA). The ANA has outlined four basic questions facing the nursing profession in the federal legislative arena:

1. What is this nation's health care policy agenda?
2. How should nursing services be organized and delivered within this nation's health care system?
3. How can the current health care system be restructured?
4. What steps can be taken to reduce health care costs (Nursing's Agenda, 1991)?

Although there are approximately 1.8 million registered nurses in the United States, a relatively small number belong to professional associations such as the ANA. Marilyn Goldwater (1984), a nurse and Representative from Maryland, believes that the reluctance of individuals within the profession to assert themselves or to align themselves with organizations that can exert the power needed to effect change is a serious roadblock to the profession.

Powerful and influential professional associations such as the ANA and AORN provide a collective voice for promoting the nursing profession and the quality of health care. The state and local affiliates of these professional associations are the "grassroots" organizations that influence the individual nurse as well as on the health care setting and the government. It is important for nurses to support these national nursing associations rather than form new associations. Nursing can develop a unified voice in dealing with political issues through this important vehicle.

Both national and state professional associations deal with issues such as rules and regulations for implementation of Medicare and Medicaid, payment equity, reimbursement for nursing services, insurance discrimination, nursing shortage, and funding for nursing education. Threats to nursing practice and the quality of care are monitored. An example of such a threat was the change in the regulations of the DHHS that allowed for a less restrictive interpretation of what type of health care provider could circulate in the operating room. Efforts by the American Medical Association (AMA) since 1988 to establish the Registered Care Technologist (RCT) as a viable health care provider is a more recent example of a threat to nursing practice.

Leah Curtin (1985) believes that unjust decisions and regulations often result because power has been vested in one group rather than another. Reasons for uneven power distribution include the economic influence of the stronger group, lack of cohesion in the weaker group, and more effective articulation by the stronger group than the weaker group.

To respond effectively, all nurses must become politically astute at the state and national levels. This requires membership in professional associations, donations to political action committees, and active and intelligent communication with local, state, and national politicians (Jordan, 1983).

One of the most important issues currently facing national nursing associations is the need to develop a unified voice for the profession. This is not an easy task, as there are more than 60 different associations. It is counterproductive for these associations to be in a power struggle among themselves. Certainly, the varied organizations have much to offer nursing's diversified profession. However, the only effective way to exercise political clout is to network, to coordinate and collaborate with other groups to achieve common goals (Maraldo and Kinder, 1985). For this reason, AORN has entered into a contract with ANA. This contract provides the basis for AORN support of the ANA legislative agenda, and in return, the ANA provides lobbying support for AORN at the federal level in Washington, DC.

Legislators expect nurses to settle their own internal differences and deliver proposals that are well coordinated and supported by their membership. It is destructive to the nursing profession to have one nursing group support a particular issue and another oppose that issue. Many nurses believe that one nursing association can negotiate a common stand for the profession; that role naturally falls to the ANA as the senior national organization (Curtin, 1985). The ANA has established itself as a political leader for years, gaining a high level of credibility, knowledge, and expertise regarding national and state policy.

Examples of efforts to unify the profession on policy issues were illustrated by the collective efforts of the ANA, the National League for Nursing (NLN), the American Association of Colleges of Nursing (AACN), and the American Organization of Nurse Executives (AONE). These four groups united under a grant from the W. K. Kellog Foundation to reach consensus throughout the nursing community on credentialing (Maraldo and Kinder, 1985). At the state level, during the 1991 legislative session, the Texas Nurses Association joined forces with several other nursing organizations to support a unified nursing legislative agenda. Efforts such as these represent an abandonment of fears and suspicions in favor of formation of effective coalitions that promote and protect the nursing profession. Nurses need to continue to find effective ways of managing conflicts and resolving opposing points of view internally. Participation in the political process means building consensus among the nursing profession.

Consumer Organizations

Consumers as well as nurses are learning the importance of collaboration and coalition building. Consumers have learned that they have considerable political power when a group with common interest and goals is formed. Examples of consumer coalitions include the Gray Panthers, the American Association of Retired Persons, and the Consumer Federation of America. Although these groups function on a national basis, coalitions are formed at the local level to address community issues such as air pollution or the handling of hazardous waste. Individuals are able to prevent duplication of efforts and maximize resources through collective behavior such as coalitions.

Nurses and other health care providers need to learn to work with consumer groups to produce change in the health care system. Frequently, health care providers have difficulty separating the role of the consumer public from that of the consumer as patient. The reluctance of some health care providers to share policy decisions about health care with the consumer public has created an opportunity for nurses to participate. Consumers generally perceive nurses as friends and allies who are supportive of their efforts to maintain some control over their own health status. This provides nursing with the opportunity to serve as a link between consumers and other providers.

Other Organizations

Professional nursing associations and consumer groups have been mentioned as having important roles within the political arena of health care. Nurses must not overlook or underestimate the role of other health care providers' professional organizations in health policy formation. One of the most politically powerful groups is the AMA, the primary professional organization for physicians. Goldwater (1984) states that one of the biggest roadblocks to nursing is the organized campaign against nursing practice by the medical profession. The medical profession has exerted unrelenting efforts to dominate all the health professions and prevent them from gaining any degree of power or control. Other disciplines and consumers tend to live with physicians' decisions and actions rather than challenge them in the political arena.

The power that physicians have created can be seen in the ability to maintain high membership levels in their professional associations. Membership in the Texas Medical Association in 1988 consisted of 86% of the licensed physicians in the state of Texas; by comparison, only 5% of licensed professional nurses belong to the Texas Nurses Association. Similarly, physicians have one of the strongest political action committees (PACs) in the nation, ranking in the top ten of all PACs based on amount of contributions.

Nurses must use effective approaches in dealing with such powerful organizations. One approach is to work with state medical associations by serving on a joint practice committee, if one exists. The National Joint Practice Commission was created to allow nurses and physicians opportunities to jointly establish and maintain standards for the care of patients in hospitals. Such committees have a powerful voice in influencing the political process.

A group's success in the process of change depends on the possession and effective use of resources greater than those of the opposing group. Because nurses make up the largest group of health care providers in the nation, the one resource nurses have that others do not is power in numbers. With increased political awareness and a larger number of nurses joining professional associations such as ANA and AORN, the nursing profession will continue to progress toward shaping the provisions of health care and defining the terms of practice of nursing professionals.

The Power of the Individual Nurse

Because people are the central element in the political process, the process begins with the individual nurse. Political networking requires the development of relationships with people in power. As in any relationship, the closer and longer the relationship, the better it will be. Nurses are continually striving to participate in decisions related to their professional destiny. The political framework of the government provides nurses the opportunity to participate in the highest levels of decision making. All it takes is commitment for individual involvement.

Most nurses believe that politicians and government officials are not interested in their opinions and input. Actually, most legislators are interested in communicating with their constituents, especially someone such as a nurse who has expertise in health care. Appendix A provides information on getting to know legislators and the legislative issues. Legislators have respect for professionals. Both individual and professional association contacts are important in the political arena. To the legislator, the individual represents a potential vote, whereas the association represents the voice of nurses. Both individual and association recommendations are sought when legislation is being considered. Both views are taken into consideration; but understandably, it is easier for a busy legislator to deal with a national or state association representative rather than with individuals or a number of specialty groups (Goldwater, 1984).

STRATEGIES FOR POLITICAL INVOLVEMENT

Joining a Professional Association

One of the most effective ways for nurses to become politically active is to join a professional nursing association. Membership in professional associations such as the AORN can be greatly enhanced when the nurse is also an active participant in a national association such as the ANA. These associations offer many benefits and opportunities for political involvement. Nurses must be socialized into the political process. This socialization

can occur within professional groups and associations (Solomon and Roe, 1986).

Nurses and professional associations need to join together to support legislative issues. Political power lies in numbers, with those numbers represented by professional nursing associations. However, nurses must not allow their subgroup or specialty group's interest to jeopardize successful legislative action. Opposing opinions by nursing groups in the legislative arena can only lead to failure (Griffith, 1981).

Individual Opportunities at Local, State, and National Levels

The most opportune way to become involved in the political arena is by way of the state or local nursing association. Most associations have governmental affairs committees that are always eager for volunteers. Even novices' energy and contributions to such committees are appreciated. By working for such an association and giving of personal time, a nurse's political network and expertise will grow.

Most governmental affairs committees provide the nurse with opportunities to learn about the political process at many different levels. Grassroots networking and involvement can be accomplished by participation in the complex communications system that most committees develop within local, state, or national regions. Most communications systems generally involve a mailing list, a telephone tree, and a telephone bank. The mailing list contains names of nurses who should receive written information concerning legislative issues. A telephone tree is a system nurses can use to notify other nurses when an issue is urgent, with no time for a mailing. A telephone bank is similar to a telethon, in which a large number of people are quickly mobilized to respond to important issues or contribute to a PAC.

More complex levels of participation in a legislative committee include serving on an interview panel that interviews political candidates during an election year regarding their positions on health care issues. Most district nursing associations are responsible for assisting state and national associations in determining endorsement of political candidates for PAC contributions. This presents an exciting opportunity for political involvement.

Nurses are often asked to provide testimony at hearings held by legislative committees regarding health care issues. These nurses are considered experts on particular issues or have had numerous encounters with particular health care situations, such as dealing with clients with Alzheimer's disease. Nursing testimony directly influences the political process, as it clarifies the issues for legislators. Most nursing associations are contacted often by legislative committees dealing with health care issues. They are often asked to provide the name of a nurse who has expertise in a certain area and would be willing to provide testimony. Maintaining contact with one's nursing association regarding current issues and offering one's expertise in testifying at the local, state, or national level is one way to become familiar with the legislative process.

Probably one of the greatest opportunities for political involvement is through a political appointment. These opportunities exist at the local, state, and national level and include paid and volunteer positions. Political appointments to health care committees and regulatory agencies are a very desirable mechanism for career and political advancement. Most political appointments stem from many years of political networking within a particular political party. For example, it is unlikely that a Republican governor would appoint a highly visible nurse to a particular committee unless she or he was also a Republican. However, a nurse who is fortunate enough to be offered a political appointment must be prepared to make a significant commitment of time and energy to become recognized as a valuable political leader in nursing.

Election to public or legislative office provides the greatest opportunity for influencing the political process. A nurse serving in any elective office, whether it be on the local school board or as a state representative, can positively influence the health care system, the nursing profession, and the political process. Many nurses are realizing this impact and have taken the challenge to seek political positions.

Communicating with a Legislator

If nurses want to significantly influence their legislator on a health care issue, contacting them once a year with their opinions will not suffice. To significantly influence any legislator or public official, they must build a long-term relationship in which they are respected for their knowledge and expertise in health care (Appendix A). This is not as difficult as it sounds, since most legislators have little, if any, knowledge about the health care system.

Nurses can begin by learning who their friends are in their state and national legislatures. They should contact their professional associations to determine past voting records of their legislators. The nurse should ask: Are they friendly to nursing and health care issues? It is important to thank a legislator for a vote on a particular issue, helping them to realize that nurses are aware of their legislative endeavors. Become familiar with the committees that handle health care legislation. Table 39–1 provides information regarding congressional committees that deal with health care legislation at the federal level. Most states have two to four primary committees in which health care legislation evolves. The members of these committees will be most interested in opinions based on professional expertise and the nurse will be better positioned to exert his or her influence.

Communicating with legislators can be done formally or informally. Sometimes, for instance, opportunities to speak with legislators present themselves unexpectedly in social settings. Nurses are often sought for their opinions on family members' health status or other similar situations. The nurse should take advantage of those times to engage in a brief, pleasant discussion of

TABLE 39–1. COMMITTEES DEALING WITH HEALTH CARE LEGISLATION		
Legislative Body	Committee	Subcommittee
Senate	Finance	Medicare and Long-Term Care
		Medicaid: Families and Uninsured
	Labor and Human Resources	
	Appropriations	Labor
	Budget	
House of Representatives	Ways and Means	Health
	Energy and Commerce	Health and Environment
	Appropriations	Labor
	Budget	

issues, conveying nursing's point of view. Formal lobbying by individual nurses, however, requires an appreciation of the critical points at which lobbying is necessary and an understanding of the legislative process.

Communication with an elected representative can be as simple as a letter or phone call or as extensive as providing testimony before a congressional committee. All legislators, whether state or federal, are extremely busy and have staff to help them deal with communications and decision making in the political process. Legislative staff therefore become very important in the political setting. Get to know a legislator's staff and administrative assistants; these are the people with whom a constituent will be dealing with in most communications. Maintain the current addresses and phone numbers for legislators. State nursing associations and the League of Women Voters maintain a current listing that can be readily obtained on request. These listings also indicate voting districts. Some common-sense rules for communicating with a legislator are included in Appendix B.

Writing a letter is the most common way in which constituents communicate with their legislators. Letters are highly effective if written properly. In fact, most legislators utilize a computer system to record responses received from constituent letters and phone calls. When the legislator needs to make a decision regarding how to vote on a particular issue, this record will be consulted to obtain an idea of constituent views.

Letters should be brief, presenting the facts, new knowledge, or your views on particular issue. Of key importance is timeliness; sending information too early or too late in the legislative process is ineffective. Never threaten a legislator, as this is disrespectful and unprofessional. The use of form letters is considered inappropriate. Legislators want to know that the ideas expressed are your opinion, not those of a large group. A simple, brief, handwritten letter is most effective. Tips on letter writing are included in Appendix C.

Not every nurse will take the time or be interested in extensive political involvement. However, there are simple ways in which every nurse can help to increase nursing's influence in the political arena:

- Register to vote, and vote in all local, state, and national elections
- Consider candidates' positions and views on health care and nursing issues before voting
- Identify yourself as a nurse when communicating with legislators or public officials
- Support and maintain memberships in national and specialty nursing associations
- Contribute to nursing political action committees

Negotiating/Lobbying

Negotiating and lobbying are two key concepts in the political process. *Negotiating* is the skill of assessing what people value and and determining how the values of various groups can be combined for mutual benefit (Stevens, 1987). It is an integral component of *lobbying*, which is the art of influencing the legislative process. Most lobbying is done by professional lobbyists who are paid by special interest groups. The ANA has several nurse lobbyists on staff at the national level; one of these lobbyists is assigned to work with the AORN. Most state associations also employ a professional lobbyist. Lobbyists, whether paid or unpaid, play a critical role in the passage or defeat of most legislation.

Not all lobbying is performed by professional lobbyists, and nurses are often asked to lobby, especially at the state level. For instance, nurses might be asked to lobby to help a particular legislative bill through the legislative process or to block its passage. Such lobbying may be as simple as a phone call to the legislator or a visit to the legislator's office to show support for a particular issue. The primary goal would be to inform the legislators and their staff on how the nursing profession or the health care system would be affected by a piece of legislation. This type of lobbying is most often called *grassroots lobbying*.

More extensive lobbying is also performed by nurse volunteers under the direction of their state specialty or professional associations. This demands a full understanding of the issues and of the arguments in favor of and against the legislation. The professional association will provide the necessary information. Often association members meet or "huddle" before lobbying, and members are updated on the issues and a strategic plan developed.

Strategy, which involves the planning and execution of a well-thought-out, purposeful goal, is very important in all forms of lobbying. Strategizing assumes working in a constantly changing environment and requires that the plan be adapted numerous times. Timing is of key importance; lobbying must be carried out before a bill is voted on. Determining when bills are scheduled for a vote is not always simple, even for a professional lobbyist. Rules may limit the amount of public notice necessary, and a vote may come up unexpectedly. In fact, the scheduling of a vote is sometimes used as a political tactic by legislators.

Lobbying and negotiating actually begin when a bill is drafted or written. Legislators are contacted by a special interest group to sponsor a bill, which involves writing the bill and introducing it into the legislative process. Nursing associations are instrumental in this process, since most legislators work with professional associations rather than individual citizens. Not only do professional associations alert members of important pending votes, but they also are instrumental in getting legislation introduced and through the legislative process by way of their lobbying efforts.

If the association was not involved in the drafting of the bill, then its initial lobbying efforts will most likely be directed toward the initial committee assigned to handling the bill. The bill is lobbied in hopes of passing it out of committee or to "kill" it in committee. It is much easier to stop a bill than to pass one, and it becomes increasingly more difficult to stop as it progresses from one level to the next. Lobbying continues even after the bill has passed the legislative branch and progressed to the executive branch, where the president or governor may veto the bill. Often, the intent of the bill will be totally changed from the original, or the bill may be "tacked" onto another piece of legislation with a better chance of passing. Negotiating and lobbying are required throughout the entire process, creating a challenge for all involved.

Political Action Committees

PACs are special committees within professional associations or special interest groups that can engage in direct, partisan, and political activities, including endorsement and financial support, without tax liability (Rouse, 1984). PACs depend on resources, which consist of money and people. PACs contribute to candidates' campaigns, and often the amount of the contributions makes a difference in the outcome of the election by gaining valuable votes for the candidate. Candidates are aware of the size of most PACs and their political clout. There are state and federal PACs, each functioning under different laws.

Nursing's PAC evolved from the ANA Nurses' Coalition for Action in Politics (N-CAP) (Rothberg, 1985). N-CAP was recently renamed as RN-PAC, so as to be more readily identified with professional nursing. More and more nurses are beginning to realize the importance of contributing to a PAC. If the approximately 1 million nurses currently practicing in the United States would each contribute only $1 to their national PAC, the nursing profession would gain sizable clout.

Not unexpectedly, physicians have one of the most powerful PACs in the nation. However, individually they do not have to contribute large sums of money, since most physicians contribute to PACs. During the 1985–1986 political campaigns, the Texas medical PAC collected more than $600,000 in contributions, which was an average of only $32 from each contributor. However, during that same election year, the Texas nursing PAC collected only $19,000; probably most nurses who contributed gave more than the average physician.

The problem is that most nurses do not consider contributing to PACs an important part of the political process. No matter how small the contribution, it is the act of contributing that is important. As more nurses begin contributing to PACs and become involved in PAC activities, nursing will continue to gain power in the political arena.

CURRENT AND FUTURE POLITICAL ISSUES FOR NURSING

Demands placed on nursing will continue to escalate as a result of the growing complexities of health care delivery (e.g., the increasing numbers of elderly members of our society, the increased acuity of patients in health care facilities and of those discharged for home health care, and and increasing numbers of AIDs patients). In July 1988, the Secretary's Commission on Nursing published a report on the state of nursing, citing 16 recommendations for strategies to address the shortage issue (Allen, 1989b). Although numerous studies have been published in the past, this particular study has the backing of an administrative agency of the executive branch of the government, perhaps lending it more influence. The commission addressed the impact of the nursing shortage on the quality of and access to health care. The report warns that ". . . if actions are not taken to reverse or moderate current trends, the shortage of RNs will extend into the future" (Allen, 1989b). The nursing shortage presents a golden opportunity for nurses to take part in shaping health care in the future by exerting their influence and working in coalition with others to develop strategies, thereby indicating their capability and willingness to participate.

Access to health care, or the ability of citizens to acquire health care at an affordable cost, will continue to be of concern. The economics of health care and the demands of society will force legislation addressing these issues. Nurses, having no vested interest in resisting changes in the health care system, have the opportunity to align with each other, as well as with consumer groups, to become leaders in the restructuring of health care (Moccia, 1989). AORN joined with more than 40 other nursing organizations in 1991 to endorse *Nursing's Agenda for Health Care Reform* (1991).

Third-party reimbursement for nurses will become a more prominent issue as the majority of health care is financed by third-party payors (Stevens, 1983). The need for increased access to health care by consumers, particularly in rural areas, will force the need for third-party reimbursement for nurse practitioners. Nurses can take advantage of the increasing health care needs of the nation by lobbying for legislation that will increase opportunities for consumers to receive health care through a variety of alternatives. Third-party reimbursement not only provides one of these alternatives, it also strengthens the autonomy of the professional nurse and provides a more accurate picture of the nursing services being contributed. Nursing needs to express its functions in terms that are marketable in the current economical climate by emphasizing cost effectiveness (Steele, 1985).

As more and more health care providers seek to secure a greater foothold in the health care system, nurses will have to increase their efforts to protect nursing practice. Refusing to accept diminishing quality in health care as a compromise to offset rising costs demands vigilance by the nursing profession. Encroachment into nursing practice by groups that would offer strategies that ultimately would compromise the quality of health care by providing a less qualified caregiver will continue to be a threat as the pressures of solving the current health care dilemmas increase.

Taking an active part in monitoring and shaping health care legislation becomes a professional responsibility of each nurse (McQuide, 1989). It is time for the "sleeping giant," as nursing has been referred to by some politicians, to awaken. The only future the nursing profession has is the one that its own members provide. Continued apathy, lack of cohesiveness, and indecisiveness lead to lack of direction, which will allow others to seize the opportunity to shape the future for health care and the nursing profession.

Bibliography

Allen, A. (1989a). Commission questions existence of RN shortage. *Journal of Postanesthesia Nursing, 4*(1), 49–52.

Allen, A. (1989b). Secretary's commission on nursing, part II: Final report. *Journal of Postanesthesia Nursing, 4*(3), 191–203.

Combs, D. (1986a). Legislation: OR circulator regs under scrutiny by Bowen. *AORN Journal, 43*(5), 976–977.

Combs, D. (1986b). Legislation: Medicare regulations on OR circulator final. *AORN Journal, 44*(2), 154–156.

Curtin, L. (1985). On the cutting edge. *Nursing Management, 16*(3), 8.

Dunn, A. (1983). Nurse activism in Oregon politics. *Nurse Practitioner, 8*(10), 54–56, 80.

Goldwater, M. (1984). Political power for nurse practitioners. *Nurse Practitioner, 9*(11), 44–45.

Griffith, H. (1981). Strategies for direct third-party reimbursement for nurses. *American Journal of Nursing, 82*(3), 408–414.

Jordan, C. (1983). The power of political activity. In K. Stevens (Ed.). *Power and influence: A source book for nurses.* New York: John Wiley & Sons.

Maraldo, P., and Kinder, J. (1985). Politics and the professional organization. In D. Mason and S. Talbott (Eds.). *Political action handbook for nurses.* Menlo Park, CA: Addison-Wesley.

Mason, D. (1988). Politics, nursing, and you. *Imprint, 35*(3), 47–52.

McQuide, P. (1989). Legislative activity is a nurse's job—let's wake up. *Journal of Neuroscience Nursing, 21*(1), 3–4.

Moccia, P. (1989). Shaping a human agenda for the nineties: Trends that demand our attention as managed care prevails. *Nursing & Health Care, 10*(1), 14–17.

Nurse Practice Act for the State of Texas. (1989). Austin, TX: Board of Nurse Examiners for the State of Texas.

Nursing's Agenda For Health Care Reform. (1991). Kansas City, MO: American Nurses Association.

Rothberg, J. (1985). The growth of political action in nursing. *Nursing Outlook, 33*(3), 133–135.

Rouse, R. (1984). Legislation: In the game of politics, do not hesitate to say 'deal me in.' *AORN Journal, 40*(4), 594–595.

Solomon, S., and Roe, S. (1986). *Key concepts in public policy.* NLN Publication 15-1995A. New York: NLN.

Steele, J. (1985). *Issues in professional nursing practice: 9. Challenges to nursing practice.* St. Louis: American Nurses Association.

Stevens, C. (1987). Reframing health policy debate: The need for public interest language. *Administration and Society, 19*(3), 309–327.

Stevens, K. (1983). Power as a positive force. In K. Stevens (Ed.). *Power and influence: A source book for nurses.* New York: John Wiley & Sons.

Wing, K. (1985). *The law and the public's health.* Ann Arbor, MI: Health Administration Press.

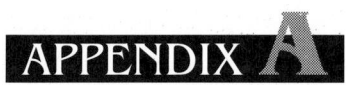

How to Get to Know Your Legislator and the Legislative Issues*

Before Elections:

1. Meet the candidates in your district and ask them about the issues of importance to you.
2. If the candidate merits your support, contribute your personal time and resources to his or her campaign.

Before a Legislative Session:

1. Contact your professional association regarding issue of importance during the upcoming legislative session and offer your support.
2. Write or phone the legislator's district office and express yourself on the issues and/or a specific bill.
3. Meet the legislative staff. It is particularly important to meet the person who handles most of the health care legislation.

---

*Adapted from *How the Texas Legislature Works*, published by The Texas Women's Commission Foundation.

During the Legislative Session:

1. Meet with the legislator in his or her office and talk about a particular bill you support or oppose.
2. Attend hearings on specific bills. Consult your professional association to offer your expertise in testifying for or against a bill.
3. Telephone, write, and send telegrams to your legislator regarding current legislative issues.
4. Contact your professional association regarding progress of legislative bills and key times to contact your legislator.
5. Subscribe to newsletters that provide updates on the status of the current legislative session.

Between Legislative Sessions:

1. Invite the legislator to speak at your professional meeting.
2. Consult your professional association regarding upcoming elections, endorsing "nurse-friendly" candidates and future legislative issues.

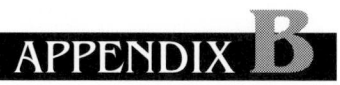

Common-Sense Rules For Communication with Legislators

1. Do your homework. Know the issues before contacting your legislator. Know the interest groups involved and how each stands to gain or lose from a change in policy.
2. Work through your professional associations. This is your best resource for current information on political issues.
3. Identify yourself as a nurse. It may or may not be appropriate to identify yourself as a member of a professional association. Your association can best advise you on this.
4. Identify yourself as a constituent if you vote in the legislator's district. Legislators are more interested in hearing from constituents than nonconstituents.
5. Identify your subject clearly and be concise. A letter should be no longer than one page (fact sheets may be attached if necessary). A phone call should be to the point and no longer than 15 minutes in duration.
6. When contacting a legislator to support or oppose a particular bill, know the bill number and name (e.g., HB 1160, the Nursing Quality Assurance Bill). All bills are identified by a prefix designating the origination of the bill (HB refers to a bill originating in the House of Representatives; S refers to a bill originating in the Senate).
7. Act in a timely fashion at the right points in the political process. Collaborate with your allies for effectiveness. Your professional nursing association will be important in helping coordinate your effort.
8. Never argue with or threaten your legislators. This is the quickest way to win disrespect for yourself and your profession.
9. Remember that listening is as important as talking, and the key lies in development of interpersonal relationships.

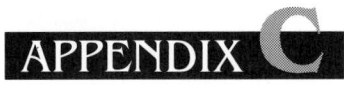

Tips for Letter Writing

1. Use the proper salutation and full name of the legislator:

   State/Federal Representatives:
   The Honorable (Full Name)
   House of Representatives
   House Office Building or State Assembly
   City, State, Zip Code
   Dear Mr./Ms. (Last Name):

   State/Federal Senators:
   The Honorable (Full Name)
   United States Senate or State Senate
   Senate Office Building
   City/State/Zip Code
   Dear Senator (Last Name):

2. Identify the bill by title and number. Address only one bill or issue per letter.

3. Briefly and courteously state the reasons for your position. Highlight any personal experience you have had with the issue.

4. Identify the effects of the bill and how they relate to health care. Key "buzzwords" to use when applicable are "cost-effectiveness," "access to health care," "quality health care."

5. The letter should be no more than one page; attach a fact sheet if necessary.

6. Request a response on how the legislator stands on the issue.

7. Include your name and address on the letter, including titles such as RN or LPN.

8. Write letters to legislators thanking them for their stand when you agree with the way they have supported or opposed a bill.

CHAPTER 40

Encroachment of Practice: Implications for the Perioperative Nurse

Suzanne Ward

It was the best of times, it was the worst of times . . .
CHARLES DICKENS

This famous phrase from *A Tale of Two Cities* (1859) describes the state of affairs in revolution-torn France. This description could also be applied to the state of affairs in the current health care system. It is the best of times in health care, particularly in nursing, because of the new challenges and opportunities. Nurses are in the unique position of becoming united, of transforming nursing's image, and of making lasting contributions to the improved health of this nation. However, it is also the worst of times because of changes in a system that has always been deemed "the best." Hospitals are in financial trouble, trauma systems are crumbling, and indigent and uncompensated care issues are reaching crisis proportions. The tenor in health care is crisis management, with various groups (physicians, nurses, and other providers) being frantic for preservation and self-survival.

During these changing times, the focus is on cost containment without sacrificing quality of care. For nursing, this offers opportunities to be creative and to demonstrate that nurses can provide significant health care and maintain costs. Groups threatened by the perspective of nursing's role expansion, coupled with threat of future economic limitations brought on by the

most severe nurse shortage this country has known, want to introduce new health care workers who will require a lower salary and "serve" other providers according to past models. The worst-of-times scenario introduces the encroachment issue.

Encroachment is defined as "the external infringement on registered nursing practice by others without the consent of the profession" (California Nurses Association, 1988). Encroachment occurs in a variety of settings. It may be debated in Washington, DC; determined by the office of state lawmakers; or permitted inside hospitals and other health care institutions.

Encroachment issues will increase as the health care system continues its evolutionary and revolutionary changes. As the health care dollar continues to shrink, all health care providers will be forced to examine all practice standards to ensure that appropriate practice parameters are in place. If any group fails to perform self-examination, others will step in to facilitate the process. This action may give focus to encroachment issues of the future.

Because encroachment issues respond constantly to a variety of stimuli, it is critical that nurses remain alert and informed at all times. Nurses must be prepared to act as individuals and collectively to ensure that nursing practice and patient safety are secure.

The intent of this chapter is to stimulate every reader to become involved with the legislative and regulatory

1011

political process and with professional associations such as the American Nurses Association (ANA) and the Association of Operating Room Nurses (AORN). Knowledge of the Nursing Practice Act in each respective state is essential. Being uninformed means that others will determine the future.

HISTORICAL REVIEW

The roots of encroachment lie in economics and power. A review of medicine's and nursing's history is important to understand current encroachment issues.

Medicine

Modern medicine is associated with power, prestige, economic success, and stability. However, this has not always been the case. Early in the 19th century, the profession was weak, divided, and unable to control entry into practice or raise the standards of medical education. Many physicians had difficulty making a respectable living (Starr, 1982).

The Flexner Report of 1910 (Schulz and Johnson, 1983) had a major impact on medicine. Sweeping changes included the development of standards for education in university settings, establishment of scientific knowledge as the basis for study, and the expansion and requirement of clinical and research experience (Dowling and Armstrong, 1980).

By the 20th century, physicians had become powerful, prestigious, and wealthy and had shaped the organization of medicine (Starr, 1982). Power and influence, for the medical profession, was birthed in dependence of the patient and exclusive knowledge of the physician. Unlike other professions, medicine enjoyed a close bond with people. The nature of an individual's illness and the physician's objective authority facilitated a high level of acceptance of the physician's judgment. Society valued health. Knowing this, physicians exercised their authority over patients, other health care workers, and the public at large (Starr, 1982).

As medicine's prominence continued to flourish, physicians' influence moved into the political arena, making it possible for them to dominate markets, policies, and programs involving the health care system. The institutional structures of medical care came completely under their dominance.

Starr (1982) states that the roots of medicine's authority lie in legitimacy and dependence. Legitimacy depends on subordinates' (i.e., patients, nurses) conviction that obedience is essential. Dependence rests on the subordinates' estimate of consequences that will befall if they are not obedient, thereby making explanations to patients and others unnecessary. At this stage in medicine's history, patients never questioned the decision of the physician, and nurses rarely questioned the practice patterns of physicians unless they were obviously harmful to patients (e.g., incorrect medication dosages).

Along with authority comes psychological dependence. Fear that the physician will withdraw from care is real. Hospital administrators and nurse managers operate under the assumption (fear) that physicians will take business elsewhere if their authority is not respected in the manner suitable to each physician.

The maturation of medicine's authority and influence in the political arena led to acquisition of economic power. Medicine was able to create a monopoly through its influence on who could enter the practice of medicine (licensure) and the numbers of physicians who could be educated (supply). This influence spread to shaping hospital and insurance company policy and achieving clout with those in the legislative arena (Starr, 1982).

As health care moved from a monopoly to a market, organized medicine was greatly influenced. Probably the most significant event in the transformation of medicine has been the conversion of health care into a market commodity (Starr, 1982). Physicians viewed this trend as a threat to their income, status, and autonomy because... "it drew no sharp boundary between the educated and uneducated, blurred lines between commerce and professionalism, and threatened to turn them into mere employees" (Starr, 1982). A battle between the philosophies of professions and markets has always been evident. The market philosophy understands the freedom of the consumer to choose, which determines the decisions of the market. Professions have placed the power of decision making in their members. "A profession who yields too much to the demands of clients violates an essential article of the professional code" (Starr, 1982).

Economics

The economic theory of supply and demand advocates that prices for goods are determined by levels of supply and demand. If this functions smoothly, buyers and sellers act independent of each other to set prices devoid of personal influences. "There are no relations of dependency in the ideal market: any individual buyer is supposed to have a free choice of sellers, and sellers a free choice of buyers, and no group of buyers or sellers is supposed to be able to force acceptance of its terms" (Starr, 1982). The buyers of health care, according to some economists, differ in that when buyers become sick, it is difficult for them to separate themselves from the physician (the seller). In a truly competitive market, power is absent.

Professions do not enjoy a true "market." At the end of the century, medicine set out to ensure control of its markets. Its established authority, stemming from legitimacy and dependence, enabled it to control supply and demand. The evolutionary process that brought licensing, control over medications, and advanced technologies helped medicine achieve its current status. Groups in power will do anything to see that power and status are maintained. Physicians have always prevented or slowed the entry of other health professionals into the arena of medicine (e.g., homeopathic physicians in the late 19th century and podiatrists, chiropractors, nurse midwives, and nurse practitioners in the 20th century).

Hospitals

Hospitals in preindustrial America were thought of as charitable religious organizations. Patients were often mentally ill, homeless, and looking for a place to die. However, the industrialization of this country transformed hospitals. People flocked to the cities, becoming less self-sufficient and gradually more dependent on medical institutions. This trend produced a change in the management of hospitals. Hospitals originally were under the management of trustees, whose focus was to raise funds to care for the poor. During the 1920s, the trustee era gave way to the physician era. As physicians became more involved in hospitals, management focused its efforts on pleasing individual physicians, with little regard to expense or duplication of services (Schulz and Johnson, 1983). A unique feature of the developing American hospital was that physicians had access to the facilities without being an employee. This was in sharp contrast to European institutions, where physicians relinquished responsibility for a patient to the staff of the hospital (Starr, 1982).

The knowledge explosion in health care continued, and the administrative period arrived in the early 1960s. Management of hospitals focused on coordinated care through the development of multisystems. Obtaining external funding was important, and application of advanced management technologies was evident (Schulz and Johnson, 1983).

The trend of the future lies in team management with consolidation of services, conservation of resources, reduction of costs, a focus on positive patient outcomes and direction toward self-care (Schulz and Johnson, 1983).

Nursing

Early nursing attracted women from the lower classes, because hospital nursing was considered menial work. Change was brought about, not by physicians, but by upperclass women who were interested in public health issues. In 1872, the New York State Charities Aid Association (NYSCAA), a women's organization, became the "watchdog" for conditions within hospitals (Starr, 1982). These organized women desired to open schools of nursing in the hope of attracting women from upperclass families. Even this early, physicians were threatened by the fact that nurses wanted to become educated. One remark made was, "Educated nurses would not do as they were told" (Starr, 1982). To establish the training programs, the NYSCAA bypassed physicians to gain the approval of hospital trustees and men of their own class.

Florence Nightingale made the largest single impact on the nursing revolution. Her suggestions for upgrading health care, work environments, and education are well known and revered.

The nurse shortage of World War II saw the development of functional nursing. Aides were given maintenance duties, while nurses were assigned specific tasks (e.g., one assigned to medications and another to treatments). Patient care became fragmented and impersonal (Schulz and Johnson, 1983). The concept of team nursing followed in an attempt to better coordinate care. Then, in the 1960s, primary nursing came on the scene. Primary nursing, along with the knowledge explosion, demanded that nurses become as specialized as physicians. The creation of the role of the Clinical Nurse Specialist met this need through advanced education at the master and doctoral levels.

Nursing has historically been plagued with recruitment and retention problems, with the late 1980s seeing the most severe shortages. In 1988, The Department of Health and Human Services (DHHS) studied the nurse shortage and made recommendations, concluding that (1) the reported shortage is real, widespread, and significant; (2) the shortage is due to an increased demand rather than a short supply; (3) there are strong indications that the registered nurse supply will not keep up with the demand; and (4) the shortage is causing deterioration of registered nurses' work environment and may also be having a negative impact on the quality of patient care and access to health services (DHHS, 1988).

As medicine became better organized and grew in power and recognition, nurses struggled with low status, confusing models of care delivery, and a fragmented education system.

DIVISION OF LABOR

Unlike medicine, most professions do not have control over the division of labor. Physicians have been able to control specialization (a division of labor) instead of having it determined by managers (hospital administrators), buyers (patients), or owners (profit organizations). Physicians wanted to use hospital facilities without being employees and also did not want to be burdened with those tasks that could be carried out by other competent individuals. The challenge was to maintain medicine's autonomy without loosing control. Therefore, medicine instituted a plan with three elements: first, the use of doctors in training; second, the encouragement of a kind of responsible professionalism among the higher ranks of subordinate health workers; and third, employment of women who, though professionally trained, would not challenge the authority or economic position of the physician (Starr, 1982). The division of labor among physicians was loosely regulated, but between physicians and other groups such as nurses and laboratory personnel, this division was hierarchical and rigid. The possibility of progressing from being a nurse to being a physician was remote, because experience at one level did not count toward qualifications at the next level.

Furthermore, while physicians resisted any division in their group, nurses divided themselves into various categories (Starr, 1982).

As nursing divided itself, it became harder to understand, thus contributing to its subservient role. Professional bickering, absent in the medical profession, became common within the nursing arena. The greatest debates have centered around entry requirements. Nursing has failed to unite, as medicine did, to advance the profession. Nursing's divisiveness has been medicine's benefit.

The legitimacy and dependence of medicine and male-vs.-female issues have historically kept nurses in a subservient role. Nursing is beginning to emerge, through a slow evolutionary process, as an autonomous profession. It is more assertive in stating that its body of scientific knowledge is an amalgamation of a variety of disciplines and is eager to point out the positive outcomes (decreased cost of care, increased patient satisfaction) of nursing practice (Fagin, 1982). New questions are being asked: What is the relationship between physicians and nurses and its effect on patient outcomes? Will the relationship between physician and nurse be colleagueal or competitive? The future must prove that nurses and physicians can work together for the good of the patient and to support each other's unique contribution.

ENCROACHMENT

The previous discussion has illustrated how physicians have dominated the health care field. Through deliberate actions, physicians have kept many groups from entering the arena traditionally considered theirs.

As nurses have gained knowledge and expertise, they have felt the need to expand their practice, which is a natural phenomenon for any occupation. Expansion into the realm of another's territory can be viewed as threatening or nonthreatening. An example of the latter occurred in the early days of medicine when only physicians measured blood pressure. As physicians' duties became more complex, they were willing to "allow" nurses to measure blood pressure, but they kept control by prohibiting nurses from informing the patient. Over time, physicians realized that measuring blood pressure would not detract from their income or status. It became routine for the nurse not only to take blood pressures, but to inform the patient and make judgments relative to the health status of the patient. Examination of this expansion into medical practice, permitted by physicians, shows that neither the status nor the income of physicians was at stake. In economic terms, the opportunity costs were low. Opportunity costs are defined as "the highest valued benefits that must be sacrificed (foregone) as a result of choosing an alternative" (Griffith, 1984). Each profession must decide what it is willing to give up in order to gain something else. An example of expansion seen as threatening to physicians (i.e., high opportunity cost) is the movement of nursing into the specialties of midwifery, nurse practitioner, and Registered Nurse First Assistant (RNFA). Legislation at the federal level that would provide direct reimbursement to nurses practicing as RNFAs has been met with great resistance on the part of physicians (i.e., American Medical Association). This is an example of encroachment of nursing practive and can be viewed as anticompetitive.

On the other hand, other health care providers (e.g., surgical technologists [STs]) want to expand their occupational horizons by moving into areas such as first assisting and the performance of circulating duties. Nurses view this as threatening. One difference is that nurses have proven they can deliver care in an expanded role both competently and at a lower cost (Diers, 1982). Another difference between expansion for nurses and expansion for STs is registered nurses' total educational preparation and the fact that the expanded functions are covered by state Nursing Practice Acts under the use of standardized procedures. (Note: please consult the individual state act for specific information on overlapping medical function and the use of standardized procedures.)

The issue of substitutability must also be considered. Substitutability can occur upward and downward. Upward substitutability (i.e., nurse replacing physician) may be one method to justify reimbursement for nurse providers (Fagin, 1982). The rationale is based on the fact that not all services provided by nurses are medical services, but some fall into the realm of overlapping practices. For example, immunizations have been the responsibility of public health nurses and are reimbursable under most insurance policies. First assisting in surgery, primarily a physician responsibility, is being eliminated for many procedures covered by Medicare reimbursement. Registered nurses, educated as first assistants and authorized by their Nursing Practice Act through use of standardized procedures, can function as qualified first assistants at a significant cost reduction. However, without reimbursement benefits, this upward substitutability will be limited.

Downward substitutability is characterized by the substitution of non-nurse providers for nurses. This is often done under the guise of cost containment. In a study of usage of RN-LPN substitution, evidence indicated that as RNs attempted to increase their salary, hospitals attempted to increase utilization of licensed practical nurses (Feldstein, 1977). Organized nursing's attempt to control substitution has consisted of establishing roadblocks or stopping attempts by other health care providers to gain legal permits to perform tasks normally performed by registered nurses.

As health care institutions struggle for financial viability, flexibility in staffing will pose an encroachment threat to nursing and will raise safe patient care issues.

SHAPERS OF NURSING PRACTICE

Nursing practice is determined by different factors. Professional organizations, educational institutions, health care institutions, physicians, and the political arena all influence nursing.

Within institutions, nurses, physicians, administrators, and patients all determine the context of nursing within an organization. Externally, professional organizations, such as the American Nurses Association, the National League for Nursing, the Association of Operating Room Nurses, and state nurses associations influence the practice of nursing. Increasingly, however, the greatest influence on nursing is coming from the political arena. It is at the legislative level where Nursing Practice Acts, regulations, and statutes are written and approved.

Nursing Practice Acts license and govern the practice of nursing within each state. While all practice acts vary, there are similarities. For example, all establish a board of nursing to screen applicants for minimal qualifications for safe practice, to set standards of safe practice, and to investigate reports of incompetent or unprofessional practice. Some states have one board that governs all of nursing, while other states have two separate boards, one for registered nurses and the other for licensed vocational/practical nurses. All practice acts establish qualifications for licensure. It is important to remember that licensure reflects minimal levels of competence (Murphy, 1989).

The scope of nursing practice is defined by the practice act. This critical portion of the act permits states to define the practice of nursing for that state. For example, in California, the Nursing Practice Act has given registered nurses the right to perform medical functions with the use of standardized procedures (Business and Professional Code, 1988).

Registered nurses must have knowledge of their state's Nursing Practice Act and use it as a template when evaluating all encroachment issues.

FACTORS THAT INFLUENCE ENCROACHMENT

The California Nurses Association (1988) has listed several factors that influence encroachment:

1. The severe shortage of registered nurses. The nurse shortage has caused bed closures and reduction or delay in scheduled surgical procedures, thereby affecting physician salaries. As physicians have more difficulty in admitting patients, they become concerned about possible litigation. However, the St. Paul Co., Inc., the nation's largest malpractice carrier for physicians and hospitals, states that the nursing shortage has yet to result in a single claim (Schutte, 1988).
2. The oversupply of physicians has led to accelerated activity to keep nurses (e.g., nurse practitioners, certified registered nurse anesthetists, and RNFAs) from expanding their practice.
3. The expansion of other health care occupations, as demonstrated by the Association of Surgical Technologists advocating the practice of the circulating

role for STs and supporting this through publication of their Standards of Practice (Association of Surgical Technologists, 1989).
4. Changes in reimbursement and resource allocation have come about with the advent of diagnosis-related groups (DRGs) and the proliferation of health maintenance organizations (HMOs) and other contracting plans. Reimbursement for health care has become prospective, with the incentive being cost cutting.
5. Competitive strategies are emerging for profit making by employers. As the health care arena becomes more of a market commodity, these influencing factors will continue to change and many will escalate nursing encroachment issues (California Nurses Association, 1988).

TYPES OF ENCROACHMENT

The most common form of encroachment is when another health care provider performs a task or function that is within the scope of practice of the registered nurse and does so with perceived authority (California Nurses Association, 1988). An example is surgical technologists who attempt to administer medications. Another form of encroachment is when another provider challenges the authority of the registered nurse to perform certain functions. For example, in California, nurses were challenged by Clinical Laboratory Technicians, who stated that registered nurses not licensed under the Clinical Laboratory Law could not lawfully perform certain standardized tests in the hospital ward or medical clinic. A ruling by the state attorney general stated clearly that nurses could lawfully perform standardized tests (California Nurses Association, 1988). This attempt at restricting nurses was economically driven.

Another form of encroachment is when the employer or other health care providers decide to add functions and responsibilities to the workload of registered nurses without the consent of those nurses or without the addition of appropriate resources. This often happens under the guise of cost-saving measures. As hospitals cut costs, layoffs occur, and nurses are expected to assume additional duties. An example of this type of encroachment is the elimination of certified registered nurse anesthetist positions, resulting in additional monitoring responsibilities for labor and delivery nurses (California Nurses Association, 1988). The change in Medicare reimbursement for anesthesiologists who monitor patients during insertion of pacemakers has eliminated this level of care, and the responsibility will fall to perioperative nurses.

Another form of encroachment is forced interchangeability or substitutability for the registered nurse (California Nurses Association, 1988). The Standards of Practice written by the Association of Surgical Technologists (1989) suggest interchangeability and substitutability for the registered nurse. The Registered Care

Technologist position proposed by the American Medical Association was the most all-encompassing attempt at substitutability.

Reallocation of function is directly related to the shrinking health care dollar. Administrators of health care institutions are attempting to achieve economic viability and are looking for ways to provide care at lower costs. Considering providers other than registered nurses is justified by economics. As the profession of nursing strives for more economic recognition, employers are looking for less costly alternatives (California Nurses Association, 1988).

Groups eager to reallocate or take on new functions operate from the misconception that a registered nurse has the authority to delegate licensed nursing functions to unlicensed personnel. It is imperative that all nurses understand the meaning of delegation and supervision in relation to their state Nursing Practice Act. Delegation is defined as the ability "to empower another to act. The person in authority, the registered nurse, confers on another licensed health care person the broad authority to perform specified functions in an autonomous manner and for which the person performing the function accepts responsibility. The person in authority, the registered nurse, also determines the level of competency and supervision required" (California Nurses Association, 1988).

Supervision is defined as the ability "to coordinate, direct, inspect and evaluate continuously and at first hand the accomplishment of; oversee with the power of direction and decision; the implementation of one's own or another's intention. The person in authority, the registered nurse, directs and controls patient care by assigning a limited or specified procedure to one who is qualified to perform the procedure. The person in authority (RN) also determines the level of competency and level of supervision required for the performance of patient care, based upon the extent of scientific knowledge and type of technical skills required" (California Nurses Association, 1988).

It is imperative that nurses understand these two important terms. Examination of daily practice settings should show that nurses are not delegating nursing practice to nonlicensed personnel and that supervising functions are clearly within nurses' pervue. Perioperative nurses perform many functions that should not be delegated to another health care provider. For example, delegation of placement of the electrocautery plate, a nursing function, to a surgical technologist may be in violation of the state's Nursing Practice Act. Delegation means that the individual accepting the delegation can also accept full responsibility, and only another registered nurse can do that. Assigning the task of electrocautery pad placement to a surgical technologist means the registered perioperative nurse must determine the qualifications of the technologist, the level of competency, and the amount of supervision needed to complete the task and then provide the supervision. The final responsibility and accountability to the patient lies with the nurse.

Without a clear understanding of their Nursing Practice Act, nurses may unknowingly be giving away important and legal portions of their practice. This sends a message to other groups of health care providers that encroachment into the arena of nursing practice is possible. Regardless of what other health providers believe, they cannot practice nursing.

ARENAS FOR ENCROACHMENT

Situations that may occur in daily practice through misuse of delegation and supervision are common arenas for encroachment. If nursing permits interchangeability and substitutability without consideration of the consequences, encroachment can occur.

The most significant encroachment issues will occur in the legislative arena. Because practice acts are statutes, they must be changed through the legislative/regulatory process. This process requires a series of steps well defined by each state. The regulations challenged may be specific components of the Nursing Practice Act or portions of licensing codes. Each perioperative nurse must know the process for changing regulations. More information can be obtained from the government relations office of the state nurses association. Proposed changes in regulations have mandatory public hearings. This forum provides nurses the opportunity to present facts in an attempt to defeat the proposed change and encroachment of nursing practice.

ORGANIZATIONS THAT AFFECT NURSING PRACTICE

Many organizations within each state can affect nursing practice. Nurses should explore information about these organizations and determine their impact on nursing practice in their state.

Such organizations differ from state to state but may include the Board of Registered Nursing, the Department of Health Services, the Industrial Welfare Commission, the Office of Administrative Law, the State Nurses Association, and the Joint Commission on Accreditation of Healthcare Organizations.

PREVENTION OF ENCROACHMENT

The protection of nursing practice is every nurse's responsibility. Being alert and informed, staying involved with professional organizations, and reacting quickly and appropriately when an encroachment issue is mounting are essential. Encroachment issues cannot be defeated by individual nurses. Nurses must be united and work together. There are three arenas in which nurses can work to ensure the protection of nursing practice.

1. *Education*: All nurses need to become as informed

about other professionals' Acts as they are about their own. Because most decisions to encroach on nursing practice are based on economics, nurses need to understand the economics of health care. Patients also must be educated about nurses' unique role and their responsibility for patient safety and well-being (California Nurses Association, 1988).

2. *Legislative/Regulatory/Judicial*: Nurses should monitor legislation and regulations that may affect nursing practice. They should be informed and proactive and know how to write a letter to their legislator (California Nurses Association, 1988).

3. *Practice*: Nurses should know state titling regulations and Joint Commission standards. Nurses should strive to eliminate non-nursing tasks from work assignments, preserve the autonomy of nursing practice, and *not give their practice away*.

CONCLUSION

Encroachment issues will continue to increase as health care completes its restructuring. Nurses must take a proactive role in initiating the examination of current nursing practice. The willingness to "let go" of many of the tasks traditionally thought of as nursing tasks and the thoughtful assignment of those tasks to other health care providers will enable nursing to provide intelligent, sophisticated, and sensitive care.

Bibliography

Association of Surgical Technologists. (1989). *Standards of practice.* Littleton, CO.

Business and Professional Code, State of California. (1988). Sacramento, CA.

California Nurses Association. (1988). *Encroachment on nursing practice.* Sacramento, CA.

California Nurses Association. (1987). *Political action: A guide for nurses.* Sacramento, CA.

Department of Health and Human Services. (1988). *Secretary's Commission on Nursing, final report. (Vol. I).* Washington D.C.: U.S. Government Printing Office.

Dickens, C. (1859). *A tale of two cities.* London: Octopus Books.

Diers, D. (1982) Future of nurse-midwives in American health care. In L. H. Aiken (Ed.). *Nursing in the 1980's: Crises, opportunities, challenges.* Philadelphia: J. B. Lippincott.

Dowling, W. L., and Armstrong, P. A. (1980). The hospital. In S. J. Williams and P. R. Torrens (Eds.). *Introduction to health services.* New York: John Wiley and Sons.

Fagin, C. M. (1982). Nursing's pivotal role in American health care. In L. H. Aiken (Ed.). *Nursing in the 1980's: Crises, opportunities, challenges.* Philadelphia: J. B. Lippincott.

Feldstein, P. J. (1977). *Health associations and the demand for legislation: The political economy of health.* Boston, MA: Ballinger Publishing.

Griffith, H. (1984). Nursing practice: Substitute or complement according to economic theory. *Nursing Economics, 2,* 105–112.

Murphy, E. K. (1989). OR nursing law: The definition and purpose of professional licensure. *AORN Journal, 4,* 1106–1109.

Salmon, M. E., and Culbertson, R. A. (1985). Health manpower oversupply: Implications for physicians, nurse practitioners and physician assistants. *Hospital and Health Services Administration 30,* 100–115.

Schulz, R., and Johnson, A. C. (1983). *Management of hospitals.* New York: McGraw-Hill.

Starr, P. (1982). *The social transformation of American medicine.* New York: Basic Books.

Webster, N. (1971). *New twentieth century dictionary of the English language unabridged.* New York: World Publishing Co.

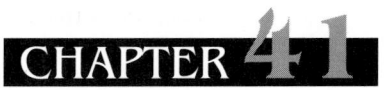

CHAPTER 41

Professional Involvement:
An Issue of Survival
for Perioperative Nursing

Jane C. Rothrock

In attempting to keep up with increasingly complex health care needs and shifting societal trends, American nursing is engaged in the excruciating task of negotiating to a higher, more uniform professional place. Its history and its future vision both support the need for nursing to continue to strive for greater professionalism, including greater autonomy, accountability, authority, and commitment to excellence if it is to thrive in the 1990s and survive into the next century. The emphasis in the marketplace will be on competition, while at the same time striving for increasing teamwork and collaboration among health care providers. Nursing will continue to build interdisciplinary and interterritorial relationships that provide flexibility and support. This will permit greater professionalism in practice and greater innovation where it is most needed, which is in the delivery of patient care (Spitzer, 1987). Building needed relationships, working toward consensus in the profession, and reaching a higher plane for the profession all require active involvement and commitment on the part of each perioperative nurse. This is an era of exciting, dynamic change for all of nursing, and the need for involvement has never been greater if nursing's agenda as a powerful, autonomous profession is to assume its rightful place in society.

The identification of professional attitudes, values, and behaviors has been an elusive and problematic area for the nursing community. Volumes have been written and spoken about nursing's quest for professional status and its attempts to professionalize. Some authors suggest that the debate be ended so that nursing can move on to other work. Others do not view the general consensus, unempirically drawn, as reason enough to abandon this focus in future work. In her 1987 keynote address to the scientific session of the American Academy of Nursing, Myrtle Aydelotte described her vision of nursing for the next 25 years. Among the attributes that she posited for this preferred vision were a well-defined knowledge base, autonomy of practice, accountability, collegiality, self-governance, a distinct public image, power, prestige, and high valuation by the public. To achieve this preferred future, one of the strategies she recommended for implementation was the clarification and definition of what makes nursing a profession.

DETERMINANTS OF PROFESSIONAL STATUS

A number of criteria for evaluation of a profession and professional status have been proposed. Greenwood (1964) described the attributes of a profession as the possession of systematic theory, authority, community sanction, ethical codes, and a culture. Having elucidated these five elements, he went on to caution that the true difference between a professional and a nonprofessional occupation was not a quantitative one but a qualitative one. Thus, Greenwood introduced the notion of professionalism occurring on a continuum wherein occupations are distributed according to the greater or lesser degrees to which they possess these five attributes. Using this model, a number of nursing authors have come to describe nursing as an emerging profession located close to the professional pole of the continuum.

Nursing is developing a systematic body of theory describing the phenomena of interest to the profession. The skills that characterize the profession flow from and are supported by this fund of knowledge. This important preoccupation with theory has resulted in treatises on nursing theory, an emphasis in nursing curricula on intellectual as well as practical skills, theory construction via research, and a validation of the move of nursing education into formal academic settings (Stevens, 1984).

The professional's authority base evolves from the knowledge base within which the professional has been educated. This authority most often manifests itself in the relationship between client and professional, wherein the client is subordinate to the professional's knowledge, and hence, the professional has authority (Light, 1979). This authority between client and professional is not the only authority invested in the profession; the community must also sanction the authority of the profession by conferring a series of powers and privileges (Moore, 1974; Wilensky, 1964). These occur primarily through the power invested in the profession for accreditation and licensing and the conferring of professional status by the profession to its members.

Because of all of the authority invested in the profession, a code of ethics becomes necessary to protect the public the profession serves. A code of ethics must also develop within the profession. Greenwood describes these ethics governing colleague relationships as demanding behavior that is cooperative, equalitarian, and supportive. Ethical codes are enforced by the profession through informal and formal sanctions.

The professional culture has both formal and informal groups through which members network (Hall, 1968). These may be the institutional settings in which the profession practices, the educational and research centers, the professional associations, and the multitudes of informally developed groups of members with common special interests. Out of this culture of the profession are born the values, norms, and symbols that characterize basic and fundamental beliefs, guide behavior, and invest meaning. These, according to Greenwood, mark the success of the professional in the chosen occupation. Mastery of the underlying body of theory and acquisition of the technical skills are in themselves insufficient guarantees of professional success (Atkinson, 1992). The transformation of a neophyte into a professional is essentially an acculturation process wherein the neophyte internalizes the social values, the behavioral norms, and the symbols of the group.

Greenwood likens the acculturation process of the professional to that of an immigrant in a relatively strange culture. There is always the ideal image of the new culture, as there is the ideal image or stereotype of the profession. This ideal usually represents a thorough adjustment to the culture. Many of the suppositions of Greenwood have led to intense study and discussion of the divergent and seemingly disconsonant values of the nursing culture and the work culture.

Corwin (1961) undertook some of the classic research that has driven current research efforts in the acculturation process and its outcomes. According to Corwin, contradictions in the occupation are countered with new and pronounced relevance at graduation. He offered several reasons for the intense realization of these contradictions. Like Greenwood, Corwin identified the ideal image of the profession that transcended the educational process as leading to an inevitable conflict between conception of the professional role and the reality of the career. Confounding the adjustment of these contradictions was the absence of the faculty persons, the ones who had guided and formed the student's self-conception of what the profession would or ought to be (Ondrack, 1975). The student, who had allegiance to the school and the values shared within that institution, moved into the workplace, where a conflicting set of values predominated, forcing new kinds of allegiance between what had been learned and valued and what was in operation and valued.

Out of this potential for conflict, Corwin conceptualized three dominant perspectives of nursing. The nurse could be seen as a responsible, independent professional (the professional perspective), a hospital employee (the bureaucratic perspective), or a public servant (the service perspective). These three perceptions of the nursing self were deemed to be incompatible with one another, dichotomously opposed to any type of mutual coexistence. In validating the types and kinds of differences that exist between the student's perspective of the nursing career and the graduate staff nurse's perspective, Corwin offers this example:

> It is in the office of the nurse rather than in the status of the student that bureaucratic and professional principles converge and conflict. . . . In the first place, their [the student's] perspectives on hospital routine may easily differ [from the graduate staff's]. The student, relatively unspecialized as yet, has direct contact with a variety of hospital situations, personnel, and supervisors, besides having the benefit of an overall perspective of the profession emphasized in many nursing programs. Contrast this with the routinization characteristic of the specialized graduate nurse, functioning not only as a surgical nurse but as a "rotating" or "scrub" surgical nurse; a perspective of her relationship to the total organization is not inherent in the office itself. Thus, the over-all aims and goals of the organization can easily become buried in a maze of specialized tasks.

Thus, even in the earliest of the research efforts and explorations of the conflicts between professional and bureaucratic conceptions of role, the operating room nurse was placed within the bureaucratic perspective, consumed by tasks, doing work that was highly standardized and governed by rules, fitting the model for resultant conflicts in loyalty. Perioperative nursing has worked hard and successfully to dispel this concept.

Corwin's research questions were primarily directed at elucidating three relationships:

1. Did bureaucratic and professional conceptions of roles conflict? The research indicated that they did, with the nurse holding both high professional and high bureaucratic ideals experiencing the most conflict and being prevented from adequately fulfilling either role.

2. Were there systematic differences in the organization of roles produced by diploma and degree programs? The research indicated that degree programs produced a product with more professional allegiance.

3. Were discrepancies between ideal roles and perceptions of reality increased after graduation? To this question the research produced less pronounced results, indicating that sometimes discrepancies intensified, and sometimes role conception was modified. The diploma graduate characteristically lowered both professional and service orientations after graduation, holding bureaucratic conceptions fairly constant. The baccalaureate graduate lowered the service ideal, increased the bureaucratic ideal, and held the professional ideal fairly constant.

The nurses in Corwin's research were not studied according to specialty areas, but the inference remains that operating room nurses, pictured as working in a highly bureaucratic role, would either capitulate professional values or experience conflict. Such an inference has permeated the thinking of nurse educators and influenced decisions about the viability of the operating room experience in a school that has as its mission the development of professional practitioners. If the operating room, and therefore the operating room nurse, conduct nursing in a value, attitude, and cultural framework diametrically opposed to professionalism, then exclusion of this practice area, both as a clinical learning laboratory and as a valid and rightful area of specialized study and acculturation, becomes a natural outcome of an educational process that desires to focus on the attitudes, values, and cultural norms of professionalism.

PERIOPERATIVE NURSING IN PROFESSIONAL EDUCATION

The excellence of educational programs that prepare nurses is defined best by what that education accomplishes in advancing knowledge, in promoting change in health care and in the health care system, and in preparing graduates who are capable of going out and implementing systems for delivery of nursing care. Excellence does not infer just the preparation of competent people to enter the profession or to specialize in it or in one of its career tracks. According to Wooley (1986), the primary objective of the nursing curriculum is to prepare students to learn what it means to be a nurse, to have the ability to use a variety of strategies to reach

a given goal, to use the resources of a variety of social systems, and to engage in effective reality testing. This is the aspiration for the professional nurse, who can teach, learn from, and respond to changing situations and advocate and help bring about social and individual change (Felton, 1986).

As the major role of nurse educators in preparing students for leading roles in nursing practice settings is elucidated and clarified, the problem of identifying the most appropriate practice settings for particular learner aspirations becomes intensified and dichotomized by discussions of professional and technical settings and general or specialized roles. Nursing leaders in a variety of practice settings are asking whether nursing education can ignore the proposition that the same tools, role models, resources, and richness of experiences may be available in specialized practice settings that contribute to the teaching, learning, advocacy, and change agentry of students. Determining the type and quality of education that will be needed for nursing's future, the nature of nursing specialization, and how specialization fits into nursing's model for professional education are complex and critical issues that will accompany nursing through the 1990s.

The forces that generated the high level of demand for nursing specialists in the 1960s have not abated. The dramatic surge in the rate of growth of biomedical technology and the increasing complexity of health care point to an increased need, well into the 21st century, for nurses who are able to specialize. The dynamics of health care are such that expectations of advanced job performance, as well as specialized knowledge bases, characterize the employment sector of the job market. Nonetheless, the dynamics of curriculum change in nursing have led to altered patterns for the preparation and implementation of the specialized role.

Along with other former areas of specialty nursing education, the operating room (OR) has been eliminated from many nursing curricula. Nurses who enter the OR as neophytes have been taught the specialty through inservice orientation and staff development programs. The emphasis of such instruction has been on the "how to" rather than the "why" of practice (Patterson, 1986). Consequently, many nursing leaders have concluded that perioperative nursing is technical nursing, focused primarily on meeting the needs of the physician. In a study to determine the priority areas for perioperative nursing research, ways in which schools of nursing can be motivated to include perioperative nursing courses in their curricula ranked ninth (Faulconer and Marchette, 1986).

The OR, as a clinical learning laboratory for acquisition of knowledge in aseptic technique, as well as a training ground for the supply of future practitioners, was used along with other clinical areas in the education of nursing students until the World War II. During that war, aggressive surgical interventions developed in response to the nature and complexity of injuries incurred by wounded patients. Intense training programs for nurses who worked in the ORs during this war evolved in response to the advances in surgical treatments and the need for highly qualified nurses to participate in the intraoperative care of the wounded. At the same time, a shortage of nurses prompted the training of civilian corpsmen to perform many of the same duties as the nurse.

At the war's conclusion, these trained corpsmen were hired into ORs to supplement the continuing shortage of nurses. Referred to as OR technicians, this group of health care workers took over many of the former duties and responsibilities of the "scrub nurse," the nurse who was a member of the sterile surgical team and intimately involved in the provision of patient care to the operative patient. As technicians gained acceptance in ORs across the country, the OR nurse was displaced from part of the nursing role that had traditionally been held as vital and necessary to the safe and smooth execution of surgical intervention. Rapid advances in modern surgical technology, accessory surgical equipment, new surgical supplies, and environmental control measures required the nurse to focus on cognitive and physical skills acquisition to master these new developments. Gradually, the circulating nurse, who was a member of the unsterile team, became viewed as primarily involved with this environment of equipment and tasks, and not primarily with patient care.

A pervasive and consistent devaluing of this type of nursing care was occurring in the field of nursing education. Beginning with the Flexner Report (1915), nursing and medicine launched a search to determine their professional status. Flexner described the attributes of professional occupations as those characterized by intellectual function with individual responsibility, based on science, and learned over a long period of study, with specialized skills and knowledge, altruistic motives, and a tendency to self-government. As nursing sought to identify a model for its professional status, elaborate and prolonged discussions took place regarding which nursing content was better (in this case, more scientific), which was more important, and which was more professional. The OR, with its seeming emphasis on tasks, surgeons, and equipment, did not fare well in these discussions of the professionalism of nursing. As concepts such as holism, total patient care, patient needs, care planning, theoretical models, and research were introduced into nursing curricula, the need for a broad professional preparation for nursing practitioners characterized educational reform.

As nursing began the move into institutions of higher education, the need for education in the planning, teaching, supervising, and administering of the increasingly complex delivery system of nursing education and nursing practice evolved. Competence in clinical specialization was superseded by competence in application of general principles and concepts to a variety of nursing situations. The OR, along with other specialty rotation areas, was viewed as a narrowly circumscribed practice area that afforded little opportunity for student mastery of these broad areas of nursing knowledge. With each new wave of curricular reform, nursing educators increasingly minimized the contribution of the OR as a learning laboratory for students of professional nursing.

Much of the literature has targeted both the inherent benefits to students of a learning experience in the OR and the barriers that prevented the integration of perioperative nursing experiences into nursing curricula. Gruendemann (1980) presented the benefits of the OR in terms of a clinical laboratory where students were afforded the opportunity to interact with other health care team members, develop critical thinking skills, use concepts from both physical and behavioral sciences, make decisions based on this nursing knowledge, and synthesize this information into independent judgments about nursing care interventions.

Koehler (1980) discussed the cost-containment benefits accruing from professional perioperative nursing care, citing earlier discharge when patients were instructed preoperatively and postoperatively by a perioperative nurse. Her emphasis was on the ability of the OR experience to provide students with many and varied opportunities for patient teaching and discharge planning. This teaching and planning were described as arising out of the implementation of the nursing process, where assessment was the key to the teaching activities undertaken by the perioperative nursing student.

Hercules (1980) listed such student opportunities as the study of humans as holistic beings in a unique situation of rapidly changing physiological and psychological needs, the study of human anatomy and physiological alterations, and the ability to work with patients in crisis situations. She went on to describe the OR as a learning laboratory wherein students could explore and apply nursing interventions based on sociocultural differences, master principles of asepsis, and begin developing organizational skills, communication skills, and skills in functioning as a team member. All of these benefits were thought to be inherently valuable in the professional education of nurses.

Sharp (1980) recognized that much of what perioperative nursing had to offer in student learning opportunities could be obtained in other clinical areas. Her position was that the OR was as viable a clinical area as any other. She cited learning theory that posited that students needed to be active participants in the learning process and afforded an opportunity to practice knowledge and skills, to see relationships, and to have more than one exposure to critical nursing material. Sharp identified learning outcomes that were relevant to the practice of nursing and related these to opportunities presented in the OR that affected such outcomes. Seeing anatomy and its subsequent surgical alteration led to improved patient teaching about the surgery; understanding the perioperative experience and what it entailed for the patient led to improved ability to provide the patient and family with explanations about the surgical experience, thereby decreasing anxiety; understanding the surgical intervention led to a reinforced comprehension of the need for preoperative measures as Foley catheter insertion and skin preparation; understanding the effects of anesthesia led to improved ability to manage the patient's pain and intervene in respiratory complications. Student learning in the OR, according to Sharp, benefited the patient in the long run, as nursing measures took on new significance and were translated into improved patient outcomes.

OR leaders recognized the need to articulate arguments about including an OR educational experience that had as its basis knowledge that was transferable and applicable to nursing in general. They also recognized the need for those employed in ORs around the country to recognize their responsibility to provide role models for students and to elevate the status of perioperative nursing from a technical perspective to one that was seen as a professional nursing practice area. In a series of published opinions about the needed relationships between practicing perioperative nurses and nurse educators (AORN, 1980), the importance of this role modeling and its relationship to professional values was presented. Nursing educators identified the barriers they perceived to placement of students in perioperative settings. One of these barriers was a lack of receptivity on the part of perioperative nurses toward students. Perioperative nurses, involved in immediate and urgent tasks, did not often make the professional nature of these nursing activities visible to students. Instead of acting as a role model in an advocacy role, a risk management role, and a quality assurance role, they continued to model the technical functions of perioperative patient care.

In addition to this lack of role modeling, a number of pragmatic issues were addressed. Educators found that ORs did not offer enough space for student placement and that, when space was available, the nursing student had to compete with medical students for learning experiences. It was difficult to schedule surgical follow-up experiences for students, in part because of faculty members' lack of experience with perioperative routines. Even when such experiences were scheduled, there was concern over how the learning objectives fit the conceptual frameworks of the curriculum. Educators did not feel that students were truly able to obtain a perspective of the patient's point of view in a perioperative rotation. Students were so overwhelmed with the activities that they were not able to integrate nursing actions and the nurse's role in the patient experience. Many educators came to the conclusion that what was learned in the OR could be learned just as well through audiovisual media and other laboratory experiences. Some admitted that when students expressed an interest in working in an OR, they were actively encouraged not to enter this specialty by faculty, who continued to see perioperative nursing from a technical rather than professional perspective.

The concepts of competency and what the outcomes of entry-level nursing curricula should be continue to raise many questions. The question of whether a nursing program should educate a student to be competent in any specialty area continues to be debated, argued, and discussed. Derdiarian's (1979) comments may shed some light on this issue. It is Derderian's position that a common goal for nursing practice is direction of education on all levels, with a common core of competencies framing the nursing component of undergraduate, graduate, and doctoral education. This core of elements, while varying in sophistication according to the level of education, should include the teaching of theories, research, and knowledge about the clinical setting for the specialization. By selecting a population that has similar characteristics or settings, practice is more controlled, more suitable for research, and has greater potential than generalist practice for contributing to the development of nursing science and the delimitation of boundaries of nursing practice. Systematizing practice enables exploration of predominant physical and psychosocial problems that are peculiar to and recur in the practice setting. Derdiarian concluded that a specialty core is important, not only in advanced levels of practice and education, but also in basic, first-level professional education as well.

Hagemeier and Hunt (1979) pose a number of questions that nurse educators must ask themselves regarding the structuring of a nursing curriculum. Educators need to know how the curriculum assists students in assimilating knowledge from a number of disciplines; how the curriculum presents information from a nursing perspective; and how that body of knowledge is articulated within a curriculum from which scientific inquiry can be pursued. The curriculum must have an inherent nursing focus, enabling the student to distinguish nursing from other health care disciplines. Most of all, according to these two authors, educators need to find ways to provide students with the opportunity to identify professional attitudes, values, and behaviors that give coherent focus and direction to the practice of nursing.

Nursing education has had a proud history of adaptation, flexibility, and responsivemenss to societal trends. The time is ripe to think again about specialty preparation to encourage the development of specialties for nursing in the emerging health care markets, specialties that will be filled by other health care providers if nursing is unable or unwilling to do so. Nursing is caught up in the turmoil of the health care delivery system, affected by supply and demand, changes in skill requirements, new patterns of education, new problems in affording opportunity, and innovation in educating those of its practitioners who seek the professional degree or who seek education in a specialty practice area. It is probable that changes in nursing will be dramatic in the next two decades, and part of that drama will be unfolding in tertiary care settings in which patients undergo complex surgical interventions. Nursing educators will need to contemplate the preparation of practitioners so that they will be ready to face this new wave of nursing.

One of the changes nurse educators will need to think about is the moving force of surgery in meeting the shifting needs of society. As technology and scientific knowledge advance, a high-tech environment will be spawned requiring competent nursing care of individuals undergoing sophisticated surgical interventions. The environment of the OR and the emerging professionalization of the perioperative nurse cannot be ignored as the roles and functions of nursing are elaborated in the reshaping and rethinking of nursing education's content and its focus.

ORGANIZATIONAL INFLUENCES ON THE NURSING PROFESSION

Nursing, as an organized occupation, began in 1873 in the United States with the formation of educational programs based on the British Florence Nightingale model. In the 1870s, women who had to work were in a very difficult position, as occupational choices were very limited. Nursing training was a reasonable alternative for women of modest means who needed or wanted a career. Although college education was beginning to become available for upperclass women, it was unaffordable and inaccessible for most women. The Nightingale model was based on the belief that nursing could provide an avenue for young women to make a meaningful contribution to society. Nightingale's thinking that nursing should be a profession for women was not philosophically based on the belief that men should be excluded, but instead was predicated on her primary concern for the plight of Victorian women.

Women in the Victorian era were either poverty stricken and forced to work at menial labor for long hours or idle, wealthy ornaments in the household of husbands or fathers, with little avenue for use of their intellectual talents (Chinn and Jacobs, 1987). Nightingale, herself a product of an upperclass English Victorian upbringing, defied her family in seeking training as a nurse and volunteering to serve in the Crimean War. Her example changed the public's image of nursing as she worked to raise the status of nursing to a trained profession. Firmly committed to the idea that nursing held specific responsibilities distinct from those of medicine, she insisted that early schools established for training nurses must be controlled and taught by women who were also trained nurses themselves (Chinn and Jacobs, 1987). Despite this initial philosophy that nursing education should be autonomous and have decision-making authority over the practice of nursing in institutions where students learned, many early forces in society opposed this tradition. It took the development and work of nursing organizations to slowly and finally effect this control.

In 1894, an organization known as the Society of Superintendents of Training Schools for Nurses of the United States and Canada was established. Within 2 years, this organization sponsored a conference for representatives of nursing school alumni associations. Subsequently, the Nurses Associated Alumnae of the United States and Canada was organized. In 1912, this association became the American Nurses Association (ANA). In the same year, the Superintendents Society became the National League of Nursing Education (NLNE), and in 1952, the National League for Nursing was founded (NLN). Its major purpose was, and continues to be, to promote improvement of nursing service and nursing education so that the nursing needs of society could be met (DeYoung, 1981). In that year, the NLN assumed responsibility for accrediting schools of nursing, an influential step in improving educational quality for nurses. In addition to its accreditation services, the League currently provides consultation services, continuing education programs, analysis of statistical data related to nursing education and nursing manpower resources, various examination and testing services, and a variety of information packages to affect recruitment, image, and legislative affairs (Leddy and Pepper, 1989). Membership is available to agencies that provide nursing education or nursing and other health care services and to individuals who are interested in nursing and the improvement of health care.

In contrast to the early efforts of the Superintendents Society, the Associated Alumnae focused on obtaining state registration for nurses who were appropriately trained. It was not uncommon in the early history of nursing for women to call themselves "nurses" and provide care to those who needed it. If care was provided in the home, it was often a female family member who did the "nursing." Much of the care of the sick in hospitals was provided by women paupers from workhouses who had neither the training nor the character and desire to be good nurses. In fact, it was not uncommon for females who had been arrested for drunkenness or vagrancy to serve their sentence as nurses in hospitals rather than in jailhouses. The early assumptions about nursing and caregiving were that they were arts possessed automatically by any woman.

The Associated Alumnae mounted registration drives in each state to differentiate nurses who were trained and therefore qualified to undertake the work of nursing. In 1903, the first registration acts were passed in North Carolina, New Jersey, New York, and Virginia. These acts defined the registered nurse as someone who had attended an approved or registered nursing program. Restrictions on the quality of those nursing programs, however, was limited, and none of the early acts defined the scope of practice for the registered nurse. It was, nonetheless, the beginning of the effort to define and differentiate professional nursing.

By 1938, the first licensing act was passed in New York; this made it illegal for anyone other than a licensed nurse to practice the work of nursing. In 1955, the ANA offered a model definition of nursing, and this language became incorporated into many state Nurse Practice Acts. The definition, however, excluded any nursing actions of diagnosis or prescription of therapeutic or corrective measures, a limitation that was soon recognized as nursing's professional role expanded and became more autonomous and responsible.

By 1971, the first Nurse Practice Act revised to include legal protection for nursing diagnostics and therapeutic responsibility was initiated in Idaho. In 1983, the National Council of State Boards of Nursing (NCSBN) published a Model Nurse Practice Act. Many states incorporated the definition of nursing offered by the NCSBN into Nurse Practice Acts, wherein the practice of nursing was defined as "assisting individuals or groups to maintain or attain optimal health status throughout the life process by assessing their health status, establishing a diagnosis, planning and implementing a strategy of care to accompany defined goals, and evaluating responses to care" (Leddy and Pepper, 1989).

Currently the ANA is the professional organization for registered nurses in the United States. Composed of constituent nurses' associations at the state level, its purposes are to "work for the improvement of health standards and the availability of health services for all people, to foster high standards of nursing, and to stimulate and promote the professional development of nurses and advance their economic and general welfare" (Leddy and Pepper, 1989). As such, the ANA accredits continuing education programs, provides for certification for individual nurses, is importantly involved in public policy analysis, maintains government relations, offers a variety of publications and member benefits, and speaks forcefully and articulately for the profession of nursing on any number of critical issues and concerns.

In 1950, the ANA developed the first Code for Nurses, setting standards for ethics for the profession. It has taken a responsive leadership role in providing input into policy making, especially in the arena of health policy. In 1980, the ANA published a document—*Nursing: A Social Policy Statement*—that gave a very specific and clear interpretation of the practice of nursing while at the same time identifying nursing's responsibilities to the public and other health professionals.

As the role of professions and professionals in society has changed, the ANA has actively and cogently identified strategies for advancing nursing's interests and the interests of the public it serves. Currently the AORN collaborates in an official, contractual relationship with the ANA in fostering a strong leadership role for both associations as organizational influences on national public policy in the United States.

Much of the work of the ANA has brought professional status to nursing. Accountability to the public it serves and responsiveness to public interest are characteristics of a profession (Flexner, 1915). To this end, the ANA has worked to enable the profession to function with autonomy in the formation of public policy and in the control of nursing's public activity. Many state nurse practice acts reinforce the premise that the public's health and welfare should be protected with a minimum of governmental regulation and that there should be checks and balances between government and professional regulation of the practice of nursing. The ANA has established Standards of Nursing Practice that identify assumptions and beliefs basic to the area of practice and provide descriptions of types of practitioners, qualifications related to educational preparation, and scope of practice. Using these standards as a guide, nurses can see clearly the scope and limits of practice and determine their own competency as well as that of others. As nursing has become more involved with its own professionalization, the development of professional standards has made it clearly evident that nursing is accountable as a profession in forming its own professional policy and controlling its own professional activity. The ANA, through individual membership, provides power to the individual nurse as a result of the collective power of the organization.

THE PROFESSIONALIZATION OF PERIOPERATIVE NURSING

A 1983 analysis of stresses experienced by 104 randomly selected OR nurses from six Seattle hospitals indicated that OR nurses experience stresses similar to those experienced by Intensive Care Unit nurses (Jacobsen and McGrath, 1983). These stresses involved nurse-physician and nurse-nurse conflicts, workload strains, knowledge base discrepancies, and philosophical problems (e.g., whether registered nurses should be phased out of the OR). The authors concluded that some of the stress of the OR nurse may be unique in the extent to which perioperative nurses must defend their specialty as a professional nursing practice area with professional contributions to patient care. Such defense of the OR as a professional practice area may be characteristic of recent nursing history but is uncharacteristic of the history of perioperative nursing in general.

It was in the late 1890s that the specialty of OR nursing evolved from surgical nursing (Lee, 1976). As advancements in the management of surgical pain, hemmorhage, and infection began to reduce operative mortality, a role began to evolve for a nurse in the OR to assist in implementing some of the environmental measures that were gaining acceptance among leaders in the surgical field. An early nursing textbook (Luckes, 1887) describes the nurse's importance in seeing that all wants of the physician are anticipated and supplied. The most important function in this nursing role was the preparation and handling of surgical sponges. Weeks (1890) describes this process in detail, and its ascendancy over other responsibilities eventually led to the description of the nurse as a "sponge" nurse.

Eventually, the nurse in the OR was given additional tasks, becoming responsible for instruments, OR tables, dressings, and preparation of the patient's postoperative bed. Checklists evolved to assist the nurse in ensuring that everything that was needed by the operating surgeon was available. While the emphasis was on tasks and the surgeon's needs, the evolving theories of antisepsis and prevention of infection were the scientific basis for many of the prescribed nursing activities. The recognition of the theoretical importance of cleanliness led to the eventual conclusion that "nurses could receive valuable training and do good service in connection with operations" (Gerster, 1888).

OR nursing as a specialty began at Johns Hopkins Hospital in Baltimore (Lee, 1976). As a result of the influence of Halsted and Robb, both of whom were physicians of prominence in the advancement of surgical techniques, a nurse was placed in a full-time position in the OR. Gradually, nurses were added to the OR team, managing instruments, sutures, and sponges as scrubbed team members and functioning as unsterile team members in the provision of additional supplies. Protecting the patient from injury by counting and being accountable for supplies used and enforcing environmental control to prevent fever and wound infections became important attributes of these nurses, and physicians soon found them indispensable to the efficient management of surgical interventions.

By 1949, the permanent and essential nature of this nursing role had been established in the United States. In an attempt to provide a forum for the exchange of knowledge and ideas about the practice of OR nursing, a group of OR supervisors from New York met together on January 28, 1949 (Driscoll, 1976). By the following month, officers and a board of directors were formed; the group applied for and was given special committee status by the ANA. Within 10 years, similar meetings were being held across the country. According to Driscoll, the New York group established six aims for this association:

1. To stimulate OR nurses in other parts of the country to form similar groups
2. To be a specialty group to pool and share nursing knowledge and technology
3. To provide the surgical patient with optimum care through a broad educational program
4. To make a body of knowledge available to OR nurses
5. To motivate experienced OR nurses to share their expertise with others
6. To be an association for the benefit of all professional OR nurses

In 1954, the New York group sponsored a national conference. In 1956, the OR nurses petitioned the ANA for permission to hold a similar national meeting annually and to develop OR nursing as a special affiliate group. The ANA, while not objecting to the affiliation of the OR nursing groups, felt that the ANA organization was meeting the needs of these OR nurse members, and special status privileges for the OR group were denied. Subsequently, at the fourth national meeting, called a Congress by the attendees, a plan to form an independent national nursing organization was presented and approved by the House of Delegates. Thus, in 1957, a constitution and bylaws were adopted and officers and a board of directors elected for the Association of Operating Room Nurses (AORN).

The AORN has grown steadily since 1949 and currently has more than 48,000 members in more than 350 local chapters who work for a positive impact on professional nurses in the OR. As the role of the professional nurse in the OR has evolved, so has the organization's attempt to take a leadership stance in clarifying the role, responsibility, aims, and purposes of the registered nurse in the OR. In 1965, a statement that included a list of the responsibilities of the OR nurse was published in the *Standards for Administrative and Clinical Practice in the Operating Room* (Lynn, 1983). These standards were elaborated in a 1969 position paper, *Definition and Objective for Clinical Practice of Professional Operating Room Nursing*, which offered a definition of professional OR nursing (AORN, 1969). This definition included nursing care measures such as identification of patient needs and development and implementation of a plan

of nursing care for the surgical patient. Intended to provide a standard of excellence in care, this position paper outlined six steps to be utilized in the implementation of the objective statement:

1. Identification of patient needs
2. Development of an individualized plan of care
3. Coordination of the plan with other health team members
4. Provision of a safe environment for patients
5. Guidance of other professional and technical personnel in the care of the patient
6. Initiation of research to develop a body of knowledge in relation to the components of professional nursing

This paper initiated a continuing effort by the AORN to promote recognition of the role of the professional OR nurse and the patient's need for nursing care by such an individual. Reaffirmed in 1971, the statement reads:

> Professional nursing in the operating room is the identification of the physiological, psychological, and sociological needs of the patient, and the implementation of an individualized program of nursing care that coordinates the nursing actions, based on a knowledge of the natural and behavioral sciences, in order to restore, or maintain, the health and welfare of the patient before, during, and after surgical intervention (AORN, 1969).

At the 1973 AORN Congress, the role of the professional nurse as the rightful care provider during a patient's surgical experience was further elaborated in the adoption of a resolution, "Necessity for the Registered Nurse in the Operating Room" (AORN, 1973). This resolution stated that because

> . . . the registered nurse has theoretical knowledge, clinical expertise, and legal responsibility pertinent to surgical intervention . . . (it is) resolved that the registered nurse is indispensible to the provision of nursing care in the operating room. . . .

This resolution established AORN's commitment to ensuring that adequate numbers of registered nurses were prepared to assume responsibility for nursing care in the OR. As a result of concern for deletion or diminution of a participative intraoperative experience for nursing students in generic nursing education programs, a second resolution, "Necessity for Nursing Student Participation in Operating Room Nursing" (AORN, 1973), was adopted. This resolution set forth AORN's position with regard to the inclusion of OR nursing in the generic curriculum, identifying those behaviors most advantageously learned through such a student experience.

In 1974, the ANA and AORN jointly adopted the *Standards of Nursing Practice: Operating Room*. Revised in 1975, the standards provided a basic model to measure the quality of nursing activities that provide continuity of care through preoperative assessment and preparation, intraoperative implementation, and postoperative evaluation in any setting for any type of physiological alteration in surgical patients. Based on the nursing process, the document outlined seven standards:

1. Collection of data about the individual
2. Derivation of a nursing diagnosis
3. Formulation of goals
4. Nursing actions prescribed for the plan of care
5. Implementation of the plan of care
6. Evaluation of the plan of care
7. Reassessment and modification of the plan of care.

The rationale for these practice standards was based on the premise that a professional nursing organization must provide measures to judge the competency of its membership and evaluate the quality of its services. If a profession's concern for the quality of its service constitutes the heart of its responsibility to the public, then it was assumed that the profession must seek control of its practice to guarantee the quality of that service.

Having endorsed these standards, the 22nd AORN Congress House of Delegates approved an additional statement of policy, the "Mandate for the Registered Nurse as Circulator in the Operating Room" (AORN, 1975). This mandate stated that only a registered nurse, having acquired the necessary knowledge and skills in nursing educational programs, was qualified to implement the Standards of Practice. The role of paraprofessionals, specifically the OR technician, was posited as one of technical assistance to the registered nurse. This marked the beginning of the recognition of the external threat posed to OR nursing by those who saw it as a technical function that did not necessitate the presence, knowledge, or skill of professional nurses.

In 1976, Project 25 was approved by the AORN Board of Directors. This task force, whose intent was to define the role of the registered nurse in the OR, evolved because of a lack of a universally accepted, operational definition of nursing practice in the OR and the past focus of OR nursing on the technical components of nursing rather than an integration of both technical and professional functions into the professional nursing role. In 1978, the report of the Project 25 Task Force was approved by the AORN House of Delegates (AORN, 1978). In that report, the role of the perioperative nurse was defined:

> The perioperative role of the operating room nurse consists of nursing activities performed by the professional operating room nurse during the preoperative, intraoperative, and postoperative phases of the patient's surgical experience. Operating room nurses assume the perioperative role at a beginning level dependent on their expertise and competency to practice. As they gain knowledge and skills, they progress on a continuum to an advanced level of practice.

The definition of the perioperative role (AORN, 1978) was further clarified as follows:

> The nurse in the operating room responsible for providing nursing care to surgical patients assumes a perioperative role. Perioperative is used as an encompassing term to incorporate the three phases of the surgical patient's experience. This includes the preoperative, in-

traoperative, and postoperative time periods. Role refers to expected behavior patterns and, in this case, the range of clinical activities performed during the preoperative, intraoperative, and postoperative phases. Those behaviors or nursing activities that the nurse performs as a part of the perioperative role are carried out using the nursing process as reflected in the Standards of Practice.

Thus, perioperative nursing was reconceptualized in terms of time rather than geographic locus of care. The preoperative phase began at the time the decision for surgical intervention was made and continued until the patient was transferred to the OR bed. The perioperative role could be actualized in the home, clinic, physician's office, patient's hospital room, or surgical holding area. The intraoperative phase began with the transfer of the patient to the OR bed and continued until the patient was admitted to a postoperative care unit. During this phase, emphasis continued to be on physical safety, physiological monitoring, and nursing management of a plan of care that had as its goal safe and effective patient outcomes. The final phase, postoperative care, began at the time the patient was admitted to a postoperative care unit and ended with a follow-up visit in the patient's hospital room, home, or clinic. During this phase, information was gathered about the intraoperative experience, nursing care was evaluated, and discharge teaching and planning took place.

With the acceptance of the Project 25 Task Force Report and the adoption of the perioperative role as the baseline along which practitioners could progress on a role continuum, the role of the OR nurse was operationalized to include both technical and professional nursing functions. Project 26, organized in 1979, developed a master plan for implementing the perioperative role. An ad hoc committee was formed to identify basic competencies in OR nursing as an integral component of implementing the perioperative role. In a discussion of the project, Dodge (1980) reported:

> Basic nursing education does not include sufficient experience in the perioperative role to insure graduating nurses' proficiency in the field. Many nursing educators view perioperative nursing as specialized practice and believe preparation for the technical and professional aspects of the role should commence after completion of a basic nursing program. They view their primary responsibility as preparing graduates for entry into an increasingly complex professional practice. Operating nursing has shown a corresponding increase in complexity—witness the change in focus to perioperative nursing and the increasing numbers of complicated surgical procedures performed. Recognizing this, AORN acknowledges its leadership role for influencing future changes in the specialty. Identification of minimal competencies is part of this responsibility. . . . Nationally, competencies might be used as . . . the basis for prototype postbasic specialty programs for implementation in colleges and universities.

As changes in technology and health care economics accelerated during the 1980s, the geographical and temporal loci of care for perioperative patients continued to shift to settings outside of the traditional inpatient operating room. The dramatic rise in outpatient surgery, laser and endoscopic interventions, and minimally invasive approaches to treatment influenced AORN to once again assume a leadership role in exploring the impact of change on perioperative nursing. A Project Team to Redefine/Reconceptualize Perioperative Nursing, part of a larger futures exploration named "Project 2000," undertook an analysis of selected definitions and concepts integral to the delivery of perioperative patient care. Research participants confirmed the increasing participation of perioperative nurses in practice settings outside of the traditional operating room (Kneedler et al., 1992). The recommendations of the Project Team were integrated into a larger work plan for the future. As this plan unfolds during the 1990s, perioperative nursing will continue to reexamine and explore the nature of nursing's work with perioperative patient populations.

Basic competencies for perioperative nursing were published in 1982 and consisted of 25 statements intended as guidelines for what a nurse who had been employed in the OR room for 6 months to 1 year could reasonably be expected to have achieved (AORN, 1982). The competency statements were offered for use in developing position descriptions for the perioperative nurse, in performance appraisal, in designing structured orientation programs, in guiding staff development activities, in peer review processes, as a means of measuring student achievement in generic curricula, and in structuring clinical ladders.

The *Standards of Nursing Practice* were also revised in 1982. Although the substantive content of the seven original statements remained the same, the terminology and organization of the standards changed. The new standards included interpretive statements that explained the standard, suggested ways this standard might be accomplished, and included criteria for determining whether the standard had been met (Harvey, 1984). Continued emphasis was on the nursing process as the conceptual basis for the perioperative role. Implementation of the revised standards and adoption of the definition of the perioperative role clearly suggested that, as members of an interdisciplinary health care team, OR nurses should be involved in professional nursing activities throughout the preoperative, intraoperative, and postoperative phases of a patient's surgical experience. The standards were intended as a vehicle to pave the way for nurses in the OR to expand their knowledge, increase their sensitivity to human needs, and be accountable to consumers. The continuing revision and clarification of AORN's *Standards of Perioperative Nursing* demonstrate the desire of the organization to professionalize perioperative nursing.

By 1992, the standards had been revised to include standards of clinical practice and standards of professional performance. The standards of professional performance included activities related to quality of care, performance appraisal, education, collegiality, ethics, collaboration, research, and resource use. Describing behaviors expected in the role of the professional, they demonstrated perioperative nursing's ongoing commitment to the professionalization of the specialty.

AORN'S RESPONSE TO THE NEED TO EDUCATE NURSES FOR PERIOPERATIVE NURSING

Metzger (1976) has tentatively identified the beginnings of OR nursing education as the introduction of pupil nurses at Massachusetts General Hospital into the OR for clinical instruction. These students were taught by Henry Bigelow, professor of surgery at Harvard Medical School, in December of 1876. The Massachusetts General Hospital was one of the first three Nightingale schools of nursing founded in this country in 1873. Although curricula in the schools were not standardized, early lecture schedules included "Surgical Instruments and Preparation for Operation," "Bandaging," and "Haemostasis" (Metzger, 1976). As Lister's influence in principles of antisepsis gained acceptance, the development of modern surgery commenced with a parallel need for nurses who were trained to assist the modern surgeon. Walsh (1929) wrote:

> Indeed, the demand for nurses, properly trained, was not felt in the hospitals generally throughout the country until Lister's revolutionary discovery of the value of antisepsis in surgery . . . made it absolutely necessary that nurses should be of such an intellectual calibre and development as would permit them to be trained in the prevention of infection through absolute cleanliness.

In the early part of the 20th century, student nurses regularly assisted with operations and the many direct and indirect patient care activities that facilitated surgery. Mastery of knowledge of administration of anesthesia, types of anesthetic agents, sterilization, preparation of instruments and supplies, and aseptic technique became regularly incorporated into nursing curricula. The 1919 Committee on Education of the National League of Nursing Education (NLNE) Standard Curriculum included 10 hours of lecture on "Operating Room Technic." It was recommended that this part of the curriculum occur in the second year of training, while students were in their OR rotation, so that classwork and practical work would complement and supplement each other.

Since that 1919 NLNE curriculum publication, numerous reports and studies of nursing education have been undertaken in the search for what is essential and what is best in nursing's preparation of its neophytes. Shifts in emphasis from technical skills to theoretical bases for nursing action emerged as significant modifiers of curriculum content. As foci on the psychological and physiological dimensions of the whole patient began to dominate curricular reform, clinical experiences for nursing students focused on situations offering opportunities for defining patient problems and developing patient care plans. The OR did not seem to offer this type of learning opportunity and was often eliminated as a clinical rotation.

In 1979, the AORN National Committee on Education (NCE) decided to undertake a project aimed at assisting OR nurses and their AORN chapters in contacting schools of nursing about integrating the perioperative role into the nursing curriculum. In 1980, Project Alpha, a model for such activity, was published (AORN, 1980). The name *Alpha*, denoting the beginning, was selected to convey the start of a plan of action that could lead to the acceptance of the essential concepts of the perioperative role by nursing faculties. The project had as its mission a conveyance of the belief that curriculum concepts could be taught effectively within the operating room.

Efforts of AORN members at the local level were dual in nature. These efforts included the formation of Project Alpha committees within chapters and chapter activities and interactions with local schools of nursing. Committees were charged with gathering data about schools' goals, philosophies, conceptual frameworks, current courses, evaluation methods, and curriculum development procedures. At the same time, committees were to gather data from local health care institutions, evaluating learning resources and opportunities for student learning experiences within perioperative settings. These data were analyzed in an attempt to identify congruence between school missions and priorities and health care institutions' abilities to incorporate missions and priorities within perioperative settings. Goals were formed to establish communication with agencies educating generic nursing students, wherein mutual identification of concepts of the perioperative nursing role might be integrated into the nursing curriculum. Contact was to be made with responsible persons in schools of nursing for dialogue. *The Surgical Experience: A Model for Professional Nursing Practice in the Operating Room* (Davis et al., 1978) provided a model for guidelines regarding the kinds of activities in ORs that could enhance student learning.

A major thrust of Project Alpha was the identification of aspects of the perioperative role appropriate for student nurses. Emphasis was placed on the professional nature of the role in an attempt to verify and validate the opportunities for professional education in specialty practice areas. The aspects of a proper role model for student nurses have been summarized by Tenzer (1986) as follows:

1. Demonstrates continuity of care through utilization of the nursing process, providing a vehicle to enhance basic competency to a level of excellence
2. Provides the student with an opportunity to identify stresses that will affect the patient and appropriately plan total care
3. Provides awareness of the patient's safety needs and risk factors
4. Allows for visualization of potential trauma related to the surgical procedure and actual intervention
5. Provides observational and experiential exposure to group dynamics, development of leadership skills, and practice in assertiveness training
6. Self-instructs students in the areas of flexibility, adaptability, and self-reliance
7. Promotes the concept of teamwork
8. Provides an arena for the application of the knowledge of medical and surgical asepsis derived from principles of microbiology
9. Provides experience in the calm, prompt management of emergencies
10. Provides a framework of knowledge for the interpretation and communication of the patient's surgical care to the patient and family

On the national level, AORN instituted a series of conferences for nurse educators and deans of nursing programs. The first of these, held in 1979, provided a forum in which AORN leaders could meet with nursing educators from around the country to encourage adding OR experience to the basic nursing curriculum (Vaiden, 1983). By 1982, the conference, renamed the Invitational Conference for Nursing Educators, had become a biennial event. Meeker (1983) reported that intraoperative clinical experiences were being implemented or reintroduced in a small but increasing number of basic nursing curricula. At the 1984 Invitational Conference, the components of perioperative nursing practice and methods of integrating those components into baccalaureate curricula were discussed. As part of an ongoing attempt to broaden the appeal of reintegration of perioperative nursing, the many benefits to institutions and to students were identified by speakers.

Benefits for the schools of nursing (Palmer, 1985) included a broader, more comprehensive view of nursing; the opening of more clinical areas for student experience; new dimensions for application of scientific knowledge; and rationales for accreditation from the NLN. Student benefits were identified in terms of a holistic perspective on patient care; opportunity to visualize surgical anatomy; opportunity to provide patient care on a wellness-illness continuum; application of principles of self-care, asepsis, and teaching-learning theories; and exposure to stages of growth and development across the life span. Benefits to surgical facilities were also identified. These included the enthusiasm and satisfaction gained from contacts with nursing students, as well as the more pragmatic potential gains in employees, reducing the institution's need to recruit and plan extensive orientation programs for new graduates.

By 1986, at the 5th Invitational Conference, an increasing emphasis was being placed on the current and highly valued aspects of professional education. One of these, nursing research, was addressed at length in terms of opportunity for student involvement, past research foci in perioperative nursing, and trends and projected influences on perioperative nursing research in the future (Palmer, 1987). When opportunities for research were placed in the context of statistics on numbers of patients admitted for surgical interventions (as they were at this conference), the availability of a pool of subjects and the identification of researchable questions about those subjects and their relationship to nursing interventions becomes impressive.

Over the past three decades, OR nurses and their professional association (AORN) have recognized the need to develop educational programs in perioperative nursing in which nurses develop the ability to identify and study professional aspects of their role. Lindeman (1975) identified the nursing process as a research priority for nursing, and perioperative nursing standards reflect this process as the conceptual basis for nursing activities with surgical patients. Faulconer and Marchette (1986) identified the top 10 priorities for perioperative research; ways in which schools of nursing can be motivated to include perioperative nursing courses in their curricula ranked ninth. AORN has pursued these same questions in initiating Project Alpha activities, Invitational Conferences for Nursing Educators, and myriad other important and consistent activities that denote the association's commitment to nursing education and perioperative nursing's place in that educational process.

PROFESSIONAL INVOLVEMENT: AN ISSUE OF SURVIVAL

Membership in a professional association provides the nurse with a sense of identity, an opportunity to work with a cadre of leaders and innovators in nursing whose ideas and careers are influential in shaping the course of the profession, a heightened awareness of current trends, and the ability to develop an informed view of contemporary issues. American nursing has reached maturity as a well-developed discipline, possessing an identifiable body of knowledge, a research orientation, sophisticated practice models and systems of care delivery, and a complex educational system. To secure the present and guarantee future progress, the important role of professional associations must be maintained through growth and member activity.

Historically, caring has been a quality that has characterized nurses and nursing. Most caring models focus on the nature of caring relationships between the nurse as care provider and the patient or client as care recipient. The nurse's individual philosophy about nursing is critical to nursing practice, as philosophy encompasses the nurse's belief system and drives her or his quest for knowledge. What one believes about nursing influences one's thinking and, ultimately, one's actions. A philosophy of nursing involves a concern with knowledge and nursing science, values regarding patient relationships, and a recognition of what it means to "be" a nurse. The nurse who philosophically believes in caring, who thinks that it is the critical component of the nursing being, must also act in a caring mode. Furthermore, caring goes beyond the strict confines of nurse-patient relationships. It must extend itself to colleague relationships and to the future of the profession.

Part of becoming a productive professional is the desire to be productive both for self and for others. For nurses, being productive for others involves contributing to the development of nursing practice, education, and research. The strength that emerges from this professional self-development is a caring that transcends individual self-concept and extends itself to the profession.

One of the actions that flows out of such broad professional caring is involvement in professional associations. Such involvement is part of the mature, productive, professional self-concept.

Professional associations, through the work of their leaders and individual members, collectively nurture and develop the nurse's ability to care about the future of the profession. The collective power and wisdom in the professional association produce a vision of the future, which is necessary if the profession is going to survive. Together, association members look for signs in the environment that indicate what form and direction nursing will take in the future. Signs are found both in the immediate work environments of the members and in the nursing literature, and these signs direct the activities of the association. It is only through the input and activities of its members that the association can stay well informed and in touch with the social, political, economic, and technical milieu of the real world of nursing. Staying in touch demands the involvement of members in the association at both the local and national levels.

Thus, participation in organized nursing activities through membership in professional associations is one way the nurse can demonstrate a commitment to caring. Through the professional association, nurses can unite to accomplish visions that they cannot achieve as individuals. The power of the nursing profession to influence events is determined by the autonomy, collaboration, and accountability of its unified members. However, individual nurses must believe that they can make a difference and can influence events. If that perception exists, the nurse is more likely to participate. The most potential power in "being for nursing" arises out of the unified power of the association; it is in that power of unified and confluent purpose that nursing can become a major force in changing the delivery of health care and collaborating in a partnership of activity that will safeguard the future of the profession.

Although differences in opinion and emphasis regarding the direction of the collective power of the associations exist in the different nursing associations and are essential to the development of ideas and progress, unity and collaboration on the major issues confronting the whole of American nursing are essential for the survival of the profession and, ultimately, the improvement of health care (Fitzpatrick, 1983). The cooperative efforts of individual nurses, harnessed by the professional association, offer a path to professionalism in nursing and securing the future of the profession.

References

American Nurses' Association/Association of Operating Room Nurses. (1975). *Standards of nursing practice: operating room.* Kansas City, MO.

Association of Operating Room Nurses. (1969). Definition and objective for clinical practice of professional operating room nursing. *AORN Journal, 10,* 43–48.

Association of Operating Room Nurses. (1973). Delegates approve statements on RN and nursing student in OR. *AORN Journal, 17,* 187, 191.

Association of Operating Room Nurses. (1975). Delegates approve statements, resolutions at 22nd Congress. *AORN Journal, 21*, 1067, 1082.

Association of Operating Room Nurses. (1978). Operating room nursing: Perioperative role. *AORN Journal, 27*, 1156–1175.

Association of Operating Room Nurses. (1980). Project alpha provides guidelines, model for chapter action. *AORN Journal, 32*, 867, 875.

Association of Operating Room Nurses. (1982). Developing basic competencies for perioperative nursing. *AORN Journal, 35*, 871–884.

Atkinson, L. J. (1992). *Berry & Kohn's operating room technique.* St. Louis: Mosby–Year Book.

Aydelotte, M. (1987, January). Academy looks at nursing's preferred future. *The American Nurse*, p. 12.

Chinn, P. L., Jacobs, M. K. (1987). *Theory and nursing: A systematic approach.* St. Louis: C. V. Mosby.

Corwin, R. G. (1961). The professional employee: A study of conflict in nursing roles. *American Journal of Sociology, 66*, 604–615.

Davis, D. L., Kneedler, J. A., Manuel, B. J. (1978). *Surgical experience: A model for professional nursing practice in the OR.* Denver: Association of Operating Room Nurses.

Derdiarian, A. K. (1979). Education: A way to theory construction in nursing. *Journal of Nursing Education, 2*, 36–47.

DeYoung, L. (1981). *Dynamics of nursing.* St. Louis: C. V. Mosby.

Dodge, G. H. (1980). Committee to identify basic competencies in OR nursing. *AORN Journal, 32*, 377–380.

Driscoll, J. (1976). AORN in retrospect: 1949–1957. *AORN Journal, 24*, 150–156.

Faulconer, D. R., Marchette, L. (1986). *Perioperative nursing research priorities study.* Research report submitted to the AORN Nursing Research Committee.

Felton, G. (1986). Nursing's future. *Nursing and Health Care, 7*, 211–213.

Fitzpatrick, M. L. (1983). *Prologue to professionalism.* Bowie, MD: Robert J. Brady Co.

Flexner, A. (1915). Is social work a profession? *Studies in Social Work, 4*, 5–10.

Gerster, A. G. (1888). *The rules of aseptic and antiseptic surgery.* New York: D. Appleton.

Greenwood, E. (1964). Attributes of a profession. *Social Work, 26*, 45–55.

Gruendemann, B. J. (1980). Educators take a new look at perioperative nursing. *AORN Journal, 32,* 448–455.

Hagemeier, D., Hunt, C. (1979). Do new graduates use conceptual frameworks? *Nursing Outlook, 33*, 545–548.

Hall, R. H. (1968). Professionalization and bureaucratization. *American Sociological Review, 33*(1), 92–104.

Harvey, C. (1984). AORN suggests tool to evaluate perioperative standards. *AORN Journal, 40*, 830–834.

Hercules, P. (1980). OR experience teaches continuity of care. *AORN Journal, 32*, 799–806.

Jacobsen, S. F., McGrath, H. M. (1983). *Nurses and stress.* New York: John Wiley.

Kneedler, J. A., Murphy E. K., Wells, M., Hercules, P., Shoup, A., Brazen, L. (1992). Reconceptualizing, redefining perioperative nursing: project team report. *AORN Journal, 56*, 688–694.

Koehler, J. (1980). Educators take a new look at perioperative nursing. *AORN Journal, 32*, 448–455.

Leddy, S., Pepper, J. M. (1989). *Conceptual bases of professional nursing.* Philadelphia: J. B. Lippincott, Co.

Lee, R. M. (1976). Early operating room nursing. *AORN Journal, 24*, 124–138.

Light, D. (1979). Uncertainty and control in professional training. *Journal of Health and Social Behavior, 20*, 310–322.

Lindeman, C. A. (1975). Delphi study of priorities in clinical nursing research. *Nursing Research, 24*, 434–441.

Luckes, E. C. E. (1887). *Lectures on general nursing.* London: Kegan Paul Trench.

Lynn, M. W. (1983). *A description of operating room registered nurses' awareness, implementation, and documentation of the perioperative role.* Unpublished master's thesis, University of South Carolina, SC.

Meeker, M. H. (1983). New regs, research support are signs of AORN's progress [President's message]. *AORN Journal, 37*, 809–812.

Metzger, R. S. (1976). The beginnings of OR nursing education. *AORN Journal, 24*, 73–90.

Moore, W. (1974). *The professions: Roles and rules.* New York: Russell Sage Foundation.

Ondrack, D. A. (1975). Socialization in professional schools: A comparative study. *Administrative Science Quarterly, 20*, 97–103.

Palmer, P. (1985). Nurse educators take some notes. *AORN Journal, 41*, 166, 168.

Palmer, P. (1987). The 5th invitational nurse educator conference. *AORN Journal, 45*, 509, 515.

Patterson, P. (1986). Shrinking pool of experienced nurses worries OR directors. *OR Manager, 2*(1), 1, 7.

Sharp, B. (1980). Student experiences: Benefits to patients. *AORN Journal, 32*, 815–817.

Spitzer, R. (1987, January). Teamwork needed for hospitals, nursing to survive. *The American Nurse*, p. 4.

Stevens, B. J. (1984). *Nursing theory: Analysis, application, and evaluation.* Boston: Little Brown.

Tenzer, I. (1986, October). *Project alpha: The beginning.* Paper presented at the Perioperative Nursing Symposium, San Francisco.

Vaiden, R. (1983). Board appoints new task forces on nursing image, first assisting [President's message]. *AORN Journal, 37*, 1260–1261.

Walsh, J. J. (1929). *History of nursing.* New York: P. J. Kenedy.

Weeks, C. S. (1890). *Textbook of nursing.* New York: D. Appleton.

Wilensky, H. L. (1964). The professionalization of everyone? *American Journal of Sociology, 70*(2), 137–158.

Wooley, A. S. (1986). From RN to BSN: Faculty perceptions. *Nursing Outlook, 26*, 103–108.

CHAPTER 42

The Entrepreneurial Nurse

Dan Sandel

Mary is a nurse who works in a large hospital in Tennessee. For years she wondered what to do with the many syringes used by the anesthesiologist; then she had an idea. She found some plastic cups with foam in them, grouped them together with tape, and offered them to the anesthesiologist as a syringe holder that provided very easy access and a safety control for his syringes. This idea is still in use at the hospital, is saving a lot of time, and has been proven to be very, very safe. However, no one else knows about it.

Karen works for a medium-sized hospital in the Midwest. It is a very friendly environment, and everyone is nice to each other. Karen had a great idea about sharps container systems. Her idea, which was conceived before the AIDS epidemic, will revolutionize the way sharps are being collected and disposed of. Happy and pleased about her innovation, she tells it to a couple of salespeople who call on her. They promise to help her develop her idea. Six months later, the product is introduced all over the country with no credit or mention of the original inventor.

Susan is an OR nurse. She is very careful and observant and has a lot of good ideas. Among her many ideas, she

came up with a unique surgical clamp. Knowing how to deal with manufacturers, she contacted a manufacturer who properly handled her idea. Susan's product is now widely used in many hospitals. It carries her name, and she shares in the financial rewards of this product's economic success.

The examples above illustrate both the tremendous opportunities for innovative nurses and the pitfalls for those who do not develop their ideas carefully. The purpose of this chapter is to identify the nature of the product development and innovation opportunities that are available to operating room nurses and provide a framework in which they can pursue these ideas.

First, this chapter will describe the environment in the health care industry. This is critical to understand the types of products the market is likely to respond to favorably. The next section examines the role of the nurse within this environment, focusing particularly on the nurse as a source of innovative ideas. The final section describes the process by which a nurse can pursue product ideas so that he or she will reap the benefits.

1031

TABLE 42–1. NATIONAL HEALTH CARE EXPENDITURES BY TYPE OF EXPENDITURE, SELECTED CALENDAR YEARS, 1965–2000 (AMOUNTS IN BILLIONS)

Type of Expenditure	2000	1995	1990	1987	1986	1985	1984	1980	1970	1965
National health expenditures	$1,529.3	$999.1	$647.3	$496.6	$458.2	$422.6	$391.1	$248.1	$75.0	$41.9
Health services and supplies	1,493.8	972.1	626.6	479.3	442.0	407.2	375.4	236.2	69.6	38.4
Personal health care	1,398.1	900.5	573.5	438.9	404.0	371.3	341.9	219.7	65.4	35.9
Hospital care	621.0	393.6	250.4	192.6	179.6	167.2	156.3	101.6	28.0	14.0
Physician services	319.6	209.0	132.6	101.4	92.0	82.8	75.4	46.8	14.3	8.5
Dentist services	89.6	62.2	41.8	32.4	29.6	27.1	24.6	15.4	4.7	2.8
Other professional services	60.4	38.1	22.9	16.2	14.1	12.4	10.9	5.7	1.6	1.0
Drugs and medical sundries	102.6	65.4	42.1	32.8	30.6	28.7	26.5	18.8	8.0	5.2
Eyeglasses and appliances	24.7	16.7	11.2	8.8	8.2	7.5	7.0	5.1	1.9	1.2
Nursing home care	129.0	84.7	54.5	41.6	38.1	35.0	31.7	20.4	4.7	2.1
Other personal health care	51.2	30.8	18.0	13.1	11.9	10.8	9.4	5.9	2.1	1.1
Program administration and net cost of private health insurance	57.7	44.4	34.6	25.9	24.5	23.6	22.6	9.2	2.8	1.7
Government public health activities	38.0	27.2	18.5	14.4	13.4	12.3	11.0	7.3	1.4	0.8
Research and construction of medical facilities	35.5	26.9	20.7	17.3	16.3	15.4	15.6	11.9	5.4	3.5
Noncommercial research*	20.2	15.3	11.5	9.0	8.2	7.4	6.8	5.4	2.0	1.5
Construction	15.3	11.6	9.3	8.3	8.0	8.1	8.9	6.5	3.4	2.0
Gross National Product	10,164	7,467	5,414	4,483	4,206	3,998	3,765	2,732	1,015	705

*Research and development expenditures of drug companies and other manufacturers and providers of medical equipment and supplies are excluded from "research expenditures," but they are included in the expenditure class in which the product falls.
Data from the Division of National Cost Estimates, Health Care Financing Administration, Office of the Actuary, Washington, D.C.

THE ENVIRONMENT IN THE HEALTH CARE INDUSTRY

The U.S. economy has undergone some fundamental changes since World War II. One of the central themes throughout this period has been the transformation from a manufacturing orientation to a service orientation. Currently, much of the Gross National Product in the United States results from the delivery of services rather than the manufacturing of products. Although this change is clearly dramatic, it is no more striking than the transformation from agriculture to manufacturing that preceded it. (Of course, manufacturing and agriculture will always play critical roles.) The trend suggests an increasing reliance on our most precious natural resource: people.

One characteristic of a service economy is a relatively slower rate of growth (only 2 to 3% annually). It is generally more difficult to develop innovations that result in a dramatically more efficient delivery of services than to improve productivity in a manufacturing environment. This is true primarily because of the dependence on people as the service delivery system. As a result, innovations most often help people to be more efficient and effective and do not replace them (as occurs, for example, in robotics). Nevertheless, to remain competitive, it is increasingly critical to develop innovations that help the service sector grow. Nowhere is this more crucial than in the health care industry.

This section will address the environment in the health care industry as it applies to entrepreneurs. In doing so, it will examine the tremendous growth that has occurred in this area as well as the regulatory changes and the types of innovations that are most common. Then the hospital will be examined as a specific market, focusing on trends there. Finally, the surgical services market will be addressed along with the opportunities for innovation and invention it presents.

CHANGE IN THE HEALTH CARE INDUSTRY

Since the 1970s, the change in the health care industry has been phenomenal. The health care sector has grown tremendously, which has led to an increasing need to regulate the industry to control skyrocketing costs. At the same time, a myriad of lifesaving innovations have emerged that, at times, exacerbate the rising cost of health care.

Growth in Health Care Expenditures

One of the clear factors in increased costs has been the phenomenal growth in the health care sector. As shown in Table 42–1, the total health care expenditures rose in the 1980s from $248 billion to an estimated $647 billion in 1990 and are predicted to be $1.529 trillion by the year 2000, an increase of 517%. During the same period (1980–2000) the gross national product (GNP) rose from $2.732 trillion to an anticipated $10.164 trillion, or an increase of 272%. The dramatic growth of health care relative to the GNP is depicted in Figure 42–1. As can be readily observed, by the year 2000, about 15% of the total output in the United States is expected to originate in the health care sector.

The growth in health care expenditures comes despite the federal and state governmental efforts to alter the trend. This rapid expansion is generally attributed to three primary factors: consumer demand for high-quality health care regardless of costs; escalating costs associ-

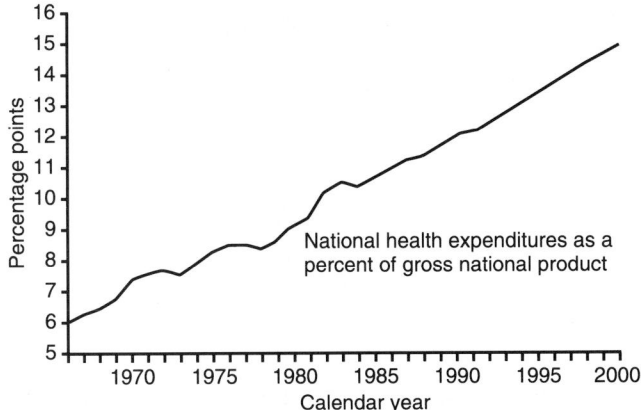

FIGURE 42–1. National health care expenditures as a percentage of the Gross National Product, 1965–2000. (From the Health Care Financing Administration, Office of the Actuary, Washington, D.C.; data from the Division of National Cost Estimates.)

ated with an aging population; and a greater utilization of technology in medicine.

At the same time, free market forces that might otherwise lead to the reduction of costs by bargain-hungry consumers are limited, because most medical bills are paid by third parties. Thus, the insurance companies and the government must sometimes work against consumer demand for quality in an effort to reduce costs.

Regulation of the Health Care Industry

This situation has left the government with the difficult problem of regulating the industry in an attempt to reverse or confine the trend. The thrust of this effort has been through Food and Drug Administration (FDA) regulations (1976), diagnosis-related group (DRG) (1983) rates, and the Doctor Cost Control Act (1991).

FDA Regulations

In the late 1970s the emphasis in the FDA has generally been to speed up the process by which drugs and products are approved. Since 1976 the FDA has been classifying products into three categories, or *classes*. These classes are general indicators of the amount of investigation, analysis, and study the FDA will require for a product before approval. Class 3 products are lifesaving and sustaining in nature. These are subject to the greatest amount of regulation, as the patient's life is directly dependent on the effectiveness of the product. Examples include pacemakers, heart valves, and implants.

Class 2 products are required to be sterile but generally do not play as critical a role in patient treatment. Thus, products such as surgical gloves or tubing are subject to less regulation and less rigorous testing.

Finally, class 1 products are those that do not easily fit into class 2 or 3 and cannot cause harm to the patient.

DRG Rates

In 1983 the standard DRG rates were developed and implemented to provide some standard frame of reference for medical expenditures. In 1990, the increase in the DRG rates was 4.3%, or about 1.5% less than the inflation rate. It is anticipated that this would result in $2.7 billion in saving from the total Medicare budget, which is about $108 billion.

The hospitals are able to shift some of the costs to private patients in the form of higher charges. In the private sector, however, the third parties who must pay the cost are shifting to lower cost Health Maintenance Organizations (HMOs) and managed care plans. There is a greater utilization of second opinions, particularly for surgical interventions, and a shifting of many types of care to outpatient settings. Insurers are also shifting to higher deductibles and other copayments so that patients will be responsible for an increasing portion of their medical bills. In addition, they are subjecting health care utilization to increasing levels of scrutiny.

Doctor Cost Control Act

This act was enacted into law in January 1992 and put restrictions on the amount of money that can be charged by doctors for many surgical procedures and other medical treatments.

Innovation in the Health Care Industry

Throughout the 1980s there was a great deal of innovation in the health care field. However, many of the innovations (e.g., magnetic resonance imaging [MRI] and lithotriptors) tend to add to the inflation problem rather than improve the situation. For example, an MRI machine costs around $1.5 million, and the procedure costs $500 to $1000. In contrast, a conventional radiograph costs about $60.

In essence, many of the innovations are still focused on improving the quality of medical care. Often the need to provide quality care at affordable prices is not recognized. Thus, although these innovations are clearly beneficial, they add to the cost containment problem.

In the coming years, the urgent need to contain costs will provide many opportunities for those who have ideas that respond to this increasing priority. Indeed, the relative lack of focus on innovations that reduce costs suggests that there is much work to be done in this area.

TABLE 42–2. **SELECTED MEASURES IN COMMUNITY HOSPITALS, 1978 AND 1987–1988**

Measure	Year			Percentage Change	
	1978	1987	1988	1978–1988	1987–1988
Hospitals	5,851	5,611	5,533	−5.4	−1.4
Beds (in thousands)	975	958	947	−2.9	−1.2
Average number of beds per hospital	167	171	171	2.6	0.2
Admissions (in thousands)	34,506	31,601	31,453	−8.8	−0.5
Average daily census (in thousands)	718	622	620	−13.6	−0.3
Average length of stay days	7.6	7.2	7.2	−5.0	0.4
Inpatient days (in thousands)	262,064	227,015	226,875	−13.4	−0.1
Occupancy percent	73.6	64.9	65.5	−11.0	0.9
Surgical operations (in thousands)	17,150	20,818	21,411	24.8	2.9
Bassinets (in thousands)*	78	73	70	−9.9	−3.0
Births (in thousands)	3,156	3,602	3,706	17.4	2.9
Outpatient visits (in thousands)†	201,931	245,524	269,129	33.3	9.6

*Based only on hospitals reporting newborn data.
†Based only on hospitals reporting outpatient visits.
From American Hospital Association. (1989–1990). *Hospital Statistics*. American Hospital Association: Chicago.

THE HOSPITAL AS A MARKET

In developing a new product, it is critical to identify the target market segment (i.e., the group of customers at whom the product is directed and who will ultimately purchase it). This enables product development efforts to be focused in such a way as to ensure that customers' needs are met. Furthermore, it draws attention to potential problems in marketing and distribution (i.e., how can you tell people about the product, and how do you get it to them?).

Within the health care industry, there are a number of interdependent markets that have different environments and different needs. Table 42–1 lists several different broad categories of health care services: personal health care, program administration and insurance, government public health care expenditures, and research and construction of medical facilities. This chapter is most interested in personal health care, which includes hospital care, physicians' services, dentists' services, other professional services, drugs and supplies, eyeglasses and appliances, and nursing home care.

Quality Verus Price

Each of these aspects of personal health care can be further delineated to reflect distinct markets. For example, hospitals can be categorized by the consumer markets that they serve. Typically, a market can be defined as falling into one of three segments that reflect varying emphases on quality and price.

Within the upper tier of the market, customers seek quality and comfort with relatively less emphasis on cost. Firms in the second tier provide services that seek to balance the concerns of price and quality. Finally, the third tier of the market centers on low-cost health care services and places somewhat less emphasis on quality. In general, most hospitals serve customers in the second tier, because people are sensitive to both the quality and the price of their health care. Clearly, however, cost is becoming an increasingly important criterion.

Product Markets

In addition to the customer markets described earlier, each department within the hospital may be examined as a separate product or service. For example, intensive care and outpatient services effectively reflect very different services and thus may be considered distinct markets.

Taken together, all of these discrete markets make up the hospital market. As Table 42–1 shows, broadly speaking, the hospital market is the largest portion of the nation's health care expenditures (about $250 million, or approximately 40% of the total), and its costs are expected to nearly triple by the year 2000.

Trends in the Hospital Services

Table 42–2 shows statistics on the changes in the community hospital market from 1978 to 1988. It can be seen that the number of hospitals is decreasing while the average number of beds per hospital is increasing and admissions are dropping slightly. It is important to note that the increase in the average number of beds is not a trend toward very large facilities. In fact, hospitals in the 400+ bed category currently supply about 30% of the total beds, rather than 33% in 1980. Thus the growth has been in 200- to 400-bed facilities, with a slight decrease in very small facilities (less than 100 beds).

Cost-cutting measures are apparent in these statistics, as the average length of stay has dropped and the number of outpatient visits has increased (currently 329 million annually). This is significant, as the number of surgical procedures is clearly on the rise (currently about 23 million annually). Thus these surgeries are being handled differently than they were in 1980 to hold down costs.

Trends in the nature of services provided and technologies used are shown in Table 42–3. Almost all facilities provide ambulatory surgical services and emergency services, and increasingly they provide birthing rooms, chemical dependency facilities, and outpatient rehabilitation facilities and have an outpatient department.

There is also an increasing reliance on medical technology. More hospitals are providing MRI scans, computed tomographic (CT) scans, and cardiac catheterization, as well as complex surgeries such as open heart and organ transplantation. However, this trend is showing signs of tapering off. For example, MRI equipment sales rose only about 6% in 1989, whereas they had increased about 20% in 1988.

Trends in Surgical Products and Services

As discussed earlier, there is a continuing trend toward the utilization of surgery (about a 2 to 3% increase each year and a 25% increase over the decade). At the same time, however, more and more surgeries are performed on an outpatient basis; outpatient visits are increasing at about 8 to 10% annually and are up 33% since the early 1980s. In addition, the average length of stay in the hospital, currently about 7.2 days, is dropping at about 0.5% annually.

These cost-cutting measures have affected the surgical instrument and supply industry considerably. The increased price sensitivity brought about by the imposition of the DRG system and other economic pressures has resulted in fierce competition, particularly in commodity or conventional type products. According to the Bureau of Labor Statistics, the price of surgical, medical, and dental instruments increased at a rate of less than 4% annually, while the price of all finished goods increased at a rate of nearly 6%. The prices of some key products such as catheters and orthopedic and prosthetic devices increased at a rate of less than 1% during the same period. The impact of this competition is clearly evident when the earnings per share within the medical supplies industry are examined.

Manufacturers and the Hospital Market

From a manufacturing standpoint, there are some fundamental differences between the hospital and medical supplies markets and oher types of product markets. The most important difference is the distance between the manufacturer and the user of the products. The easiest way to understand this is to compare this industry with others such as consumer goods or high technology.

In consumer goods, members of senior management are generally also users of the product and can well understand what they expect it to do and what standards it should meet. For example, the president of Ford Motor Company drives the cars he sells and regularly

TABLE 42–3. **TRENDS IN SELECTED SERVICES AND TECHNOLOGIES IN COMMUNITY HOSPITALS, 1984 AND 1987–1988**

	1984		1987		1988	
	No. of Hospitals	*Percent*	*No. of Hospitals*	*Percent*	*No. of Hospitals*	*Percent*
Selected services						
Ambulatory surgery	4,836	90.7	4,959	94.5	4,989	95.1
Birthing rooms	2,449	45.9	2,897	55.2	3,322	63.3
Blood bank	3,923	73.6	3,724	71.0	3,675	70.1
Emergency department	5,064	95.0	4,977	94.9	4,935	94.1
Outpatient alcoholism/chemical dependency	767	14.4	985	18.8	990	18.9
Physical therapy	4,830	90.6	4,593	87.6	4,486	85.5
Trauma care	938	17.6	1,026	19.6	703	13.4
Volunteer services	3,712	69.6	3,236	61.7	3,477	66.3
Outpatient rehabilitation	1,939	36.4	2,149	41.0	2,408	45.9
Outpatient department	2,634	49.4	3,671	70.0	4,064	77.5
Number of hospitals reporting	5,331		5,246		5,244	
Technologies						
Cardiac catheterization	942	17.7	1,152	22.0	1,229	23.4
CT scanner	2,555	47.9	3,169	60.4	3,347	63.8
Lithotripsy	N/A	N/A	196	3.7	255	4.9
Magnetic resonance imaging	166	3.1	487	9.3	656	12.5
Megavoltage radiation therapy	898	16.8	928	17.3	963	18.4
Open heart surgery	631	11.8	743	14.2	789	15.0
Organ transplantation	244	4.6	305	5.8	392	7.5
Number of hospitals reporting	5,331		5,246		5,244	

N/A, Data not available.
From American Hospital Association. (1989–1990). *Hospital Statistics*. American Hospital Association: Chicago.

provides feedback into the manufacturing and design process.

A different feedback process prevails in high-technology industries. Here, there are engineers and technicians in both the customer and the manufacturing firms. The design specifications are provided in detailed engineering terms. These generally ensure that the product is measured against design specifications that both firms understand at the outset.

In contrast, medical and hospital supplies most often are not produced by health care practitioners. As such, the manufacturers may not fully understand the way in which the product will be applied. In addition, there is no common dialect to convey technical design standards; engineering terminology is used, but the health care practitioner rarely communicates ideas in that fashion.

The problem is exacerbated by the salesperson, who acts as an intermediary between the manufacturer and the practitioner. These salespeople are often independent contractors with little loyalty toward one product. Even those who serve one manufacturer may be more anxious to make their sale and move on than to listen to complaints or suggestions. The result is that manufacturers are greatly insulated from the markets they serve and are starved for feedback and ideas.

Entrepreneurial Opportunities

Clearly there are always opportunities for products that improve the quality of health care services. As described earlier, technology continues to be applied to enhance critical care. However, there are increasing opportunities for products that streamline medical care and thus contribute to the drive for cost reduction. Indeed, the environment has become more challenging at the same time new opportunities have opened up (i.e., new products are more likely to be scrutinized to compare their costs and benefits than in the past). Nonetheless, products that justifiably reduce costs will be in high demand.

Thus, in spite of the competitive pressures in the medical supplies industry, analysts project a growth rate in the earnings per share of nearly 16%. This is double the growth rate anticipated for Standard & Poor's 500 largest firms (7.7%).

At the same time, some good ideas may be deemed unprofitable because competition will drive prices down. Ultimately the idea must not only be effective, it must deliver margins to the manufacturer as well.

THE ROLE OF THE NURSE

The role of the nurse has expanded considerably over time. While nurses will always serve as caregivers, they are increasingly serving as managers and administrators. These roles give nurses a unique vantage point from which they can identify unmet or partially met needs in the various markets.

In this respect the market for hospital and surgical supplies is very different from that for consumer goods. That is, the manufacturer of hospital supplies does not generally consume the end product and is thus less able to meet the market's needs without the help of others who are closer to the market. The manufacturer may make a blunder that is obvious to the nurse but not to the manufacturer. This section, then, will examine how these roles facilitate nurses' ability to identify important new products.

Administrative Roles and Purchasing Power

Nurses are increasingly accepting management and administrative roles in addition to or instead of roles in direct patient care. Thus, registered nurses have become supervisors, managers, department heads, and vice presidents.

Many of the organizational skills that make nurses successful in patient care also make them excellent administrators. These skills in interpersonal relationships, negotiation, budgeting, decision making, leadership, and planning are critical to the success of the hospital as well.

As nurses gravitate toward more managerial and administrative roles in the system, their power and influence over purchasing decisions are enhanced. As shown previously, health care expenditures are a tremendous portion of the gross national product. Table 42–4 shows total expenditures and expenditures by hospital size. As shown, hospitals spend an average of $30 million each annually. Even the smallest hospitals operate on budgets of $2 million or more. An average of about $4 million per hospital is spent annually on equipment and supplies.

This purchasing power grants nurses considerable leverage, if they choose to use it, in dealing with vendors and manufacturers. That is, if they are dissatisfied with a given product, they can seek out alternatives or go straight to the manufacturer and ask for modifications. As a general rule, manufacturers will seek and appreciate input from nurses even from the smallest hospitals.

Nurses as Plant Managers

The various departments in a hospital have considerable budgets to manage, and the administrative nurse directing a department can be compared to a plant manager in a manufacturing firm. Although there are guidelines within which the administrator must operate, there generally is latitude for decisions that may make the department run more efficiently (especially in this cost-conscious environment). Like most plant managers, nurses are under considerable pressure to contain costs.

Proximity to the Product

Because nurses are in a position to be familiar with many different aspects of the whole system and because

	Total Expenditures (Millions)*			Average Expenditures per Hospital (Millions)
	1987	1988	Percent Change	1988
Total community hospitals	$152,585	$168,723	10.6	$30
Urban community	132,578	146,900	10.8	49
Rural community	20,007	21,823	9.1	9
Bed size category (number of beds)				
6–24	354	375	5.9	2
25–49	3,121	3,431	9.9	4
50–99	9,970	10,820	8.5	8
100–199	24,856	27,887	12.2	21
200–299	28,579	31,916	11.7	43
300–399	25,583	27,962	9.3	68
400–499	17,612	19,043	8.1	92
500 or more	42,510	47,288	11.2	160

*Figures have been rounded to the nearest million; therefore, entries in vertical columns will not necessarily add to the total given.
From American Hospital Association. (1989–1990). *Hospital Statistics*. American Hospital Association: Chicago.

they are skilled at identifying more efficient means of accomplishing tasks, they are an ideal source of innovation in medical supplies. As discussed earlier, they are proximal to the process in a way that manufacturers are not. Thus, rather than wondering why many products are not sufficient and choosing to live with them, nurses are in a unique position to improve the nature of the products available to them.

When identifying products that are substandard or when delineating new needs, nurses often complain to the sales representative. This feedback, however, often never reaches the manufacturer, because the salesperson is generally an independent contractor who has little stake in improving the product.

PURSUING ENTREPRENEURIAL IDEAS

Once you have an idea, you must go through several basic steps. It is critical to consider each step carefully to ensure that you have thought through your idea and have guarded your rights at each phase of the process. First, you must develop a proposal for your product. There are a number of options for pursuing your developed idea. You may take your idea to an engineering firm and commission them to make a prototype. You may go to a patent attorney to file an application for a patent, or you may wish to take the product idea directly to a manufacturer. These phases of the process are described below.

Nurturing Your Idea

The first step in the process is to recognize the value associated with your ideas. Many ideas occur while you are in the middle of something else or when you must hurry to meet a deadline. These may be lost if they are not written down and considered later. They should not be brushed off as being impractical, since many others

may perceive the same market need (i.e., they would buy the product).

Often ideas are lost in the waking hours of the morning, and a simple note pad can preserve them for later examination. These creative impulses, whimsical though they may seem at the time, may serve a critical unmet need in the market.

You may also take a hard look at your work environment and the various "jury-rigged" systems and implements used to get through the day. You may take them for granted, but these reflect opportunities to develop products that serve the need better than the improvised tool.

Developing a Proposal

The written proposal for the product must answer several basic questions that will allow you and others to assess the viability of your product idea. Thus, it should not only describe your product, but should also indicate who will purchase it and the approximate price range envisioned. It should include options for the distribution channels for the product, as well as ideas for marketing the product to the end user. In addition, the proposal should include manufacturing standards and problems that have been identified a priori and some rough projections of sales and costs.

Identifying Market Need

The first and foremost step is to identify who you expect to buy the product and why they would choose your product over others that serve similar functions. As discussed earlier, there are a number of different ways to identify a market. The product may be directed toward a specific department in hospitals or toward certain types of hospitals. It may be so specialized that the market reflects an area of specialization within the health care field.

The proposal must identify a need in this market that is either not met or not met adequately. This market and perceived need must be identified in as detailed a fashion as possible, because a myriad of other decisions rest on the nature of the target market.

Impact on Patient Care and Staff Safety. Perhaps the most fundamental concern in introducing a new product in the health care industry is the extent and manner in which the product influences patient care and staff safety. Even though cost control has become a major concern, the ultimate objective is to provide quality health care services.

Universality of the Product. One critical consideration is the size the potential market is. For example, is the product for use in performing one specific type of surgery, or is it applicable to all surgeries? Does it resolve a problem that all operating room teams are experiencing, or is the problem relatively rare? Developing a product to solve an unusual problem that others do not experience will not be very profitable to the manufacturer.

Product Description

The description of the product must be very detailed with respect to both design and function. It should include the diagrams and exhibits necessary to make its use understood. The product description follows the delineation of the market and should demonstrate how the product meets the market need. Because many of the readers will not be technical experts in the health care field or in the specific area in which the product will be used, technical jargon should be applied sparingly.

The product description should classify the product into one of several categories. For example, the proposal should clearly state the FDA product class that the proposed product fits in. This will give readers a sense of how much testing and development will be required to bring the product to market.

The proposal must make it clear whether the product would be considered capital equipment or a supplies expense from the perspective of the target market. This, of course, is related to the target market, the pricing, and the fundamental nature of the product.

If the product falls into the category of medical supplies, the proposal should examine whether the product will be reusable or disposable. This is critical to determine the nature of the manufacturing process, the product's profitability, and the anticipated sales volume. Specifically, although disposable products are often almost identical to reusable products, the anticipated volume is generally much higher, and different manufacturing techniques may be appropriate.

Marketing

Once the market and product have been identified, the proposal should examine the potential means of reaching that market and present evidence as to how successful each alternative is likely to be. Ultimately, even when a market and product have been successfully identified, the product may be deemed not to be viable if the market is very difficult to reach.

Manufacturing

As discussed earlier, the product description provides most of the information that the manufacturer will need to set up the production process. Although many of the basic manufacturing decisions are best left to the manufacturer, it is critical that specifications and standards be clearly stated in the proposal. In addition, if any manufacturing problems are anticipated, they should be discussed here. Remember, however, that the manufacturer is not a user, and concepts and issues that are obvious to you may not be clear to the manufacturer.

Distribution

The proposal should also examine several alternative distribution channels. That is, it should consider which vendors might be suited to sell the product to the target market. Among the various distribution channels, the following should be considered:

- National distributors
- Regional distributors
- Local distributors
- Manufacturing representatives
- Direct mail

You can start by identifying which vendors already sell products that are commonly used in the target market.

Pricing

As suggested earlier, the market segment generally reflects a trade-off between price and quality. Thus, you must examine which segment you will pursue and price your product to meet the expectations of that market.

Sales and Cost Projections

Finally, the proposal must include some projections of the profitability of the product. You should present multiple scenarios while maintaining some degree of conservatism. Those who will evaluate your proposal must gain confidence in your understanding of the market and product. If the projections appear unreasonable or are otherwise not sufficiently defensible, the credibility of the entire proposal will be brought into question.

PURSUING YOUR DEVELOPED IDEA

When you have developed your idea, you want to ultimately bring it to a manufacturer and negotiate an agreement. However, you may wish to refine the presentation of the idea and ensure your own protection before presenting the idea to a manufacturer.

Obtaining a Patent

To determine whether you should pursue a patent, you must first examine the nature of your idea. If it reflects an innovation or improvement on an existing idea or product, it is probably not eligible for a patent. On the other hand, if it is a new product that did not exist before your effort, you should consider filing a patent application. Broadly speaking, the patent office will award patents when the product is perceived as useful and novel.

A patent provides some degree of protection from others claiming rights to the same innovation. However, the patent must be approached cautiously to ensure that the maximum degree of protection is obtained. As such, the best way to proceed is through an attorney who specializes in patent applications. In this way you can be assured that you will gain the greatest possible protection.

The attorney will help you follow the guidelines and meet the deadlines imposed by the U.S. Patent Office. In addition, he or she will help you formulate the characterization of your product to maximize the protection the patent will provide. For example, if possible, you should seek a patent on the function of the product rather than its design. This way others cannot make minor changes in your product design and effectively exempt themselves from the patent.

The patent, however, will not provide protection by itself. It may provide a legal course of action, but that is of little value unless you are willing to pursue such action to protect your rights. Because this can be costly (and others are aware of the cost), you should still be careful, even when you have obtained a patent.

Developing a Prototype

If the product is fairly complex and/or you are uncertain that laypersons will fully comprehend its use and value, you may consider developing a prototype to help with your presentation. Generally, small engineering or design firms are well equipped to perform this function in a timely manner.

When pursuing this avenue, you should be careful to have the engineering firm sign a nondisclosure agreement. This will prevent the firm from releasing the information in a damaging fashion or pursuing development of the product on their own.

Presenting the Product to a Manufacturing Firm

Once you have a proposal, you may wish to proceed directly to a manufacturer and present your idea. You must determine not only who to go to, but also how and when to proceed.

Selecting a Manufacturer. Generally, manufacturers are receptive to ideas, but you may find that the very largest firms are less receptive and may not even want to hear your idea. This is because they have internal research and development departments that may or may not be working on similar ideas. If they view your idea and have a similar one in development, they may be opening themselves to a lawsuit. Smaller firms, however, make a business out of acting on these ideas and will tend to be very receptive.

You must also find a firm that is familiar with the specific market you wish to target. This will help you in a number of ways. First, the firm will understand the market and its needs. This means that it is better able to produce products that meet the standards of this market. Second, the firm will have a better understanding of the potential value of your product to the market and will be able to evaluate the product quickly. This will allow you to bring the product to market in a more timely fashion. Finally, the manufacturer that already serves the target market will have a distribution system and marketing program in place to provide information to the market and deliver the product to them.

When to Approach the Manufacturer. You may approach the manufacturer at any time. If your idea is in rough form but is easily understandable, the manufacturer can help you fill out the details of your proposal. If the idea is complex or has nuances that require some explanation or justification, it would probably be better to proceed with a more formalized proposal.

Making Contact With the Manufacturer. As discussed earlier, manufacturers are generally receptive to ideas for new products. If you find that you have difficulties getting a given manager interested, you should not hesitate to contact senior management in the firm.

In initiating discussions with the firm, you must follow the formality of having them sign a nondisclosure agreement before your presentation. While most manufacturers conscientiously guard the rights of those who bring them ideas (since it is the source of their business), some misunderstandings do occur. In general, the manufacturer should view the nondisclosure agreement as a standard procedure.

Your presentation to the manufacturer can reflect varying degrees of formality but must address each of the major issues identified in the proposal. In many cases, the manufacturer will wish to study the prospects for the product further and hold additional discussions after a brief examination. Occasionally, the manufacturer will have access to information about the market or the manufacturing problems raised that will make the product impractical to pursue. If the manufacturer has such an opinion, you may wish to proceed to another firm or re-evaluate the efficacy of your idea.

When the manufacturer expresses interest, you are ready to begin the negotiation phase of the process. Here, you are probably better off if you seek representation from an experienced attorney or negotiator. You should recognize, however, that the manufacturer, in the interest of a potential long-term business relationship, wants both you and the company to reap benefits from the product. Thus, you should not have much difficulty in settling on a reasonable agreement for compensation and other issues that may arise.

THE ENTREPRENEURIAL NURSE

When you have a good idea, you should be able to let the idea work *for* you. This means that the idea has the potential to change your life in a very positive way. To understand and appreciate the process, you should consider what expectations you can realistically foster. You should also examine how you anticipate that the product development effort will affect your life-style and your future.

Expectations

A product idea can be likened to a child. The child's parents have a great emotional investment in the child's success, and they agonize over any failures. While you must have confidence in the value of your idea, you should be aware that many ideas are unsuccessful as a result of problems in timing or technical issues. A failed product does not imply that the idea was ill conceived. Furthermore, it may take several "misses" before a "hit" can be achieved—but all it takes is one hit!

Time Frame for Results

As discussed throughout, the process does take time to reach maturity and may require some patience on your part. It takes time to develop the idea and examine its true potential. It takes even more time to develop a manufacturing process to produce enough of the product to make a profit. Additional time passes as you and the manufacturer develop and implement a marketing plan to reach the target customers. Finally, there is generally some lag time between when customers hear about the product and when they actually buy it. The bottom line, then, is that you may have to wait some time to see any profit. In fact, the process often requires some up-front investment on your part.

What It Means for Day-to-Day Activities

As you resolve yourself to pursue your own ideas and dreams, you need to recognize some fundamental changes that may occur in the way you function on a day-to-day basis.

Learning to Play. First, many ideas are the result of creative play. That is, ideas reflect a creative examination of what could exist and how things could be different. Often the first step here is to step back from the day-to-day aggravation long enough to see how the situation could be different and what would make things easier. In many cases we become so familiar with our jobs and the way work is completed that we go about our tasks in habitual fashion, taking for granted that we are doing things in the best possible way. A little creative play may change the way in which you look at your job and generate numerous product ideas. These ideas must then be nurtured and developed.

A Change in Life-style. Once you have decided to follow up on an idea, you should be aware of the time commitment. It may not be encouraging to know that most entrepreneurs work very long days. However, it is important also to be aware that entrepreneurs tend to be happier and feel more fulfilled, because they are creating something that reflects their efforts and dreams.

Index

Note: Page numbers in *italics* refer to illustrations; page numbers followed by t refer to tables.